PEDIATRIC NURSING

CARING FOR
CHILDREN

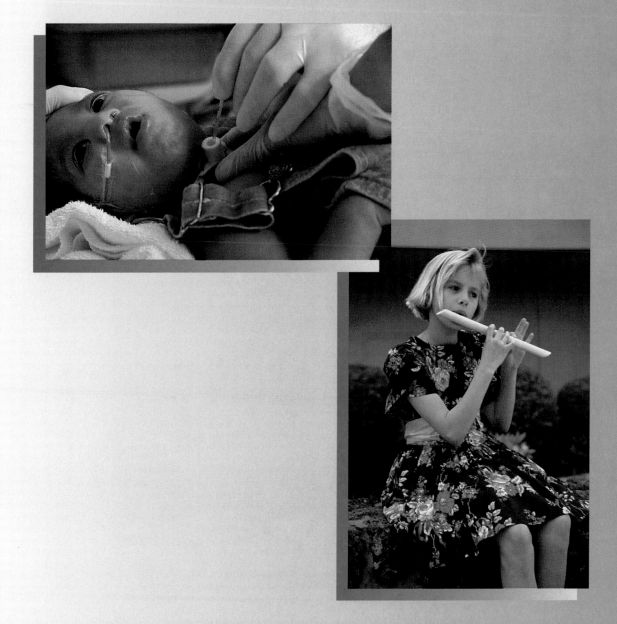

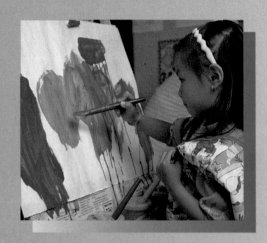
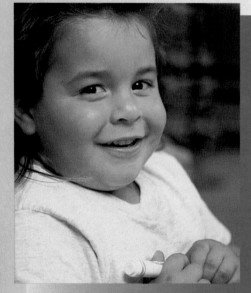
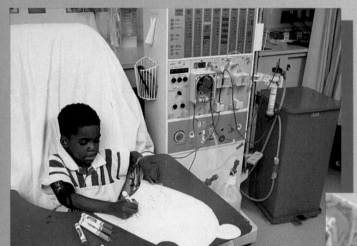
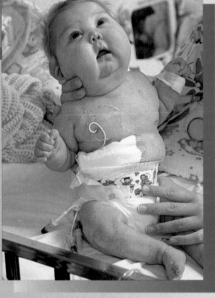

PEDIATRIC NURSING

CARING FOR CHILDREN

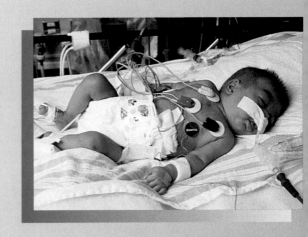

JANE BALL, RN, CPNP, DrPH

Program Director
Pediatric Emergency Education and Research Center
Emergency Trauma Services
Children's National Medical Center
Washington, DC

RUTH BINDLER, RNC, MS

Associate Professor
Intercollegiate Center for Nursing Education
Washington State University
Spokane, Washington

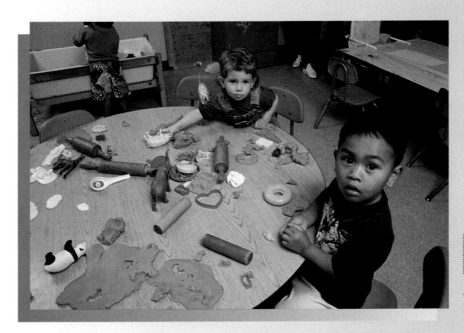

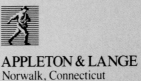

APPLETON & LANGE
Norwalk, Connecticut

Copyright © 1995 by Appleton & Lange
Paramount Publishing Business and Professional Group

95 96 97 98 99 / 10 9 8 7 6 5 4 3 2 1

Prentice Hall International (UK) Limited, *London*
Prentice Hall of Australia Pty. Limited, *Sydney*
Prentice Hall Canada, Inc., *Toronto*
Prentice Hall Hispanoamericana, S.A., *Mexico*
Prentice Hall of India Private Limited, *New Delhi*
Prentice Hall of Japan, Inc., *Tokyo*
Simon & Schuster Asia Pte. Ltd. *Singapore*
Editora Prentice Hall do Brasil Ltda., *Rio de Janeiro*
Prentice Hall, *Englewood Cliffs, New Jersey*

Library of Congress Cataloging-in-Publication Data
Pediatric nursing: caring for children / [edited by] Jane Ball, Ruth Bindler.
    p.   cm.
  Includes index.
  ISBN 0-8385-8018-1
  1. Pediatric nursing.   I. Ball, Jane.   II. Bindler, Ruth
McGillis.
  [DNLM: 1. Pediatric Nursing. 2. Critical Care—in infancy &
childhood. 3. Acute Disease—in infancy & childhood. 4. Acute
Disease—therapy. 5. Wounds and Injuries—in infancy & childhood.
  6. Wounds and Injuries—therapy.   WY 159 P3733 1994]
RJ245.P414 1994
610.73'62—dc20
DNLM/DLC
for Library of Congress   93-38642
                                                              CIP

Editor-in-Chief: Sally J. Barhydt
Production: CRACOM Corporation
Development: CRACOM Corporation
Cover Design: Michael J. Kelly
Interior Design: Diane Beasley

ISBN: 0-8385-8018-1
PRINTED IN THE UNITED STATES OF AMERICA

ISBN 0-8385-8018-1

9 780838 580189

CONTRIBUTORS

Jane Ball, RN, CPNP, DrPH
(Chapters 1, 3, 4, 5, & 12)

Ruth Bindler, RNC, MS
(Chapters 1, 2, 4, 5, & 12)

Jan Dalby, RNC, MS
Maternal Clinical Nurse Specialist
St. Mary's Hospital
Richmond, Virginia
(Chapter 18)

Linda Felver, RN, PhD
Associate Professor
School of Nursing
Oregon Health Sciences University
Portland, Oregon
(Chapters 7 & 8)

Darla Gowan, RN, FNPC, MN
Nurse Practitioner
Kosair Children's Hospital
Louisville, Kentucky
(Chapter 20)

Joyce Griffin, RN, OCN, PhD
Associate Professor
Nursing Department
Fairleigh Dickinson University
Teaneck, New Jersey
(Chapters 9 & 13)

Sandra Jo Hammer, RN, MPH, MSN
Nursing Supervisor
Children's Hospital, Oakland
Oakland, California
(Atlas of Infectious and Communicable Diseases)

Linda Kinrade, RN, PNP, MN
Professor
Department of Nursing
California State University
Hayward, California
(Chapter 16)

Katherine Morris, RN, CPNP
Nurse Clinician
Department of Pediatrics
Endocrinology & Metabolic Division
Medical College of Virginia
Richmond, Virginia
(Chapter 19)

Jean Moss, ARNP, CPNP, PhD
Pediatric Nurse Practitioner
Planned Parenthood
Child Health Clinic
Claremont, New Hampshire
(Chapter 11)

Ruth Novitt-Schumacher, RN, MSN
Pediatric Nursing Instructor
Maternal Child Department
University of Illinois at Chicago
Chicago, Illinois
(Chapter 15)

Nan Peterson, RN, MS
Clinical Nurse Manager
Pediatric Intensive Care Program
University of Wisconsin Children's Hospital
Madison, Wisconsin
(Chapter 6)

Deborah Thomas, RNC, MSN
Pediatric Psychiatric Clinical Nurse Specialist
Kosair Children's Hospital
Louisville, Kentucky
(Chapter 21)

Robert Wayner, MD
Neurosurgeon
The Neurological Clinic
Laguna Hills, California
(Chapter 14)

Amy Weigelt-Leinweber, RN, BSN
Staff Nurse
Shriners Hospital for Crippled Children
Spokane, Washington
(Chapter 17)

Marcia Wellington, RN, MS
Education Coordinator
Emergency Trauma Services
Children's National Medical Center
Washington, D.C.
(Chapter 14 & Atlas of Pediatric Procedures)

Rosemarie C. Westberg, RN, MSN
Associate Professor, Nursing
Northern Virginia Community College
Annandale, Virginia
(Chapter 10)

REVIEWERS & CONSULTANTS

PREFACE

This book, like clinical pediatric nursing, is about tough choices. Practicing nurses must make tough choices every day in caring for patients. Faculty members must make similar choices in preparing students to practice safely and effectively in the clinical setting. What information must students have to provide care? What is the best way to prepare students to practice in the clinical setting?

The answers to these questions have been, and will continue to be, debated. This book reflects how students learn and apply information and is structured to reflect clinical and academic realities.

- The first reality is that faculty have 4 to 9 weeks to prepare students to become clinically safe pediatric nurses.
- The second reality is that most graduates will work in the acute care setting.
- The third reality is that if students learn how to make decisions about what is important, they will be able to adapt to future changes in clinical practice.
- The fourth reality is that there are defined, acceptable standards of care for specific problems.

The goal of this book is to provide a core of pediatric nursing content that will prepare students for practice and provide them with the tools for continued self-learning. Students who learn which questions to ask, when to ask them, how to evaluate the answers, and how to think from a multidisciplinary perspective in the clinical setting will be able to learn and adapt to a changing health care system.

■ The Focus of This Book Is on Nursing Care of Children and Their Families in an Acute Care Environment

Because the vast majority of graduating nurses go on to practice in acute care facilities, this book emphasizes the information necessary to prepare students to work in that setting. Students who understand how to effectively care for and communicate with children and families in an acute care setting where children are extremely ill can readily transfer these skills to other nursing situations and environments.

There is solid coverage of long-term management of complex conditions as well as the nurse's role in preparing families for the child's discharge from the acute care facility. Selected ambulatory pediatric conditions are included because students will see these conditions in everyday life and in the hospital where these conditions are secondary to the presenting problem.

■ The Book Is Organized by Body System, with the Nursing Process as the Framework for Care

The book is organized by body system rather than age group for several reasons: this approach makes it easier for students to find information, study, prepare for clinical experiences, and review for the National Council of State Boards of Nursing Licensure Examination (NCLEX). The key to this book is integration. No child is treated in isolation, so the emphasis throughout is on the child and family. The nursing process provides the underlying structure for the book.

■ Six Themes Are Integrated throughout the Book in the Narrative, Art, Legends, Labels, and Margin Notes

Critical thinking and problem solving, communication, cultural diversity, growth and development, assessment, and legal and ethical concerns are six themes fundamental to daily nursing practice. These themes are interwoven through narrative, margin notes, and art, resulting in a unique, integrated presentation that engages students and makes them active participants in the material, rather than passive recipients of information. Students and faculty can therefore make use of important applied information where and when it is most appropriate.

- **Critical thinking** principles are integrated in the organization, pedagogy, writing style, and art program. Students practice critical thinking and problem-solving skills in their everyday lives. Many students have not, however, learned to apply these skills to the practice of nursing. This book will help students understand how their normal curiosity and problem-solving skills can be applied to pediatric nursing. They will learn, by example, which questions to ask, when, and why.
- **Communication** is one of the most important skills that students need to learn. Effective communication is the very fiber of nursing practice. This book integrates communication skills in an applied manner where students can most benefit.
- Current demographic trends demand that nurses be culturally sensitive. **Cultural considerations,** like the other five themes, are integrated throughout the book where appropriate. The information is presented in a manner that is both applied and engaging to the student. Students must deal with cultural differences as part of everyday practice and need to know when and why these differences are important in the care of children. Cultural information appears in the body of the text and in the art and is highlighted in margin notes.
- Knowledge of **growth and development** and **assessment** are central to the effective practice of pediatric nursing. A separate review chapter is devoted to each area. In addition, both topics are integrated where appropriate in the narrative, art, labels, and legend copy and are highlighted in the margin as applied information where necessary. This supports students' need to know relevant information associated with a specific topic or concept to help them apply theoretical information to clinical nursing practice.
- Throughout the book, **legal and ethical concerns** are provided in margin notes. This material is designed to sensitize students to thinking about the implications of what they do on a daily basis and to consider whether or not there are legal and ethical repercussions to their actions.

■ The Four-Color Text and Art Program Enhance Learning and Engage the Instructor and Student

The unique handling of narrative, art, figure labels, and legend copy prevents duplication of information in text and art unless there is a reason to provide additional reinforcement. Photographs are used whenever possible. This prepares students for the realities of the clinical setting and reinforces the focus on a child and family with a problem and not on a problem that happens to be associated with a child. Numerous four-color illustrations are included to reinforce students' understanding of anatomy and procedures. Line drawings superimposed over photographs enable students to learn the relationship of internal structures to surface anatomy.

The art, labeling, and legend copy take on an active and untraditional teaching role by engaging the student directly with strong visual images. For this reason, you will notice that sometimes labels contain descriptive and applied information. This approach ties explanations directly to the art rather than forcing the student to move back and forth between text and art. Some of the labels ask a question of the student that is then answered either in the legend or in the body of the text. This encourages students to think about what they are seeing and to test their knowledge, rather than passively absorb information.

Emphasis Is on Recognition of Injuries and Prevention in Each Age Group

Most unique to this book is the emphasis throughout on injury and safety precautions. It is especially important to recognize the impact that injuries have on childhood mortality, hospitalization, and the general care of children. In this book, an effort is made to present injuries by body system and by age group.

Pediatric Procedures and Infectious and Communicable Diseases Are Presented Using an Illustrated Atlas Format

Many areas of pediatric nursing at the introductory level lend themselves to a visual approach. Pediatric procedures and communicable diseases are two such areas. The Atlas of Pediatric Procedures allows students to quickly learn and review what they need to do and when. The Atlas of Infectious and Communicable Diseases provides an easy-to-use reference to these diseases. This approach facilitates learning and comprehension.

Student and Faculty Material

The student resource guide has been coordinated closely with this text. It will help students to improve their communication skills and will assist them in reviewing the material covered in both the text and lectures. The resource guide includes a combination of exercises that will reinforce students' critical thinking skills while helping them to learn pediatric nursing.

Faculty material includes an instructor's manual, containing additional critical thinking exercises and learning resources; a testbank of NCLEX-format questions; and a transparency package.

■ ■ ■

We made the tough choices about what to include, but our decisions were made with extensive input from faculty and students over a 2-year period before writing this book. Our emphasis is clearly on nursing care in the acute care setting and the most common problems that students will see. The material is applied and designed to make students think in the same way that they will need to think in clinical practice. The interplay between the art and text is unique, interesting, and designed to engage students and make them active participants in learning.

Is this book a unique learning tool for students and an innovative teaching tool for faculty? Yes! We are confident that this book represents a solid core of essential information that will prepare students for the realities of clinical practice in pediatrics.

Jane Ball
Ruth Bindler

ACKNOWLEDGMENTS

Although it is exciting to be offered an opportunity to write a new textbook, it is a major undertaking. The planning and effort involved in making a textbook creative, useful for students, and marketable requires an enormous investment of time and talent by many persons. CRACOM Corporation envisioned, researched, and directed the development and production of this text. Barbara Norwitz interpreted and implemented the vision, ensuring that the conceptual design and content were expressed on each page. Without her dedication and management, this book would never have happened. We are thrilled that Appleton & Lange recognized the promise of this textbook and boldly chose to become its publisher.

Pediatric nursing has become so specialized that a comprehensive textbook would not have been possible without our contributing authors. Several other individuals made major contributions to the textbook. Donna Frassetto's developmental editing and revisions clarified the chapter organization plan and ensured that each chapter was complete and conformed to the design. The talent of photographer George Dodson and his partner Katie Lawyer is easy to recognize. Their ability to make children comfortable and to capture their images in all types of settings is unsurpassed. We are also appreciative of the photographs contributed by Roy Ramsey. Diane Beasley, who created the book's design, provided an opportunity to make the presentation of content exciting and stimulating for students. The artist team of Nadine Sokol, Jeanne Robertson, George Caras, and Judy Schmitt helped complete the visual design of the book. Many other individuals at CRACOM Corporation worked behind the scenes to manage the book's editing and production details. Special thanks go to Mary Espenschied, Carlotta Seely, Martha Cushman, Bette Russ, Jeanne Gulledge, and Melinda Philbrook.

Several hospitals gave us the opportunity to photograph children being cared for on their pediatric units. In Spokane, Washington, children were photographed in Shriners Hospital, Sacred Heart Medical Center, and Deaconess Medical Center. In Washington, D.C., children were photographed in several units of the Children's National Medical Center. We are grateful for the opportunity to use the skills laboratory at the Intercollegiate Center for Nursing Education in Spokane, Washington, and for the assistance of Neysa Dobson in providing needed equipment and verifying the appropriateness of techniques demonstrated in many photographs. The Head Start Center in Spokane and day care provider Linda Berna also facilitated our photographing of children. We sincerely thank all the parents and children who allowed us to illustrate development, pediatric health care conditions, and nursing care with their pictures.

Finally, we must acknowledge the support and sacrifices of our families. They made it possible to dedicate endless hours to writing, reviewing, and editing the chapters of this book.

Jane Ball
Ruth Bindler

BRIEF CONTENTS

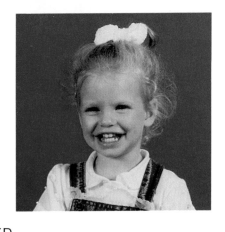

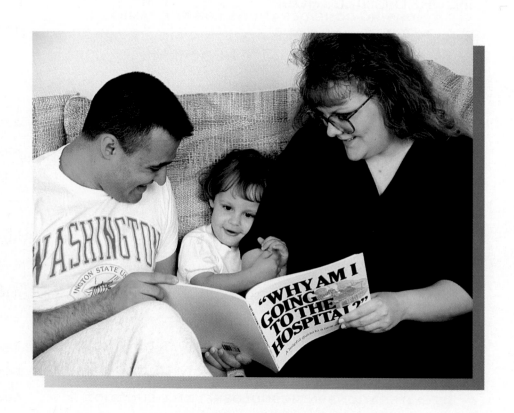

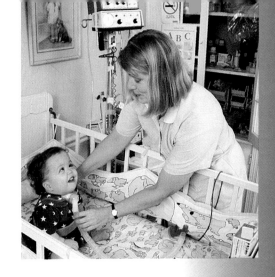

CONTENTS

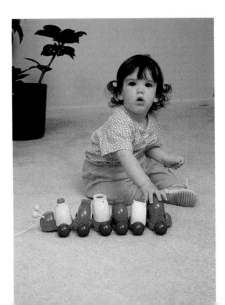

CHAPTER 3

PEDIATRIC ASSESSMENT   75

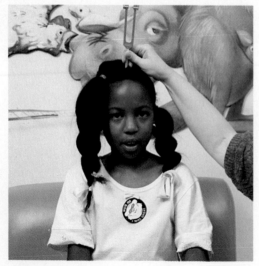

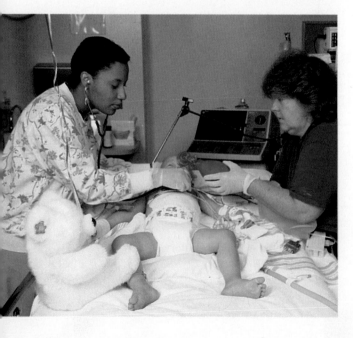

CHAPTER 16

ALTERATIONS IN CELLULAR GROWTH   541

CHAPTER 17

ALTERATIONS IN MUSCULOSKELETAL FUNCTION   583

CHAPTER 18

ALTERATIONS IN GENITOURINARY FUNCTION   619

CHAPTER 19

ALTERATIONS IN ENDOCRINE FUNCTION   653

CHAPTER 20

ALTERATIONS IN SKIN INTEGRITY   689

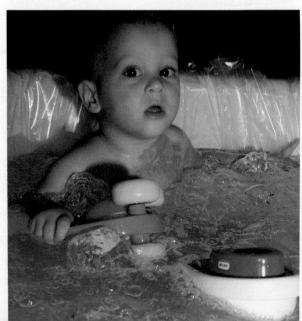

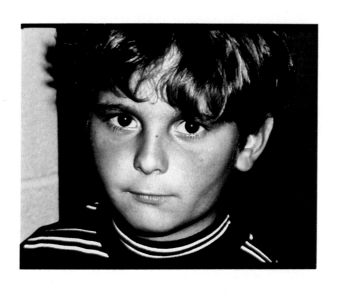

CHAPTER 21

ALTERATIONS IN PSYCHOSOCIAL FUNCTION 723

ATLAS OF INFECTIOUS AND COMMUNICABLE DISEASES 765

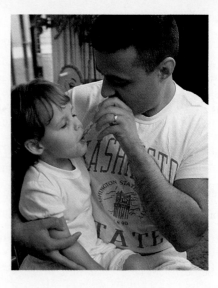

NURSING CARE PLANS

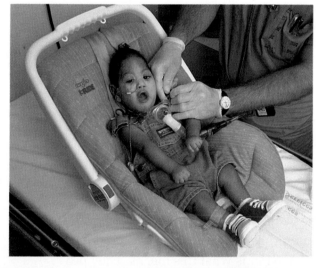

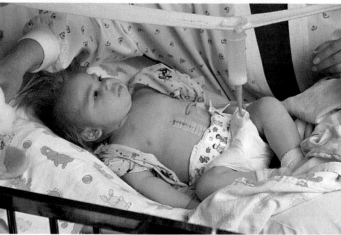

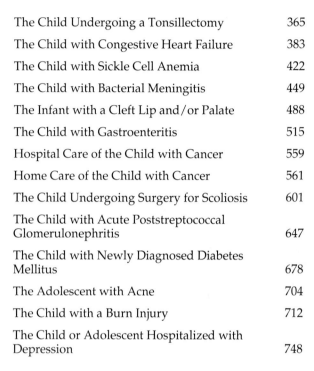

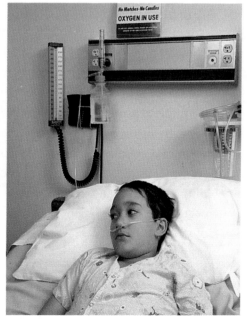

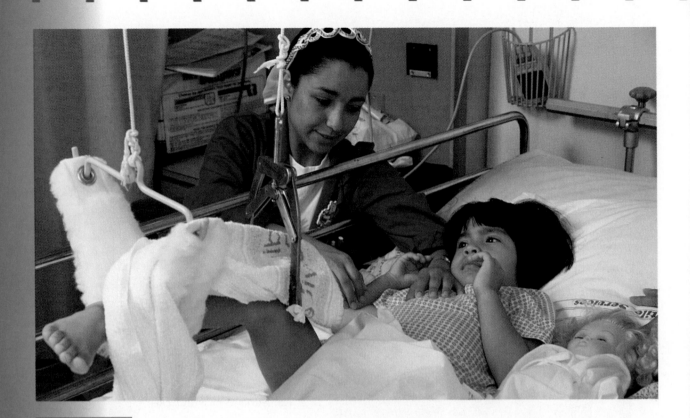

Juanita chased a ball out into the street and was struck by a car. She is awake and crying on arrival at the hospital emergency department. Physicians and nurses assess Juanita for life-threatening injuries and begin treatment for shock. One nurse talks to her continuously while monitoring her vital signs and level of consciousness.

Juanita's mother, who came to the hospital with her, waits anxiously. A physician tells her that Juanita has a mild head injury and a fractured femur. The nurses make sure her mother understands what this means. They provide support in several ways: they help her notify family members about Juanita, they prepare her daughter for the operating room, and they arrange her admission to the pediatric inpatient unit.

Juanita spends the next 2 weeks in traction, and she has difficulty being confined to bed. The nurses and child life workers engage her in therapeutic play (play that allows children to deal with their fears and concerns) to help occupy her time. The nurses also teach Juanita's mother about the importance of good nutrition and skin care because of the complications that immobilization can cause.

After 2 weeks Juanita is discharged in a hip spica cast. To make sure Juanita's parents know how to care for their daughter at home, the nurses teach them how to take care of the cast, how to watch for skin breakdown, and what to do if other problems arise. The nurses give Juanita's parents the phone number of the pediatric inpatient unit in case they have any questions about their daughter's care.

NURSE'S ROLE IN CARE OF THE ILL AND INJURED CHILD: HOSPITAL AND HOME

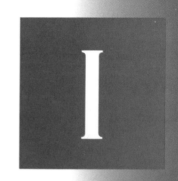

TERMINOLOGY

advance directives A patient's living will or appointed durable power of attorney for health care decisions.

assent A child's voluntary agreement to participate in a research project or to accept treatment.

continuum of care The system of care for ill and injured children that includes each of the following elements: illness or injury prevention, acute care in the hospital, and restorative care in either the home or a rehabilitation center until the child is reintegrated into the family, school, and community.

culture The socially learned beliefs, life-styles, and values that are characteristic of the family and community.

emancipated minors Self-supporting adolescents under 18 years of age who are not subject to parental control.

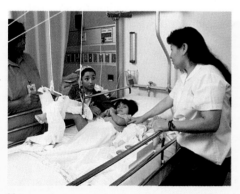

❝ I wonder how hard it will be to take care of Juanita when her cast is on? She won't be able to move around and help herself. Who can I get to come in during the day to take care of her while I'm at work? Can I afford it? ❞

ethics The philosophic study of morality, moral judgments, and moral problems.

family-centered care A philosophy of care that integrates the family's values and potential contributions in the plans for and provision of care to the child.

infant mortality Deaths of infants during the first year of life.

informed consent A formal preauthorization for an invasive procedure or participation in research.

mature minors Adolescents of 14 and 15 years of age who are able to understand treatment risks and who in some states can consent to or refuse treatment.

moral dilemma A conflict of social values and ethical principles that supports different courses of action.

morbidity An illness or injury that limits activity, requires medical attention or hospitalization, or results in a chronic condition.

quality assurance A process for monitoring the procedures and outcomes of care that uses indicators to measure compliance with standards of care.

risk management A process established by a health care institution to ensure compliance with standards of care and thereby reduce the institution's liability.

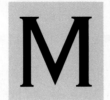

Many nurses come in contact with Juanita and her family during her hospital stay and transition to home care. Nurses are important members of the team during all phases of the **continuum of care** (the system of care for ill and injured children that includes each of the following elements: illness or injury prevention, acute care in the hospital, and restorative care in either the home or rehabilitation center until the child is reintegrated into the family, school, and community). In what settings is pediatric nursing care provided? What are the different roles of nurses in caring for children throughout the continuum of care? This chapter reviews concepts important to pediatric nursing: the role of the nurse in pediatrics, the contemporary climate of pediatric health care, and legal and ethical issues.

Role of the Nurse in Pediatrics

Clinical Practice

Pediatric nursing focuses on protecting children from illness and injury, assisting them to attain optimal levels of health, regardless of health problems, and rehabilitating them. These aims fit the American Nurses Association definition of the scope of nursing practice, "the nursing diagnosis and treatment of human responses to health and to illness."[1] The nursing roles in caring for children and their families include direct care, patient education, advocacy, and case management.

Direct Nursing Care

The primary role of pediatric nurses is to provide direct nursing care to children and their families. The nursing process provides the framework for delivery of direct pediatric nursing care. The nurse assesses the child, identifies the nursing diagnoses that describe the responses of the child and family to the illness or injury, and implements nursing care. This care is designed to meet the child's physical and emotional needs. It is tailored to the child's developmental stages, giving the child additional responsibility for self-care with increasing age.

Nurses also attempt to minimize the psychologic and physical distress experienced by children and families. Providing support to children and their families is one component of direct nursing care. This often involves listening to the concerns of children and parents and simply being present during stressful or emotional experiences. Nurses also help families by suggesting ways to support their children in the hospital and home care setting.

Patient Education

Patient education improves treatment results. In pediatric nursing, patient education is especially difficult because you must be prepared not only to work with children at various levels of understanding but also to change the behavior of family members.

As patient educators, nurses help children adapt to the hospital setting and prepare them for procedures (Fig. 1–1). Most hospitals encourage a parent to stay with the child and provide much of the direct and the supportive care. Nurses teach parents to watch for important signs, to increase the child's comfort, and even to provide advanced care. Taking an active role prepares the parent to assume total responsibility for care after the child leaves the hospital.

Counseling is another form of patient education. Counseling may involve guidance, such as injury prevention strategies. Nurse specialists or other ex-

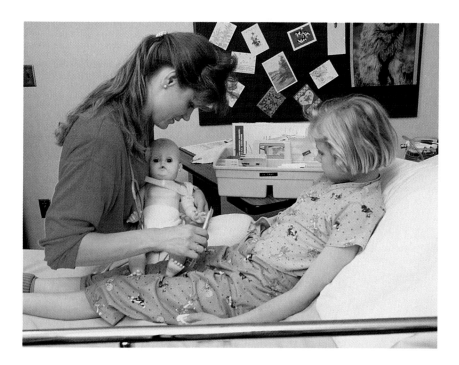

FIGURE 1-1 In patient education you can reduce the patient's and family's fears and anxieties about what to expect as well as instruct them in procedures and proper care at home.

perienced nurses are often responsible for counseling that is directed to helping the child or family solve a problem.

Patient Advocate

To be an effective advocate, the nurse must be aware of the child's and the family's needs, the family's resources, and the health care services available in the hospital and the community. The nurse informs parents about these services and the child's rights to use them. As advocates, nurses also ensure that the hospital's policies and resources meet the psychosocial needs of children and their families.

Case Management

What happens when a child has significant health problems? Can you handle it all?

When a child has a significant health problem or handicapping condition, health care professionals (physicians, nurses, social workers, physical and occupational therapists, and other specialists) create an interdisciplinary plan to meet the child's medical, nursing, developmental, educational, and psychosocial needs. Because nurses spend large amounts of time providing nursing care for the child and family, they often know more than other health care professionals about the family's wishes and resources. The nurse often becomes the child's case manager, coordinating the implementation of the interdisciplinary care plan. The nurse also serves as an advocate to ensure that the care plan considers the family's wishes and contains appropriate services.

Discharge planning is another form of case management. Good discharge planning promotes a smooth, rapid, and safe transition into the community and improves results of treatment begun in the hospital. To be a discharge planner the nurse needs to know about community medical resources, home care agencies qualified to care for children, educational interventions, and financial resources.

Nursing Process in Pediatric Care

Can you name the five steps of the nursing process? Pediatric nurses use the nursing process to identify and solve problems and to plan patient care. The systematic framework for practice that the nursing process provides is the same for pediatric patients as for other patients.

- *Assessment* involves collecting patient and family data and performing physical examinations at admission and periodically during the child's hospitalization. The nurse analyzes and synthesizes data to make a judgment about the patient's problems.
- *Nursing diagnoses* describe the health promotion and dysfunctional health patterns that nurses may manage. Once health patterns have been identified, specific nursing actions can be planned.
- *Nursing care plans* are based on goals that will improve the child's or family's dysfunctional health patterns. Specific planned outcomes should be realistic. The family and the nurse (and the child, when old enough) should agree to the care plan.

    Standard care plans for specific diagnoses are often used in the pediatric unit of the hospital. The nurse is responsible for individualiz- ing the standard care plans based on data from patient assessment and on evaluation of the patient's responses to care. Individualized nursing action plans provide directions for nursing care.
- *Implementation* is the carrying out of interventions outlined in the nurs- ing care plan. Interventions may be modified if the child's responses are undesirable.
- *Evaluation* is the use of specific objective and subjective measures to assess the child's and family's progress in reaching the goals defined in the nursing care plan. Following evaluation of the child's and family's progress toward the goals, the nursing care plan may be modified. For example, as the child's condition improves and goals are attained, new goals and nursing action plans must be defined.

Settings for Pediatric Nursing Care

Pediatric nurses function in many different settings. Within the hospital, acute care may be provided in the emergency department, postanesthesia unit, intensive care unit, and general pediatric inpatient unit. Pediatric nurses, working with children and families on a general pediatric hospital unit, promote health improvement in several ways:

- By gathering data and assessing health of children and families
- By providing ordered medical therapies
- By providing nursing care in a manner that preserves as many normal routines as possible while maintaining the family unit
- By working with the family and health care team to develop an indi- vidualized health care plan and a discharge plan

Pediatric nurses assist families in making the transition from the acute hos- pital setting to:

- The home, for a short recuperation
- A rehabilitation center or long-term care hospital
- A nurse-managed home care or hospice program

Managing the child's transition from acute care to another setting involves planning the discharge, implementing interdisciplinary plans, and collabo- rating with a broad range of health care professionals.

Pediatric nurses also work in several other health care settings.

- In *pediatricians' offices* and *health maintenance organizations* nurses assess children, provide telephone counseling, and support and counsel families regarding growth and development and nutrition.
- In *home health agencies* nurses provide home care to children with acute and chronic conditions. Children need medical treatment and nursing care for acute, self-limited conditions, chronic conditions, and terminal conditions.
- In *rehabilitation centers* nurses provide inpatient care to restore children to an optimal state.
- In *schools* nurses assess children, monitor their health status, and provide health education to teachers and children.

Contemporary Climate for Pediatric Nursing Care

More than 80 million children under the age of 21 live in the United States. They account for 31.8% of the population.[2] (See Figure 1–2 for a distribution of the population by age group.) At one time children were valued primarily as laborers. Over the past century, however, the unique needs and qualities of children have been recognized. In today's society, children are considered to have special value; they are vulnerable and need protection.

■ CULTURAL CONSIDERATIONS

Conflicts can occur within a family when traditional rituals and practices of the family elders do not conform with current health care practices. Nurses must be sensitive to such potential implications for the child's health care, especially after the child is discharged from the hospital. Parents may be forced to decide whether the family's beliefs take priority over the health care professional's guidance when cultural values are not part of the nursing care plan.

Culturally Sensitive Care

The U.S. population has a varied mix of cultural groups. **Culture** develops from socially learned beliefs, life-styles, and values that are characteristic of the family and community. The cultural background and values of children and their parents are often quite different from those of the nurse.

Specific elements that contribute to a family's value system include the following:

- Religion and social beliefs
- Presence and influence of the extended family, as well as socialization within the ethnic group
- Communication patterns
- Beliefs and understanding about the concepts of health and illness
- Permissible physical contact with strangers
- Education

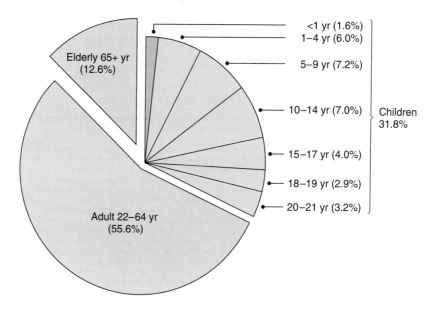

FIGURE 1–2 In 1990 children from birth to 21 years of age accounted for about one third of the population in the United States, with slightly over one fourth of the total population being under 17.

From U.S. Bureau of the Census. (1992). *Statistical Abstract of the United States,* 112th ed. Washington, DC: Author.

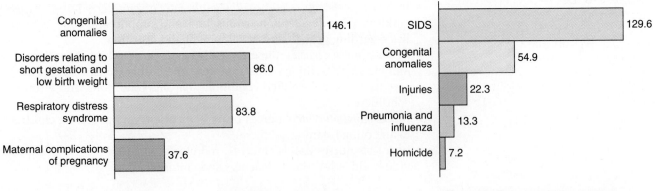

Number of deaths per 100,000 live births   Number of deaths per 100,000 live births

FIGURE 1–3 Leading causes of death in the United States in 1989 in infants up to 28 days old **(A)** and in infants 1 to 12 months old **(B).**

From National Center for Health Statistics. (1989). *Vital Statistics of the United States, vol 2: Mortality.* Part A. Hyattsville, MD: Public Health Service.

These elements in differing degrees influence the cultural beliefs and values of an ethnic group, making the group unique. Misunderstandings may occur when the health care professional and the family come from different cultural groups.[3]

When the family's cultural values are incorporated into the care plan, the family is more likely to accept and comply with care needed, especially for the child's home care. Avoid imposing your personal cultural values on the children and families in your care. By learning about the values of the different ethnic groups in the community—their religious beliefs that have an impact on health care practices, their beliefs about common illnesses, and their specific healing practices—you can develop an individualized nursing care plan for each child and family.

Pediatric Health Statistics

Children have different health care problems than adults, and the problems may depend on age and development. For example, the leading causes of **infant mortality** (death occurring during the first year of life) vary according to the age of the infant (Fig. 1–3).

The leading causes of death in neonates (birth to 28 days of age) are congenital anomalies, low birth weight, respiratory distress syndrome, and maternal complications of pregnancy. Sudden infant death syndrome accounts

FIGURE 1–4 Age-specific death rate per 100,000 children in the United States in 1990. The leading cause of death in children between the ages of 1 and 9 years was unintentional injury. Why do you think that is? Do you think this data still applies today? Which type of unintentional injury has the highest rate of death? Firearms? Fires? Motor vehicle accidents? Falls? See Figure 1–5 for the answer.

From National Center for Health Statistics. (1993). National Vital Statistics System, unpublished data.

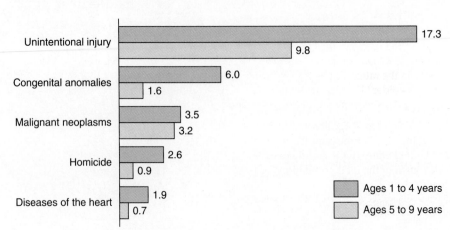

PEDIATRIC NURSING

FIGURE 1–5 Death rates from unintentional injuries per 100,000 children ages 1 to 9 years in the United States in 1988. Which type of unintentional injury is the most common?

From Children's Safety Network. (1991). *A Data Book of Child and Adolescent Injury.* Washington, DC: National Center for Education in Maternal and Child Health.

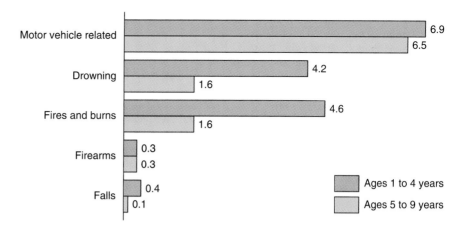

for nearly 67% of deaths to infants in the postneonatal period (between 1 and 12 months of age). Figure 1–3 shows the relative frequency of other major causes of death in the postneonatal age group.[4]

The most common cause of death for children between 1 and 9 years of age is unintentional injury. Congenital anomalies, cancer, homicide, and diseases of the heart are the other major causes. Figure 1–4 shows the distribution of these causes by age group. The major causes of death from unintentional injury in childhood include motor vehicle crashes (passengers and pedestrians), drowning, fires and burns, firearms, and falls (Fig. 1–5).[4] Deaths from homicide and firearms have increased so dramatically over the past decade that they are now the fourth leading cause of mortality.

Unintentional injury continues to be the leading cause of death in adolescents. Homicide, suicide, cancer, and diseases of the heart are other major causes of death (Fig. 1–6). Of all deaths from unintentional injury, motor vehicle crashes are the leading cause, followed by drowning, fires and burns, firearms, and falls (Fig. 1–7).

The U.S. government has set objectives to improve the health of children and young adults in the 1990s. These objectives focus on reducing the incidence of death and disability from the major causes of death shown in Figure 1–6. Federal funding is available to health care institutions for the development of programs aimed at reducing the number of deaths from these factors in specific high-risk groups.

Morbidity (an illness or injury that limits activity, requires medical attention or hospitalization, or results in a chronic condition) also varies according to the age of the child. Figure 1–8 shows the leading causes of hospitalization of children by age group. Respiratory diseases are the leading cause of hospitalization in children between 1 and 9 years of age, accounting for

FIGURE 1–6 Death rates per 100,000 adolescents in the United States in 1990. Do you notice any difference in the rates of homicide as the child gets older? Do you think that these numbers would vary between socioeconomic and cultural groups? Why do you think there are differences? Are your conclusions supported by fact or are they influenced by your personal bias?

From National Center for Health Statistics. (1993). *National Vital Statistic System.* Personal communication, Ken Kochanek.

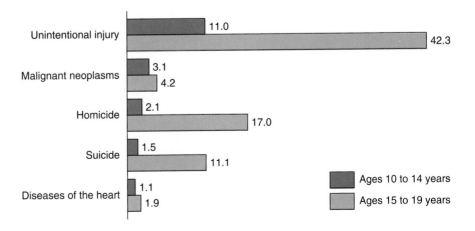

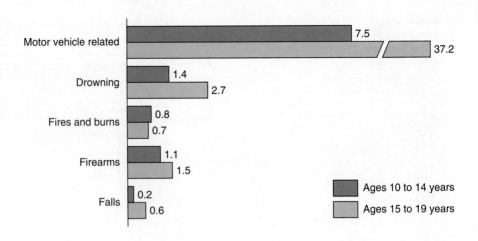

FIGURE 1–7 Death rates from unintentional injuries per 100,000 adolescents in the United States in 1988. Why do you think that motor vehicle–related accidents jump so significantly in the 15- to 19-year age group? Can you see ways to use these data with patients and families during patient teaching and when talking with them while providing care?

From Children's Safety Network. (1991). *A Data Book of Child and Adolescent Injury.* Washington, DC: National Center for Education in Maternal and Child Health.

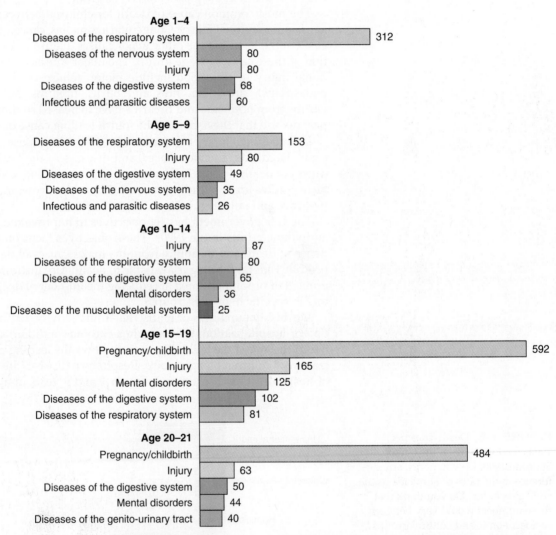

FIGURE 1–8 The leading causes of hospitalization in 1989 in the United States in those 21 and under present some interesting summary data for comparison (number of hospital discharges [in 1000's]). How can you apply this information when providing care and patient education?

From National Center for Health Statistics. (1990). Hospital discharge survey, 1989. In Maternal and Child Health Bureau. (1991). *Child Health USA '91.* (DHHS Publication No. HRS-M-CH 91-1). Washington, DC: National Center for Education in Maternal and Child Health.

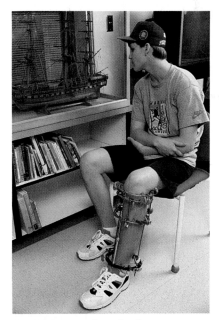

FIGURE 1-9 Joey has been at Shriner's Hospital for over 8 months undergoing external fixation (lengthening the leg), which is a long and painful process. It is important that children undergoing long-term care continue their schooling, develop friendships with other children in the hospital, maintain contact with their friends at home, and learn self-care.

35% of hospital discharges in this age group. Injury is among the top three causes of hospitalization in all age groups between 1 and 21 years of age. Another important cause of hospitalization is diseases of the digestive system. Pregnancy and childbirth are the leading causes of hospitalization in adolescents from 15 to 21 years of age.[4]

In 1990 chronic illnesses and impairments limited the activities of more than 3.5 million children between 1 and 19 years of age. More boys than girls had activity limitations before age 15.[4]

Health Care Issues

Health Care Technology

Research and technology have enabled many children with congenital anomalies and low birth weight to survive, with and without chronic conditions. Lifesaving technology has also created such burdens as high costs of health care and stresses on the functioning of the child's family. Many children with chronic conditions or complications of acute illnesses and injuries are managed in long-term care hospitals, rehabilitation centers, or home care programs (Fig. 1–9). Approximately 400,000 children in the United States are unable to engage in normal childhood activities or depend on some form of medical technology (Fig. 1–10).[5]

Health Care Financing

Not all children in the United States have access to health care. In 1989, 9.5 million children, nearly 15% of those below 18 years of age, had no health insurance and 11% were covered by public insurance programs such as Medicaid. Of all children who lived in poverty in 1989, 32.5% had no health insurance and 46.7% were covered by public insurance.[4] Most of these children had difficulty obtaining the most basic preventive health care, including immunizations (Fig. 1–11).

Many children with severe chronic illnesses can be treated at home rather than by continued hospitalization. A 1989 study reported that more than 1 million children had a severe chronic illness that required ongoing home care.[6] After studies found that home health care was substantially less ex-

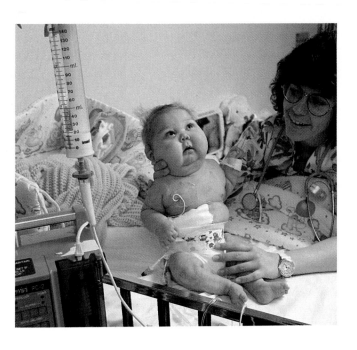

FIGURE 1-10 This child is dependent on the latest technology for necessary nutrients.

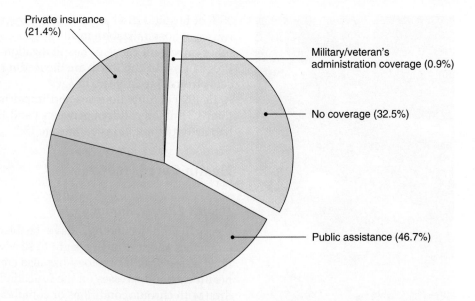

FIGURE 1-11 In the United States, who pays for the health care of children under 18 years living in poverty? This data from 1989 shows that our taxes support nearly 80% of the costs. What can you do to help? Something as simple as counseling parents on proper immunizations while a child is under care for other problems can prevent potential health problems. Part of good nursing care is supporting the well-being of the child in addition to caring for the presenting problem.

From National Center for Health Statistics. Ries, P. Characteristics of persons with and without health coverage, U.S. 1989. *Advance Data from Vital and Health Statistics*, 201, Hyattsville, MD: Public Health Service.

Private insurance (21.4%)

Military/veteran's administration coverage (0.9%)

No coverage (32.5%)

Public assistance (46.7%)

pensive than hospital care,[6] Congress amended laws to permit payment of home care services with federal funds. Technologic advances have enabled the design of portable medical and infusion therapy equipment for home care. Some families have regained control over their lives by creating intensive care units in their homes (Fig. 1–12). Children who 10 years ago would have died of respiratory, neurologic, or other medical conditions are thriving with home care and are participating in family, community, and school life.[7]

Legal Concepts and Responsibilities

Regulation of Nursing Practice

Because nurses are accountable for their professional actions, each state regulates nursing practice with a Nurse Practice Act. In many states nursing is defined as "the nursing diagnosis and treatment of human responses to health and to illness."[1] A state's Nurse Practice Act defines the legal roles and responsibilities of nurses. Become familiar with the Nurse Practice Act in your state.

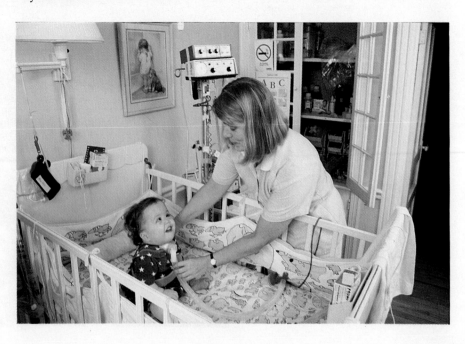

FIGURE 1-12 It is often desirable from a family and cost perspective to provide health care in the home, and the advance in technology has made it possible.

As professionals, nurses set standards for education and practice that conform to state regulations. Professional nursing organizations and state agencies that accredit nursing programs modify the standards for nursing education as the science of nursing progresses. Nurses in professional organizations develop Standards of Nursing Practice. These standards describe the public and patient responsibilities for which nurses are accountable.

Standards of Clinical Nursing Practice developed by the American Nurses Association define standards for both nursing care and performance.[8] Standards of Care describe the competent level of nursing care using the nursing process and form the foundation of clinical decision making. Standards of Performance describe the nurse's behavior in the professional role and include such criteria as quality of care, ethics, research, education, and collaboration. Specific standards have also been developed for maternal and child nursing practice (Table 1–1).

Accountability and Risk Management

Accountability

The family entrusts the child's care to the health care team. Family members expect this team to provide good medical and nursing care and not to make mistakes that cause harm. Nurses are personally accountable for expanding their knowledge base, for recognizing important changes in the child's condition that require intervention, and for taking action as necessary to protect the child.

Because the child is influenced by and is dependent on the family, the pediatric nurse is accountable to both the family and the child for nursing care provided. **Family-centered care** (a philosophy of care that integrates the family's values and potential contributions when planning and providing care to the child) has become an important concept in pediatric nursing.

TABLE 1–1 Professional Practice Standards for Maternal and Child Nursing

   I. The nurse helps children and parents attain and maintain optimal health.

  II. The nurse assists families to achieve and maintain a balance between the personal growth needs of individual family members and optimal family functioning.

 III. The nurse intervenes with vulnerable clients and families at risk to prevent potential developmental and health problems.

 IV. The nurse promotes an environment free of hazards to reproduction, growth and development, wellness, and recovery from illness.

  V. The nurse detects changes in health status and deviations from optimal development.

 VI. The nurse carries out appropriate interventions and treatment to facilitate survival and recovery from illness.

VII. The nurse assists clients and families to understand and cope with developmental and traumatic situations during illness, childbearing, childrearing, and childhood.

VIII. The nurse actively pursues strategies to enhance access to and utilization of adequate health care services.

 IX. The nurse improves maternal and child health nursing practice through evaluation of practice, education, and research.

From American Nurses Association. (1983). Standards of maternal and child health nursing practice (MCH-3). Washington, DC: Author.

Risk Management

Health care institutions make every effort to promote optimal patient care and reduce liability by various activities of **risk management** (a process established by a health care institution to ensure compliance with standards of care to reduce the institution's liability), **quality assurance** (a process used to monitor the procedures and outcomes of care using indicators to measure compliance with standards of care), or quality improvement. Nurses participate in development of institutional standards of nursing practice. Hospitals and home health agencies encourage development of diagnosis-specific nursing care plans that serve as minimal institutional standards of care. After development of institutional standards of care, indicators of effective nursing care are identified. These indicators may measure either the process or the outcome of nursing care. Patient records are regularly reviewed to ensure compliance with institutional standards, as measured by the indicators. When cases of noncompliance are found, the nursing staff is educated about standards and methods for improving nursing practice. Recommendations for revision of institutional standards to further improve nursing care in the institution often result.

Documentation of nursing care is an essential part of risk management and quality assurance. If a patient record is subpoenaed, documented care is considered the only care provided, regardless of the quality of undocumented care. The patient assessment, the nursing care plan, and the child's responses to medical therapies and nursing care, including the regularly scheduled evaluation of the patient's progress toward nursing goals, must all be documented accurately and sequentially. Nurses must also report any untoward incidents that could inhibit the patient's recovery.

■ LEGAL AND ETHICAL CONSIDERATIONS

The patient's record is a legal document that is admissible evidence in court. Information in the patient's record must be legibly written in objective terms. When recording patient responses to therapies, the nurse includes physiologic responses and exact quotes. The date, time, and nurse's signature and title are required.

■ Legal and Ethical Issues in Pediatric Care

Shanti, a 15-year-old with acute myelocytic leukemia, has come out of her second remission with an acute onset of fever, joint pain, and petechiae. A bone marrow transplant is one of the few remaining therapeutic options. While Shanti has agreed to a transplant if a suitable donor is found, she does not want to be resuscitated and placed on life support equipment should she have a cardiac arrest. She has talked extensively with the hospital chaplain and social worker and feels comfortable with her decision. Her parents want an all-out effort to sustain her life until a donor is located.

Shanti's case illustrates the legal and ethical dilemmas in caring for children. At what age can children make an informed decision about whether to accept or refuse treatment? What happens when the parents and child have contrasting opinions about treatment? How are ethical decisions resolved?

Informed Consent

Informed consent is a formal preauthorization for an invasive procedure or participation in research. Consent must be given voluntarily. Parents, as the legal custodians of minor children, are customarily requested to give informed consent on behalf of a child. When parents are divorced, either may give informed consent. Both children and parents must understand that they have the right to refuse treatment at any time. In an emergency, consent for treatment to preserve life or limb is not required.

Children under 18 or 21 years of age, depending on state law, can legally give informed consent in the following circumstances[9]:

- When they are minor parents of the child patient

■ LEGAL AND ETHICAL CONSIDERATIONS

Information that the physician must provide to obtain informed consent includes a detailed description of the treatment, possible benefits and significant risks associated with the proposed treatments, possible alternative treatments, and notification of a parent's or guardian's right to refuse treatment in behalf of the child.

The physician is legally responsible for obtaining informed consent. The nurse's role in obtaining informed consent includes the following:
- Alerting physicians to the need for informed consent
- Responding to questions asked by parents and children
- Serving as a witness when parents sign consent forms or give verbal consent by telephone

■ GROWTH AND DEVELOPMENT CONSIDERATIONS

By 7 or 8 years of age a child is able to understand concrete explanations about informed consent for research participation. By age 11 a child's abstract reasoning and logic are advanced. By age 14 an adolescent can weigh options and make decisions regarding consent as capably as an adult.

■ LEGAL AND ETHICAL CONSIDERATIONS

Jehovah's Witnesses oppose blood transfusions for themselves and their children because they believe transfusions are equivalent to the oral intake of blood, which is morally and spiritually wrong according to their interpretation of the Bible (Leviticus 17:13-14). A Jehovah's Witness who receives a transfusion has committed a sin and may have forfeited everlasting life. Transfusions of any blood products, including plasma and the patient's own blood, are forbidden.

FIGURE 1-13 Children need to be actively involved in decisions regarding their care when appropriate. The nurse (behind bed) has brought the entire family together to discuss the child's care in a positive and honest manner.

- When they are **emancipated minors** (self-supporting adolescents under 18 years of age, not subject to parental control)
- When they are adolescents between 16 and 18 years of age seeking birth control, an abortion, mental health counseling, or substance abuse treatment

Mature minors (14- and 15-year-old adolescents who are able to understand treatment risks) can give consent for treatment or refuse treatment in some states.

Children should become more actively involved in decision making about treatment procedures as their reasoning skills develop. Children too young to give informed consent can be given age-appropriate information about their condition and asked about their care preferences. Their parents, however, make ultimate decisions regarding their care (Fig. 1–13).

With regard to participation in research, federal guidelines state that children 7 years and older must receive information about a research project and give **assent** (the child's voluntary agreement to participate in a research project or to accept treatment) before they are enrolled. Children should be given adequate time to ask questions and told that they have the right to refuse to participate in the study.[10,11]

Child's Rights Versus Parent's Rights

Parents have absolute authority to make choices about their child's health care except in specific cases:

- When the child and parents do not agree on major treatment options
- When the parent's choice of treatment does not permit lifesaving treatment for the child

In either case the court may be requested to appoint a proxy decision maker for the child or to determine that the child is capable of making a major treatment decision.

Confidentiality

When the child is an emancipated or mature minor, the physician may provide birth control and substance abuse treatment without informing the

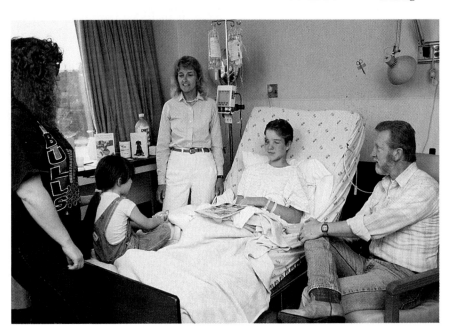

child's parents. If the child has a reportable disease, confidentiality may create a public health hazard. In such cases the health care professional is obligated to report the presence of the disease to the appropriate state or county agency.[12,13] Suspected cases of child abuse must be reported to the appropriate agency specified by state law.

Patient Self-Determination Act

The federal Patient Self-Determination Act directs health care institutions to inform hospitalized patients about their rights, which include expressing a preference for treatment options and making **advance directives** (writing a living will or authorizing a durable power of attorney for health care decisions on the patient's behalf). Nurses often discuss these issues with patients and their families.[14] Minor children and their parents should also be informed of their rights.

Ethical Issues

Ethics is the philosophical study of morality, moral judgments, and moral problems. Ethical issues may arise from a **moral dilemma** (a conflict of social values and ethical principles that support different courses of action). Technology makes it possible to sustain the lives of children who previously would have died, which creates many ethical issues. Problems sometimes develop because physicians and nurses have differing opinions about treatments for an infant or child with a serious or fatal condition. Nurses often face ethical dilemmas when providing care to such a child. They witness parents struggling to decide among treatment options.[15]

Ethical decision making is based on respect for persons and their ability to make decisions independently. All individuals must be treated without prejudice, regardless of race, gender, religious preference, cultural or educational background, financial status, or sexual orientation.[16] Health care professionals may have different values than patients, based on culture and life experiences.

Certain principles guide decision making about treatment when moral dilemmas exist. A major principle is to avoid harm and provide beneficial care to the child. When making treatment decisions in pediatrics, health care professionals must determine whether their responsibility is limited to the child or includes the interests of the parents. The health care institution's ethics committee should make treatment decisions using the process of data collection and evaluation outlined in Table 1–2. Courts should make ethical decisions only when health care professionals and parents are unable to agree about providing or withholding treatment.

Terminating Life-Sustaining Treatment

Baby Joe at 1 day of age has severe myelomeningocele with hydrocephalus. His physicians are seeking his parents' consent for surgical placement of a shunt to control the progression of hydrocephalus. Regardless of medical care and surgical intervention, the infant is expected to have a severe handicap. The parents, after much consideration and discussions with their family and pastor, have requested that life-sustaining treatment be withheld.

What happens when the parents' request differs from the opinion of physicians? How do federal regulations for care of infants with severe defects affect current health care practice?

Federal "Baby Doe" regulations were developed to protect the rights of infants with severe defects. Parents of such infants are usually the ultimate decision makers about the child's care. They may want to terminate treatment

TABLE 1-2 Steps in Making Ethical Decisions

Collect Information

What decisions are needed?
Who are the key persons involved?
What information will help make the situation more clear?
Are there any legal constraints?

Identify the Ethical Issues or Concerns of the Situation

What are their historical roots, the religious and philosophical positions?
What are the current societal views of each issue?

Define the Personal and Professional Moral Positions on the Issues

What personal constraints are raised by the issues?
What is the professional code for guidance?
Are there any conflicting loyalties or obligations?
What are the moral positions of the key individuals involved?

Identify Any Value Conflicts

What is the basis for the conflict?
What is the possible resolution?

Decision Making

Who should make the decision?
What are the possible actions and their anticipated outcome?
What is the moral justification for each action?
Which action fits the criteria for this situation?
Decide on a course of action and carry it out.

Evaluate the Results of the Decision Action

Did the expected outcome occur?
Is a new decision needed?
Is the decision process complete?

Adapted from Thompson, J.B., & Thompson, H.O. (1981). *Ethics in nursing*. New York: Macmillan Publishing.

because of the tremendous social, emotional, and financial burden.[17] Physicians may believe treatment will help the child and improve the quality of life (sometimes defined as a meaningful existence or an ability to develop human relationships). Federal regulations require a formalized ethical decision-making process before physicians accept or reject a parent's wishes.

Justifications for withholding, withdrawing, or limiting therapy include the following[18]:

- The treatment in question will not work.
- The burdens of the treatment outweigh the benefits, or the quality of life is poor after treatment.
- The burdens of the disease outweigh the benefits of continued survival, or the quality of life is poor before the treatment.

Treatment to save the infant's life is elected if it has the potential for improving the quality of life as well. Physicians are not obligated to offer interventions that cause extreme pain and suffering when there is no or limited potential benefit. Treatments that only prolong life represent a misuse of expensive health care resources.

Organ Transplantation Issues

The death of a child can benefit another child through organ transplantation. The National Organ Transplant Act (PL98-507) generated laws, regulations, and guidelines for organ collection and transplantation.[19] Regulations are important because too few organs are available for patients needing transplantation. The limited supply of organs has created numerous ethical issues. Which patients on the waiting list should receive the organs available? Should families be permitted to pay donor families for organs? Should the family's ability to pay for an organ transplant give a child higher priority for an organ? What are the brain death criteria for infants that enables organ collection to proceed?

Summary

Many topics discussed in this chapter are serious and may be distressing when applied to children. Fortunately, pediatric nursing more often involves caring for children who have episodes of acute illness or injury and who recover quickly without serious consequences. The challenge and gratification of pediatric nursing are to provide appropriate care in a supportive environment that promotes the family unit and the child's development.

REFERENCES

1 American Nurses Association. (1987). *The Scope of Nursing Practice* (NP-72 15M). Kansas City, MO: Author.

2 U.S. Bureau of the Census. (1992). *Statistical Abstract of the United States, 1992* (112th ed.). Washington, DC: Author.

3 Neiderhauser, V.P. (1989). Health care of immigrant children: Incorporating culture into practice. *Pediatric Nursing, 15,* 569–574.

4 Maternal and Child Health Bureau. (1991). *Child Health USA '91* (DHHS Publication No. HRS-M-CH 91-1). Washington, DC: National Center for Education in Maternal and Child Health.

5 Klug, R.M. (1992). Selecting a home care agency. *Pediatric Nursing, 8,* 504–506.

6 U.S. General Accounting Office. (1989a). *Home care experiences of families with chronically ill children.* Washington, DC: Author.

7 Grammatica, G. (1989). Developing a quality home care program for children. *Pediatric Nursing, 15,* 33–35.

8 American Nurses Association. (1991). *Standards of Clinical Nursing Practice* (NP-79). Washington, DC: Author.

9 Hogue, E.E. (1989). Consent for minors. *Pediatric Nursing, 15,* 404.

10 U.S. Department of Health and Human Services. (1983). *Protection of Human Subjects: Code of Federal Regulations, 45 CFR #46, Subpart D.*

11 Thurber, F.W., Deatrick, J.A., & Grey, M. (1992). Children's participation in research: Their right to consent. *Journal of Pediatric Nursing, 7,* 165–170.

12 King, N.M.P., & Cross, A.W. (1989). Children as decision makers: Guidelines for pediatricians. *Journal of Pediatrics, 115,* 10–16.

13 Fiesta, J. (1992). Protecting children: A public duty to report. *Nursing Management, 23,* 14–15.

14 Badzek, L.A. (1992). What you need to know about advance directives. *Nursing '92, 22,* 58–59.

15 Smith, J. (1989). Ethical issues raised by new treatment options. *Maternal Child Nursing, 14,* 183–187.

16 Fowler, M.D.M. (1989). Ethical decision making in clinical practice. *Nursing Clinics of North America, 24,* 955–965.

17 Schlomann, P. (1992). Ethical considerations of aggressive care of the very low birth weight infant. *Neonatal Network, 11,* 31–36.

18 Tomlinson, T., & Brody, H. (1988). Ethics and communication in do-not-resuscitate orders. *New England Journal of Medicine, 318,* 43–46.

19 Davis, F.D. (1989). Organ procurement and transplantation. *Nursing Clinics of North America, 24,* 823–826.

SUGGESTED READINGS

Crummette, B.D., & Boatwright, D.N. (1991). Case management in inpatient pediatric nursing. *Pediatric Nursing, 17,* 469–473.

Davis, B.D., & Steele, S. (1991). Case management for young children with special health care needs. *Pediatric Nursing, 17,* 15–19.

Erlen, J.A., & Holzman, I.R. (1988). Anencephalic infants: Should they be organ donors? *Pediatric Nursing, 14,* 60–63.

Everson-Bates, S. (1988). Research involving children: Ethical concerns and dilemmas. *Journal of Pediatric Nursing, 2,* 234–239.

Jones, N.E. (1992). Childhood injuries: An epidemiologic approach. *Pediatric Nursing, 18,* 235–239.

Malloy, C. (1992). Children and poverty: America's future at risk. *Pediatric Nursing, 18,* 553–557.

McClowry, S.G. (1993). Pediatric nursing psychosocial care: A vision beyond hospitalization. *Pediatric Nursing, 19,* 146–148.

Rushton, C.H., & Hogue, E.E. (1993). When parents demand "everything." *Pediatric Nursing, 19,* 180–183.

Selekman, J. (1991). Pediatric rehabilitation: From concepts to practice. *Pediatric Nursing, 17,* 11–14.

Spector, R.E. (1991). *Cultural Diversity in Health and Illness.* 3rd ed. Norwalk, CT: Appleton & Lange.

Thurber, F., Berry, B., & Cameron, M.E. (1991). The role of school nursing in the United States. *Journal of Pediatric Nursing, 5,* 135–140.

Vikell, J.H. (1991). The process of quality management. *Pediatric Nursing, 17,* 618–619.

Zagorsky, E.S. (1993). Caring for families who follow alternative health care practices. *Pediatric Nursing, 19,* 71–75.

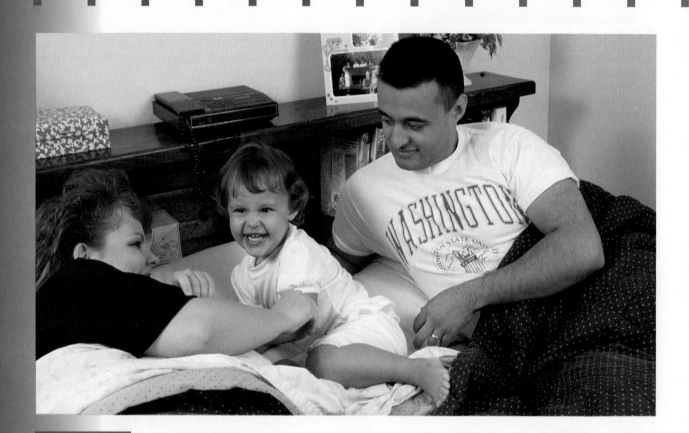

Three-and-a-half-year-old Jasmine wakes up and runs into her parents' room. She jumps onto their bed and tickles them, giggling. They soon join in the fun and return her tickles, laughing and playing. Everyone then quiets briefly, cuddles, rubs backs, and talks about the plans for the day.

While her parents get dressed, Jasmine goes to the kitchen. She plays with her toy dishes on the kitchen floor. Later, as she eats a breakfast of dry cereal, cheese slices, banana, and orange juice, she imagines that her slices of cheese are people walking. She blows bubbles in her juice. When she begins playing with her food, her mother decides she has had enough, picks up the left-overs, and directs her to go play.

Jasmine asks to watch *Sesame Street* on television, sings along with several of the songs, and answers the questions out loud. Although she cannot read the word "camel," she learns to count to three each time three objects are shown. After the show, Jasmine opens "her" kitchen drawer, gets out play-dough, and starts modeling worms and balls at the kitchen counter. After about 20 minutes she notices neighbor children outside swinging and riding Big Wheels and joins them. When Jasmine's mother looks out the window, she notices that although all these children are preschoolers, their sizes are quite different, even among those of the same age. Jasmine is small for her age in comparison with her friends, but her ability to perform motor activities is about the most advanced in the group.

GROWTH AND DEVELOPMENT

TERMINOLOGY

anticipatory guidance The process of understanding upcoming developmental needs and then teaching caretakers to meet those needs.

associative play A type of play that emerges in preschool years when children interact with one another, engaging in similar activities and participating in groups.

cephalocaudal development The process by which development proceeds from the head downward through the body and toward the feet.

collective monologue A type of speech demonstrated when two people talk about separate subjects, wait for each other to speak, and do not respond to each other's topics; common during preschool years.

cooperative play A type of play that emerges in school years when children join into groups to achieve a goal or play a game.

defense mechanisms Techniques used by the ego to unconsciously change reality, thereby protecting itself from excessive anxiety.

development An increase in capability or function.

dramatic play A type of play in which a child lives out the drama of daily life.

ego The realistic part of the personality that struggles for acceptable behavior and balances the id and superego.

expressive jargon Use of unintelligible words with normal speech intonations as if truly communicating in words; common in toddlerhood.

growth An increase in physical size.

id A basic sexual energy that is present at birth and drives the individual to seek pleasure.

nature The genetic or hereditary capability of an individual.

nurture The effects of the environment on an individual's performance.

object permanence The knowledge that an object or person continues to exist when not seen, heard, or felt.

parallel play A type of play that emerges in toddlerhood when children play side by side with similar or different toys, demonstrating little or no social interaction.

physiologic anorexia A decrease in appetite manifested when the extremely high metabolic demands of infancy slow to keep pace with the more moderate growth rate of toddlerhood.

proximodistal development The process by which development proceeds from the center of the body outward to the extremities.

puberty The age at which sexual maturity is attained.

superego A moral system that develops in childhood and includes a set of values and a conscience.

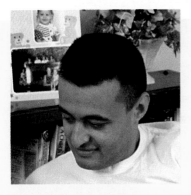

❝ Watching Jasmine grow is fascinating and scary. She is changing so fast, learning new things. It is hard to keep up with her. It is an exciting time. **❞**

What Is Accomplished by Play?

To understand the important facets of development that are explored in this chapter, you need to examine what was accomplished and demonstrated during Jasmine's activity in the morning (Fig. 2–1).

Physical Growth and Development

Jasmine is smaller than many of her peers. However, her gross or large motor skills of running and jumping are well developed. Fine motor skills are evident in her ability to feed herself, manipulate toy dishes, and sculpt with playdough.

Cognitive Development

Jasmine's morning activity demonstrates and enhances her cognitive learning. She learns new words and grammar by speaking with others and by watching *Sesame Street*. She learns that a symbol such as the number "3" represents three objects. By manipulating playdough, she forms concepts that are the basis for learning about matter and its qualities when she is older.

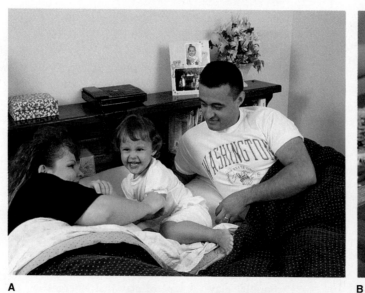
A

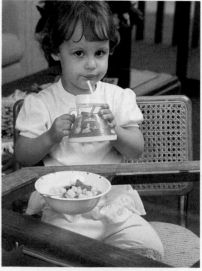
B

FIGURE 2–1 Carefully observing all of a child's activities helps determine what stage of growth and development the child has reached. **A,** Jasmine's play with her parents is indicative of physical and social skills. **B,** Children gradually learn how to take care of themselves and develop psychosocial and motor skills. **C,** Children need to be nurtured and to develop trust. **D,** Napping gives children the added rest they need.

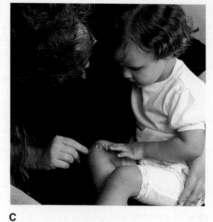
C

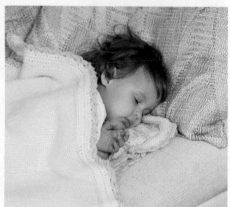
D

Play

Jasmine's play is typical of preschoolers in that she enjoys a mixture of solitary play and associative play with other young children. She is too young to engage in cooperative play such as ball sports and board games.

Nutrition

Jasmine eats foods from all the food groups similar to those enjoyed by the rest of her family. Smaller servings and more frequent meals are the norm for preschoolers. At this age children can be given limited choices in the foods they eat. Meal manners typical of the culture are taught, as when Jasmine begins to play with her food and her mother stops the meal.

Injury Prevention

Cognitive and physical development mirror the changing hazards to the health and well-being of children. Jasmine jumps from a picnic table, presenting an obvious potential for injury. She might just as easily be injured on her Big Wheels or when playing with other toys. Although Jasmine's physical skills are well developed, she does not yet understand the hazards present; therefore she needs close supervision. The nurse uses **anticipatory guidance** to discuss safety hazards and injury prevention with her parents.

Personality and Temperament

Jasmine has always had what experts term an "easy" temperament; that is, she readily chooses a regular schedule for eating and sleeping, her mood is generally pleasant, and she is easily comforted when upset. These temperamental characteristics form a critical link to communication with family, teachers, and friends.

Communication

Jasmine has learned words from television and contact with other people. She understands most speech and uses complete, short sentences. She has refined her social skills and is able to cooperate with others. Feedback from others has helped to form her self-image and promote learning.

Principles of Growth and Development

Growth and development are essential concepts when one is seeking to understand and care for children. **Growth** refers to an increase in physical size. **Development** refers to an increase in capability or function. These quantitative changes in functioning of body organs, ability to communicate, and performance of motor skills unfold over time.

Each child displays a unique maturational pattern during the process of development. Although the exact age at which skills emerge differs, the sequence or order of skill performance is uniform among children. Skill development proceeds according to two processes: from the head down and from the center of the body out to extremities. Development that proceeds from the head downward through the body and toward the feet is termed **cephalocaudal development** (Fig. 2–2). Thus an infant learns to hold up its head before holding a rattle with its hands. Skills, such as walking, that involve the legs and feet develop last in infancy. Similarly, development proceeds from the center of the body outward to the extremities, a process called

FIGURE 2–2 In normal *cephalocaudal* growth the child gains control of her head and neck before the trunk and the limbs. In normal *proximodistal* growth and development the child controls her arm movements before the hand movements; that is, the child reaches for objects before she can grasp them. Children gain control of their hands before their fingers; that is, they can hold things with the entire hand before they can pick something up with just their fingers.

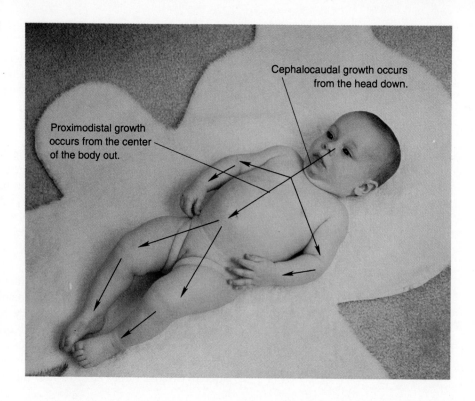

Cephalocaudal growth occurs from the head down.

Proximodistal growth occurs from the center of the body out.

proximodistal development (Fig. 2–2). For example, an infant is first able to control the trunk, then the arms; only later are fine motor movements of the fingers possible.

There is controversy among the experts concerning the relative importance of heredity and environment—nature and nurture—in human development. **Nature** refers to the genetic or hereditary capability of an individual. The ability to learn and the sequence of skill acquisition are inborn qualities. **Nurture** refers to the effects of the environment on a person's performance (Fig. 2–3). Stimulating experiences can improve the speed and level of skill performance. In reality, the influences of both nature and nurture play a role in determining the child's developmental potential.

During childhood years, extraordinary changes occur in all aspects of development. Physical size, motor skills, cognitive ability, language, sensory ability, and psychosocial patterns all undergo major transformations. Nurses study normal developmental patterns so that they can perform thorough pediatric assessments and identify children who demonstrate abnormal development. Such assessments can guide the nurse in planning interventions for the child and family, such as referring the child for diagnosis and rehabilitation or teaching the parents how to provide adequate stimulation for the child. When development is proceeding normally, the nurse uses that knowledge to plan teaching approaches based on the child's cognitive and language ability, to offer appropriate toys and activities during illness, and to respond therapeutically during interactions with the child.

Influences on Development

Development appears to unfold in a predictable pattern as the individual matures. Why then are there differences among individuals? Why do the time frames for acquisition of skills vary? Why do identical twins and close siblings show so much variation?

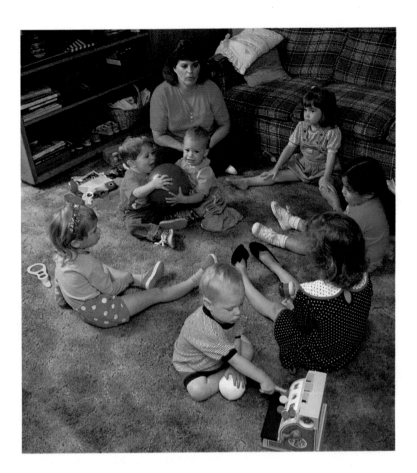

FIGURE 2–3 Children exposed to pleasant stimulation and who are supported by an adult will develop and refine their skills faster. Group play such as this provides an environment for both motor skill and psychosocial development. Can you identify which skills are being developed?

Although an inborn pattern of development is present, many factors influence these innate qualities. Taken together, the forces of nature and nurture create uniqueness among children. Let us look at some of the factors that lead to individual differences.

Genetics

Each child inherits 23 chromosomes from the mother's egg and 23 from the father's sperm, resulting in a unique individual with 46 chromosomes. Every chromosome carries many genes that determine physical characteristics, intellectual potential, personality type, and other traits (Table 2–1). A child is born with certain potential features; however, interaction with the environment influences how and to what extent particular traits are manifested. For

---

TABLE 2–1 Laws of Mendelian Inheritance

dominant inheritance A gene that produces a trait whenever it is present. Achondroplasia dwarfism is one example.

recessive inheritance A gene that produces a trait only when paired with another like gene. Examples include cystic fibrosis, Tay Sachs disease, and phenylketonuria.

X-linked inheritance A disease carried in either a dominant or recessive fashion on the X chromosome. Hemophilia is a common example of an X-linked disease.

chromosome defect Diseases caused by nondisjunction or translocation of chromosomes. Down syndrome is usually caused by a trisomy of chromosome 21.

---

example, a child may have potential for a high level of intellectual performance, but because that child lives in an unstimulating environment, he or she may not reach that potential.

Chromosomal abnormalities that lead to such conditions as Down syndrome may result from such factors as radiation exposure, parental age, or parental disease states. Some children also inherit genes that lead to such diseases as cystic fibrosis. A family history of these diseases is usually present, although they may appear without an identifiable history. This is because genes sometimes mutate, leading to an initial incidence of a genetic disorder.

Prenatal Influences

Some Asian cultures calculate age from the time of conception. This practice acknowledges the profound influence of the prenatal period.

The mother's nutrition and general state of health play a part in pregnancy outcome. Poor nutrition can lead to small infants, compromised neurologic performance, or low maternal stores of iron and resultant anemia in the newborn[1]. Maternal smoking is associated with low-birth-weight infants. Ingestion of alcoholic beverages, including beer and wine, during pregnancy may lead to fetal alcohol syndrome. Illicit drug use by the mother may result in neonatal addiction, convulsions, hyperirritability, poor social responsiveness, and other neurologic disturbances.

Even prescription drugs may adversely affect the fetus. An example is the drug thalidomide, commonly used in pregnancy during the 1950s, which resulted in the birth of infants with limb abnormalities. Other drugs may lead to bleeding, stain teeth, injure hearing, or cause a variety of other defects in the infant.[2]

Some maternal illnesses are harmful to the developing fetus. An example is rubella (German measles), which is rarely a serious disease for adults but which can cause deafness, vision defects, heart defects, and mental retardation in the fetus if it is acquired by a pregnant woman. A fetus can also acquire diseases, such as AIDS (HIV infection) or hepatitis B from the mother.

Radiation, chemicals, and other environmental hazards may adversely affect a fetus when the mother is exposed to these influences during her pregnancy. The best outcomes for infants occur when mothers eat well, exercise regularly, seek early prenatal care, refrain from use of drugs, alcohol, tobacco, and excessive caffeine, and follow general principles of good health.

Family Structure

The families into which children are born influence them profoundly. Children are supported in different ways and acquire different world views depending on such factors as whether one or both parents work, how many siblings are present, and whether an extended family is close by. Note should be made of variations in family structure such as single-parent, homosexual parents, extended family, and step parents.

First-born children tend to be concerned with achievement and grades, often become leaders, and more commonly obtain advanced degrees. Last-born children more often demonstrate a relaxed approach to school and achievements.[3]

Nearly half of all marriages in the United States end in divorce. Divorce has a profound effect on children, varying with the child's age and cognitive stage. Young children who have limited ability to understand divorce may show such behavioral manifestations as crying, sleep disturbance, regression, and aggressive behavior[4] (see Table 2–2). Remarriage, single parenting, and joint custody arrangements all create special challenges for families.

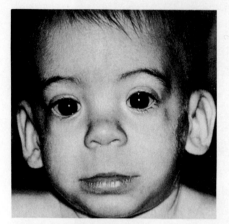

Fetal alcohol syndrome.
From Rudolph, A.M., Hoffman, J.I.E., & Rudolph, C.D. (Eds.). (1991). *Rudolph's Pediatrics*. Norwalk, CT: Appleton & Lange, p. 438.

TABLE 2–2 Effects of Divorce

Age (years)	Behavior
3–5	Fear, anxiety, and dread in daily life events Regression Searching and questioning Self-blame Increased aggression
6–8	Extreme sadness Fantasies and panic Worries about lack of food, money, caretaking
9–12	Intense anger Somatic complaints Confused self-identity
13–18	Withdrawal from family Concern about sex and marriage Loss Anger

Adapted from Wallerstein, J., and Kelly, J. (1980). *Surviving the breakup*. New York: Basic Books.

Socioeconomic Influences

Basic financial stability contributes much to the general health and well-being of children. The United States has the world's largest gross national product but does not meet the needs of many of its children. One quarter of all women in the United States receive no prenatal care in the first trimester of pregnancy, which contributes to a high infant mortality rate. One in four children in the United States is born into poverty, increasing the child's risk of prematurity, health problems, and abuse.[5]

Low socioeconomic status and unemployment are associated with a number of risk factors for children's development, such as poor nutrition, lack of immunization, increased injuries, and a high rate of teenage pregnancy.[6] Homelessness is one example of an economic problem that places children at risk. Families are the fastest growing group of homeless people. Homeless children do not usually have health insurance. They are more likely to lack immunizations, proper nutrition, safe environment, and stable school and family situations.[7]

Culture

The traditional customs of the many cultural groups represented in North American society influence the development of the children in these groups. Foods commonly eaten vary among people with different cultural backgrounds (Table 2–3) and influence the incidence of health problems such as cardiovascular disease in the groups. The Native American practice of carrying infants on boards often delays walking when it is measured against the norm for walking on some developmental tests. Children who are carried by straddling the mother's hips or back for extended periods have a low incidence of developmental hip dislocation since this keeps their hips in an abducted position.

All cultural groups have rules regarding patterns of social interaction. Schedules of language acquisition are determined by the number of languages spoken and the amount of speech in the home. The particular social roles assumed by men and women in the culture affect school activities and ultimately career choices. Attitudes toward touching and other methods of encouraging developmental skills vary among cultures.

Environment

Media

The violence on television and in video games has been associated with aggressive behavior in children[8] (Fig. 2–4). An increased amount of television viewing time is associated with above-normal weight, lower reading and intellectual test scores, and poorer sports performance.[9] Parents at home and nurses in the hospital should be aware of the shows children are watching, make decisions about their suitability, and be available to discuss the content with children.

School

Once a child is 5 or 6 years of age, several hours daily are spent in a school setting. Physical education and sports develop their physical skills. Psychosocial stages are met as the child interacts with children and adults and learns social interaction patterns and pride in accomplishments. Presentation of concepts that challenge thought processes enhance cognitive development.

TABLE 2-3 Traditional Foods of Various Cultures

Culture	Traditional Foods	Special Notes
African American	Okra, kale, collard, and other greens; red and lima beans; black eyed peas; corn bread; grits; pork products; tongue; chitterlings	Foods are similar to those common to all Southerners.
Orthodox Jewish	Kosher foods	Pork products and shell fish are avoided. Milk and meat are not mixed or eaten at the same meal.
Native American	Blue corn meal, meats, fish, fruits, berries, greens	Practices vary among tribes. Milk products may not be widely used.
Mexican American	Beans, rice, cheese, corn, tortillas, enchiladas, burritos, avocados, chilies, melons, tomatoes	All meats and foods are labeled as "hot" or "cold," which does not relate to temperature. "Hot" foods such as cheese, eggs, onions, peppers, and beef are used to treat "cold" diseases such as cancer, teething, colds, and stomach cramps. "Cold" foods such as fruits and vegetables, dairy products, or chicken are used to treat "hot" diseases such as fever, rashes, or constipation.
Chinese American	Rice, tofu, bok choy, bean sprouts, water chestnuts, bamboo shoots, snow peas, melons, pineapple, duck, shellfish, thinly sliced beef, pork, or chicken	Special seasonings such as soy sauce and oyster sauce are used. Monosodium glutamate (MSG) used for cooking can increase salt intake. Lactose intolerance is frequent.
East Indian American	Wheat, rice, barley, chick peas, leafy green vegetables, potatoes, melons, berries	East Indian Hindus are vegetarians. Special spices are used for flavoring.

Although the primary role of schools is educational, they also perform several health-related functions. School health screening programs play an important role in identifying children with such health problems as hearing loss, visual impairment, and scoliosis.

Many schools teach good nutrition, healthful living and sexuality practices, and other health-related topics. A school nurse may be present, at least part time, to plan these educational offerings, as well as to provide emergency health care when needed. With the increase in mainstreaming, schools now have the responsibility for administering medications, maintaining urinary catheters and respiratory care, and for other treatments to ensure the child's proper growth and development.

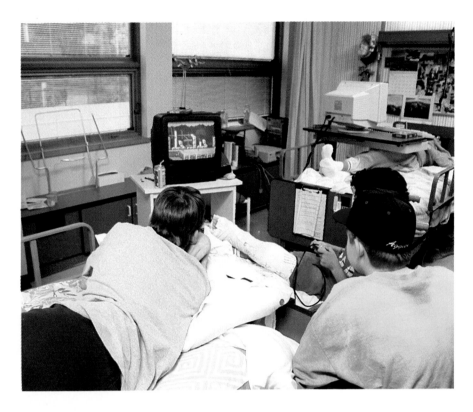

FIGURE 2-4 Some research suggests a correlation between violence on TV, in the movies, and in video games and aggressive behavior in children. Nurses should determine the parents' preference for what their child should watch when they are not with the child.

Community

The community in which a child lives may support the child's development or, conversely, expose the child to hazards. Social programs such as Head Start preschools, sports activities, after-school programs, and child abuse treatment centers offer valuable services that improve the experiences of growing children. On the other hand, an economically depressed community with scant services and a high homicide rate is unsupportive and hazardous for growing children.[10]

The physical environment is supportive when the child is provided with sidewalks on which to walk to school, open spaces in which to learn and play, and clean air to breathe. Children who must walk to school on unsafe roads, have access to contaminated water supplies, or live near polluting manufacturing companies or in crowded housing or old structures are at risk for injuries and health problems such as lead poisoning.

Stress

The adverse effect of stress on adults is well documented. More recently the impact of stress on children has been recognized. Children manifest stress in a variety of ways, including regressive behavior, interrupted sleep, hyperactive behavior, gastrointestinal symptoms, crying, and withdrawal from normal events. Common stressful events for children include moving to a new home or school, marital difficulties in the family, abuse, and being expected to achieve at an extremely high level in school or sports[11] (Fig. 2–5).

The child experiencing stress has more frequent respiratory and gastrointestinal illnesses and is more likely to be the victim of an accident. The negative long-term effects of stress on body organs and systems suggest that children under stress are more likely to develop illnesses such as strokes, hypertension, and heart attacks later in life.

FIGURE 2–5 Sports can be an excellent way for children to develop their psychosocial, cognitive, and motor skills. When coaches and parents make demands of children beyond their developmental capabilities, the resultant stress can be manifested in respiratory and gastrointestinal disorders.
Courtesy Rebecca Scheirer, Kensington, Maryland.

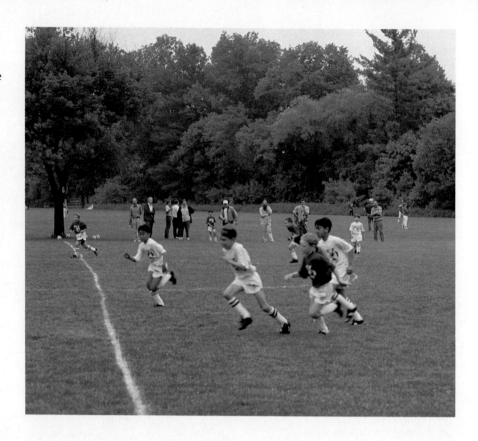

Major Theories of Development

Child development is a complex process. Many theorists have attempted to organize their observations of behavior into a description of principles or a set of stages. Each theory focuses on a particular facet of development. Most developmental theorists group children in age groups by common characteristics (Table 2–4).

Freud's Theory of Psychosexual Development

Theoretical Framework

The psychoanalytic techniques used by Freud led him to believe that early childhood experiences form the unconscious motivation for actions in later

---

TABLE 2–4 Developmental Age Groups

infancy Birth to 12 months. This stage includes infants or babies up to one year of age who require a high level of care in daily activities.

toddlerhood 1 to 3 years. This stage encompasses about two years and is characterized by increased motor ability and independent behavior.

preschool 3 to 6 years. This stage encompasses about three years. The preschooler refines gross and fine motor ability and language skills and often participates in a preschool learning program.

school age 6 to 12 years. This stage begins with entry into a school system and is characterized by growing intellectual skills, physical ability, and independence.

adolescence 12 to 18 years. This stage begins with entry into the teen years. Mature cognitive thought, formation of identity, and influence of peers are important characteristics of adolescence.

TABLE 2-5 Common Defense Mechanisms Used by Children

Defense Mechanism	Definition	Example
Regression	Return to an earlier behavior	A previously toilet trained child becomes incontinent when separated from parents during a hospitalization.
Repression	Involuntary forgetting of uncomfortable situations	An abused child cannot consciously recall episodes of abuse.
Rationalization	An attempt to make unacceptable feelings acceptable	A child explains hitting another because "he took my toy."
Fantasy	A creation of the mind to help deal with unacceptable fear	A hospitalized child who is weak pretends to be Superman.

■ SIGMUND FREUD (1856–1939)

Freud was a physician in Vienna, Austria. His work with adults who were experiencing a variety of nervous disorders led Freud to develop the approach called psychoanalysis, which explored the driving forces of the unconscious mind.[12]

life. He developed a theory that sexual energy is centered in specific parts of the body at certain ages. Unresolved conflict and unmet needs at a certain stage lead to a fixation of development at that stage.

Freud viewed the personality as a structure with three parts: the **id** is the basic sexual energy that is present at birth and drives the individual to seek pleasure; the **ego** is the realistic part of the person that develops during infancy and searches for acceptable methods of meeting sexual needs; and the **superego** is the moral system that develops in childhood and contains a set of values and conscience.[12] The ego protects itself from excess anxiety by use of **defense mechanisms**, including regression to earlier stages and repression or forgetting of painful experiences such as child abuse (Table 2–5).

Stages

Oral (birth–1 year). The infant derives pleasure largely from the mouth, with sucking and eating as primary desires.

Anal (1–3 years). The young child's pleasure is centered in the anal area, with control over body secretions as a prime force in behavior.

Phallic (3–6 years). Sexual energy becomes centered in the genitalia as the child works out relationships with parents of the same and opposite sexes (Oedipus and Electra complexes).

Latency (6–12 years). Sexual energy is at rest in the passage between earlier stages and adolescence.

Genital (12 years–adulthood). Mature sexuality is achieved as physical growth is completed and relationships with others occur.

Nursing Application

Freud emphasized the importance of meeting the needs of each stage in order to move successfully into future developmental stages. The crisis of illness can interfere with normal developmental processes and add challenges for the nurse striving to meet an ill child's needs. For example, the importance of sucking in infancy guides the nurse to provide a pacifier for the infant who cannot have oral fluids. The preschool child's concern about sexuality guides the nurse to provide privacy and clear explanations during any procedures involving the genital area. It may be necessary to teach parents that masturbation by the young child is normal and to help them deal with it. The adolescent's focus on relationships suggests that the nurse should include questions about significant friends during history taking. Table 2–6 summarizes ways in which the nurse can apply these theoretical concepts to the care of children.

TABLE 2–6 Nursing Application of Theories of Freud, Erikson, Piaget

Age Group	Developmental Stages	Nursing Application
Infant (birth–1 year)	Oral stage (Freud): The baby obtains pleasure and comfort through the mouth.	When a baby is NPO, offer a pacifier if not contraindicated. After painful procedures, offer a baby a bottle or pacifier or have the mother breast feed.
	Trust vs. mistrust stage (Erikson): The baby establishes a sense of trust when basic needs are met.	Hold the hospitalized baby often.(1) Offer comfort after painful procedures. Meet the baby's needs for food and hygiene. Encourage parents to room in. Manage pain effectively.
	Sensorimotor stage (Piaget): The baby learns from movement and sensory input.	Use crib mobiles, manipulative toys, wall murals, and bright colors to provide interesting stimuli and comfort. Use toys to distract the baby during procedures and assessments.
Toddler (1–3 years)	Anal stage (Freud): The child derives gratification from control over bodily excretions.	Ask about toilet training and the child's rituals and words for elimination during admission history. Continue child's normal patterns of elimination in the hospital. Do not begin toilet training during illness or hospitalization. Accept regression in toileting during illness without reprimand. Make potty chairs available in hospital. Allow self-feeding opportunities.
	Autonomy vs. shame and doubt stage (Erikson): The child is increasingly independent in many spheres of life.	Encourage child to remove and put on own clothes, brush teeth, or assist with hygiene. (2) If restraint for a procedure is necessary, proceed quickly, providing explanations and comfort.
	Sensorimotor stage (end); preoperational stage (beginning) (Piaget): The child shows increasing curiosity and explorative behavior. Language skills improve.	Keep surroundings safe to allow opportunities to manipulate objects. Name objects and give simple explanations.

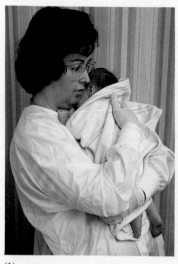

(1)

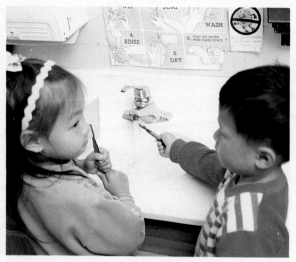

(2)

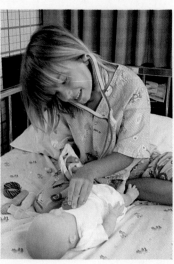

(3)

Age Group	Developmental Stages	Nursing Application
Preschooler (3–6 years)	Phallic stage (Freud): The child initially identifies with the parent of the opposite sex but by the end of this stage has identified with the same-sex parent. Initiative vs. guilt stage (Erikson): The child likes to initiate play activities. Preoperational stage (Piaget): The child is increasingly verbal but has some limitations in thought processes. Causality is often confused, so the child may feel responsible for causing an illness.	Be alert for children who appear more comfortable with male or female nurses, and attempt to accommodate them. Encourage parental involvement in care. Plan for play time and offer a variety of materials from which to choose. Offer medical equipment for play to lessen anxiety about strange objects. (3) Assess children's concerns as expressed through their drawings. Accept the child's choices and expressions of feelings. Offer explanations about all procedures and treatments. Clearly explain that the child is not responsible for causing the illness.
School age (6–12 years)	Latency stage (Freud): The child places importance on privacy and understanding the body. Industry vs. inferiority stage (Erikson): The child gains a sense of self-worth from involvement in activities. Concrete operational stage (Piaget): The child is capable of mature thought when allowed to manipulate and see objects.	Provide gowns, covers, and underwear. Knock on door before entering. Explain treatments and procedures. Continue school work while hospitalized. Encourage child to bring favorite pastimes to the hospital. (4) Help child adjust to limitations on favorite activities. Give clear instructions about details of treatment. Provide equipment for the child to see that is used in treatment.
Adolescent (12–18 years)	Genital stage (Freud): The adolescent's focus is on genital function and relationships. Identity vs. role confusion stage (Erikson): The adolescent's search for self-identify leads to independence from parents and reliance on peers. Formal operational stage (Piaget): The adolescent is capable of mature, abstract thought.	Ensure access to gynecologic care for adolescent girls. Provide information on sexuality. Ensure privacy during health care. Have brochures and videos available for teaching issues of sexuality. Provide a separate recreation room for teens who are hospitalized. (5) Take health history and perform examinations without parents present. Introduce adolescent to other teens with same health problem. Give clear and complete information about health care and treatments. Offer both written and verbal instructions. Reeducate the adolescent with a chronic illness about the disease, since mature thought now leads to greater understanding.

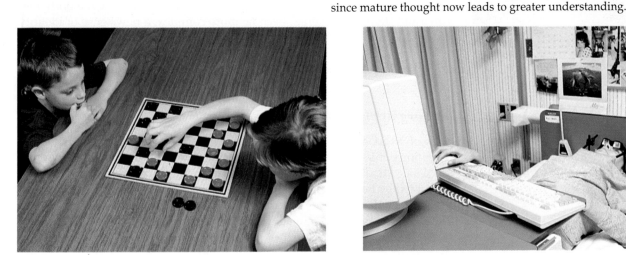

(4)

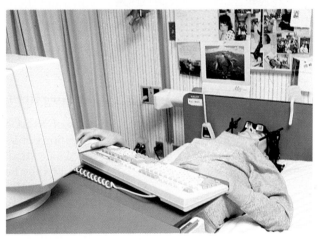

(5)

Erikson studied Freud's theory of psychoanalysis under Freud's daughter Anna but later established his own developmental theory emphasizing the psychosocial nature of individuals. Erikson's is one of the few theories that addresses development over the entire life span.[13]

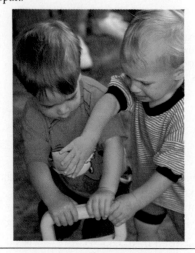

Autonomy vs. shame and doubt.

Erikson's Theory of Psychosocial Development

Theoretical Framework

Erikson's theory establishes psychosocial stages during eight periods of human life. For each stage Erikson identifies a crisis, that is, a particular challenge that exists for healthy personality development to occur.[13] The word "crisis" refers to normal maturational social needs rather than to a single critical event. Each developmental crisis has two possible outcomes. When needs are met, the consequence is healthy and the individual moves on to future stages with particular strengths. When needs are not met, an unhealthy outcome occurs that will influence future social relationships.

Stages

Trust vs. Mistrust (birth–1 year). The task of the first year of life is to establish trust in the people providing care. Trust is fostered by provision of food, clean clothing, touch, and comfort. If basic needs are not met, the infant will eventually learn to mistrust others.

Autonomy vs. Shame and Doubt (1–3 years). The toddler's sense of autonomy or independence is shown by controlling body excretions, saying no when asked to do something, and directing motor activity. Children who are consistently criticized for expressions of autonomy or for lack of control—for example, during toilet training—will develop a sense of shame about themselves and doubt in their abilities.

Initiative vs. Guilt (3–6 years). The young child initiates new activities and considers new ideas. This interest in exploring the world creates a child who is involved and busy. Constant criticism, on the other hand, leads to feelings of guilt and a lack of purpose.

Industry vs. Inferiority (6–12 years). The middle years of childhood are characterized by development of new interests and involvement in activities. The child takes pride in accomplishments in sports, school, home, and community. If the child cannot accomplish what is expected, however, the result will be a sense of inferiority.

Identity vs. Role Confusion (12–18 years). In adolescence, as the body matures and thought processes become more complex, a new sense of identity or self is established. The self, family, peer group, and community are all examined and redefined. The adolescent who is unable to establish a meaningful definition of self will experience confusion in one or more roles of life.

A child takes pride in accomplishments in sports.

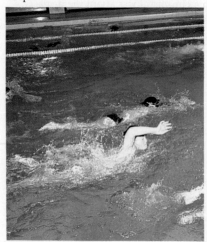

Nursing Application

Erikson's theory is directly applicable to nursing care of children. The social situations created by health care provide opportunities for meeting children's needs. The child's usual support from family, peers, and others is interrupted by hospitalization. The challenge of hospitalization also adds a situational crisis to the normal developmental crisis a child is experiencing. Although the nurse may meet many of the hospitalized child's needs, continued parental involvement is needed to ensure progression through expected developmental stages (see Table 2–6).

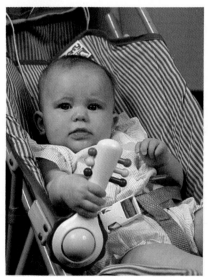

Piaget's Theory of Cognitive Development

Theoretical Framework

Based on his observations and work with children, Piaget formulated a theory of cognitive (or intellectual) development. He believed that the child's view of the world was influenced largely by age and maturational ability. Given nurturing experiences, the child's ability to think matures naturally.[14]

Stages

Sensorimotor (birth–2 years). Infants learn about the world by input obtained through the senses and by their motor activity. Six substages are characteristic of this stage.

USE OF REFLEXES (BIRTH–1 MONTH). The infant begins life with a set of reflexes such as sucking, rooting, and grasping. By using these reflexes, the infant receives stimulation via touch, sound, smell, and vision. The reflexes thus pave the way for the first learning to occur.

PRIMARY CIRCULAR REACTIONS (1–4 MONTHS). Once the infant responds reflexively, the pleasure gained from that response causes repetition of the behavior. For example, if a toy grasped reflexively makes noise and is interesting to look at, the infant will grasp it again.

SECONDARY CIRCULAR REACTIONS (4–8 MONTHS). Awareness of the environment grows as the infant begins to connect cause and effect. The sounds of bottle preparation will lead to excited behavior. If an object is partially hidden, the infant will attempt to uncover and retrieve it.

COORDINATION OF SECONDARY SCHEMES (8–12 MONTHS). Intentional behavior is observed as the infant uses learned behavior to obtain objects, create sounds, or engage in other pleasurable activity. **Object permanence** (the knowledge that something continues to exist even when out of sight) begins when the infant remembers where a hidden object is likely to be found; it is no longer "out of sight, out of mind."

TERTIARY CIRCULAR REACTIONS (12–18 MONTHS). Curiosity, experimentation, and exploration predominate as the toddler tries out actions to learn results. Objects are turned in every direction, placed in the mouth, used for banging, and inserted in containers as their qualities and uses are explored.

MENTAL COMBINATIONS (18–24 MONTHS). Language provides a new tool for the toddler to use in understanding the world. Language enables the child to think about events and objects before or after they occur. Object permanence is now fully developed as the child actively searches for objects in various locations and out of view.

Preoperational (2–7 years). The young child thinks by using words as symbols, but logic is not well developed. During the preconceptual substage (2–4 years), vocabulary and comprehension increase greatly but the child is egocentric (that is, unable to see things from the perspective of another). In the intuitive substage (4–7 years) the child relies on transductive reasoning (that is, drawing conclusions from one general fact to another). For example, when a child disobeys a parent and then falls and breaks an arm that day, the child may ascribe the broken arm to bad behavior. Cause-and-effect relationships are often unrealistic or a result of "magical thinking."

Concrete Operational (7–11 years). Transductive reasoning has given way to a more accurate understanding of cause and effect. The child can reason quite well if concrete objects are used in teaching or experimentation. The concept of conservation (that matter does not change when its form is altered) is learned at this age.

Formal Operational (11 years–adulthood). Fully mature intellectual thought has now been attained. The adolescent can think abstractly about objects or concepts and consider different alternatives or outcomes.

Nursing Application

Piaget's theory is essential to the pediatric nurse. The nurse must understand a child's thought to design stimulating activities and meaningful, appropriate teaching plans. Understanding a child's concept of time suggests to the nurse how far in advance to prepare that child for procedures. Similarly, whether the nurse offers manipulative toys, reads stories, draws pictures, or gives the child reading matter to explain health care measures depends on the child's cognitive stage of development (Table 2–6).

■ **LAWRENCE KOHLBERG (B. 1927)**

Kohlberg used Piaget's cognitive stage theory as the basis for his theory of moral development. He worked with children in his native Germany and in many other countries, including Kenya, Taiwan, and Mexico.[15]

Kohlberg's Theory of Moral Development

Theoretical Framework

Kohlberg focused on a particular type of cognitive development, that concerned with moral decisions. He presented stories involving moral dilemmas to children and adults and asked them to solve the dilemmas. Kohlberg then analyzed the motives they expressed when making decisions about the best course to take. Based on the explanations given, Kohlberg established three levels of moral reasoning. Although he provided age guidelines, he stated that they are approximate and that many people never reach the highest (postconventional) stage of development.[15]

Stages

Preconventional (4–7 years). Decisions are based on the desire to please others and to avoid punishment.

Conventional (7–11 years). Conscience or an internal set of standards becomes important. Rules are important and must be followed to please other people and "be good."

Postconventional (12 years and older). The individual has internalized ethical standards on which to base decisions. Social responsibility is recognized. The value in each of two differing moral approaches can be considered and a decision made.

Nursing Application

Decision making is required in many areas of health care. Children can be assisted to make decisions about health care and to consider alternatives when available. The nurse should keep in mind that young children may agree to participate in research simply because they want to comply with adults and appear cooperative.

Bandura is a Canadian who has conducted psychologic research at Stanford University for many years. He believes that children learn from their social environment, particularly by modeling the observed behaviors of others.[16]

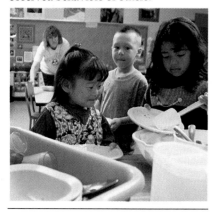

Social Learning Theory

Theoretical Framework

Bandura, a contemporary psychologist, believes that children learn through their social contacts with adults and other children. Children imitate (or model) the behavior they see, and if they are positively reinforced, this behavior tends to recur. The external environment and the child's internal processes are key elements in social learning theory.[16]

Nursing Application

The importance of modeling behavior can readily be applied in health care. Children are more likely to cooperate if they see adults or other children performing a task willingly. A frightened child may watch another child perform vision screening or have blood drawn and then decide to allow the procedure to take place. Contact with positive role models is useful when teaching children and adolescents care for diseases such as diabetes. Positive reinforcement should be used intentionally to give feedback for desired activity.

Behaviorism

Watson was an American scientist who applied the work of animal behaviorists, such as Ivan Pavlov and B.F. Skinner, to children.[17]

Theoretical Framework

Watson studied the research of Pavlov and Skinner, who demonstrated that actions are determined by responses from the environment. Pavlov and Skinner worked with animals, presenting a stimulus such as food and pairing it with another stimulus such as a ringing bell. Eventually the animal they were feeding began to salivate when the bell rang. As Skinner and then Watson began to apply these concepts to children, they showed that behaviors can be elicited by positive reinforcement, such as a food treat, or extinguished by negative reinforcement, such as by scolding or withdrawal of attention. Watson believed that he could take any child and make of that person anyone he desired—from a professional to a thief or beggar—simply by reinforcing behavior in certain ways.[17]

Nursing Application

Behaviorism has been criticized for its simplicity and its denial of the inherent capability of persons to respond willfully to events in the environment. This theory does, however, have some use in health care. When particular behaviors are desired, positive reinforcement can be established to encourage these behaviors. Behavioral techniques are also used to alter behavior of misbehaving children or to teach skills to handicapped children. Parents often use reinforcement in toilet training and other skills learned in childhood.

Chess and Thomas are psychiatrists who began a landmark study in 1956 with 141 children, which they expanded in 1961 with 95 additional children. Most of these individuals are still being assessed periodically as adults. Their research has identified characteristics of personality and provides a basis for the ongoing study of temperament.[19]

Temperament Theory

Theoretical Framework

In contrast to behaviorists such as Watson, Chess and Thomas recognized the innate qualities of personality that each individual brings to the events of daily life. Chess and Thomas looked at a wide spectrum of behaviors and identified nine parameters of response to daily events (Table 2–7). Infants

TABLE 2-7 Nine Parameters of Personality

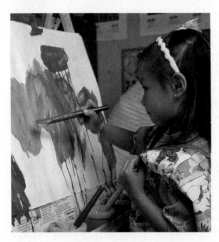

1. **Activity level:** The degree of motion during eating, playing, sleeping, bathing. Scored as high, medium, or low.
2. **Rhythmicity:** The regularity of schedule maintained for sleep, hunger, elimination. Scored as regular, variable, or irregular.
3. **Approach or withdrawal:** The response to a new stimulus such as a food, activity, or person. Scored as approachable, variable, or withdrawal.
4. **Adaptability:** The degree of adaptation to new situations. Scored as adaptive, variable, or nonadaptive.
5. **Threshold of responsiveness:** The intensity of stimulation needed to elicit a response to sensory input, objects in the environment, or people. Scored as high, medium, or low.
6. **Intensity of reaction:** The degree of response to situations. Scored as positive, variable, or negative.
7. **Quality of mood:** The predominant mood during daily activity and in response to stimuli. Scored as positive, variable, or negative.
8. **Distractability:** The ability of environmental stimuli to interfere with the child's activity. Scored as distractible, variable, or nondistractible.
9. **Attention span and persistence:** The amount of time devoted to activities (compared with other children of the same age) and the degree of ability to stick with an activity in spite of obstacles. Scored as persistent, variable, or nonpersistent.[8]

generally displayed clusters of responses, which Chess and Thomas classified into three major personality types (Table 2–8). Although most children do not demonstrate all behaviors described for a particular type, they usually show a grouping indicative of one personality type.[18,19]

Recent research demonstrates that personality characteristics displayed during infancy are often consistent with those seen later in life. The ability to predict future characteristics is not possible, however, because of the complex and dynamic interaction of personality traits and environmental reactions.

Many other researchers have expanded the work of Chess and Thomas, developing assessment tools for temperament types. The concept of "goodness of fit" is an outgrowth of the theory. Goodness of fit refers to whether parents' expectations of their child's behavior are consistent with the child's temperament type. For example, an infant who is very active and reacts strongly to verbal stimuli may be unable to sleep well when placed in a room with older siblings. A child who is slow to warm up may not perform well in the first few months at a new school, much to parents' disappointment. When parents understand a child's temperament characteristics, they are better able to shape the environment to meet the child's needs.

Nursing Application

The concept of personality type or temperament is a useful one for nurses. Nurses can assess the temperament of young children and alter the environment to meet their needs. This may involve moving a hospitalized child to a single room to ensure adequate rest if the child is easily stimulated, or allowing a shy child time to become accustomed to new surroundings and equipment before beginning new procedures or treatments.

Parents are often relieved to learn about temperament characteristics. They learn to appreciate their children's qualities and to adapt the environment to meet the children's needs. A burden of guilt can also be lifted from parents who feel that they are responsible for their child's actions. The nurse can teach parents ways of enhancing goodness of fit between the child's personality and the environment (Table 2–9).

TABLE 2-8 Patterns of Temperament

The **"easy" child** is generally moderate in activity; shows regularity in patterns of eating, sleeping, and elimination; and is usually positive in mood and when subjected to new stimuli. The easy child adapts to new situations and is able to accept rules and work well with others. About 40% of children in the New York Longitudinal Study displayed this personality type.

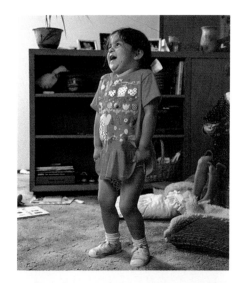

The **"difficult" child** displays irregular schedules for eating, sleeping, and elimination; adapts slowly to new situations and persons; and displays a predominantly negative mood. Intense reactions to the environment are common. About 10% of children in the New York Longitudinal Study displayed this personality type.

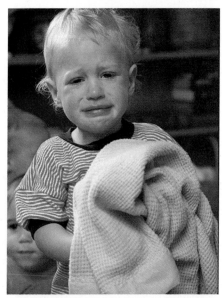

The **"slow-to-warm-up" child** has reactions of mild intensity and slow adaptability to new situations. The child displays initial withdrawal followed by gradual, quiet, and slow interaction with the environment. About 15% of children in the New York Longitudinal Study displayed this personality type.
The remaining 35% of children studied showed some characteristics of each personality type.[19]

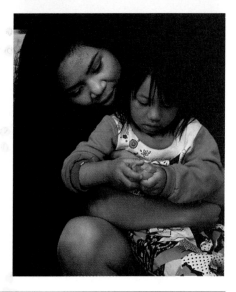

TABLE 2-9 Ways to Improve Goodness of Fit Between Parents and Child

Child's Behavior	Parent's Activity
Extremely active	Plan periods of active play several times in day. Have restful periods before bedtime to foster sleep.
Shy	Allow time to adapt at own pace to new people and situations.
Easily stimulated	Have quiet room for sleeping as an infant. Have quiet room for homework as a school-age child.
Short attention span	Provide projects that can be completed in a short period. Gradually encourage longer periods at activities.

✓ Infant (Birth–1 Year)

Can you imagine tripling your present weight in one year? Or becoming proficient in understanding fundamental words in a new language and even speaking a few? These and many more accomplishments take place in the first year of life. Starting the year as a mainly reflexive creature, the infant can walk and communicate by the year's end. Never again in life is development so swift (Fig. 2–6).

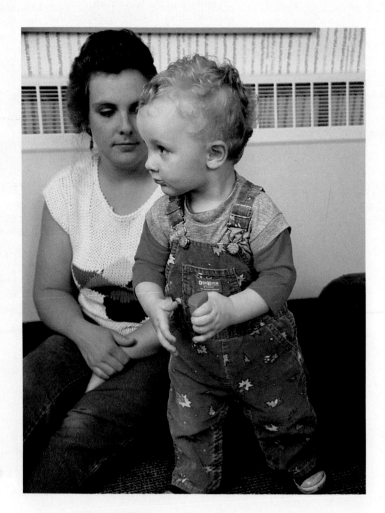

FIGURE 2-6 A 12-month-old child will have tripled his birth weight, learned to walk, and will be beginning to talk.

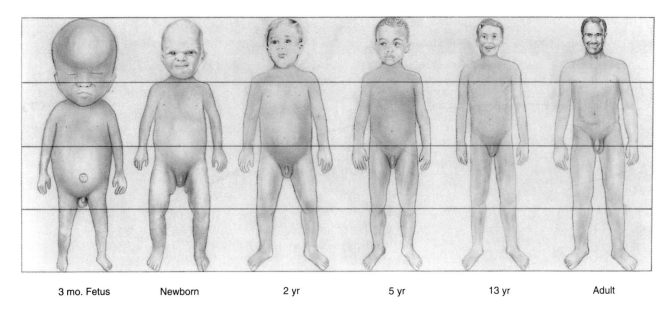

FIGURE 2-7 Body proportions at various ages.

| 3 mo. Fetus | Newborn | 2 yr | 5 yr | 13 yr | Adult |

■ CULTURAL CONSIDERATIONS

Health care providers in the United States use one set of growth charts for all children, but these charts do not take into account variations related to hereditary differences. Black infants generally weigh less at birth than white infants but grow faster during childhood, thereby attaining a larger size. Some Asian groups have a hereditary predisposition to short stature. A review of parental and sibling size provides important data about the effects of cultural heritage. When height and weight are assessed, it is most important that growth follows the same percentile curve.[20]

Physical Growth and Development

The first year of life is one of rapid change for the infant. The birth weight usually doubles by about 5 months and triples by the end of the first year (Fig. 2–7). Height increases by about a foot during this year. Teeth begin to erupt at about 6 months, and by the end of the first year the infant has six to eight deciduous teeth (see Chapter 3).

Body organs and systems, although not fully mature at 1 year, function differently than they did at birth. Kidney and liver maturation helps the 1-year-old excrete drugs or other toxic substances more readily than in the first weeks of life. The changing body proportions mirror changes in developing internal organs. Maturation of the nervous system is demonstrated by increased control over body movements, enabling the infant to sit, stand, and walk. Sensory function also increases as the infant begins to discriminate visual images, sounds, and tastes (Table 2–10).

Cognitive Development

The brain continues to increase in complexity during the first year. Most of the growth involves maturation of cells, with only a small increase in number of cells. This growth of the brain is accompanied by development of its functions. One has only to compare the behavior of an infant shortly after birth with that of a 1-year-old to understand the incredible maturation of brain function. The newborn's eyes widen in response to sound; the 1-year-old turns to the sound and recognizes its significance. The 2-month-old cries and coos; the 1-year-old says a few words and understands many more. The 6-week-old grasps a rattle for the first time; the 1-year-old reaches for toys and feeds himself or herself.

The infant's behaviors provide clues about thought processes. Piaget's work outlines the infant's actions in a set of rapidly progressing changes in the first year of life. The infant receives stimulation through sight, sound, and feeling, which the maturing brain interprets. This input from the environment interacts with internal cognitive abilities to enhance cognitive functioning.

TABLE 2-10 Growth and Development Milestones During Infancy

Age	Physical Growth	Fine Motor Ability	Gross Motor Ability	Sensory Ability	Nutrition
Birth–1 month	Gains 5–7 ounces/week Grows 1.5 cm in first month Head circumference increases 1.5 cm/month	Holds hand in fist (1) Draws arms and legs to body when crying	Inborn reflexes such as startle and rooting are predominant activity May lift head briefly if prone (2) Alerts to high pitched voices Comforts with touch (3)	Prefers to look at faces and black and white geometric designs Follows objects in line of vision (4)	Eats every 2–3 hours, breast or bottle, 2–3 ounces per feeding

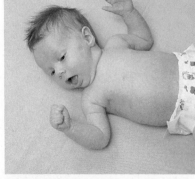

(1) Holds hand in fist

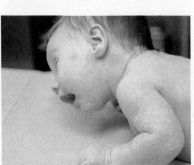

(2) May lift head

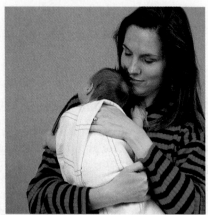

(3) Comforts with touch

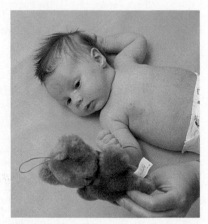

(4) Follows objects

2–4 months	Gains 5–7 ounces/week Grows 1.5 cm/month Head circumference increases 1.5 cm/month Posterior fontanel closes Eats 120 mL/kg/24 hr	Holds rattle when placed in hand (5) Looks at and plays with own fingers Readily brings objects from hand to mouth	Moro reflex fading in strength Can turn from side to back and then return (6) Decrease in head lag when pulled to sitting; sits with head held in midline with some bobbing When prone, holds head and supports weight on forearms (7)	Follows objects 180° Turns head to look for voices and sounds	Has coordinated suck-swallow Establishes regular eating pattern of 3–4 ounces every 3–4 hours

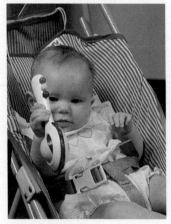

(5) Holds rattle

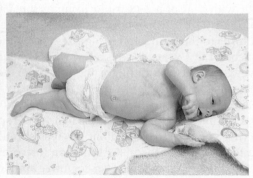

(6) Can turn from side to back

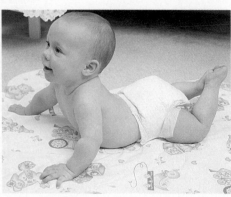

(7) Holds head up and supports weight with arms

TABLE 2-10 Growth and Development Milestones During Infancy Continued

Age	Physical Growth	Fine Motor Ability	Gross Motor Ability	Sensory Ability	Nutrition
4–6 months	Gains 5–7 ounces/week Doubles birth weight by 5–6 months Grows 1.5 cm/month Head circumference increases 1.5 cm/month Teeth may begin erupting by 6 months Eats 100 mL/kg 24 hr	Grasps rattles and other objects at will; drops them to pick up another offered object (8) Mouths objects Holds feet and pulls to mouth Holds bottle Grasps with whole hand (palmar grasp) Manipulates objects (9)	Head held steady when sitting No head lag when pulled to sitting Turns from abdomen to back by 4 months and then back to abdomen by 6 months When held standing supports much of own weight (10)	Examines complex visual images Watches the course of a falling object Responds readily to sounds	Eats 4–5 ounces four or more times/day Begins baby food, usually rice cereal

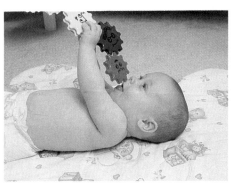

(8) Grasps objects at will

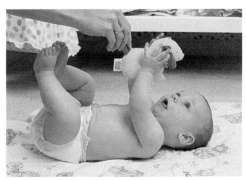

(9) Manipulates objects

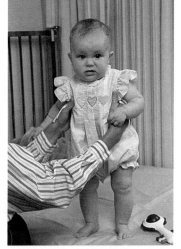

(10) Supports most of weight when held standing

Age	Physical Growth	Fine Motor Ability	Gross Motor Ability	Sensory Ability	Nutrition
6–8 months	Gains 3–5 ounces/week Grows 1 cm/month Growth rate slower than first 6 months	Bangs two objects held in hands Transfers objects from one hand to the other Beginning pincer grasp at times	Most inborn reflexes extinguished Sits alone steadily without support by 8 months (11) Likes to bounce on legs when held in standing position	Recognizes own name and responds by looking and smiling Enjoys small and complex objects at play	Eats 6–8 ounces four times/day Eats baby food such as rice cereal, fruits, and vegetables

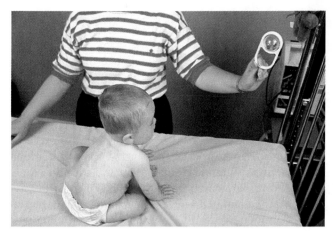

(11) Sits alone without support

Continued.

Age	Physical Growth	Fine Motor Ability	Gross Motor Ability	Sensory Ability	Nutrition
8–10 months	Gains 3–5 ounces/week Grows 1 cm/month	Picks up small objects (12) Uses pincer grasp well (14)	Crawls or pulls whole body along floor by arms (13) Creeps by using hands and knees to keep trunk off floor Pulls self to standing and sitting by 10 months Recovers balance when sitting	Understands words such as "no" and "cracker" May say one word in addition to "mama" and "dada" Recognizes sound without difficulty	Eats 6 ounces four times/day Enjoys soft finger foods (15)

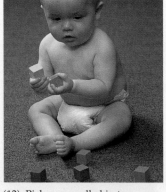

(12) Picks up small objects

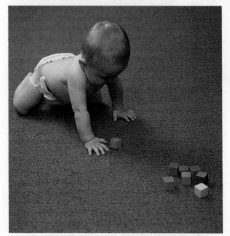

(13) Crawls or pulls body by arms

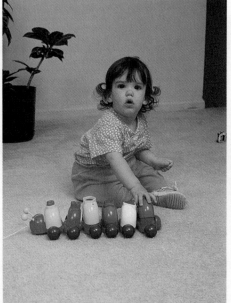

(14) Uses pincer grab well

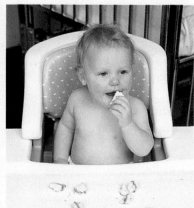

(15) Enjoys soft finger foods

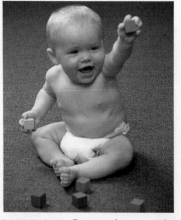

FIGURE 2-8 Garrett shows us that an 8-month-old child can play with blocks, demonstrating physical, cognitive, and social capabilities.

Play

An 8-month-old infant is sitting on the floor, grasping blocks and banging them on the floor. When a parent walks by, the infant laughs and waves hands and feet wildly (Fig. 2–8). Physical capabilities enable the infant to move toward and reach out for objects of interest. Cognitive ability is reflected in manipulation of the blocks to create different sounds. Social interaction enhances play. The presence of a parent or other person increases interest in surroundings and teaches the infant different ways to play.

The play of infants begins in a reflexive manner. When an infant moves extremities or grasps objects, the foundations of play are established. Pleasure is gained from the feel and sound of these activities, and they gradually are performed purposefully. For example, when a parent places a rattle in the hand of a 6-week-old infant, the infant grasps it reflexively. As the hands move randomly, the rattle makes an enjoyable sound. The infant learns to move the rattle to create the sound and then finally to grasp the rattle at will to play with it.

TABLE 2-10 Growth and Development Milestones During Infancy Continued

Age	Physical Growth	Fine Motor Ability	Gross Motor Ability	Sensory Ability	Nutrition
10–12 months	Gains 3–5 ounces/week Grows 1 cm/month Head circumference equals chest circumference Triples birth weight by 1 year	May hold crayon or pencil and make mark on paper Places objects into containers through holes (16)	Stands alone (17) Walks holding onto furniture Sits down from standing (18)	Plays peek-a-boo and patty cake	6–8 ounces four times/day Uses cup with lid and attempts to feed self with spoon though spills often (19) Eating most soft table foods with family

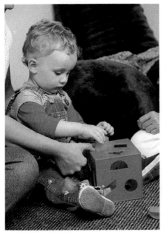

(16) Places objects in container through holes

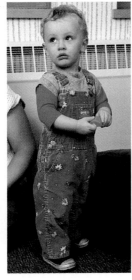

(17) Stands alone

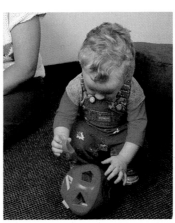

(18) Sits down from standing

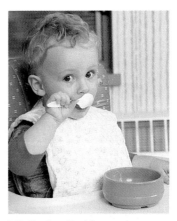

(19) Feeds self with spoon

The next phase of infant play focuses on manipulative behavior. The infant examines toys closely, looking at them, touching them, and placing them in the mouth. The infant learns a great deal about texture, qualities of objects, and all aspects of the surroundings. At the same time, interaction with others becomes an important part of play. The social nature of play is obvious as the infant plays with adults and other children.

Toward the end of the first year the infant's ability to move in space enlarges the sphere of play (Fig. 2–9). Once the infant is crawling or walking, he or she can get to new places, find new toys, discover forgotten objects, or seek out other people for interaction. Play is a reflection of every aspect of development, as well as a method for enhancing learning and maturation (Table 2–11).

Nutrition

From the first feeding of a few ounces of breast milk or formula to a meal of soft table foods with the family at 1 year of age, the infant demonstrates an amazing growth in ability to ingest and digest a wide variety of foods. Never again will the individual have such a high metabolic rate, intake requirements in relation to size, or such a change in the types of food eaten. Meeting these needs is made difficult by the small size of the infant's stomach and the immaturity of the digestive system. The great physical activity necessitates a high caloric intake. Nutrient demands for protein and vitamins must be met for the cells of the nervous system and body organs to develop properly.

■ **SAFETY PRECAUTIONS**

Formula can be mixed with tap water but must be refrigerated once mixed. Formula that the baby does not drink should be discarded after use and not kept for future feedings. This minimizes the chance for bacteria to grow and to cause illness in the baby.

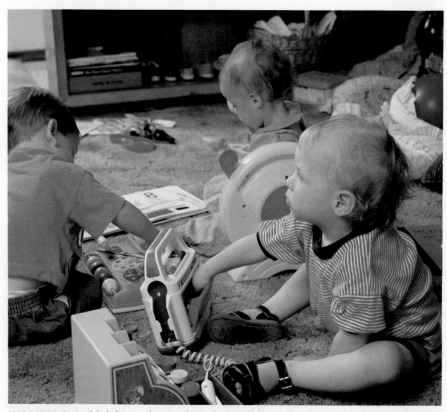

FIGURE 2–9 Mobility enlarges the sphere of play, allowing the child to seek new toys and spaces and to seek out people for interaction. Which psychosocial, cognitive, and motor skills do you see taking place in this photograph?

TABLE 2-11 Favorite Toys and Activities in Infancy

Birth–2 months

Mobiles, black and white patterns, mirrors
Music boxes, singing, tape players, soft voices
Rocking and cuddling
Moving legs and arms while singing and talking
Varying stimuli—different rooms, sounds, visual images

3–6 months

Rattles
Stuffed animals
Soft toys with contrasting colors
Noise-making objects that are easily grasped

6–12 months

Large blocks
Teething toys
Toys that pop apart and back together
Nesting cups and other objects that fit into one another or stack
Surprise toys such as jack-in-the-box
Social interaction with adults and other children
Games such as peek-a-boo
Soft balls
Push and pull toys

■ CLINICAL TIP

Nursing bottle mouth syndrome occurs when an infant is allowed to nurse or drink from a bottle for long periods, especially when sleeping. The milk, juice, or other fluid pools around the upper anterior teeth, salivary flow decreases, and acid buffering is decreased, resulting in tooth decay.

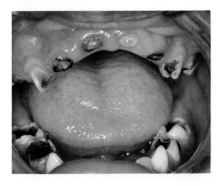

Teach parents to avoid putting the child to bed with a bottle. Encourage pacifier use or a bottle of water instead. Mothers who breast feed should also be cautioned to limit nursing to specific feeding times so that milk will not pool in the mouth during sleep.[22]

Courtesy Dr. Lezley McIlveen, Department of Dentistry, Children's National Medical Center, Washington, D.C.

Early Breast or Bottle Feeding. The first decision parents have to make about their infant's food intake is whether to breast feed or bottle feed. Citing the nutritional, immunologic, and psychosocial benefits of breast feeding, the American Academy of Pediatrics encourages mothers to breast feed for the first few months of life. Breast milk naturally provides all necessary nutrients for the infant, as well as immunity against several diseases.[21]

Providing breast-feeding information and instruction positively influences the number of women who decide to breast feed and increases the number of months mothers choose to breast feed. Some hospitals have lactation specialists who assist breast-feeding mothers; in others the staff nurses provide this service. Home visits or phone calls from the hospital nursing staff and telephone numbers for support organizations such as LaLeche League can provide mothers with needed breast-feeding information or problem-solving suggestions. Support programs are especially helpful to mothers who have difficulty breast feeding, feel unsure how it will fit into family and work life, or have an infant with problems related to feeding, such as prematurity. The mother of a hospitalized child will need special support to continue breast feeding. The mother should be encouraged to come to the hospital to feed her baby on the same schedule as at home. If the infant cannot breast feed, many hospitals have electric pumps so the mother can maintain lactation. Often hospitals provide some meals for the mother to help maintain quality nutrition for the baby.

Some women decide against breast feeding or are unable to breast feed. Nurses can provide these mothers with information about formula feeding. Three types of infant formula are available—ready to feed, concentrate, and powder. All are nutritionally adequate for infants. The nurse helps the parents decide which preparation of formula is best suited for their infant (Table 2–12). Breast or bottle feeding is assessed at each contact with health professionals to identify potential teaching needs.

TABLE 2-12 Advantages and Disadvantages of Formula Preparations

Formula Preparation	How Packaged	Advantages	Disadvantages
Ready to feed	Bottles or cans	No preparation needed	Most expensive formula type
Concentrate	Cans of concentrated liquid	Easy to add equal amounts of formula concentrate and water directly into bottle and shake	Is sometimes incorrectly measured, leading to inadequate or unsafe nutrition for infant; requires access to clean water supply such as city tap water or bottled water; well water may have too high a mineral concentration
Powder	Cans	Least expensive	Is sometimes incorrectly measured, leading to inadequate or unsafe nutrition for infant; requires shaking to mix thoroughly; requires access to clean water supply such as city tap water or bottled water; well water may have too high a mineral concentration

Introduction of Other Foods. When should other foods be added to the infant's diet? Although some parents add other foods when the infant is only days or weeks old, it is best to take cues from the infant's developmental milestones. The American Academy of Pediatrics recommends introducing semisolid food at 4 to 6 months. At this age the protrusion reflex (or tongue thrust) decreases and the infant can sit well with support.[23]

The first food added to the infant's diet is usually rice cereal. The advantage of introducing cereal first is that it provides iron at an age when the infant's prenatal iron stores begin to decrease, seldom causes allergy, and is easy to digest. A tablespoon or two is fed to the infant once or twice daily, just before formula or breast feeding. The infant may appear to spit out the food at first because of the natural in-and-out movement of the tongue. Parents should not interpret this early feeding behavior as indicating dislike for the food. With a little practice the infant becomes adept at spoon feeding.

Once the infant eats ¼ cup cereal twice a day, usually at 6 to 8 months of age, vegetables or fruits can be introduced (Table 2–13). By 8 to 10 months of age, most fruits and vegetables have been introduced and strained meats can be added to the infant's diet. Finger foods are introduced during the second half of the first year as the infant's palmar and then finger grasp develops and as teeth begin to erupt. Infants enjoy toast, O-shaped cereal, finely sliced meats, and small pieces of cooked, softened vegetables. Advise parents to use caution in providing finger foods to the infant. Hard foods slip easily into the throat and may cause choking. As food and juice intake increases, breast or formula feedings decrease in amount and frequency (Table 2–14).

■ FOODS THAT COMMONLY CAUSE CHOKING

Hot dogs
Nuts
Popcorn
Hard candy
Ice cubes
Grapes
Uncooked vegetable chunks
Lumps of peanut butter

TABLE 2-13 Introduction of Solid Foods in Infancy

Recommendation	Rationale
Introduce rice cereal at 4–6 months.	Rice cereal is easy to digest, has low allergenic potential, and contains iron.
Introduce fruits or vegetables at 6–8 months.	Fruits and vegetables provide needed vitamins.
Introduce meats at 8–10 months.	Meats are harder to digest, have high protein load, and should not be fed until close to 1 year of age.
Use single-food prepared baby foods rather than combination meals.	Combination meals usually contain more sugar, salt, and fillers.
Introduce one new food at a time, waiting at least 3 days to introduce another.	If a food allergy develops, it will be easy to identify.
Avoid carrots, beets, and spinach before 4 months of age.	Their nitrates can be converted to nitrite by young infants, causing methemoglobinemia.
Infants can be fed mashed portions of table foods such as carrots, rice, and potatoes.	This is a less expensive alternative to jars of commercially prepared baby food; it allows parents of various cultural groups to feed ethnic foods to infants.
Avoid adding sugar, salt, spices when mixing own baby foods.	Infants need not become accustomed to these flavors; they may get too much sodium from salt or develop gastric distress from some spices.
Avoid honey until at least 1 year of age.	Infants cannot detoxify *Clostridium botulinum* spores sometimes present in honey and can develop botulism.

PEDIATRIC NURSING

TABLE 2–14 Typical Daily Intake at Various Ages

	Breakfast	Snack	Lunch	Snack	Dinner	Snack
Infant 6 months	2 T. rice cereal with 60 ml (2 oz) formula	120 ml (4 oz) formula or breast milk	180 ml (6 oz) formula or breast milk	180 ml (6 oz) formula or breast milk	2 T. rice cereal with 60 ml (2 oz) formula, then 180 ml (6 oz) formula or breast milk	120 ml (4 oz) formula or breast milk
12 months	180 ml (6 oz) apple juice 4 T. rice cereal with 120 ml (4oz) milk	3 crackers ½ cup milk	1 thin slice (14 g [½ oz]) of turkey ½ cup soft cooked carrots 1 cup milk	½ slice of cheese ½ cup juice	¼ cup plain pasta ¼ cup thin sliced apple chunks ½ cup milk	½ cup yogurt
Toddler	¼ cup orange juice ¼ cup cereal with ½ cup milk ¼ banana	5 crackers ½ cup milk	2 thin slices (28g [1 oz]) of turkey with ½ slice of bread ½ cup cooked carrots 1 cup milk	1 slice cheese ½ cup juice	¼ cup plain pasta ¼–½ cup thin sliced apple chunks ½ cup milk	½ cup yogurt
Preschooler	½ cup orange juice ⅓ cup cereal with ¾ cup milk ½ banana	5 crackers ½ orange ½ cup milk	3 thin slices (42 g [1½ oz]) of turkey with ½ slice bread ¼ cup cooked carrots ¾ cup milk	1 slice cheese ½ cup juice	¼ cup plain pasta with meat sauce ½ cup thin sliced apple chunks ½ cup milk	½ cup yogurt
School age child	½ cup orange juice ¾ cup cereal with 1 cup milk ½ bagel with jam		4 thin slices (56 g [2 oz]) of turkey with 1 slice bread and condiments Apple 1 cup milk 1 oatmeal cookie	1½ cups popcorn 1 cup lemonade	½ cup pasta with meat sauce Dinner salad 1 slice garlic bread 1 cup milk	1 cup pudding or yogurt
Adolescent	½ cup orange juice 1 cup cereal 1 cup milk 1 bagel with 1 T. peanut butter and jam		84 g (3 oz) meat with 2 slices of bread plus condiments Apple 1 cup milk 1 oatmeal cookie	3 cups popcorn 1 cup lemonade	1½ cup pasta with meat sauce 1 slice garlic bread Salad with dressing 1 cup milk	1 cup pudding Fruit

■ SAFETY PRECAUTIONS

The American Academy of Pediatrics reviewed data from available studies and found an association between prone sleeping position and sudden infant death syndrome (SIDS). They therefore recommend supine or side-lying positioning for babies.[24]

Injury Prevention

Injuries are a major cause of death in childhood. The infant is particularly vulnerable to injuries when not adequately supervised. Increasing mobility during the second half of the first year challenges parents to childproof the home and environment. The nurse can provide anticipatory guidance to help prevent unintentional injuries (Table 2–15).

Personality and Temperament

Why does one infant frequently awaken at night crying while another sleeps for 8 to 10 hours undisturbed? Why does one infant smile much of the time

TABLE 2–15 Injury Prevention in Infancy

Hazard	Developmental Characteristics	Preventive Measures
Falls	Infant is increasingly mobile in first year of life, progressing from squirming movements to crawling, rolling, and standing.	Do not leave infant unsecured in infant seat, even in newborn period. Do not place on high surfaces such as tables or beds unless holding child. (1) Once mobile by crawling, keep doors to stairways closed or use gates. Standing walkers have led to many injuries and are not recommended.
Burns	Infant is dependent on caretakers for environmental control. The second half of the first year is marked by crawling and increased mobility. Objects are explored by touching and placing in mouth.	Check temperature of bath water and food/liquids for drinking. Cover electrical outlets. Supervise infant so that play with electrical cords cannot occur.
Motor vehicle crashes	Infant is dependent on caretakers for placement in car. On impact with another motor vehicle, an infant held on a lap acts as a torpedo.	Use only approved restraint systems (according to Federal Motor Vehicle Safety Standards). The seat must be used for every trip, even if very short. The seat must be properly buckled to the car's lap belt system. (2)
Drowning	Infant cannot swim and is unable to lift head.	Never leave infant alone in a bath of even 2.5 cm (1 in.) of water. Supervise when in water even when a life preserver is worn. Flotation devices such as arm inflatables are not certified life preservers.

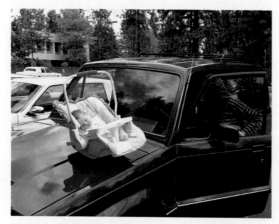

(1) Never leave infant unsecured or on high surface.

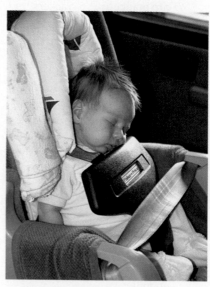

(2) Always use approved restraint system.

and react positively to interactions while another is withdrawn with unfamiliar people and frequently frowns and cries? Such differences in responses to the environment are believed to be inborn characteristics of temperament. Infants are born with a tendency to react in certain ways to noise, interact differently with people, display varying degrees of regularity in activities of eating and sleeping, and manifest a capacity for concentrating on tasks for different amounts of time.

Nursing assessment identifies personality characteristics of the infant that the nurse can share with the parents. With this information the parents can appreciate the uniqueness of their infant and design experiences to meet the infant's needs. Parents can learn to modify the environment to promote adaptation. For example, an infant who does not adapt easily to new situations may cry, withdraw, or develop another way of coping when adjusting

TABLE 2–15 **Injury Prevention in Infancy** Continued

Hazard	Developmental Characteristics	Preventive Measures
Poisoning	Infant is dependent on caretakers to keep harmful substances out of reach. The second half of infancy is marked by exploratory reaching and mouthing of objects.	Keep medicines out of reach. Teach proper dosage and administration of medicines to parents. Cleaning products and other harmful substances should not be stored where the infant can reach them. Remove plants from play areas. Have poison control center number by telephone.
Choking	Infant explores objects by placing them in the mouth. (3)	Avoid foods that commonly cause choking. Keep small toys away from infants, especially toys labeled "not intended for use in those under 3 years."
Suffocation	Young infant has minimal head control and may be unable to move if vomiting or having difficulty breathing.	Position infant on side for sleep, particularly after feeding. Do not place pillows, stuffed toys, or other objects near head. Do not use plastic in crib. Avoid latex balloons. (4)
Strangulation	Infant is able to get head into railings or crib slats but cannot remove it.	Be sure older cribs have slats spaced 6 cm (2⅜ in.) or less apart. The mattress must fit tightly against the crib rails.

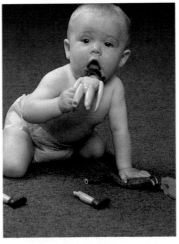

(3) Explores objects with mouth.

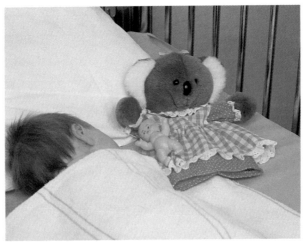

(4) Place infant on side after eating, keep toys clear.

to new people or places. Parents might be advised to use one or two baby-sitters rather than engaging new sitters frequently. If the infant is easily distracted when eating, parents can feed the infant in a quiet setting to encourage focus on eating. Although the infant's temperament is unchanged, the ability to fit with the environment is enhanced.

Communication

Even at a few weeks of age, infants communicate and engage in two-way interaction. Comfort is expressed by soft sounds, cuddling, and eye contact. The infant displays discomfort by thrashing the extremities, arching the back, and crying vigorously. From these rudimentary skills, communication ability continues to develop until the infant speaks several words at the end of the first year of life (Table 2–16).

Nurses assess communication to identify possible abnormalities or developmental delays. Language ability may be assessed with the Denver II[25] and other developmental screening tools (see Table 3–29 and Appendix B). Normal infants understand (receptive speech) more words than they can speak (expressive speech). Abnormalities may be caused by a hearing deficit, de-

TABLE 2-16 Patterns of Infant Communication

Age	Behavior
Birth–2 months	Coos
	Babbles
	Comfort sounds
	Cries
3–6 months	Vocalizations with play and favorite people
	Laughs
	Less crying
	Squeals and pleasure sounds
	Multisyllable babbling
6–9 months	Increasing vowel and consonant sounds
	Links syllables together
	Rhythm of speech when "talking" with adult
9–12 months	Understands "no" and other simple commands
	Says dada and mama to identify parents
	Learns one or two other words
	Receptive speech surpasses expressive speech

■ **COMMUNICATION STRATEGIES: INFANT**

Hold for feedings.
Hold, rock, and talk to infant often.
Talk and sing frequently during care.
Tell names of objects.
Use high-pitched voice with newborns.
Swaddle and hold infant securely when he or she is upset.

velopmental delay, or lack of verbal stimulation from caretakers. Further assessment may be required to pinpoint the cause of the abnormality.

Nursing interventions focus on providing a stimulating environment. Parents are encouraged to speak to infants and teach words. Hospital nurses should include the infant's known words when providing care.

✓ Toddler (1–3 Years)

Toddlerhood is sometimes called the first adolescence. An infant only months before, the child from 1 to 3 years is now displaying independence and negativism. Pride in newfound accomplishments emerges.

Physical Growth and Development

The rate of growth slows during the second year of life. By age 2 the birth weight has usually quadrupled and the child is about one half of the adult height. Body proportions begin to change, with legs longer and head smaller in proportion to body size than during infancy (Fig. 2–7). The toddler has a pot-bellied appearance and stands with feet apart to provide a wide base of support. By approximately 33 months, eruption of deciduous teeth is complete, with 20 teeth present.

Gross motor activity develops rapidly (Table 2–17), as the toddler progresses from walking to running, kicking, and riding a Big Wheel tricycle (Fig. 2–10). As physical maturation occurs, the toddler develops the ability to control elimination patterns (Table 2–18).

Cognitive Development

During the toddler years the child moves from the sensorimotor to the preoperational stage of development. The early use of language awakens in the

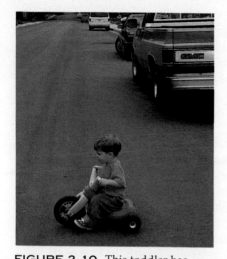

FIGURE 2-10 This toddler has learned to ride the Big Wheel, which he is doing right into the street. Toddlers must be closely watched to prevent injury.

TABLE 2-17 Growth and Development Milestones During Toddlerhood

Age	Physical Growth	Fine Motor Ability	Gross Motor Ability	Sensory Ability	Nutrition
1–2 years	Gains 227 g (½ lb) or more per month Grows 9–12 cm during this year Anterior fontanel closes	By end of 2nd year, builds a tower of four blocks (1) Scribbles on paper (2) Can undress self (3) Throws a ball	Runs Walks up and down stairs (7) Likes push and pull toys (5)	Visual acuity 20/50	Eats three meals per day with snacks Drinks regular milk or follow-up formula Uses cup and spoon but often prefers finger foods
2–3 years	Gains 1.4–2.3 kg (3–5 lb)/year Grows 5–6.5 cm/year	Draws circle and other rudimentary forms Learns to pour Learning to dress self (4)	Jumps Kicks balls (6) Throws ball over-hand		May begin to use fork but still needs food cut into bite-size pieces

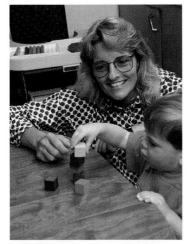

(1) Second year tower of 4 blocks

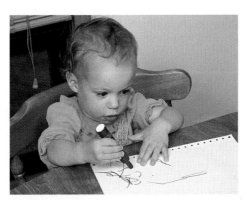

(2) Scribbles on paper

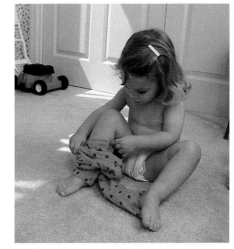

(3) Can undress self

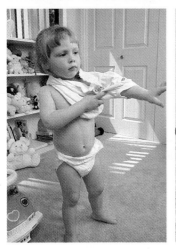

(4) Learning to dress self

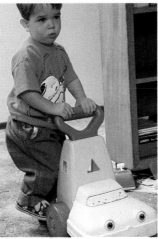

(5) Likes push and pull toys

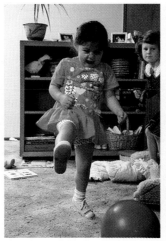

(6) Jumps and kicks balls

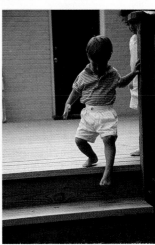

(7) Walks up and down stairs

■ CULTURAL CONSIDERATIONS

In traditional Native American families, a child is allowed to unfold and develop naturally at his or her own pace. Children thus wean and toilet-train themselves at their own pace with little interference or pressure from parents.

1-year-old the ability to think about objects or people when they are absent. Object permanence is well developed.

At about 2 years of age the increasing use of words as symbols enables the toddler to use preoperational thought. Rudimentary problem solving, creative thought, and an understanding of cause-and-effect relationships are now possible.

TABLE 2–18 Toilet Training

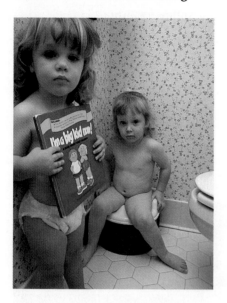

When are children ready to learn toileting? Are parents responsible for the differences in ages at which toilet training is accomplished? Does toilet training provide clues to a child's intellectual ability?

We know that children are not ready for toilet training until several developmental capabilities exist: to stand and walk well, to pull pants up and down, to recognize the need to eliminate and then to be able to wait until in the bathroom. Once this readiness is apparent, the child can be given a small potty chair and the procedure explained.

Children often prefer their own chair on the floor to using the large toilet. The child should be placed on the chair at regular intervals for a few moments and can be given reward or praise for successes. If the child seems not to understand or does not wish to cooperate, it is best to wait a few weeks and then try again. Just as all of development is subject to individual timetables, toilet training occurs with considerable variability from one child to another. Identify for parents the developmental characteristics of their child and encourage them to appreciate without anxiety the unfolding of skills. These timetables are not predictive of future development.

The child who is ill or hospitalized or has other stress often regresses in toilet training activities. It is best to quietly reinstitute attempts at training after the trauma. Potty chairs should be available on pediatric units and toileting habits identified during initial assessment so that regular routines can be followed and the child's usual words for elimination can be used.

Play

Many changes in play patterns occur between infancy and toddlerhood. The toddler's motor skills enable him or her to bang pegs into a pounding board with a hammer. The social nature of toddler play is also readily seen. Toddlers find the company of other children pleasurable, even though socially interactive play may not occur. Two toddlers tend to play with similar objects side by side, occasionally trading toys and words. This is called **parallel play.** This play time with other children assists toddlers to develop social skills. Toddlers engage in play activities they have seen at home, such as pounding with a hammer and talking on the phone. This imitative behavior teaches them new actions and skills (Fig. 2–11).

Physical skills are manifested in play as toddlers push and pull objects, climb in and out and up and down, run, ride a Big Wheel, turn the pages of books, and scribble with a pen. Both gross motor and fine motor abilities are enhanced during this age period.

Cognitive understanding enables the toddler to manipulate objects and learn about their qualities. Stacking blocks and placing rings on a building tower teach spatial relationships and other lessons that provide a foundation for future learning.

Various kinds of play objects should be provided for the toddler to meet play needs. These play needs can easily be met whether the child is hospitalized or at home (Table 2–19).

Nutrition

Why do parents of toddlers frequently become concerned about the small amount of food their children eat? Why do toddlers seem to survive and even thrive with minimal food intake? The toddler often displays the phenomenon of **physiologic anorexia,** caused when the extremely high metabolic demands of infancy slow to keep pace with the more moderate growth rate of toddlerhood. Although it can appear that the toddler eats nothing at times, intake over days or a week is generally sufficient and balanced enough to meet the body's demands for nutrients and energy.

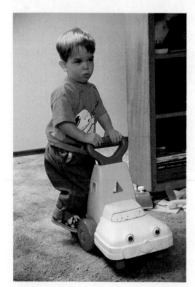

FIGURE 2–11 Imitative play such as pushing and pulling allows the toddler to develop gross and fine motor skills.

TABLE 2-19 Favorite Toys and Activities in Toddlerhood

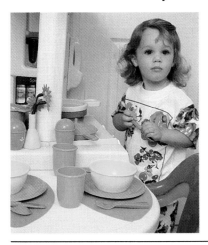

Play Need	Types of Toys and Activities
Facilitate imitative behavior	Play kitchen Grocery carts Pounding board Toy phone
Encourage gross motor activity and provide an outlet for stress	Big Wheel tricycle Soft ball and bat Water and sand Bean bag toss
Foster fine motor skills	Cloth books Large pencil and paper Wooden puzzles
Facilitate cognitive growth	Educational television shows Music Stories and books

Advise parents to offer a variety of nutritious foods several times daily (three meals and two snacks) and let the toddler make choices from the foods offered. Small portions are also more appealing to the toddler. A general rule of thumb for food quantity at a meal is one tablespoon of each food per year of age (see Table 2–14). The toddler should drink 16 to 24 ounces of milk daily. Caution parents against giving the toddler more than a quart of milk daily, since this interferes with the desire to eat other foods, leading to an unbalanced diet.

The toddler displays characteristic autonomy (independence) during mealtime. Advise parents to provide opportunities for self-feeding with food and fingers and to allow some simple choices, such as type of juice. Because social skills are developing, the hospitalized toddler may eat better if allowed to have meals with parents or other hospitalized children.

Injury Prevention

By 1 year of age, unintentional injuries are by far the leading cause of death in children.[26] Injuries also cause disfigurement and other ongoing health problems. Nurses intervene to care for injured children in the hospital and are responsible for making sure that the hospital environment is free from safety hazards. Nurses are also instrumental in teaching parents how to make the toddler's environment safe (Tables 2–20 and 2–21).

Personality and Temperament

The toddler retains most of the temperamental characteristics identified during infancy but may demonstrate some changes. The normal developmental progression of toddlerhood also plays a part in responses. For example, the infant who previously responded positively to stimuli, such as a new babysitter, may appear more negative in toddlerhood. The increasing independence characteristic of this age is shown by the toddler's use of the word no. The parent and child constantly adapt their responses to each other and learn anew how to communicate with each other.

Communication

Because of the phenomenal growth of language skills during the toddler period, adults should communicate frequently with children in this age group.

TABLE 2–20 Injury Prevention in Toddlerhood

	Hazard	Developmental Characteristics	Preventive Measures
	Falls	Gross motor skills improve. Toddler is able to move chairs to counters and can climb up ladders.	Supervise toddler closely. Provide safe climbing toys. Begin to teach acceptable places for climbing.
	Poisoning	Gross motor skills enable toddler to climb onto chairs and then cabinets. Medicine chests, cosmetics, and other poisonous substances are easily reached.	Keep medicines and other poisonous materials locked. Use child-resistant containers and cupboard closures. Have poison control center number by telephone. Keep syrup of ipecac in home.
	Burns	Toddler is tall enough to reach stove top. Toddler can walk to fireplace and may reach into fire.	Keep pot handles turned inward on stove. Do not burn fires without close supervision. Use a fire screen.
	Motor vehicle crashes	Toddler may be able to undo seat belt, may resist using car seat, demonstrating characteristic negativism and autonomy.	Insist on safety seat use for all trips. Use approved safety seats only, such as forward-facing convertible seat. Toddler is not large enough to use car seat belts.
	Drowning	Toddler can walk onto docks or pool decks. Toddler may stand on or climb seats on boat. Toddler may fall into buckets, toilets, and fish tanks and be unable to get top of body out.	Supervise any child near water. Swimming classes do not protect a toddler from drowning. Use child-resistant pool covers. Use approved child life jackets near water and on boats. Empty buckets when not in use.

TABLE 2-21 Parent Teaching: Use of Infant and Child Car Seats [27]

Weight below 9 kg (20 lb)
Use infant or convertible seat in backward-facing position.
Do not place in front passenger seat if an air bag is present.
Fasten seat securely to car using car seat belt.
Adjust harnesses to fit snugly at shoulders and legs.

9–18 kg (20–40 lb)
Use convertible seat in front-facing position.
Fasten seat securely to car using car seat belt.
Adjust harnesses to fit snugly at shoulders and legs; readjust as child grows.

18–29.5 kg (40–65 lb)
Use shield booster seat if child has outgrown convertible seat.
Adjust shield to fit over child's lap and use car seat belt to secure.

Toddlers imitate words and speech intonations, as well as the social interactions they observe.

At the beginning of toddlerhood the child may use four to six words in addition to "mama" and "dada." Receptive speech (the ability to understand words) far outpaces expressive speech. By the end of toddlerhood, however, the 3-year-old has a vocabulary of almost 1000 words and uses short sentences.

Communication occurs in many ways, some of which are nonverbal. Toddler communication includes pointing, pulling an adult over to a room or object, and speaking in expressive jargon. **Expressive jargon** is using unintelligible words with normal speech intonations as if truly communicating in words. Another communication method occurs when the toddler cries, pounds feet, displays a temper tantrum, or uses other means to illustrate dismay. These powerful communication methods can upset parents, who often need suggestions for handling them. It is best to verbalize the feelings shown by the toddler, for example, by saying, "You must be very upset that you cannot have that candy. When you stop crying you can come out of your

■ COMMUNICATION STRATEGIES: TODDLER

Give short, clear instructions.
Do not give choices if none exist.
Offer a choice of two alternatives when possible.
Approach positively.
Tell toddler what you are doing, names of objects.

TABLE 2-22 Communicating with a Toddler

Procedures such as drawing blood can be frightening for a toddler. Effective communication minimizes the trauma caused by such procedures:

Avoid telling toddlers about the procedure too far in advance. They do not have an understanding of time and can become quite anxious.
Use simple terminology. "We need to get a little blood from your arm. It will help us to find out if you are getting better. Your Mom will hold your arm still so we can do it quickly."
Allow the toddler to cry. Acknowledge that it must be frightening and that you understand.
Perform the procedure in a treatment room so that the toddler's bed and room are a safe haven.
Be sure the toddler is restrained, with the joints above and below the procedure immobilized.
Use a Band-Aid to cover up the site. This can reassure the toddler that the body is still intact.
Allow the toddler to choose a reward such as a sticker after the procedure.
Praise the toddler for cooperation and acknowledge that you know this was difficult.
Comfort the toddler by rocking, offering a favorite drink, playing music, and holding. If parents are present, they can offer the comfort needed.

room," and then to ignore further negative behavior. The toddler's search for autonomy and independence creates a need for such behavior. Sometimes an upset toddler responds well to holding, rocking, and stroking.

Parents and nurses can promote a toddler's communication by speaking frequently, naming objects, explaining procedures in simple terms, expressing feelings that the toddler seems to be displaying, and encouraging speech. The toddler from a bilingual home is at an optimal age to learn two languages. If the parents do not speak English, the toddler will benefit from a day care experience so that both languages can be learned.

The nurse who understands the communication skills of toddlers is able to assess expressive and receptive language and communicate effectively, thereby promoting positive health care experiences for these children (Table 2–22).

✓ Preschool Child (3–6 Years)

The preschool years are a time of new initiative and independence. Most children are in a day care center or school for part of the day and learn a great deal from this social contact. Language skills are well developed, and the child is able to understand and speak clearly. Endless projects characterize the world of busy preschoolers. They may work with playdough to form animals, then cut out and paste paper, then draw and color (Fig. 2–12).

Physical Growth and Development

Preschoolers grow slowly and steadily, with most growth taking place in long bones of the arms and legs. The short, chubby toddler gradually gives way to a slender, long-legged preschooler.

FIGURE 2–12 Preschoolers have well-developed language, motor, and social skills, and they can work creatively together on an art project such as this group is doing at a day care center in Spokane.

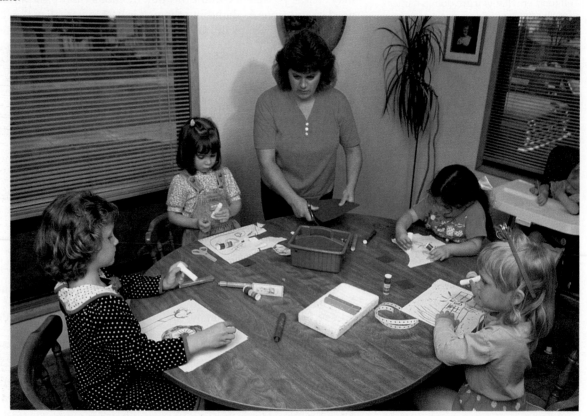

PEDIATRIC NURSING

FIGURE 2–13 Preschoolers continue to develop more advanced skills, such as kicking a ball without falling down.

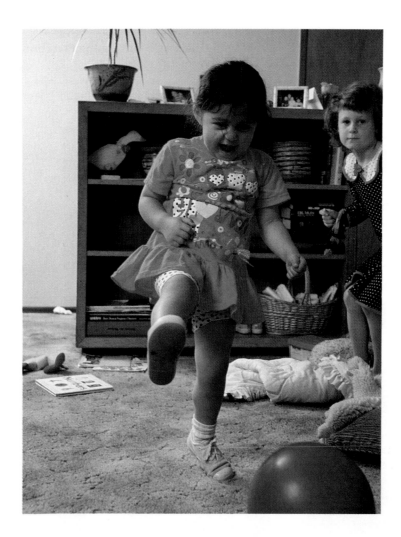

Physical skills continue to develop (Fig. 2–13). The preschooler runs with ease, holds a bat, and throws balls of various types. Writing ability increases, and the preschooler enjoys drawing and learning to write a few letters (Table 2–23).

Cognitive Development

The preschooler exhibits characteristics of preoperational thought. Symbols or words are used to represent objects and people, enabling the young child to think about them. This is a milestone in intellectual development; however, the preschooler still has some limitations in thought (Table 2–24).

Play

The preschooler has begun playing in a new way. Toddlers simply play side by side with friends, each engaging in his or her own activities, but preschoolers interact with others during play. One child cuts out colored paper while her friend glues it on paper in a design. This new type of interaction is called **associative play** (Fig. 2–14).

In addition to this social dimension of play, other aspects of play also differ. The preschooler enjoys large motor activities such as swinging, riding a tricycle, and throwing a ball. Increasing manual dexterity is demonstrated in greater complexity of drawings and manipulation of blocks and modeling. These changes necessitate planning of playtime to include appropriate activ-

TABLE 2–23 Growth and Development Milestones During the Preschool Years

Physical Growth		Fine Motor Ability

Physical Growth

Gains 1.5–2.5 kg (3–5 lb)/year

Grows 4–6 cm (1½–2½ in)/year

Fine Motor Ability

Uses scissors (1)
Draws circle, square, cross (2)
Draws at least a six-part person
Enjoys art projects such as pasting, stringing beads, using clay
Learns to tie shoes at end of preschool years (3)
Buttons (4)
Brushes teeth (5)

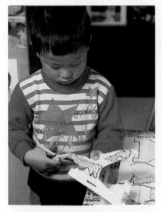

(1) Uses scissors (fine motor)

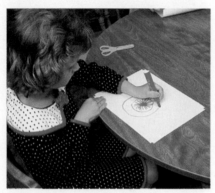

(2) Draws circle, square, cross (fine motor)

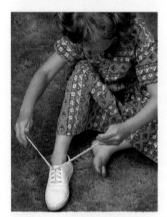

(3) Ties shoes (fine motor)

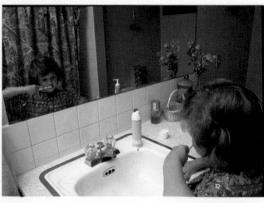

(4) Buttons clothes (fine motor)

(5) Brushes teeth (fine motor)

Gross Motor Ability

Throws a ball overhand
Climbs well (6)
Rides tricycle (7)

Sensory Ability

Visual acuity continues to improve
Can focus on and learn letters and numbers (8)

Nutrition

Eats three meals with snacks
Uses spoon, fork, and knife

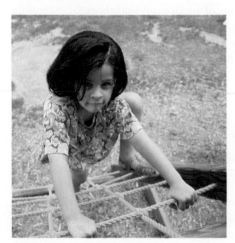

(6) Climbs well (gross motor)

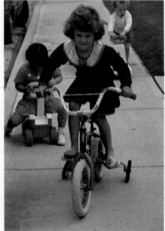

(7) Rides tricycle or bicycle with training wheels (gross motor)

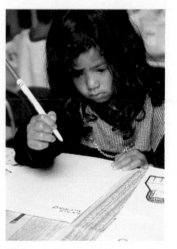

(8) Learns letters and numbers (sensory)

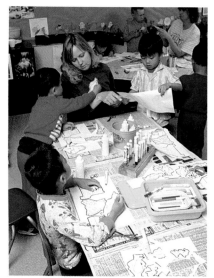

FIGURE 2-14 These preschoolers are participating in associative play, which means they can interact. One child is cutting out shapes, and the other is gluing them in place.

TABLE 2-24 Characteristics of Preoperational Thought [28]

Characteristic	Definition	Example
Egocentrism	Ability to see things only from one's own point of view	The child who cannot understand why parents may need to leave the hospital for work when the child wishes them to be present
Transductive reasoning	Connecting two events in a cause-effect relationship simply because they occur together in time	A child who, awakening after surgery and feeling pain, notices the intravenous infusion and believes that it is causing the pain
Centration	Focusing on only one particular aspect of a situation	The child who is concerned about breathing through an anesthesia mask and will not listen to any other aspects of preoperative teaching
Animism	Giving lifelike qualities to nonliving things	The child who views a monitoring machine as alive because it beeps

ities. Preschool programs and child life departments in hospitals help meet this important need.

Materials provided for play can be simple but should guide activities in which the child engages. Since fine motor activities are popular, paper, pens, scissors, glue, and a variety of other such objects should be available. The child can use them to create important images such as pictures of people, hospital beds, or friends. A collection of dolls, furniture, and clothing can be manipulated to represent parents and children, nurses and physicians, teachers, or other significant people. Because fantasy life is so powerful at this age, the preschooler readily uses props to engage in **dramatic play,** that is, the living out of the drama of human life (Fig. 2–15).

The nurse can use playtime to assess the preschool child's developmental level, knowledge about health care, and emotions related to health care experiences. Observations about objects chosen for play, content of dramatic play, and pictures drawn can provide important assessment data. The nurse can also use play periods to teach the child about health care procedures and offer an outlet for expression of emotions (Table 2–25).

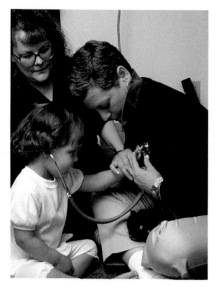

FIGURE 2-15 Jasmine is participating in dramatic play with a nurse while the mother looks on. In dramatic play the child uses props to live out the drama of human life. It can be an excellent way for a nurse to assess the developmental level of children and to talk to them. Notice that the child and the nurse are on the floor at the same level and the informal atmosphere. Why is it important to be at the same level as the child?

TABLE 2-25 Favorite Toys and Activities in the Preschool Years

Play Need	Types of Toys and Activities
Facilitate associative play	Simple games
	Puzzles
	Nursery rhymes, songs
Promote dramatic play	Dolls and doll clothes
	Play houses and hospitals
	Dress-up clothes
	Puppets
Encourage outlet for stress	Pens, paper
	Glue, scissors
Facilitate cognitive growth	Educational television shows
	Music
	Stories and books

Nutrition

The diet of the preschooler is similar to that of the toddler, but mealtime is now a more social event. Preschoolers like the company of others while they eat, and they enjoy helping with food preparation and table setting. Involving them in these tasks can provide a forum for teaching about nutritious foods and principles of preparation such as the need for refrigeration, safety around stoves, and cleanliness.

Although the rate of growth is slow and steady during the preschool years, the child has periods of food jags (eating only a few foods for several days or weeks) and greater or lesser intake. Parents should be advised to assess food intake over a 1- or 2-week period rather than at each meal to obtain a more accurate impression of total intake. Food jags can be handled by providing the desired food along with other foods to foster choice. The child who chooses not to eat at snacktime or mealtime should not be given other foods in between. Three meals and two or three snacks daily are the norm (Table 2–14).

The preschool period is a good time to encourage good dental habits. Children can begin to brush their own teeth with parental supervision and help to reach all tooth surfaces. Parents should floss their children's teeth, give fluoride as ordered if the water supply is not fluoridated (Table 2–26), and schedule the first dental visit so the child can become accustomed to the routine of periodic dental care.[20]

Injury Prevention

The increasing independence of preschool children puts them at risk of injury. The 3- to 7-year-old group is at highest risk of pedestrian injury from motor vehicle crashes, with many of these crashes occurring as the child plays in unsafe locations.[20] Nurses can teach parents preventive measures and can also begin to include preschoolers in safety teaching (Table 2–27).

Personality and Temperament

Characteristics of personality observed in infancy tend to persist over time. The preschooler may need assistance as these characteristics are expressed in the new situations of preschool or nursery school. An excessively active child, for example, will need gentle, consistent handling to adjust to the structure of a classroom. Parents should be encouraged to visit preschool programs to choose the one that would best foster growth in their child. Some preschoolers enjoy the structured learning of a program that focuses on cognitive skills, whereas others are happier and more open to learning in a small group that provides much time for free play. Nurses can help parents

---

TABLE 2-26 Recommended Daily Fluoride Dosages [29]

Age	Amount of Fluoride in Water Supply		
	Under 0.3 ppm	0.3–0.7 ppm	Above 0.7 ppm
Birth–2 years	0.25 mg	0	0
2–3 years	0.50 mg	0.25 mg	0
3–13 years	1.00 mg	0.50 mg	0

ppm, parts per million.
NOTE: Fluoride is available as a liquid to be mixed in a small amount of food or fluid for the infant and toddler and as a chewable tablet for the older child. It acts both systemically to promote strong teeth before they erupt and topically to strengthen tooth surfaces it comes in contact with.

PEDIATRIC NURSING

TABLE 2–27 Injury Prevention in the Preschool Years

	Hazard	Developmental Characteristics	Preventive Measures
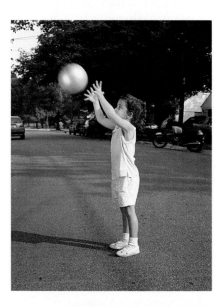	Motor vehicle crashes	Older preschooler independently gets into car and puts on seat belt. Child may forget to belt up or may do so incorrectly.	Teach parents to verify that child is belted in properly before starting car. Child restraint systems must be used until child weighs 18 kg (40 lb) and is 100 cm (40 in) tall.
	Motor vehicle and pedestrian accidents	Preschooler increasingly plays outside alone or with friends. Preschooler assumes driver of a car knows that he or she is present and is unable to judge speed of moving car.	Parents should teach child never to go into road. A safe, preferably enclosed, play yard is recommended.
	Drowning	Preschooler may choose to go into a lake or pool, since he or she has had swimming lessons.	Parents should teach child never to go into water without an adult. They should provide supervision whenever child is near water.
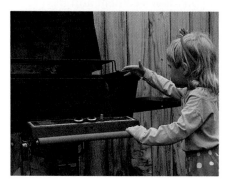	Burns	Preschooler can understand the hazards of fire.	Parents should teach child to stop, drop, and roll if clothes are on fire. Practice escapes from home are useful. A visit to a fire station can reinforce the preschooler's learning. Teach child how to call 911.
	Needle sticks in hospital	Preschooler can ambulate and is interested in new objects.	Keep needles out of reach. Remove from unit immediately after use.
	Electrical injury in hospital	Preschooler is mobile and may trip over cords and equipment or may choose to examine them.	Avoid use of electrical cords if possible. Keep equipment out of major traffic areas. Keep beds away from electrical outlets. Monitor child closely.

to identify their child's personality or temperament characteristics and to find the best environment for growth.

Communication

Language skills blossom during the preschool years. The vocabulary grows to over 2000 words, and children speak in complete sentences of several words and use all parts of speech. They practice these newfound language skills by endlessly talking and asking questions.

The sophisticated speech of preschoolers mirrors the development occurring in their minds and helps them to learn about the world around them. However, this speech can be quite deceptive. Although preschoolers use many words, their grasp of meaning is usually literal and may not match that of adults. These literal interpretations have important implications for health care providers. For example, the preschooler who is told she will be "put to sleep" for surgery may think of a pet recently euthanised; the child who is told that a dye will be injected for a diagnostic test may think he is going to die; mention of "a little stick" in the arm can cause images of tree branches rather than of a simple immunization.

The child may also have difficulty focusing on the content of a conversation. The preschooler is egocentric and may be unable to move from individual thoughts to those the nurse is proposing. Read the following conversation:

Nurse: I'd like to tell you about the operation that you will have tomorrow.
Sharisse: OK. Did you know my brother just got a new squirt gun?
Nurse: That's nice. Now, first thing in the morning you will wake up early and your foot will be scrubbed with a special soap.
Sharisse: The gun can spurt for about 40 feet—you have to pump it up.
Nurse: We'll talk about that later. Let me tell you about your operation now. After your foot is scrubbed, the nurse will measure your blood pressure and temperature and feel the pulse in your arm. Do you remember my doing those things today?
Sharisse: Yes. And I got a sticker when I came into the hospital today, too. Do you know that my Mom is going to stay here tonight?

In this interchange Sharisse is engaging in **collective monologue,** in which separate conversations occur even though each person waits for the other to speak. While waiting for the nurse to speak, Sharisse is not generally responding to the nurse's content but is instead focusing on content from her own mind. The nurse needs to respond to Sharisse's content and then reinsert more facts about the preparations for surgery.

Concrete visual aids such as pictures of a child undergoing the same procedure or a book to read together enhance teaching by meeting the child's developmental needs. Handling medical equipment such as intravenous bags and stethoscopes increases interest and helps the child to focus. Teaching may have to be done in several short sessions rather than one long session.

✓ School-Age Child (6–12 Years)

Errol, 10 years old, arrives home from school shortly after 3 PM each day. He immediately calls his friends and goes to visit one of them. They are building models of cars and collecting baseball cards. Endless hours are spent on these projects and on discussions of events at school that day (Fig. 2–16).

Nine-year-old Karen practices soccer two afternoons a week and plays in

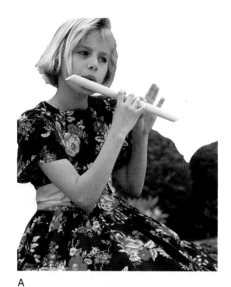

A

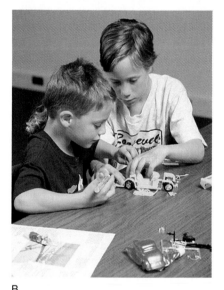

B

FIGURE 2-16 A, School-age children may take part in activities that require practice. This is a consideration when children are hospitalized and unable to practice or perform. Why? **B,** School-age children enjoy spending time with others the same age on projects and discussing the activities of the day. This is an important consideration when they are in an acute-care setting. When you are in the clinical setting, look for facilities where this type of interaction is taking place.

games each weekend. She also is learning to play the flute and spends her free time at home practicing. Although practice time is not her favorite part of music, Karen enjoys the performances and wants to play well in front of her friends and teacher. Her parents now allow her to ride her bike unaccompanied to the store or to a friend's house.

These two school-age children demonstrate common characteristics of their age group. They are in a stage of industry in which it is important to the child to accomplish good work. Meaningful activities take on great importance and are usually carried out in the company of peers. A sense of achievement in these activities is important to develop self-esteem and to prevent a sense of inferiority or poor self-worth.

Physical Growth and Development

School age is the last period in which girls and boys are close in size and body proportions. As the long bones continue to grow, leg length increases (Fig. 2–7). Fat gives way to muscle, and the child appears leaner. Jaw proportions change as the first deciduous tooth is lost at 6 years and permanent teeth begin to erupt. Body organs and the immune system mature, resulting in fewer illnesses among school-age children. Medications are less likely to cause serious side effects, since they can be metabolized more easily. The urinary system can adjust to changes in fluid status. Physical skills are also refined as children begin to play sports, and fine motor skills are well developed through school activities (Table 2–28 and Fig. 2–17).

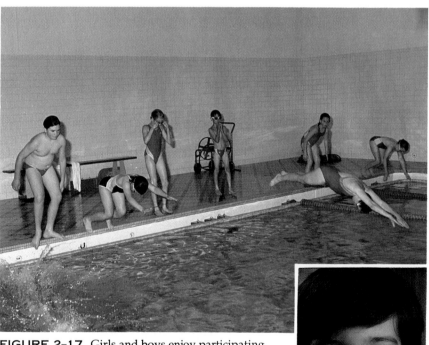

FIGURE 2-17 Girls and boys enjoy participating in sports. They begin to lose fat while developing their muscles, so they appear leaner. *Inset,* Front teeth are lost around age 6. The family may have rituals associated with the loss of teeth that could affect the child's behavior if he loses a tooth while in the hospital.

TABLE 2-28 Growth and Development Milestones During the School-Age Years

Physical Growth	Fine Motor Ability	Gross Motor Ability	Sensory Ability	Nutrition
Gains 1.4–2.2 kg (3–5 lb)/years Grows 4–6 cm (1½–2 ½ in)/year	Enjoys craft projects Plays card and board games	Rides two-wheeler (1) Jumps rope (2) Roller skates or ice skates	Can read Able to concentrate for longer periods on activities by filtering out surrounding sounds (3)	Eats three meals per day Enjoys food prepar--ation; may prepare own snacks

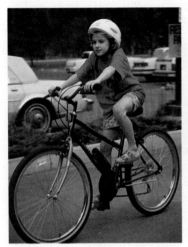

(1) Rides two-wheeler

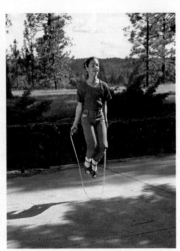

(2) Jumps rope

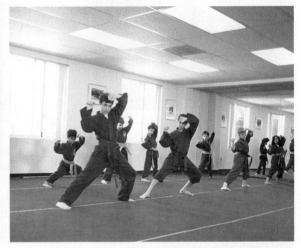

(3) Concentrates on activities for longer periods

Cognitive Development

The child enters the stage of concrete operational thought at about 7 years. This stage enables school-age children to consider alternative solutions and solve problems. However, school-age children continue to rely on concrete experiences and materials to form the content of thought.

During the school-age years the child learns the concept of conservation (that matter is not changed when its form is altered). At earlier ages a child believes that when water is poured from a short, wide glass into a tall, thin glass, there is more water in the taller glass. The school-age child recognizes that although it may look like the taller glass holds more water, the quantity is the same. The concept of conservation is helpful when the nurse explains medical treatments. The school-age child understands that an incision will heal, that a cast will be removed, and that an arm will look the same as before once the intravenous infusion is removed.

Play

When the preschool teacher tries to organize a game of baseball, both the teacher and the children become frustrated. Not only are the children physically unable to hold a bat and hit a ball, but they seem to have no understanding of the rules of the game and do not want to wait for their turn at bat. By 6 years of age, however, children have acquired the physical ability to hold the bat properly and may occasionally hit the ball. School-age children also understand that everyone has a role—the pitcher, the catcher, the batter, the outfielders. They cooperate with one another to form a team, are eager to

TABLE 2-29 Favorite Play Activities of School Age Children

Play Need	Types of Activities
Foster gross motor activity	Ball sports
	Skating
	Water and snow skiing
	Biking
Promote sense of industry	Musical instrument
	Collections
	Hobbies
	Board and video games
Facilitate cognitive growth	Reading
	Crafts
	Word puzzles

learn the rules of the game, and want to ensure that these rules are followed exactly (Table 2–29).

The characteristics of play exhibited at school age, then, are cooperation with others and the ability to play a part in order to contribute to a unified whole. This type of play is called **cooperative play.** The concrete nature of cognitive thought leads to a reliance on rules to provide structure and security. Children have an increasing desire to spend much of playtime with friends, which demonstrates the social component of play. Play is an extremely important method of learning and living for the school-age child.

When a child is hospitalized, the separation from playmates can lead to sadness and purposelessness. School-age children often feel better when placed in multibed units with other children. Games can be devised even when children are wheelchair bound (Fig. 2–18). Normal, rewarding parts of play should be integrated into care. Friends should be encouraged to visit or call a hospitalized child. Discharge planning for the child acquiring a cast or brace should address the activities the child can engage in and those the child must avoid. Involvement in games with friends is important.

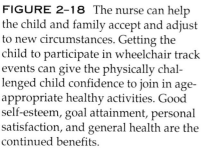

FIGURE 2–18 The nurse can help the child and family accept and adjust to new circumstances. Getting the child to participate in wheelchair track events can give the physically challenged child confidence to join in age-appropriate healthy activities. Good self-esteem, goal attainment, personal satisfaction, and general health are the continued benefits.
Courtesy Gail C. Weyant, Parallax Productions, Inc., Centreville, Virginia.

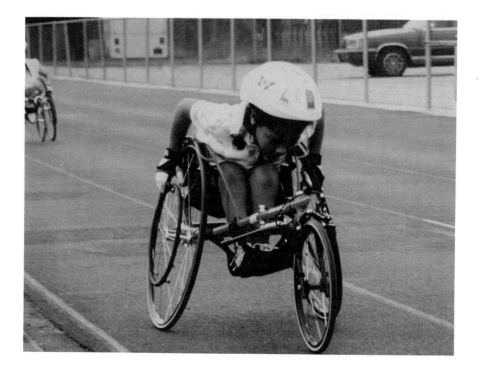

Nutrition

The school-age years are a period of gradual growth when energy requirements remain at a steady level. The child is increasingly responsible for preparing snacks and even some parts of the meal. This makes school age an appropriate time to teach children how to choose nutritious foods and how to plan a well-balanced meal (Table 2–14). Because school-age children still operate at the concrete level of cognitive thought, nutrition teaching is best presented by using pictures, samples of foods, videotapes, handouts, and hands-on experience.

School-age children often prefer the types of food eaten at home and may be resistant to new food items. A hospitalized child may refuse to eat, slowing the recuperative process. Family members can be encouraged to bring favorite foods from home that meet nutritional requirements. This can be especially helpful for children from different cultural groups. A child accustomed to a diet of rice, tofu, marinated chicken, and vegetables may not enjoy a hamburger and fries. Many hospitals have children plan a pizza night or sponsor other events to encourage eating. By school age, food has become strongly associated with social interaction, so it is beneficial to have children eat together or to encourage family members to take the child off the unit to eat or to bring in food from home and eat with their child.

The start of adolescence (age 12) generally begins a rapid increase in growth (the so-called adolescent growth spurt). However, growth spurts sometimes occur before that time. Girls may begin a growth spurt by 9 or 10 years and boys a year or so later (Fig. 2–19). Nutritional needs increase dramatically with this spurt, as discussed in the following section on the adolescent.

The loss of the first deciduous teeth and the eruption of permanent teeth usually occur at about age 6, or at the beginning of the school-age period. Of the 30 permanent teeth, 22 to 26 erupt by age 12 and the remaining molars follow during the teenage years. The school-age child should be closely monitored to ensure that brushing and flossing are adequate, that fluoride is taken if the water supply is unfluoridated, that dental care is obtained to provide for examination of teeth and alignment, and that loose teeth are identified before surgery or other events that may lead to loss of a tooth.

Injury Prevention

School-age children play in unsupervised settings for longer periods and are therefore at risk for different types of injuries than younger children (Table 2–30). Motor vehicle crashes are still common, but firearm and burn injuries increase in incidence.[20] Safety teaching should be an integral part of each school's curriculum.

Personality and Temperament

The enduring aspects of temperament continue to be manifested during the school years. The child classified as "difficult" at an earlier age may now have trouble in the classroom. Parents can be advised to provide a quiet setting for homework and to reward the child for concentration. Creative efforts and alternative methods of learning should be valued. The "slow-to-warm-up" child may need encouragement to try new activities and to share experiences with others.

Communication

During the school-age years the child corrects any lingering pronunciation or grammatical errors. Vocabulary increases, and the child is taught about parts

TABLE 2-30 Injury Prevention in the School-Age Years

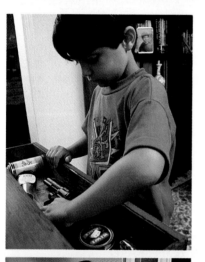

	Hazard	Developmental Characteristics	Preventive Measures
	Motor vehicle/ pedestrian/ biking crashes	Child plays outside; may follow balls into road; rides two-wheeler.	Teach child safe outside play, especially near streets. Expect use of bike helmet. Teach biking safety rules and provide safe places for riding.
	Firearms	Child may have been shown location of guns; is interested in showing them to friends.	Child should be taught never to touch guns without parent present. Guns should be kept unloaded and locked away. Guns and ammunition should be stored in different locations.
	Burns	Child may perform experiments with flames or toxic substances.	Teach child what to do in case of fire or if toxic substances touch skin or eyes. Reinforce teaching about 911.
	Assault	Child may be left alone after school and may walk or bike or take public transportation alone.	Provide telephone numbers of people to contact in case of an emergency or loneliness. Leave child alone for brief periods initially, and evaluate child's success in managing time. Teach child not to accept rides or talk to strangers. Teach child not to open doors at home and how to answer the phone.

of speech in school. School-age children enjoy writing and can be encouraged to keep a journal of hospitalization experiences as a method of dealing with anxiety. The literal translation of words characteristic of preschoolers is uncommon among school-age children.

Adolescent (12–18 Years)

Adolescence is a time of passage signaling the end of childhood and the beginning of adulthood. Adolescents differ in behaviors and accomplishments;

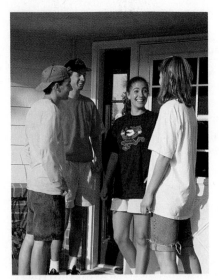

FIGURE 2–19 Because girls have a growth spurt earlier than boys, girls often are taller than boys of the same age. Remember what it was like at your first dance?

however, all are in a period of identity formation. If a healthy identity and sense of self-worth are not developed in this period, role confusion and purposeless struggling will ensue. The adolescents in your care will represent various degrees of identity formation and each will offer unique challenges.

Physical Growth and Development

The physical changes ending in **puberty,** or sexual maturity, begin near the end of the school-age period. The prepubescent period is marked by a growth spurt at an average age of 10 years for girls and 13 years for boys. The increase in height and weight is generally remarkable and is completed in 2 to 3 years (Table 2–31). The growth spurt in girls is accompanied by an increase in breast size and growth of pubic hair. Menstruation occurs last and signals achievement of puberty. In boys the growth spurt is accompanied by growth in size of the penis and testes and by growth of pubic hair. Deepening of the voice and growth of facial hair occur later, at the time of puberty. See Chapter 3 for a description of the pubertal stages.

During adolescence children grow stronger and more muscular and establish characteristic male and female patterns of fat distribution. The apocrine and eccrine glands mature, leading to increased amount and distinct odor to perspiration. All body organs are now fully mature, enabling the adolescent to take adult doses of medications.

The adolescent must adapt to a rapidly changing body for several years. These physical changes and hormonal variations offer challenges to identity formation.

TABLE 2–31 Growth and Development Milestones During Adolescence (12–18 Years of Age)

Physical Growth	Fine Motor Ability	Gross Motor Ability	Sensory Ability	Nutrition
Variation in age of growth spurt During growth spurt, girls gain 7–25 kg (15–55 lb) and grow 2.5–20 cm (2–8 in); boys gain approximately 7–29.5 kg (15–65 lb) and grow 11–30 cm (4½–12 in)	Skills are well developed (1)	New sports activities attempted and muscle development continues (2) Some lack of coordination common during growth spurt	Fully developed	Large appetite, which increases during growth spurt Eats many meals with friends; food choices influenced by peers (3)

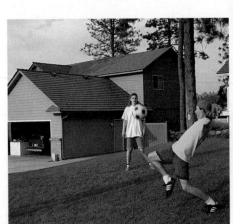

(1) Skills are well developed

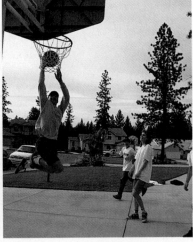

(2) New sports activities attempted

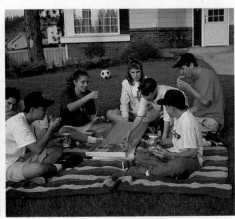

(3) Eats many meals with friends

TABLE 2-32 Favorite Activities in Adolescence

Sports

Ball sports
Gymnastics
Water and snow skiing
Swimming
School team sports

School Activities

Drama
Yearbook
Class officer
Committee participation

Peer Group Activities

Movies
Dances
Driving
Eating out

Quiet Activities

Reading
School work
Television and video games
Music

Cognitive Development

Adolescence marks the beginning of Piaget's last stage of cognitive development, the stage of formal operations. The adolescent no longer depends on concrete experiences as the basis of thought but develops the ability to reason abstractly. Such concepts as justice, truth, beauty, and power can be understood. The adolescent revels in this newfound ability and spends a great deal of time thinking, reading, and talking about abstract concepts.

The ability to think and act independently leads many adolescents to rebel against parental authority. Through these actions, adolescents seek to establish their own identity and values.

Activities

Maturity leads to new activities. Adolescents may drive, ride buses, or bike independently. They are less dependent on parents for transportation and spend more time with friends. Activities include participation in sports and extracurricular school activities, as well as "hanging out" and attending movies with friends (Table 2–32). The peer group becomes the focus of activities (Fig. 2–20), regardless of the teen's interests. Peers are important in establishing identity and providing meaning. Although same-sex interactions predominate, boy-girl relationships are more common than at earlier stages. Adolescents thus participate in and learn from social interactions fundamental to adult relationships.

Nutrition

Most adolescents need well over 2000 calories daily to support the growth spurt, and some adolescent boys require nearly 3000 calories daily. When teenagers are active in a variety of sports, these requirements increase further. Because adolescents prepare much of their own food and often eat with friends, they need nutritional knowledge. Developing a diet that includes a large number of calories, meets other requirements for vitamins and minerals, and is acceptable to the teen may be a challenge (Table 2–14). Small improvements can be viewed positively and may lead to further changes. An adolescent who does not like the hospital lunch and reaches into a bag for a soft drink and chips may be receptive to offers of juice and pizza, a more nutritionally beneficial meal.

FIGURE 2-20 Social interaction between children of same and opposite sex is as important inside the acute care setting as it is outside.

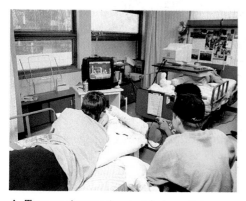

A, Teenage interaction inside hospital.

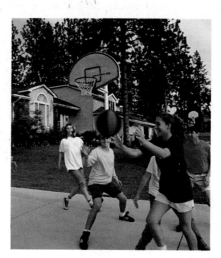

B, Teenagers enjoy playing together.

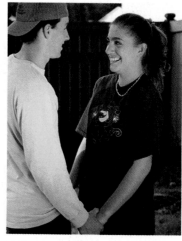

C, Emotional relationships form during adolescence.

TABLE 2-33 Injury Prevention in Adolescence

Hazard	Developmental Characteristics	Preventive Measures
Motor vehicle crashes	Adolescents learn to drive, enjoy new independence, and often feel invulnerable.	Insist adolescent take driver's education classes. Enforce rules about safe driving. Seat belts should be used for every trip. Discourage drug and alcohol use. Get treatment for teenagers who are known substance abusers.
Sporting injuries	Adolescents may engage in physically challenging sports such as soccer, gymnastics, or football. They may be allowed to drive motorboats.	Encourage use of protective sporting gear. Have injuries evaluated by health care professionals. Teach safe boating practices. Perform teaching related to hazards of drug and alcohol use, especially when using motorized equipment.
Drowning	Adolescents overestimate endurance. They take risks diving.	Encourage swimming only with friends. Enforce rules and inform them of risks.

Some common deficits in diets of adolescents are iron, calcium, and zinc. Iron and calcium deficiencies are often greater problems for girls. Nutritional teaching and offerings of snacks can help to provide for these needs. The adolescent who restricts food intake because of a disease process such as anorexia nervosa or bulimia is at high risk for these and other nutritional deficits. Health care visits for any purpose should incorporate assessment of height and weight and patterns of food intake. Because the peer group influence is important, group sessions in which adolescents eat lunch together while nutritional information is presented provide a forum for influencing food habits.

Injury Prevention

Injuries cause about 70% of deaths during adolescence.[20] Teenagers have access to potentially harmful objects, such as firearms, motor vehicles, and boats. They often think that no harm can come to them. This encourages adolescents to put themselves at high risk from dangerous behaviors (Table 2–33).

Suicide among adolescents has increased by 300% over the past two decades.[30] The high rate of stress experienced by today's teenagers coupled with easy access to harmful substances promotes death by suicide.

Nurses can be instrumental in assessing the potential for injury of adolescents seen in practice. Teaching about prevention is most successful when young people who have been injured share their experiences with other adolescents.

Violence is an increasingly important factor in adolescent injury. Homicide is the number one cause of death for young black males. The environment should be assessed for factors contributing to violence, and adolescents at risk can be referred to special programs for violence prevention. Abuse in homes and schools must be reported to law enforcement agencies when nurses are aware that it may have occurred.

Personality and Temperament

Characteristics of temperament manifested during childhood usually remain stable in the teenage years. For instance, the adolescent who was a calm, scheduled infant and child often demonstrates initiative to regulate study times and other routines. Similarly, the adolescent who was an easily stimulated infant may now have a messy room, a harried schedule with assignments always completed late, and an interest in many activities. It is also common for an adolescent who was an easy child to become more difficult because of the psychologic changes of adolescence and the need to assert independence.

As at the child's earlier ages the nurse's role may be to inform parents of different personality types and to help them support the teen's uniqueness while providing necessary structure and feedback. Nurses can help parents to understand their teen's personality type and to work with the adolescent to meet expectations of teachers and others in authority.

Communication

All parts of speech are used and understood by the adolescent. Colloquialisms or slang is commonly used with the peer group. The adolescent often studies foreign language in school, having the ability to understand and analyze grammar and sentence structure.

The adolescent increasingly leaves home base and establishes close ties with peers. These relationships become the basis for identity formation. There is generally a period of stress or crisis before a strong identity can emerge. The adolescent may try out new roles by learning a new sport or other skills, experimenting with drugs or alcohol, wearing different styles of clothing, or other activities. It is important to provide positive role models and a variety of experiences to help the adolescent make wise choices.

The adolescent also has a need to leave the past, to be different, and to change from former patterns in order to establish his or her own identity. Rules that are repeated constantly and dogmatically will probably be broken in the adolescent's quest for self-identity. This poses difficulties when the adolescent has a health problem, such as diabetes or a heart problem, that requires ongoing care. Introducing the adolescent to other teens who manage the same problem appropriately is usually more successful than telling the adolescent what to do.

Privacy should be ensured during the taking of health histories or interventions with teens. Even if a parent is present for part of a history or examination, the adolescent should be given the opportunity to relay information or ask questions alone with the health care provider. The adolescent should

☐ COMMUNICATION STRATEGIES: ADOLESCENT

Provide written as well as verbal explanations.

Direct history and explanations to teen alone; then include parent.

Allow for safe exploration of topics by suggesting that teen is similar to other teens. ("Many teens with diabetes have questions about.... How about you?")

Arrange meetings for discussions with other teens.

be given a choice of whether to have a parent present during an examination or while care is provided. Most information shared by an adolescent is confidential. Some states mandate disclosure of certain information to parents such as an adolescent's desire for an abortion. In these cases the adolescent should be informed of what will be disclosed to the parent.

Setting up teen rooms (recreation rooms for use only by adolescents) or separate adolescent units in hospitals can provide necessary peer support during hospitalization. Most adolescents are not pleased when placed on a unit or in a room with young children. Choices should be allowed whenever possible. These might include preference for evening or morning bathing, the type of clothes to wear while hospitalized, when a treatment will be given, and who should be allowed to visit and for how long. Use of contracts with adolescents may increase compliance. Firmness, gentleness, choices, and respect must all be balanced during care of adolescent patients.

Sexuality

With maturation of the body and hormones the adolescent achieves sexual maturity. This is a complex process involving growing interactions with members of the opposite sex, an interplay of the forces of society and family, and identity formation. The early adolescent progresses from dances and other social events with members of the opposite sex to the late adolescent who is mature sexually and may have regular sexual encounters. About half of all teens in the United States have had intercourse by the age of 16 years.

Teenagers need much information about their bodies and emerging sexuality. They should understand the interests and forces they experience. Including sex education in school classes and health care encounters is important. Information on methods to prevent sexually transmitted diseases is given, with most school districts now providing some teaching on AIDS. Far more common risks to teens, however, are diseases such as gonorrhea and herpes. Health histories must include questions on sexual activity, sexually transmitted diseases, and birth control use and understanding. Most hospitals routinely perform pregnancy screening on adolescent girls before elective procedures.

Adolescents will benefit from clear information about sexuality, an opportunity to develop relationships with adolescents in various settings, an open home and school where problems and issues can be discussed, and previous experience in problem solving and self–decision making. Sexual issues should be open topics that adolescents can discuss in a variety of settings. Alternatives and support for their decisions should be available.

REFERENCES

1 Worthington-Roberts, B., Vermeersch, J., & Williams, S. (1985). *Nutrition in pregnancy and lactation*. St. Louis: C. V. Mosby, p. 21–44.

2 Briggs, G., Freeman, R., & Yaffe, S. (1986). *Drugs in pregnancy and lactation* (2nd ed.). Baltimore: Williams & Wilkins, p. xii–xix.

3 Zajonc, R. B. (1983). Validating the confluence model. *Psychological Bulletin*, 93(3), 457–480.

4 Wallerstein, J. S. & Kelly, J. B. (1980). *Surviving the breakup: How children actually cope with divorce*. New York: Basic Books.

5 Hughes, D., Johnson, K., Rosenbaum, S., & Liu, J. (1989). *The health of America's children*. Washington, DC: Children's Defense Fund.

6 Johnson, C., Miranda, L., Sherman, A., & Weill, J. (1991). *Child poverty in America*. Washington, DC: Children's Defense Fund.

7 Murata, J., Mace, J. P., & Strehlow, A. et al. (1992). Disease patterns in homeless children: A comparison with national data. *Journal of Pediatric Nursing*, 7(3), 196–204.

8 Groer, M. et al. (1990). Autonomic and cardiovascular responses of preschool children to television programs.

Journal of Child and Adolescent Psychiatric Mental Health Nursing, 3(3), 134–138.

9 Dietz, W. H. & Gortmaker, S. L. (1985). Do we fatten our children at the television set? Obesity and television viewing in children and adolescents. *Pediatrics, 75*, 807–812.

10 Higgs, Z. & Gustafson, D. (1985). *Community as a client: Assessment and diagnosis.* Philadelphia: F. A. Davis.

11 Elkind, D. (1981). *The hurried child.* Menlo Park, CA: Addison-Wesley, p. 3–22.

12 Mussen, P. (ed.). (1983). *Handbook of child psychology, Volume I, History, theory and methods.* New York: John Wiley & Sons, p. 58–60.

13 Erikson, E. (1963). *Childhood and society.* New York: W. W. Morton, p. 247-273.

14 Ginsburg, H. & Opper, S. (1969). *Piaget's theory of intellectual development.* Englewood Cliffs, NJ: Prentice Hall, p. 1–25.

15 Eisenberg, N. (Ed.). (1987). *Contemporary topics in developmental psychology.* New York: John Wiley & Sons, p. 171.

16 Mussen, P. (Ed). (1983). *Handbook of child psychology, Volume IV, Socialization, personality and social development.* New York: John Wiley & Sons, p. 336.

17 Papalia, D. & Olds, S. (1990). *A child's world.* New York: McGraw-Hill.

18 Chess, S. & Thomas, A. (1986). *Temperament in clinical practice.* New York: Guilford Press.

19 Thomas, A. & Chess, S. (1979). *Temperament and development.* New York: Brunner/Mazel.

20 Behrman, R. (1992). *Nelson textbook of pediatrics.* Philadelphia: W. B. Saunders, p. 216–217.

21 Worthington-Roberts, G., Vermeersch, J., & Williams, S. (1985). *Nutrition in pregnancy and lactation.* St. Louis: C. V. Mosby, p. 304–321.

22 Barnes, G. P. et al. (1992). Ethnicity, location, age and fluoridation factors in baby bottle tooth decay and caries prevalence of Head Start children. *Public Health Report,* 10(2), 167–73.

23 Pipes, P. & Trahms, C. (1993). *Nutrition in infancy and childhood* (5th ed.). St. Louis: C. V. Mosby, p. 101–102.

24 American Academy of Pediatrics Task Force on Infant Positioning and SIDS. (1992). *Pediatrics,* 89(6), 1120–1126.

25 Frankenberg, W. (1990). *Denver II manual.* Denver, CO: Denver Developmental Materials.

26 Behrman, R. (1992). *Nelson textbook of pediatrics.* Philadelphia: W. B. Saunders, p. 923.

27 Joones, N. E. (1992). Prevention of childhood injuries: Motor vehicle injuries. *Pediatric Nursing,* 18(4), 380–382.

28 Piaget, J. (1972). *The child's conception of the world.* Totowa, NJ: Littlefield, Adams & Co.

29 Bindler, R. & Howry, L. (1991). *Pediatric drugs and nursing implications.* Norwalk, CT: Appleton & Lange, p. 231.

30 American Academy of Pediatrics, Committee on Adolescence. (1988). Suicide and suicide attempts in adolescents and young adults. *Pediatrics,* 81(2), 322–324.

SUGGESTED READINGS

Brenner, A. (1984). *Helping children cope with stress.* Lexington, MA: Lexington Books.

Cross cultural medicine. (1992). *Western Journal of Medicine,* 157(3), 248–373.

Edelman, M. (1991). *The measure of our success.* Boston: Beacon Press.

Elkind, D. (1987). *Miseducation.* New York: Alfred Knopf.

Family Service America. (1987). *The state of families.* Milwaukee: Family Service America.

Flavell, J. (1963). *The developmental psychology of Jean Piaget.* New York: D. Van Nostrand Co.

Institute of Medicine. (1992). *Nutrition during pregnancy and lactation.* Washington, DC: National Academy Press.

Lawrence, R. (1989). *Breastfeeding: A guide for the medical profession.* St. Louis: C. V. Mosby.

Mohrbacher, N., & Stock, J. (1991). *The breastfeeding answer book.* Franklin Park, IL: LaLeche League International.

Piaget, J. (1969). *The child's conception of physical causality.* Totowa, NJ: Littlefield, Adams & Co.

Piaget, J. (1973). *The psychology of intelligence.* Totowa, NJ: Littlefield, Adams & Co.

Spector, R. (1991). *Cultural diversity in health and illness.* Norwalk, CT: Appleton & Lange.

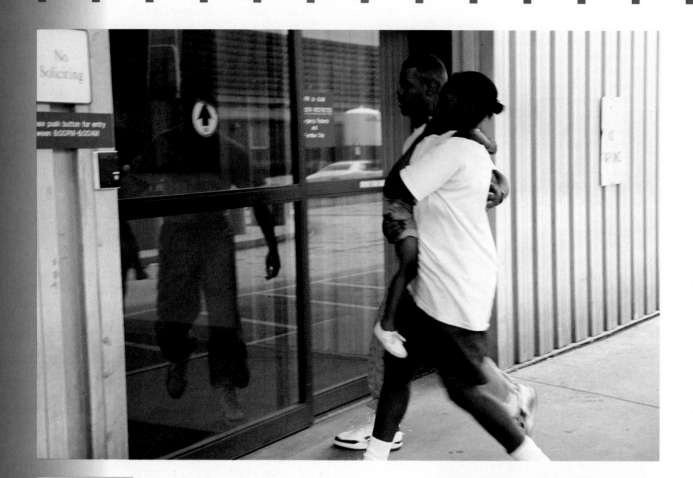

Kimberly, 3 years old, is brought by her mother and father to the emergency room. She is an emergency admission from the local pediatrician's office with a diagnosis of croup. As Kimberly's nurse, you are responsible for assessing her condition after she arrives on the pediatric nursing unit.

What information do you look for, and in what order do you gather this information? What techniques can you use to obtain information about Kimberly's condition? How do you organize your findings to make sense of them? The patient history and physical examination provide a structure and a sequence for collecting and analyzing relevant **assessment** data. The initial physical examination findings provide the baseline for monitoring Kimberly's response to treatment. Analysis of the assessment data also enables you to form nursing diagnoses and to develop a nursing care plan to direct the nursing care that Kimberly will receive.

PEDIATRIC ASSESSMENT

3

TERMINOLOGY

assessment The process of collecting information about a child and family to develop the nursing diagnoses. The assessment process includes the patient history, physical examination, and analysis of the collected data to identify relevant information.

auscultation The technique of listening to sounds produced by the airway, lungs, stomach, heart, and blood vessels to identify their characteristics. Auscultation is usually performed with the stethoscope to enhance the sounds heard.

clinical judgment Analyzing and synthesizing data from the patient history, physical examination, screening tests, and laboratory studies to make decisions about the child's health problems. This is also called diagnostic reasoning.

effective communication Information exchanged between the nurse, parent, and child that is clearly understood by all persons involved in the conversation.

inspection The technique of purposeful observation by carefully looking at the characteristics of the child's physical features and behaviors. Physical feature characteristics include size, shape, color, movement, position, and location.

nonverbal behavior The use of facial expression, eye contact, touch, tone of voice, posture, and body movements that communicate feelings during a conversation.

palpation The technique of touch to identify characteristics of the skin, internal organs, and masses. Characteristics include texture, moistness, tenderness, temperature, position, shape, consistency, and mobility of masses and organs.

percussion The technique of striking the surface of the body, either directly or indirectly, to set up vibrations that reveal the density of underlying tissues and borders of internal organs.

range of motion The direction and extent to which a particular joint is capable of moving, either independently or with assistance.

review of systems A comprehensive interview to identify and record the parent's or child's health concerns and health problems by body system that provides an overview of the child's health status.

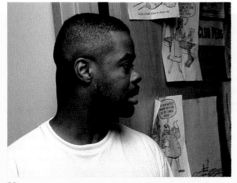

❝ I was scared when we brought Kimberly to the hospital. Kimberly looked helpless, afraid, and sick. The nurses and doctors took over when we got to the hospital, and I felt better because they seemed to know what to do. ❞

Anatomic and Physiologic Characteristics of Children

It is readily apparent that infants and children are smaller than adults. Significant differences in physiology also normally exist between children and adults. Knowledge of pediatric anatomic and physiologic differences will aid in recognizing normal variations found during the physical examination. It also assists with understanding the different physiologic responses children have to illness and injury. Figure 3–1 provides an overview of important anatomic and physiologic differences between children and adults.

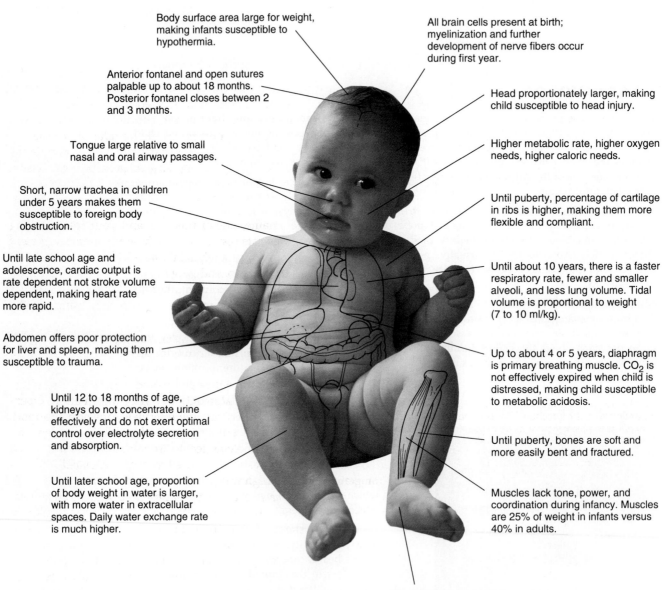

Body surface area large for weight, making infants susceptible to hypothermia.

Anterior fontanel and open sutures palpable up to about 18 months. Posterior fontanel closes between 2 and 3 months.

Tongue large relative to small nasal and oral airway passages.

Short, narrow trachea in children under 5 years makes them susceptible to foreign body obstruction.

Until late school age and adolescence, cardiac output is rate dependent not stroke volume dependent, making heart rate more rapid.

Abdomen offers poor protection for liver and spleen, making them susceptible to trauma.

Until 12 to 18 months of age, kidneys do not concentrate urine effectively and do not exert optimal control over electrolyte secretion and absorption.

Until later school age, proportion of body weight in water is larger, with more water in extracellular spaces. Daily water exchange rate is much higher.

All brain cells present at birth; myelinization and further development of nerve fibers occur during first year.

Head proportionately larger, making child susceptible to head injury.

Higher metabolic rate, higher oxygen needs, higher caloric needs.

Until puberty, percentage of cartilage in ribs is higher, making them more flexible and compliant.

Until about 10 years, there is a faster respiratory rate, fewer and smaller alveoli, and less lung volume. Tidal volume is proportional to weight (7 to 10 ml/kg).

Up to about 4 or 5 years, diaphragm is primary breathing muscle. CO_2 is not effectively expired when child is distressed, making child susceptible to metabolic acidosis.

Until puberty, bones are soft and more easily bent and fractured.

Muscles lack tone, power, and coordination during infancy. Muscles are 25% of weight in infants versus 40% in adults.

Blood volume is weight dependent: 80 ml/kg.

FIGURE 3–1 Children are not just small adults. There are important anatomic and physiologic differences between children and adults that will change based on a child's growth and development. Can you identify which of these differences are of greatest concern for the hospitalized child and why?

Communication Strategies

What makes communication effective? What does it mean when a parent or caretaker will not look you in the eye when speaking with you? What types of cues indicate that a parent may be withholding historical information?

The health history interview is a very personal conversation with a parent, caretaker, or adolescent during which private concerns and feelings are shared. Try to ensure that this exchange of information with the parent or the child is clearly understood by both parties, that it is an **effective communication.** Effective communication is difficult to accomplish because parents and children often do not correctly interpret what the nurse says, just as you may not understand completely what the parent or child says. People base their interpretation of information on their life experiences and the influences of culture and education.

Strategies to Build a Rapport with the Family

As you begin the history, make sure the parents understand the purpose of the interview and that the information will be used appropriately. To develop rapport, demonstrate your interest in and concern for the child and family during the interview. This rapport forms the foundation for the collaborative relationship between the nurse and parent that will provide the best nursing care for the child. The following strategies help to establish a rapport with the child's family during the nursing history:

- *Introduce yourself* (your name, title or position, and your role in caring for the child). To demonstrate respect, ask each family member present what name they prefer you to use when talking with them.
- *Explain the purpose of the interview* and why the nursing history is different from the information collected from other health professionals. For example, "The nurses will use this information to plan nursing care for your child."
- *Provide privacy* and remove as many distractions as possible during the interview. If the patient's room does not offer privacy, attempt to find a vacant patient room or lounge.
- *Direct the focus of the interview* with open-ended questions. Use close-ended questions or directing statements to clarify information. Open-ended questions are useful to initiate the interview, develop a rapport, and understand the parent's perceptions of the child's problem; for example, "Tell me what problems led to Roberto's admission to the hospital?" Close-ended questions are used to obtain detailed information; for example, "How high was Tommy's fever this morning?"
- *Ask one question at a time* so that the parent or child understands what piece of information you want and so that you know which question the parent is answering. "Does any member of your family have diabetes, heart disease, or sickle cell anemia?" is a multiple question. Ask about each disease separately to ensure the most accurate response.
- *Involve the child in the interview* by asking age-appropriate questions. Young children can be asked "What is your doll's name?" or "Where does it hurt?" Demonstrating an interest in the child initiates development of rapport with both the child and parents. Ask older children and teens questions about their illness or injury. Offer them an opportunity to privately discuss their major concerns when their parents are not present.

■ **CULTURAL CONSIDERATIONS**

Some cultural groups, particularly Asians, try to anticipate the answers you want to hear or say yes even if they do not understand the question. This is done in an effort to please you or as an expression of politeness. Remember to phrase your questions in a neutral manner.

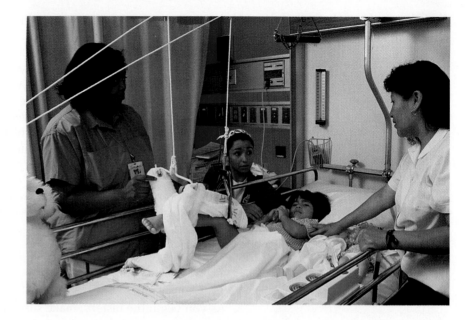

FIGURE 3–2 Selecting and using an interpreter. Most hospitals have designated interpreters that you should use. If not, find a professional interpreter whom you have identified beforehand and who knows medical terms and the typical cultural norms of the family. The interpreter (*center*) should be positioned to improve communication. Maintain eye contact with the parent or patient, not the interpreter. To ensure confidentiality of information for the parents, avoid using a family member for history taking.

- *Be honest* with the child when answering questions or when giving information about what will happen. Children need to learn they can trust you.
- *Choose the language style* best understood by the parent and child. Commonly used phrases can have different meanings to persons in various regions of the country or ethnic groups. To improve communication, request frequent feedback from the parents or child to ensure that their interpretation of phrases is accurate.
- *Use an interpreter to improve communication* when you are not fluent in the family's primary language (Fig. 3–2).

Careful Listening

Complete attention is necessary to "hear" and accurately interpret information the parents and child give during the nursing history. Carefully *listen* to the information provided by the parent, as well as how it is expressed, and *observe behavior* during the interaction.

- Does the parent hesitate or avoid answering certain questions?
- Pay attention to the parent's attitude or tone of voice when the child's problems are discussed. Determine if it is consistent with the seriousness of the child's problem. The tone of voice can reveal anxiety, anger, or lack of concern.
- Be alert to any underlying themes. For example, the parent who talks about the child's diagnosis, but repeatedly refers to the impact of the illness on the family's finances or on meeting the needs of other family members, is requesting that these issues be addressed.
- Observe the parent's **nonverbal behavior** (posture, gestures, eye contact, and facial expression) for consistency with the words and tone of voice used. Is the parent interested in and appropriately concerned about the child's condition? Behaviors such as sitting up straight, making eye contact, and appearing apprehensive reflect appropriate concern for the child. Physical withdrawal, failure to make eye contact, or a happy expression could be inconsistent with the child's serious condition.

Subtle nonverbal and verbal cues often indicate that the parent has not provided complete information about the child's problem. Observe for be-

■ CULTURAL CONSIDERATIONS

Eye contact with the interviewer may be avoided by many cultural groups (Asian, Native American, and Middle Eastern patients) because it is considered impolite, aggressive, or a sign of disrespect.[1]

haviors such as avoiding eye contact, change in voice pitch, or hesitation when responding to a question. Being supportive and asking clarifying questions encourage description or the expression of information that is difficult for the parent or child to share; for example, "It sounds like that was a very difficult experience. How did Latasha react?"

Encourage parents to share information, even if it is private or sensitive, especially when it influences nursing care planning. Often parents avoid sharing some information because they want to make a good impression, or they do not understand the value of the missing information. If a hesitation to share information is detected, briefly explain why the question was asked, for example, to make their child's hospital experience more pleasant or to begin planning for the child's discharge and home care.

In some cases the parent becomes too agitated, upset, or angry to continue responding to questions. When the information is not needed immediately, move on to another portion of the history to determine if the parent is able to respond to other questions. Depending on the emotional status of the parent, it may be more appropriate to collect the remaining historical data at a later time.

Data to Be Collected

The child's health, medical, and personal-social history is collected and organized to plan the child's nursing care. The Burns Classification System is the data collection framework selected for this text.[2] Physiologic, psychosocial, and developmental data are organized to help develop the nursing diagnoses and the nursing care plan. Be alert for nonverbal cues (Fig. 3–3).

Patient Information

Obtain the child's name and nickname, age, sex, and ethnic origin. The child's birth date, race, religion, address, and phone number can be obtained from the admission form. Ask the parent for an emergency contact address and phone number, as well as a work phone number. The person providing the patient history and that person's relationship to the patient are recorded.

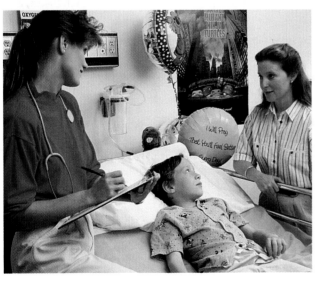

FIGURE 3–3 While you are collecting physiologic data, you should be observing patient behavior.

Physiologic Data

Information about the child's health problems and diseases is collected chronologically in a format similar to the traditional medical history.

- The *chief complaint* is the child's primary problem or reason for hospital admission, stated in the parent's or child's exact words.
- The *history of the present illness or injury* is a detailed description of the current health problem. This includes the onset and sequence of events, characteristics and changes in symptoms over time, influencing factors, and the current status of the problem. Each problem is described separately. Table 3–1 lists the specific data to be collected about each illness and injury.
- The *past history* is a more detailed description of the child's prior health problems. It includes the birth history and all major past illnesses and injuries. A detailed and complete birth history is obtained when the child's present problem may be related to the birth history (Table 3–2). Record the child's age at the

TABLE 3-1 History of Present Illness or Injury

Characteristic	Defining Variables
Onset	Sudden or gradual, previous episodes, date and time began
Type of symptom	Pain, itching, cough, vomiting, runny nose, diarrhea, rash, etc.
Location	Generalized or localized—anatomically precise
Duration	Continuous or episodic, length of episodes
Severity	Effect on daily activities, e.g., interrupts sleep, decreased appetite, incapacitating
Influencing factors	What relieves or aggravates symptoms, what precipitated the problem, recent exposure to infection or allergen
Past evaluation for the problem	Laboratory studies, physician's office or hospital where done, results of past examinations
Previous and current treatment	Prescribed and over-the-counter drugs used, other measures tried (heat, ice, rest), response to treatments

time of each illness, injury, related surgery, or hospitalization. Obtain information about each specific diagnosis, treatment, outcomes, complications or residual problems, and the child's reaction to the event (Table 3–3).

- The **review of systems** provides a comprehensive overview of the child's health. This is an opportunity to identify additional signs and symptoms associated with the child's admission problem or to identify other problems that have no relationship to the child's significant health problem. For example, asking about any urinary problems may reveal that a child still wets the bed at 7 years of age, but the admission is for a femur fracture. For each problem, obtain the treatment, outcomes, residual problems, and age at time of onset. Data collection guidelines are given in Table 3–4.
- The *familial and hereditary diseases* summarize the major familial and

TABLE 3-2 Birth History

Prenatal

Mother's age, health during pregnancy, prenatal care, weight gained, special diet, expected date of delivery
Details of illnesses, x-ray findings, hospitalizations, medications, complications, and timing during pregnancy
Prior obstetrical history

Antenatal—Description of Delivery

Site of delivery (hospital, home, birthing center)
Labor induced or spontaneous
Vaginal or cesarean-section, forceps or suction used, vertex or breech position
Single or multiple birth

Condition of Baby at Birth

Weight, Apgar score, cried immediately
Need for incubator, oxygen, suctioning, ventilator
Any abnormalities detected, meconium staining

Postnatal

Difficulties in the nursery—feeding, respiratory difficulties, jaundice, cyanosis, rashes
Length of hospital stay, special nursery, home with mother
Breast or bottle fed, weight gained in hospital

TABLE 3-3 Past Illnesses and Injuries

Illnesses	Major illnesses including common communicable diseases
Injuries	Major injuries, their mechanism (cause) and severity
Surgery	Specific type, day surgery or hospitalized
Hospitalizations	Reason and length of hospitalization
Allergies	To food, medication, animals, insect bites, environment, etc.
Immunizations	Types received, dates, unexpected reactions
Transfusions	Circumstances, reactions

TABLE 3-4 Review of Systems

Body Systems	Examples of Problems to Identify
General	General growth pattern, overall health status, ability to keep up with other children or tires easily with feeding or activity, fever, sleep patterns.
	Allergies, type of reaction (hives, rash, respiratory difficulty, swelling, nausea), seasonal or with each exposure
Skin and lymph	Rashes, dry skin, itching, skin color or texture changes, tendency for bruising, swollen or tender lymph glands
Hair and nails	Hair loss, color, or texture change, use of dye or chemicals on hair
	Abnormalities of nail growth or color
Head	Headaches, head injuries
Eyes	Vision problems, squinting, crossed eyes, lazy eye, wears glasses, eye infections, redness, tearing, burning, rubbing, swelling eyelids
Ears	Ear infections, frequent discharge from ears, or tubes in ears
	Hearing loss (no response to loud noises or questions, inattentiveness, hearing test ever done)
Nose and sinuses	Nosebleeds, nasal congestion, colds with runny nose, sinus pain or infections
	Nasal obstruction, difficulty breathing, snoring at night
Mouth and throat	Mouth breathing, difficulty swallowing, sore throats, strep infections
	Tooth eruption, cavities, braces
	Voice change, hoarseness, speech problems
Cardiac and hematologic	Heart murmur, anemia, hypertension, cyanosis, edema, rheumatic fever, chest pain
Chest and respiratory	Trouble breathing, choking episodes, cough, wheezing, cyanosis, exposure to tuberculosis, other infections
Gastrointestinal	Bowel movements, frequency, color, regularity, consistency, discomfort, constipation or diarrhea, abdominal pain, bleeding from rectum, gas or flatulence
	Nausea or vomiting, appetite
Urinary	Frequency, urgency, dysuria, dribbling, enuresis, strength of urinary stream
	Toilet trained—age when day and night dryness attained
Reproductive	For pubescent children
Female	Menses onset, amount, duration, frequency, discomfort, problems; vaginal discharge, breast development
Male	Puberty onset, emissions, erections, pain or discharge from penis, swelling or pain in testicles
Both	Sexual activity, use of contraception, sexually transmitted diseases
Musculoskeletal	Weakness, clumsiness, poor coordination, balance, tremors, abnormal gait, painful muscles or joints, swelling or redness of joints, fractures
Neurologic	Seizures, fainting spells, dizziness, numbness, learning problems, attention span, hyperactivity, memory problems

hereditary diseases in family members, including the parents, grandparents, aunts, uncles, and siblings. Collect information about the health status of each parent. Record information in either a pedigree or a narrative format. Specific diseases the nurse inquires about are listed in Table 3–5.

Psychosocial Data

Obtain the following information about family composition to establish a socioeconomic and sociologic context within which to plan the child's care in the hospital and home.

TABLE 3-5 Familial or Hereditary Diseases

Infectious diseases	Tuberculosis, HIV, or hepatitis
Heart disease	Heart defects, myocardial infarctions, hypertension, hypercholesterolemia
Allergic disorders	Eczema, hay fever, or asthma
Eye disorders	Glaucoma or cataracts
Hematologic disorders	Sickle cell anemia, thalassemia, G6PD deficiency, leukemia
Lung disorders	Cystic fibrosis
Cancer	Type
Endocrine disorders	Diabetes mellitus
Mental disorders	Mental retardation, epilepsy, Huntington chorea, psychiatric disorders
Musculoskeletal disorders	Arthritis, muscular dystrophy
Gastrointestinal disorders	Ulcers, colitis, kidney disease

- Family composition, including family members in the home, their relationship to the child, marital status of parents or other family structure, and persons participating in the care of the child
- Household members employed, family income, and financial resources or agencies used such as health insurance, food stamps, Aid to Families with Dependent Children (AFDC), or the Easter Seals Society

TABLE 3-6 Daily Living Patterns

Health Maintenance

Name of health care provider	Last visit
Name of dentist	Last visit
Other health care professionals	

Safety Measures Used

Car restraint	Smoke detectors
Window guards	Bicycle helmet
Medication storage	Other

Activities

Physical mobility
Play activities
Limitations and adaptive equipment

Elimination Habits

Potty training, toilet habits, and ability for self-care
Bed wetting
Bowel patterns

Sleep

Sleep and rest pattern
Disturbances
Bedtime rituals

Role Relationships

Family relationships/alterations in family process
Peer relationships
Social interactions: e.g., day care, preschool, school
Communication

Self-Perception/Self-Concept

Personal identity and role identity
Self-esteem
Body image/nonvisible disorder

Coping/Stress Tolerance

Temperament
Coping behaviors
Discipline
Any substance abuse

Values and Beliefs

Religion
Personal values/beliefs

Home Care Provided for Child's Condition

Resources needed/available
Knowledge and skills of parents, other family members

Sensory/Perceptual Problems

Adaptations to daily living for any sensory loss (vision, hearing, cognitive, or motor)

Adapted from Burns, C. (1992). *Journal of Pediatric Health Care 6*, 73–81.

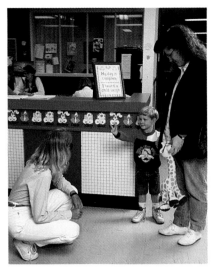

FIGURE 3–4 Examination of child begins from the first contact. You must be observing behavior of child and parent and using your visual cues to make a proper assessment. Does the child appear properly nourished? Does the child appear secure with the parent?

- Description of the housing and home environment (atmosphere, emotional stresses, family activities); safe play area; use of city or well water; and availability of electricity, heat, and refrigeration
- School or day care arrangements; description of the neighborhood, including playgrounds, transportation, and proximity to stores

Information about daily routines, psychosocial data, and other living patterns forms the basis for many nursing diagnoses and development of an individualized nursing care plan. Collection of information should focus on issues that have an impact on the quality of daily living, even if some data seem to overlap with disease data (Table 3–6).

Developmental Data

Information about the child's motor, cognitive, language, and social development is recorded. The parent is asked about the child's milestones and current fine and gross motor skills. The age at which the child first used words appropriately and the current words used or language ability are obtained. For children in school the nurse asks about academic performance to assess cognitive development. The parent is asked about the child's manner of interaction with other children, family members, and strangers.

The developmental data will help the nurse plan nursing care appropriate for the child. Guidelines for a nursing assessment of development can be found in Chapter 2.

General Appraisal

The examination begins when you first meet the child, either when admitting the child to the nursing unit or in the patient's room (Fig. 3–4). Measure the infant's weight, length, and head circumference. If the child can stand, a standing height measurement is substituted for length. Take the child's temperature, heart rate, respiratory rate, and blood pressure. Refer to the Atlas of Pediatric Procedures at the end of this text for technique.

Observe the child's general appearance and behavior. The child should appear well nourished and well developed. Infants and young children are often fearful and seek reassurance from their parents. The child may resist interacting with you until a rapport is established.

Observe the behavior and tone of voice used by the parent when he or she is talking to the child. Is the child encouraged to speak? Is the child appropriately reassured or supported by the parent? The child should feel secure with the parent and perceive permission to interact with the nurse.

Assessing Skin and Hair Characteristics and Integrity

What is indicated when the child's skin is not uniform in color or when it feels spongy to the touch? What are each of the primary skin lesions called, and what characteristics are used to describe each of them? How can cyanosis and jaundice be detected in dark-skinned children? Why is skin turgor assessed? How is the presence of head lice identified in a child?

Examination of the skin requires good lighting to detect variations in skin color and to identify lesions. Daylight is preferred, but it is not always available. Rather than inspecting the entire skin surface of the child at one time, the nurse examines the child's skin simultaneously with other body systems as each region of the body is exposed.

Gloves

The color of the bruise provides clues to its age.[3]

Color	Age of Bruise
Reddish blue	Up to 48 hours
Brownish blue	2 to 3 days
Brownish green	4 to 7 days
Greenish yellow	7 to 10 days
Yellow-brown	More than 8 days
Normal skin color	2 to 4 weeks

Inspection of the Skin

The child's skin is inspected for color and the presence of imperfections, elevations, or other lesions.

Skin Color

The color of the child's skin usually has an even distribution. The skin is inspected for color variations, such as increased or decreased pigmentation, pallor, mottling, bruises, erythema, cyanosis, or jaundice, that may be associated with local or generalized conditions. Some variations in skin color are common and normal, such as freckles found in the white population and Mongolian spots found on dark-skinned infants (Fig. 3–5). Bruises are common on the knees, shins, and lower arms as children stumble and fall. Bruises on other parts of the body, especially in various stages of healing, should raise a suspicion of child abuse.

When a skin color abnormality is suspected, the buccal mucosa and tongue should be inspected to confirm the color change. This is especially important in darker skinned children because the mucous membranes are usually pink, regardless of skin color. The gums are pressed lightly for 1 to 2 seconds. Any residual color, such as jaundice or cyanosis, is more easily detected in blanched skin. Jaundice may also be noticed in sclerae of the eyes. Generalized cyanosis is associated with respiratory and cardiac disorders. Jaundice is associated with liver disorders.

Palpation of the Skin

Palpation of the skin provides a sense of its characteristics: temperature, texture, moistness, and resilience or turgor. To evaluate these characteristics, the nurse lightly touches or strokes the skin surface. The nurse follows Universal Precautions by wearing gloves when palpating mucous membranes, open wounds, and lesions.

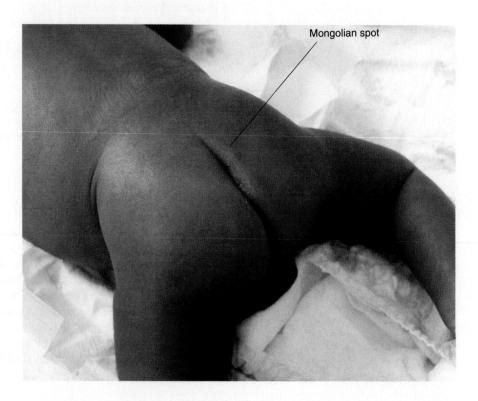

Mongolian spot

FIGURE 3–5 Mongolian spots are large patches of bluish skin on the buttocks. They are a normal occurrence in dark-skinned infants but are sometimes incorrectly thought to be bruises.

Temperature

The child's skin normally feels cool to the touch. A general evaluation of skin temperature can be obtained by placing the wrist or dorsum of the hand against the child's skin. Excessively warm skin may indicate the presence of fever or inflammation, while abnormally cool skin may be a sign of shock or cold exposure.

Texture

Children have soft, smooth skin over the entire body. Any areas of roughness, thickening, or induration (area of extra firmness with a distinct border) should be identified. Abnormalities in texture are associated with endocrine disorders, chronic irritation, and inflammation.

Moistness

The child's skin is normally dry to the touch. The skin may feel slightly damp when the child has been exercising or crying. Excessive sweating without exertion is associated with a fever, an uncorrected congenital heart defect, or cystic fibrosis.

Resilience (Turgor)

The child's skin is taut, elastic, and mobile because of the balanced distribution of intracellular and extracellular fluids. To evaluate skin turgor, the examiner pinches a small amount of skin on the abdomen between the thumb and forefinger, releases the skin, and watches the speed of recoil (Fig. 3–6). If the skin rapidly returns to its previous contour, good skin turgor is indicated. When poor skin turgor is present, the skin tents or stands up rather than resuming its previous contour. Poor skin turgor is commonly associated with dehydration.

If *edema*, an accumulation of excess fluid in the interstitial spaces, is present, the skin feels doughy or boggy. To test for the degree of edema present, the examiner presses for 5 seconds against a bone beneath the area of puffy skin, releases the pressure, and observes how rapidly the indentation disappears. If the indentation disappears rapidly, the edema is "nonpitting." Slow

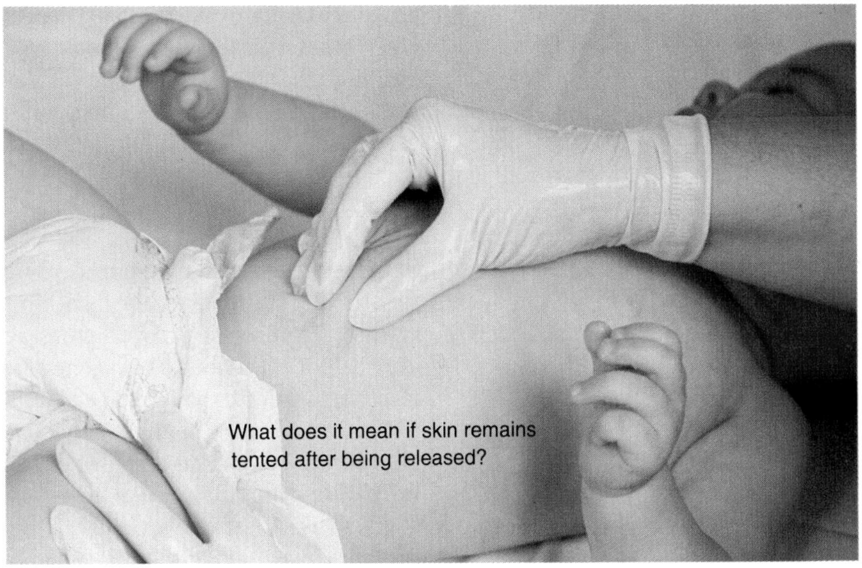

■ CLINICAL TIP

The degree of dehydration, or weight loss caused by dehydration, can be estimated from the time tented skin takes to return to its natural configuration.[4]

Weight Loss from Dehydration	Time to Return to Normal
<5 %	<2 sec
5%–8%	2–3 sec
9%–10%	3–4 sec
>10%	>4 sec

What does it mean if skin remains tented after being released?

FIGURE 3–6 Tenting of the skin is associated with poor skin turgor. Skin with normal turgor will return to flat position quickly.

FIGURE 3–7 Capillary refill technique. **A,** Pinch the end of a finger until the skin is blanched. **B,** Release your grip and color should return promptly. Technique for small-vein filling time. **C,** Using the index finger, milk a vein on the dorsum of the hand or foot from distal to proximal. **D,** Quickly release the finger and count the seconds it takes the vein to fill. Slow filling could relate to shock or restriction due to a tight bandage or cast.

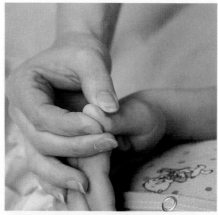
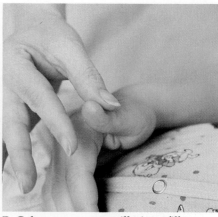

A, Skin will lose color as capillaries are closed off.

B, Color returns as capillaries refill.

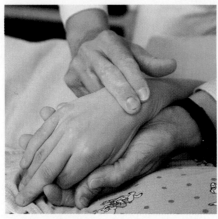
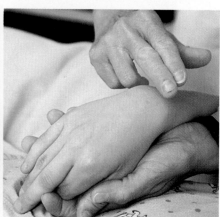

C, Blood returns to the heart in veins, so you must move index finger down.

D, Remove finger; blood returns to vein.

■ COMMON PATTERNS OF SKIN LESIONS

Annular: Circular, begins in center and spreads to periphery
Polycyclic: Annular lesions running together
Linear: In a row or stripe
Groups: Clustered
Gyrate: Twisted, spiral, coiled

disappearance of the indentation indicates "pitting" edema, which is commonly associated with kidney or heart disorders.

Capillary Refill and Small-Vein Filling Times

Two techniques are used to determine the adequacy of tissue perfusion (oxygen circulating to the tissues). When tissue perfusion is inadequate, immediately assess the child for shock or a physical constriction such as a cast or bandage that is too tight. The capillary refill time is normally less than 2 seconds (Fig. 3–7A and B). The small-vein filling time is normally less than 4 seconds (Fig. 3–7C and D).

Skin Lesions

Skin lesions are usually an indication of an abnormal skin condition. Characteristics of these lesions—location, size, type of lesion, pattern, and discharge, if present—provide clues about the cause of the condition. Inspect and palpate the isolated or generalized skin color abnormalities, elevations, lesions, or injuries to describe all characteristics present.

Primary lesions (such as macules, papules, and vesicles) are often the skin's initial response to injury or infection. Mongolian spots and freckles are normal findings also classified as primary lesions. Secondary lesions (such as scars, ulcers, fissures) are the result of irritation, infection, and delayed healing of primary lesions. Table 3–7 describes common primary lesions.

TABLE 3-7 Common Primary Skin Lesions and Associated Conditions

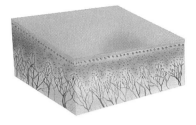

Lesion Name: Macule
Description:
Flat, nonpalpable, diameter <1 cm
Example: Freckle, rubella, rubeola, petechiae

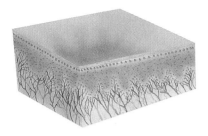

Lesion Name: Patch
Description:
Macule, diameter >1 cm
Example: Vitiligo, Mongolian spot

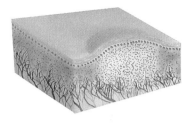

Lesion Name: Papule
Description:
Elevated, firm, diameter <1 cm
Example: Warts, pigmented nevi

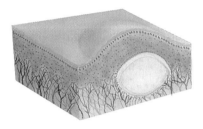

Lesion Name: Nodule
Description:
Elevated, firm, deeper in dermis than papule, diameter 1–2 cm
Example: Erythema nodosum

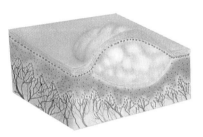

Lesion Name: Tumor
Description:
Elevated, solid, diameter >2 cm
Example: Neoplasm, hemangioma

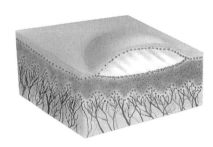

Lesion Name: Vesicle
Description:
Elevated, filled with fluid, diameter <1 cm
Example: Early chicken pox, herpes simplex

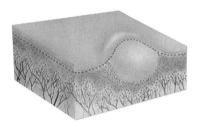

Lesion Name: Pustule
Description:
Vesicle filled with purulent fluid
Example: Impetigo, acne

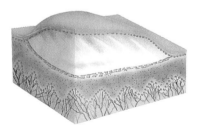

Lesion Name: Bulla
Description:
Vesicle diameter >1 cm
Example: Burn blister

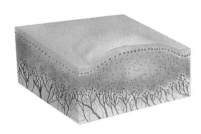

Lesion Name: Wheal
Description:
Irregular elevated solid area of edematous skin
Example: Urticaria, insect bite

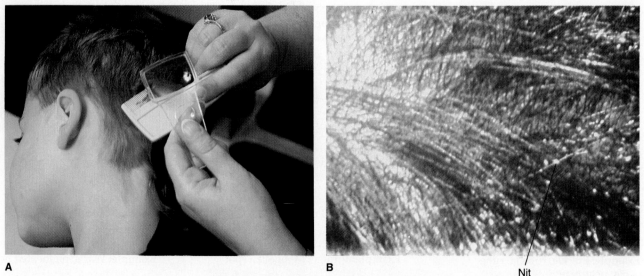

A

B

Nit

FIGURE 3-8 A, Inspecting for head lice with a magnifying glass. **B,** Nits on hair.
B courtesy of Reed and Carnrich Pharmaceuticals.

Inspection of the Hair

Inspect the scalp hair for color, distribution, and cleanliness. The hair shafts should be evenly colored, shiny, and either curly or straight. Variation in hair color not caused by bleaching can be associated with a nutritional deficiency. Normally, hair is distributed evenly over the scalp. Investigate areas of hair loss. Hair loss in a child may result from tight braids or skin lesions such as ringworm. Notice any unusual hair growth patterns. An unusually low hairline on the neck or forehead may be associated with a congenital disorder such as hypothyroidism.

Children are frequently exposed to head lice. Inspect the individual hair shafts for small nits (lice eggs) that adhere to the hair (Fig. 3-8). None should be present.

Observe the distribution of body hair as other skin surfaces are exposed during examination. Fine hair covers most areas of the body. The presence of body hair in unexpected places should be noted. For example, a tuft of hair at the base of the spine often indicates a spine defect.

It is important to note the age at which pubic and axillary hair develops in the child. Development at an unusually young age is associated with precocious puberty.

Palpation of the Hair

Palpate the hair shafts for texture. Hair should feel soft or silky with fine or thick shafts. Endocrine conditions such as hypothyroidism may result in coarse, brittle hair.

Part the hair in various spots over the head to inspect and palpate the scalp for crusting or other lesions. If lesions are present, describe them using the characteristics in Table 3-7.

Assessing the Head for Skull Characteristics and Facial Features

What can cause a child's head or face to be asymmetric? How does a normal fontanel feel? What does an unusually large or small head suggest in an infant? What is the ping-pong phenomenon and what does it indicate?

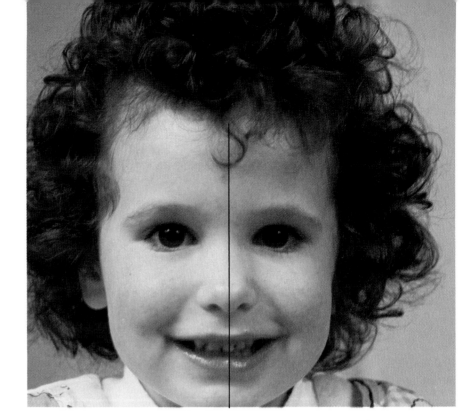

FIGURE 3-9 Draw an imaginary line down the middle of the face over the nose and compare the features on each side. Significant asymmetry may be caused by cranial nerve V or VII paralysis, in utero positioning, swelling from infection, allergy, or trauma.

Inspection of the Head and Face

Head

During early childhood the skull's sutures permit expansion for brain growth. Infants and young children normally have a rounded skull with a prominent occipital area. The shape of the head changes during childhood, and the occipital area becomes less prominent. An abnormal skull shape can result from premature closure of the sutures.

The head circumference of infants and young children is routinely measured until 5 years of age to ensure that adequate growth for brain development has occurred. The Atlas of Pediatric Procedures describes the proper technique. A larger than normal head is associated with hydrocephalus, and a smaller than normal head suggests microcephaly.

Face

Inspect the child's face for symmetry during several facial expressions such as resting, smiling, talking, and crying (Fig. 3–9). Significant asymmetry may result from paralysis of trigeminal or facial nerves (cranial nerves V or VII), in utero positioning, and swelling from infection, allergy, or trauma.

Next inspect the face for unusual facial features such as coarseness, wide eye spacing, or disproportionate size. Tremors, tics, and twitching of facial muscles are often associated with seizures.

Palpation of the Skull

Palpate the skull in infants and young children to assess the sutures and fontanels and to detect soft bones (Fig. 3–10).

■ **EQUIPMENT NEEDED**

Tape measure

■ **CLINICAL TIP**

Children who were low-birth-weight infants often have a flat, elongated skull because the soft skull bones were flattened by the weight of the head early in infancy.

■ **CULTURAL CONSIDERATIONS**

The head is a sacred part of the body to Southeast Asians. Ask for permission before touching the infant's head to palpate the sutures and fontanels.[1] When a Hispanic child is examined, however, not touching the head is considered bad luck.

FIGURE 3–10 The sutures are separations between the bones of the skull that have not yet joined. The fontanels are formed at the intersection of these sutures where bone has not yet formed. Fontanels are covered by tough membranous tissue that protects the brain. Posterior fontanel closes between 2 and 3 months. Anterior fontanel and sutures are palpable up to 18 months.

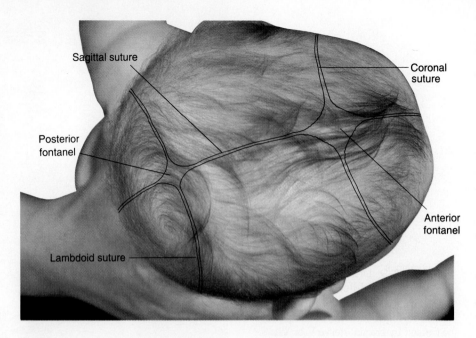

■ GROWTH AND DEVELOPMENT CONSIDERATIONS

The suture lines of the skull are seldom palpated after 2 years of age. After that time the sutures rarely split.

Sutures

Use the fingerpads to palpate each suture line. The edge of each bone in the suture line is felt but normally there is no separation of the two bones. If additional bone edges are felt, it may indicate a skull fracture.

Fontanels

At the intersection of the sutures, palpate the anterior and posterior fontanels. The fontanel should feel flat and firm inside the bony edges. The anterior fontanel is normally smaller than 5 cm in diameter at 6 months of age and then becomes progressively smaller. It closes between 12 and 18 months of age. The posterior fontanel closes between 2 and 3 months of age.

A tense fontanel, bulging above the margin of the skull, is an indication of increased intracranial pressure. A soft fontanel, sunken below the margin of the skull, is associated with dehydration.

Craniotabes

Craniotabes is a snapping, ping-pong sensation associated with soft bones. Press firmly above and behind the ears. If craniotabes is present, a small section of bone suddenly sinks and then snaps back up when compression is lifted. Craniotabes is an abnormal finding associated with hydrocephalus and rickets.

Assessing Eye Structures, Function, and Vision

What is one of the most common eye problems that occurs during childhood? What do bulging or sunken eyeballs look like? What is the red reflex and what does it indicate? How is eye muscle balance tested? Is it normal for a child's visual acuity to differ at certain ages?

■ EQUIPMENT NEEDED

Ophthalmoscope
Vision chart
Penlight or small toy
Index card or paper cup

Inspection of the External Eye Structures

The function of the external and internal eye structures and related cranial nerves makes vision possible. The external eye structures, including the eye-

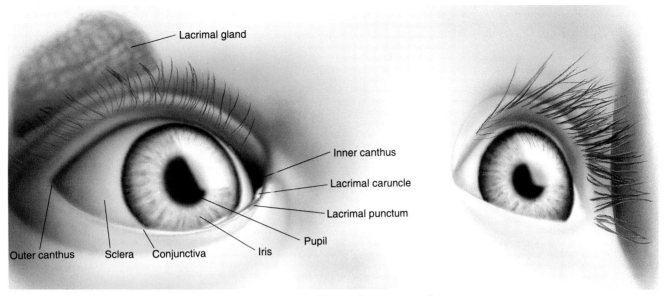

FIGURE 3-11 External structures of the eye.

balls, eyelids, and eye muscles, are inspected. The function of cranial nerves II, III, IV, and VI, which innervate the eye structures, is also tested (Fig. 3–11).

Eye Size and Spacing

Inspect the eyes and surrounding tissues simultaneously when examining facial features. The eyes should be the same size but not unusually large or small. Observe for eye bulging, which can be identified by retracted eyelids or a sunken appearance. Bulging may be associated with a tumor, and a sunken appearance may reflect dehydration.

Next inspect the eyes to see if they are appropriately distanced from each other. *Hypertelorism,* or widely spaced eyes, is often a normal variation in children (Fig. 3–12).

Eyelids

Inspect the eyelids for color, size, position, mobility, and condition of the eyelashes. Eyelids are the same color as surrounding facial skin and are free of swelling or inflammation along the edges. Sebaceous glands that look like yellow striations are often present near the hair follicles. Eyelashes curl away from the eye to prevent irritation of the conjunctivae.

Inspect the conjunctivae lining the eyelids by pulling down the lower lid and then everting the upper lid. The conjunctivae should be pink and glossy. The lacrimal punctum, the opening for the lacrimal gland on each lid, is located near the **medial canthus.** No redness or excess tearing should be present.

When the **eyes are** open, inspect the level at which the upper and lower lids cross the eye. Each lid normally covers part of the iris but not any portion of the pupil. The lids should also close completely over the iris and cornea. Ptosis, drooping of the lid over the pupil, is often associated with injury to the oculomotor nerve, cranial nerve III. Sunset sign, in which sclera is seen between the upper lid and the iris, may indicate retracted eyelids or hydrocephalus.

Inspect the eyes for the palpebral slant (Fig. 3–13). The eyelids of most people open horizontally. An upward or Mongolian slant is a normal finding in Asian children; however, children with Down syndrome also often have a

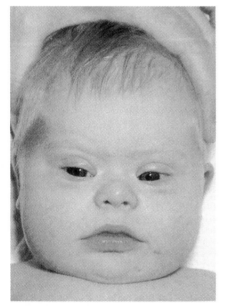

FIGURE 3-12 Hypertelorism is an extra-wide distance between the medial canthi of the eyes. Widely spaced eyes are the most common sign of Down syndrome along with epicanthal folds.

From Zitelli, B.J., & Davis, H.W. (Eds). (1987). *Atlas of pediatric physical diagnosis.* New York: Mosby–Year Book Europe Ltd.

■ CLINICAL TIP

The eyelids of newborns are often swollen and difficult to open after antibiotics are instilled at birth to prevent infection.

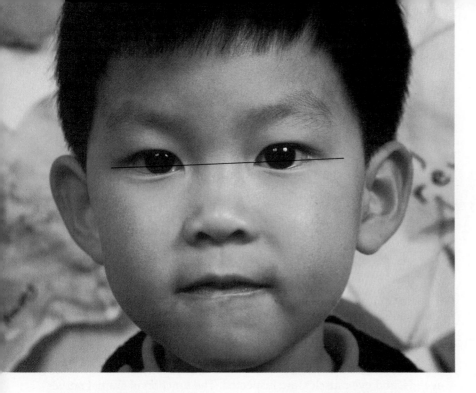

FIGURE 3–13 Draw an imaginary line across the medial canthi and extend it to each side of the face to identify the slant of the palpebral fissures. When the line crosses the lateral canthi, the palpebral fissures are horizontal and no slant is present. When the lateral canthi fall above the imaginary line, the eyes have an upward or Mongolian slant. A downward or anti-Mongolian slant is present when the lateral canthi fall below the imaginary line. Epicanthal folds are present when an extra fold of skin partially or completely covers the caruncles in the medial canthi. Which type of slant does this child have?

Mongolian slant. A downward or anti-Mongolian slant is seen in some children as a normal variation.

Eye Color

Inspect the color of each sclera, iris, and bulbar conjunctiva. The sclera is normally white or ivory in darker skinned children. Sclerae of another color suggest the presence of an underlying disease. For example, yellow sclerae indicate jaundice. Typically the iris is blue at birth and becomes pigmented within 6 months. Inspect the iris for the presence of Brushfield spots, white specks in a linear pattern around the iris circumference, often associated with Down syndrome. The bulbar conjunctivae, which cover the sclera to the edge of the cornea, are normally clear. Redness can indicate eyestrain, allergies, or irritation.

Pupils

Inspect the pupils for size and shape. Normally the pupils are round, clear, and equal in size. Some children have a coloboma, a keyhole-shaped pupil caused by a notch in the iris. The presence of this sign can indicate that the child has other congenital anomalies.

To test the pupillary response to light, shine a bright light into one eye. A brisk constriction of the pupil exposed to direct light and the other pupil is a normal finding.

To test pupillary response to accommodation, ask the child to look first at a near object (for example, a toy) and then at a distant object (for example, a picture on the wall). The expected response is pupil constriction with near objects and pupil dilation with distant objects. This procedure tests the optic nerve, cranial nerve II.

Inspection of the Eye Muscles

One of the most common pediatric eye disorders is strabismus, or crossed eyes. This condition is important to detect because, if uncorrected, it can cause vision impairment. Several tests are used to detect the presence of a

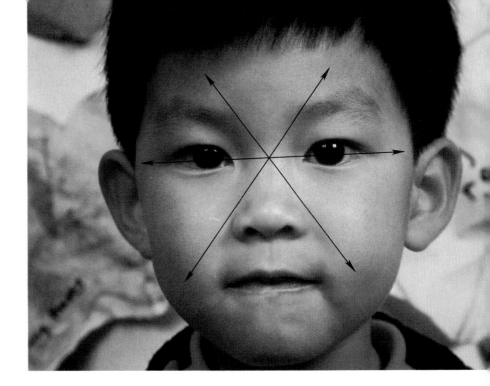

FIGURE 3-14 Begin the eye muscle examination with inspection of the extraocular movements. Have the child sit at your eye level. Hold a toy or penlight about 12 inches from the child's eyes and move it through the six cardinal fields of gaze. Both eyes should move together tracking the object. This procedure tests cranial nerves III, IV, and VI.

muscle imbalance that can result in strabismus. These tests include the evaluation of extraocular movements, the corneal light reflex, and the cover-uncover test.

Extraocular Movements

Seat the child at your eye level to evaluate the extraocular movements. Hold a toy or penlight 30 cm from the child's eyes and move it through the six cardinal fields of gaze. Both eyes should move together, tracking the object. This procedure tests the oculomotor, trochlear, and abducens nerves (cranial nerves III, IV, and VI) (Fig. 3–14).

Corneal Light Reflex

To test the corneal light reflex, shine a light on the child's nose, midway between the eyes. Identify the location where the light is reflected on each eye. The light reflection is normally symmetrical, at the same spot on each cornea. An asymmetric corneal light reflex indicates strabismus.

Cover-Uncover Test

The cover-uncover test can be used only for older, cooperative children. Standing slightly to one side but still able to see the child's eyes, ask the child to look at a picture on the wall. Cover one eye with an index card and simultaneously inspect the uncovered eye for movement as it focuses on the picture. Then remove the card from the covered eye and inspect it for movement as it focuses on the picture. The procedure is repeated with the other eye covered. No obvious movement of either eye is expected because the eyes work together. Eye movement indicates a muscle imbalance.

Vision Assessment

Because vision is such an **important sense** for learning, assessment is essential to detect any serious problems. Vision is evaluated using an age-appro-

Research has discovered that newborns
have vision good enough at birth to prefer faces to other patterns and to follow a
moving object. The child's visual acuity
develops during early childhood.[4]

Age	Visual Acuity
3 years	20/50
4 years	20/40
5 years	20/30
6 years	20/20

priate vision testing, but no simple method exists. It is possible to assess the presence of vision in infants and children by observing their behavior in response to certain maneuvers and during play.

Infants and Toddlers

When the infant's eyes are open, test the blink reflex by moving your hand quickly toward the infant's eyes. A quick blink is the normal response. Absence of the blink reflex can indicate that the infant is blind.

To test an infant's ability to visually track an object, hold a light or toy about 15 cm from the infant's eyes. When the infant has fixated on or is staring at the object, move it slowly to each side. The infant should follow the object with the eyes and by moving the head.

Once an infant has developed skills to reach for and then pick up objects, observe play behavior to evaluate vision. The ability to easily find and pick up small toys is a good indicator of vision in children under 3 years of age.

Standardized Vision Charts

Standardized vision charts cannot be used to test vision until the child can understand directions and cooperate, usually about 3 or 4 years of age. The Snellen E chart or Picture chart can be used to test visual acuity of preschool-aged children just as the Snellen Letter chart is used for school-aged children and adolescents. The Atlas of Pediatric Procedures describes the use of these charts.

Inspection of the Internal Eye Structures

The funduscopic examination permits **inspection** of internal eye structures—the retina, optic disc, arteries and veins, and macula (Fig. 3–15). This examination takes extensive practice because the ophthalmoscope is a complex instrument to master and because the examination is hard to perform on uncooperative children. Most often it is performed by experienced examiners.

Darkening the room will cause the child's pupils to dilate. Explain the procedure to the child to gain cooperation. Have a picture on the wall or have the parent or assistant hold a toy for the child to stare at so that the child's eye will not have to be held open forcibly.

FIGURE 3–15 Normal fundus.

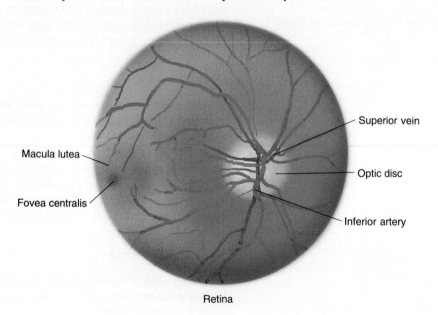

FIGURE 3-16 Ophthalmoscope.

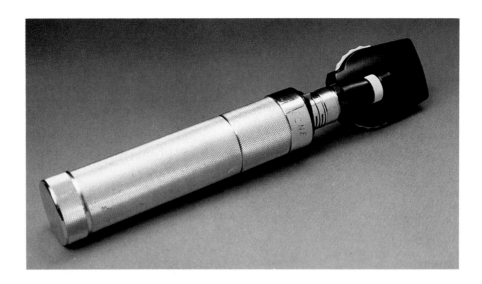

Using the Ophthalmoscope

The ophthalmoscope has a lens and mirror system and a bright light for inspection of structures of the internal eye (Fig. 3–16). Different lens powers are arranged on the rotating disk of the ophthalmic head. This system permits compensation for vision difference between the child and the examiner. The black-numbered plus lenses magnify images, and the red-numbered minus lenses reduce them in a range of powers. The lenses can be changed by turning the disk with the forefinger.

Turn the ophthalmoscope on and set the lens power at 0. Keep your forefinger on the disk to change the lens power as needed. Hold the ophthalmoscope so you can see through the lens. Rest the top against your eyebrow and the handle against your cheek to keep the instrument stabilized. The right eye is used to examine the child's right eye and the left eye to examine the child's left eye. This position is best for visualizing the eye, and it reduces direct exposure to infection. Place a hand on the child's head for stabilization.

■ CLINICAL TIP

Keep the red reflex in view to make sure your head and the ophthalmoscope move as one unit. If you lose the red reflex when moving closer to the child, move back, find the red reflex, and start again.

Red Reflex. Shine the ophthalmoscope light at the child's eye from a distance of 30 cm. The first image seen is the red reflex, the red glow of the vascular retina. When the red reflex is seen, the ophthalmoscope is being used correctly and the child's lens is clear. Black spots or opacities within the red reflex are abnormal and may indicate congenital cataracts. If a white reflex is seen rather than a red reflex, a retinoblastoma may be present. The red reflex can also be tested by shining a small flashlight into the eye.

Visualizing the Internal Eye Structures. Slowly move closer to the child. Deeper levels of the vitreous humor are inspected before the pink retina comes into view. The retina is a deeper pink in dark-skinned children. A blood vessel is the first retinal structure usually seen. Continue moving closer to the child's eye and adjust the plus or minus lenses to focus on this blood vessel. Retinal arteries appear smaller and brighter red than veins. The blood vessels branch to spread and cover the retina.

Inspect and follow the branching of the blood vessels toward the nose until they merge into the optic disc. Dark areas along the blood vessels may indicate retinal hemorrhages. Carefully inspect sites where arteries and veins cross. Notches and indentations at these sites are associated with hypertension.

The **optic disc margin** is normally sharply defined, round, and yellow to **creamy pink**. Blurring of the disc margins or bulging of the optic disc is a sign of increased intracranial pressure. The diameter of the optic disc is used to identify the location of other landmarks on the retina.

The macula is located approximately 2 disc diameters lateral to the optic disc. To see the macula, ask the child to look at the light. It appears as a yellow dot surrounded by deep pink. The macula is inspected last because the bright light causes the child to blink and look away.

Assessing the Ear Structures and Hearing

How do you identify proper ear placement on the head? What is the significance of low-set ears? Why is otitis media the most common ear problem during early childhood? What play activities can be used to test hearing in young children? How do you evaluate the hearing of an older child?

▓ EQUIPMENT NEEDED

Otoscope
Noisemakers (bell, rattle, tissue paper)
Tuning fork, 500–1000 Hz

Inspection of the External Ear Structures

The position and characteristics of the pinna, the external ear, are inspected as a continuation of the head and eye examination. The pinna is considered "low set" when the top lies completely below an imaginary line. Low-set ears are often associated with congenital renal disorders (Fig. 3–17).

Inspect the pinna for any malformation. The pinna should be completely formed with an open auditory canal. Next, inspect the tissue around the pinna for abnormalities. A pit or hole in front of the auditory canal may indicate the presence of a sinus. If the pinna protrudes outward, there may be swelling behind the ear, a sign of mastoiditis.

Inspect the external auditory canal for any discharge. A foul-smelling, purulent discharge may indicate the presence of a foreign body or an infection in the external canal. Clear fluid or a blood-tinged discharge may indicate a cerebrospinal fluid leak caused by a basilar skull fracture.

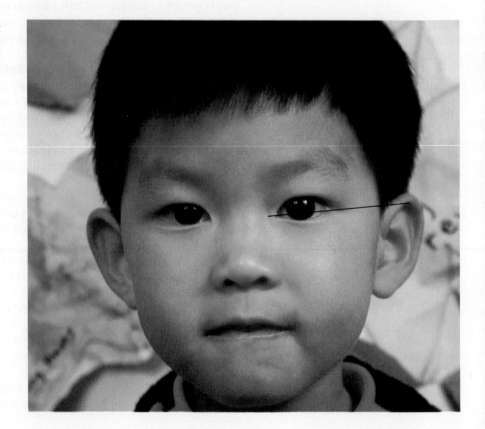

FIGURE 3–17 To detect the correct placement of the external ears, draw an imaginary line through the medial and lateral canthus of the eye toward the ear. This line normally passes through the upper portion of the pinna. The pinna is considered "low set" when the top lies completely below the imaginary line. Low-set ears are often associated with renal disorders. Is this a normal ear placement? Yes, it is.

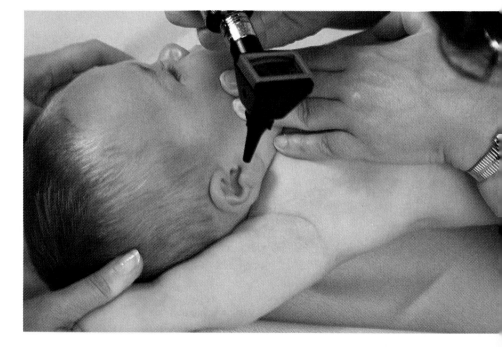

FIGURE 3–18 To restrain an unco-operative child, place the child prone on the examining table. Have an assistant hold the child's arms over the head to restrain the child's head movements. Restrain the child's body movements by lying across the child's body. Keep your hands free to hold the otoscope and position the external ear.

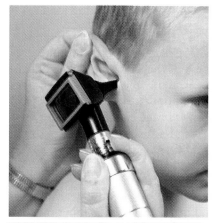

FIGURE 3–19 To straighten the auditory canal, pull the pinna up and back for children over 3 years of age. Pull the pinna back and down for children under 3 years of age.

■ SAFETY PRECAUTIONS

Never irrigate the canal if any discharge is present. Cold water should never be used for irrigation.

Inspection of the Tympanic Membrane

Examination of the tympanic membrane is important in infants and young children because they are prone to otitis media, a middle ear infection. The eustachian tubes are shorter, wider, and more horizontally positioned in infants and young children. This positioning enables bacteria to move up the eustachian tube from the pharynx, causing an infection.

The otoscope, an instrument with a magnifying lens, bright light, and speculum, is used to examine the internal auditory canal and tympanic membrane.

Infants and young children often resist having their ears inspected with the otoscope because of past painful experiences. The otoscopic examination is often delayed until portions of the assessment requiring cooperation are completed. Use simple explanations to prepare the child. Let the child play with the otoscope or demonstrate how it is used on the parent or a doll. Figure 3–18 illustrates one method that can be used to restrain an uncooperative child.

Using the Otoscope

To begin the otoscopic examination, hold the handle in the palm of your hand with your thumb pointed toward the base of the handle. If a pneumatic squeeze bulb is used, hold it between the index finger and the handle. Choose the largest ear speculum that fits into the auditory canal to form a seal for testing tympanic membrane movement. A large speculum is also less likely to injure the auditory canal if the child moves suddenly.

Hold the otoscope in the hand closest to the child's face and rest the back of your hand against the child's head to stabilize it. Use your other hand to pull the pinna toward the back of the head and either up or down. Pulling the pinna straightens the auditory canal and improves inspection of the tympanic membrane (Fig. 3–19).

Slowly insert the speculum into the auditory canal, inspecting the walls for signs of irritation, discharge, or a foreign body. The walls of the auditory canal are normally pink, and some cerumen is present. Children often put

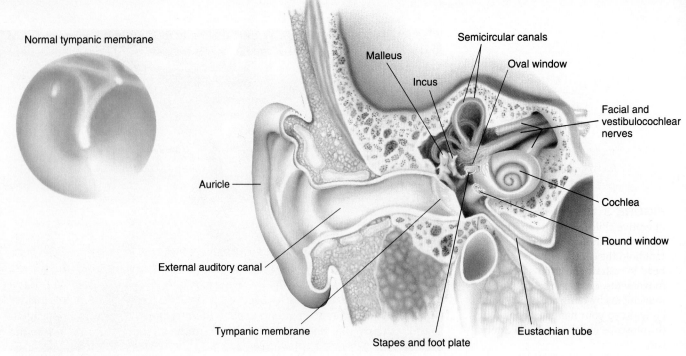

Normal tympanic membrane

Semicircular canals
Malleus
Incus
Oval window
Facial and vestibulocochlear nerves
Cochlea
Round window
Auricle
External auditory canal
Tympanic membrane
Stapes and foot plate
Eustachian tube

FIGURE 3–20 Cross section of the ear. The tympanic membrane normally has a triangular light reflex with the base on the nasal side pointing toward the center. The bony landmarks, the umbo and handle of malleus, are seen through the tympanic membrane.

beads, peas, or other small objects into their ears. If the auditory canal is obstructed by cerumen or a foreign body, irrigation can be used to clean the canal.

The tympanic membrane, which separates the outer ear from the middle ear, is usually pearly gray and translucent. It reflects light, and the bones (ossicles) in the middle ear are normally visible. When the pneumatic attachment is squeezed, the tympanic membrane normally moves in and out in response to the positive and negative pressure applied (Fig. 3–20). Table 3–8 lists the abnormal findings of a tympanic membrane examination and their associated conditions.

Hearing Assessment

Hearing evaluation is important in children of all ages because hearing is essential for normal speech development and learning. Often hearing must be evaluated by inspection of the child's responses to various auditory stimuli.

■ GROWTH AND DEVELOPMENT CONSIDERATIONS

Indicators of hearing loss in an infant:
- No startle reaction to loud noises
- Does not turn toward interesting sounds by 4 months of age
- Babbles as a young infant but does not keep babbling or develop speech sounds after 6 months of age

Indicators of hearing loss in a young child:
- No speech by 2 years of age
- Speech sounds are not distinct at appropriate ages

TABLE 3–8 Unexpected Findings on Examination of the Tympanic Membrane and Their Associated Conditions

Characteristics of Tympanic Membrane	Unexpected Findings	Associated Conditions
Color	Redness	Infection in middle ear
	Slight redness	Prolonged crying
	Amber	Serous fluid in middle ear
	Deep red or blue	Blood in middle ear
Light reflex	Absent	Bulging tympanic membrane, infection in middle ear
	Distorted, loss of triangular shape	Retracted tympanic membrane, serous fluid in middle ear
Bony landmarks	Extra prominent	Retracted tympanic membrane, serous fluid in middle ear
Movement	No motility	Infection or fluid in middle ear
	Excess motility	Healed perforation

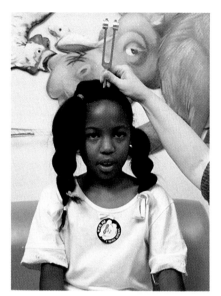

A, Weber test.

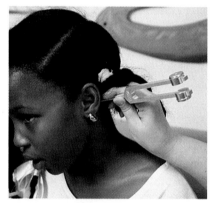

B, Rinne test, step 1.

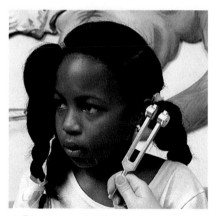

C, Rinne test, step 2.

FIGURE 3–21 **A,** Weber test. Place vibrating tuning fork on midline of child's head. **B,** Rinne test. Place vibrating tuning fork on mastoid process. **C,** Reposition the still vibrating tines between 2.5 to 5 cm from ear.

Hearing loss may occur at any time during early childhood as the result of birth trauma, frequent otitis media, meningitis, or antibiotics that damage cranial nerve VIII.

Use hearing and speech articulation milestones as an initial hearing screen. Select an age-appropriate method to screen hearing. When a hearing deficiency is suspected as a result of screening, the child is referred for audiometry, tympanometry, or evoked response to obtain the most accurate evaluation of hearing.

Infants and Toddlers

Select noisemakers with different frequencies, such as a rattle, bell, and tissue paper, that will attract the young child's attention. Ask the parent or an assistant to entertain the infant with a quiet toy, such as a teddy bear. Stand behind the infant, about 2 feet away from the infant's ear but outside the infant's field of vision, and make a soft sound with the noisemaker. Have the parent or your assistant observe the child for any of the following responses when the noisemaker is used: widening the eyes, briefly stopping all activity to listen, or turning the head toward the sound. Repeat the test in the other ear and with the other noisemakers.

Preschool and Older Children

Whispered words are used to evaluate the hearing of children over 3 years of age. Position your head about 12 inches away from the child's ear, but out of the range of vision so the child cannot read your lips. Use words easily recognized by the child, such as Mickey Mouse, hot dog, and Popsicle, and ask the child to repeat the words. Repeat the test with different words in the opposite ear. The child should correctly repeat the whispered words.

An alternative procedure is used to assess hearing when the child will not cooperate by repeating the whispered words. In a whisper, direct the child to point to different parts of the body or objects, for example, "Show me your eyes" and "Point to your mouth." Children should point to the correct body part each time.

Bone and Air Conduction of Sound

A tuning fork is used to evaluate the hearing of school-aged children who can follow directions. Stroke the tines of the tuning fork to begin the vibration. Avoid touching the vibrating tines, which will dampen the sound. Bone conduction is tested when the handle of the tuning fork is placed on the child's skull. Air conduction is tested when the vibrating tines are held close to the child's ear (Fig. 3–21).

To perform the *Weber test* place the vibrating tuning fork on top of the child's skull in the midline. Ask the child to tell you where the sound is heard the best, either in both ears equally or in one ear. The sound should be heard equally in both ears.

To perform the *Rinne test* place the vibrating tuning fork handle on the mastoid process behind an ear. Ask the child to tell you when the sound is no longer heard. Immediately move the tuning fork, holding the vibrating tines about 2.5 to 5 cm from the same ear. The child again says when the sound is no longer heard. The child normally hears the air-conducted sound twice as long as the bone-conducted sound. The Rinne test is repeated on the other ear. Table 3–9 provides an interpretation of the Weber and Rinne tests.

TABLE 3-9 Interpretation of the Weber and Rinne Tests of Hearing

Test and Result	Associated Condition
Weber Test	
Sound heard equally in both ears	No hearing loss
Sound heard better in one ear (lateralized)	Conductive hearing loss if sound lateralized to deaf ear
	Sensorineural hearing loss if sound lateralized to good ear
Rinne Test	
Sound heard by air conduction twice as long as bone conduction	No hearing loss
Sound heard longer by bone conduction than air conduction	Conductive hearing loss in affected ear
Sound heard longer by air conduction than bone conduction, but less than twice as long	Sensorineural hearing loss in affected ear

Assessing the Nose and Sinuses for Airway Patency and Discharge

What is the most common cause of a nasal obstruction in children? What does nasal flaring indicate? What signs indicate that a foreign body might be lodged in the nose? What does it mean if the child frequently wipes the nose upward with a hand?

EQUIPMENT NEEDED

Otoscope with nasal speculum
Penlight

Inspection of the External Nose

The external nose characteristics and placement on the face are examined simultaneously with the facial features. Inspect the external nose for size, shape, symmetry, and midline placement on the face. The nose should be proportional in size to other facial features and positioned in the middle of the face. A flattened nasal bridge is the expected finding in Asian and black children.

The nasolabial folds are normally symmetric. Asymmetry of the nasolabial folds may be associated with injury to the facial nerve (cranial nerve VII). A saddle-shaped nose is associated with congenital defects such as cleft palate.

Inspect the external nose for the presence of unusual characteristics. For example, a crease across the nose between the cartilage and bone is often caused by the allergic child's wiping an itchy nose upward with a hand.

Palpation of the External Nose

When a deformity is noted, gently palpate the nose to detect any pain or break in contour. No tenderness or masses are expected. Pain and a contour deviation are usually the result of trauma.

Nasal Patency

The child's airway must be patent to ensure adequate oxygenation. To test for nasal patency, occlude one nostril and observe the child's effort to breathe through the open nostril with the mouth closed. Repeat the procedure with the other nostril. Breathing should be noiseless and effortless. *Nasal flaring*, an effort the child makes to widen the airway, is a sign of respiratory distress and should not be present.

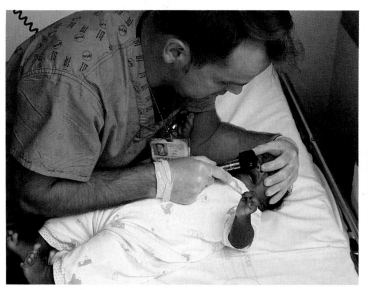

A, Technique for infant or small child.

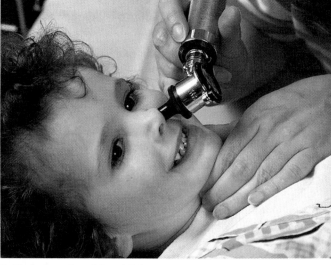

B, Technique for older child.

FIGURE 3–22 Techniques for examining nose.

■ GROWTH AND DEVELOPMENT CONSIDERATIONS

Infants under 6 months of age will not automatically open their mouths to breathe when their nose is occluded, such as by mucus.

If the child struggles to breathe, a nasal obstruction may be present. Nasal obstruction may be caused by a foreign body, congenital defect, dry mucus, discharge, polyp, or trauma. Newborns may have respiratory distress because of *choanal atresia*, a congenital membranous or bony obstruction between the nose and the nasopharynx. Young children commonly place objects up their nose, and unilateral nasal flaring is a sign of such an obstruction.

Assessment of Smell

The olfactory nerve (cranial nerve I) is rarely tested in preschool children, but it can be tested in school-aged children and adolescents. When testing smell, choose scents the child will easily recognize such as orange, chocolate, and mint. When the child's eyes are closed, occlude one nostril and hold the scent under the nose. Ask the child take a deep sniff and identify the scent. Alternate odors between the nares. The child normally identifies common scents.

Inspection of the Internal Nose

Inspect the internal nose for color of the mucous membranes and the presence of any discharge, swelling, lesions, or other abnormalities. Use a bright light, such as the otoscope light or penlight. For infants and young children, push the nose tip upward and shine the light at the end of the nose (Fig. 3–22). The nasal speculum for the otoscope can be used in older children. Avoid touching the septum of the nose with the speculum. Injury to the septum can cause a nosebleed.

Mucous Membranes

The mucous membranes should be dark pink and glistening. A film of clear discharge may also be present. Turbinates, if visible, should be the same color as the mucous membranes and have a firm consistency. When the turbinates are pale or bluish gray, the child may have allergies. A polyp, a rounded mass projecting from the turbinate, is also associated with allergies.

TABLE 3-10 Nasal Discharge Characteristics and Associated Conditions

Discharge Description	Associated Condition
Watery	
Clear, bilateral	Allergy
Serous, unilateral	Spinal fluid from fracture of cribriform plate
Mucoid or purulent	
Bilateral	Upper respiratory infection
Unilateral	Foreign body
Bloody	Nose bleed, trauma

Nasal Septum

Inspect the nasal septum for alignment, perforations, bleeding, or crusting. The septum should be straight. Crusting will be noted over the site of a nosebleed.

Discharge

Observe for the presence of nasal discharge, noting if the drainage is from one or both nares. Nasal discharge is not a normal finding unless the child is crying. Discharge may be watery, mucoid, purulent, or bloody. The character of the discharge depends on the condition present. A foul smelling discharge in only one nostril is often associated with a foreign body. Table 3–10 lists conditions associated with nasal discharges.

Inspection of the Sinuses

The maxillary and ethmoid sinuses develop during early childhood (Fig. 3–23). Sinus infections are rare in young children but occasionally can occur in school-aged children. Suspect a sinus problem when the child has a headache or pain and swelling around one or both eyes.

Inspect the face for any puffiness around one or both eyes. Puffiness and swelling are not normally present. To palpate over the maxillary sinuses, press up under both zygomatic arches with the thumbs. To palpate the ethmoid sinuses, press up against the bone above both eyes with the thumbs. No swelling or tenderness is expected. Tenderness may be an indication of sinusitis.

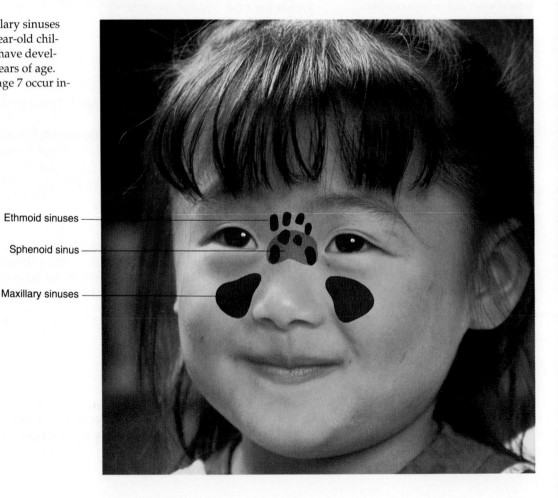

FIGURE 3–23 Maxillary sinuses can be identified in 1-year-old children. Ethmoid sinuses have developed in children by 6 years of age. Sinus problems under age 7 occur infrequently.

Ethmoid sinuses

Sphenoid sinus

Maxillary sinuses

Assessing the Mouth and Throat for Color, Function, and Signs of Abnormal Conditions

What is the best site to evaluate cyanosis in children? What is the expected sequence of tooth eruption? How is it determined that the tongue has adequate movement for all speech sounds? How can the throat be inspected without gagging the child?

Inspection of the Mouth

Young children often need coaxing and simple explanations before they will cooperate with the mouth and throat examination. Most children readily show their teeth. If the child resists by clenching the teeth, they can be gently separated with the tongue blade. According to Universal Precautions, gloves are worn when examining the mouth because of contact with mucous membranes (Fig. 3–24).

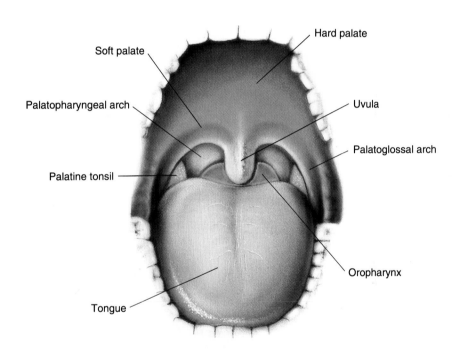

FIGURE 3–24 Structures of the mouth.

Soft palate
Hard palate
Palatopharyngeal arch
Uvula
Palatine tonsil
Palatoglossal arch
Oropharynx
Tongue

Lips

Inspect the lips for color, shape, symmetry, moisture, and lesions. The lips are normally symmetric without drying, cracking, or other lesions. Lip color is normally pink in white children and more bluish in darker skinned children. Pale, cyanotic, or cherry-red lips are indicators of poor tissue perfusion caused by various conditions.

Teeth

Inspect and count the child's teeth. The timing of tooth eruption is often genetically determined, but there is a regular sequence of tooth eruption. Figure 3–25 presents the typical sequence of tooth eruption for both deciduous and permanent teeth.

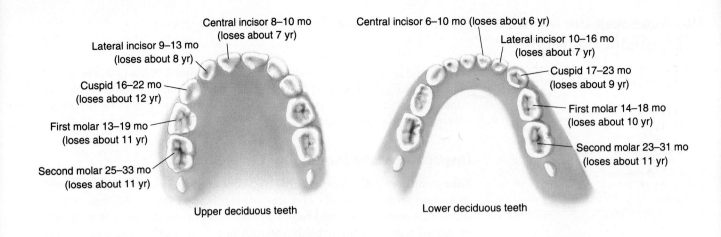

Lateral incisor 9–13 mo
(loses about 8 yr)

Central incisor 8–10 mo
(loses about 7 yr)

Central incisor 6–10 mo (loses about 6 yr)

Lateral incisor 10–16 mo
(loses about 7 yr)

Cuspid 16–22 mo
(loses about 12 yr)

Cuspid 17–23 mo
(loses about 9 yr)

First molar 13–19 mo
(loses about 11 yr)

First molar 14–18 mo
(loses about 10 yr)

Second molar 25–33 mo
(loses about 11 yr)

Second molar 23–31 mo
(loses about 11 yr)

Upper deciduous teeth

Lower deciduous teeth

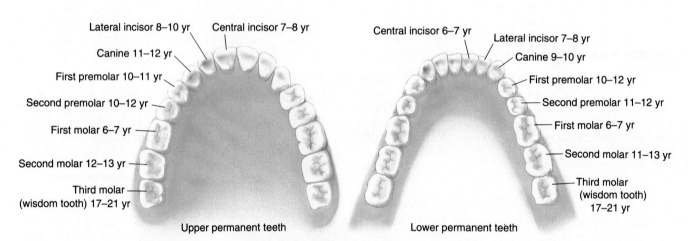

Lateral incisor 8–10 yr

Central incisor 7–8 yr

Central incisor 6–7 yr

Lateral incisor 7–8 yr

Canine 11–12 yr

Canine 9–10 yr

First premolar 10–11 yr

First premolar 10–12 yr

Second premolar 10–12 yr

Second premolar 11–12 yr

First molar 6–7 yr

First molar 6–7 yr

Second molar 12–13 yr

Second molar 11–13 yr

Third molar
(wisdom tooth) 17–21 yr

Third molar
(wisdom tooth)
17–21 yr

Upper permanent teeth

Lower permanent teeth

FIGURE 3–25 Typical sequence of tooth eruption for both deciduous and permanent teeth. Notice that bottom teeth come in first for each kind of tooth, incisors, cuspids, and molars. They lose them in the same pattern.

Inspect the condition of the teeth, look for loose teeth, and note any spaces where teeth are missing. Compare empty tooth spaces with the child's developmental stage of tooth eruption. Once the permanent teeth have erupted, none should be missing. Teeth are normally white without a flattened, mottled, or pitted appearance. Discolorations on the crown of a tooth may indicate caries.

Mouth Odors

During inspection of the teeth, be alert to any abnormal odors that may indicate problems such as diabetic ketoacidosis, infection, or poor hygiene.

Gums

Inspect the gums for color and adherence to the teeth. The gums are normally pink with a stippled or dotted appearance. Use a tongue depressor to help visualize the gums around the upper and lower molars. No raised or receding gum areas should be apparent around the teeth. When inflammation, swelling, or bleeding is observed, palpate the gums to detect tenderness. Inflammation and tenderness are associated with infection and poor nutrition.

Buccal Mucosa

Inspect the mucous membrane lining the cheeks for color and moisture. The mucous membrane is usually pink, but patches of hyperpigmentation are commonly seen in darker skinned children. The Stensen duct, the parotid gland opening, is opposite the upper second molar bilaterally. Normally pink, the duct opening becomes red when the child is infected with mumps. Small pink sucking pads can be present in infants. No areas of redness, swelling, or ulcerative lesions should be present.

Tongue

Inspect the tongue for color, moistness, size, tremors, and lesions. The child's tongue is normally pink and moist, without a coating. The tongue's size permits it to fit easily into the mouth. A pattern of gray, irregular borders that form a design (geographic tongue) is often normal, but it may be associated with fever, allergies, or drug reactions. Tremors are abnormal. A white adherent coating on an infant's tongue may be caused by thrush, a *Candida* infection.

Observe the mobility of the tongue. The child should be able to touch the gums above the upper teeth with the tongue. This tongue movement is adequate to enunciate all speech sounds clearly. Ask the child to stick out the tongue and lift it so the underside of the tongue and the floor of the mouth can be inspected for distended veins.

Palate

Inspect the hard and soft palate to detect any clefts or masses or an unusually high arch. The palate is normally pink with a dome-shaped arch and no cleft. The uvula hangs freely from the soft palate. Newborns often have Epstein pearls, white papules in the midline of the palate that disappear in a few weeks. A high-arched palate can be associated with sucking difficulties in young infants.

Palpation of the Mouth Structures

Palpate any masses seen in the mouth to determine their characteristics, such as size, shape, firmness, and tenderness. No masses should be found.

Tongue

To assess the tongue's strength, simultaneously testing the hypoglossal nerve (cranial nerve XII), place the index finger against the child's cheek and ask the child to push against your finger with the tongue. Some pressure against the finger is normally felt.

Palate

To palpate the palate, insert the little finger, with the fingerpad upward, into the mouth. While the infant sucks against your finger, palpate the entire palate. This procedure also tests the strength of the sucking reflex, innervated by the hypoglossal nerve (cranial nerve XII). No clefts should be palpated.

Inspection of the Throat

Inspect the throat for color, swelling, lesions, and the condition of the tonsils. Ask the child to open the mouth wide and stick out the tongue. A flashlight is used to illuminate the throat. A tongue blade can be used, if needed, to visualize the posterior pharynx. Moistening the tongue blade may decrease the child's tendency to gag. The throat is normally pink without lesions, drainage, or swelling. Swelling in the posterior pharynx may be associated with a peritonsillar abscess.

Tonsils

During childhood the tonsils are large in proportion to the size of the pharynx because lymphoid tissue grows fastest in early childhood. The tonsils should be pink without exudate, but *crypts* (fissures) may be present as a result of prior infections.

Gag Reflex

Use a tongue blade when you are unable to see the posterior pharynx or need to test the gag reflex. The gag reflex is tested at the end of the examination because children dislike the gagging sensation. Prepare the child for what will happen. Ask the child to say "Ah" and watch for the symmetric rising movement of the uvula. This reflex tests the glossopharyngeal and vagal nerves (cranial nerves IX and X). If the uvula does not rise or rises to one side, cranial nerves IX and X may be paralyzed. The epiglottis lies behind the tongue and is normally pink like the rest of the buccal mucosa.

Assessing the Neck for Characteristics, Range of Motion, and Lymph Nodes

What does it mean when the child's head is tilting to one side? By what age should the infant be able to control his or her head? What does a lymph node feel like? What does an enlarged lymph node feel like?

Inspection of the Neck

Inspect the neck for size, symmetry, swelling, and any abnormalities. A short neck with skin folds is normal for infants. The neck is normally symmetric. No swelling should be present. Swelling may be caused by local infections such as mumps or a congenital defect. The neck lengthens between 3 and 4 years of age.

Inspect the child's neck for any *webbing*, an extra skin fold on each side of the neck. Webbing is commonly associated with Turner syndrome.

Infants develop head control by 2 months of age. By this age an infant can lift the head up and look around when lying on the stomach. A lack of head control can result from neurologic injury, such as an anoxic episode.

Palpation of the Neck

Face the child and use the fingerpads to simultaneously palpate both sides of the neck for lymph nodes, as well as the trachea and thyroid.

Lymph Nodes

To palpate the lymph nodes, slide the fingerpads gently over the lymph node chains in the head and neck. The sequence for lymph node palpation is as fol-

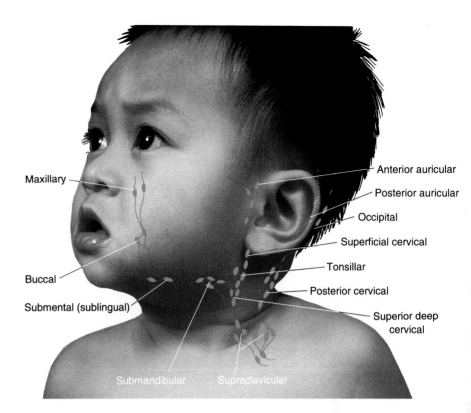

Maxillary

Buccal

Submental (sublingual)

Submandibular

Anterior auricular

Posterior auricular

Occipital

Superficial cervical

Tonsillar

Posterior cervical

Superior deep cervical

Supraclavicular

FIGURE 3–26 The neck is first palpated for enlarged lymph nodes around the ears, under the jaw, in the occipital area, and in the cervical chain of the neck.

lows: around the ears, under the jaw, the occipital area, and the cervical chain in the neck (Fig. 3–26). Firm, clearly defined, nontender, movable lymph nodes up to 1 cm in diameter are common in young children. Enlarged, firm, warm, tender lymph nodes indicate the presence of local infection.

Trachea

Palpate the trachea to determine its position and to detect the presence of any masses. The trachea is normally in the midline of the neck. It is difficult to palpate in children less than 3 years of age because of their short neck. To palpate the trachea, place the thumb and forefinger on each side of the trachea near the chin and slowly slide them down the trachea. Any shift to the right or left of midline may indicate a tumor or a collapsed lung.

Thyroid

As the fingers slide over the trachea in the lower neck, attempt to feel the isthmus of the thyroid, a band of glandular tissue crossing over the trachea. The lobes of the thyroid wrap behind the trachea and are normally covered by the sternocleidomastoid muscle. Because of anatomy, the lobes of the thyroid are not usually palpable in the child unless they are enlarged.

Range of Motion Assessment

To test the neck's **range of motion,** ask the child to touch the chin to each shoulder and to the chest and then to look at the ceiling. Move a light or toy in all four directions when assessing infants. Children should freely move the neck and head in all four directions without pain.

When the child is unable to move the head voluntarily in all directions, passively move the child's neck through the expected range of motion. Limited horizontal range of motion may be a sign of *torticollis*, persistent head tilting. Torticollis results from a birth injury to the sternocleidomastoid muscle or from unilateral vision or hearing impairment. Pain with flexion of the neck toward the chest (Brudzinski sign) may indicate meningitis.

▢ Assessing the Chest for Shape, Movement, Respiratory Effort, and Lung Function

FIGURE 3–27 Intercostal spaces and ribs are numbered to describe the location of findings. **A,** To determine the rib number on the anterior chest, palpate down from the top of the sternum until a horizontal ridge, the angle of Louis, is felt. Directly to the right and left of that ridge is the second rib. The second intercostal space is immediately below the second rib. Ribs 3 to 12 and the corresponding intercostal spaces can be counted as the fingers move toward the abdomen. **B,** To determine the rib number on the posterior chest find the protruding spinal process of the seventh cervical vertebra at the shoulder level. The next spinal process belongs to the first thoracic vertebra, which is attached to the first rib.

What terms are used to describe the location of specific sounds heard when auscultating the chest? What is indicated when the child's chest is rounded in shape? What are retractions and what do they indicate? How can normal and adventitious breath sounds be distinguished when auscultating the lungs?

Examination of the chest includes the following procedures: inspecting the size and shape of the chest, palpating chest movement that occurs during respiration, observing the effort of breathing, and auscultating breath sounds.

Topographic Landmarks of the Chest

The chest skeleton provides most of the landmarks used to describe the location of findings during examination of the chest, lungs, and heart. The intercostal spaces are the horizontal markers used to describe the location of a finding on the chest. The sternum and spine are the vertical landmarks. When both a horizontal and a vertical landmark are used, the location of findings can be precisely described (Figs. 3–27 and 3–28). Be sure to indicate whether the finding is on the right or left side of the patient's chest (Table 3–11).

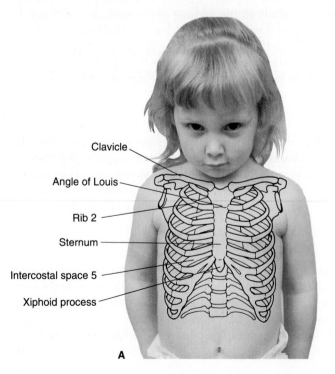

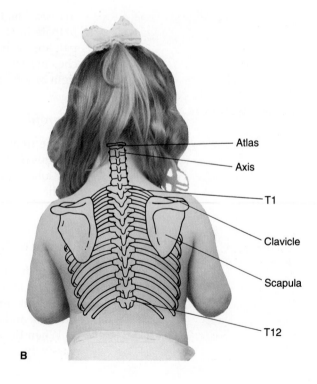

A

B

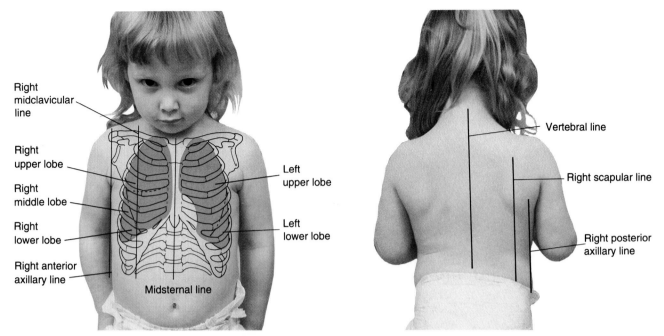

Right
midclavicular
line

Right
upper lobe

Right
middle lobe

Right
lower lobe

Right anterior
axillary line

Midsternal line

Left
upper lobe

Left
lower lobe

Vertebral line

Right scapular line

Right posterior
axillary line

FIGURE 3–28 The sternum and spine are the vertical landmarks used to describe the anatomic location of findings. The distance between the finding and the center of the sternum (midsternal line) or the spinal line can be measured with a ruler. Imaginary vertical lines, parallel to the midsternal and spinal lines, are used to further describe the location of findings.

TABLE 3-11 Vertical Landmarks of the Chest

Vertical Lines for Examining the Chest	Location of Verticle Lines
Midsternal	Through the middle of the sternum
Midclavicular	From the middle of the clavicle
Anterior axillary	From the anterior axillary fold
Midaxillary	From the middle of the axilla
Posterior axillary	From the posterior axillary fold
Spinal	Through the spinous processes of the vertebrae

EQUIPMENT NEEDED

Stethoscope

GROWTH AND DEVELOPMENT CONSIDERATIONS

In infants the chest is rounded with the anteroposterior diameter approximately equal to the lateral diameter. The chest becomes more oval with growth and by 2 years of age the lateral diameter is greater than the anteroposterior diameter.

Inspection of the Chest

Position the child on the parent's lap or on the examining table with all clothing above the waist removed to inspect the chest. The thoracic muscles and subcutaneous tissue are less developed in children than in adults, so the chest wall is thinner. As a result the rib cage is more prominent.

Size and Shape of the Chest

Inspect the chest for any irregularities in shape. A rounded chest is present when the anteroposterior diameter is approximately equal to the lateral diameter. If a rounded chest is found in a child over 2 years of age, a chronic obstructive lung condition such as asthma or cystic fibrosis may be present.

An abnormal chest shape results from three different structural deformities. If the sternum protrudes, increasing the anteroposterior diameter, pi-

TABLE 3-12 Normal Respiratory Rate Ranges for Each Age Group

Age	Respiratory Rate per Minute
Newborn	30–80
1 year	20–40
3 years	20–30
6 years	16–22
10 years	16–20
17 years	12–20

■ GROWTH AND DEVELOPMENT CONSIDERATIONS

Infants and children have a faster respiratory rate than adults because of a higher metabolic rate and need for oxygen. Young children are also unable to increase the depth of respirations because not all the alveoli are developed.[5]

■ CLINICAL TIP

To get the most accurate reading of a newborn's respiratory rate, wait until the baby is sleeping or resting quietly. Use the stethoscope to auscultate the rate or place your hand on the abdomen. Count the number of breaths for an entire minute, because newborns often have irregular respirations.

geon chest (pectus carinatum) may be present. If the lower portion of the sternum is depressed, decreasing the anteroposterior diameter, funnel chest (pectus excavatum) may be present. *Scoliosis*, curvature of the spine, causes a lateral deviation of the chest.

Chest Movement and Respiratory Effort

Inspect for simultaneous chest expansion and abdominal rise. Chest movement is normally symmetric bilaterally, rising with inspiration and falling with expiration. The chest movement of infants and young children is less pronounced than the abdominal movement. The diaphragm is the primary breathing muscle in infants and children under 6 years. The thoracic muscles are less developed and serve as accessory muscles in cases of respiratory distress. As the thoracic muscles develop, they assume a primary ventilatory role. On inspiration the chest and abdomen should rise simultaneously. Asymmetric chest rise is associated with a collapsed lung. Retractions, depression of sections of the chest wall with each inspiration, are seen when the accessory muscles are used for breathing in cases of respiratory distress.

Respiratory Rate

Because young children use the diaphragm as the primary breathing muscle, observe or feel the rise and fall of the abdomen to count the respiratory rate in children under 6 years. Table 3–12 gives the normal respiratory rates for each age group. Make every effort to count the respiratory rate when the child is quiet. The respiratory rate rises in response to excitement, fear, respiratory distress, fever, and other conditions that increase oxygen needs.

A sustained respiratory rate greater than 60 breaths per minute is an important sign in respiratory distress. At that rate, children develop hypoxemia if treatment is not started. The child's airway is very narrow, resulting in higher airway resistance than occurs in adults. When the respiratory rate exceeds 60 breaths per minute, inspired oxygen does not reach the alveoli for gas exchange because air moves no farther than the upper airway.[6]

Palpation of the Chest

Palpation is used to evaluate chest movement, respiratory effort, deformities of the chest wall, and tactile fremitus.

Chest Wall

To palpate the chest motion with respiration, place the palms of your hands with fingers spread on each side of the child's chest. Confirm the bilateral symmetry of chest motion. Use your fingerpads to palpate any depressions, bulges, or unusual chest wall shape that might indicate abnormal findings such as tenderness, cysts, other growths, crepitus, or fractures. None should be found. *Crepitus*, a crinkly sensation palpated on the chest surface, is caused by air escaping into the subcutaneous tissues. It often indicates a serious injury to the upper or lower airway. Crepitus may also be felt near a fracture.

Tactile Fremitus

Crying and talking produce vibrations, known as *tactile fremitus*, that can be palpated on the chest. Place the palms of your hands on each side of the chest to evaluate the quality and distribution of these vibrations. Ask the child to repeat a series of words or numbers, such as Mickey Mouse or ice cream. As

■ **CLINICAL TIP**

Auscultation of breath sounds is difficult when an infant is crying. First, try to quiet the infant with a pacifier, bottle, or toy. If the infant continues to cry, all is not lost. At the end of each cry the infant takes a deep breath, which you can use to assess breath sounds, vocal resonance, and tactile fremitus. Encourage toddlers and preschoolers to take deep breaths by providing a pinwheel or mobile to blow.

■ **GROWTH AND DEVELOPMENT CONSIDERATIONS**

Infants and young children have a thin chest wall because of immature muscle development. The breath sounds of one lung are heard over the entire chest. It takes practice to accurately identify absent or diminished breath sounds in infants and young children. Carefully auscultate at the apices and midaxillary areas, comparing the quality of breath sounds heard bilaterally. These are the best sites at which to identify absent or diminished breath sounds in young children, because the distance between the lungs is greatest at these locations.

the child repeats the words, move your hands systematically over the anterior and posterior chest, comparing the quality of findings side to side. The vibration or tingling sensation is normally palpated over the entire chest. Decreased sensations indicate that air is trapped in the lungs, as occurs with asthma. Increased sensations indicate lung consolidation, as occurs with pneumonia.

Auscultation of the Chest

Auscultate the chest with a stethoscope to assess the quality and characteristics of breath sounds, to identify abnormal breath sounds, and to evaluate vocal resonance. Use an infant or pediatric stethoscope when available to help you localize any unexpected breath sounds. Use the stethoscope diaphragm because it transmits the high-pitched breath sounds better.

Breath Sounds

Evaluate the quality and characteristics of breath sounds over the entire chest, comparing sounds between the sides. Select a routine sequence for auscultating the entire chest so you will consistently assess all lobes of the lungs. Figure 3–29 shows one suggested chest **auscultation** sequence. Listen to an entire inspiratory and expiratory phase at each spot on the chest before you move to the next site.

Three types of normal breath sounds are usually heard when the chest is auscultated. *Vesicular* breath sounds are low-pitched, swishing, soft, short expiratory sounds. They are usually heard in older children but not in infants and young children. *Bronchovesicular* breath sounds are medium-pitched, hollow, blowing sounds heard equally on inspiration and expiration in all age groups. The location of these sounds on the chest is related to the child's age. *Bronchial/tracheal* breath sounds are hollow and higher pitched than vesicular breath sounds.

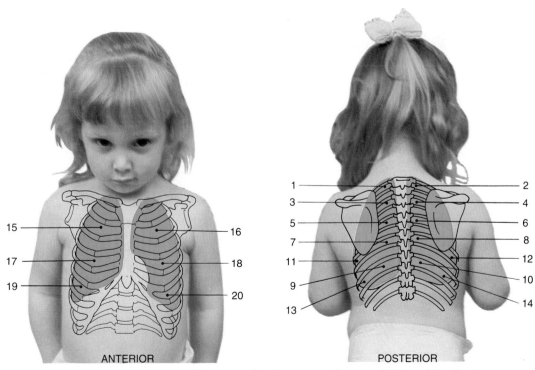

FIGURE 3–29 One example of a sequence for auscultation of the chest.

Breath sounds normally have equal intensity, pitch, and rhythm bilaterally. Absent or diminished breath sounds generally indicate a partial or total obstruction, such as from a foreign body or mucus, that does not permit airflow.

Vocal Resonance

Auscultate the chest to evaluate how well voice sounds are transmitted, just as vibrations from voice sounds are transmitted. Have the child repeat a series of words, either the same as or different from those used for evaluating tactile fremitus. Use the stethoscope to auscultate the chest, comparing the quality of sounds from side to side and over the entire chest. Voice sounds, with words and syllables muffled and indistinct, are normally heard throughout the chest.

If voice sounds are absent or more muffled than usual, an airway obstruction condition such as asthma may be present. When a lung consolidation condition such as pneumonia is present, the vocal resonance quality changes in characteristic ways. These abnormal characteristics are called whispered pectoriloquy, bronchophony, and egophony. *Whispered pectoriloquy* is present when syllables are heard distinctly in a whisper. *Bronchophony* is the increased intensity and clarity of sounds while the words remain indistinct. *Egophony* is the transmission of the "eee" sound as a nasal "ay" sound.

Abnormal Breath Sounds

Abnormal breath sounds, also called adventitious sounds, generally indicate the presence of a disease process. Examples of abnormal breath sounds are crackles, rhonchi, and friction rubs. To further assess abnormal breath sounds, the examiner determines their location, the respiratory phase in which they are present, and whether they change or disappear when the child coughs or shifts position. To routinely identify these adventitious sounds takes practice. Table 3–13 describes adventitious sounds.

Audible Voice Sounds

Observing the quality of the voice and other audible sounds is also important during an examination of the lungs. Examples of these sounds are hoarse-

---

TABLE 3-13 Description of Selected Adventitious Sounds and Their Cause

Type	Description	Cause
Fine crackles	High pitched, discrete, noncontinuous sound heard at end of inspiration *Rub pieces of hair together beside your ear to duplicate the sound.*	Air passing through watery secretions in the smaller air ways (alveoli and bronchioles)
Sibilant rhonchi	Musical, squeaking or hissing noise heard during inspiration or expiration, but generally louder on expiration	Bronchospasm or an anatomic narrowing of the trachea, bronchi, or bronchioles
Sonorous rhonchi	Coarse, low-pitched sound like a snore, heard during inspiration or expiration; may clear with coughing	Air passing through thick secretions that partially obstruct the larger bronchi and trachea

FIGURE 3-30 Normal resonance patterns expected over the chest. *Tympany* is a loud, high-pitched sound, like a drum. It is usually heard over an air-filled stomach. *Flatness* is a soft, dull sound, like the sound made when percussing your thigh. It is heard over dense muscles and bone. *Dullness* is a moderately loud, thudlike sound. It is heard when percussing over the liver and heart and at the base of the lungs (level of the diaphragm). *Resonance* is a loud, low-pitched, hollow sound, like the sound made when percussing a table. It is heard over the lungs. *Hyperresonance* is a loud, very low-pitched, booming sound. It is usually heard over superinflated lungs. However, because of the thin chest wall in young children, hyperresonance may be a normal finding.

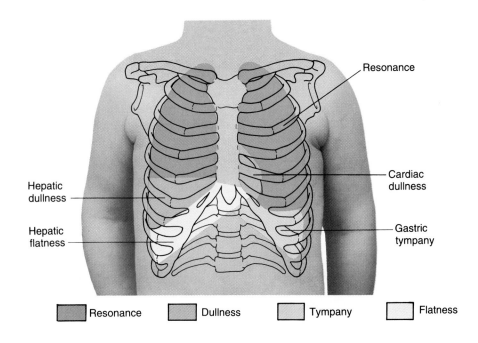

ness, stridor, and cough. *Stridor*, noise resulting from air movement in a narrowed trachea and larynx, is associated with croup. *Wheezing*, passage of air through mucus or fluids in the lower airway, is associated with asthma. A *cough* is a reflexive clearing of the airway associated with a respiratory infection. *Hoarseness* is associated with inflammation of the larynx.

Percussion of the Chest

Percussion is a method sometimes used to assess the resonance of the lungs and the density of underlying organs, such as the heart and liver. Today there is less reliance on percussion to evaluate the lungs because of the frequent use of x-ray examination.

When percussing the anterior and posterior chest, choose a sequence that covers the entire chest and permits comparison bilaterally. The sequence used for auscultation is effective. To perform *indirect percussion*, lay the middle finger of your nondominant hand on the child's chest, keeping the other fingers off the chest. With a springlike motion, use the fingertip of your other hand to tap the finger in contact with the chest. *Direct percussion* is a technique effective for infants. Tap the chest at an intercostal space with a fingertip to elicit the quality of resonance.

Characteristic patterns of percussion resonance are expected (Fig. 3–30). Characteristic descriptions of sounds heard with percussion of the chest include tympany, flatness, dullness, resonance, and hyperresonance.

Assessing the Breasts for Development and Masses

What is the first stage of breast development in girls? Do boys have breast development during puberty? What does breast tissue feel like?

Inspection of the Breasts

Stage of Development

Inspect the breasts for stage of development (Fig. 3–31). Breast development in girls precedes other pubertal changes. Breast budding, the first stage of pubertal development in girls, normally occurs between 10 and 14 years of age. Breast development before 8 years of age is abnormal. Figure 3–31 shows normal breast development. A girl's breasts may develop at different rates and appear asymmetric. Boys often have unilateral or bilateral breast enlargement during adolescence. This enlargement can occur as breast buds

FIGURE 3–31 Normal stages of breast development.

From Van Wieringen, J.C., et al (1971). *Growth diagrams 1965 Netherlands*. Groningen: Wolters-Noordhoff.

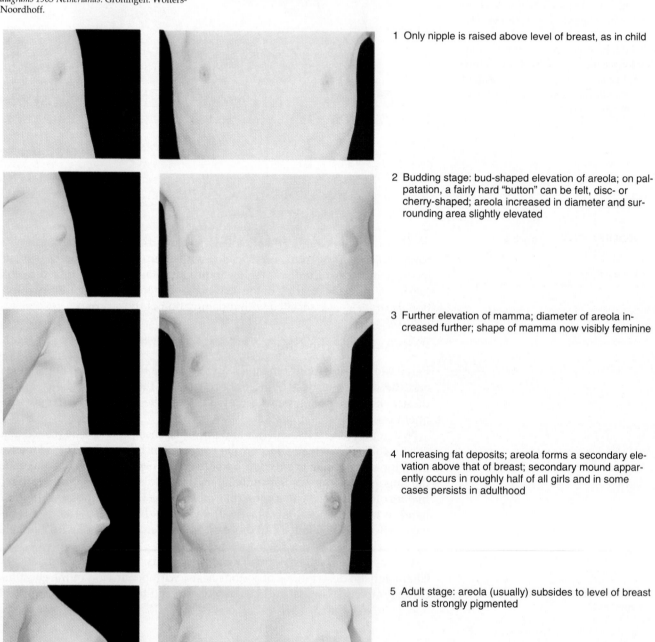

1 Only nipple is raised above level of breast, as in child

2 Budding stage: bud-shaped elevation of areola; on palpatation, a fairly hard "button" can be felt, disc- or cherry-shaped; areola increased in diameter and surrounding area slightly elevated

3 Further elevation of mamma; diameter of areola increased further; shape of mamma now visibly feminine

4 Increasing fat deposits; areola forms a secondary elevation above that of breast; secondary mound apparently occurs in roughly half of all girls and in some cases persists in adulthood

5 Adult stage: areola (usually) subsides to level of breast and is strongly pigmented

or actual breast tissue (gynecomastia). Breast development generally disappears without treatment, usually within a year. Some boys are very distressed by the breast enlargement.

Nipples

The nipples of prepubertal boys and girls are symmetrically located near the midclavicular line at the fourth to sixth ribs. The areola is normally round and more darkly pigmented than the surrounding skin. Inspect the anterior chest for other dark spots that may be *supernumerary nipples*, which are small, undeveloped nipples and areola that may be mistaken for moles. Their presence may be associated with congenital renal or cardiac anomalies.

Palpation of the Breasts

The developing breasts of adolescent females are palpated for abnormal masses or hard nodules. Breast tissue normally feels dense, firm, and elastic.

Assessing the Heart for Heart Sounds and Function

What is the point of maximum intensity and where is it located? Where are the pulse points to assess pulse quality? What heart sounds are associated with systole and diastole? What is the normal heart rate of infants and children? What is the difference between heart sounds and murmurs?

EQUIPMENT NEEDED

Stethoscope
Sphygmomanometer

Inspection of the Precordium

Begin the heart examination by inspecting the *precordium*, or anterior chest. Place the child in a reclining or semi-Fowler's position, either on the parent's lap or on the examining table. Inspect the shape and symmetry of the anterior chest from the front and side views. The rib cage is normally symmetrical. Bulging of the left side of the chest wall may indicate an enlarged heart.

Observe for any chest movement associated with the heart's contraction. The *apical impulse*, sometimes called the point of maximum intensity, is located where the left ventricle taps the chest wall during contraction. The apical impulse can normally be seen in thin children. A *heave*, an obvious lifting of the chest wall during contraction, may indicate an enlarged heart.

Palpation of the Precordium

Place the entire palmar surface of the fingers together on the chest wall to palpate the precordium. Systematically palpate the entire precordium to detect any pulsations, heaves, or vibrations. Palpating with minimal pressure increases the chance of detecting abnormal findings.

GROWTH AND DEVELOPMENT CONSIDERATIONS

The location of the apical impulse changes as the child's rib cage grows. In children under 7 years, it is located in the fourth intercostal space just lateral to the left midclavicular line. In children over 7 years, it is located in the fifth intercostal space at the left midclavicular line.

Apical Impulse

The apical impulse is normally felt as a slight tap against one fingertip. Use the topographic landmarks of the chest to describe its location (Figs. 3–27 and 3–28). Any other sensation palpated is usually abnormal.

Abnormal Sensations

A *lift* is the sensation of the heart lifting up against the chest wall. It may be associated with an enlarged heart or a heart contracting with extra force. A *thrill* is a rushing vibration that feels like a cat's purr. It is caused by turbulent blood flow from a defective heart valve and a heart murmur. If present, the thrill is palpated in the right or left second intercostal space. To describe a thrill's location, use the topographic landmarks of the chest (Figs. 3–27 and 3–28) and estimate the diameter of the thrill palpated.

Percussion of the Heart Borders

Percussion to detect the borders of the heart is rarely used during physical examination because that information is better identified by x-ray examination. Percussion of the heart should be performed by an experienced examiner.

Auscultation of the Heart

Auscultation is used to count the apical pulse, to assess the characteristics of the heart sounds, and to detect abnormal heart sounds. Use the bell of the stethoscope to detect these higher pitched sounds.

To assess the heart sounds completely, auscultate the heart with the child in both sitting and reclining positions. Differences in heart sounds caused by a change in the child's position or by a change in the position of the heart near the chest wall can then be detected. If differences in heart sounds are detected with a position change, place the child in the left lateral recumbent position to auscultate again.

■ GROWTH AND DEVELOPMENT CONSIDERATIONS

The child's heart rate varies with age, decreasing as the child grows older. The heart rate also increases in response to exercise, excitement, anxiety, and fever. Such stresses increase the child's metabolic rate creating a simultaneous need for more oxygen. Children respond to the need for more oxygen by increasing their heart rate, called sinus tachycardia. They cannot increase their cardiac stroke volume to deliver more oxygen to the tissues as adults do.

Heart Rate and Rhythm

The apical heart rate can be counted at the site of the apical impulse, either by palpation or by auscultation. Count the apical rate for 1 minute in infants and in children who have an irregular rhythm. The brachial or radial pulse rate should be the same as the auscultated apical heart rate. Table 3–14 gives normal heart rates in children of different ages.

Listen carefully to the heart rate rhythm. Children often have a normal cycle of irregular rhythm associated with respiration called *sinus arrhythmia*. With sinus arrhythmia the child's heart rate is faster on inspiration and slower on expiration. When any rhythm irregularity is detected, ask the child to take a breath and hold it while you listen to the heart rate. The rhythm should become regular during inspiration and expiration. Other rhythm irregularities are abnormal.

Differentiation of Heart Sounds

Heart sounds are due to the closure of the valves and vibration or turbulence of blood produced by that valve closure. Two primary sounds, S_1 and S_2, are heard when the chest is auscultated.

TABLE 3-14 Normal Heart Rates for Children of Different Ages

Age	Heart Rate Range	Average Heart Rate
Newborns	100–170	120
Infants to 2 years	80–130	110
2 to 6 years	70–120	100
6 to 10 years	70–110	90
10 to 16 years	60–100	85

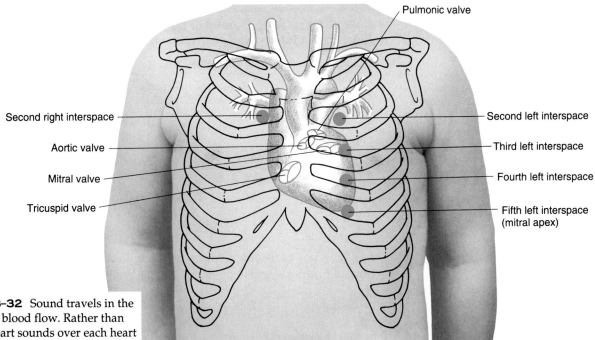

Pulmonic valve

Second right interspace

Aortic valve

Mitral valve

Tricuspid valve

Second left interspace

Third left interspace

Fourth left interspace

Fifth left interspace
(mitral apex)

FIGURE 3–32 Sound travels in the direction of blood flow. Rather than listen for heart sounds over each heart valve, auscultate heart sounds at specific areas on the chest wall away from the valve itself. These areas are named for the valve producing the sound. *Aortic:* Second right intercostal space near the sternum. *Pulmonic:* Second left intercostal space near the sternum. *Tricuspid:* Fifth right or left intercostal space near the sternum. *Mitral (apical):* In infants—third or fourth intercostal space, just left of the left midclavicular line. In children—fifth intercostal space at the left midclavicular line.

■ **CLINICAL TIP**

Palpate the carotid pulse when auscultating the heart to distinguish between the two heart sounds. The heart sound heard simultaneously with the pulsation is S_1.

S_1, the first heart sound, is produced by closure of the tricuspid and mitral valves when the ventricular contraction begins. The two valves close almost simultaneously, so only one sound is normally heard.

S_2, the second heart sound, is produced by the closure of the aortic and pulmonic valves. Once blood has reached the pulmonic and aortic arteries, the valves close to prevent leakage back into the ventricles during diastole. The timing of the valve closure varies with respirations. Sometimes S_2 is heard as a single sound and at other times as a *split sound*, that is, two sounds heard a fraction of a second apart.

Sound is easily transmitted in liquid, and it travels best in the direction of blood flow. Auscultate heart sounds at specific areas on the chest wall in the direction of blood flow, just beyond the valve (Fig. 3–32). The sounds produced by the heart valves or blood turbulence are heard throughout the chest in thin infants and children. Both S_1 and S_2 can often be heard in all listening areas.

Auscultate heart sounds for quality (distinct versus muffled) and intensity (loud versus weak). First, distinguish between S_1 and S_2 in each listening area. Heart sounds are usually distinct and crisp in children because of their thin chest wall. Muffling or indistinct sounds may indicate a heart defect or congestive heart failure. Document the area where heart sounds are heard the best. Table 3–15 and Figure 3–32 review the location where each sound is normally heard the best for assessment of quality and intensity.

Splitting of the Heart Sounds

After the first and second heart sounds are successfully distinguished, try to detect *physiologic splitting*. The split second heart sound is more apparent during inspiration when the child takes a deep breath. More blood returns to the right ventricle, causing the pulmonic valve to close a fraction of a second later than the aortic valve. To detect physiologic splitting, auscultate over the pulmonic area while the child breathes normally and then while the child takes a deep breath. Splitting is normally more easily detected after a deep breath. The splitting returns to a single sound with regular breathing. If split-

TABLE 3-15 Identification of the Listening Sites for Auscultation of the Quality and Intensity of Heart Sounds

Heart Sound	Locations Best Heard	Where Heard Softly
S_1	Apex of the heart Tricuspid area Mitral area	Base of the heart Aortic area Pulmonic area
S_2	Base of the heart Aortic area Pulmonic area	Apex of the heart Tricuspid area Mitral area
Physiologic splitting	Pulmonic area	
S_3	Mitral area	

ting does not vary with respiration, it is called fixed splitting. This is an abnormal finding associated with an atrial septal defect.

Third Heart Sound

A third heart sound, S_3, is occasionally heard in children as a normal finding. S_3 is caused when blood rushes through the mitral valve and splashes into the left ventricle. It is heard in diastole, just after S_2. It is distinguished from a split S_2 because it is louder in the mitral area than in the pulmonic area.

Murmurs

Occasionally abnormal heart sounds are auscultated. These sounds are produced by blood passing through a defective valve, great vessel, or other heart structure.

To hear murmurs in children takes practice. Often murmurs must be very loud to be detected. For softer murmurs, normal heart sounds must be distinguished before an extra sound is recognized. Once a murmur is detected, define the characteristics of the extra sound.

Murmurs are classified by the following characteristics:

- *Intensity.* How loud is it? Can a thrill also be palpated?
- *Location.* Where is the murmur the loudest? Identify the listening area and precise topographic landmarks. Is the child sitting or lying down?
- *Radiation.* Is the sound transmitted over a larger area of the chest, to the axilla, or to the back?
- *Timing.* Is the murmur heard best after S_1 or S_2? Is it heard during the entire phase between S_1 and S_2?
- *Quality.* Describe what the murmur sounds like, for example, machine-like, musical, or blowing.

Completing the Heart Examination

A complete assessment of the cardiac function also involves measurement of the blood pressure, palpation of the pulses, and evaluation of signs from other systems.

Blood Pressure

Assessment of blood pressure is important to detect conditions of hypertension or hypovolemic shock. The technique for obtaining the blood pressure

▪ GUIDELINES FOR GRADING THE INTENSITY OF A MURMUR

Intensity	Description
Grade I	Barely heard in a quiet room
Grade II	Quiet, but clearly heard
Grade III	Moderately loud, no thrill palpated
Grade IV	Loud, a thrill is usually palpated
Grade V	Very loud, a thrill is easily palpated
Grade VI	Heard without the stethoscope in direct contact with the chest wall

PEDIATRIC NURSING

Infants have a low systolic blood pressure, and detecting the distal pulses is often difficult. Use the brachial artery in the arms and the popliteal or femoral artery in the legs to evaluate the pulses. The radial and distal tibial pulses are normally palpated easily in older children.

TABLE 3-16 Median Systolic and Diastolic Blood Pressure Values for Children of Different Ages

Age	Systolic (mmHg) 50th Percentile Readings	Diastolic (mmHg) 50th Percentile Readings
Newborn	73	55
1 month	86	52
6 months	90	53
1 year	90	56
3 years	92	55
6 years	96	57
9 years	100	61
12 years	107	64
15 years	114	65
18 years	121	70

Adapted from the Normal Blood Pressure Readings for Boys from the Second Task Force on Blood Pressure Control in Children, National Heart, Lung, and Blood Institute, Bethesda, MD. Normal blood pressure readings for girls are very similar to those for boys at all age groups.

in children can be found in the Atlas of Pediatric Procedures. Table 3–16 gives average blood pressure readings of children at different ages.

Palpation of the Pulses

Palpate the characteristics of the pulses in the extremities to assess the circulation. The technique and sites for palpating the pulse are the same as those used for adults (Fig. 3–33). Evaluate the pulsation for rate, regularity of rhythm, and strength in each extremity and compare your findings bilaterally. The femoral and brachial pulses are the most important pulses to evaluate.

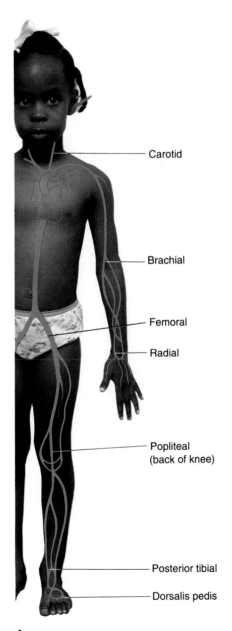

— Carotid

— Brachial

— Femoral

— Radial

— Popliteal (back of knee)

— Posterior tibial

— Dorsalis pedis

A

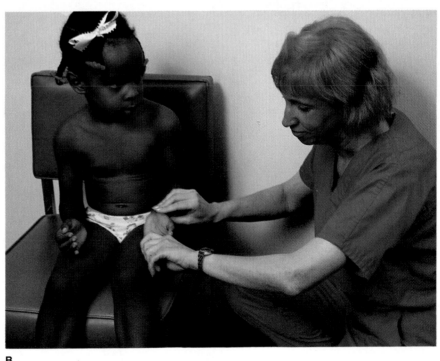

B

FIGURE 3–33 **A,** The sites used to assess pulses in children. **B,** Place your fingerpads firmly over each pulse point to evaluate the pulsation.

Palpate the femoral arteries and compare their strength with the strength of the brachial pulse. The femoral pulsations are usually stronger than or as strong as the brachial pulsations. A weaker femoral pulse is associated with coarctation of the aorta.

Other Signs

To assess the heart and tissue perfusion, other signs should be considered. These signs include skin color, capillary refill, and respiratory distress. The mucous membranes are usually pink. Cyanosis is most commonly associated with a congenital heart defect in children. Capillary refill is normally less than 2 seconds, indicating good circulation and perfusion of the tissues. Signs of respiratory distress, such as tachypnea, flaring, and retractions, may be associated with the child's attempts to compensate for hypoxemia caused by a congenital heart defect.

Assessing the Abdomen for Shape, Bowel Sounds, and Underlying Organs

What does a sunken abdomen indicate? What do bowel sounds normally sound like? How frequently should bowel sounds be heard in children? What do the various percussion tones indicate? What does a rigid abdomen indicate?

Topographic Landmarks of the Abdomen

The location of underlying organs and structures of the abdomen must be considered when the abdomen is examined. The abdomen is commonly divided by imaginary lines into quadrants for the purpose of identifying underlying structures (Fig. 3–34).

FIGURE 3–34 Topographic landmarks of the abdomen. The abdomen is commonly divided by imaginary lines into quadrants for the purpose of identifying underlying structures.

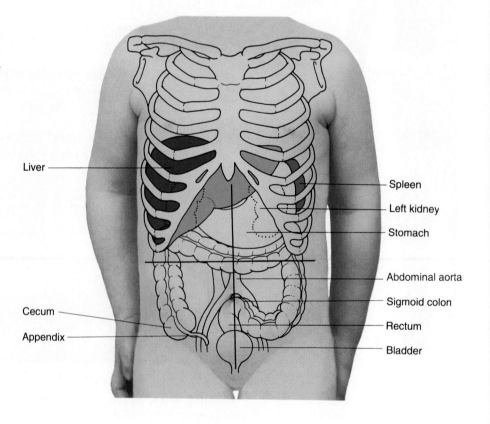

Liver

Cecum

Appendix

Spleen

Left kidney

Stomach

Abdominal aorta

Sigmoid colon

Rectum

Bladder

Inspection of the Abdomen

Begin the examination of the abdomen by inspecting the shape and contour, condition of the umbilicus and rectus muscle, and abdominal movement. Inspect the child's abdomen from the front and side with good lighting.

Shape

Inspect the shape of the abdomen to identify an abnormal contour. The child's abdomen is normally symmetric and rounded or flat when the child is supine. A scaphoid or sunken abdomen is abnormal and may indicate dehydration.

Umbilicus

Observe the newborn's umbilical stump for color, bleeding, odor, and drainage. The stump becomes black, dry, and hard within a couple of days after birth. It normally falls off between 7 and 14 days after birth. After the stump falls off, inspect the umbilicus for complete healing. Continued drainage may indicate an infection or a granuloma.

Inspect the umbilicus in older infants and toddlers. Children in these age groups often have an umbilical hernia, a protrusion of abdominal contents through an open umbilical muscle ring.

Rectus Muscle

Inspect the abdominal wall for any depression or bulging at midline above or below the umbilicus, indicating separation of the rectus abdominis muscles. The depression may be up to 5 cm wide. Measure the width of the separation to monitor change over time. As abdominal muscle strength develops, the separation usually becomes less prominent. However, the splitting may persist if congenital muscle weakness is present.

Abdominal Movement

Infants and children up to 6 years of age breathe with the diaphragm. The abdomen rises with inspiration and falls with expiration, simultaneously with the chest rise and fall. When the abdomen does not rise as expected, peritonitis may be present.

Other abdominal movements such as peristaltic waves are abnormal. Their presence generally indicates an intestinal obstruction, such as pyloric stenosis.

■ CLINICAL TIP

Inspection and auscultation are performed before palpation and percussion because touching the abdomen may change the characteristics of bowel sounds.

Auscultation of the Abdomen

To evaluate bowel sounds, auscultate the abdomen with the diaphragm of the stethoscope. Bowel sounds normally occur every 10 to 30 seconds. They have a high-pitched, tinkling, metallic quality. Loud gurgling (borborygmi) is heard when the child is hungry. Listen in each quadrant long enough to hear at least one bowel sound. Before determining that bowel sounds are absent, auscultate at least 5 minutes. Absence of bowel sounds may indicate peritonitis. Hyperactive bowel sounds may indicate gastroenteritis or a bowel obstruction.

Next auscultate over the abdominal aorta and the renal arteries for a vascular hum or murmur. No murmur should be heard. A murmur may indicate a narrowed or defective artery.

■ CLINICAL TIP

Expected pattern of percussion tones over the abdomen: *Dullness* is found over organs such as the liver, spleen, and full bladder. *Tympany* is found over the stomach or the intestines when an obstruction is present. Tympany may be found over areas beyond the stomach in infants because of air swallowing. A *resonant tone* may be heard over other areas.

■ CLINICAL TIP

When children are ticklish, some special approaches are needed to gain their cooperation. Use a firm touch and do not pretend to tickle the child at any point in the examination. Alternatively, put the child's hand on the abdomen and place your hand over the child's. Let your fingertips slide over to touch the abdomen. The child has a sense of being in control, and you may be able to palpate directly.

Percussion of the Abdomen

Use indirect percussion to evaluate borders and sizes of abdominal organs and masses. Percussion is performed with the child supine. Choose a sequence that permits you to systematically percuss the entire abdomen (Fig. 3–35).

Different tones are expected when the abdomen is percussed, depending on the underlying structures. Organ size can be identified by listening for a percussion tone change at the border of an organ. For example, when you percuss down the chest, the upper edge of the liver is usually detected by a tone change from resonant to dull near the fifth intercostal space at the right midclavicular line. The lower liver edge is usually detected 2 to 3 cm below the right costal margin in infants and toddlers, but closer to the costal margin in older children.

Palpation of the Abdomen

Both light and deep palpation are used to examine the abdomen's organs and to detect any masses. *Light palpation* is used to evaluate the tenseness of the abdomen (how soft or hard it is), the liver, the presence of any tenderness or masses, and any defects in the abdominal wall. *Deep palpation* is used to detect masses, define their shape and consistency, and identify tenderness in the abdomen.

To make the most accurate interpretation, perform the abdominal examination when the child is calm and cooperative. Organs and other masses are more easily palpated when the abdominal wall is relaxed. Infants and toddlers often feel more secure lying supine across both the parent's and the examiner's laps. A bottle, pacifier, or toy may distract the child and improve cooperation for the examination.

To begin palpation, position the child supine with knees flexed. Stand beside the child and place your warmed fingertips across the child's abdomen. Palpate with the edge of your fingers, not just your fingerpads and palpate in

FIGURE 3–35 Sequence for indirect percussion of the abdomen.

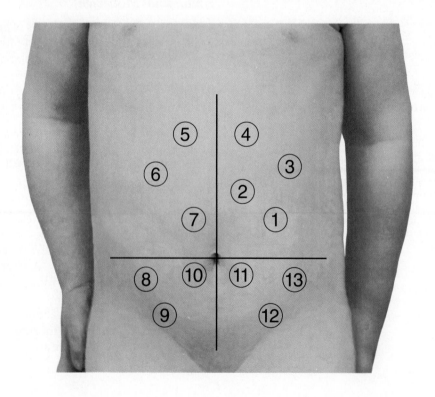

a sequence to examine the entire abdomen. Watch the child's face as you palpate for a grimace or constriction of the pupils, which indicates the presence of pain.

Light Palpation

For light palpation, use a superficial, gentle touch that slightly depresses the abdomen. Usually the abdomen feels soft and no tenderness is detected. Palpate any bulging along the abdominal wall, especially along the rectus muscle and umbilical ring, which indicates the presence of a hernia. Measure the diameter of the muscle ring, rather than the protrusion, to monitor change over time. The muscle ring normally becomes smaller and closes by 4 years of age. An umbilical hernia persisting beyond this age may need surgical repair.

Liver. Locate and lightly palpate the lower liver edge. Place the fingers in the right midclavicular line at the level of the umbilicus and gently move them toward the costal margin during expiration. As the liver edge descends with inspiration, a flat, narrow ridge is usually felt by your finger. Measure the distance of the liver edge from the right costal margin at the right midclavicular line. The liver edge is normally palpated 2 to 3 cm below the right costal margin in infants and toddlers. It may not be palpable in older children. The liver is enlarged when the edge is more than 3 cm below the right costal margin. An enlarged liver may be associated with congestive heart failure or hepatic disease.

Deep Palpation

To perform deep palpation, press the fingers of one hand (for small children) or two hands (for older children) more deeply into the abdomen. Because the abdominal muscles are most relaxed when the child takes a deep breath, ask the child to take regular deep breaths when each area of the abdomen is palpated.

Spleen. Palpate for the spleen at the left costal margin in the midclavicular line. The spleen tip may be felt when the child takes a deep breath. The spleen is enlarged when it can be easily palpated below the left costal margin.

Kidneys. Palpate for the kidneys deep in the abdomen along each side of the spinal column. The kidneys are difficult to palpate in all children, except newborns, because of the deep layer of abdominal muscles and intestines. If a kidney is actually palpated, an abnormal mass may be present.

Other Masses. Occasionally other masses, both normal and abnormal, can be palpated in the abdomen. A tubular mass commonly palpated in the lower left or right quadrant is often an intestine filled with feces. A distended bladder is often palpated as a firm, central, dome-shaped mass above the symphysis pubis in young children. Any fixed mass that moves laterally, pulsates, or is located along the vertebral column may be a neoplasm.

Assessment of the Inguinal Area

The inguinal area is inspected and palpated during the abdominal examination to detect enlarged lymph nodes or masses. The femoral pulse, a part of the heart examination, may be assessed simultaneously with the abdominal examination.

■ **CLINICAL TIP**

Older children often need distraction, especially when there is a question of abdominal tenderness and guarding or when the child is ticklish. Have the child perform a task that requires some concentration, such as pressing the hands together or pulling locked hands apart.

■ **NURSING ALERT**

If an enlarged kidney is detected, do not continue to palpate the kidney. Pressure on the mass may release cancerous cells.

Inspection

Inspect the inguinal area for any change in contour, comparing sides. A small bulging noted over the femoral canal in girls is associated with a femoral hernia. A bulging in the inguinal area in boys may be associated with an inguinal hernia.

Palpation

Palpate the inguinal area for lymph nodes and other masses. Small lymph nodes, less than 1 cm in diameter, are often present in the inguinal area because of minor injuries on the legs. Any tenderness, heat, or inflammation in these palpated lymph nodes may be associated with a local infection.

Assessing the Genital and Perineal Areas for Pubertal Development and External Structural Abnormalities

How is the stage of pubertal development determined in girls and boys? What can a vaginal discharge indicate in a preadolescent girl? Is swelling in a newborn's scrotum normal? Where is the proper location of the urethral meatus on the penis?

■ EQUIPMENT NEEDED

Gloves
Lubricant
Penlight

Preparation of Children for the Examination

Examination of the genitalia and perineal area can cause stress in children because they sense their privacy has been invaded. To make young children feel more secure, position them on the parent's lap with their legs spread apart. Children can also be positioned on the examining table with their knees flexed and the legs drawn back toward the hips like a frog.

In younger children the genital and perineal examination is performed immediately after assessment of the abdomen. The genitals and perineum may be examined last in older children and adolescents.

■ GROWTH AND DEVELOPMENT CONSIDERATIONS

Preschool-aged children are often taught that strangers are not permitted to touch their "private parts." When a child this age actively resists examination of the genital area, ask the parent to tell the child you have permission to look and touch these parts of the body. Some children develop modesty during the preschool period. Briefly explain what you need to examine and why. Then calmly and efficiently examine the child.

Inspection of the Female Genitalia

The external genitalia of girls are inspected for color, size, and symmetry of the mons pubis, labia, urethra, and vaginal opening (Fig. 3–36). The stage of pubertal maturation is also determined. Simultaneously look for any abnormal findings such as swelling, inflammation, masses, lacerations, or discharge.

Mons Pubis

Inspect the mons pubis for pubic hair. The presence, amount, and distribution of pubic hair indicates the sexual maturation stage in the girl. Preadolescent girls have no pubic hair. Initial pubic hair is lightly pigmented, sparse, and straight. Pubic hair develops in consistent stages for all girls, but the timing of pubic hair stages is individually determined.[7] Figure 3–37 illustrates the normal stages of female pubic hair development. Breast development usually precedes pubic hair development. The presence of pubic hair before 8 years of age is unusual.

FIGURE 3-36 Anatomic structures of the female genital and perineal area.

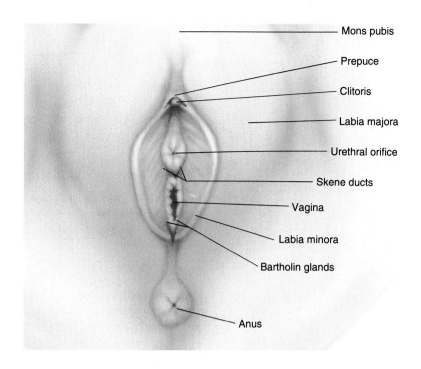

- Mons pubis
- Prepuce
- Clitoris
- Labia majora
- Urethral orifice
- Skene ducts
- Vagina
- Labia minora
- Bartholin glands
- Anus

▪ GROWTH AND DEVELOPMENT CONSIDERATIONS

The newborn's external genital structures are strongly influenced by maternal hormones. The labia majora are swollen and the labia minora may be more prominent. The clitoris is relatively large. A white mucoid vaginal discharge can also be seen. As the hormonal influence decreases over a few weeks, these structures attain normal size.

Labia

The labia minora are usually thin and pale in preadolescent girls but become dark pink and moist after puberty. In young infants the labia minora may be fused and cover the structures in the vestibule. These adhesions may need to be separated.

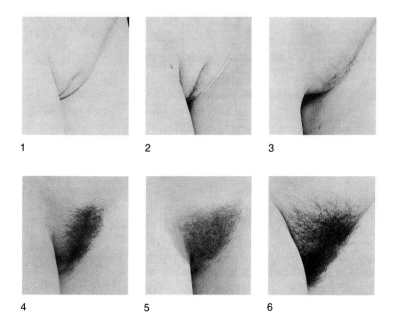

1 No growth of pubic hair

2 Initial, scarcely pigmented hair, especially along labia

3 Sparse, dark, visibly pigmented, curly pubic hair on labia

4 Hair "adult" in type but not in extent

5 Lateral spreading; type and spread of hair adult

6 Further extension laterally, upward, or disperse (apparently occurs in only 10% of women)

FIGURE 3-37 The stages of female pubic hair development with sexual maturation. Soft downy hair along the labia majora is an indication that sexual maturation is beginning. Hair grows progressively coarse and curly as development proceeds.
From Van Wieringen, et al (1971). *Growth diagrams 1965 Netherlands.* Groningen: Wolters-Noordhoff.

Hymen

Use the thumb and forefinger of one hand to separate the labia minora for viewing structures in the vestibule. The hymen is just inside the vaginal opening. In preadolescents it is usually a thin membrane with a crescent-shaped opening. The vaginal opening is usually about 1 cm in adolescents when the hymen is intact. Sexually active adolescents may have a vaginal opening with irregular edges.

Urethral and Vaginal Openings

Inspect the vestibule for lesions. No lesions or signs of inflammation are expected around the urethral or vaginal opening. Redness and excoriation are often associated with an irritant such as bubble bath.

Vaginal Discharge

Preadolescent girls do not normally have a vaginal discharge. Adolescents often have a clear discharge without a foul odor. Menses generally begin approximately 2 years after breast bud development. A foul-smelling discharge in preschool-aged children may be associated with a foreign body. Various organisms may cause a vaginal infection in older children.

An internal vaginal examination is indicated when abnormal findings such as a vaginal discharge or trauma to the external structures is noted. The vaginal examination of the child should be performed by an experienced examiner.

Palpation of the Female Genitalia

Palpate the vaginal opening with a finger of your free hand. The Bartholin and Skene glands are not usually palpable. Palpation of these glands in preadolescent children indicates enlargement because of an infection such as gonorrhea.

Inspection of the Male Genitalia

The male genitalia are inspected for the structural and pubertal development of the penis, scrotum, and testicles. Boys are placed in tailor position, seated with their legs crossed in front of them. This position puts pressure on the abdominal wall to push the testicles into the scrotum.

Penis

The penis is inspected for size, foreskin, hygiene, and position of the urethral meatus. The length of the nonerect penis in the newborn is normally 2 to 3 cm. The penis enlarges in length and breadth during puberty. The penis is normally straight. A penis with a downward bowing may be caused by a *chordee*, a fibrous band of tissue associated with hypospadias.

When the penis is circumcised, the glans penis is exposed. To inspect the glans penis of an uncircumcised boy, ask the child or parent to pull the foreskin back. Alternatively, the examiner may retract the foreskin. The foreskin of children over 6 years of age normally retracts easily. If the foreskin is tight and cannot be retracted, phimosis is present.

The glans penis is normally clean and smooth without inflammation or ulceration. The urethral meatus is a slit-shaped opening near the tip of the

---

■ **NURSING ALERT**

Signs of sexual abuse in young children include bruising or swelling of the vulva, foul-smelling vaginal discharge, enlarged opening of the vagina, and rash or sores in the perineal area.

■ **GROWTH AND DEVELOPMENT CONSIDERATIONS**

The foreskin is usually not completely separated from the glans at birth. Separation is normally completed by 3 to 6 years of age. A foreskin opening large enough for a good urinary stream is normal, even when the foreskin does not fully retract.

■ SAFETY PRECAUTIONS

When the boy's foreskin does not easily retract, do not forcefully pull it back. Force may result in torn tissues that heal with adhesions between the foreskin and the glans.

■ GROWTH AND DEVELOPMENT CONSIDERATIONS

The stage of pubertal maturation is determined by inspecting the amount of pubic hair, size of the penis, and development of the testicles and scrotum. Pubic hair usually appears after the scrotum and testicles start to grow but before the penis begins enlarging.[7]

FIGURE 3–38 The stages of male pubic hair and external genital development with sexual maturation.
From Van Wieringen, J.C., et al (1971). *Growth diagrams 1965 Netherlands*. Groningen: Wolters-Noordhoff.

glans. No discharge should be present. A round, pinpoint urethral meatus may indicate meatal stenosis. Location of the urethral meatus at another site on the penis is abnormal, indicating hypospadias or epispadias. Inspect the urinary stream. The stream is normally strong without dribbling.

Scrotum

Inspect the scrotum for size, symmetry, presence of the testicles, and any abnormalities. The scrotum is normally loose and pendulous with rugae, or wrinkles. The scrotum of infants often appears large in comparison to the penis. A small, undeveloped scrotum that has no rugae indicates that the testicles are undescended. Enlargement or swelling of the scrotum is abnormal. It may indicate an inguinal hernia, hydrocele, torsion of the spermatic cord, or testicular inflammation. A deep cleft in the scrotum may indicate ambiguous genitalia.

Pubic Hair

Inspect the presence, amount, and distribution of pubic hair. Straight, downy pubic hair first develops at the base of the penis. The hair becomes darker, dense, and curly, extending over the pubic area in a diamond pattern by the completion of puberty. The presence of pubic hair before 9 years of age is uncommon. Stages of pubic hair development follow a standard pattern, as illustrated in Figure 3–38.

Palpation of the Male Genitalia

Penis

Palpate the shaft of the penis for nodules and masses. None should be present.

Testicles

Palpate the scrotum for the presence of the testicles. Make sure your hands are warm to avoid stimulating the cremasteric reflex that causes the testicles

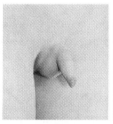
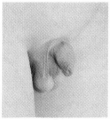

1

2

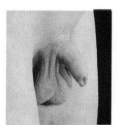
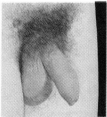
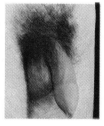

3

4

5

1 Testis, scrotum, and penis are same size and shape as in young child

2 Enlargement of scrotum and testis; skin of scrotum becomes redder, thinner, and wrinkled; penis no larger or scarcely so

3 Enlargement of penis, especially in length; further enlargement of testis; descent of scrotum

4 Continued enlargement of penis and sculpturing of glans; increased pigmentation of scrotum; this stage is sometimes best described as "not quite adult"

5 Adult stage: scrotum ample, penis reaching nearly to bottom of scrotum

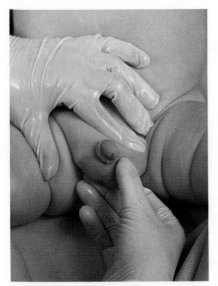

FIGURE 3–39 Palpating the scrotum for descended testicles and spermatic cords.

to retract. Place your index finger and thumb over both inguinal canals on each side of the penis. This keeps the testicles from retracting into the abdomen (Fig. 3–39).

Gently palpate each testicle with only enough pressure to identify the shape and size. The testicles are normally smooth and equal in size. They are approximately 1 to 1.5 cm in diameter until puberty when they increase in size. A hard, enlarged, painless testicle may indicate a tumor.

If a testicle is not palpated in the scrotum, the examiner palpates the inguinal canal for a soft mass. When the testicle is found in the inguinal canal, try to move it to the scrotum to palpate the size and shape. The testicle is descendable when it can be moved into the scrotum. An undescended testicle is one that does not descend into the scrotum or cannot be palpated in the inguinal canal.

Spermatic Cord

Palpate the length of the spermatic cord between the thumb and forefinger from the testicle to the inguinal canal. It normally feels solid and smooth. No tenderness is expected.

Enlarged Scrotum

When bulging or swelling of the scrotum is present, palpate the scrotum to identify the characteristics of the mass. Try to determine whether the mass is unilateral or bilateral and attempt to reduce the mass by pushing it back through the external inguinal ring. A mass that decreases may indicate an inguinal hernia. A mass that does not decrease may indicate a hydrocele or an incarcerated hernia.

Inguinal Canal

Attempt to insert your little finger into the external inguinal canal to determine whether the external inguinal ring is dilated. The inguinal ring is normally too small for the finger to pass into the canal. If the finger passes into the inguinal canal, ask the child to cough. A sensation of abdominal contents coming down to touch the fingertip may indicate an inguinal hernia.

Cremasteric Reflex

Stroke the inner thigh of each leg to stimulate the cremasteric reflex. The testicle and scrotum normally rise on the stroked side. This response indicates intact function of the spinal cord at the T12, L1, and L2 levels.

Inspection of the Anus and Rectum

Inspect the anus for sphincter control and any abnormal findings such as inflammation, fissures, or lesions. The external sphincter is usually closed. Inflammation and scratch marks around the anus may be associated with pinworms. A protrusion from the rectum may be associated with a rectal wall prolapse or a hemorrhoid.

Palpation of the Anus and Rectum

Lightly touching the anal opening should stimulate an anal contraction or "wink." Absence of a contraction may indicate the presence of a lower spinal cord lesion.

Patency of the Anus

Passage of meconium by newborns indicates a patent anus. When passage of meconium is delayed, a lubricated catheter can be inserted 1 cm into the anus. Resistance in passage of the catheter may indicate an obstruction.

Rectal Examination

A rectal examination is not routinely performed on children. It is indicated for symptoms of intraabdominal, rectal, bowel, or stool abnormalities. The rectal examination should be performed by an experienced examiner.

Assessing the Musculoskeletal System for Bone and Joint Structure, Movement, and Muscle Strength

What do extra skin folds on an arm or leg indicate? What causes poor muscle tone? What condition does a rib hump indicate? At what age is it normal for children to be knock-kneed and bow-legged?

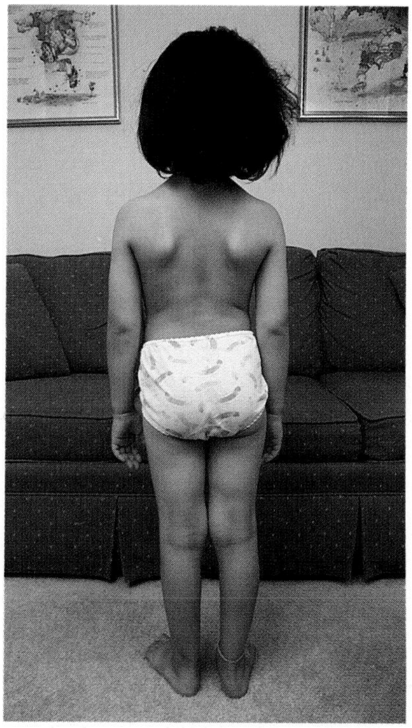

Inspection of the Bones, Muscles, and Joints

Bones and Muscles

Inspect and compare the arms and then the legs for differences in alignment, contour, skin folds, length, and deformities. The extremities normally have equal length, circumference, and numbers of skin folds bilaterally. Extra skin folds and a larger circumference may indicate a shorter extremity (Fig. 3–40).

Joints

Inspect and compare the joints bilaterally for size, discoloration, and ease of voluntary movement. Joints are normally the same color as surrounding skin with no sign of swelling. Children should voluntarily flex and extend joints during normal activities without pain. Redness, swelling, and pain with movement may indicate injury or infection.

Palpation of the Bones, Muscles, and Joints

FIGURE 3–40 Asymmetric extremities.

Bones and Muscles

Palpate the bones and muscles in each extremity for muscle tone, masses, or tenderness. Muscles normally feel firm, and bony masses are not normally present. Doughy muscles may indicate poor muscle tone. Rigid muscles, or *hypertonia,* may be associated with an active seizure or cerebral palsy. A mass over a long bone may indicate a recent fracture or bone cancer.

■ GROWTH AND DEVELOPMENT CONSIDERATIONS

Palpate the clavicles of the newborn from the sternum to the shoulder. These bones are often fractured during delivery. A mass and crepitus may indicate a fracture.

Joints

Palpate each joint and surrounding muscles to detect any swelling, masses, heat, or tenderness. None is expected when the joint is palpated. Tenderness, heat, swelling, and redness can result from injury or a chronic joint inflammation such as juvenile rheumatoid arthritis.

Range of Motion and Muscle Strength Assessment

GROWTH AND DEVELOPMENT CONSIDERATIONS

Newborns typically have a limited extension of the hips, knees, and elbows resulting from their flexed fetal position. When the newborn's arms and legs are extended and released, the extremities rapidly return to flexed fetal positioning.

CLINICAL TIP

To check the muscle strength in a newborn, hold the infant upright with your hands under the infant's arms. When the chest is lightly held, the infant normally does not slip through the hands. Muscle weakness is present when the infant slides through the hands.

Active Range of Motion

Observe the child during typical play activities, such as reaching for objects, climbing, and walking, to assess range of motion of all major joints. Children spontaneously move their joints through the full normal range of motion with play activities when no pain is present. Limited range of motion may indicate injury, inflammation of a joint, or a muscle abnormality.

Passive Range of Motion

When a joint is suspected of having limited active range of motion, perform passive range of motion. Flex and extend, abduct and adduct, or rotate the affected joint cautiously to avoid causing extra pain. Full range of motion without pain is normal. Limitations in movement may indicate injury, inflammation, or malformation.

Muscle Strength

Observe the child's ability to climb onto an examining table, throw a ball, clap the hands, or move around on the bed. The child's ability to perform age-appropriate play activities indicates good muscle tone and strength. Attainment of age-appropriate motor development is another indicator of good muscle strength (Table 3–17).

To assess the strength of specific muscles in the extremities, engage the child in some games. Muscle strength is compared bilaterally to identify muscle weakness. For example, ask the child to squeeze the examiner's fingers tightly with each hand; push against and pull the examiner's hands with the hands, lower legs, and feet; and resist extension of a flexed elbow or knee by the examiner. Children normally have good muscle strength bilaterally. Unilateral muscle weakness may be associated with a nerve injury. Bilateral muscle weakness may result from hypoxemia or a congenital disorder such as Down syndrome.

When generalized muscle weakness is suspected in a preschool or school-aged child, ask the child to stand up from the supine position. Children are normally able to rise to a standing position without using their arms as levers. Children who push their body upright with the arms and hands have generalized muscle weakness, a *positive Gower sign*. This may indicate muscular dystrophy.

TABLE 3–17 Selected Gross Motor Milestones for Age

Gross Motor Milestones	Age Attained
Rolls over from prone to supine position	4 months
Sits without support	8 months
Pulls self to standing position	10 months
Walks around room holding on to objects	11 months
Walks alone well	15 months
Kicks ball	24 months
Throws ball overhand	30 months
Jumps in place	36 months

From Frankenburg, W.K., Sciarillo, W., & Burgess, D. (1981). *Journal of Pediatrics, 99,* 995.

After beginning to walk, young children often have a pot-bellied stance because of a lumbar lordosis. This posture generally disappears by 5 years of age.

Posture and Spinal Alignment

Posture

Inspect the child's posture when standing from a front, side, and back view. The shoulders and hips are normally level. The head is held erect without a tilt, and the shoulder contour is symmetric. The spine has a normal thoracic convex and lumbar concave curves after 6 years of age. Table 3–18 shows normal posture and spinal curvature development.

TABLE 3-18 Normal Development of Posture and Spinal Curves

Infants

2 to 3 months

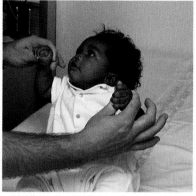

Holds head erect when held upright; thoracic kyphosis when sitting.

6 to 8 months

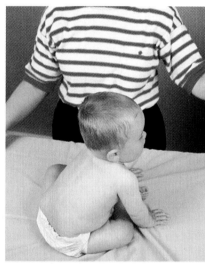

Sits without support; spine is straight.

10 to 15 months

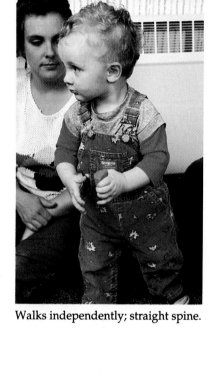

Walks independently; straight spine.

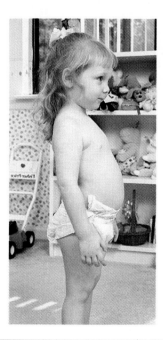

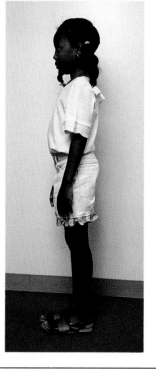

Toddler

Protruding abdomen; lumbar lordosis.

School-age child

Height of shoulders and hips is level; balanced thoracic convex and lumbar concave curves.

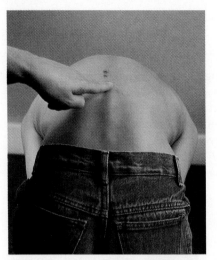

FIGURE 3-41 Inspection of the spine for scoliosis. Ask the child to slowly bend forward at the waist, with arms extended toward the floor. Run your forefinger down the spinal processes, palpating each vertebra for a change in alignment. A lateral curve to the spine or a one-sided rib hump is an indication of scoliosis.

Spinal Alignment

Assess the school-age child and adolescent for *scoliosis*, a lateral spine curvature. Stand behind the child, observing the height of the shoulders and hips. Ask the child to bend forward slowly at the waist, with arms extended toward the floor. No lateral curve should be present in either position. The ribs normally stay flat bilaterally. The lumbar concave curve should flatten with forward flexion (Fig. 3-41). A lateral curve to the spine or a one-sided rib hump is an indication of scoliosis. (See also Chapter 17.)

Inspection of the Upper Extremities

Arms

The alignment of the arms is normally straight with minimal angle at the elbows where the bones articulate.

Hands

Count the fingers. Extra finger digits (*polydactyly*) or webbed fingers (*syndactyly*) are abnormal. Inspect the creases on the palmar surface of each hand. Multiple creases across the palm are normal. A single crease that crosses the entire palm of the hand, a simian crease, is associated with Down syndrome (Fig. 3-42).

Nails

Inspect the nails for size, shape, and color. Nails are normally convex, smooth, and pink. *Clubbing*, widening of the nailbed with an increased angle between the proximal nail fold and nail, is abnormal. Clubbing is associated with chronic respiratory and cardiac conditions.

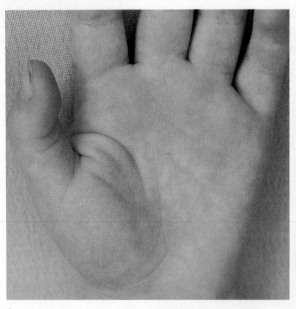
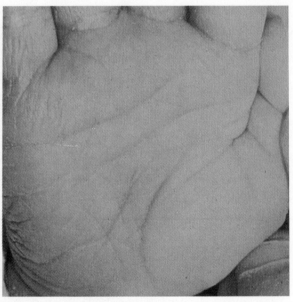

A   B

FIGURE 3-42 **A,** Normal palmar creases; **B,** Simian crease is associated with Down syndrome.

B from Zitelli, B.J., & Davis, H.W. (Eds.). (1987). *Atlas of pediatric physical diagnosis*. New York: Mosby–Year Book Europe Ltd.

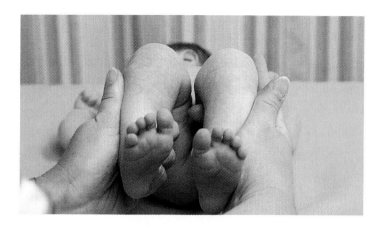

FIGURE 3–43 Flex the infant's hips and knees at a 90-degree angle. The knees are usually the same height. A difference in knee height (Allis sign) is an indicator of hip dislocation. (See also Chapter 17.)

Inspection of the Lower Extremities

Hips

Assess the hips of newborns and young infants for dislocation or subluxation. The skin folds on the upper legs are inspected first. The same number of skin folds should be present on each leg. Uneven skin folds may indicate a hip dislocation or difference in leg length. Then check for a difference in knee height symmetry (Fig. 3–43). The Ortolani-Barlow maneuver is used to assess an infant's hips for dislocation or subluxation (Fig. 3–44).

The child is asked to stand on one leg and then the other. The iliac crests should stay level. A lower iliac crest opposite the weight-bearing leg may indicate dislocation of the hip bearing weight.

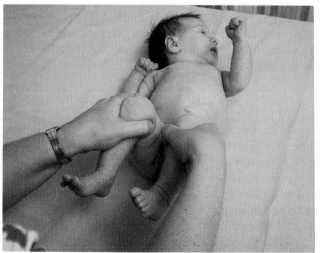

A

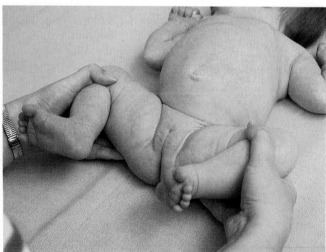

B

FIGURE 3–44 Ortolani-Barlow maneuver. **A,** With the infant on his or her back, flex the hips and knees at a 90-degree angle. Place a hand over each knee with the thumb over the inner thigh, and the first two fingers over the upper margin of the femur. Move the infant's knees together until they touch, and then put downward pressure on the femurs to see if the hips easily slip out of joint or dislocate. **B,** Slowly abduct the hips, moving each knee toward the examining table. Keep pressure on the hip joint with the fingers in a lever-type motion. Equal hip abduction, with the knees nearly touching the examining table, is normal. Any resistance to abduction or a clunk felt on palpation may indicate a congenital hip dislocation.

FIGURE 3–45 To evaluate the child with knock knees, have the child stand on a firm surface. Measure the distance between the ankles when the child stands with the knees together. No more than 2 inches (5 cm) between the ankles is normal.

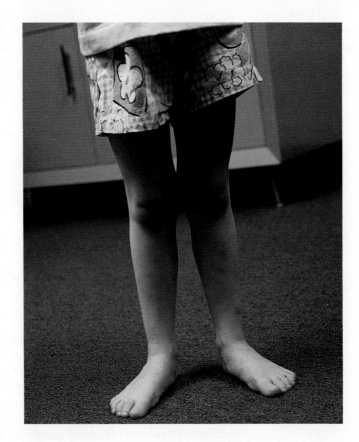

■ GROWTH AND DEVELOPMENT CONSIDERATIONS

Infants are often born with a twisting of the tibia caused by positioning in utero (tibial torsion). The infant's toes turn in as a result of the tibial torsion. Toddlers go through a skeletal alignment sequence of bow legs (genu varum) and knock knees (genu valgum) before the legs assume a straight alignment.

Legs

Inspect the alignment of the legs. After a child is 4 years of age the alignment of the long bones is straight with minimal angle at the knees and feet where the bones articulate. Alignment of the lower extremities in infants and toddlers is assessed to ensure that normal changes are occurring. To evaluate the toddler with bowlegs, have the child stand on a firm surface. Measure the distance between the knees when the child's ankles are together. No more than 1.5 inches (3.5 cm) between the knees is normal (Fig. 3–45).

Feet

Inspect the feet for alignment, the presence of all toes, and any deformities. The weight-bearing line of the feet is usually in alignment with the legs. Many newborns have a flexible forefoot inversion, metatarsus adductus, that results from uterine positioning. Any fixed deformity is abnormal.

Inspect the feet for the presence of an arch when the child is standing. Children up to 3 years of age normally have a fat pad over the arch, giving the appearance of flat feet. Older children normally have a longitudinal arch. The arch is usually seen when the child stands on tiptoe or is sitting.

Assessing the Nervous System for Cognitive Function, Balance, Coordination, Cranial Nerve Function, Sensation, and Reflexes

■ EQUIPMENT NEEDED

Reflex hammer	Penlight
Cotton balls	Tongue blades

What aspects of developmental information are useful for assessment of cognitive function? How is the infant's and child's level of consciousness evaluated? How are cranial nerves assessed in infants? A scissoring gait is associated with what condition? At what age does a Babinski response become abnormal? What response is expected when a deep tendon reflex is stimulated?

Cognitive Function

Observe the child's behavior, facial expressions, gestures, communication skills, activity level, and level of consciousness to assess cognitive functioning. Match the neurologic examination to the child's stage of development. For example, cognitive function is evaluated much differently in infants than in older children because infants cannot use words to communicate.

Behavior

The alertness of infants and children is indicated by their behavior during the assessment. Infants and toddlers are curious but seek the security of the parent, either by clinging or by making frequent eye contact. Older children are often anxious and watch all of the examiner's actions. Lack of interest in assessment or treatment procedures may indicate a serious illness. Excessive activity or an unusually short attention span may be associated with an attention deficit disorder.

Communication Skills

Speech, language development, and social skills provide good clues to cognitive functioning. Listen to speech articulation and words used, comparing the child's performance with standards of social development and speech articulation for the child's age (Table 3–19). Toddlers can normally follow simple directions such as "Show me your mouth." By 3 years of age the child's speech should be easily understood. Delay in language and social skill development may be associated with mental retardation.

Memory

Immediate, recent, and remote memory can be tested in children starting at approximately 4 years of age. To evaluate recent memory, ask the child to remember a special name or object. Then later during the examination, have the child recall the name or object. To evaluate remote memory, ask the child to repeat his or her address or birth date or a nursery rhyme. By 5 or 6 years of age, children are normally able to recall this information without difficulty.

TABLE 3-19 Expected Language Development for Age

Language Milestones	Age Attained
Understands Mama and Dada	10 months
Says Mama, Dada, 2 other words; imitates animal sounds	12 months
4–6 word vocabulary, points to desired objects	13–15 months
7–20 word vocabulary, points to 5 body parts	18 months
2 word combinations	20 months
3 word sentences, plurals	36 months

From Capute, A.J., Shapiro, B.K., & Palmer, R.B. (1987). *Contemporary Pediatrics, 4*, 24–41.

Level of Consciousness

When approaching the infant or child, observe the level of consciousness and activity, including facial expressions, gestures, and interaction. Children are normally alert, and sleeping children arouse easily. The child who cannot be awakened is unconscious. A lowered level of consciousness may be associated with a number of neurologic conditions such as a head injury, seizure, infection, or brain tumor.

Cerebellar Function

Observe the young child at play to assess coordination and balance. Development of fine motor skills in infants and preschool children provides clues to cerebellar function.

Balance

Observe the child's balance during play activities such as walking, standing on one foot, and hopping (Table 3–20). The Romberg procedure can also be used to test balance in children over 3 years of age (Fig. 3–46). Once balance and other motor skills are attained, children do not normally stumble or fall when tested. Poor balance may indicate cerebellar dysfunction or an inner ear disturbance.

TABLE 3-20 Expected Balance Development for Age

Balance Milestones	Age Attained
Stands without support briefly	12 months
Walks alone well	15 months
Walks backwards	2 years
Balances on 1 foot for 5 seconds	4 years
Hops on 1 foot, heel-toe walking	5 years
Heel-toe walking backwards	6 years

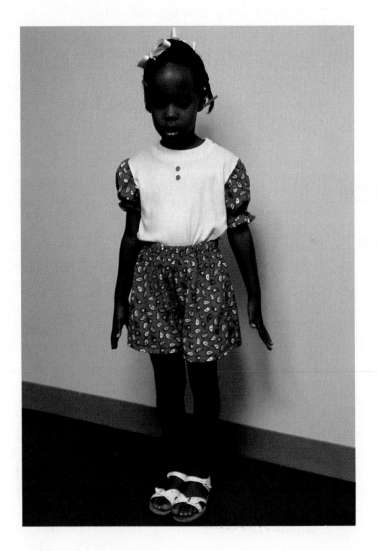

FIGURE 3-46 Romberg procedure. Ask the child to stand with feet together and eyes closed. Protect the child from falling by standing close. Preschool-aged children may extend their arms to maintain balance, but older children can normally stand with arms at their sides. Leaning or falling to one side is abnormal and indicates poor balance.

PEDIATRIC NURSING

TABLE 3-21 Expected Fine Motor Development for Age

Fine Motor Milestones	Age Attained
Transfers objects between hands	7 months
Picks up small objects	10 months
Feeds self with cup and spoon	12 months
Scribbles with crayon or pencil	18 months
Builds 2 block tower	24 months
Builds 4 block tower	30 months
Unfastens front buttons	36 months

From Frankenburg, W.K., Sciarillo, W., & Burgess, D. (1981). *Journal of Pediatrics, 99,* 995.

Coordination

Tests of coordination assess the smoothness and accuracy of movement. Development of fine motor skills can be used to assess coordination in young children (Table 3–21). After 6 years of age the tests for adults (finger-to-nose, finger-to-finger, heel-to-shin, and alternating motion) can be used. The child usually responds enthusiastically when these tests are presented as games. Jerky movements or inaccurate pointing *(past pointing)* indicates poor coordination, which can be associated with delayed development or a cerebellar lesion (Fig. 3–47).

FIGURE 3–47 Tests of coordination. **A,** *Finger-to-nose test.* Ask the child to close the eyes and touch the nose, alternating the index fingers of the hands. **B,** *Finger-to-finger test.* Ask the child to alternately touch the nose and the examiner's index finger with the index finger. The examiner's hand is moved to several positions within the child's reach to test pointing accuracy. Repeat the test with the child's other hand. **C,** *Heel-to-shin test.* Ask the child to rub the leg from the knee to the ankle with the heel of the other foot. Repeat the test with the other foot. This test is normally performed without hesitation or inappropriate placement of the foot. **D,** *Rapid alternating motion test.* Ask the child to rapidly rotate the wrist so the palm and dorsum of the hand alternately pat the thigh. Repeat the test with the other hand. Hesitating movements are abnormal. Mirroring movements of the hand not being tested indicates a delay in coordination skill refinement.

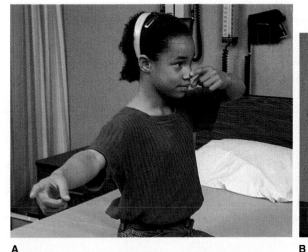

A

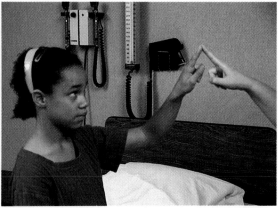

B

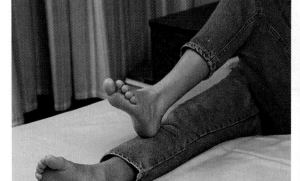

C

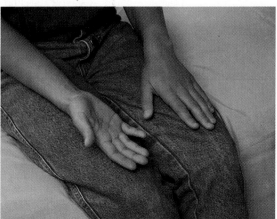

D

Gait

A normal gait requires intact bones and joints, muscle strength, coordination, and balance. Inspect the child when walking from both a front and a rear view. The iliac crests are normally level during walking, and no limp is expected. A limp may indicate injury or joint disease. Staggering or falling may indicate cerebellar ataxia. *Scissoring*, in which the thighs tend to cross forward over each other with each step, may be associated with cerebral palsy or other spastic conditions.

Cranial Nerve Function

To assess the cranial nerves in infants and young children, make some modifications in procedures used for school-aged children and adults (Table 3–22). Abnormalities of cranial nerves may be associated with compression on an individual nerve, head injury, or infections.

Sensory Function

To assess sensory function, compare the responses of both sides to various types of stimulation. Equal responses bilaterally are normal. Loss of sensation may indicate a brain or spinal cord lesion.

Superficial Tactile Sensation

Stroke the skin on the lower leg or arm with a cotton ball or a finger while the child's eyes are closed. Cooperative children over 2 years of age can normally point to the location touched.

TABLE 3–22 Age-Specific Procedures for Assessment of Cranial Nerves in Infants and Children

Cranial Nerve*	Assessment Procedure and Normal Findings†
I Olfactory	Infant—Not tested.
	Child—Not routinely tested. Give familiar odors to child to smell, one naris at a time. *Identifies odors such as orange, peanut butter, and chocolate.*
II Optic	Infant—Shine a bright light in eyes. *A quick blink reflex and dorsal head flexion indicates light perception.*
	Child—Test vision and visual fields if cooperative. *Visual acuity appropriate for age.*
III Oculomotor	Infant—Shine a penlight at the eyes and move it side to side. *Focuses on and tracks the light to each side*
IV Trochlear	Child—Move an object through the 6 cardinal points of gaze. *Tracks object through all fields of gaze.*
VI Abducens	All Ages—Inspect eyelids for drooping. Inspect pupillary response to light. *Eyelids do not droop and pupils are equal sized and briskly respond to light.*
V Trigeminal	Infant—Stimulate the rooting and sucking reflex. *Turns head toward stimulation at side of mouth and sucking has good strength and pattern.*
	Child—Observe the child chewing a cracker. Touch forehead and cheeks with cotton ball when eyes are closed. *Bilateral jaw strength is good. Child pushes cotton ball away.*
VII Facial	All Ages—Observe facial expressions when crying, smiling, frowning, etc. *Facial features stay symmetric bilaterally.*
VIII Acoustic	Infant—Produce a loud sound near the head. *Blinks in response to sound, moves head toward sound, or freezes position.*
	Child—Use a noisemaker near each ear or whisper words to be repeated. *Turns head toward sound and repeats words correctly.*
IX Glossopharyngeal	Infant—Observe swallowing during feeding. *Good swallowing pattern.*
X Vagus	All Ages—Elicit gag reflex. *Gags with stimulation.*
XI Spinal accessory	Infant—Not tested.
	Child—Ask child to raise the shoulders and turn the head side to side against resistance. *Good strength in neck and shoulders.*
XII Hypoglossal	Infant—Observe feeding. *Sucking and swallowing are coordinated.*
	Child—Tell the child to stick out the tongue. Listen to speech. *Tongue is midline with no tremors. Words are clearly articulated.*

*Bracketed nerves are tested together.
†Italic indicates normal findings.

Superficial Pain Sensation

Break a tongue blade to get a sharp point. After asking the child to close the eyes, touch the child in various places on each arm and leg, alternating the sharp and dull ends of the tongue blade. Children over 4 years of age can normally distinguish between a sharp and dull sensation each time. To improve the child's accuracy with the test, let the child practice telling you the difference between the sharp and dull stimulation.

An inability to identify superficial touch and pain sensation may indicate sensory loss. Identify the extent of sensory loss, such as all areas below the knee. Other sensory function tests (temperature, vibratory, deep pressure pain, and position sense) are performed when sensory loss is found. Refer to other texts for description of these procedures.

Infant Primitive Reflexes

Evaluate the movement and posture of newborns and young infants by the Moro, palmar grasp, plantar grasp, placing, stepping, and tonic neck primitive reflexes (Table 3–23). These reflexes appear and disappear at expected intervals in the first few months of life as the central nervous system develops. Movements are normally equal bilaterally. An asymmetric response may indicate a serious neurologic problem on the less responsive side.

Superficial and Deep Tendon Reflexes

Evaluate the superficial and deep tendon reflexes to assess the function of specific segments of the spine.

Superficial Reflexes

Assess superficial reflexes by stroking a specific area of the body. The plantar reflex, testing spine levels L4 to S2, is routinely evaluated in children (Fig. 3–48). Assess the cremasteric reflex in boys (see p. 128).

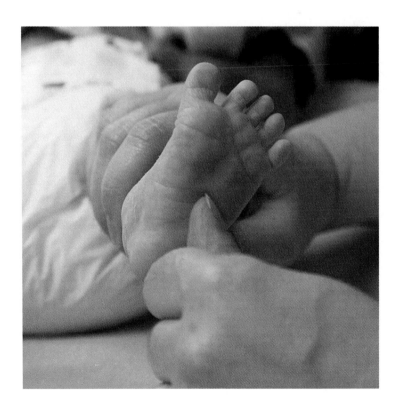

FIGURE 3–48 To assess the plantar reflex, stroke the bottom of the foot in the direction of the arrow. Watch the toes for plantar flexion or the Babinski response, fanning and dorsiflexion of the big toe. The Babinski response is normal in children under 2 years of age. Plantar flexion of the toes is the normal response in older children. A Babinski response in children over 2 years of age may indicate neurologic disease.

TABLE 3-23 Techniques for Assessing Selected Primitive Reflexes, with Normal Findings and Their
Expected Age of Occurrence

Primitive Reflex	Technique and Normal Findings*	Normal Appearance and Disappearance
Moro 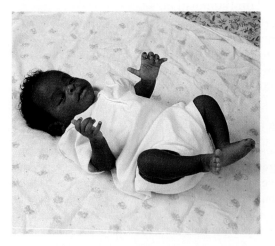	Startle the infant with a sudden noise or change in position. *The arms extend and the fingers form a C as they spread. The arms slowly move together as in a hug. The legs may make a similar motion.*	Present at birth. Decreases in strength by 4 months of age. Disappears by 6 months of age.
Palmar grasp 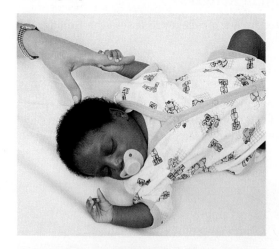	Place finger across the palm and avoid touching the thumb. *A strong grip around the finger is normal.*	Present at birth. Disappears by 3 months of age.
Plantar grasp 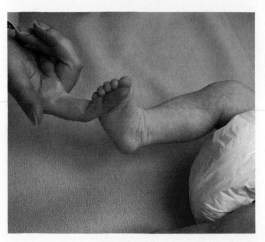	Place finger across the foot at the base of the toes. *The toes normally curl as if gripping the finger.*	Present at birth. Disappears at about 8 months of age.

*Italics indicate normal findings.

Primitive Reflex	Technique and Normal Findings*	Normal Appearance and Disappearance
Placing 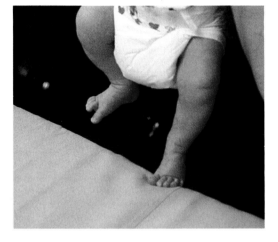	Hold the infant erect and touch the top of one foot with the edge of a table or chair. *The infant normally lifts the foot, as if to step up onto the surface.*	Present within days of birth. Disappears at various times.
Stepping 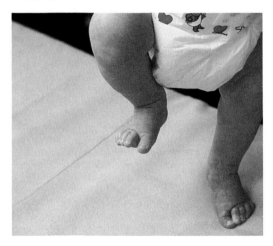	Hold the infant erect and touch the bottom of one foot on the surface of a table or chair. *The feet lift in an alternating pattern as if to walk.*	Present at birth. Disappears between 4 and 8 weeks of age.
Tonic neck 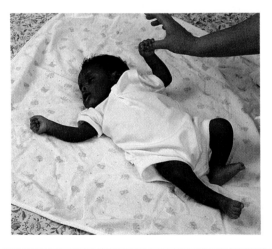	Place the infant in a supine position and, when relaxed, turn the head to one side. Repeat by turning the head to the opposite side. *The arm and leg on the face side normally extend and the opposite arm and leg flex, as if to assume a fencing position.*	Appears about 2 months of age. Deceases by 4 months of age. Disappears no later than 6 months of age. This reflex must disappear before the infant can turn over.

TABLE 3–24   Assessment of Deep Tendon Reflexes and the Spinal Segment Tested with Each

Deep Tendon Reflex	Technique and Normal Findings*	Spine Segment Tested
Biceps 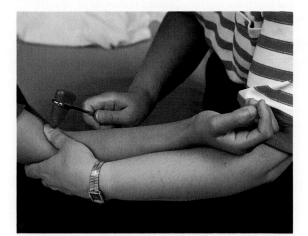	Flex the arm at the elbow, and place a thumb over the biceps tendon in the antecubital fossa. Tap the thumb. *Elbow flexion as the biceps muscle contracts.*	C5 and C6
Triceps 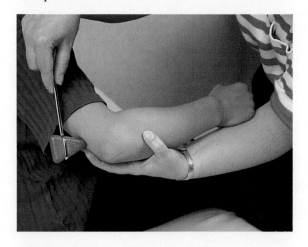	With the arm flexed, tap the triceps tendon above the elbow. *Elbow extension as the triceps muscle contracts.*	C6, C7, and C8
Brachioradialis 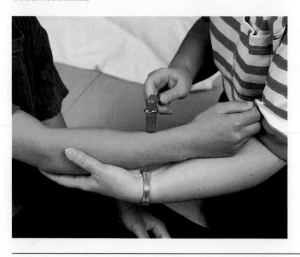	Lay the child's arm with the thumb upright over the examiner's. Tap the brachioradial tendon 2.5 cm (1 in) above the wrist. *Forearm pronation (palm facing downward) and elbow flexion.*	C5 and C6

*Italics indicate normal findings.

Deep Tendon Reflex	Technique and Normal Findings*	Spine Segment Tested
Patellar 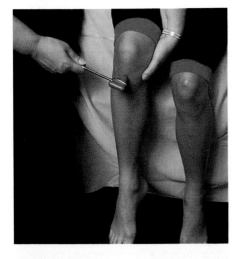	Flex the child's knees, and when the legs are relaxed, tap the patellar tendon just below the knee. *Knee extension (knee jerk) as the quadriceps muscle contracts.*	L2, L3, and L4
Achilles 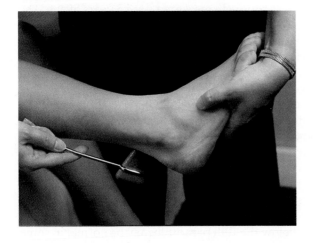	While the legs are flexed, support the foot and tap the Achilles tendon. *Plantar flexion (ankle jerk) as the gastrocnemius muscle contracts.*	S1 and S2

■ CLINICAL TIP

The best response to deep tendon reflex testing is achieved when the child is relaxed or distracted. Children often anticipate the knee jerk and either tighten up or exaggerate the response. Making the child focus on another set of muscles may provide a more accurate response. When testing the reflexes on the lower legs, have the child press the hands together or try to pull them apart when gripped together.

Deep Tendon Reflexes

To assess the deep tendon reflexes, tap a tendon near specific joints with a reflex hammer (or with the index finger for infants), comparing responses bilaterally. The biceps, triceps, brachioradialis, patellar, and Achilles tendons are usually evaluated in children. Inspect for movement in the associated joint and palpate the strength of the expected muscle contraction (Table 3-24). Table 3-25 outlines the numeric scoring of deep tendon reflexes. Responses are normally symmetric bilaterally. Absence of response is associated with decreased muscle tone and strength. Hyperactive responses are associated with muscle spasticity.

TABLE 3-25 Numeric Scoring of Deep Tendon Reflex Responses

Grade	Response Interpretation
0	No response
1+	Slow, minimal response
2+	Expected response, active
3+	More active or pronounced than expected
4+	Hyperactive, clonus may be present

Assessing Nutritional Status by Measuring Growth and Evaluating Dietary Intake

What is the best indication that the child's nutrition is adequate? Which data collection tools provide good information about a child's dietary intake?

CULTURAL CONSIDERATIONS

Although growth curves have been standardized on the U.S. population, they can be used on children of different ethnic groups. Children of first- or second-generation immigrants to the United States follow patterns of growth similar to those of the children whose families have been in the United States longer, but often at a lower percentile.

CULTURAL CONSIDERATIONS

Each culture has eating practices that influence dietary intake. It is important to understand the foods commonly eaten by each cultural group and their contribution to the total nutrition of the child.

Growth Measurements

The infant's weight, length, and head circumference are measured to assess growth. A standing height is substituted for the length measurement in children. The head circumference is routinely measured until 5 years of age. The Atlas of Pediatric Procedures presents techniques used to measure the weight, length, standing height, and head circumference.

Once the measurements are collected for the child, plot the readings on the appropriate standardized growth curves for weight, length or height, head circumference, and weight for length for the child's age and sex. For example, to plot the length measurement, mark an X on the spot where the child's age and length intersect. Appendix A gives standardized growth curves for infants, children, and adolescents by sex. Identify the percentile of weight, length or height, weight for length, and head circumference for age. The child normally falls between the 10th and 90th percentiles for weight, length or height, and weight for length. A measurement below the 10th percentile of weight for length may indicate undernutrition, whereas a measurement over the 90th percentile may indicate overnutrition. Measurements of weight, length, or height below the 10th percentile may be normal in some cultural groups.

When measurements of the child's weight and length at earlier ages are available, plot them on the same growth curve. Growth measurements following a same percentile curve for weight and length or height over time are normal, indicating that the child has adequate nutrition. A sudden or sustained drop below a previously established percentile for weight or length may indicate inadequate dietary intake or a chronic disorder.

Dietary Intake

Obtain detailed information about the child's dietary intake when there is a potential for nutritional deficiency because of disease, knowledge deficit, or socioeconomic status. After the information is collected, compare the dietary intake to the energy and recommended daily nutritional needs of the child. (See Appendix C for the Recommended Dietary Allowances chart.) The 24-hour recall of food intake and the dietary screening history provide a good overview of the infant's or child's dietary intake and eating patterns. A food diary provides information about the child's precise food intake.

24-Hour Recall of Food Intake

Ask the parent to list all foods eaten by the infant or child during the past 24 hours. Make sure the 24-hour period is an example of the child's typical dietary intake. For example, when the child is ill, food intake changes. In such a case a recent, more typical 24-hour period should be used for data collection. When obtaining the information, ask the parent specifically about the following food intake:

- All meals and between meal snacks
- Approximate amounts (for example, tablespoon, half cup) of each food eaten at each feeding
- What was added to foods, such as cereal mixed with formula
- How the food was prepared
- Vitamins or other food supplements (iron, fluoride) given

Dietary Screening History

Ask the parent about the infant's or child's eating habits using questions in Tables 3–26 and 3–27. These responses provide additional information about the family's eating habits and food beliefs beyond that collected on the 24-hour dietary recall.

TABLE 3-26 Dietary Screening History for Infants

Overview Questions

What was the infant's birth weight?
At what age was the birth weight doubled and tripled?
Was the infant premature?
Does the infant have any feeding problems such as difficulty sucking and swallowing, spitting up, or fussiness?

If Infant Is Breast Fed

How long does the baby nurse at each breast?
What is the usual schedule for nursing?
Does the baby also take any milk or formula? Amount and frequency? What type?

If Infant Is Fed Other Foods

What formula is used? Is it iron fortified?
   How is it prepared?
Do you hold or prop the bottle for feedings?
How much formula is taken at each feeding?
How many bottles are taken each day?
Does the baby take a bottle to bed for naps or nighttime? What is in the bottle?

If Infant Is Formula Fed

At what age did the baby start eating other foods?
   Cereal   Finger foods
   Fruit/juices   Meats
   Vegetables   Other protein sources
Do you use commercial baby food or make your own?
Does the baby eat any table foods?
How often does the baby take solid foods?
How is the baby's appetite?
Do you have any concerns about the baby's feeding habits?
Does the baby take a vitamin supplement?
Have there been any allergic reactions to foods? Which ones?
   Does the baby spit up frequently?
   Have there been any rashes?
What types of stools does the baby have? Frequency? Consistency?

TABLE 3-27 Dietary Screening History for Children

What foods or beverages does the child dislike?
What types of food or beverage does the child especially like?
What is the child's typical eating schedule? Meals and snacks?
Does the child eat with the family or at separate times?
   Where does the child eat each meal?
Who prepares the food for the family?
   What method of cooking is used? Baking? Frying? Broiling?
   What ethnic foods are commonly eaten?
Does the family eat in a restaurant frequently? What type?
   What type of food does the child usually order?
Is the child on a special diet?
Does the child need to be fed, feed himself, need assistance eating, or need any
   adaptive devices for eating?
What is the child's appetite like?
Does the child take any vitamin supplements? (iron, fluoride)?
Does the child have any allergies? What types of symptoms?
What types of regular exercise does the child get?
Are there any concerns about the child's eating habits?

■ CLINICAL TIP

Parents seldom control all of the food a child eats. To help parents record the most complete food diary, remind them about all places a child might be fed or obtain food. Older children often get snacks independently. Younger children may be fed in day care centers. Parents must plan to obtain information from the child and all persons feeding the child.

Food Diary

Parents are asked to keep a food diary when the child has a nutrition problem, such as malnutrition, obesity, or a disorder like diabetes mellitus that requires dietary management. All meals and snacks, with food preparation method and quantities eaten, over a 3- to 7-day period are recorded. Eating patterns change significantly for holidays or family gatherings, so ask parents to select typical days for the food diary or to record specific events affecting food intake.

Assessing the Adequacy of Intake

Review the overall pattern of food intake to ensure that the child is getting some foods from all the basic food groups (milk, meat, fruits, vegetables, and grains or bread). A good mix of protein, carbohydrates, and fats is also im-

TABLE 3-28 Signs of Inadequate Nutrition in Children

Nutrient Deficiency	Physical Signs of Malnutrition
Protein and calorie	Poor growth Hair: dull, dry, thin Mouth: enlarged parotid glands Skin: depigmentation, pretibial edema Musculoskeletal: muscle weakness Neurologic: listlessness Abdomen distended
Minerals	Enlarged thyroid Heart: murmur, tachycardia, arrhythmias Musculoskeletal: muscle weakness, bony overgrowth, bending
Vitamins	Skin: rough, dry, lesions, pallor Eyes: night blindness, light sensitivity, dull, dark circles Mouth: cracking, scaling lips; spongy, swollen, bleeding gums; smooth or fissured tongue; poor tooth development Musculoskeletal: soft bones, bowing or knock-knees, bony overgrowth Neurologic: depressed deep tendon reflexes, motor weakness, lethargy

portant. Estimate the daily caloric intake by using a calorie chart. Various physical signs of malnutrition from protein, calorie, and specific nutrients may be detected in various body systems (Table 3–28). A nutritionist can perform a more detailed nutritional assessment.

Assessing Motor Skills, Personal-Social Skills, Language Skills, and Behavior with Developmental Screening Tests

◼ EQUIPMENT NEEDED

Selected screening tool
Forms, testing equipment, and manual

◼ CULTURAL CONSIDERATIONS

Many developmental screening tests are not standardized on children of lower socioeconomic and ethnic groups. For example, Southeast Asian parents are often more protective of their children and may not provide opportunities to learn the self-help skills included on the Denver II.[8] Some children fail a test item because the language is different from what is used at home. Consider these cultural differences when administering and scoring developmental screening tests.

What interpretation is made when a hospitalized child performs below age level on a screening tool? What differences in the child's development can result from culture?

It is important to identify young children with developmental delays early, so that appropriate support and treatment can be provided. The same tools may also be used to monitor developmental progress as the child ages. Standardized screening tools are available to evaluate various aspects of development, such as fine and gross motor skills, social skills, language, behavior, and temperament. Another tool evaluates how the child's environment supports development. Select a screening tool appropriate for the child's age and the evaluation purpose (Table 3–29).

Carefully follow the instructions for administration and interpretation of the child's responses when using any screening tool to obtain reliable and valid results. The child's responses to screening tests can be affected by fatigue, illness, or separation anxiety. Responses are also affected by physical conditions such as visual, hearing, and neurologic problems. Ask parents whether the child's performance is typical of his or her usual behavior and skills. Special interpretation guidelines may be provided for children of various ethnic groups and premature infants.

Analyzing Data from the Physical Examination

◼ LEGAL CONSIDERATIONS

Be sure to record all findings from the physical assessment legibly, in detail, and in the format approved by your institution.

Once the physical examination has been completed, the abnormal examination findings for each system are grouped with those of other systems. **Clinical judgment** is used to identify common patterns of physiologic responses associated with medical conditions. Individual abnormal physiologic responses are also the basis of many nursing diagnoses.

Let's return to the vignette at the beginning of the chapter. Your thorough physical assessment of Kimberly has revealed signs of respiratory distress and inadequate tissue perfusion from several body systems. These signs include mottled skin color, an increased resting respiratory rate, retractions, increased respiratory effort, nasal flaring, stridor, tachycardia, and agitation. These signs represent the integumentary, respiratory, cardiac, and neurologic systems. Based on these findings, you would be able to select nursing diagnoses appropriate to a child with croup, for example, Altered Tissue Perfusion, Cardiopulmonary, related to upper airway obstruction and hyp-oxia; and Ineffective Breathing Pattern related to respiratory distress. These diagnoses, in turn, would direct your nursing care of this child.

TABLE 3-29 Developmental Screening Tools for Infants and Young Children

Test Name and Age Group	Test Methods and Features Evaluated	Available From:
Denver II; birth–6 years	Observation of child; personal-social, fine motor–adaptive, language, and gross motor *Standardized for whites, Afro-Americans, and Hispanics*	Denver Developmental Materials, Inc., P.O. Box 6919, Denver, CO 80206-0919
Revised Prescreening Developmental Questionnaire (R-PDQ); birth–6 years	Parent questionnaire; gross motor, personal-social, fine motor–adaptive, language *Determines need for DDST II administration*	Denver Developmental Materials, Inc., P.O. Box 6919, Denver, CO 80206-0919
Washington Guide for Promoting Development in the Young Child; birth–5 years	Observation of child; feeding, sleep, play, language, motor activities, discipline, toilet training, and dressing *Useful for examining handicapped child's functional skills*	Powell, M. (1981): *Assessment and management of developmental changes and problems in children.* St. Louis, CV Mosby
McCarthy Scales of Children's Abilities; 2.5–8.5 years	Observation of child; motor, verbal, perceptual-performance, quantitative, general cognition, and memory *Useful when child is suspected of having retarded development*	Psychological Corp., 757 3rd Ave., New York, NY 10017
Developmental Profile; birth–9 years	Parent interview; provides general developmental level of function in physical, self-help, social, academic, and communication sections. *Lacks referral criteria.*	Psychological Development Publications, Box 3198, Aspen, CO 81612
Goodenough-Harris Drawing Test; 5–15 years	Observation of the child; child draws a picture of a person which is analyzed for body parts, clothing details, proportion, and perspective. *An intellectual age is obtained*	Psychological Corporation, 757 3rd Ave., New York, NY 10017
Carey-Revised Infant Temperament Questionnaire; 4–8 months	Parent questionnaire; patterns of feeding, sleeping, elimination, playing, and responses to different situations *Looks at infant's responses that influence relationship with parents and caregivers*	William B. Carey, MD, 319 W. Front St., Media, PA 19063
HOME (Home Observation Measurement of the Environment); birth–3 years, 3–6 years	Observation of child; age-specific subscales such as organization, play materials, stimulation, avoiding restriction or punishment, parental control *Designed to identify characteristics of the social, emotional, and cognitive environment*	Dr. Bettye Caldwell, Center for Child Development and Education, Univ. of Arkansas, 33rd & Univ. Ave., Little Rock, AR 77204
Denver Articulation Screening Exam (DASE); 2.5–6 years	Observation of child; articulation of 30 sound elements, and intelligibility *For English-speaking children only*	Denver Developmental Materials, Inc., P.O. Box 6919, Denver, CO 80206-0919
Early Language Milestone Scale (ELM); birth–3 years	Observation of the child; assesses auditory expressive, auditory receptive, and visual components of speech. *Screens children for potential language problems*	Modern Education Corporation, Box 721, Tulsa, OK 74101

REFERENCES

1 Spector, R.E. (1991). *Cultural diversity in health and illness.* Norwalk, CT: Appleton & Lange.
2 Burns, C. (1992). A new assessment model and tool for pediatric nurse practitioners. *Journal of Pediatric Health Care, 6,* 73–81.
3 Wilson, E.F. (1977). Estimation of the age of cutaneous contusions in child abuse. *Pediatrics, 60,* 750.
4 Seidel, H.M., Ball, J.W., Dains, J., & Benedict, G.W. (1991). *Mosby's guide to physical examination* (2nd ed.). St. Louis: Mosby–Year Book.
5 Smith, J. (1988). Big differences in little people. *American Journal of Nursing, 88,* 458–462.
6 Eichelberger, M.R., Ball, J.W., Pratsch, G.S., & Runion, E.F. (1992). *Pediatric emergencies: A manual for prehospital care providers.* Englewood Cliffs, NJ: Prentice Hall.
7 Tanner, J.M. (1962). *Growth at adolescence.* (2nd ed.). Oxford: Blackwell Scientific Publications, Inc.
8 Miller, V., Onotera, R., & Deinard, A. (1984). Denver Developmental Screening Test: Cultural variations in Southeast Asian children. *Journal of Pediatrics, 104,* 481–482.

SUGGESTED READINGS

Barness, L. (1991). *Manual of pediatric physical diagnosis.* (6th ed.). St. Louis: Mosby–Year Book.
Bradley, J.C., & Edinberg, M.A. (1990). *Communication in the nursing context.* (3rd ed.). Norwalk, CT: Appleton & Lange.
Calhoun, M. (1986). Providing health care to Vietnamese in America: What practitioners need to know. *Home and Healthcare Nurse, 4,* 14–19,22.
Castiglia, P.T. (1989). Ambiguous genitalia. *Journal of Pediatric Health Care, 3,* 319–321.
Curry, L.C., & Gibson, L.Y. (1992). Congenital hip dislocation: The importance of early detection and comprehensive treatment. *Nurse Practitioner, 17,* 49–52, 55.
Elvik, S.L. (1990). Vaginal discharge in the prepubertal girl. *Journal of Pediatric Health Care, 4,* 181–185.
Engel, J. (1993). *Pocket guide to pediatric assessment.* (2nd ed.). St. Louis: Mosby–Year Book.
Finelli, L. (1991). Evaluation of the child with acute abdominal pain. *Journal of Pediatric Health Care, 5,* 251–256.
Fung, K., & Lau, S. (1985). Denver Developmental Screening Test: Cultural variables. *Journal of Pediatrics, 106,* 343.
Henry, J.J. (1992). Routine growth monitoring and assessment of growth disorders. *Journal of Pediatric Health Care, 6,* 291–301.
Lippe, B.M. (1987). Short stature in children: Evaluation and management. *Journal of Pediatric Health Care, 1,* 313–322.
Litt, I.F. (1990). *Evaluation of the adolescent patient.* Philadelphia: Hanley & Belfus, Inc.
Olade, R.A. (1984). Evaluation of the Denver Developmental Screening Test as applied to African children. *Nursing Research, 33,* 204–207.
Pipes, P.L. (1989). *Nutrition in infancy and childhood.* (4th ed.). St. Louis: Times Mirror/Mosby College Publishing.
Rudy, E.C. (1991). Hair loss in children and adolescents. *Journal of Pediatric Health Care, 5,* 245–250.
Wade, G.H. (1992). Update on the Denver II. *Pediatric Nursing, 18,* 140–141.

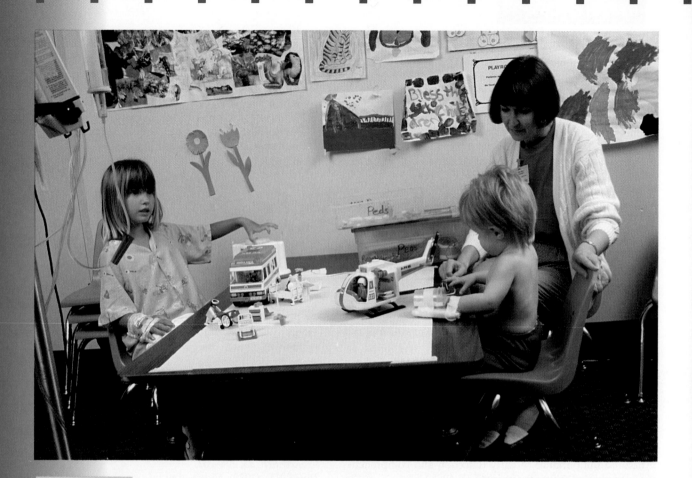

Four-year-old Sabrina has had several nosebleeds and fainting spells recently. After examination by her physician and a number of diagnostic studies such as chest x-ray examination, echocardiography, and electrocardiography, coarctation of the aorta is diagnosed. Sabrina will come in this week for a cardiac catheterization. In 2 weeks she is scheduled to have open heart surgery.

Sabrina and her family live about 50 miles from the medical center. Her parents have three other children, ages 9, 7, and 2. The parents are both employed, but Sabrina's mother plans to take several days off at the time of surgery. Sabrina attends preschool, and she is used to spending time with other children.

Sabrina has had few health problems, and her experiences with health care professionals are limited. Her parents, who are anxious about the heart surgery, are concerned about how their daughter will adapt to hospitalization.

How should you prepare Sabrina for the cardiac catheterization and for the surgery? How far in advance should teaching take place? What teaching aids are helpful? How can Sabrina's parents be involved in and reinforce the teaching? What kind of support do her parents, siblings, and friends need during hospitalization?

NURSING CONSIDERATIONS FOR THE FAMILY: HOSPITAL AND HOME

4

TERMINOLOGY

case manager Person who coordinates health care to prevent gaps or overlaps.

child life specialist Trained professional who plans therapeutic activities for hospitalized children.

individualized education plan Assessment of a child and formulation of a specific learning approach for a child with a physical or mental handicap.

rehabilitation Treatment and education of a disabled child to maximize function.

rooming in Practice in which parents stay in the child's hospital room and care for the child.

separation anxiety Behaviors observed in young children separated from their parents.

therapeutic play Planned play techniques that provide an opportunity for children to deal with their fears and concerns related to illness or hospitalization.

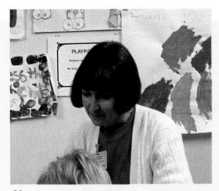

66 As a child life teacher, my job is to ensure that the child understands what is involved in hospitalization. Like the nurse and the other team members, I strive to make the child feel comfort and trust in what is sometimes a stressful environment. Therapeutic play is one of the tools I use to help children understand and work through their feelings about hospitalization. 99

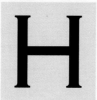

Hospitalization, whether elective, planned in advance, or a result of emergency or trauma, is stressful for children of all ages and their families. Children are in an unfamiliar environment, surrounded by strange people, equipment, and frightening sights and sounds. They are subjected to various routine and invasive procedures, possibly even surgery. For both children and families, routines are disrupted and normal coping strategies are tested.

To minimize the stress of hospitalization, nurses provide support to children and their families before, during, and after hospitalization. Through preadmission preparation, children and their families are introduced to the acute care setting. During hospitalization, various strategies may be used to promote coping and adaptation and prepare children for procedures and surgery. Nurses are instrumental in ensuring that the developmental and educational needs of children are met, especially when hospitalization is long term. Nurses also help prepare children and their families for discharge or for transfer to a long-term care or rehabilitation facility.

Effects of Illness and Hospitalization on Children and Families

Children's Understanding of Health and Illness

Can you remember as a child thinking that yelling at your mother caused your strep throat? Or perhaps as an adolescent you believed that you would never become ill or have an accident. Maybe you feared being in a car crash like that of a friend.

Children have limited knowledge about the body and its relation to health and illness. Their understanding is based primarily on their cognitive ability at various developmental stages and on previous experiences with health care professionals.

Infant

By about 6 months of age, infants have developed awareness of themselves as separate from their mother or father. They are able to identify primary caretakers and to feel anxious when in contact with strangers. Hospitalization can be a traumatic time for the infant, particularly if the parents are not staying with the child.

The three phases of **separation anxiety** were first identified in young children who were separated from parents for long periods or permanently and lacked a close relationship with one caretaker before separation.[1] Characteristic behaviors of children in the three phases of separation anxiety are listed in Table 4–1. Infants and young children who are hospitalized often display these behaviors.

Before the 1970s, health care professionals assumed that the despair and denial manifested by infants and young children after prolonged separation were signs of positive adaptation. They observed that infants protested when parents visited and sometimes advised parents not to visit often. However, the protest phase is now viewed as a healthy response to separation from loved ones and as an indication that the infant has meaningful close relationships. Parents should be encouraged to remain with and provide care to the hospitalized infant.

Toddler and Preschooler

Toddlers and preschoolers are beginning to understand illness but not its cause. Two unrelated events may appear to have a cause-and-effect relation-

TABLE 4-1 Stages of Separation Anxiety in Young Children

Protest

Screaming, crying
Clinging to parents
Withdrawal from other adults

Despair

Sadness, depression
Withdrawal or compliant behavior
Crying when parents appear

Denial

Lack of protest when parents leave
Appearance of being happy and content with everyone
Close relationships not established
Developmental delay possible

Based on Bowlby, J. (1960). *International Journal of Psychoanalysis, 41*, 89–113.

ship for young children, who may consider the sun, an animal, bad behavior, or even magic to be the cause of illness. These children may blame other people, events, or themselves for illness.[2] This is especially true if the other event occurs shortly before the illness.

The child's concept of the body usually is limited to names and locations of some body parts. Toddlers and preschoolers are not likely to understand how lungs, heart, bones, or other body parts function.[3]

Separation from parents remains the major stressor for the child. When a parent cannot be present, reminders can be left with the child. These might include a piece of cloth saturated with the mother's favorite perfume or father's cologne, an object belonging to the parent, or an audiotape with messages from the parents. Toddlers and preschoolers fear bodily mutilation and change. If, like Sabrina, the child is undergoing an operation, the nurse should explain to the child that surgery will fix the body. The nurse should encourage the parents to be present as much as possible for important rituals such as toileting, carrying out bedtime routines, and singing favorite nursery rhymes.

■ GROWTH AND DEVELOPMENT CONSIDERATIONS

School-age children between the ages of 5 and 8 years believe that the internal body consists of heart and bones. They view the digestive system as having two parts, the mouth and the stomach.

■ GROWTH AND DEVELOPMENT CONSIDERATIONS

Young adolescents, aged 11 to 13 years, can describe the location and function of major organs such as the brain, nose, eyes, heart, and stomach.

School-Age Child

Older children have a more realistic understanding of the reasons for illness and are able to comprehend explanations. The child's concept of body parts and function is maturing. Concepts of time are well formed, and parents should be encouraged to tell the child when they will return. Parents should also be available for telephone calls to provide support and comfort.

Adolescent

After 11 years of age, adolescents become increasingly aware of physiologic and then psychologic and behavioral causes of illness and injury. Adolescents are preoccupied with appearance. Illness or injury may interfere with body image, and adolescents perceive illness in terms of its effect on their body image. Privacy and modesty are major concerns of adolescents because their physical characteristics are rapidly changing. Nurses should respect their feelings. Adolescents are in the process of becoming independent of their parents' influence, and the peer group is a major influence in their lives. Separation from peers may be difficult.

Family Responses to Hospitalization

The illness and hospitalization of a child disrupt a family's usual routines.[4] Sometimes roles are altered as one parent stays at the hospital while the other parent or siblings take on additional tasks at home. Family members may be anxious and fearful, especially when the outcome is unknown or potentially serious. Watching a child in pain is difficult for a parent. Adjustment is made more difficult by a lengthy illness, chronic condition, poor prognosis, lack of family support, and lack of financial or community services.[4]

The siblings of an ill child often receive little attention from the parents. Parents are preoccupied and may not think to take the siblings to visit the child in the hospital. The siblings may fantasize about the illness or injury and the appearance of their brother or sister. Siblings who are not adequately informed about the hospitalized child's condition may fear that the child will be disabled or even die, even when this is unlikely. They may feel guilty about fighting with or being mean to their brother or sister in the past and believe that they played a role in causing his or her illness.

As family roles and routines change, siblings may feel insecure and anxious. Behavioral problems may develop, or school performance may deteriorate. Siblings may feel jealous because the ill brother or sister seems to monopolize the parents' attention. Given support, however, the siblings of an ill child manage well. Chapter 6 describes strategies for working with siblings of a hospitalized child.

Preparation for Hospitalization

Hospitalization may be planned or unexpected. A child may be hospitalized for one of the following reasons:

- The child who has been ill at home gradually or suddenly becomes worse.
- The child needs diagnostic or treatment procedures or requires elective surgery.
- The child who was previously healthy suffers an injury, necessitating unexpected hospitalization.

When hospitalization is planned, both children and their parents have time to prepare for the experience. The nurse first assesses the family's knowledge and expectations and then provides information about what is likely to happen. A variety of approaches can be used to provide information and allay fears.

- Tours of the hospital unit or surgical area are helpful. During tours preschoolers and school-age children should be allowed to see and touch items with which they will come in contact. The surgical team's attire is less frightening if the child has had a chance to try it on (Fig. 4–1). Medical equipment is not as scary when the child learns what it does and sees how it is used, for example, through demonstration on a doll (Fig. 4–2).
- If a tour is not possible, photographs or a videotape can be used to show the medical setting and procedures.
- Many hospitals offer health fairs to explain health procedures to children. The Association for the Care of Children's Health (ACCH) sponsors a "National Children and Hospital Week" each spring.
- During a tour, while hospitalized, or at home, the child can be exposed to books or films that explain in age-appropriate terms what to expect

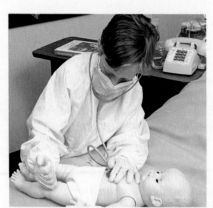

FIGURE 4–1 Allowing the child to dress up as a doctor or a nurse helps prepare the child for hospitalization. This helps the child adjust to treatment, care, and the recovery process. Why? What might the child's concerns be? Can you think of any concerns that could be related to cultural background?

FIGURE 4-2 The child's anxiety and fear often will be reduced if the nurse explains what is going to happen and demonstrates how the procedure will be done by using a doll. Based on your experience, can you list five things you can do to prepare a school-age child for hospitalization?

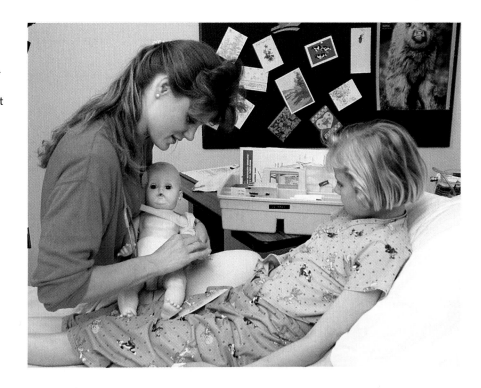

during various procedures (Table 4-2). Use coloring books or other methods to reinforce teaching.

Parents can be instrumental in preparing children for hospitalization. They reinforce and strengthen material presented, are available when questions arise, and are trusted, familiar adults (Table 4-3, Fig. 4-3).

Different approaches are useful when adolescents are being prepared for hospitalization. They learn not only from written materials, models, and

---

TABLE 4-2 Sample Teaching Materials for Children Requiring Hospitalization

Videotapes

Clean Intermittent Catheterization. Learner Managed Designs, Inc.
I Have Epilepsy Too. Epilepsy Foundation.
What Do I Tell My Children? How to Help a Child Cope with the Death of a Loved One.
  Life Cycle Productions.

Books

Becky's Story. Baznick, Donna. Association for the Care of Children's Health.
Curious George Goes to the Hospital. Rey, M. & Rey, H.A. Houghton Mifflin Company.
Doctors and Nurses: What Do They Do? Green, C. Harper & Row Junior Books.
The Fall of Freddie the Leaf. Buscaglia, L.
First Time at the Hospital. Burton, Nita & Burton, Terry. Macdonald Educational Ltd.
Having an Operation. Greenwald, Arthur & Head, Barry. Family Communications.
The Hospital Book. J. Howe. Crown Publishers.
Hospitals. Fisher, Leonard E. Holiday House.
No Measles, No Mumps for Me. Showers, Paul. Thomas Y. Crowell.
The Operation. Anderson, Penny. Children's Press.
Richard Scarry's Nicky Goes to the Doctor. Scarry, R. A Golden Book.
Wearing a Cast. Greenwald, Arthur & Head, Barry. Family Communications.
Why Am I Going to the Hospital? Cilliota, Claire & Livingston, Carole. Lyle Stuart.

TABLE 4–3 Parental Preparation of Children for Hospitalization

- Read stories to the child about the experience.
- Talk about going to the hospital, what it will be like, about coming home.
- Encourage the child to ask questions.
- Encourage the child to draw pictures of what it will be like.
- Visit the hospital unit if possible.
- Let the child touch or see equipment if possible.
- Plan for support via parents' presence, telephone calls, special items of the parents which child can keep during the stay.
- Be honest.

FIGURE 4–3 Jasmine's parents are taking the time to prepare her for hospitalization by reading a book recommended by the nurse. Such material should be appropriate to the child's age and culture. Why do you think that having the parents read this material to and with the child is valuable? How would you have related to this approach when you were Jasmine's age?

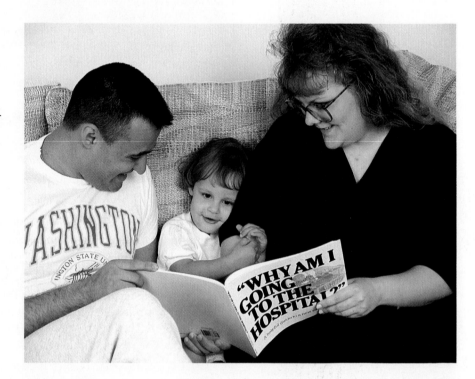

videotapes, but also from talking with peers who have had similar experiences. A forum for asking questions without parents present should be provided.

Adaptation to Hospitalization

Special Units and Types of Care

Children who are admitted to a hospital may be cared for in one or more of the following units: emergency department, intensive care unit, or short stay unit. They may require surgical treatment involving preoperative and postoperative care. Children with infectious diseases may require isolation precautions. Other children may need rehabilitative care to achieve or restore maximum potential.

Emergency Care

When a child is brought to an emergency department, the parents are usually frightened and insecure and may even be in a state of shock. The fast pace and critical nature of the unit create an atmosphere in which parents are hesitant to ask questions and are anxious about the outcome. Nurses should keep both the child and the family informed about what is being done and when more news may be available. The parents and child should remain together as much as possible.

Intensive Care

Parents of a child in an intensive care unit are also likely to be anxious, particularly since the child's illness may be severe and the prognosis may be guarded. The unfamiliar equipment may create an atmosphere of fear. Numerous health care professionals come and go, and parents may not know who to turn to or even what questions to ask. Nurses should provide emotional support, explain the purpose of treatments and machines, help parents to hold or touch their child, and provide support and referral to other services if appropriate. (See Chapter 6 for a discussion of stressors in parents and children in an intensive care unit and the nursing strategies intended to address these stressors.)

Preoperative and Postoperative Areas

Many hospitals now allow parents to be with their child right up until surgery begins and again in the postanesthesia recovery area. Parents often want to be with and support their child before and immediately after surgical procedures, and their presence may offer reassurance and comfort to the child.

Nurses should prepare family members for what will happen and what is expected of them. In some hospitals only one or two close family members are allowed to see the child. They may need to wear special gowns, shoes, or hats, and they may be restricted to certain areas. Special equipment such as intravenous setups and monitoring devices should be explained.

Short Stay Units

Hospitalizations are becoming shorter for many reasons. Often minor surgery, diagnostic tests such as radiology studies, and treatments such as chemotherapy are performed in one day. The child may be admitted in the morning and go home in the afternoon. These short stays are beneficial because they cause minimal disruption of family patterns. Nurses can help parents prepare the child properly for the admission, monitor the child during the procedures, and keep families well informed (Table 4–4).

TABLE 4-4 Preparation for Planned Short Stay Admission

- Are there special requirements, such as not being permitted food or drink or needing extra fluid intake?
- What time and where must the child appear?
- Are any special forms, insurance numbers, or previous records needed?
- How long will the child stay in the hospital?
- Are parents expected or encouraged to be with the child or stay in the health facility?
- Is there a chance the child may need to remain longer than expected?
- What will the child's condition be for transfer home?
- Will special equipment or care be needed?
- What symptoms can indicate problems?
- Where can the family go or who can they call in case of problems or questions?

Isolation

Children who are placed in isolation may suffer lack of stimulation because of limited contact with other children. Frequent family visits are important and should be encouraged. Family members may be reluctant to wear protective garments either out of fear of using them incorrectly or a belief that they are unnecessary. The family needs to understand the reason for isolation and any special procedures. Having contact with and holding the child should be encouraged whenever possible. (Isolation precautions are described in the Atlas of Pediatric Procedures.)

Rehabilitation

Rehabilitation units provide children with ongoing care and support to continue recovery beyond the initial period of illness or injury. These may be separate units within a hospital or independent centers. The objective of **rehabilitation** is to help the child reach his or her maximum potential and to promote achievement of developmentally appropriate skills. Parental involvement is essential.

Family Assessment

To develop a plan of care that involves all family members, the nurse needs to assess the impact of the child's illness or hospitalization on the family (Table 4–5). Teaching the child and family, providing support, and referring them to community resources are key elements of the plan.

The family's resources should be assessed frequently. These resources include the coping strategies of family members, financial resources, access to

---

TABLE 4–5 Family Assessment

Family Roles
- What changes will the child's illness create in the family?
- Will household tasks need to be reallocated?
- Will a burden be placed on certain family members?
- Will one parent room in or spend a great deal of time in the hospital?

Knowledge
- What knowledge does the family have about the child's condition and treatment? Do they need further information?
- Is there a need to start discharge planning and teaching early?

Support Systems
- Does the family have medical insurance? What percentage of costs will it cover? Will other financial support be needed?
- Are close friends or family available to provide child care for other children, assist with family tasks, or help in other ways?
- Are there community services such as support groups, camps for children with disabilities, education sessions, or equipment and financial resources to which the nurses can refer the family?

Siblings
- Have they been informed of the ill child's condition and the expected outcome?
- Have they been reassured that they did not cause the illness?
- Do they understand the change in roles and family routines?
- Are they able to visit the ill child?
- Have their teachers been informed of the family stress?
- If the hospitalized child's life is threatened, are the siblings involved in a therapy plan to assist them in dealing with that stress?

---

health care, and availability of community services. One family may manage quite well with limited financial support because they have good coping strategies, while another family with greater financial resources may have difficulty caring for an ill child.

It is important for the nurse to assess the family dynamics. The nurse evaluates the quality of communication, methods of handling problems, and sources of strength. Referrals to family service agencies or other community organizations may be needed. Support groups in the community or agencies that provide medical equipment can also be helpful.

Child and Family Teaching

Teaching is an essential part of the nurse's role in care of the hospitalized child and his or her parents. Teaching may be informal, as when the nurse provides an explanation during routine care, or structured, as when the nurse plans and implements a formal teaching program.

Teaching directed at children must take into account their developmental level and cognitive abilities. Learning is easier when teaching involves more than one sense (such as hearing, vision, and touch). Teaching directed at parents must be geared to their level of understanding. If English is the parents' second language, a translator may be necessary.

Timing is a critical factor in teaching. Parents and children are less receptive to teaching when they are preoccupied with other thoughts or activities. Scheduling specific times for teaching sessions may be helpful.

Depending on the information to be presented, teaching may use the cognitive, psychomotor, or affective domains of learning. Teaching that includes all three domains is more effective.

Teaching Plans

A teaching plan is a written plan that includes outcome objectives, interventions needed to achieve specified goals, and a method and time for evaluation. The teaching plan may also specify teaching methods and types of materials to be used. Developing a teaching plan helps to ensure that all the necessary information is included and makes teaching more efficient.

The child's primary caretaker should participate in the teaching. The primary caretaker is most often a parent but may be a close family member (uncle, aunt, grandparent). The first step in establishing a teaching plan is to assess the child's or parent's knowledge, skills, and feelings by asking the following questions:

- What does the parent or child know about the health issue?
- What is the cognitive level or ability to learn?
- Is there a desire to learn?
- What previous experiences affect the learning experience, either positively or negatively?
- Are there feelings or beliefs that might interfere with the learning process?

The second step involves deciding what knowledge, skill, or change in attitude is desired. Outcome criteria or objectives are established for the parent and child. A learning objective for a parent might be: The parent states the importance of checking the child's toes in the casted leg twice daily for temperature, movement, sensations, color, and edema (cognitive domain). An objective for a child might be: The child self-catheterizes using correct technique and records the amount of urine in a log (psychomotor domain). An objective for an adolescent might be: The adolescent explores methods of managing feelings of loss of control related to diabetes management (affective domain).

Possible teaching methods and approaches should be explored. A variety of sources, including written materials (books, pamphlets, handouts, and stories), computer software, audiovisual presentations, and others, are available (Table 4–2). In some settings, audiovisual and computer resources may be limited. Small group teaching sessions (for example, for children with recently diagnosed diabetes or cystic fibrosis) may be another option. Gathering two or three parents or children together on a unit to learn and share experiences may be helpful.

For some conditions, standardized teaching plans are available in books and from health care agencies. These plans can serve as a guide to the nurse in developing an individualized teaching plan.

Children with Special Needs

Children with disabilities may have special learning needs.[5] If they have visual impairment or visual perceptual difficulty, material must be presented in auditory and tactile ways. Children with hearing deficits need visual and tactile presentations. Children with learning disabilities may need more frequent reinforcement and shorter teaching sessions. They should be evaluated for comprehension often so teaching can be adjusted as necessary. When psychomotor skill performance is needed, special aids may be necessary so the child can hold a syringe, draw up a liquid, or perform other tasks. Adequate assessment of the child's strengths and disabilities, along with consultation with parents and the child's teachers, can help the nurse plan teaching methods.

Strategies to Promote Coping and Normal Development

During hospitalization, care of the child focuses not only on meeting physiologic needs, but also on meeting psychosocial and developmental needs. Several strategies may be used to help children adapt to the hospital environment, promote effective coping, and provide developmentally appropriate activities. These strategies include child life programs, rooming in, therapeutic play, and therapeutic recreation.

Child Life Programs

Many hospitals have child life programs that focus on the psychosocial needs of hospitalized children. Professional child life specialists, paraprofessionals, and volunteers staff these departments. A **child life specialist** plans activities to provide age-appropriate playtime for children either in the child's room or in a playroom. Some of the planned activities are designed to assist children in working through feelings about illness. Examples include playing with medical equipment or drawing pictures about hospital treatments (Fig. 4–4). A trusted child life specialist may stay with a child during a particularly frightening procedure such as a venipuncture or bone marrow aspiration.

Both the child life department and the nursing staff focus on the emotional needs of hospitalized children. Child life specialists and nurses may formulate a plan together to assist children with particular needs.

Rooming In

Rooming in is the practice of having a parent stay in the child's hospital room and care for the hospitalized child. Some hospitals provide cots, others

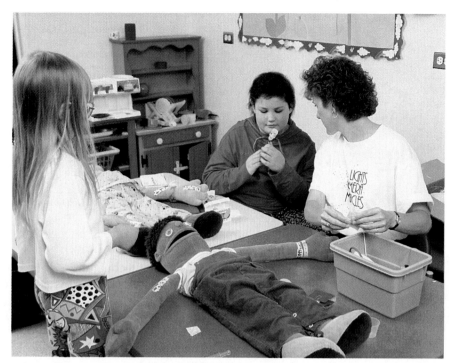

FIGURE 4–4 At Deaconess Hospital in Spokane, Washington, the child life specialist works with children being treated for cancer. Special dolls are used to familiarize children with the procedures that they will undergo.

have special built-in beds on pediatric wards, and in some institutions a parent stays in a separate room on the unit. A parent who is rooming in may want to perform all of the child's basic care or help with some of the medical care. Communication between the nurse and parent is important so that the parent's desire for involvement is supported.

Therapeutic Play

Play is an important part of childhood. The stress of illness and hospitalization increases the value of play. Not only is normal development facilitated by play, but play sessions can provide a means for the child to learn about health care, to express anxieties, to work through feelings, and to achieve a sense of mastery or control over frightening or little understood situations. Play that presents an opportunity to deal with the fears and concerns of health experiences is called **therapeutic play**.[6]

Through therapeutic play the nurse may assess the child's knowledge of his or her illness or injury. A common technique involves using body line drawings (Fig. 4–5) or stories and asking the child to draw in or talk about what the illness or injury means to him or her.[7] Alternatively, the child may be asked to draw a picture[8] or make up a story, enabling the nurse to assess fears and other emotions. The Goodenough-Draw-A-Person test helps the nurse assess the cognitive level of children between 3 and 13 years of age (Table 4–6). The Gellert Index is another tool that helps the nurse assess the child's knowledge of the body. The same techniques may be used in a slightly different way to teach the child about surgery or plan activities that allow the child to express fears and gain mastery over the situation.

FIGURE 4–5 The nurse can use a simple gender-specific line drawing of a child's body to encourage children to draw what they think about their medical problem. Such drawings reveal a child's interpretation, which you can work with to provide appropriate care.

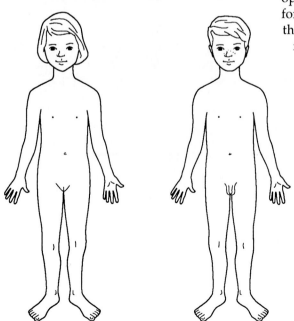

TABLE 4-6 Goodenough Draw-A-Person Test

- The child is asked to draw a picture of a person and to do so carefully and completely, taking his or her time. It is preferable to have the child take the test alone, away from parents.
- Points are assigned for specific details included in the drawing, for example, 1 point each for the presence of head, legs, arms, trunk, and eyes. Additional points are assigned depending on the complexity of details.
- For every 4 points assigned, another year is added to a baseline age of 3 years. For example, a child who scores 24 points (by including 24 details) would have a total score of 9 years (6 plus 3 baseline years). This number is compared to the child's chronologic age to determine his or her cognitive level.

The Goodenough Test may be obtained from the Psychological Corporation, 555 Academic Court, San Antonio, TX 78204.

A variety of techniques may be used to promote therapeutic play (Table 4–7). Specific techniques are chosen to reflect the child's developmental stage.

*Toddler.** Play is important for toddlers. Through play they explore the environment and learn to identify with significant people in their lives. Play is also an acceptable way for toddlers to release tensions caused by stress or aggressive impulses.

Toddlers should be approached slowly, and the initial approach should be made in their parents' presence, if possible, to decrease feelings of stranger anxiety (wariness of strangers). Playing a variation of peek-a-boo or

*Therapeutic play strategies for the toddler, preschooler, and school-age child were provided by Nan Peterson, RN, MS.

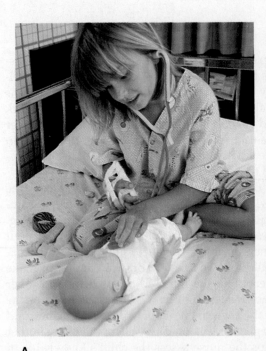

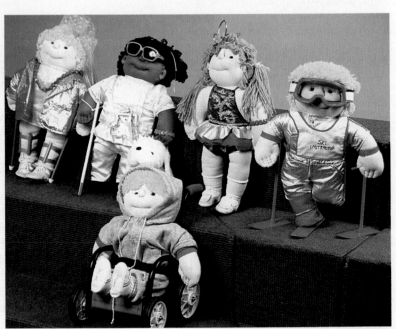

FIGURE 4-6 A, Age-appropriate play will help the child adjust to hospitalization and care. **B,** Having the child play with dolls that have "disabilities" similar to his or her own will help the child adjust. Such play helps the child realize what activities are possible.

TABLE 4-7 Therapeutic Play Techniques

Technique	Assessment	Intervention
Stories	Have the child make up a story about a picture. Analyze content and emotional clues in the story. Have children tell a story about an important experience in a group of other children.	Read or make up stories to explain illness, hospitalization, or other specific aspects of health care. Emotions such as fear can be included.
Drawings	Administer Goodenough Draw-A-Person test (see Table 4–6) to evaluate cognitive level. Consider subject matter, size and placement of items in drawings, colors used, presence or absence of physical barriers, and general emotional feeling. Administer Gellert Index to learn about the child's knowledge of the body and its functioning before planning teaching.	Use the child's drawings or body line drawings to explain care, procedures, or conditions. Provide opportunity for child to draw pictures of his or her choice or directed topics such as a picture of child's family or health care encounter. Ask the child: "Tell me about your picture." Sense child's emotions: "This child must be frightened by the big x-ray machine."
Music	Observe types of music chosen and effects of played music on behavior.	Encourage parents and children to bring favorite tapes to the hospital for stress relief. Have tapes playing during tests and procedures. Parents can tape their voices to play for infants and young children during separations. During longer hospitalizations children can tape messages for siblings or classmates, who are then encouraged to retape their messages. Playtime can include opportunity to play instruments and sing.
Puppets	The puppets can ask questions of young children, who are often more likely to answer the puppet than a person.	Perform short skits to teach children necessary health care information. Include emotional content when appropriate.
Dramatic play	Provide dolls and medical equipment, and analyze the roles assigned to dolls by the child, the behavior demonstrated by the dolls in the child's play, and the apparent emotions. Dolls with handicaps like those of the child are especially helpful (Fig. 4–6).	Provide dolls and equipment for play sessions. To ensure safety, supervise closely when actual equipment is used. Respond to emotions and behavior shown. Use dolls and equipment such as casts, nebulizer, intravenous apparatus, and stethoscope to explain care. Use dolls with problems or handicaps similar to those of the child when available. Provide toys that foster expression of emotion such as pounding board and indoor darts.

Additional techniques, such as sand or water play or pet therapy, may be appropriate in specific situations.

hide-and-seek using the curtain surrounding the toddler's crib or bed helps promote the realization that objects out of sight, such as parents, do return. The use of transitional objects, such as a familiar blanket or stuffed animal, can temporarily substitute for the security of parents. The toddler who is restrained can be read familiar stories. Repetition of stories promotes a sense of stability in the unfamiliar hospital environment.

A doll is a familiar toy that can be used to recreate a stressful environment, thereby providing an opportunity for the child to express and work through feelings. Other developmentally appropriate toys for toddlers include familiar objects from home such as measuring cups or spoons, wooden puzzles, building blocks, and push-and-pull toys. Playing with safe hospital equipment (bandages, syringes without needles, and stethoscopes) helps toddlers to overcome the anxiety associated with these items.

Preschooler. The nurse can intervene to reduce the stress produced by preschoolers' fears through the use of some kinds of play. A simple body outline or doll can be used to address the child's fantasies and fears of bodily harm. Playing with safe hospital equipment may help preschoolers to work through feelings such as aggression.

Preschoolers like crayons and coloring books, puppets, felt and magnetic boards, play dough, books, and recorded stories. Both preschool and school-age children may enjoy playing with a toy hospital (Fig. 4–7).

School-Age Child. Although play begins to lose its importance in the school-age years, the nurse can still use some techniques of therapeutic play to help the hospitalized child deal with stress. School-age children often regress developmentally during hospitalization, demonstrating behaviors characteristic of an earlier state, such as separation anxiety and fear of bodily injury. Body outlines and occasionally dolls can be used to illustrate the cause and treatment of the child's illness. Terms for body parts that are suitable for

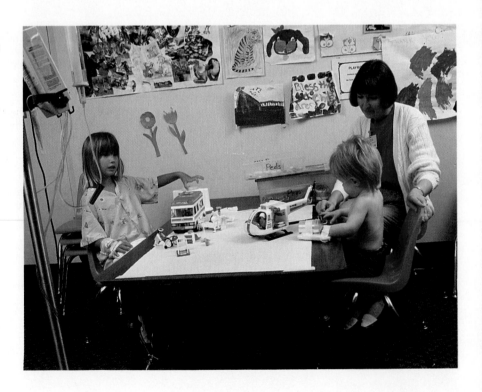

FIGURE 4–7 Children who are at different developmental levels often play together in the hospital setting.

FIGURE 4-8 Having interaction with other hospitalized adolescents and maintaining contact with friends outside the hospital are very important so that the teenager does not feel isolated and alone. A friendly yet competitive video game helps to stimulate this group and allows for self-expression. What are the other benefits?

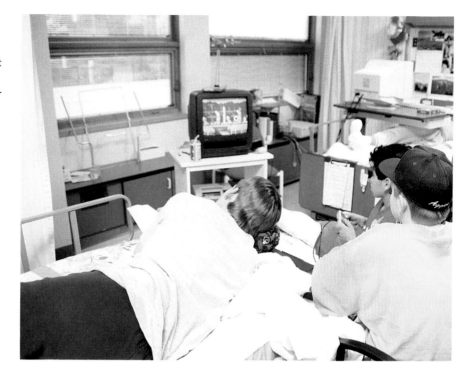

older children should be used. Drawings provide an outlet for expression of fears and anger.

School-age children enjoy collecting and organizing objects and often ask to keep disposable equipment that has been used in their care. They may use these items later to relive the experience with their friends. Games, books, schoolwork, crafts, tape recordings, and computers provide an outlet for aggression and increase self-esteem in the school-age child. The type of play used should promote a sense of mastery and achievement.

Therapeutic Recreation

Many of the special play techniques used with younger children are not suitable for adolescents. However, adolescents do need a planned recreation program to assist them in meeting developmental needs during hospitalization. Peers are important, and the isolation of hospitalization can be difficult. Telephone contact with other teenagers and visits from friends should be encouraged. Interactions with other teenagers at a pizza party or a video game or movie night can help adolescents feel normal (Fig. 4–8). Physical activities that provide an outlet for stress are recommended. Even adolescents on bed rest or in wheelchairs can play a modified form of basketball.

The independence of adolescence is interrupted by illness. Nurses can provide choices for teenagers to assist them in regaining control. Giving them options and letting them choose an evening recreational activity can promote their feelings of independence. Passes to leave the hospital for special activities may be possible.

Strategies to Meet Educational Needs

Some hospitalizations are so short that the absence of the child or adolescent from school and peers is of minimal concern. However, if hospitalization is expected to last longer than a few days or if the child's condition will change,

▪ LEGAL CONSIDERATIONS

The Joint Commission on Accreditation of Healthcare Organizations (1992) mandates provision for schooling of the child in a health care facility for an extended period.

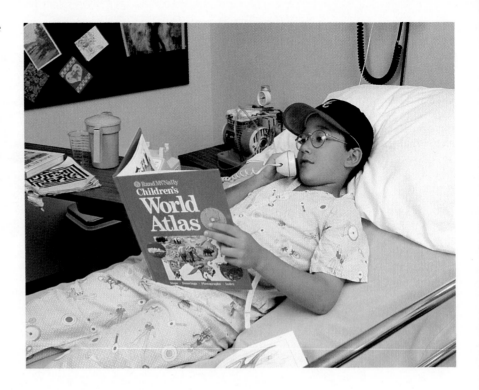

FIGURE 4-9 It is important that the hospitalized child not fall behind in schoolwork. As soon as the child is able, schoolwork should be resumed. If the child is unable to get out of bed, all necessary study materials need to be brought to the child.

necessitating special school arrangements, the nurse should assess the effects of hospitalization on the child's education.

When an elective procedure occurs, families are encouraged to arrange the extended school absence with teachers. The child can then be provided with schoolwork to do in the hospital or at home when well enough. This minimizes educational deficits and future problems for the child. Pencils, paper, comfortable work areas, and quiet work times should be provided. Telephone calls with teachers can be arranged as needed (Fig. 4-9).

The social aspects of school and peers should also be considered. Peers can be encouraged to visit a hospitalized classmate, send cards and letters, or call on the phone. When the child returns to school, the nurse can visit the classroom to provide classmates with information about the child's medical condition.

The hospital nurse may contact the child's school nurse when special arrangements are necessary. For example, the child who is wearing a large cast or who requires medications or other treatments may offer challenges in a traditional school setting.

The child with chronic health problems or in long-term hospitalization has other needs regarding school. Hospitals or rehabilitation units may have classrooms, teachers, and facilities to promote learning (Fig. 4-10). Many school districts provide tutors for students who are hospitalized or receiving home care for long periods. Telephone or computer contacts with the classroom may be necessary. Teachers can visit children at the hospital or at home. Parents are often pivotal in making arrangements to meet the child's educational needs, since they interact with the child, the school, and the health care team.

Preparation for Procedures

A number of procedures take place during hospitalization, from collection of urine or blood specimens to spinal taps and surgery. Special techniques can

PEDIATRIC NURSING

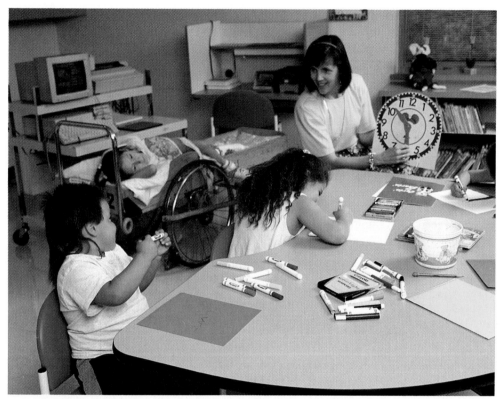

FIGURE 4–10 Shriners Hospital in Spokane, Washington, has a special classroom and teacher for children who require a long hospital stay so that they can remain current with their schoolwork. The child who falls behind other students might not fit in when he or she returns to school or might be required to repeat a grade. What are the potential consequences of these situations?

help the child to understand and cope with feelings about these procedures. Nurses should never assume that a procedure will not be traumatic for the child. Even providing urine in a specimen cup or undergoing x-ray examination can be frightening if the child does not understand the reason for the procedure or what to expect.

To assess the child's feelings about the procedure, ask the following questions:

- Does the child know the purpose of the procedure?
- Has the child experienced this procedure before? Was the experience painful, frightening, or reassuring?
- What does the child think will happen? Are the child's beliefs accurate?
- Is the procedure painful?
- What techniques does the child use to gain control in challenging situations?
- Will the parents or adult friends be present to provide support?

Preparation may begin a few moments to several days before the procedure, depending on the child's age. Use words that the child understands to describe the procedure and its purpose (refer to Chapter 2). Older children need explanations geared to their cognitive level and previous experiences. They will want to know what is happening, why, and what they can do to cope during the procedure (Table 4–8).

TABLE 4-8 Assisting Children Through Procedures

Developmental Stage	Before Procedure	During Procedure
Infant	None for infant. Explain to parents the procedure, the reason for it, and their role.	Restrain infant securely and gently. Perform procedure quickly. Use touch, voice, pacifier, and bottle as distractions. Have parent hold, rock, and sing to infant after procedure.
Toddler	Give explanation just before procedure, since toddler's concept of time is limited. Explain that child did nothing wrong; the procedure is simply necessary.	Perform in treatment room. Give short explanations and directions in a positive manner. Avoid giving choices when none are available. For example, "We are going to do this now" is better than "Is it okay to do this now?" Allow child to cry or scream. Comfort child after procedure. Give child a choice of favorite drink or special sticker.
Preschool child	Give simple explanations of procedure. Basic drawings may be useful. While providing supervision, allow the child to touch and play with equipment to be used if possible. Since any entry into the body is viewed as a threat, state that the child's body will remain the same, and use Band-Aids to reassure the child that the body is intact and parts will not "fall out."	Perform in treatment room. Restrain securely. Give short explanations and directions in a positive manner. Encourage control by having the child count to 10 or spell name. Allow child to cry. Give positive feedback for cooperation and getting through procedure. Encourage the child to draw afterward to explore the experience.
School-age child	Clear, thorough explanations are helpful. Use drawings, pictures, books, and contact with equipment. Teach stress reduction techniques such as deep breathing and visualization. Offer a choice of reward after procedure is completed.	Be ready to restrain child if needed. Allow child to remain in position by self if child is able to be still. Explain throughout procedure what is happening. Facilitate use of stress control techniques. Praise cooperative efforts.
Adolescent	Give clear explanations orally and in writing. Teach stress reduction techniques. Explore fear of certain procedures, such as staple removal or venipuncture.	Assist adolescent in self-control. Avoid using restraints. Assist with use of stress control techniques. Explain expected outcome and tell when results of test will be completed.

TABLE 4-9 Communication Strategy: Preparing a Toddler for Venipuncture

Twenty-eight-month-old Clarissa needs to have her blood drawn. How can the nurse best communicate with her?

1. Avoid telling Clarissa about the procedure in advance, since she has no concept of time and may become quite anxious. Tell her about the procedure just before it occurs and in simple terms: "We need to get a little blood from your arm. It will help us to find out if you are getting better. Your Mom will hold your arm real still so we can do it quickly."
2. Allow Clarissa to cry. Tell her it must be frightening and that you understand.
3. Perform the procedure in a treatment room so that Clarissa's bed and room are a safe haven.
4. Be sure Clarissa is restrained securely. Keep the joints above and below the area where blood is to be drawn immobilized. This way the procedure can be done quickly with the least trauma possible. Be sure the parent who is helping to restrain the child knows how to do this.
5. Use a Band-Aid to cover up the site. This may reassure Clarissa that her body is still intact.
6. Praise Clarissa's cooperation and acknowledge that the venipuncture is difficult.
7. Comfort Clarissa by holding, rocking, offering a favorite drink, and playing music. If her parents are present, they can comfort her.

Provide written information for adolescents, and schedule time for questions and discussions. Adolescents can make many choices about their own health care. They can be asked such questions as, "Do you want a local or general anesthetic?" or "Do you want your hand numbed for the intravenous start?" Some adolescents want their parents involved in their care, while others prefer to minimize the parents' role.

The procedure should be performed as quickly and efficiently as possible. Parents may wish to be involved or may prefer to be available afterward to comfort the child.

The parents or nurse can be designated to support the child. This may involve gentle touch, talking, singing, reassurance, or a stress reduction technique.

Procedures on young children are generally performed in a treatment room so the child's own room is viewed as a "safe" and relatively pain-free site. After the procedure the child can be taken back to his or her room for comfort and reassurance. A choice of reward often soothes the young child. Table 4–9 describes strategies for preparing a toddler for venipuncture.

Preparation for Surgery

A child's surgical experience can be elective, planned in advance, or a result of an emergency or trauma. How the child responds to the experience depends on the psychologic and physical preparation that he or she receives.

Preoperative Care

Preoperative care of the child includes both psychosocial and physical preparation for surgery. See the Nursing Care Plan for the Child Undergoing Surgery, which summarizes preoperative care.

Psychosocial Preparation. The goal of preoperative teaching is to reduce the fear associated with the unknown and decrease stress and anxiety associated with surgery. Teaching should be geared to the child's developmental level. If child life teachers are available, they can play an important role in preparing the child for surgery.

If the child will be in an intensive care unit or recovery room after surgery, a visit there before surgery can reduce the fear and anxiety associated with waking up in a strange environment filled with frightening sights, sounds, and smells. The use of tapes, anatomically correct puppets and dolls, drawings, and models is encouraged to teach the child about the surgical procedure. Playing with stethoscopes, gowns, masks, and syringes without needles also helps the child feel more in control.

Children should be reassured that their parents can accompany them to the operating room floor and will be waiting when they awaken from surgery.

Physical Preparation. Preoperative procedures and guidelines vary among hospitals and outpatient surgical centers. Preoperative checklists are used in ambulatory and acute care settings to ensure proper physical preparation of patients for surgery. A sample checklist is provided in Table 4–10.

TABLE 4–10 Preoperative Checklist

____ Check that consent forms are witnessed and signed and in the patient's chart.
____ Be sure the child's name band is in place.
____ Be sure any allergies are prominently noted in the child's chart.
____ Remove any prosthetic devices, including orthodontic appliances.
____ Check the child's mouth for loose teeth.
____ Remove eyeglasses.
____ Bathe and cleanse operative site if ordered.
____ Put the child in an operating room gown, allowing the child to wear underwear.
____ Check that all special tests have been completed and the results are in the child's chart.
____ Have the child void before surgery.
____ Keep the child NPO before surgery.
____ Give the child prescribed medications.
____ Transport the child safely to the operating room.

Postoperative Care

Postoperative care of the child includes both physical and psychologic care. The child's level of consciousness is evaluated, and vital signs are taken frequently. The surgical site is observed for drainage, and dressings are checked. The nurse monitors the child's intake and output and provides comfort and pain relief. (See Chapter 5 for details concerning pain management.) Parents should be allowed to visit with the child as soon after surgery as possible (Fig. 4–11). Refer to the Nursing Care Plan for the Child Undergoing Surgery, which summarizes postoperative care.

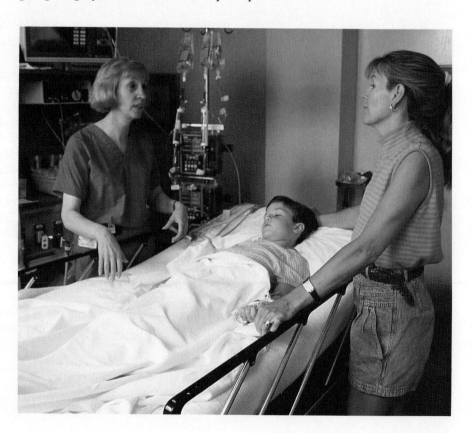

FIGURE 4–11 This child has just undergone cardiac surgery and is in the PICU. Although the child's physical care is immediate and important, remember that both the child and the family have strong psychosocial needs that need to be addressed concurrently. It is important to reunite the family as soon as possible after surgery.

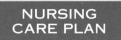

THE CHILD UNDERGOING SURGERY

GOAL	INTERVENTION	RATIONALE	EXPECTED OUTCOME

Preoperative Care

1. Knowledge Deficit related to preoperative and postoperative events

Child and family will verbalize procedures and events related to operation.	Ask questions of parent and child about surgery.	Prior knowledge and understanding can be reinforced and used to guide nurse's presentation.	Child and family are able to verbalize details about expected preoperative and postoperative events. They ask questions that demonstrate understanding.
	Teach about preoperative and postoperative events using appropriate developmental methods such as dolls, drawings, stories, and tours.	Developmental level determines the cognitive approach that works best for teaching.	
	Reinforce information family has received about purpose of surgery.	Physician may have explained operation.	
	Have child demostrate postoperative events that pertain to his or her case such as deep breathing, putting bandage on doll, taping intravenous line on doll, and pressing patient-controlled analgesia button.	Concrete experience promotes learning.	Child demonstrates skills needed in postoperative period.
	Allow parents and child to ask questions.	Learners must have opportunity to ask questions.	

2. Anxiety related to preoperative and postoperative events

Child and family will show decreased behavior indicating anxiety.	Question child about expectations of hospitalization and previous experiences.	Previous experiences can influence present anxiety level.	Child and family demonstrate less anxiety. They verbalize understanding and comfort in hospital routines.
	Orient child to hospital setting, routines, staff, and other patients.	Familiarity with the setting and people can decrease anxiety by removing unknown factors.	
	Institute age-appropriate play and interactions with the child.	Play can increase trust level and decrease anxiety.	Parents support child for traumatic procedures.
	Explain procedures and prepare for those that might cause trauma. Encourage parents to support the child.	Child is more likely to trust caregivers if they are truthful and if parents are present.	
	Allow parents and child to ask questions.	Questioning provides an opportunity to explain the unknown, which decreases anxiety.	

3. High Risk for Injury related to exposure to nosocomial infection and use of preoperative medication

Child will show no signs of infections.	Monitor vital signs at least every 4 hours. Inspect skin and respiratory status each shift.	Increase in vital sign levels, skin lesions, nasal drainage, or adventitious breath sounds can indicate signs of infection in the child.	Child's vital signs and assessment are within normal limits.

Continued.

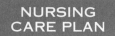
THE CHILD UNDERGOING SURGERY—CONTINUED

GOAL	INTERVENTION	RATIONALE	EXPECTED OUTCOME
Child will remain free of injury.	Report any variations from expected vital signs.	Symptoms are reported so surgery can be cancelled if necessary.	
	Keep side rails up after preoperative medication is given. Maintain NPO status when ordered. Transport the child to operating room safely secured.	Preoperative medication can alter level of consciousness. NPO status prevents aspiration.	The child is transported safely to the operating room.

Postoperative Care

4. High Risk for Infection related to surgical procedure and intravenous line

Child will be free of infection.	Monitor vital signs per hospital routine. Record and report changes from baseline.	Changes in vital signs, especially increased temperature and pulse, can indicate infection.	Child shows no signs of infection.
	Monitor surgical dressing and drains every hour. Change or reinforce dressings when wet.	Excess drainage may indicate infection. Wet dressing can allow organisms to come into contact with surgical wound.	Surgical wound heals without infection.
	Check intravenous site every 2 hours for redness, swelling, pain, or pallor.	Intravenous lines may become infiltrated or cause thrombophlebitis.	Intravenous line remains patent without signs of infection.
	Teach parents signs of infection before discharge. Teach parents aseptic technique for dressing change and wound care.	Parents report signs of infection and perform home care as needed.	Child continues to demonstrate no signs of infection at home.

5. High Risk for Constipation related to surgical procedure and anesthetics

Child will achieve and maintain normal bowel functioning by fourth postoperative day.	Auscultate bowel sounds every 4 hours. Offer liquids only when bowel sounds are present. Assess abdomen for distention.	Restricting fluids avoids distention if peristalsis is not normal.	Child has bowel movement within 2 to 3 days after surgery with normal pattern by fourth postoperative day.
	Document character and frequency of bowel movements. Advance diet as tolerated.	Knowledge of bowel status ensures early identification of constipation. Fluids and roughage promote normal bowel functioning.	
	Increased activity as ordered and tolerated.	Physical activity promotes peristalsis.	

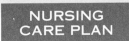

GOAL	INTERVENTION	RATIONALE	EXPECTED OUTCOME
6. Fluid Volume Excess or Deficit related to intravenous infusion and NPO status			
Child will achieve and maintain proper circulating volume. Child will tolerate oral intake when started with no nausea, vomiting, or dehydration present.	Monitor vital signs per hospital routines.	Changes in vital signs, especially pulse or blood pressure, can indicate fluid imbalance.	Child remains in fluid balance with no vomiting in postoperative period.
	Record intake and output. Be alert for fluid loss via dressings or watery stools. Evaluate hydration status by skin turgor and mucous membranes.	Intake and output are roughly equivalent. Urinary retention sometimes occurs postoperatively as a result of anesthesia. Fluid status can be assessed by skin and mucous membrane hydration.	
	Monitor laboratory values of hematocrit and hemoglobin.	Increased hematocrit and hemoglobin can indicate hemoconcentration and underhydration. Decreased serum values can indicate hemodilution or overhydration.	
	Begin oral intake after assessment of bowel sounds. Record vomiting. Administer antiemetics if indicated.	Vomiting can cause fluid loss.	
7. Ineffective Airway Clearance related to anesthetics and pain			
Child will maintain adequate ventilation with no respiratory impairment.	Auscultate lungs every 2 hours. Record rate, rhythm, and quality of respiration. Evaluate respiratory rate after analgesics. Administer oxygen if ordered.	Early identification of respiratory difficulty aids early treatment. Analgesics, especially morphine, may slow respiratory rate. Oxygen may facilitate breathing status postoperatively.	Child remains free of respiratory complications.
	Reposition child every 2 hours. Encourage deep breathing and coughing every 2 hours. Use incentive spirometer, pinwheels, or other blow toys appropriate for developmental level of child.	Repositioning ensures expansion of all lung fields. All areas of lungs must be expanded. Mucus is expectorated.	
	Ensure proper intake and output.	Balanced fluid status ensures liquification of secretions and prevents excess fluid accumulation.	

Continued.

GOAL	INTERVENTION	RATIONALE	EXPECTED OUTCOME
8. Pain related to surgical procedure			
Child will maintain adequate comfort level.	Assess behavioral cues (e.g., crying, movement, guarding).	Behavior of preverbal children provides clues to pain experience.	The child's pain is controlled as demonstrated by a low number on the pain control scale (behavioral or verbal).
	Use appropriate pain scale with verbal children.	Pain scales allow children to quantify amount of pain (see Chapter 5).	
	Administer prescribed pain medications on a regular basis.	Narcotics and non-narcotic analgesics alter pain perception.	
	Use age-appropriate non-pharmacologic methods of pain control (e.g., distraction, repositioning).	Nonpharmacologic interventions interfere with pain perception.	
9. High Risk for Impaired Skin Integrity related to limited mobility after surgery			
Child's skin will remain intact.	Turn and reposition child every 2 hours.	Repositioning takes pressure off skin and allows increased circulation.	Child develops no pressure areas.
	Keep linens clean and dry.	Clean linen decreases chance of skin breakdown.	Wound heals without complication.
	Check pressure areas when turning and rub erythematous areas with lotion.	Rubbing increases circulation.	
	Get child up and ambulate when ordered.	Movement decreases pressure on skin.	
	Check incision for drainage, redness, and intactness of staples or stitching every 4 to 8 hours.	Early identification of infection or problems with wound healing can ensure fast treatment.	
10. Anxiety (Child and Family) related to equipment and surgical outcome			
Child and family will verbalize comfort with postoperative care and outcome.	Explain monitors, drains, dressings, intravenous lines, and procedures.	Knowledge of purpose decreases anxiety.	Child and family demonstrate coping skills to deal with hospitalization.
	Reassure child and family that anxiety is a normal response to the stressful event of surgery.	Knowledge of what is expected decreases anxiety.	
	Encourage parental presence and care of the child.	Child's anxiety decreases with parental presence.	
11. Knowledge Deficit (Child and Family) related to needed home care			
Child and family will verbalize self-care required at home.	Provide oral and written home care instructions regarding surgical wound care, medications, activities, and diet.	Teaching regarding home care is necessary early in hospitalization.	Child and family demonstrate skills needed for home care following discharge. They verbalize plans for future care.
	Provide a number to call for questions or concerns. Instruct on follow-up visits.	Parents need to know emergency information and that follow-up care is required.	

Preparation for Long-Term Care

When ill or injured children require long-term care, they are often transferred from an acute care hospital to a rehabilitation center or other long-term care facility. The rehabilitation phase of the treatment does not begin at the time of discharge from the acute care hospital but early in the hospitalization phase. The plan of care is instituted in the hospital, interventions and therapies are begun, and plans are made for continued care.

When it becomes apparent that a child will need long-term care, the health care team explores with the family the options and resources available to provide such care:

- Home care with support services such as visiting nurses and physical therapists
- A long-term care facility
- A specialized rehabilitation center that can provide care for an extended period

The family should make the decision about which option will work best, considering the needs of the child, the financial implications, the roles and supports available to the family unit, and the resources available in the community. Guidelines to assist parents in evaluating rehabilitation centers are available from the National Head Injury Foundation (see Appendix F).

Nurses in acute care hospitals frequently coordinate services when transfer to another facility occurs. This involves giving information about the child's history, plan of care, and treatment to the new facility. Forms are available to assist the person responsible for coordinating the transfer. Families will need support and assistance in dealing with the transfer from the acute care setting to another facility.

Preparation for Home Care

Nurses play an important role in preparing the child and family for discharge home. When care will continue, the nurse works with the social service department, home care agencies, and the family to plan for equipment, procedures, and other home care needs. Home care nurses then take over the child's care and assist families to meet the child's health care needs.

Assessing the Child in Preparation for Discharge

Discharge plans should begin early in the child's hospitalization. A health care team, including physician, nurse, social worker, discharge planner, and family, works together to ensure a smooth transition home. An assessment of the family's ability to manage the child's care and of the appropriateness of the home for providing care must be made.[9]

Children with multisystem problems may require home care involving specialized equipment and personnel. Early planning gives the family time to investigate health insurance benefits, support services in the community, and other needs before discharge.

When a child is to be discharged home, the school district should be contacted and plans for education made. This involves an assessment of the child by the school district and formulation of an **individualized education plan** (IEP). The IEP may include home tutors, specialized services from persons such as physical or speech therapists, or arrangements for transport of the handicapped child to the school and provisions for special medical care as needed.

LEGAL CONSIDERATIONS

The Education for All Handicapped Children Act, P.L. 94-142, mandates that public education be provided for all handicapped children from 2 to 21 years of age.

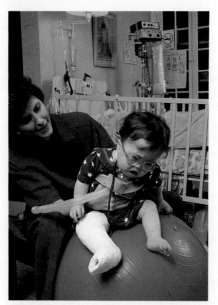

FIGURE 4-12 This child with chronic medical problems is being cared for at home. Are there any legal implications for the hospital and the nurse associated with the preparation of the child and family for home care?

Home Care Teaching

The family may need to learn physical and rehabilitative procedures for the child's care. Short-term care may be necessary until the child regains full function. In other situations care may be required throughout the child's life. This may involve measuring vital signs or determining blood glucose levels. For the child requiring complex long-term care, parents may need to learn about intravenous lines, medications, oxygen administration, or ventilators (Fig. 4–12). The machinery used for care must be explained and demonstrated, and the parents must show that they can use it correctly. They must understand and be able to identify symptoms of distress and report them immediately to the health care provider. The education provided and the parents' ability to perform care are discussed with a visiting nurse or individual who manages the home care program. Parents should be encouraged to learn cardiopulmonary resuscitation.

Help parents explore options for respite. If they cannot provide daily care or need a break, they should be able to rely on others for a short period. Some agencies are available to provide respite care.

Preparing Parents to Act as Case Managers

The family is an integral part of the plan of care for an ill or hospitalized child. The child with a chronic illness or an injury requiring long-term care will probably require the services of numerous health care personnel or health care agencies. One person needs to be identified as a **case manager** to coordinate health care and to prevent gaps and overlaps. In some hospitals nurses act as case managers. They may organize a patient care conference while the child with a chronic condition is hospitalized. Management goals are set and decisions are made about which health care provider or agency is responsible for helping the child meet each goal.

Parents can also be case managers. The parent as case manager coordinates medical care, hospital stays, and visits to specialists; meets with school district representatives to plan the individualized education program for the child; finds equipment, personnel, and other services for home care; and manages the child's overall care.

Nurses should strongly encourage parents who want to take over case management to do so. They can be assisted to learn the management skills required. Many communities have workshops for parents who are managing the complex care of their children.

REFERENCES

1 Bowlby, J. (1960). Separation anxiety. *International Journal of Psychoanalysis, 41*, 89–113.

2 Bibace, R., & Walsh, M. (1981). Children's conceptions of illness. In Bibace, R., & Walsh, M. (Eds.). *Children's conceptions of health, illness, and bodily function.* San Francisco: Jossey-Bass.

3 Logsdon, D.A. (1991). Conceptions of health and health behaviors of preschool children. *Journal of Pediatric Nursing, 6*(6), 396–405.

4 Knafl, K., Cavallari, K., & Dixon, D. (1988). *Pediatric hospitalization.* Boston: Scott, Foresman & Co.

5 Greenberg, L.A. (1991). Teaching children who are learning disabled about illness and hospitalization. *American Journal of Maternal-Child Nursing, 16*(5), 260–263.

6 Schaefer, G., & O'Connor, K. (1983). *Handbook of play therapy.* New York: John Wiley & Sons.

7 Kreitmeyer, B., & Heiney, S. (1992). Storytelling as a therapeutic technique in a group for school-aged oncology patients. *Children's Health Care, 21*(1), 14–20.

8 Furth, G. (1988). *The secret world of drawings: Healing through art.* Boston: Sigo Press.

9 McCoy, P., & Votroubek, W. (1990). *Pediatric home care: A comprehensive approach.* Rockville, MD: Aspen Publications.

SUGGESTED READINGS

Abbot, K. (1990). Therapeutic use of play in psychological preparation of preschool children undergoing cardiac therapy. *Issues in Comprehensive Pediatric Nursing, 13*(4), 265–277.

Azarnoff, P. (1990). Teaching materials for pediatric health professionals. *Journal of Pediatric Health, 4*(6), 282–289.

Azarnoff, P. (1983). *Health, illness, and disability: A guide to books for children and young adults.* New York: R.R. Bowker Co.

Azarnoff, P. (Ed.). (1983). *Preparation of young healthy children for possible hospitalization: The issues.* Santa Monica, CA: Pediatric Projects.

Azarnoff, P., & Flegal, S. (1980). *A pediatric play program.* Springfield, IL: Charles C Thomas.

Byers, M.L. (1987). Same day surgery: A preschooler's experience. *American Journal of Maternal-Child Nursing, 16*(3), 277–282.

Jones, E., Badger, T., & Moore, I. (1992). Children's knowledge of internal anatomy: Conceptual orientation and review of research. *Journal of Pediatric Nursing, 7*(4), 262–268.

Oster, G., & Gould, P. (1987). *Using drawings in assessment and therapy.* New York: Brunner/Maazel.

Petrillo, M., & Sanger, S. (1980). *Emotional care of hospitalized children.* Philadelphia: J.B. Lippincott.

Ramsey, A.M., & Siroky, A. (1988). The use of puppets to teach school-age children with asthma. *Pediatric Nursing, 14*(3), 187–190.

Redman, B.K. (1993). *The process of patient education* (7th ed.). St. Louis: Mosby–Year Book.

Riddle, I. (1990). Reflections on children's play. *American Journal of Maternal-Child Nursing, 19*(4), 271–279.

Schaefer, G., & O'Connor, K. (1983). *Handbook of play therapy.* New York: John Wiley & Sons.

Smallwood, S. (1988). Preparing children for surgery. *AORN, 47*(1), 177–185.

Woldum, K., Ryan-Morrell, V., Towson, M., Bower, K., & Zander, K. (1985). *Patient education.* Rockville, MD: Aspen Publications.

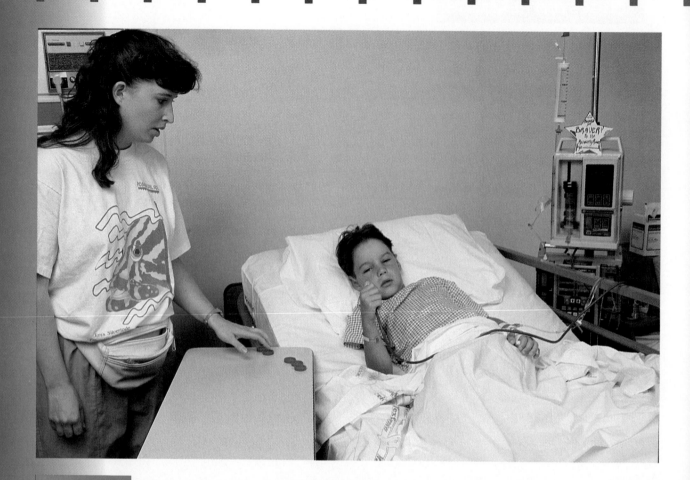

M anuel, who is 4 years old, was struck by a car. Six hours ago he had surgery to repair a liver laceration. After spending 3 hours in the recovery room, he was moved to the pediatric inpatient unit. He has an intravenous line in place, as well as a nasogastric tube for suction. His abdominal dressing is clean and dry.

Manuel's mother is rooming in with him during his hospital stay. She thinks her son is in pain because he is thrashing around, and she asks the nurse to give him some pain medication. When the nurse enters Manuel's room, he is napping and his facial expression indicates that he is not in pain. When the nurse attempts to straighten his position in bed, he moans. The nurse asks Manuel if he hurts, and he shakes his head no. According to Manuel's chart, he received pain medication just before his transfer from the recovery room. His physician has ordered pain medication every 3 to 4 hours as needed. How do you know whether Manuel is in pain? Can you expect him to tell you if he feels pain? Is any additional assessment needed to justify giving Manuel more pain medication? What other pain relief measures could reduce or help to control his pain?

PAIN ASSESSMENT AND MANAGEMENT

TERMINOLOGY

acute pain Sudden pain of short duration that is associated with a tissue-damaging stimulus.

chronic pain Persistent pain lasting longer than 6 months, generally associated with a prolonged disease process.

conscious sedation Light sedation during which the child maintains airway reflexes and responds to verbal stimuli.

deep sedation A controlled state of depressed consciousness or unconsciousness in which the child may experience partial or complete loss of protective reflexes.

distraction The ability to focus attention on something other than pain, such as an activity, music, or a story.

electroanalgesia Transcutaneous electrical nerve stimulation (TENS), which competes with pain stimuli for transmission to the spinal cord.

equianalgesic dose The amount of drug, whether administered orally or parenterally, needed to produce the same analgesic effect.

NSAIDs The nonsteroidal antiinflammatory drugs used for pain treatment.

opioids Natural and synthetic narcotic drugs used for pain treatment.

pain An unpleasant sensory and emotional experience associated with actual or potential tissue damage. Pain exists when the patient says it does.

patient-controlled analgesia A method for administration of an intravenous analgesic, such as morphine, using a computerized pump that the patient controls.

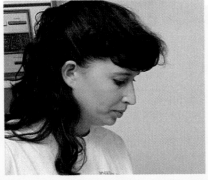

❝ Perhaps the most difficult part of working with children is seeing them in pain. They try to be brave and often handle it better than adults, but it is still difficult as a health care professional.❞

Pain, a neurologic response to tissue injury, is an unpleasant sensory and emotional experience associated with actual or potential tissue damage. It exists when the patient says it does, and everyone has his or her own perceptions of pain.

Pain may be either acute or chronic. **Acute pain,** which is sudden pain of short duration, may be associated with a single event, such as surgery, or an acute episode of a condition such as sickle cell disease. **Chronic pain,** which is persistent pain lasting longer than 6 months, is generally associated with a prolonged disease process such as juvenile rheumatoid arthritis.

Outdated Beliefs About Pain in Children

In the past, children did not receive adequate treatment for pain. Undertreatment still occurs. Health care professionals once believed that children feel less pain than adults (Table 5–1). In fact, most physicians did not prescribe pain medication for children or ordered it only as needed. This undertreatment was based on the attitudes of health care professionals about pain, the difficulty and complexity of pain assessment in children, and inadequate research.[1]

Research has shown that past beliefs about children's perception of pain were incorrect. Neonates and infants do feel and remember pain. By 6 months of age, children demonstrate anticipatory fear of pain when taken to a location where they once experienced pain.[2] Health care professionals now recognize that children do not complain of pain because they are afraid that the injection to relieve pain will hurt more than the pain already does.

Pain Indicators

Physiologic Indicators

Acute pain stimulates the adrenergic nervous system and results in physiologic changes, including tachycardia, tachypnea, hypertension, pupil dilation, pallor, and increased perspiration. As the body adapts physiologically,

---

TABLE 5-1 Outdated Beliefs About Pain and Pain Medication in Children

- Children without obvious physical reasons for pain are not likely to have pain.
- Neonates do not feel pain.
- Children do not feel pain with the same intensity as adults because a child's nervous system is immature.
- Children tolerate discomfort well. They become accustomed to pain after having it for a while.
- Children tell you if they are in pain. They do not need medication unless they appear to be in pain.
- Children are not in pain if they can be distracted or they are sleeping.
- Children recover more quickly than adults from painful experiences such as surgery.
- Parents exaggerate or aggravate their child's pain.
- Children have no memory of pain.
- Narcotics are dangerous for children because they can cause respiratory depression and addiction.
- The best route for giving analgesics is intramuscular.
- After surgery, children should not receive the next analgesic dose until they show obvious signs of pain.
- As-needed medication orders mean that medication should be given as infrequently as possible.

PEDIATRIC NURSING

vital signs return to near normal and perspiration decreases after several minutes. Thus changes in vital signs are not a reliable indicator of pain in children because they last such a short time.

Chronic pain may be associated with signs of vagal stimulation such as a fall in heart rate, respiratory rate, and blood pressure (Fig. 5–1).

Behavioral Indicators

Children in acute pain behave in many of the same ways as children who show signs of fear and anxiety.[3] These behaviors include the following:

- Restless and agitated or hyperalert and vigilant
- Short attention span (child is difficult to distract)
- Irritability (child is difficult to comfort)
- Facial grimacing, posturing (guarding a painful joint by avoiding movement), or protecting the painful area
- Anorexia
- Lethargy
- Sleep disturbances

Children often suffer additional emotional distress and fear that the discomfort will worsen. Depression and aggressive behavior are frequently overlooked as indicators of pain.

Behavioral indicators of chronic pain and pain of long duration include posturing and inactivity, restricted activities of daily living, and no anxiety about pain.[4]

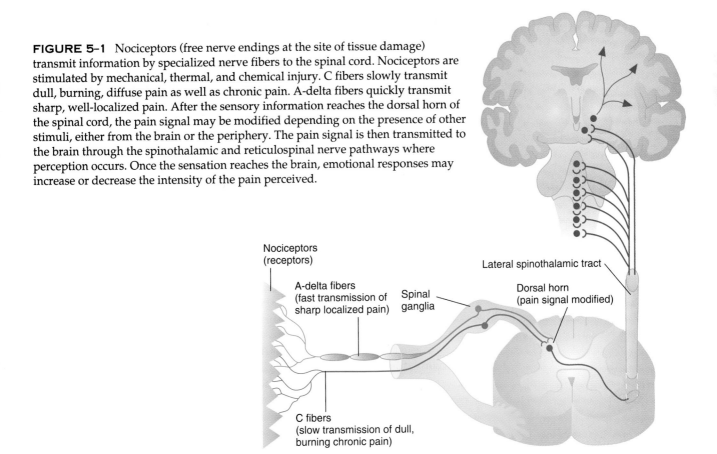

FIGURE 5–1 Nociceptors (free nerve endings at the site of tissue damage) transmit information by specialized nerve fibers to the spinal cord. Nociceptors are stimulated by mechanical, thermal, and chemical injury. C fibers slowly transmit dull, burning, diffuse pain as well as chronic pain. A-delta fibers quickly transmit sharp, well-localized pain. After the sensory information reaches the dorsal horn of the spinal cord, the pain signal may be modified depending on the presence of other stimuli, either from the brain or the periphery. The pain signal is then transmitted to the brain through the spinothalamic and reticulospinal nerve pathways where perception occurs. Once the sensation reaches the brain, emotional responses may increase or decrease the intensity of the pain perceived.

Nociceptors (receptors)

A-delta fibers (fast transmission of sharp localized pain)

Spinal ganglia

Lateral spinothalamic tract

Dorsal horn (pain signal modified)

C fibers (slow transmission of dull, burning chronic pain)

TABLE 5-2 Physiologic Consequences of Unrelieved Pain in Children

Responses to Pain	Potential Physiologic Consequences
Respiratory Changes	
Rapid shallow breathing	Alkalosis
Inadequate lung expansion	Atelectasis, bronchiectasis
Inadequate cough	Retention of secretions
Cardiovascular Changes	
Tachycardia	Tissue ischemia
Metabolic Changes	
Increased metabolic rate with increased perspiration	Increased fluid and electrolyte losses

Modified from Eland, J.M. (1990). Pain in children. *Nursing Clinics of North America, 25,* 871–884.

■ **CLINICAL TIP**

The presence of physiologic symptoms such as nausea, fatigue, dyspnea, bladder and bowel distention, and fever may influence the intensity of pain felt by a child. The child's behavior or responses to pain stimuli may also be affected by fear, anxiety, separation from parents, anger, culture, age, or a previous pain experience.

Consequences of Pain

Unrelieved pain is stressful and has many undesirable physiologic consequences (Table 5–2). For example, the child with acute postoperative pain takes shallow breaths and suppresses coughs to avoid more pain. These self-protective actions increase the potential for respiratory complications. Unrelieved pain may also delay the return of normal gastric and bowel functions. Anorexia associated with pain may delay the healing process. The long-term effects of pain on the child's physical or psychologic condition are unknown.

■ Pain Assessment

No laboratory tests are routinely used to assess pain. Prolonged, severe pain produces a physiologic stress response that includes the chemical release of catecholamines, cortisol, aldosterone, and other corticosteroids. In some cases increased levels of these chemicals may be detected by routinely ordered laboratory tests,[5] and untreated pain should be considered a potential explanation. Insulin secretion also decreases, leading to increased amounts of glucose and severe hyperglycemia.[3] Existing conditions such as infection, trauma, and anemia may also cause the vital sign changes seen with sudden pain.

The goal of pain assessment is to provide accurate information about the location and intensity of pain and its effects on the child's functioning. When assessing pain in children, keep the following questions in mind:

- What is happening in tissues that might cause pain? Assume that children who have had surgery, injury, or illness are experiencing pain, since these events also cause pain in adults.
- What external factors could be causing pain? For example, is the cast too tight or is the child poorly positioned in bed?
- Are there any indicators of pain, either physiologic or behavioral?
- How is the child responding emotionally? For example, is the child anxious, fearful, depressed, or angry?[6]
- How does the child or parent rate the pain?

Pain History

Parents can provide a great deal of information about the child's response to pain, such as the following:

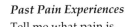

TABLE 5-3 Pediatric Pain History for Children and Parents

Questions for Children	Questions for Parents
Past Pain Experiences	
Tell me what pain is.	What word(s) does your child use to describe pain?
Tell me about the hurt you have had before.	Describe pain experiences your child has previously had.
Do you tell others when you hurt? Who?	Does your child tell you or others when he or she is in pain?
What do you do for yourself when you are hurting?	How do you know when your child is in pain?
What do you want others to do for you when you hurt?	How does your child usually react to pain?
What don't you want others to do for you when you hurt?	What do you do for your child when he or she is in pain?
What helps the most to take your hurt away?	What does your child do to manage his or her pain?
Is there anything special you want me to know about you when you hurt? What?	What works best to reduce or take away your child's pain?
	Is there anything special you would like me to know about your child and pain?
Present Pain Experiences	
Where is the pain?	Tell me about the pain your child is now having. Where is it and what does it feel like?
What does it feel like?	
What do you think is causing the pain?	What would you like me to do for your child?
What would you like me to do for you?	

Modified from Hester, N.O., & Barcus, C.S. (1986). Assessment and management of pain in children. *Pediatrics: Nursing Update, 1,* 2–8.

By using patient-controlled analgesia, the older child is able to regulate the intake of an intravenous analgesic such as morphine.

- How the child typically expresses pain, both verbally and behaviorally. Children and parents use similar terms to describe pain.[7] Some examples of words used are a hurt, stinging, sore, cutting, burning, itching, hot, and tight.[8] Knowing the appropriate word to use makes communicating with the child easier.
- The child's previous experiences with painful situations.
- How the child copes with pain. The child with several past pain experiences may not exhibit the same types of stressful behaviors as the child with few pain experiences.
- The parent's and child's preferences for analgesic use.

Older children may also be able to give a history of painful procedures. When attempting to obtain information about the child's pain experiences and present level of pain, ask the child and parent similar open-ended questions. Sample questions are given in Table 5–3. Many children modify their pain descriptions depending on the type of questions asked and what they expect will happen as a result of their response.

Cultural Influences on Pain

Children's culture and social learning have a tremendous influence on their expression of pain. Cultural traditions often guide children about self-control, coping, and enlisting the assistance of others.[8,9] Children learn di-

■ CULTURAL CONSIDERATIONS

Some ethnic groups, such as Asian, Anglo-Saxon-Germanic, and Irish, do not openly express pain. People of Italian and Jewish descent are more likely to use both verbal and nonverbal methods to express pain freely. However, children have individualized responses, and younger children have had less time to acquire culturally learned behaviors.

rectly and indirectly from their parents about how to respond to pain. By showing approval and disapproval, parents teach their children how to behave when in pain. This instruction includes the following:

- How much discomfort justifies a complaint
- How to express the complaint
- How and when to stop complaining
- Whom to approach for pain relief

For example, boys in the United States are usually encouraged to hide their pain by acting brave and not crying. Girls are often encouraged to express their pain openly. Children also observe other family members in pain and imitate their responses.[10]

TABLE 5-4 Behavioral Responses and Verbal Descriptions of Pain by Children of Different Developmental Stages

Age Group	Behavioral Response	Verbal Description
Infants		
< 6 months	Generalized body movements, chin quivering, facial grimacing, poor feeding	Cries
6–12 months	Reflex withdrawal to stimulus, facial grimacing, disturbed sleep, irritability, restlessness	Cries
Toddlers		
1–3 years	Localized withdrawal, resistance of entire body, aggressive behavior, disturbed sleep	Cries and screams, cannot describe intensity or type of pain
Preschoolers		
3–6 years (preoperational)	Active physical resistance, directed aggressive behavior, strikes out physically and verbally when hurt, low frustration level	Can identify location of pain, denies pain, may believe his or her pain is obvious to others
School-Age Children		
7–9 years (concrete operations)	Passive resistance, clenches fists, holds body rigidly still, suffers emotional withdrawal, engages in plea bargaining	Can specify location of pain and describe its physical characteristics
10–12 Years		
(transitional)	May pretend comfort to project bravery, may regress with stress and anxiety	Able to describe intensity and location with more characteristics, able to describe psychologic pain
Adolescents		
12–18 years (formal operations)	Want to behave in a socially acceptable manner (like adults), show a controlled behavioral response	More sophisticated descriptions as experience is gained

Pain Assessment Scales

Various pain scales have been developed to assess pain in children (Figs. 5–2 to 5–6). A child's responses to and understanding of pain depend on the child's age and stage of development (Tables 5–4 and 5–5).[11] For example, neonates cannot anticipate pain and may not demonstrate typical behavior associated with a painful response. Young children are unable to give a detailed description of their pain because of their limited vocabulary and pain experiences. Depending on their developmental stage, children use different coping strategies, such as escape, postponement or avoidance, diversion, and imagery, to deal with pain.

Physical and behavioral indicators are used to quantify pain in children. Some pain assessment scales rely on the nurse's observation of the child's behavior if the child is nonverbal. The Children's Hospital of Eastern Ontario Pain Scale (CHEOPS) (Table 5–6) and the Objective Pain Scale (Table 5–7) are examples of behavioral assessment tools developed to quantify pain in nonverbal postoperative children.[12,13] Most scales depend on the child's report of pain intensity (Table 5–7). These assessment tools cannot determine whether children feel the same amount of pain as adults who undergo similar procedures.

■ GROWTH AND DEVELOPMENT CONSIDERATIONS

Identify the child's stage of development for readiness to use pain scales.

- Assess the child's language skills (ability to use words in sequence, follow simple directions, and answer simple questions).
- Ask the child to count his or her fingers or up to 20.
- Determine whether the child can understand concepts such as more or less and higher or lower.

TABLE 5-5 Children's Understanding of Pain by Developmental Stage

Developmental Stage	Understanding of Pain
Infants	
< 6 months	No apparent understanding of pain; infants do have memory of pain; neonates exposed to repeated painful experiences in intensive care unit demonstrate memory of pain by breathholding when approached by care providers
6–12 months	Anticipate a painful event such as an immunization with fear
Toddlers	
1–3 years	Demonstrate a fear of painful situations; use common words for pain such as "owie" and "boo-boo"
Preschoolers	
3–6 years (preoperational)	Pain is a hurt; do not relate pain to illness but may relate pain to an injury; often believe pain is punishment; do not believe an injection takes pain away
School-Age Children	
7–9 years (concrete operations)	Can understand simple relationships between pain and disease but have no clear understanding of the cause of pain; can understand the need for painful procedures to monitor or treat disease; may recognize psychologic pain related to grief and hurt feelings
10–12 years (transitional)	Have a more complex awareness of physical and psychologic pain, such as moral dilemmas and mental pain
Adolescents	
12–18 years (formal operations)	Have a capacity for sophisticated and complex understanding of the causes of physical and mental pain; can relate to the pain experienced by others; pain has both qualitative and quantitative characteristics

TABLE 5–6 Pain Assessment Scales

Scale and Age Group	Administration	Use
Objective Pain Scale <7 years	Observe the child's crying, movement, agitation level, blood pressure, and body language or verbal evaluation, and rate according to scale	Behavioral assessment for postoperative pain or painful procedures; does not require patient participation; scale may identify nonspecific stress in preverbal as well as verbal children
CHEOPS 1–7 years	Observe the child's cry, facial expression, torso position, leg position, touch-painful area, and verbal complaints; select the numerical score for each category after 5 seconds	Primarily behavioral assessment for postoperative pain or following painful procedures; researchers have no specific score indicating pain in need of medication; in preverbal children scale may measure nonspecific stress rather than only pain
Eland Color Tool 4–9 years	Child picks a crayon color representing the most pain, then color of next most pain, etc. until four crayons selected; then child colors the body outline to indicate the location of the areas of hurt by level of pain	You need six crayons: black, purple, blue, red, green, and orange; no one color is most often selected by children as representing the most pain; limited reliabilty and validity data*
Oucher Scale 3–7 years (Fig. 5–2)	Child selects face that best fits his or her level of pain; older child can select a number between 0 and 100	Useful in hospital settings; child must understand concepts of higher/lower and more/less; cultural versions available; tool has been successfully tested for reliability and validity in some age groups*

FIGURE 5–2†

A   B   C

*Reliability is the extent to which the same score is obtained when an instrument or scale is used either by different persons or by the same person at different times. Validity is the extent to which an instrument or scale measures what it is supposed to measure.

†Source: **A,** The Caucasian version of the Oucher, developed and copyrighted by Judith E. Beyer, RN, PhD, 1983. **B,** The African-American version of the Oucher, developed and copyrighted by Mary J. Denyes, RN, PhD, and Antonia M. Villarruel, RN, PhD, 1990. **C,** The Hispanic version of the Oucher, developed and copyrighted by Antonia M. Villarruel, RN, PhD, and Mary J. Denyes, RN, PhD, 1990.

TABLE 5-6 Pain Assessment Scales—*Continued*

Scale and Age Group	Administration	Use
Poker Chip Scale 3–7 years (Fig. 5–3)	Child selects the number of chips or checkers (0–5) that matches level of hurt (1 = a little hurt, 5 = the most hurt)	Useful in hospital settings; child must have number concepts from 1 to 5; then get the child's perception of pain

FIGURE 5–3

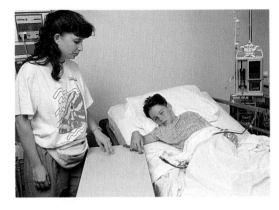   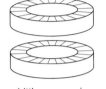

A tiny bit of hurt   Little more pain   Still more pain   Most hurt of all

Faces Pain Scale (pre-school children) (Fig. 5–4)	Child selects from one of several pictures of faces from happy to sad; child selects one most like his or her pain	Provides a global index of how the child perceives pain; reliable and valid for children over 5 years

FIGURE 5–4*

Numeric Pain Scale 9 years–adult (Fig. 5–5)	Ask child to rate pain felt on a line with 10 marks (1 = a little pain, 10 = the most pain)	Child must be verbal; easy to carry tool to patient

FIGURE 5–5

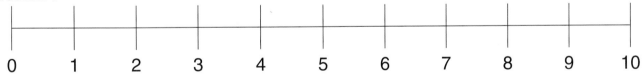

0   1   2   3   4   5   6   7   8   9   10

Pediatric Pain Questionnaire	Child selects pain descriptors from checklist, rates current and average pain intensity with visual analogue scale (Fig. 5–6), and uses own color choices to identify different pain intensities on pain map of body	Parent, child, and adolescent forms exist; parent form provides information about history of pain problem and its management; useful for chronic pain

FIGURE 5–6†

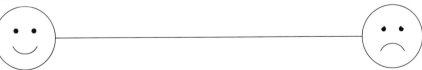

*From McGrath, P.A., deVeber L., & Hearn, M.: Multidimensional pain assessment in children. In Fields, H., Dubner R., & Cervero, F. (Eds.). (1985). *Advances in pain research and therapy.* New York: Raven Press, pp. 387–393.
†From Varni, J.W., Thompson, K.L., & Hanson V. (1987). *Pain 28,* 27–38.

Surgery and trauma result in multiple sites of pain (incision or laceration, cut or bruised muscles, interrupted blood supply, nasogastric tube placement, insertion sites of intravenous lines). When using pain scales in the assessment of a verbal child, attempt to identify all sites of pain. Then evaluate the intensity of pain at each site.

TABLE 5–7 Objective Pain Scale*

Categories and Criteria	Definitions	Score
Blood Pressure		
Systolic change	≤10% of preoperative value	0
	11%–20% of preoperative value	1
	≥21% of preoperative value	2
Crying		
Not crying	Awake and not crying	0
Crying but responds when touched, reassured, or helped by parent or nurse (TLC)	Crying but responds to TLC	1
Crying and does not respond to TLC	Crying uncontrollably; no response to TLC	2
Movement		
None	Asleep, or if awake, lying or playing quietly	0
Restless	Unable to sit or lie still; frequent position change; no threat of self-harm	1
Thrashing	Kicking or squirming; potential for self-harm; has to be protected or restrained for safety	2
Agitation		
Asleep or calm	Asleep or awake and calm	0
Mild	Tense; voice quivering; responds rationally to questions or attempts to console	1
Hysterical	Does not appear rational; eyes wide; cannot be consoled; may cling to nurse or parent	2
Verbal Evaluation or Body Language in Preverbal Child		
Asleep or states no pain, or no special posture		0
Mild pain or cannot localize, flexing extremities	Complains of general feeling of discomfort, but unable to describe location of pain, or states pain is mild in nature; legs drawn up; arms may be folded across body	1
Moderate pain, can localize, holding location of pain	Complains of pain that is bothersome; is able to point to or describe location of pain; holding, guarding, or touching location of pain; infants with legs drawn up, fists clenched	2

A score of ≥6 signifies significant pain, and the child should receive a narcotic analgesic.

*For explanation of how this scale is used, see Table 5–6.
TLC, tender loving care.
From Norden, J., Hannallah, R., & others. (1990). Reliability of an objective pain scale in children. *Anesthesia Analgesia*, 72, Abstract No. S199. Copyright © International Anesthesia Research Society, Williams & Wilkins.

▨ Medical Management of Pain

The U.S. government recently published guidelines for management of pain in all age groups, including children.[14] The recommendations for pain management include both drug and nondrug measures. Drug interventions include the use of **opioids** (narcotics) and nonsteroidal antiinflammatory drugs **(NSAIDs)**.

TABLE 5-8 Opioid Analgesics and Recommended Doses for Children and Adolescents

Drug	Approximate Equianalgesic Oral Dose	Approximate Equianalgesic Parenteral Dose	Recommended Starting Dose (Adults >50 kg Body Weight)		Recommended Starting Dose (Children and Adults <50 kg Body Weight*)	
			Oral	Parenteral	Oral	Parenteral
Opioid Agonist						
Morphine†	30 mg q 3–4 hr (around-the-clock-dosing) 60 mg q 3–4 hr (single dose or intermittent dosing)	10 mg q 3–4 hr	30 mg q 3–4 hr	10 mg q 3–4 hr	0.3 mg/kg q 3–4 hr	0.1 mg/kg q 3–4 hr
Codeine‡	130 mg q 3–4 hr	75 mg q 3–4 hr	60 mg q 3–4 hr	60 mg q 2 hr (intramuscular/ subcutaneous)	1 mg/kg q 3–4 hr§	NR
Hydromorphone† (Dilaudid)	7.5 mg q 3–4 hr	1.5 mg q 3–4 hr	6 mg q 3–4 hr	1.5 mg q 3–4 hr	0.06 mg/kg q 3–4 hr	0.015 mg/kg q 3–4 hr
Hydrocodone (in Lorcet, Lortab, Vicodin, others)	30 mg q 3–4 hr	NA	10 mg q 3–4 hr	NA	0.2 mg/kg q 3–4 hr§	NA
Levorphanol (Levo-Dromoran)	4 mg q 6–8 hr	2 mg q 6–8 hr	4 mg q 6–8 hr	2 mg q 6–8 hr	0.04 mg/kg q 6–8 hr	0.02 mg/kg q 6–8 hr
Meperidine (Demerol)	300 mg q 2–3 hr	100 mg q 3 hr	NR	100 mg q 3 hr	NR	0.75 mg/kg q 2–3 hr
Methadone (Dolophine, others)	20 mg q 6–8 hr	10 mg q 6–8 hr	20 mg q 6–8 hr	10 mg q 6–8 hr	0.2 mg/kg q 6–8 hr	0.1 mg/kg q 6–8 hr
Oxycodone (Roxicodone, also in Percocet, Percodan, Tylox, others)	30 mg q 3–4 hr	NA	10 mg q 3–4 hr	NA	0.2 mg/kg q 3–4 hr§	NA
Oxymorphone† (Numorphan)	NA	1 mg q 3–4 hr	NA	1 mg q 3–4 hr	NR	NR
Opioid Agonist-Antagonist and Partial Agonist						
Buprenorphine (Buprenex)	NA	0.3–0.4 mg q 6–8 hr	NA	0.4 mg q 6–8 hr	NA	0.004 mg/kg q 6–8 hr
Butorphanol (Stadol)	NA	2 mg q 3–4 hr	NA	2 mg q 3–4 hr	NA	NR
Nalbuphine (Nubain)	NA	10 mg q 3–4 hr	NA	10 mg q 3–4 hr	NA	0.1 mg/kg q 3–4 hr
Pentazocine (Talwin, other)	150 mg q 3–4 hr	60 mg q 3–4 hr	50 mg q 4–6 hr	NR	NR	NR

From Acute Pain Management Guideline Panel. (1992). *Acute pain management in infants, children, and adolescents: Operative and medical procedures. Quick reference guide for clinicians.* (AHCPR Pub. No. 92-0020). Rockville, MD: Agency for Health Care Policy and Research, U.S. Public Health Service, Department of Health and Human Services.

Note: Published tables vary in the suggested doses that are equianalgesic to morphine. Clinical response is the criterion that must be applied for each patient; titration to clinical response is necessary. Because there is not complete cross tolerance among these drugs, it is usually necessary to use a lower than equianalgesic dose when changing drugs and to retitrate to response.

NA, not available; NR, not recommended.

Caution: Recommended doses do not apply to patients with renal or hepatic insufficiency or other conditions affecting drug metabolism and kinetics.

*Caution: Doses listed for patients with body weight less than 50 kg cannot be used as initial starting doses in babies less than 6 months of age. Consult the *Clinical Practice Guideline for Acute Pain Management: Operative or Medical Procedures and Trauma* section on management of pain in neonates for recommendations.

†For morphine, hydromorphone, and oxymorphone, rectal administration is an alternate route for patients unable to take oral medications, but equianalgesic doses may differ from oral and parenteral doses because of pharmacokinetic differences.

‡*Caution:* Codeine doses above 65 mg often are not appropriate because of diminishing incremental analgesia with increasing doses but continually increasing constipation and other side effects.

§*Caution:* Doses of aspirin and acetaminophen in combination opioid/NSAID preparation must also be adjusted to the patient's body weight.

Opioids

Narcotics such as morphine and codeine may be administered by oral, subcutaneous, intramuscular, and intravenous routes. Administration of opioids by an oral route is as effective as by intramuscular and intravenous routes when the drug is given in an **equianalgesic dose** (the amount of drug, whether given by oral or parenteral routes, needed to produce the same analgesic effect) (Table 5–8). Rectal preparations of some opioids are also available.

Potential complications of opioids include respiratory depression, cardiovascular collapse, and addiction. When the child's condition is unstable, as in trauma or critical illness, the dosage of opioids must be carefully calculated to match the child's cardiorespiratory status. Infants and children are no more likely than adults to develop respiratory depression following administration of a weight-specific dose of narcotics.[15] Addiction is a rare complication in adults treated for painful conditions, and the same holds true for children.

Nonsteroidal Antiinflammatory Drugs

NSAIDs such as aspirin and acetaminophen, which are primarily given orally, are effective for relief of mild to moderate pain and chronic pain. Table 5–9 presents recommended dosages of these drugs. They are most commonly used for bone, inflammatory, and rheumatoid conditions. An NSAID may be prescribed in combination with an opioid to increase the effectiveness of the narcotic drug. This combination may ultimately reduce the amount of opioids needed for pain relief.

Drug Administration

Pain from surgery, major trauma, or cancer will be present for predictable periods because of the effects of tissue damage. Pain relief should be provided around the clock. Every effort should be made to give analgesic drugs without causing the child more pain. The preferred routes of administration are intravenous and oral.

Continuous infusion analgesia, which eliminates the peaks and valleys in pain control, is recommended to keep the drug level constant in children in

■ NURSING ALERT

Respiratory depression (a respiratory rate less than 20 breaths per minute in infants, 16/min in children, and 12/min in adolescents that may progress to respiratory arrest) is the major life-threatening complication of opioid administration. Identify the time interval before drug-specific peak respiratory depression occurs, and then carefully monitor the child's vital signs during that period.

TABLE 5-9 Recommended Doses of NSAIDs for Children and Adolescents

Oral NSAID	Usual Adult Dose	Usual Pediatric Dose*	Comments
Acetaminophen	650–975 mg q 4 hr	10–15mg/kg q 4 hr	Acetaminophen lacks the peripheral antiinflammatory activity of other NSAIDs
Aspirin	650–975 mg q 4 hr	10–15 mg/kg q 4 hr†	Standard against which other NSAIDs are compared; inhibits platelet aggregation; may cause postoperative bleeding
Choline magnesium trisalicylate (Trilisate)	1000–1500 mg bid	25 mg/kg bid	May have minimal antiplatelet activity; also available as oral liquid
Ibuprofen (Motrin, others)	400 mg q 4–6 hr	10 mg/kg q 6–8 hr	Available as several brand names and as generic; also available as oral suspension
Naproxen (Naprosyn)	500 mg initial dose followed by 250 mg q 6–8 hr	5 mg/kg q 12 hr	Also available as oral liquid

Modified from Acute Pain Management Guideline Panel. (1992). *Acute pain management in infants, children, and adolescents: Operative and medical procedures. Quick reference guide for clinicians.* (AHCPR Pub. No. 92-0020). Rockville, MD: Agency for Health Care Policy and Research, U.S. Public Health Service, Department of Health and Human Services.
*Drug recommendations are limited to NSAIDs where pediatric dose experience is available.
†Contraindicated in presence of fever or other evidence of viral illness.

FIGURE 5–7 Child receiving patient-controlled analgesia.

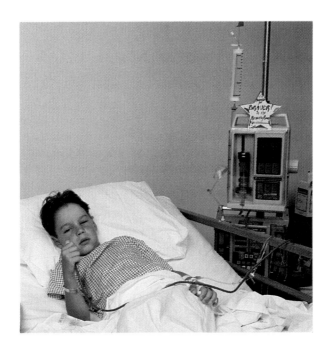

acute pain. Analgesics may also be given intravenously on a scheduled basis, that is, every 3 to 4 hours. Any delay in giving the analgesic when ordered on a scheduled basis increases the chances of breakthrough pain. Once the effects of analgesia wear off, more medication is often needed to regain pain relief. Giving analgesics on an as-needed basis for acute pain also results in loss of pain control. Often more analgesia is needed to restore pain control than would have been required for continuous infusion analgesia.

Patient-controlled analgesia (PCA) is a method of administering an intravenous analgesic, such as morphine, using a computerized pump that is programmed by the health care professional and controlled by the child (Fig. 5–7).[12,13] This technique is especially useful for pain control in the first 48 hours after surgery. PCA is prescribed mostly for school-age children and adolescents, but some preschool children have used it successfully.[16] Children selected for PCA should be able to push the injection button and should understand that pushing the button will give medication to relieve pain (Table 5–10).

■ SAFETY PRECAUTIONS

To prevent overdoses, the PCA computerized pump has safety features that include the ability to set the maximum number of infusions per hour and the maximum amount of drug received in a given time period.

TABLE 5–10 Patient Education Guidelines for Patient-Controlled Analgesia (PCA)

- What is PCA? Analgesia means pain relief: you get to control the amount of medicine you get with the machine.
- The machine gives the medicine by passing it through the tube that is connected to your intravenous line. When you push the button, the machine pumps pain medicine into the intravenous line to make you feel better.
- The machine limits the amount of medicine you can get to what the doctor orders. You can get any amount up to the maximum by pushing the button repeatedly. The push button will not let you make a mistake if you drop it or roll on it.
- Whenever you feel pain, hurt, or discomfort, push the button to get more medicine. Only you should push the button.
- No pain shots are needed as long as the intravenous line is in place.
- The PCA may not relieve all of your pain, but you should feel comfortable. Let the nurse know if you think your PCA is not working.
- The PCA will be used until you can take pills or drink pain medicine.

After initial pain control has been achieved with an IV infusion by the nurse, the child presses a button to receive a smaller analgesic dose for episodic pain relief. The PCA monitor can be set up with or without a continuous infusion of opioid drug in addition to the dose administered when the child pushes the button. A continuous infusion prevents a recurrence of pain during long sleeping periods. Additional pain medication is often ordered as needed to supplement the continuous and patient-administered infusion when pain control is not maintained.

Children and adolescents benefit from PCA by receiving continuous pain control and having the ability to control their comfort level with no trauma from injections. Several studies have documented the occurrence of pain relief without an increase in narcotic side effects.[17] Once children can take oral analgesics, PCA is discontinued.

Nursing Management of Pain

To provide effective nursing management of children in pain, anticipate the presence of pain and recognize the child's right to pain control. Nurses have an ethical obligation to relieve a child's suffering not only because of the consequences of unrelieved pain but also because appropriate pain management may have further benefits such as earlier mobilization, shortened hospital stays, and reduced costs. Nursing management involves the following:

- Recognition of pain and formulation of a nursing diagnosis
- Pharmacologic intervention
- Nonpharmacologic intervention
- Monitoring the effectiveness of pain control measures to provide optimal comfort
- Patient education

Examples of nursing diagnoses for children in pain include the following:

- Pain related to surgery, injury, invasive procedure, nerve compression from tumor growth
- Chronic Pain related to joint degeneration, inflammatory process
- Anxiety related to anticipation of pain from an invasive procedure, pain recurrence
- Sleep Pattern Disturbance related to inadequate pain control
- Knowledge Deficit related to self-management of pain control, use of nonpharmacological pain control measures
- Inability to Sustain Spontaneous Ventilations: Potential for, related to opioid overdose
- Constipation: Potential for, related to side effect of pain medication and limited activity

Increase and Maintenance of Patient Comfort

Pharmacologic Intervention

Give analgesics as ordered by the physician, ensuring that the dose is appropriate for the child's weight. When administering an opioid by intravenous infusion or PCA, monitor the intravenous rate and the intravenous site for

Box 2000, Station 'A', Hamilton, Ontario L8N 3Z5 (416) 521-2100

CHEDOKE HOSPITAL	McMASTER UNIVERSITY
Sanatorium Road	MEDICAL CENTRE
	Main Street, West

PEDIATRIC PAIN MANAGEMENT SHEET

	19 Month Date							
	Time							
Intensity	Worst pain imaginable 10 9 8 7 child O 6 parent ☐ 5 nurse * 4 3 2 1 0							
Location	Incisional							
	Other							
Aggravating Factors	Movement/positioning							
	Coughing/Deep breathing							
	Anxiety/Fear							
	Parents — not present							
	Treatments/procedures							
	Other							
Alleviating Factors	Repositioning							
	Toileting/Feeding							
	Parents — present							
	Verbal support							
	Play							
	Holding/Rocking							
	Other							
ADL	Hygiene							
	Movement/Walking							
	Playing/Schoolwork							
Medications	Drug, Dose, Route 1. 2.							
	Effectiveness Yes No							
	SIGNATURES							

FIGURE 5–8 Sample pain flowsheet.
Copyright Chedoke-McMaster Hospitals, Hamilton, Ontario, Canada.

infiltration. Make sure analgesic antagonists such as naloxone are available should complications develop.

Monitor the child's vital signs for complications related to opioids, such as respiratory depression. Naloxone may be used to treat the respiratory depression caused by an opioid drug at a dose that does not reverse the pain control effects of the narcotic. Other vital signs (heart rate and blood pressure) may not change in response to effective analgesia when infection, trauma, or other stressors keep them elevated. Check for the presence of other side effects of analgesics, such as sedation, nausea, and constipation.

Evaluate the child's level of pain at frequent intervals to determine whether the analgesic eliminated pain and to identify any increase in pain intensity. Use information collected from the child and parent, as well as an appropriate pain scale. Dramatic reductions in pain should occur, although not all pain may disappear. Many children sleep after receiving an analgesic. This sleep is not a side effect of the drug or a sign of an overdose, but the result of pain relief. Pain interrupts sleep, and once pain is relieved, the child can sleep comfortably. On the other hand, sleep does not always indicate pain control. A child in pain may fall asleep in exhaustion. Other symptoms of pain, such as excess movement or moaning, are present. A flowsheet may be used to document assessments and medication administration during the postoperative period (Fig. 5–8).

Become an advocate for children when the dose or type of analgesic ordered is inadequate. Tolerance to the ordered drug dose may occur when children with severe pain have been taking narcotics for several days. Breakthrough pain occurs, and an increase in dosage is needed to achieve the previous level of pain relief. Before asking the physician to change the analgesia, review the child's record for documentation that the prescribed drugs have been given at the appropriate dose and frequency and that pain relief is ineffective in spite of the drug administration. After verifying the record, provide the physician with information about the characteristics of the child's pain and ask for the medication change.

Oral NSAIDs are generally ordered for less severe pain or chronic pain. These drugs may mask fever. Be alert to the potential complication of gastrointestinal hemorrhage in critically ill children who have a physiologic stress response of increased gastric acids.

Nonpharmacologic Intervention

Use nonpharmacologic methods of pain control with or without analgesics. One or more of these methods may provide adequate pain relief when the child has low levels of pain. When used with analgesics, nonpharmacologic techniques often increase the effectiveness of the analgesic or reduce the dosage required.

Parental Involvement. Parents are the single most powerful nonpharmacologic method of pain relief available to children.[3] Parental presence greatly reduces the anxiety associated with pain and hospitalization. Children often feel more secure telling their parents about their pain and anxiety. Even children recognize the importance of their parents' presence in reducing their pain and anxiety.[18]

Distraction. **Distraction** involves engaging children in a wide variety of activities that help them focus attention on something other than pain. Examples of distracting activities are listening to music, singing a song, playing a game, watching television or a video, and focusing on a picture while counting. Select activities that are developmentally appropriate for the child. Do not assume the pain is gone if a child can be distracted. Children in severe pain cannot be distracted.

Cutaneous Stimulation. Cutaneous stimulation involves rubbing the painful area, massaging the skin gently, and holding or rocking the child. Infants require firm stroking to soothe their pain. The touching provides a stimulus to compete with pain stimuli that are transmitted from the peripheral nerves to the spinal cord. These actions may reduce the pain felt by the child.

Electroanalgesia. Also known as transcutaneous electrical nerve stimulation (TENS), **electroanalgesia** delivers small amounts of electrical stimulation to the skin by electrodes. This stimulation may interfere with transmission of pain from the peripheral nerves to the spinal cord.

Relaxation Techniques. Relaxation techniques are used to reduce muscle tension. Pain is often aggravated when muscles are tensed. Relaxation methods include rhythmic breathing (repeatedly taking a deep breath and slowly releasing it), alternately tensing and relaxing selected muscle groups, and focusing attention on something the child likes.

Hypnosis. An altered state of consciousness occurs when appropriate suggestions distort perception, memory, and mood in the child. Children who respond to hypnotic suggestions are often more relaxed and experience less pain.

Imagery. Imagery is a cognitive process that encourages the child to focus on and explore a favorite place, event, or funny story unrelated to the pain process. This method is most effective in children over 6 years of age. Ask the child to think about all the sights, sounds, smells, tastes, and feelings that will help him or her to experience the favorite place. Imagery is a form of self-hypnosis, and it is most effective when preceded by a relaxation exercise.

Application of Heat and Cold. Heat application promotes dilation of blood vessels. The increased blood circulation permits the removal of debris of cell breakdown from the site. Heat also promotes muscle relaxation, breaking the pain-spasm-pain cycle. To reduce edema, avoid applying heat in the first 24 hours after injury.

The application of cold is believed to slow the ability of pain fibers to transmit pain impulses. Cold also controls pain by decreasing edema and inflammation. When cold is applied, care should be taken to avoid causing thermal injury.

Discharge Planning and Family Home Care Teaching

Children are frequently discharged from the hospital with oral analgesics following surgery, injury, or treatment of acute medical conditions. Teach parents and children about the dosage and frequency of administration and the side effects of the analgesic ordered. Make sure parents know that a sudden increase in pain intensity indicates the development of a complication requiring medical attention.

Educate school-age children and adolescents about pain that may occur with elective procedures, the use of pain scales, and the methods available for pain relief, both pharmacologic and nonpharmacologic. Encourage children and parents to use the techniques that work best for them.

■ **GROWTH AND DEVELOPMENT CONSIDERATIONS**

Methods of distraction for pain control vary according to the child's developmental stage and individual interests.
- Infants: holding, cuddling, sucking a pacifier
- Preschoolers: engaging in therapeutic play, watching television or a video
- School-age children: talking about pleasant experiences, listening to radio, watching television or a video
- Adolescents: having visitors, playing games, watching television, listening to radio or tape player

Children with chronic conditions often need long-term pain control. For example, children with severe, long-term pain that is associated with cancer may be cared for at home with intravenous analgesics. Care of these children is usually managed by a home health care team. Educate parents thoroughly regarding intravenous care and analgesic administration.

Pain Associated with Medical Procedures

Children undergo a wide variety of painful diagnostic and treatment procedures in the hospital. Procedures rated the most painful by children in one study included chest tube insertion, arterial puncture, lumbar puncture, bone marrow aspiration, insertion of an intravenous line, and venipuncture.[19] Anticipation of such procedures causes anxiety and emotional distress that can lead to greater pain intensity. Children who have experienced severe pain in the past may be unwilling to cooperate with health care personnel.

Medical Management

Such procedures as burn debridement, laceration repair, bone marrow aspiration, and fracture reduction are associated with so much pain and anxiety that children need premedication with analgesics and sedatives.

A local anesthetic such as lidocaine is often injected subcutaneously in a small area to reduce the pain of deeper needle insertion. Topical anesthetics in the form of a patch or spray can be used to reduce the pain associated with the first needle stick.

Conscious sedation is a light sedation during which the child maintains airway reflexes and responds to verbal stimuli (Table 5–11). Conscious sedation can be used on a cooperative child. With conscious sedation, children have minimal anxiety, less pain, and often no memory of the procedure.[20] Conscious sedation is produced with various drugs, including midazolam, fentanyl, and a combination of meperidine, promethazine, and chlorpromazine.

Nursing Management

Increase Comfort During Painful Procedures

Help the child cope with a painful procedure by telling the child what sensations to expect and what will happen during the procedure. This reduces

TABLE 5–11 Characteristics of Conscious Sedation and Deep Sedation

Assessment Factors	Conscious Sedation	Deep Sedation
Airway	Able to maintain airway independently and continuously	Unable to maintain airway independently or continuously
Cough and gag reflexes	Reflexes are intact	Partial or complete loss of reflexes
Level of consciousness	Easily aroused with verbal or gentle physical stimulation	Not easily aroused, may not respond purposefully to verbal or gentle physical stimulation

From Zimmerman, S. (1993). *Conscious sedation in the Emergency Medical Trauma Center.* Washington, DC: Children's National Medical Center.

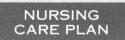

THE CHILD WITH POSTOPERATIVE PAIN

GOAL	INTERVENTION	RATIONALE	EXPECTED OUTCOME
1. Pain related to surgery and injury			
Child will state reduced pain	Give analgesic by a pain-free method.	Child may deny pain to avoid analgesia by painful route.	Child reports reduced pain after administration of analgesia.
	Have child select a pain scale and rate amount of pain perceived before and 30–60 minutes after analgesic is given to ensure pain relief.	The child's pain rating is the best indicator of pain. Maintenance of pain control requires less analgesia than treating each acute pain episode.	Child's rating of pain stays at 0 or a low level.
2. Sleep Pattern Disturbance related to inadequate pain control			
Child will experience fewer disruptions of sleep by pain	Give analgesia by continuous infusion or every 3–4 hours around the clock.	Pain breakthrough occurs even during sleep	Child sleep undisturbed by pain for age-appropriate number of hours per day.
3. Anxiety related to anticipation of a pain recurrence			
Child will state reduced concern about pain recurrence	Reposition child every 2 hours and maintain good body alignment. Provide therapeutic touch or massage.	Anxiety increases perception of pain. New positions decrease muscle cramping and skin pressure.	Child expresses no anxiety about pain management.
4. Knowledge Deficit related to self-management of pain control and use of nondrug pain control measures			
Child and family will understand use of patient-controlled analgesia (PCA) and nondrug pain control measures by patient and family	Teach child how the PCA works and when to push the button. Teach family and child how to use age-appropriate imagery, distraction, relaxation techniques, and other nondrug pain relief measures.	Child must know pushing PCA button will keep pain under control. Nondrug pain control measures reduce amount of analgesia needed.	Child's pain rating stays low. Child and family independently use nondrug pain control measures.
Child and family will use appropriate analgesia after discharge	Discuss appropriate pain control for use at home after discharge.	Family and child may be anxious about pain management at home.	Family understands pain relief measures for use at home and knows where to call if help is needed.
5. High Risk for Inability to Sustain Ventilations related to opioid overdose			
Child will maintain adequate respirations	Verify that correct dose of opioid analgesic is given. Monitor vital signs before analgesic is administered and at time of peak drug action. Calculate antagonist dose ordered by physician to be sure it will reverse respiratory depression, not counteract effect of analgesia.	Respiratory depression is a significant complication of opioid analgesics.	There is no episode of respiratory depression associated with analgesic. Respiratory depression episode does not progress to respiratory arrest.

stress more effectively than just providing information about the procedure.[21] Chapter 4 gives methods for preparing children of different developmental ages for procedures.

Drugs are not often used for quick procedures, such as dressing changes, injections, intravenous insertions, and venipunctures. Nonpharmacologic measures, especially imagery, relaxation techniques, and distraction, may reduce the anxiety associated with the anticipation of the procedure. Teach parents and children to use these interventions before the procedure. Help children to control their anxiety through therapeutic play.

When pharmacologic pain management is used for a procedure, the nurse's responsibilities include the following:

- Treat anticipated procedure-related pain prophylactically. For example, give an analgesic before a bone marrow aspiration or fracture reduction. Permit time for the drug to become effective.
- Manage preexisting pain before beginning a procedure such as scrubbing a burn.
- Whenever possible, administer drugs by a nonpainful route (oral, transmucosal, intravenous). Avoid intramuscular injections.
- When procedures must be repeated (for example, bone marrow aspirations for children with leukemia), give optimal analgesia for the first procedure to reduce anxiety about future procedures.
- To prevent increased anxiety, avoid delays in performing procedures.

When the child receives conscious sedation, monitoring the child's status is important. Nursing assessments include heart and respiratory rates, blood pressure, pulse oximetry, level of consciousness (response to verbal and physical stimulation), and color. Vital signs must be checked every 15 minutes until the child regains full consciousness and level of functioning. If conscious sedation progresses to **deep sedation** (a controlled state of depressed consciousness or unconsciousness), vital signs should be checked every 5 minutes.

REFERENCES

1 Schecter, N.L. (1989). The undertreatment of pain in children: An overview. *Pediatric Clinics of North America, 36*, 781–794.

2 Lutz, W.J. (1986). Helping hospitalized children and their parents cope with painful procedures. *Journal of Pediatric Nursing, 1*, 24–32.

3 Eland, J.M., & Banner, W., Jr. (1992). Assessment and management of pain in children. In Hazinski, M.F. (Ed.), *Nursing care of the critically ill child* (2nd ed.). (pp. 79–100). St. Louis: Mosby–Year Book.

4 Page, G.G. (1991). Chronic pain and the child with juvenile rheumatoid arthritis. *Journal of Pediatric Health Care, 5*, 18–23.

5 McGrath, P.A. (1987). An assessment of children's pain: A review of behavioral, physiological and direct scaling techniques. *Pain, 31*, 147–176.

6 Olsson, G., & Parker, G., (1987). A model approach to pain assessment. *Nursing 87, 17*, 52–57.

7 Varni, J.W., Thompson, K.L., & Hanson, V. (1987). The Varni/Thompson pediatric pain questionnaire: Chronic musculoskeletal pain in juvenile rheumatoid arthritis. *Pain, 28*, 27–38.

8 Abu-Saad, H. (1984). Cultural group indicators of pain in children. *Maternal-Child Nursing Journal, 13*, 187–196.

9 McGrath, P.J., & Craig, K.D. (1989). Developmental and psychological factors in children's pain. *Pediatric Clinics of North America, 36*, 823–836.

10 Abu-Saad, H. (1984). Cultural components of pain: The Asian-American child. *Children's Health Care, 13*, 11–14.

11 Bradshaw, C., & Zeanah, P.D. (1986). Pediatric nurses' assessment of pain in children. *Journal of Pediatric Nursing, 1*, 314–322.

12 Norden, J., Hannallah, R., Getson, P., O'Donnell, R., Kelliher, G., & Walker, N. (1991). Concurrent validation of an objective pain scale for infants and children, *Anesthesiology, 75*, Abstract No. 934.

13 Norden, J., Hannallah, R., Getson, P., O'Donnell, R., Kelliher, G., & Walker, N. (1991). Reliability of an Objective Pain Scale in children. *Anesthesia Analgesia, 72*, Abstract No. S199.

14 Acute Pain Management Guideline Panel. (1992). *Acute pain management in infants, children, and adolescents: Operative and medical procedures. Quick reference guide for clinicians.* (AHCPR Pub. No. 92-0020). Rockville, MD: Agency

of Health Care Policy and Research, Public Health Service, U.S. Department of Health and Human Services.

15 Lau, N. (1992). Pediatric pain management, Part 1. *Journal of Pediatric Health Care, 6*, 87–92.

16 Gureno, M.A. & Reisinger, C.L. (1991). Patient controlled analgesia for the young pediatric patient. *Pediatric Nursing, 17*, 251–254.

17 Berde, C.B., Lehn, B.M., Yee, J.D., Sethna, N.F., & Russo, D. (1991). Patient-controlled analgesia in children and adolescents: A randomized, prospective comparison with intramuscular administration of morphine for postoperative analgesia. *Journal of Pediatrics, 118*, 460–466.

18 Rogers, A.G. (1984). Children in pain. *American Journal of Nursing, 84*, 247.

19 Wong, D.L., & Baker, C.M. (1988). Pain in children: Comparison of assessment scales. *Pediatric Nursing, 14*, 9–16.

20 Stroud, S. & Dyer, J. (1992). Premedication takes the pain out of painful procedures for children. *American Journal of Nursing, 92*, 66.

21 Broome, M.E. (1990). Preparation of children for painful procedures. *Pediatric Nursing, 16*, 537–541.

SUGGESTED READINGS

Bender, L.H., Weaver, K., & Edwards, K. (1990). Postoperative patient-controlled analgesia in children. *Pediatric Nursing, 16*, 549–554.

Beyer, J.E., & Wells, N. (1989). The assessment of pain in children. *Pediatric Clinics of North America, 36*, 837–854.

Jones, M.A. (1989). Identifying signs that nurses interpret indicating pain in newborns. *Pediatric Nursing, 15*, 76–79.

McCready, M., MacDavitt, K., & O'Sullivan, K.K. (1991). Children and pain: Easing the hurt. *Orthopaedic Nursing, 10*, 33–42.

Morrison, R.A., & Vedro, D.A. (1989). Pain management in the child with sickle cell disease. *Pediatric Nursing, 15*, 595–599.

Ross, D.M., & Ross, S.A. (1988). *Childhood pain: Current issues, research, and management.* Baltimore: Urban & Schwarzenberg.

Stevens, B. (1990). Development and testing of a pediatric pain management sheet. *Pediatric Nursing, 16*, 543–548.

Tyler, D.C., Tu, A., Douthit, J., & Chapman, C.R. (1993). Toward validation of pain measurement tools for children: A pilot study. *Pain, 52*, 301–309.

Yaster, M., Bean, J.D., Tremlett, M., Nicholas, E., & Rogers, M.C. (1992). Pain, sedation, and postoperative anesthetic management in the pediatric intensive care unit. In Rogers, M.C. (Ed.), *Textbook of pediatric intensive care, Vol. 2* (2nd ed.). (pp. 1518–1567). Baltimore: Williams & Wilkins.

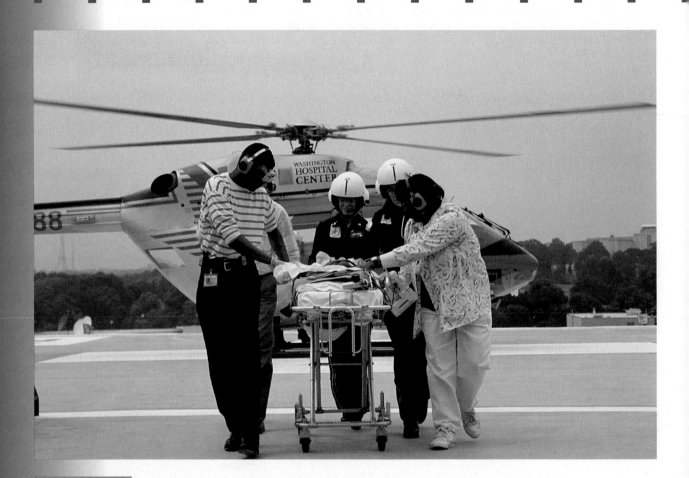

T he telephone in the pediatric intensive care unit (PICU) rings at 10:30 PM. A referring hospital is calling to request helicopter transport of an unstable 13-year-old girl, Allison, who was injured when a car in which she was a passenger was struck head on by another vehicle. Allison's parents have two other children, ages 6 and 9 years.

The transport team is in the air within minutes and arrives at the rural community hospital 25 minutes later. After stabilizing Allison and receiving reports from the medical and nursing team, the transport team meets briefly with her parents, answers a few questions, and is back in the air.

Allison is admitted directly to the PICU, where the unit team has been preparing for her arrival. She is connected to cardiorespiratory and noninvasive blood pressure monitors, while her existing intravenous lines, nasogastric tube, and urinary catheter are evaluated for patency. Team members quickly complete a head-to-toe assessment. The unit clerk enters Allison's room to say that her parents have arrived in the emergency department and are being escorted to the PICU.

THE CHILD WITH A LIFE-THREATENING ILLNESS OR INJURY

6

TERMINOLOGY

death anxiety A feeling of apprehension or fear of death.

death imagery Any reference to death or death-related topics, such as going away, separation, funerals, and dying, given in response to a picture or story that would not usually stimulate other children to discuss death-related topics.

family crisis An event occurring when a family encounters problems that for a time seem insurmountable and with which the family is unable to cope in its usual ways.

hospice A philosophy of care that focuses on helping persons with short life expectancies to live their remaining lives to the fullest—without pain and with choices and dignity.

stranger anxiety Wariness of strange people and places, often shown by infants between 6 and 12 months of age.

support systems The extended network of family, friends, and religious and community contacts that provide nurturance, emotional support, and direct assistance to parents.

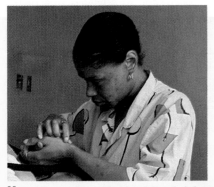

❝ I was never more afraid or felt so helpless with everybody running around, doing all those things to Allison. I just wanted someone to tell me that she was going to be OK. Now I'm sitting here watching her, and I wonder if she will really be OK. I've heard that sometimes head injuries cause problems years later. I just want her to be OK like she was before. ❞

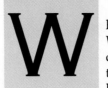

hat stressors do children like Allison face after admission to the PICU? What strategies can you use to help such critically ill or injured children cope with the experience? What stressors will parents face during the initial period when you work with them? How can you intervene to help them in this crisis? What strategies should be used to help siblings understand what has happened to their brother or sister? This chapter will enable you to answer these questions and will assist you to provide supportive care to critically ill and injured children like Allison and to their families.

The intense emotional and physical demands placed on the critically ill or injured child present a challenge to nurses' attempts to provide developmentally appropriate care. The child's parents and siblings are confronted with a stressful situation. A family-centered model of nursing practice offers a framework for performing interventions that help to minimize stress and enhance coping by parents, siblings, and the ill or injured child.

Life-Threatening Illness or Injury

A threat to a child's life may be expected, as in a chronic illness or progressive disabling disease, or unexpected, as in an unintentional injury. How children, parents, and siblings cope with the threat will depend on the anticipated or unanticipated nature of the event and the conditions surrounding the child's admission to the hospital.

When death results from a chronic disease or terminal illness, the child and family have time to adjust to the impending death. Parents can become involved in the child's therapy as integral members of the treatment team. Emergency admission for an acute illness or unintentional injury, on the other hand, brings with it sudden stressors as the child and family are thrust into an unfamiliar environment, confronted with frightening or invasive procedures, and faced with an uncertain outcome.

Nursing care of children and families coping with specific chronic diseases or terminal illnesses such as cancer, cystic fibrosis, or muscular dystrophy is discussed elsewhere in this book. The following discussion focuses on care of children with life-threatening illnesses or injuries.

Child's Experience

Admission to the hospital, emergency department, or PICU is one of the most frightening experiences a child can have. The critically ill child may appear extremely anxious and fearful, or withdrawn, solemn, and preoccupied with his or her physical condition. The illness or injury often brings pain, decreases energy, and changes the child's level of consciousness. Younger children may be unable to understand what is happening to them. The environment appears overwhelming, fast paced, and frightening. The child's normal sleep patterns can be disrupted because of the lack of day-night patterns in many intensive care units. Being cared for by strangers produces anxiety in the child. The child's limited ability to move intensifies his or her feelings of powerlessness and vulnerability.

Children's responses to stress are influenced by their developmental level, past experience, type of illness, coping mechanisms, and available emotional support. Nurses must take into consideration how the child's developmental level and coping skills will influence his or her ability to deal with the PICU experience. Successful coping can provide the child with the skills to handle difficult situations in the future.

Stressors to the Child

The four most significant stressors for hospitalized children of all ages are (1) separation from parents or the primary caretaker, (2) loss of self-control, autonomy, and privacy, (3) being subjected to painful and invasive procedures, and (4) fear of bodily injury and disfigurement.[1] Table 6–1 highlights key stressors of hospitalization for children at each developmental stage.

In addition to dealing with these stressors, the critically ill child experiences an intense emotional and physical threat to his or her well-being.

An unanticipated admission places the child at emotional risk for several reasons, including the lack of preparation for the experience, the uncertainty and unpredictability of events that follow, the unfamiliarity of the environment, and the heightened anxiety of parents. An admission for exacerbation of a disease such as cystic fibrosis or leukemia can bring a feeling of depression or hopelessness.

Infant

After 3 months of age, most infants have started to develop a sense of object permanence (the knowledge that an object or person continues to exist when not seen, felt, or heard) and corresponding trust in parents and familiar caretakers. This makes separation from parents an anxiety-producing experience (see Chapter 4). In addition to separation anxiety, infants between 6 and 12 months of age may display **stranger anxiety** (wariness of strangers) when

---

TABLE 6–1 Stressors of Hospitalization for Children in Various Developmental Stages

Infant

Separation anxiety
Stranger anxiety
Painful, invasive procedures
Immobilization

Toddler

Separation anxiety
Loss of self-control
Painful, invasive procedures
Bodily injury
Fear of the dark

Preschooler

Separation anxiety and fear of abandonment
Loss of self-control
Bodily injury
Painful, invasive procedures
Fears of the dark, ghosts, and monsters

School-Age Child

Loss of control
Bodily injury
Painful, invasive procedures
Fear of death

Adolescent

Loss of control
Altered body image, disfigurement
Separation from peer group

Modified from Smith, J.B. (1983). *Pediatric critical care.* New York: Wiley & Sons; and Stevens, K.R. (1981). *Nursing Clinics of North America, 16*(4), 611–622.

FIGURE 6–1 Jooti feels pain, hears noises, has her sleep disrupted, and has limited mobility because of all the equipment attached to her. What care and comfort can you offer parents who see their child like this?

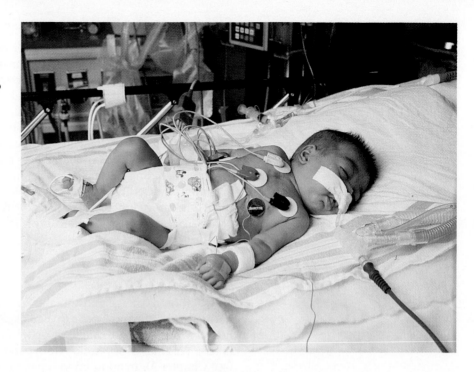

confronted with health care professionals. Other stressors to the infant include painful procedures, immobilization of extremities, and sleep deprivation caused by disruption of normal rhythms and patterns (Fig. 6–1).

Toddler

Toddlers are the group most at risk for a stressful experience as a result of illness. Separation from parents is extremely distressing to toddlers, and they protest vigorously when their parents depart. The toddler often becomes upset when known routines are altered. Being placed in restraints and confined is especially threatening to children in this age group. Fear of pain, invasive procedures, and mutilation are common.

Preschooler

The greatest stressors to preschoolers are fear of being alone, fear of abandonment, fear of loss of self-control related to the body and emotions, and fear of bodily injury or dismemberment. Waking up restrained in the PICU and feeling the presence of an endotracheal, nasogastric, or chest tube, along with intravenous, arterial, and urinary catheters, are terrifying to the preschooler.

School-Age Child

Major sources of stress for school-age children are loss of control related to bodily functions, privacy issues, fear of bodily injury, and concerns related to death. School-age children attempt to maintain their composure during painful or invasive procedures but generally still require a great deal of support.

Adolescent

Major stressors to adolescents are separation from the peer group, issues of control and related dependency, privacy, changes in body image, disability, and death. Adolescents often try to maintain rigid self-control when undergoing painful and invasive procedures.

Coping Mechanisms

The child may mirror the parents' behaviors and responses, which may help or hinder the child's response to stress. The child's temperament, previous coping experiences, and availability of support systems all combine to influence his or her ability to cope with the current experience.

The nature and severity of the illness and an emergency admission to the hospital stress a child's coping capabilities. Defense mechanisms displayed by children in these situations include regression, or return to an earlier behavior (a common reaction to stress), denial, repression (involuntary forgetting), postponement, and bargaining.

Nursing Assessment

Nursing assessment involves, in addition to physiologic parameters, skilled observation of the child's psychosocial and emotional needs. It is important for the nurse to understand normal psychosocial and cognitive development in order to plan developmentally appropriate interventions. Assessment should include the child's response to illness, the environment, coping strategies, and the need for information and support.

Nursing Diagnoses

The accompanying Nursing Care Plan gives common nursing diagnoses for the child coping with a critical illness or injury. The following nursing diagnoses may also be appropriate:

- Impaired Verbal Communication related to the effects of mechanical ventilation
- Impaired Social Interaction related to separation from family and friends
- Social Isolation related to the critical care environment
- Altered Sexuality Functions related to the effects of acute illness or change in a body part
- Spiritual Distress related to the crisis of illness or suffering
- Ineffective Individual Coping related to changes in body integrity, separation from family and friends, or critical illness
- Impaired Physical Mobility related to trauma, pain, or use of physical restraints
- Fatigue related to illness, crisis, or sensory overload
- Sleep Pattern Disturbance related to medications, pain, fear, or critical care unit environment
- Diversional Activities Deficit related to the monotony of confinement
- Altered Growth and Development related to critical illness or injury, the critical care environment, or separation from family and friends
- Body Image Disturbance related to loss of body function, severe trauma, or invasive procedures
- Self-Esteem Disturbance related to loss of body function, hospitalization, or loss of independence and autonomy
- Hopelessness related to critical illness, deteriorating condition, prolonged pain, altered body image, or separation from family and friends
- Anticipatory Grieving related to actual or perceived loss of function or impending death

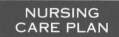
THE CHILD COPING WITH A LIFE-THREATENING ILLNESS OR INJURY

GOAL	INTERVENTION	RATIONALE	EXPECTED OUTCOME

1. Fear or Anxiety (Child) related to separation from parents, foreign environment, strangers as caretakers, invasive procedures

Child will exhibit or express an increased sense of security.	Encourage parents to remain at the bedside (open visitation) and to participate in the child's care by touching, talking to, reading to, and singing to the child.	Presence of parents is comforting to child.	Child appears more relaxed, acknowledges parents' presence, and allows staff to be supportive.
	Talk with the child. Avoid discussions at bedside that the child should not overhear.	Child may overhear and remember, even if unconscious.	
	Provide the child with developmentally appropriate explanations when possible, encourage the child to ask questions, and express concerns.	Information reduces anxiety and builds trust.	
	Prepare the child in advance for procedures using developmentally appropriate techniques.	Preparation decreases anxiety related to the unknown.	
	Make the child's bedside more personal and familiar by encouraging parents to bring in security objects, family photos, and favorite toys from home.	Security objects decrease foreignness of hospital environment. Child derives comfort from presence of personal items.	
	Involve the child in play appropriate to developmental age (see Chapter 4).	Play provides familiarity, decreases fantasy, and provides motor activity.	
	Provide care using a primary nursing care model.	Consistency in caregivers helps to build child's trust.	

2. Powerlessness related to inability to communicate, lack of privacy, control relinquished to the health care team

Child or adolescent will have an increased sense of control over situation.	Provide opportunities for choices when possible. Encourage participation in self-care.	Provides sense of control and autonomy through decision making.	Child or adolescent expresses satisfaction over ability to control some element of situation.
	Prepare the child or adolescent in advance (timing dependent on developmental level) for procedures. Describe the sensations that will be experienced. Allow some choice in timing or method of pain relief.	Information provides anticipatory guidance and a sense of involvement and value to the child.	
	Provide coverage of private body areas. Use curtains around bed when feasible.	Privacy lessens feelings of vulnerability.	

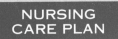

THE CHILD COPING WITH A LIFE-THREATENING ILLNESS OR INJURY—CONTINUED

GOAL	INTERVENTION	RATIONALE	EXPECTED OUTCOME
2. Powerlessness related to inability to communicate, lack of privacy, control relinquished to the health care team—continued			
	Provide routines for the child, both within a 24-hour period and for scheduled care. Tell the child before (timing dependent on developmental level), repeat explanation of why necessary, complete procedure in a consistent manner, and offer praise or a special story when completed. When possible, incorporate rituals from home.	Self-control is maintained through rituals.	
	Encourage play as a means of expression of feelings.	Play is a normal activity for children and provides freedom of expression.	
	Provide other means of communication to the intubated child (e.g., a word board or finger board).	Provides autonomy and independence for the child.	
	For the child requiring restraints, use as seldom as possible, provide appropriate explanations, and release at regular intervals. Wrapping IV lines well and using armboards can help maintain lines and avoid restraints.	Helps to diminish sense of powerlessness that accompanies use of restraints.	
3. Pain related to injuries, invasive procedures, surgery			
Child will experience reduced pain and improved comfort.	Assess child's pain: location, intensity, what makes it better or worse.	Assessment provides baseline information from which a plan of care can be developed.	Child experiences a perceived or actual improvement in comfort level.
	If appropriate, use pain assessment scale (see Chapter 5).	Use of scale provides continuity and consistency in monitoring of child's pain.	
	Prepare the child for procedures. Be honest in explanations and use developmentally appropriate language and format. Describe the sensations that the child will feel, smell, taste, or see. Comfort the child after the procedure. Provide rest periods between procedures.	Information reduces anxiety and fear associated with the unknown and helps child maintain self-control.	
	Provide optimal pain relief with prescribed analgesics. Provide diversional activities as appropriate or possible.	Physiologic and psychologic methods of pain control can be used in combination to maximally improve outcome.	

Nursing Management

Nursing care focuses on promoting a sense of trust, providing education about the illness or injury and preparing the child for procedures, facilitating the use of play, and promoting a sense of control. Children admitted to a PICU are presented with a traumatic experience for which they need support. Nurses play a key role in providing developmentally appropriate support to the child. Nursing interventions are directed at building a trusting relationship, minimizing the stresses experienced by the child, and promoting coping. Ongoing reassessment of progress in meeting the child's needs is critical. Honesty in all discussions is key to building trust with the child. The accompanying Nursing Care Plan summarizes nursing care for the child coping with a life-threatening illness or injury.

Promote a Sense of Security

For children of all ages, feeling secure depends on a sense of physical and psychologic safety.[2] A sense of physical safety is difficult to attain within the PICU because of the constant barrage of procedures that are part of the child's treatment plan. A sense of psychologic safety is best achieved by the presence of parents. An open visitation policy that enables parents to be at the bedside is optimal. Including parents as partners in the child's care provides comfort and reassurance to the child. Consistency of staff is invaluable in developing familiarity and a trusting relationship with the child.

Personalizing the child's bedside can promote comfort and a sense of security for the child. Pictures from home, a favorite blanket or toy, music tapes, or posters can make the environment friendlier and more familiar to the child (Fig. 6–2).

Provide Education About the Illness or Injury and Prepare the Child for Procedures

A child's ability to understand the cause of the illness and its therapy depends on his or her cognitive abilities. Help younger children to understand that illness and hospitalization are not a punishment.

Preparation for procedures is important at all ages, even for the unconscious or sedated child. The time for this preparation depends on the child's cognitive level. Generally, the younger the child, the shorter the interval between teaching and procedure (see Chapter 4).

Children often feel and hear even when unconscious, so touch and verbal interchanges are important. The toddler will benefit from being talked to, soothed, and touched during and after the procedure. Provide the preschooler, school-age child, and adolescent with an explanation of how the experience will feel. In any explanations to the child, avoid medical jargon and use simple language appropriate to the child's developmental level.

Facilitate the Use of Play

The use of play is important in alleviating stress and helping children to prepare for procedures. It is also another way for the nurse to assess the child's developmental level. Therapeutic play adds familiarity, diminishes fantasies, provides motor activity, and helps the child develop a sense of mastery (see Chapter 4). Children who are immobilized by tubes and restraints can still feel a sense of accomplishment by completing a puzzle, even if the nurse needs to point to each piece and, through nods and gestures, indicate where it should be placed. Play can help children work through a painful situation, making it more tolerable.

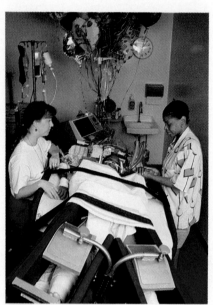

FIGURE 6–2 By their very nature, PICUs are ominous and sterile. To lessen this effect, it can help to personalize the child's space. Being there with the child and parent, answering questions, or just talking can be a comfort to both.

Promote a Sense of Control

Children between toddlerhood and adolescence experience a loss of control during a life-threatening illness. This loss of control may be related to the body, emotions, normal routines, or privacy. Nursing interventions should promote a sense of control over these areas.

Give choices to the child whenever possible. Even the simple choice of which arm will receive a new intravenous line can help the child feel in control. Scheduling routine activities and treatments at the same time each day adds predictability and lessens anxiety. Limited mobility and the use of restraints, although often necessary, contribute to the child's sense of powerlessness. Plan to release the child's restraints regularly for short periods. Restrain the toddler and preschooler as little as possible, and explain the rationale for restraints, emphasizing that they are not a punishment. Provide diversional activities for the child, for example, by reading stories, playing music, or watching videotapes (see Chapter 4).

Parents' Experience

Families have different reactions and coping mechanisms when challenged. Children who are hospitalized for a critical illness cannot be adequately cared for if their families' needs are not met. Not only will parents find it difficult to support the child if their own needs are not met, but also they can transmit their anxiety to the child, who then becomes even more anxious.

What Makes a Problem a Crisis?

A **family crisis** occurs when a family encounters a problem that seems insurmountable and that the family cannot cope with in its usual ways.[3] The critical care environment and the implications of a life-threatening illness or injury are far removed from the everyday experiences of most families. The unfamiliarity of the environment and the uncertainty and seriousness of the illness or injury create a crisis for the family.

Unexpected illness or injury adds another dimension of stress, since families have little time to prepare for the experience. A sudden admission threatens family integrity, causing enormous stress and separation from loved ones.

Reactions to Life-Threatening Illness or Injury

How do parents react to a threat to their child's life? What parental behaviors might nurses see when a child is critically ill or injured? Parents typically progress through five stages: (1) shock and disbelief, (2) deprivation and loss, (3) anger and guilt, (4) anticipatory waiting, and (5) elation or mourning.[4-6]

Shock and Disbelief

The universal reaction of parents is shock and disbelief. As the familiar is disrupted, parents experience a loss of control, inability to regain their bearings, and feelings of immobility. The hospital environment, the emergency department, or PICU may seem unreal. The emotions parents experience initially are intensified by the physical appearance of their child (particularly after traumatic injury); the presence of monitors, tubing, and equipment; and the actual injury or illness (Fig. 6–3). As the mother of a 5-year-old trauma

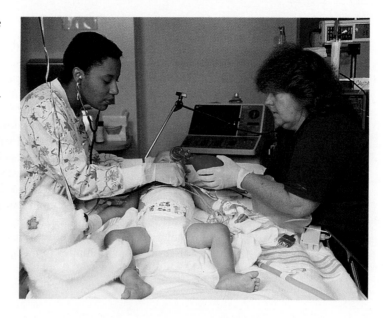

FIGURE 6–3 Procedures done in the PICU, such as mechanical ventilation, are frightening for parents. Treat the child first, but also remember the needs, fears, and anxieties of the parents and other family members. Anticipating the family's needs and keeping them informed will help them adjust.

patient said, "I felt distanced, in a daze, in and out of it that first day after the accident."

The stage of shock and disbelief begins in the first few moments after hearing the "news" and can last for days. For most parents, however, the overwhelming sense of shock passes during the first 24 hours. During this period, parents grope for answers and explanations about the illness or injury. Information must be repeated many times to parents, since in this stage they are often unable to assimilate information easily.

Deprivation and Loss

As the shock slowly recedes, parents enter a stage of deprivation and loss related to their parental role. Within minutes or hours, parents have gone from the familiar role of being a parent of a healthy child to the unexpected and unfamiliar role of being a parent of a critically ill child. Parents have compared this deprivation and loss to that experienced when a family member dies.

Parents' difficulties and ambivalence in releasing to strangers a part of their responsibility as the child's primary caretakers can threaten their self-esteem and self-control. Moreover, if parents cannot participate in the child's care, they may feel helpless or worthless.

Anger and Guilt

Anger and guilt surface as parents become more aware of their child's illness or injury. Their anger may be directed toward themselves, each other, health care providers, or other children or parents, as in the case of a motor vehicle crash involving a group of teenagers. Parents may also be angry with their child. This anger may be a result of injuries the child sustained when breaking known rules such as drinking and driving, playing with matches, or riding a bike without a helmet. Lastly, the anger may not be directed at anyone specifically. Injuries caused by natural disasters such as an earthquake, flood, or hurricane provoke just as much anger as those that result from the actions of people. This may create a challenge to the parents' spiritual beliefs.

Parents typically react to their child's illness or injury with some degree of guilt. This reaction may be magnified in the intensive care environment. The fact that the guilt usually has no basis in real events does not lessen the feeling. A question parents frequently ask at this stage is, "Why not me instead of my child?" Parents' feelings of guilt may have one of two causes:

1. *They may feel responsible for causing the illness or injury.* Statements such as, "If only I hadn't sent him to the store on his bike, this wouldn't have happened," or, from the father of a 2-year-old who nearly drowned, "Maybe if I hadn't been working, he would have been in my care and this wouldn't have happened," reflect feelings of guilt for causing or failing to prevent the injury.
2. *They may feel guilty about not noticing the onset of an illness or disregarding earlier symptoms of an illness.* The mother of a 1-year-old with *Haemophilus influenzae* meningitis repeatedly said, "I shouldn't have waited so long to take her to the doctor!"

Anticipatory Waiting

Once the child's condition is stabilized and survival seems likely, parents often move into a period of anticipatory waiting. This stage is characterized as "life suspended in time." Parents spend a great deal of time waiting: for test results, for explanations, for their child to become conscious, or for surgery to be over.

During this period parents pose questions about the long-term effects of the illness or injury on the child, about the potential for brain damage, or about the need for additional surgeries. Parents may place demands on staff and be frustrated when the child's progress is slow.

Elation or Mourning

The last stage that parents experience is elation or mourning. Elation is experienced as the child recovers, improves steadily, and prepares for transfer and discharge. In contrast, parents of the child who dies reenter the cycle of emotions characteristic of grief. Mourning also occurs when the child re-

---

TABLE 6–2 Parental Needs During Hospitalization of a Critically Ill or Injured Child

Information (the most important identified need)
- To be informed about the child's condition
- To be given explanations they can understand
- To talk with a physician daily
- To be called regarding changes in the child's condition

Proximity
- To remain at the bedside
- To have open, flexible visiting hours

Reestablishment of the parental role
- To be recognized as important to the child's recovery

Participation in the child's care (bathing, diaper changes, feeding, range-of-motion exercises, massages, hair care, reading, singing, telling stories, touching, talking)

Confidence in the treatment plan and caregivers
- To have continuity in staffing and health care contacts
- To know that staff care about the child
- To know that the child is receiving the best care possible

Rest and nutrition
- To maintain physical resources necessary for coping

Hope (an essential component of coping)

Modified from Jay, S.S., & Youngblut, J.M. (1991). *AACN Clinical Issues in Critical Care Nursing*, 2(2), 276–284; Kasper, J.W., & Nyamathi, A.M. (1988). *Heart & Lung*, 17(5), 574–581; and Philichi, L.M. (1989). *Journal of Pediatric Nursing*, 4(4), 268–276.

mains seriously ill or unresponsive, when the outcome remains uncertain for an extended period, or when long-term care is required.

■ ■ ■

Table 6–2 lists the most important needs of parents during a child's critical illness or injury.

Nursing Assessment

Nurses who work with families of critically ill children have a unique opportunity to help them adapt and to promote family functioning. They begin by assessing the family's reaction to the illness, coping skills, stressors, and needs. This initial assessment provides a baseline of information for developing a care plan and strategies to meet the psychosocial as well as physiologic needs of families.

Nursing Diagnosis

Several nursing diagnoses may apply to parents who are dealing with their child's critical illness or injury. They include:

- Knowledge Deficit related to the child's critical condition and uncertain prognosis
- Altered Parenting related to the child's critical illness or injury
- Altered Family Processes related to the impact of a critically ill child on the family system
- Parental Role Conflict related to the child's critical illness or injury
- Spiritual Distress related to the child's critical illness, suffering, or death
- Ineffective Individual or Family Coping related to the child's severe or fatal illness
- Family Coping: Potential for Growth related to constructive crisis management
- Fatigue related to extreme stress, crisis, and sensory overload
- Hopelessness related to the child's deteriorating physiologic condition
- Powerlessness related to relinquishment of control to the health care team
- Anticipatory Grieving related to perceived loss of the child or the child's impending death

Nursing Management

Nursing care focuses on providing information and building trust, promoting parental involvement, providing for physical and emotional needs, facilitating positive staff-parent relationships and communication, and maintaining or strengthening family support systems. Ongoing reassessment provides a measure with which to evaluate the family's ability to manage the crisis. The best way to meet the needs of families, minimize stress, and enhance family coping is to provide care using a family-centered approach. Table 6–3 lists the eight essential elements of family-centered care as set forth by the Association for the Care of Children's Health.[7] The challenge to nurses is to blend and balance technology with caring.

Provide Information and Build Trust

The information given to parents must be provided frequently and accurately. Information on the child's illness, condition, and plan of care should be delivered in a manner and language readily understandable to parents.

TABLE 6-3 Key Elements of Family-Centered Care

- Recognizing that the family is the constant in a child's life while the service systems and personnel within those systems fluctuate.
- Facilitating parent-professional collaboration at all levels of health care: care of an individual child; program development, implementation, and evaluation; and policy formation.
- Honoring the racial, ethnic, cultural, and socioeconomic diversity of families.
- Recognizing family strengths and individuality and respecting different methods of coping.
- Sharing with parents, on a continuing basis and in a supportive manner, complete and unbiased information.
- Encouraging and facilitating family-to-family support and networking.
- Understanding and incorporating the developmental needs of infants, children, and adolescents and their families into health care systems.
- Implementing comprehensive policies and programs that provide emotional and financial support to meet the needs of families.
- Designing accessible health care systems that are flexible, culturally competent, and responsive to family-identified needs.

From National Center for Family-Centered Care (1990). *What is family-centered care?* [brochure]. Bethesda, MD: Association for the Care of Children's Health.

Upon admission, parents need to be given an idea of what to expect in the days ahead and prepared for special procedures or major changes in therapy that may become necessary.

Honesty in discussions with parents is extremely important. If parents feel misled or that information is being withheld, a trusting relationship will be impossible. Informed parents, on the other hand, will feel that they are active participants in decision making and care planning for their child. Trust is facilitated when parents believe that the staff truly cares about the child and sees him or her as an individual, special child.

Promote Parental Involvement

An important role of nurses is to encourage and strengthen parents in their parenting role. The parents' place when possible is at the bedside—their very presence can comfort the child and minimize fears. Parents' needs are best met when they are encouraged to participate in their child's care.

If the child is in the PICU, parents need to be prepared before they see their child for the first time. Throughout the child's hospitalization, parents will continue to need reassurance and encouragement. Open visitation by parents is less stressful than structured, time-limited visitation when the child is in the PICU.[8,9]

Provide for Physical and Emotional Needs

The experience of having a child with a critical illness drains parents' physical and emotional reserves. Parents often need encouragement to take care of themselves. A statement such as, "It is important for you to eat and rest because Allison's really going to need you when she wakes up," helps parents to realize that becoming exhausted benefits neither them nor the child.

Orienting parents to the hospital, as well as to the unit routines, helps them to adapt to their surroundings. Many communities now have Ronald McDonald houses—an inexpensive but warm and supportive environment for parents of ill children (see Appendix F). When financial burdens are a consideration, family and social service referrals may be needed.

Parents are often at different levels of coping during a crisis. The child's critical illness may foster cohesion between the couple and build a stronger

■ **CLINICAL TIP**

Encourage parents to take time for themselves to be alone. Provide parents with a beeper, if possible, to reduce anxiety when they are away from the unit.

relationship. Unfortunately, the reverse may also be true—differences in levels of coping may foster a sense of isolation, placing a strain on the couple's relationship. Nurses may need to refer the family for counseling or therapy.

Facilitate Positive Staff-Parent Relationships and Communication

Given the intensity of the parents' experience when their child is critically ill, it is easy to see how problems can arise between staff and parents. Each health care team member must be aware of the child's current status so that parents receive the same information from all staff. Consistency in the message can instill confidence. Provide explanations geared to parents' level of understanding, using language that parents can understand.

Parents need to know who has the overall responsibility for the care of their child. They should be introduced to the nurse and physician responsible for the child's care. This is especially important in teaching hospitals that have rotating staff. The staff physician with the overall responsibility should meet with parents as often as necessary to talk about changes in the child's condition or treatment plan and to allow time for parents to ask questions (Fig. 6–4). Encourage parents to keep a daily log or notebook to record information on the child's care, progress, and needs. Family care conferences can be helpful when a large number of team members provide care.

Maintain or Strengthen Family Support Systems

Support systems are the extended network of family, friends, and religious and community contacts that provide nurturance, emotional support, and direct assistance to parents, enabling them to cope with overwhelming problems and crises. Most parents indicate that having family or friends nearby is crucial as a support system.

Parents may need to be reassured that it is all right to ask for help from family, friends, or community services. They may be uncomfortable asking for help, instead attempting to handle multiple responsibilities themselves,

■ CULTURAL CONSIDERATIONS

As in many other cultural groups, Mexican-American families have close kinship ties with an extended network of relatives, including grandparents, uncles, aunts, cousins, and *compadres* (children's godparents). The extended family is a source of strength and can provide much-needed emotional and physical support during crises.

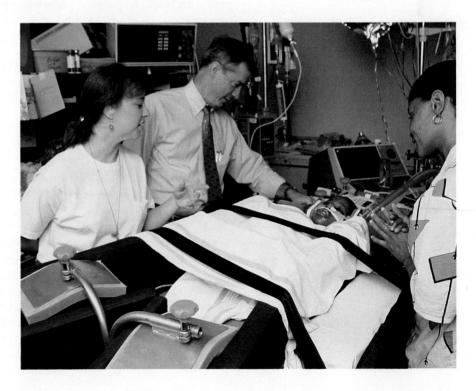

FIGURE 6–4 In times of crisis, everyone likes to know that someone is in charge and who that person is. The parents should meet and talk with the staff physician in charge and the nurses as often as possible. Parents need to know that someone is responsible, even if different people are providing care.

often to the point of exhaustion. Some parents are unable to respond to offers of help because it requires too great a mental effort on their part.

Nurses may need to intervene on parents' behalf when they have inappropriate support.[10] Parents may be frustrated by people who come to visit unannounced, stay too long, or visit too often, and may find it difficult to tell well-meaning but insensitive friends that they cannot deal with visitors right now. In these situations, offering to serve as a gatekeeper may be helpful.

Families of critically ill or dying children often have emotional needs beyond the support capabilities of the nurse caring for the child. Referrals to family and support services or pastoral care may be beneficial in these instances.

Siblings' Experience

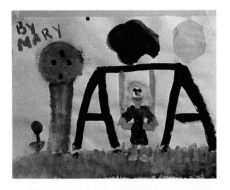

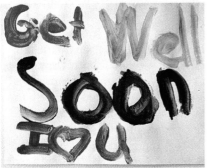

FIGURE 6–5 It is important that parents and siblings feel comfortable communicating with the seriously ill child. If siblings cannot visit, they should be encouraged to paint or record messages. They need to be able to express themselves and to feel that they are helping.

As parents' focus shifts to the critically ill child, they may need support in dealing with the healthy siblings. Siblings also need care and may feel left out when the attention is focused on the ill child. Siblings of critically ill children may demonstrate behaviors ranging from jealousy or envy to resentment, guilt and hostility, anger, insecurity, and fear. Recognize that siblings may fear becoming ill themselves or believe that they played a role in the child's illness. Siblings often have nightmares about the illness or injury their brother or sister has sustained and about the ill child dying.

Tell siblings about their brother or sister using language and concepts appropriate to their age and developmental level. As appropriate, siblings should be allowed to visit. These visits often help to lift the spirits of the ill child. Because children's fantasies are often worse than reality, unfounded fears may be relieved by a visit.

Preparation for the visit is important. Before the visit, talk with the siblings about what to expect and describe how their brother or sister will look. If the ill child acts, moves, talks, or looks different than usual, provide an explanation beforehand. Describe the hospital environment, including equipment, sounds, and smells. Using a doll, drawing pictures, or showing an actual picture of the child can help prepare the siblings. Table 6–4 summarizes strategies for working with siblings of an ill or injured child.

During the visit, demonstrate how to talk to and touch the ill child and encourage the siblings to do the same. After the visit, discuss with siblings what they saw and felt, and answer any questions they may have. When a sibling cannot visit, contact with the ill child can be maintained by sending pictures, drawings, cards, and messages on audiotapes or videotapes (Fig. 6–5).

TABLE 6–4 Strategies for Working with Siblings of an Ill or Injured Child

- Be truthful. Tell why the child is hospitalized, what the treatment involves, and how long the hospitalization is expected to last.
- Assure siblings that they did not cause the illness and that the ill child did nothing wrong.
- Allow siblings to ask questions and state fears and other feelings.
- Allow siblings to visit if possible. Prepare them for any equipment, dressing, and procedures they might see. Warn them if the ill child is not speaking. Say something like, "John can't talk now. He seems to be sleeping deeply. He may be able to hear, though, so you can touch him and talk to him."
- Encourage siblings to express their feelings related to the disruptive effect of the child's hospitalization on family life.

If parents are staying at the hospital with the ill child, encourage them to call the siblings at home at a regular time each night. Allowing the siblings at home the opportunity to share their day as well as to receive an update on the ill child provides a feeling of connectedness. The phone call offers siblings a consistent link to the parent as well as the reassurance that they are important and loved.

Bereavement

Parents' Reactions

The death of one's child is probably the most painful experience for a parent. When the loss is sudden and unexpected, the abruptness adds a dimension of shock. The goal of the nurse in these situations is to provide comfort and support for the dying child and the family. Staff education must be built on the premise that grief and mourning are normal, necessary processes.

Grief is painful, individualized, and exhausting. Many factors influence parents' grief responses, including their perception of the preventability of the illness or injury, the circumstances of the death, the nature of their attachment to the child, previous losses, spiritual or religious orientation, and culture.

Although parents progress through distinct stages of grief, the timeline and nature of the grief process differ for each individual. The intense pain and shock initially felt by parents gradually give way to feelings of anger, guilt, depression, and loneliness. Very slowly, and with much support, energy returns and parents again begin to enjoy life experiences. Spouses may need additional support when they are at different levels of grieving to prevent a sense of loneliness and isolation.

Work closely with the family when the child's death is imminent, since they will remember the experience for the rest of their lives. Prepare the family for changes in the child's appearance and the events to follow. Providing parents with a room in which to be alone with the child ensures privacy at this extremely personal time. Ask the family what is important to them in the last moments or hours of their child's life. Certain religious or cultural practices may need to be planned. Holding the child is a universal request and should be permitted. Many families find that saying good-bye as a group is helpful. Allowing the family to hold, kiss, and talk to the dying child can help grieving.[11] Encourage parents to continue in their parental role by continuing with caregiving activities such as bathing or dressing the child for the last time.

After the child's death, allow the family to spend as much time as they need with the child's body. Never rush family members who are saying good-bye to the child. Save all of the child's personal items—especially in the case of an infant, whose parents may have few mementos. A lock of hair, hand or foot prints, the infant's identification band, or a picture of the infant can be sources of comfort and remembrance for families.

Parents may need direction about resources available to help with a memorial service or funeral. Information about organ and tissue donation, as well as the need for an autopsy, if required, needs to be discussed. Acknowledge with parents that certain dates—such as the day of the week the child died, the child's birthday, or family holidays—will be difficult and may trigger intense sadness again. Parents may benefit from keeping a journal of their thoughts and memories, or writing letters or poems to or about their child.

Emphasize to parents that although the period surrounding their child's death is difficult, caring for themselves physically and mentally is important. A list of appropriate support groups, books, and articles can be given to par-

■ CULTURAL CONSIDERATIONS

Many culturally influenced rules and customs surround dying. The Hmong belief system holds that children will live in eternity in the same state in which they existed at the time of death. Therefore it is important that the child's body be intact at death.

ents for later use. Parents can be referred to national organizations, such as the Candlelighters Foundation or Compassionate Friends, and to local support groups for bereaved parents or siblings (refer to Appendix F). Some institutions have formal follow-up programs for bereaved parents to encourage a healthy progression through the grieving process.

Siblings' Reactions

Siblings experiencing the death of a brother or sister require supportive and compassionate care. In the course of the child's illness the siblings probably will have received less attention from parents. They may fear that they caused their brother or sister to be injured or become ill, or worry that bad thoughts on their part brought on the illness. They need help in adapting to their parents' distraction, grief, and increased protectiveness of them.[12]

A sibling's reaction to a brother's or sister's death often may be observed through behavior and play. The sibling may display anger, fear, or denial; become more "clingy"; or regress to earlier behaviors. Table 6–5 highlights children's understanding of death at different developmental stages.

When talking to the siblings of a dying child, honesty is most important. Provide explanations in language that is developmentally appropriate. Reassure siblings that they did not cause their brother or sister to die. Acknowledge the emotions they are feeling, and emphasize that it is all right for them to be angry, frightened, or tearful. Ask how they feel about saying good-bye to the dying child, and provide physical and emotional support. Preparation of the siblings before seeing the dying child involves a brief explanation of

---

TABLE 6-5 Children's Understanding of Death

Infant
- Lacks understanding of concept of death
- May sense caregivers are tense, routines are altered

Toddler
- Unable to distinguish fact from fantasy
- No understanding of true concept of death

Preschooler
- Believes death is reversible, temporary
- Displays anger at failure to keep person "alive"
- Believes bad thoughts cause death
- Believes magical thinking can bring the dead person back
- May see death as punishment
- May fear going to sleep
- Is developing a sense of past, present, future
- Has beginning experience with death of animals and plants

School-Age Child
- Acquires more realistic understanding of death
- By 8 to 10 years understands that death is permanent and irreversible
- Believes that death is universal and will happen to him or her
- May have exaggerated concerns about death

Adolescent
- Intellectually capable of understanding death
- Has a better grasp of association between illness and death
- Sense of invincibility conflicts with fear of death

From Krulik, T., Holaday, B., & Martinson, I.M. (Eds.) (1987). *The child and family facing life-threatening illness.* Philadelphia: J.B. Lippincott.

what they will see, feel, hear, and smell. Answer questions truthfully. You may have to repeat information several times.

As appropriate and comfortable, siblings should be permitted to participate in planning the child's memorial or funeral service. Being able to grieve as a family provides siblings with a sense of connectedness to parents and provides security at a vulnerable time.

■ Dying Child*

Care of the dying child presents one of the greatest challenges to the nurse, requiring the utmost sensitivity and compassion. Children's understanding of death varies according to developmental stages, as described in Table 6–5.

Children as young as 5 years of age can sense when they are seriously ill. Children's awareness of death develops more rapidly when they are experiencing the progression of a disease and related medical treatment. Children with life-threatening illnesses often learn about death and their own illness from exposure to other seriously ill and dying children when they are receiving treatment during hospitalization or clinic visits.

Preschool children can see their body deteriorate and feel the toxic effects of chemicals during disease progression and treatment. Changes in self-concept occur as they perceive these body changes. They often describe their illness in terms of mutilation to their body. They may realize that they are dying because of these physical changes.

School-age children also have subtle fears about body integrity and anxieties about the seriousness of their illness. This greater preoccupation with illness is considered by many professionals as the child's version of **death anxiety,** a feeling of apprehension or fear of death. Death anxiety occurs in children even though they are unable to conceptualize or describe death at an adult's level of understanding. It can develop from the perception of loneliness associated with a separation from the known world. Children may express death anxiety as a concern with treatments that invade the body or interfere with normal body functions.

Children intuitively know when they are dying, and they usually do not have the same fears that adults do. Some children keep most of their thoughts about death to themselves. They may fear that the family members will abandon them emotionally. Displays of anger often are avoided, since children fear desertion more than death. They may also believe that expressing their awareness of death and their fears will place added emotional burdens on family members that could be unbearable to the family. Parents may not recognize the child's death anxiety because of their own fears, concerns, and feelings of helplessness.

Waechter's study of hospitalized and fatally ill children revealed that children who were given an opportunity to discuss issues related to death openly did not have greater anxiety about death. The permission to discuss any aspect of the illness made the child feel less isolated and alienated from the parents. The child felt that the illness was not too terrible to discuss.[13]

Adolescents have a mature understanding of death, but the normal developmental milestones of adolescence add to their problems in facing a terminal illness. They are struggling with establishing their own identity and plans for the future. At a time when body image is extremely important, they may be faced with the possibility of mutilation and disfigurement. Dying teens are often isolated from their peers during a period when peers are the most essential social group. Adolescents with terminal illnesses may be angry because they recognize their loss when the whole world is opening up to them.

*This section and the following one were provided by Jane Ball, RN, CPNP, DrPH.

Do not expect adolescents to handle feelings in the same way that adults do. Adolescents often avoid expressing anger against the family, seeking to control and direct these feelings elsewhere. They often become angry at changes in treatment procedures, lack of explanations, and threats to their independence. As death nears, the adolescent may permit comforting and support and may accept care from warm and loving family members, as long as he or she is not treated disrespectfully.

Nursing Management

Make a commitment to children while they are living—to promote growth and development and to foster relationships with family and peers. Help children maintain contact with peers on the hospital unit as long as the child has energy to benefit from the companionship. The comfort of peers reduces the child's feelings of isolation.

Provide opportunities for fantasy play, drawings, and storytelling, without emphasizing or reinforcing death themes. Listen to what children tell you about themselves and their lives. **Death imagery,** references to death or death-related topics (going away, separation, and funerals), or anticipated experiences with treatment may be themes of their stories. These themes are expected and do not reflect repression or other pathology.

Parents may feel incapable of dealing directly with the child's questions about dying. They may fear that they will be unable to cope with their own feelings during a frank discussion of the possibility of the child's imminent death. The types of questions that children most frequently ask include the following:

- What will death be like?
- What will happen to me when I die?
- Will I be punished for the bad things I have done?
- When will I be with [person(s) closest to child] again?
- Will my parents be all right?
- Will I experience much pain?

Some parents need help in understanding and answering the child's questions at a developmentally appropriate level for the child. Provide guidance about appropriate methods and words to use that will support the child. Some parents may prefer that the child's questions be answered honestly by another professional. A professional who has faced personal anxieties about death can assist children and families with discussions.

When caring for adolescents, remember that outbursts of anger are common but not personally directed at you. Provide activities to help teens channel their feelings. Continue providing support in spite of their behavior. This approach may encourage teens to accept comfort without losing face. Be available to listen when the teen wants to talk and express feelings and frustrations. Promote friendships with other teens having similar interests or problems.

Provide teens with as much independence and control over their situation as possible. Give them a voice in decisions. Answer questions honestly without using a condescending tone.

Hospice care helps persons with short life expectancies to live their remaining lives to the fullest—without pain and with choices and dignity. In pediatric hospice, the family is helped to focus on the quality of life by facilitating communication between the child and family. Families need help to focus on the time left with the child. Encourage the family to participate in the child's physical and emotional care. Families need to cry together and to

■ CULTURAL CONSIDERATIONS

Depending on the family's cultural and religious beliefs, a chaplain or other health care professional who specializes in working with terminally ill children and families may help reduce a child's spiritual fears and promote peace and comfort among family members.

■ LEGAL CONSIDERATIONS

The Patient Self-Determination Act of 1990 (PSDA) supports the rights of persons 18 years of age or older in decisions about their medical care and when to be admitted to a medical facility. Although many adolescents younger than age 18 have the cognitive skills necessary for decision making and are involved in decisions concerning their care, the PSDA limits their legal rights. Creative strategies are needed to develop a model of adolescents' decision-making rights and responsibilities built on the PSDA.

tell each other how much they will miss each other. They need to be assured that the vigil with the child is important so the child does not feel isolated or abandoned as death approaches.

Staff Reactions to the Death of a Child

Children are highly valued by society because of their potential future contributions. Children are expected to have a normal life span, and the death of a child is often viewed as a tragedy. Caring for dying children is especially stressful and demanding for health care professionals. Nurses often cope by distancing themselves socially from the dying child and family to maintain composure and a professional demeanor. Waechter reported that the total time nurses spent with children decreased as death became more imminent.[14]

Caring for the dying child may be especially difficult for nurses with young children of their own. They tend to identify with the child, making it more likely that they will have difficulty dealing with the death in a professional manner. Nurses also may not identify the dying child's anxiety and fears because of their own personal defenses against their sense of helplessness to alter the course of the child's disease.

Nurses who work with terminally ill children and their families need special preparation to meet the needs of the patients and to manage personal stress simultaneously. Additional educational experiences and discussion and support following encounters with death in the hospital may help promote professional nursing care. Nurses who work with dying children and families must develop confidence, empathy, and competence in their ability to provide more humane and effective nursing care.

Nurses working in hospice settings or hospital units that care for terminally ill children need support systems to help balance the stresses of working with dying children. These supports may be discussions with peers or group sessions with mental health professionals that provide an opportunity to discuss their feelings and concerns.

REFERENCES

1 Smith, J.B. (1983). *Pediatric critical care.* New York: Wiley & Sons.

2 Jacobson, S.F. (1981). Stress: Child, family, and staff. In Vestal, K.W. (Ed.), *Pediatric critical care nursing.* New York: Wiley & Sons.

3 Redmond, G. (1992). Family health. In Berger, K.J., & Williams, M.B. (Eds.), *Fundamentals of nursing: Collaborating for optimal health.* Norwalk, CT: Appleton & Lange.

4 Miles, M.S., & Carter, M.C. (1982). Sources of parental stress in pediatric intensive care units. *Children's Health Care, 11*(2), 65–69.

5 Miles, M.S. (1979). Impact of the intensive care unit on parents. *Issues in Comprehensive Pediatric Nursing, 3*(7), 72–90.

6 Etzler, C.A. (1984). Parents' reactions to pediatric critical care settings: A review of the literature. *Issues in Comprehensive Pediatric Nursing, 7,* 319–331.

7 Shelton, T., Jeppson, E., & Johnson, B. (1987) *Family-centered care for children with special health care needs.* Washington, D.C.: Association for the Care of Children's Health.

8 Henneman, E.A., McKenzie, J.B., & Dewa, C.S. (1992). An evaluation of interventions for meeting the information needs of families of critically ill patients. *American Journal of Critical Care, 1*(3), 85–93.

9 Proctor, D.L. (1987). Relationship between visitation policy in a pediatric intensive care unit and parental anxiety. *Children's Health Care, 16*(1), 13–17.

10 Tomlinson, P.S., & Mitchell, K.E. (1992). On the nature of social support for families of critically ill children. *Journal of Pediatric Nursing, 7*(6), 386–394.

11 Chard, P.S. (1987). Grief: Handling theirs and yours. *Emergency Medical Services, 16*(1), 36–41.

12 Shonkoff, J.P. (1987). Family transitions, crises, and adaptations. *Current Problems in Pediatrics, 17,* 503–553.

13 Waechter, E.H. (1987). Children's reactions to fatal illness. In Krulik, T., Holaday, B., & Martinson, I.M. (Eds.), *The child and family facing life-threatening illness,* Philadelphia: Lippincott.

14 Davies, B., & Eng, B. (1993). Factors influencing nursing care of children who are terminally ill: A selective review. *Pediatric Nursing, 19,* 9–14.

Anderson, A.H., Bateman, L.H., Ingallinera, K.L., & Woolf, P.J. (1991). Our caring continues: A bereavement follow-up program. *AACN, 18*(6), 523–526.

Armstrong-Dailey, A. (1990). Children's hospice care. *Pediatric Nursing, 16,* 337–339, 409.

Broome, M.E. (1985). Working with the family of a critically ill child. *Heart & Lung, 14*(4), 368–372.

Carpenito, L.J. (1992). *Nursing diagnosis: Application to clinical practice.* Philadelphia: Lippincott.

Curley, A.Q. (1988). Effects of the nursing mutual participation model of care on parental stress in the pediatric intensive care unit. *Heart & Lung, 17*(6), 682–688.

Fiser, D.H., Stanford, G., & Dorman, D.J. (1984). Services for parental stress reduction in a pediatric ICU. *Critical Care Medicine, 12*(6), 504–507.

Hazinski, M.F. (1992). *Nursing care of the critically ill child* (2nd ed.). St. Louis: Mosby–Year Book.

Hedenkamp, E.A. (1980). Humanizing the intensive care unit for children. *Critical Care Quarterly, 3*(1), 63–73.

Hersch, S.P., & Wiener, L.S. (1993). Psychosocial support for the family of the child with cancer. In Pizzo, P.A., & Poplack, D.G. (Eds.), *Principles and practice of pediatric oncology,* ed. 2. Philadelphia: Lippincott.

Jay, S.S. (1977). Pediatric intensive care: Involving parents in the care of their child. *American Journal of Maternal-Child Nursing, 6,* 195–203.

Krulik, T., Holaday, B., & Martinson, I.M. (Eds.) (1987). *The child and family facing life-threatening illness.* Philadelphia: Lippincott.

Kubler-Ross, E. (1983). *On children and death.* New York: Collier/Macmillan.

LaMontagne, L.L., Hepworth, J.T., Pawlak, R., & Chiafery (1992). Parental coping and activities during pediatric critical care. *American Journal of Critical Care, 1*(2), 76–80.

Leske, J.S. (Ed.) (1991). Family interventions. *AACN Clinical Issues in Critical Care Nursing, 2*(2), 181–355.

Lewandowski, L. (1980). Stress and coping styles of parents of children undergoing open-heart surgery. *Critical Care Quarterly, 3*(1), 75–84.

Miles, M.S., & Carter, M.C. (1985). Coping strategies used by parents during their child's hospitalization in an intensive care unit. *Children's Health Care, 14*(1), 14–21.

Miles, M.S., & Carter, M.C. (1983). Assessing parental stress in intensive care units. *American Journal of Maternal-Child Nursing, 8*(5), 354–359.

Mishel, M. (1983). Parents' perceptions of uncertainty concerning their hospitalized child. *Nursing Research, 32,* 324–330.

Parkman, S.E. (1992). Helping families say good-bye. *American Journal of Maternal-Child Nursing, 17,* 14–17.

Petrillo, M., & Sanger, S. (1980). *Emotional care of hospitalized children.* Philadelphia: Lippincott.

Philichi, L.M. (1989). Family adaptation during a pediatric intensive care hospitalization. *Journal of Pediatric Nursing, 4*(4), 268–276.

Rothstein, P. (1980). Psychological stress in families of children in a pediatric intensive care unit. *Pediatric Clinics of North America, 27*(3), 613–620.

Rushton, C.H. (1990). Family-centered care in the critical care unit: Myth or reality? *Children's Health Care, 19*(2), 68–70.

Rushton, C.H. (1990). Strategies for family-centered care in the critical care setting. *Pediatric Nursing, 16*(2), 195–199.

Rushton, C.H., & Lynch, M.E. (1992). Dealing with advance directives for critically ill adolescents. *Critical Care Nurse, 12*(5), 31–37.

Stevens, K.R. (1981). Humanistic nursing care for critically ill children. *Nursing Clinics of North America, 16*(4), 611–622.

Tichy, A.M., Braam, C.A., Meyer, T.A., & Rattan, N.S. (1988). Stressors in pediatric intensive care units. *Pediatric Nursing, 14*(1), 40–42.

Tse, A.M., Perez-Woods, R.C., & Opie, N.D. (1987). Children's admissions to the intensive care unit: Parents' attitudes and expectations of outcome. *Children's Health Care, 16*(2), 68–75.

Vachon, M.L.S., & Pakes, E. (1985). Staff stress in the care of the critically ill and dying child. *Issues in Comprehensive Pediatric Nursing, 8,* 151–182.

Vestal, K.W. (1981). *Pediatric critical care nursing.* New York: Wiley & Sons.

Wyckoff, P.M., & Erickson, M.T. (1987). Mediating factors of stress on mothers of seriously ill, hospitalized children. *Children's Health Care, 16*(1), 4–12.

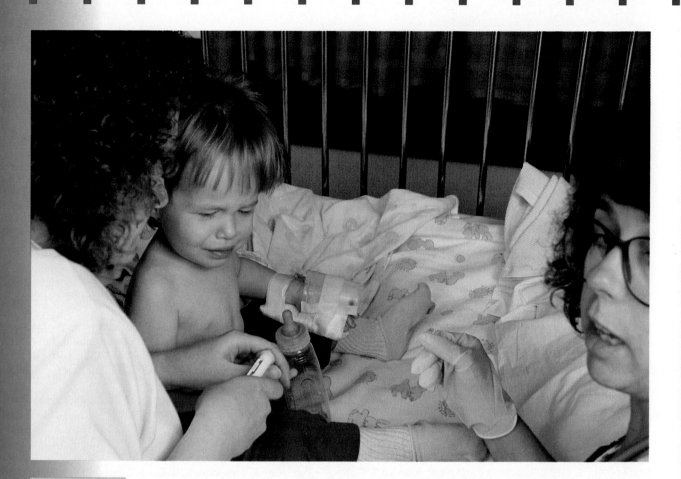

S eth is 2 years old. Several days ago he developed diarrhea. His parents tried to get him to eat, but he had little appetite. He drank a little water and a few sips of diet cola, but the next morning he was listless and would not drink anything. The diarrhea continued. His mother brought him to the emergency room. Seth was unresponsive. His eyes appeared sunken. His tongue was dry. His pulse was weak and rapid. The skin over Seth's sternum stayed pinched up for 5 seconds after the nurse tested his skin turgor. In response to the nurse's question, his mother says Seth weighed 13 kg (29 lb) at the clinic last week. However, when the nurse weighed him, the scale read only 11 kg (24½ lb). Seth had clinical dehydration. He needed rapid replacement of the proper type of fluids.

What happens inside the body when clinical dehydration occurs? How can a nurse recognize clinical dehydration? What type of fluids does Seth need? What nursing management is important for his recovery? What do Seth's parents need to be taught to prevent him from becoming dehydrated the next time he develops diarrhea?

ALTERATIONS IN FLUID AND ELECTROLYTE BALANCE

TERMINOLOGY

aldosterone A hormone secreted by the adrenal cortex that causes the renal tubules to reabsorb saline (sodium and water) and retain it in the body.

antidiuretic hormone A hormone released by the posterior pituitary gland that causes the renal tubules to reabsorb water and retain it in the body.

body fluid The body water with substances (solutes) dissolved in it.

electrolytes Substances that are charged particles when they are dissolved.

extracellular fluid The fluid in the body that is outside the cells.

filtration Movement into or out of capillaries as the net result of several opposing forces.

hypertonic fluid Fluid that is more concentrated than normal body fluid.

hypotonic fluid Fluid that is more dilute than normal body fluid.

interstitial fluid That portion of the extracellular fluid that is between the cells and outside the blood and lymphatic vessels.

intracellular fluid The fluid in the body that is inside the cells.

isotonic fluid Fluid that has the same osmolality as normal body fluid.

osmolality The "concentratedness" of a fluid; technically, the number of moles of particles per kilogram of water.

osmosis Movement of water across a semipermeable membrane into an area of higher particle concentration.

vascular fluid That portion of the extracellular fluid that is in the blood vessels.

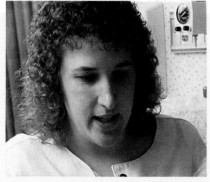

❝ So few parents realize how important proper hydration is in children. Such a large percentage of children's body weight is water that when they become dehydrated it can cause serious problems. ❞

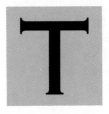

This chapter presents information about normal fluid and electrolyte homeostasis and imbalances. It provides guidance for nursing management of pediatric patients, like Seth, who have fluid and electrolyte imbalances. Using the information in this chapter, you would be able to assist in restoring Seth's fluid and electrolyte balance and help prevent similar imbalances in the future.

Body Fluid Compartments

More than half of a child's body weight is due to the water that is in the body. Body water is important because the biochemical reactions that enable the cells to function take place among the substances (solutes) dissolved in body water. The term **body fluid** is used to describe body water that has solutes dissolved in it. Some of these solutes, called **electrolytes**, are charged particles, or ions, in solution. These electrolytes, such as sodium (Na^+), potassium (K^+), calcium (Ca^{++}), magnesium (Mg^{++}), chloride (Cl^-), and inorganic phosphorus (Pi) ions, must be present in the proper concentration for the cells to function effectively. This chapter discusses body fluids and electrolytes and the alterations they may undergo in children.

In persons of all ages, body fluid is located in several compartments.[1] The two major fluid compartments contain the **intracellular fluid** (fluid inside the cells) and the **extracellular fluid** (fluid outside the cells) (Fig. 7–1).

FIGURE 7–1 The major body fluid compartments. Extracellular fluid is composed mainly of *vascular fluid* (fluid in blood vessels) and *interstitial fluid* (fluid between the cells and outside the blood and lymphatic vessels).

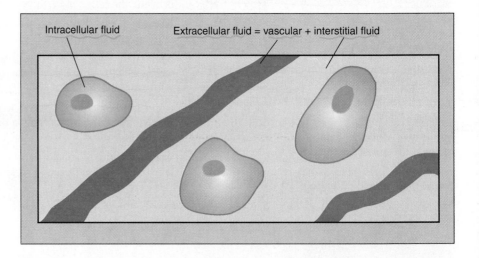

The concentrations of electrolytes differ in the fluid in the various body fluid compartments. For example, extracellular fluid is rich in sodium ions; intracellular fluid, by contrast, is low in sodium ions but rich in potassium ions (Table 7–1).

Fluid moves between the vascular and interstitial compartments (the two divisions of the extracellular fluid) by the process of filtration. Water moves into and out of the cells by the process of osmosis. These processes are discussed later in the chapter in the sections on edema and osmolality imbalances.

The percentage of body weight that is water varies with age. This percentage is highest at birth and decreases with age (Fig. 7–2). Neonates and young infants have a proportionately larger **interstitial fluid** volume than older children or adults because their brain and skin (both rich in interstitial fluid)

TABLE 7-1 Electrolyte Concentrations in Body Fluid Compartments

Components	Extracellular Fluid (ECF)		Intracellular Fluid
	Vascular	Interstitial	
Na^+	High	High	Low
K^+	Low	Low	High
Ca^{++}	Low	Low	Low (higher than ECF)
Mg^{++}	Low	Low	High
Pi	Low	Low	High
Cl^-	High	High	Low
Proteins	High	Low	High

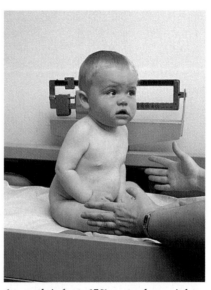

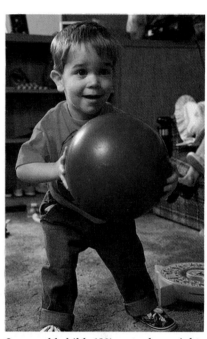

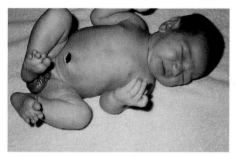

Full-term neonate, 75% water by weight

6-month infant, 65% water by weight

2-year-old child, 60% water by weight

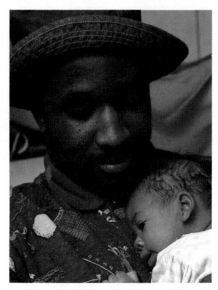

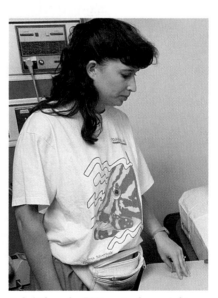

Adult male, 55% water by weight

Adult female, 50% water by weight

FIGURE 7-2 The percentage of water in the body varies with age.

FIGURE 7-3 The proportion of extracellular fluid and intracellular fluid varies with age.

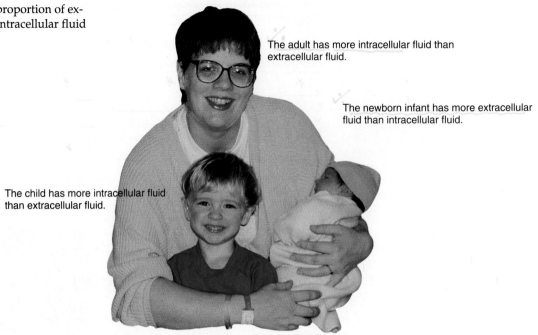

The adult has more intracellular fluid than extracellular fluid.

The newborn infant has more extracellular fluid than intracellular fluid.

The child has more intracellular fluid than extracellular fluid.

occupy a greater proportion of their body weight. As infants grow, the proportion of water inside the cells increases (Fig. 7–3).

Principles of Body Fluid Homeostasis

The fluid in the body is in a dynamic state. In persons of all ages, fluid is continuously leaving the body through the skin, during breathing, in the feces, and in the urine (Fig. 7–4). To offset this continuous fluid excretion, fluid intake must occur. If fluid intake falls below fluid excretion, the body fluid volume can become too low (Fig. 7–5).

Some children lose fluid by abnormal routes in addition to their normal fluid excretion. These abnormal routes include fever, vomiting, diarrhea, removal through tubes, fistula drainage, and hemorrhage. These children need

FIGURE 7-4 Normal routes of fluid excretion from infants and children: *skin:* insensible perspiration (greatly increased in low-birthweight infants) and sweating (reduced or absent in premature infants); *lungs:* water is excreted during exhalation (increased with increased respiratory rate, as in respiratory distress); *feces:* amount of fluid excreted in feces increases dramatically with diarrhea; *urine:* neonate has limited ability to concentrate or dilute urine.

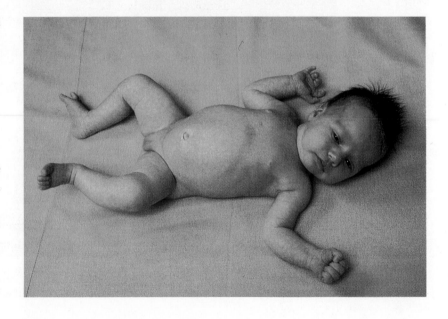

PEDIATRIC NURSING

FIGURE 7-5 Use of an overhead warmer or phototherapy increases insensible fluid excretion through the skin and thus increases the fluid intake needed.

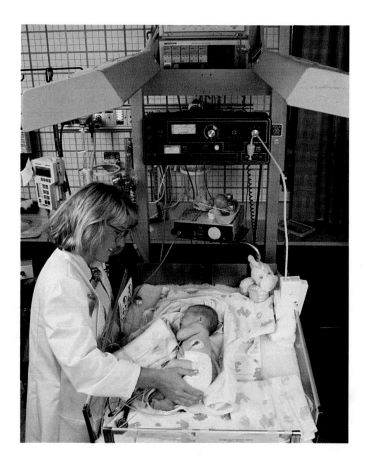

additional fluid intake to prevent a decrease in their body fluid volume. Oral fluid intake occurs by both drinking and eating because most foods contain water. In addition to the oral route, fluid may be given intravenously, through tubes into the gastrointestinal tract, rectally, or by emergency routes such as infusion into the bone marrow.

If fluid excretion and losses are balanced by the proper volume and type of fluid intake, normal fluid balance will be maintained. If, however, fluid output and intake are not matched, fluid imbalance may occur rapidly. The two major types of fluid imbalances are extracellular volume imbalances and osmolality imbalances.

Extracellular Fluid Volume Imbalances (Saline Imbalances)

Extracellular fluid volume imbalances are often called saline imbalances or **isotonic fluid** imbalances. They occur when there is too much or too little fluid in the extracellular fluid compartment. Fluid has weight (1 L of water weighs 1 kg [2.2 lb]); therefore, extracellular fluid volume imbalances can be detected by rapid changes in body weight. They also cause changes in vein filling and in interstitial volume that may be seen clinically. In their most severe forms, they can lead to death.

Extracellular Fluid Volume Excess (Saline Excess)

As the name implies, extracellular fluid volume excess occurs when there is too much fluid in the extracellular compartment (vascular and interstitial). This imbalance may also be called saline excess or extracellular volume overload. If this disorder occurs by itself (without a concurrent osmolality disorder), the serum sodium concentration will be normal. There is simply too much extracellular fluid, even though it has a normal concentration.

Clinical Manifestations

Since fluid has weight, extracellular fluid volume excess is characterized by weight gain. You can tell if a weight gain is due to normal growth or to development of extracellular fluid volume excess by looking at the speed with which the increase develops. Sudden weight gain (for example, 0.5 kg [1 lb] in one day) is due to accumulation of fluid. Gain of 0.5 kg overnight is due to retention of about 500 mL of saline.

The other clinical manifestations of extracellular fluid volume excess—bounding pulse, distended neck veins (older children), hepatomegaly, crackles, dyspnea, orthopnea—are due to overload of fluid in the blood vessels and in the interstitial spaces. In older children distention of neck veins may be visible when the child is sitting upright. Distended neck veins are usually not visible in infants.

Edema is the sign of overload of the interstitial fluid compartment. In an infant, edema is often generalized. Edema in children with extracellular fluid volume excess occurs in the dependent portions of the body, that is, the parts closest to the ground. Thus edema occurs first in the sacral area in a child with extracellular fluid volume excess who is supine in bed. Edema may also arise from other causes, which are described later in this chapter.

Etiology and Pathophysiology

Infants and children who develop an extracellular fluid volume excess have a condition that causes them to retain saline or else they have been given an overload of intravenous sodium-containing isotonic fluid (Fig. 7–6). What conditions cause retention of saline? The hormone **aldosterone** is secreted by the adrenal cortex. One of its normal functions is to cause the kidneys to retain sodium and water (saline) in the body (Fig. 7–7). Saline excess can be caused by any condition that results in excessive aldosterone secretion, such as adrenal tumors that secrete aldosterone, congestive heart failure, liver cirrhosis, and chronic renal failure. Most glucocorticoid medications (such as prednisone) have a mild saline-retaining effect when taken on a long-term basis.

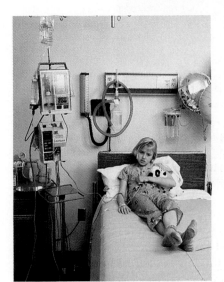

FIGURE 7–6 If isotonic fluid containing sodium is given too rapidly or in too great an amount, an extracellular fluid volume excess will develop. It is important to monitor fluid intake, excretion, and retention in children.

FIGURE 7–7 Aldosterone has a saline-retaining effect. Increased aldosterone secretion can be caused by adrenal tumors or congestive heart failure.

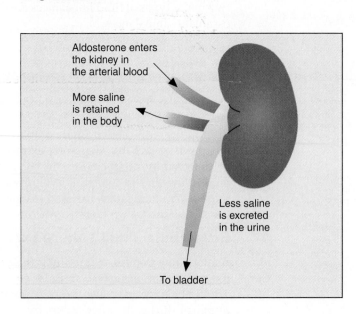

Aldosterone enters the kidney in the arterial blood

More saline is retained in the body

Less saline is excreted in the urine

To bladder

Medical Management

The medical management of extracellular fluid volume excess focuses on treating the underlying cause of the disorder. For example, a child who has congestive heart failure is given medications to strengthen the heart's ability to contract. Managing the underlying cause also helps to reduce the extracellular fluid volume excess. Diuretics may be given to remove fluid from the body, thus reducing the extracellular fluid volume directly.

Nursing Assessment

Rapid weight gain is the most sensitive index of extracellular fluid volume excess.[2] Therefore daily weighing is an important nursing assessment. Measurement of intake and output is also important; when monitored accurately, intake will be greater than output. The volume excess in the vascular compartment can be assessed by noting the character of the pulse (bounding) and observing for distention of the neck veins when the child is upright (usually visible only in older children). A severe imbalance will cause pulmonary edema, which should be monitored by listening to lung sounds in the dependent lung fields (crackles) and assessing for respiratory distress (rapid respiratory rate, dyspnea, use of accessory muscles of respiration). The volume excess in the interstitial compartment is assessed by looking for edema.

The presence of edema, especially in an older child, may lead to social embarrassment or altered body image. If a child has a condition that causes a prolonged extracellular fluid volume excess with edema, nursing assessment needs to include the areas of self-concept and interaction with other children (as appropriate to developmental level).

Nursing Diagnosis

The most obvious nursing diagnosis for a child with extracellular fluid volume excess is Fluid Volume Excess. Several other nursing diagnoses may be appropriate, depending on the severity of the imbalance and the age of the child. Specific examples include:

- Fluid Volume Excess manifested by (patient's signs and symptoms)
- High Risk for Altered Peripheral Tissue Perfusion related to exchange problems
- High Risk for Altered Skin Integrity related to presence of edema
- Knowledge Deficit (Parent) regarding home management of sodium restriction
- Impaired Social Interaction with peers related to embarrassment about edema

Nursing Management

The potential for causing an extracellular fluid volume excess is present whenever an isotonic intravenous fluid containing sodium is being administered. Therefore monitor the infusion rate frequently and carefully (Fig. 7–8).

If an extracellular fluid volume excess has already developed, it is important to administer the medical therapy as prescribed and to monitor for the complications of medical therapy. For example, many diuretics increase potassium excretion in the urine, which may lead to an abnormally low plasma potassium concentration unless potassium intake is increased. This is discussed in the section on hypokalemia in this chapter. It is also important to monitor for the development of extracellular fluid volume deficit from diuretic therapy.

■ ISOTONIC INTRAVENOUS FLUIDS CONTAINING SODIUM

Normal saline (0.9% NaCl)
Ringer solution
Lactated Ringer solution

If edema is present, provide careful skin care and protection for edematous areas. Parents will need to be taught how to provide skin care at home.

If a child has a long-term condition such as chronic renal failure that predisposes to extracellular fluid volume excess, a dietary sodium restriction may be prescribed. A nurse has a valuable role in teaching the parents how to manage sodium restriction at home. This teaching should include practice in planning low-sodium meals that fit the family's cultural practices. If the child is old enough to participate, games can be incorporated into the teaching sessions. The parents (or other caregivers) also need to be taught to record the child's weight daily.

Extracellular Fluid Volume Deficit (Saline Deficit)

Extracellular fluid volume deficit occurs when there is not enough fluid in the extracellular compartment (vascular and interstitial). This situation may also be called saline deficit or isotonic dehydration. The serum sodium concentration is normal unless an osmolality imbalance is also present.

Clinical Manifestations

A child who has an extracellular fluid volume deficit will have a rapid weight loss, except with third space accumulation (e.g., fluid in the peritoneal cavity), when the weight will not decrease. The other clinical manifestations are due to the decreased vascular volume and the decreased interstitial fluid volume (Table 7–2). A severe extracellular fluid volume deficit will cause hypovolemic shock.[3]

How many of the signs of extracellular fluid volume deficit did Seth have in the case study at the beginning of this chapter? Seth had clinical dehydration, which is a combination of extracellular fluid volume deficit and hypernatremia. Clinical dehydration is discussed later in this chapter.

Etiology and Pathophysiology

Extracellular fluid volume deficit is usually caused by loss of a sodium-containing fluid from the body. Conditions that cause loss of fluid containing

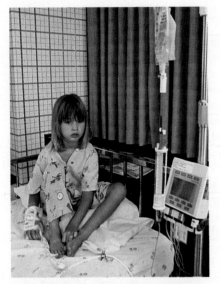

FIGURE 7–8 The use of a volume control device with an intravenous saline infusion is important to prevent a sudden extracellular fluid volume overload.

TABLE 7–2 Clinical Manifestations of Extracellular Fluid Volume Deficit

Signs and Symptoms	Physiologic Basis
Weight loss	Decreased fluid volume; 1 L of fluid weighs 1 kg
Postural blood pressure drop (older children)	Inadequate circulating blood volume to offset the force of gravity when in upright position
Increased small vein filling time	Decreased vascular volume
Delayed capillary refill time	Decreased vascular volume
Flat neck veins when supine (older children)	Decreased vascular volume
Dizziness, syncope	Inadequate circulation to brain
Oliguria	Inadequate circulation to kidneys
Thready, rapid pulse	Cardiac reflex response to decreased vascular volume
Sunken fontanel (infants)	Decreased fluid volume
Decreased skin turgor	Decreased interstitial fluid volume

sodium include adrenal insufficiency, bedrest, overuse of diuretics, emesis, diarrhea, nasogastric suction, burns, and hemorrhage. Extracellular fluid volume deficit may also occur if extracellular fluid accumulates in a "third space" such as the peritoneal cavity.

Medical Management

The treatment for extracellular fluid volume deficit is administration of intravenous fluid that contains sodium. This fluid may be isotonic saline (normal saline), lactated Ringer solution (especially with older children), half-normal, or quarter-normal saline (especially with infants or with concurrent hypernatremia). The original cause is also treated.

■ **CLINICAL TIP**

To obtain urine from an infant for testing specific gravity, place two cotton balls in a test tube (males) or in the diaper. When they are wet, push them into a 10 mL syringe and squeeze out the urine.

Nursing Assessment

Weighing the child daily is essential. Other useful assessments are intake and output measurements, character of heart rate, filling of neck veins, small vein filling time (see Fig. 3–7), capillary refill time, urine specific gravity, postural blood pressure measurements, and skin turgor. Compare the blood pressure when the child is supine with the pressure when the child is sitting with legs hanging down or is standing. If the extracellular fluid volume is decreased, the sitting or standing blood pressure will be less than the supine blood pressure because blood accumulates in the dependent legs.

Nursing Diagnosis

The nursing diagnosis Fluid Volume Deficit applies to all children who have an extracellular fluid volume deficit. Other diagnoses depend on the severity of the condition and the age of the child. Specific examples include:

- Fluid Volume Deficit manifested by (patient's specific signs and symptoms)
- High Risk for Altered Peripheral Tissue Perfusion related to exchange problems
- High Risk for Injury related to postural hypotension
- Activity Intolerance related to weakness and dizziness
- Knowledge Deficit (Parent) regarding home management of diarrhea and vomiting

Nursing Management

Because dizziness is one manifestation of extracellular fluid volume deficit, interventions to promote safety are important. The side rails of the bed are kept in the up position. When intravenous isotonic fluid replacement is being given, monitor for saline overload by listening for crackles in the dependent portions of the lungs.

A mild extracellular fluid volume deficit occurs after about 4 days of bedrest. Use caution in helping a sick or weak child to sit in a chair and provide assistance when the child walks after prolonged bedrest.

Teach parents to replace a child's fluid losses from vomiting and diarrhea with both salt and water. Commercial preparations of oral electrolyte solution are now preferred for initial management of mild or moderate extracellular fluid volume deficit.

Osmolality Imbalances (Serum Sodium Imbalances)

135–145 mEq/L (except newborns)
139–162 mEq/L (newborns)

The serum sodium concentration reflects the **osmolality** ("concentrated-ness") of body fluids. It indicates the degree of concentration or dilution of body fluids. The serum sodium concentration does not indicate how much sodium is in the body. Rather, it reflects the relative proportion of sodium and water. When the osmolality of body fluids becomes abnormal, the cells swell or shrink. These cell size changes are due to **osmosis**, the movement of water across a semipermeable membrane into an area of higher particle concentration. Swelling or shrinking of brain cells alters the level of consciousness and may be fatal. The two osmolality imbalances are hypernatremia (body fluids too concentrated) and hyponatremia (body fluids too dilute).

Hypernatremia

Hypernatremia indicates increased osmolality of the blood. The body fluids contain excess salt relative to water. In other words, they are too concentrated.

Clinical Manifestations

A serum sodium level above 145 mEq/L (162 mEq/L in newborns) is diagnostic of hypernatremia. An infant or child who has hypernatremia will be thirsty. The urine output is usually small unless the hypernatremia is caused by diabetes insipidus. A decreased level of consciousness—confusion, lethargy, and coma—results from shrinking of the brain cells. Seizures may occur when hypernatremia arises rapidly or is severe. Severe hypernatremia may be fatal.

What signs of hypernatremia did Seth have in the case study at the beginning of this chapter? Hypernatremia is one component of clinical dehydration, which is discussed below.

Etiology and Pathophysiology

Hypernatremia is caused by conditions that make body fluid too concentrated. These conditions cause loss of relatively more water than salt or gain of relatively more salt than water. Causes of hypernatremia are presented in Table 7–3. Special circumstances in which a high solute intake may occur without adequate water are giving an infant formula that is too concentrated or a formula mistakenly prepared with salt instead of sugar.[4]

TABLE 7-3 Causes of Hypernatremia

Loss of Relatively More Water Than Salt	Gain of Relatively More Salt Than Water
Diabetes insipidus (not enough antidiuretic hormone)	Inability to communicate thirst
Diarrhea or vomiting without fluid replacement	Limited or no access to water
Excessive sweating without fluid replacement	High solute intake without adequate water (e.g., tube feedings)
High solute intake without adequate water (causes kidneys to excrete water)	Intravenous hypertonic saline

---

Medical Management

Hypernatremia is treated by intravenous administration of **hypotonic fluid.** This therapy dilutes the body fluids back to normal concentration. The nurse should watch for rebound hyponatremia while monitoring the fluid replacement for treatment of hypernatremia. If the child has a coexisting extracellular fluid volume deficit, administration of isotonic fluids may be ordered first to replenish the volume, followed by hypotonic fluid to correct the osmolality.

Nursing Assessment

Monitor serum sodium level and measure intake and output and urine specific gravity. Frequent assessment of level of consciousness is necessary to monitor the hypernatremic child's response to therapy. As the concentration of body fluids returns to normal, the child will become more alert and responsive. The urine specific gravity will also decrease.

Water deprivation is one form of child abuse. A small child who is hospitalized with hypernatremia that does not have a detectable cause may have been subjected to such "thirsting."[5] Careful assessment of the child's physical condition and of family dynamics should follow.

Nursing Diagnosis

For the child who has hypernatremia, the following nursing diagnoses may apply:

- High Risk for Injury related to decreased level of consciousness
- Self-Care Deficit related to lethargy
- Knowledge Deficit (Parent) regarding home management of diarrhea and vomiting

Nursing Management

Teaching can prevent hypernatremia. When an infant is sick or developing slowly, sometimes the parents want to "feed up" the baby to make it stronger. Parents and other caregivers of bottle-fed babies should be taught never to give undiluted evaporated milk or double-strength formula because this concentrated fluid can actually harm infants instead of making them stronger. Parents should be cautioned to keep salt out of reach, since eating handfuls of salt has caused hypernatremia. Nursing interventions to prevent hypernatremia also include administering water between tube feedings, keeping water available, and offering it frequently to hospitalized infants and children.

A child who has hypernatremia needs safety interventions, such as raised bedrails, for protection. Administration of the prescribed water replacement for hypernatremia is also a nursing function. When water is to be replaced orally, creative interventions, for example, making a game of the activity, may be necessary.

When hypernatremia results from diarrhea and vomiting, the parents need to be taught home management of diarrhea and vomiting. This topic is discussed in the section on oral rehydration below.

Clinical Dehydration

The case study at the beginning of this chapter is a typical scenario for the development of clinical dehydration. Clinical dehydration occurs when hypotonic body fluids containing sodium are lost and not replaced. In infants

TABLE 7–4 Severity of Clinical Dehydration

	Mild	Moderate	Severe
Percent of body weight lost	Up to 5%	5%–9%	10% or more
Level of conciousness	Alert, restless, thirsty	Restless or lethargic (infants and very young children); alert, thirsty, restless (older children and adolescents)	Lethargic to comatose (infants and young children); often conscious, apprehensive (older children and adolescents)
Blood pressure	Normal	Normal or low; postural hypotension (older children and adolescents)	Low to undetectable
Rapid pulse	Normal	Rapid	Rapid, weak to nonpalpable
Skin turgor	Normal	Poor	Very poor
Mucous membrane	Moist	Dry	Parched
Urine	May appear normal	Decreased output, dark color	Very decreased or absent output

TABLE 7–5 Manifestations of Clinical Dehydration

Clinical Observation	Cause	Findings in the Case Study
Weight loss	Extracellular volume deficit	10% (severe dehydration)
Rapid pulse	Cardiac response to extracellular volume deficit	Pulse weak and rapid
Dry mucous membranes	Extracellular volume deficit	Tongue dry
Decreased skin turgor	Extracellular volume deficit	Skin tented for 5 seconds
Absence of tears	Extracellular volume deficit	
Sunken eyeballs	Extracellular volume deficit	Eyes appeared sunken
Sunken fontanel (infants)	Extracellular volume deficit	Fontanel closed
Lethargic to comatose	Hypernatremia	Unresponsive

■ GROWTH AND DEVELOPMENT CONSIDERATIONS

Infants and young children are at high risk for clinical dehydration because of their higher percentage of body water by weight, proportionately large body surface area, and frequent gastrointestinal illness.

and children, clinical dehydration arises most commonly from gastroenteritis, repeated vomiting, and diarrhea. Clinical dehydration is the combination of extracellular fluid volume deficit and hypernatremia. The body fluid volume is too low; the body fluids are also too concentrated (Table 7–4).

Table 7–5 presents the manifestations of clinical dehydration. Severe clinical dehydration causes death from hypovolemic shock. In the case study, Seth was brought to the hospital in time for satisfactory treatment.

Oral Rehydration

A child who has clinical dehydration needs fluid replacement. The fluid used for replacement is isotonic saline with extra water added (e.g., half-normal or quarter-normal saline). This fluid combination replenishes the extracellular fluid volume (isotonic saline) and dilutes the body fluid back to normal (extra water). In developed countries a child who has severe clinical dehydration (weight loss of 10% or more) is usually given intravenous fluid replacement. In developing countries oral rehydration therapy is used for treatment of severe dehydration. Fluids used for oral rehydration should contain salt (sodium chloride), sugar, and potassium. Bicarbonate or citrate (which is metabolized to bicarbonate by the liver) is also present in commercially available solutions. The salt with the water replaces extracellular fluid volume. The sugar is necessary for gastrointestinal absorption of sodium. The potassium helps to replace potassium lost in the emesis or diarrhea fluid. Bicarbonate helps to prevent metabolic acidosis that is associated with diarrhea. Commercial oral rehydration solutions (e.g., Rehydralyte) are available in drugstores in the United States without a prescription. Oral rehydration solution may be prepared at home.

Nursing Management

The accompanying Nursing Care Plan summarizes care of the child with severe clinical dehydration. Rehydration fluid should be given frequently in small amounts. For example, 1 to 3 teaspoons of fluid every 10 to 15 minutes is a useful guideline for starting oral rehydration. Parents need to know that if a child vomits, current recommendations are to continue with oral rehydration because usually some of the fluid is retained and absorbed.[6] Repeated vomiting of large volumes of fluid may indicate the need for intravenous therapy, and the parents should contact a health care professional.

Less severe dehydration can be managed (and severe dehydration prevented) with oral rehydration therapy. Teaching parents what fluids to give at home when a child has diarrhea or vomiting is a vital nursing intervention because it can prevent the need for hospitalization. In the case study Seth was given inappropriate fluids in small quantities when he had diarrhea. The result was severe dehydration and hospitalization.

Another important nursing intervention is to teach the parents the signs of clinical dehydration. They need to know that if the child's condition becomes worse or is not improved after 4 hours of oral rehydration therapy, they should contact a health care professional. As the child becomes rehydrated, fluids can be given more slowly for maintenance, rather than for replacement (Table 7–6).

TABLE 7-6 Rehydration and Maintenance Fluids for Clinical Dehydration

Maintenance Solutions to Prevent Clinical Dehydration from Diarrhea

Pedialyte
Infalyte
Lytren
Resol

Replacement Solutions to Treat Clinical Dehydration

Rehydralyte
WHO solution (90 mEq Na^+/L; 20 mEq K^+/L; 80 mEq Cl^-/L; 30 mEq HCO_3^-/L; 20 g glucose/L)

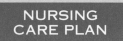

THE CHILD WITH SEVERE CLINICAL DEHYDRATION

GOAL	INTERVENTION	RATIONALE	EXPECTED OUTCOME
1. Fluid Volume Deficit manifested by poor skin turgor, delayed capillary refill and small vein filling times, and high urine specific gravity			
The child will return to normal hydration status. The child will not develop hypovolemic shock.	Monitor weight daily. Assess intake and output every shift. Assess heart rate, postural blood pressure, skin turgor, small vein filling time, capillary refill time, fontanel (infant), neck vein filling (older child), and urine specific gravity every 4 hours or more frequently as indicated.	Frequent assessment of hydration status facilitates rapid intervention and evaluation of effectiveness of fluid replacement.	The child has signs of normal hydration.
	Administer IV fluids as ordered. Monitor for crackles in dependent portions of the lungs.	Replace fluid lost from the body. Excessive replacement of sodium-containing fluids could cause extracellular fluid volume excess.	
2. High Risk for Injury related to decreased level of consciousness or to postural hypotension			
The child will not experience injury.	Raise side rails of bed. Ensure that a small child does not become tangled in bedcovers.	Safety measures protect the child.	The child does not fall or suffer other injury.
	Monitor level of consciousness every 2 to 4 hours or more often as indicated.	Frequent assessment provides evidence of need for safety interventions and of effectiveness of therapy.	
	Monitor serum sodium concentration daily or more often.	Elevated serum sodium concentration causes brain cell shrinking and decreased level of consciousness.	
	Have child sit before rising from bed and assist to stand slowly.	Slow adjustment to upright posture reduces lightheadedness from decreased blood volume.	
3. Knowledge Deficit (Parent) regarding home management of diarrhea and vomiting			
The parent or other caregiver will describe appropriate home management of fluid replacement for diarrhea and vomiting.	Explain how to replace body fluid with sodium, some sugar, and water, using oral rehydration solution (infants and young children) or bouillon and other fluids (older children).	Anticipate potential for recurrence and assist preparedness. Explain rationale for type of fluids to assist understanding.	The parent (and older child) describes home management of fluid replacement after teaching.
	Emphasize avoidance of diet soda and need to dilute apple juice or cola.	Sugar facilitates absorption of sodium from the gastrointestinal tract and provides calories. Fluid with high osmolality may cause more diarrhea.	
	Provide written summary.	Written instructions reinforce verbal teaching and provide a reference for future use.	The parent takes the instruction sheet home.

Hyponatremia

Hyponatremia indicates decreased osmolality of the blood. The body fluids contain excess water relative to salt. In other words, they are too dilute.

Clinical Manifestations

A serum sodium level below 135 mEq/L (139 mEq/L in newborns) is diagnostic of hyponatremia. A child who has hyponatremia has a decreased level of consciousness, which results from swelling of brain cells. This can be seen as lethargy, confusion, or coma. If hyponatremia arises rapidly or is extreme, seizures may occur. Nausea and vomiting also occur in some children. Severe hyponatremia may be fatal.

Etiology and Pathophysiology

Hyponatremia is caused by conditions that make body fluids too dilute. These conditions cause gain of relatively more water than salt or loss of relatively more salt than water. Examination of the causes of hyponatremia (Table 7–7) shows that several involve excessive administration of dilute fluids. These include tap water enemas, intravenous D5W, and distilled water as an irrigating solution. Oral intake of water causes hyponatremia only under unusual conditions such as forced fluid intake (child abuse)[7] or feeding an infant only water instead of formula or breast milk. Some "water babies" have developed hyponatremia after swallowing water from a swimming pool.[8]

Medical Management

In most cases, hyponatremia is treated by restricting the intake of water (Table 7–8). This therapy allows the kidneys to correct the imbalance by ex-

---

TABLE 7–7 Causes of Hyponatremia

Gain of Relatively More Water Than Salt	Loss of Relatively More Salt Than Water
Excessive intravenous D5W (5% dextrose in water)	Diarrhea or vomiting with replacement by tap water only instead of fluid containing sodium
Excessive tap water enemas	
Irrigation of body cavities with distilled water	
Excessive antidiuretic hormone	
Forced excessive oral intake of tap water	

TABLE 7–8 Nursing Interventions for a Child Who Has a Fluid Restriction

(Modify according to child's developmental level)

- Give cold rather than lukewarm fluids.
- Use an insulated glass that looks bigger than it is.
- Be sure that extra fluids are removed from meal trays before the child sees them.
- Have the child swish fluids around in the mouth before swallowing, to relieve thirst.
- Provide frequent oral care.
- Suggest eating meals dry and drinking between meals.
- Provide a chart so an older child can keep intake records.

creting excess water from the body. If a child is having seizures from hyponatremia, intravenous hypertonic saline may be administered. Use of this concentrated fluid is a rapid way to make body fluids more concentrated but must be monitored carefully because it can easily cause rebound hypernatremia.

Nursing Assessment

Monitor serum sodium level and measure intake and output. Since hyponatremia is characterized by decreased level of consciousness, frequent assessment of level of consciousness will be necessary to monitor the response to therapy. The child will become more alert and responsive as the concentration of body fluids returns to normal.

Nursing Diagnosis

As with hypernatremia, the highest priority nursing diagnosis for hyponatremia addresses the potential for injury caused by the child's decreased level of consciousness. The following diagnoses may apply:

- High Risk for Injury related to decreased level of consciousness
- Self-Care Deficit related to lethargy
- Knowledge Deficit (Parents) regarding home management of diarrhea and vomiting
- Knowledge Deficit (Parents) regarding home management of constipation

Nursing Management

Nurses can prevent hyponatremia in hospitalized children by using normal saline instead of distilled water for irrigations and by avoiding repetitive tap water enemas.

The most important nursing interventions for a child who already has hyponatremia are providing a safe environment and helping the child to comply with the prescribed fluid restriction. A child on a fluid restriction should be allowed to choose favorite fluids. Visual aids help young children to choose favorite fluids.

Parents of a child whose hyponatremia is caused by replacing fluids lost through diarrhea or vomiting with just tap water (and no salt) need to be taught to replace body fluid with oral electrolyte solutions rather than tap water.

Hyponatremia that occurs without a detectable cause in a child who does not have abnormally high levels of **antidiuretic hormone** (ADH) may be due to unusual circumstances that require skillful nursing intervention. Perhaps the family has no money and the hungry infant is being fed water instead of formula. A toddler or young school-age child may be subjected to forced fluid intake as a form of child abuse. Careful questioning may lead the family to disclose such a situation, which can then be managed appropriately.

■ Edema

Edema is an abnormal increase in the volume of the interstitial fluid. It may be caused by an extracellular fluid volume excess or it may be due to other causes.[9] Edema pushes the cells farther apart than normal. Thus edematous tissue is fragile.

Clinical Manifestations

Edema causes swelling, which may be localized or generalized. The swelling of tissue may cause pain and restrict motion. For example, a child will have difficulty bending an edematous finger. Edema that is due to extracellular fluid volume excess or right-sided heart failure usually occurs in the dependent portion of the body. In a child who is walking, dependent edema is observed in the ankles; in a bedfast supine child it is in the sacral area. The skin over an edematous area may appear thin and shiny.

Etiology and Pathophysiology

The causes of edema are best understood in the context of normal capillary dynamics. As mentioned previously, fluid moves between the vascular and interstitial compartments by the process of **filtration**. Filtration is the net result of forces that tend to move fluid in opposing directions. The direction with the strongest forces will be the direction of fluid movement. At the capillary level, two forces (blood hydrostatic pressure and interstitial fluid osmotic pressure) tend to move fluid from the capillary into the interstitial fluid, while two other forces (blood colloid osmotic pressure and interstitial fluid hydrostatic pressure) tend to move fluid in the opposite direction (from the interstitial fluid into the capillary) (Fig. 7–9).

The net result of these forces usually moves fluid from the capillaries into the interstitial compartment at the arterial end of the capillaries and fluid from the interstitial compartment back into the capillaries at the venous end of the capillaries. This process brings oxygen and nutrients to the cells and removes carbon dioxide and other waste products.

If the balance of these four forces is altered so that excess fluid enters the interstitial compartment, edema occurs. Edema also occurs if the balance of forces is altered so that too little fluid leaves the interstitial compartment (Fig. 7–10).

The four causes of edema are increased blood hydrostatic pressure, decreased blood osmotic pressure, increased interstitial fluid osmotic pressure, and blocked lymphatic drainage (Table 7–9). Many different clinical condi-

FIGURE 7–9 Normal capillary dynamics. Edema is not present. Fluid moves out of the compartment by the force of hydrostatic pressure in the blood vessel and is pulled out by interstitial osmotic pressure. Fluid moves into the compartment by being forced in by interstitial hydrostatic pressure and pulled in by compartment osmotic pressure.

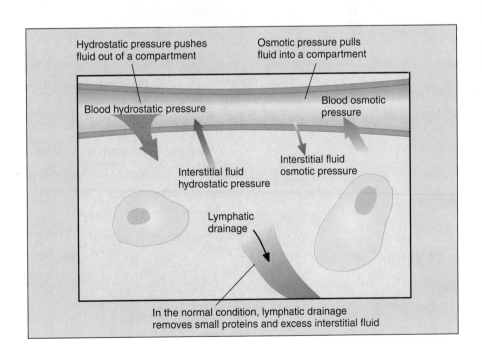

Hydrostatic pressure pushes fluid out of a compartment

Osmotic pressure pulls fluid into a compartment

Blood hydrostatic pressure

Blood osmotic pressure

Interstitial fluid hydrostatic pressure

Interstitial fluid osmotic pressure

Lymphatic drainage

In the normal condition, lymphatic drainage removes small proteins and excess interstitial fluid

FIGURE 7-10 Abnormal capillary dynamics that cause edema.

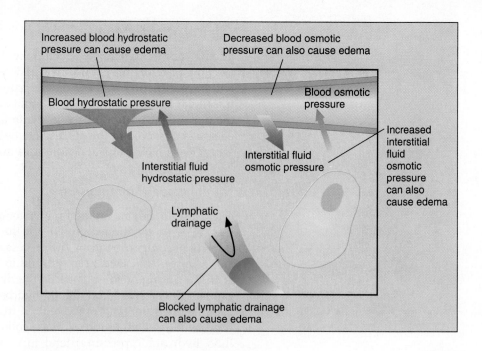

Increased blood hydrostatic pressure can cause edema

Decreased blood osmotic pressure can also cause edema

Blood hydrostatic pressure

Blood osmotic pressure

Interstitial fluid hydrostatic pressure

Interstitial fluid osmotic pressure

Increased interstitial fluid osmotic pressure can also cause edema

Lymphatic drainage

Blocked lymphatic drainage can also cause edema

TABLE 7-9 Clinical Conditions That Cause Edema

Edema Due to Increased Blood Hydrostatic Pressure

Increased Capillary Blood Flow

Inflammation
Local infection

Venous Congestion

Extracellular fluid volume excess
Right heart failure
Venous thrombosis
External pressure on vein
Muscle paralysis

Edema Due to Decreased Blood Osmotic Pressure

Increased Albumin Excretion

Nephrotic syndrome (albumin leaks into urine)
Protein-losing enteropathies (much albumin in feces)

Decreased Albumin Synthesis

Kwashiorkor (low-protein, high-carbohydrate starvation diet provides too few
    amino acids for liver to make albumin)
Liver cirrhosis (diseased liver unable to make enough albumin)

Edema Due to Increased Interstitial Fluid Osmotic Pressure

Increased Capillary Permeability

Inflammation
Toxins
Hypersensitivity reactions
Burns

Edema Due to Blocked Lymphatic Drainage

Tumors
Goiter
Parasites that obstruct lymph nodes
Surgery that removes lymph nodes

tions are associated with these altered forces. The edema that occurs with extracellular fluid volume excess is caused by *increased blood hydrostatic pressure*. The increased fluid volume in the vascular compartment congests the veins. The pressure against the sides of the capillary is increased and more fluid then enters the interstitial compartment.

The osmotic pressure of the blood is important in pulling fluid into the capillaries. Much of this osmotic pressure is due to the presence of albumin and other plasma proteins made by the liver. The part of the blood osmotic pressure that is due to plasma proteins is often called oncotic pressure or blood colloid osmotic pressure. Any condition that decreases plasma proteins will *decrease blood colloid osmotic pressure* and cause edema. For example, if a clinical condition causes large amounts of albumin to leak into the urine, the liver is unable to make albumin fast enough to replace it. Thus the plasma protein level will fall, decreasing the blood osmotic pressure. Without this pulling force to return fluid to the capillaries, edema will occur. This is the cause of the edema that occurs in children who have nephrotic syndrome.

Increased interstitial fluid osmotic pressure is caused by increased capillary permeability, which allows large amounts of plasma proteins to leak into the interstitial fluid. Ordinarily, only a few small proteins enter the interstitial fluid and the interstitial fluid osmotic pressure is small. If the capillary becomes abnormally permeable to proteins, the influx of proteins into the interstitial fluid causes a dramatic increase in interstitial fluid osmotic pressure. This increased pulling force keeps an abnormal amount of fluid in the interstitial compartment. This mechanism plays an important part in the edema caused by a bee sting or a sprained ankle.

The fourth cause of edema is *blocked lymphatic drainage*. The lymph vessels normally drain small proteins and excess fluid from the interstitial compartment and return them to the blood vessels. If this process is blocked, fluid accumulates in the interstitial compartment.

Medical Management

The main focus of medical management of edema is to treat the underlying condition that caused the edema. Such conditions are discussed elsewhere in this book. For example, medical management of nephrotic syndrome is discussed in Chapter 18. The inflammation-produced local edema from an injury is treated initially with application of cold to reduce capillary blood flow and thus reduce blood hydrostatic pressure.

Nursing Assessment

A child or parent may make comments that will alert the nurse to the development of edema. Shoes may become too tight by the end of the day (dependent edema); the waistband of pants or skirt may be "outgrown" suddenly (generalized edema or ascites [accumulation of fluid in the peritoneal cavity]); the eyes may be "puffy" (periorbital edema); a ring may be too tight in an older child; fingers may "feel like sausages."

In many cases visual inspection is sufficient to recognize the swelling of edema. The nurse can also observe for the presence of pitting edema (Fig. 7–11). To detect changes in the amount of swelling, measure around the edematous body part (Fig. 7–12). If the edema is caused by extracellular fluid volume excess, daily measurements of weight and intake and output are a useful part of the daily assessment.

In addition to assessment of the location and extent of the edema and changes from day to day, nursing assessment of edema should focus on the integrity of the skin, pain, restricted motion, and alterations in the child's body image (if appropriate for age).

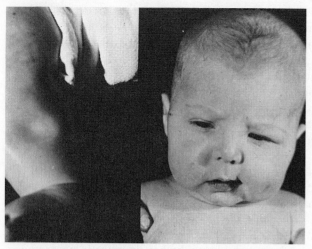

FIGURE 7–11 Pitting edema is detected by pushing the thumb gently into the tissue and watching for an indentation that remains after the thumb is removed.
Copyright ©1975 by MEDCOM, Inc.

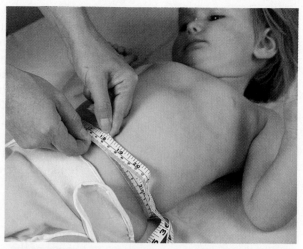

FIGURE 7–12 Finding the same location each day for measuring circumference to assess edema can be accomplished by use of a reference point. An indelible marker may be used to mark the measurement location on the skin, if this is acceptable to the child and parents.

Nursing Diagnosis

High Risk for Altered Skin Integrity is an important nursing diagnosis that will guide nursing care and teaching for the parents. Other nursing diagnoses may be appropriate, depending on the location, severity, and expected duration of the edema and the age of the infant or child. Specific examples include:

- High Risk for Altered Skin Integrity related to presence of edema
- Impaired Physical Mobility related to presence of edema
- Pain related to presence of edema
- Knowledge Deficit (Parent) regarding home management of edema
- Body Image Disturbance related to presence of edema
- Impaired Social Interaction with peers related to embarrassment about edema

Nursing Management

Elevation of an area of localized edema helps to reduce the swelling. The skin over an edematous area needs extra care because it is fragile (Fig. 7–13). An infant or bedfast child should be positioned carefully and turned frequently to prevent a pressure sore. Turning must be performed carefully to avoid causing sheet burns. Frequent cleansing with patting dry, rather than rubbing, is appropriate. The child's fingernails should be trimmed smooth so the skin will not easily be broken from scratching. Parents should be taught skin care so that they can care for the child at home. Older children can participate actively in this aspect of their own care.

If restricted mobility is a problem, specific plans to help the child manage activities are needed. For example, if edematous fingers restrict the motion of a hand, food can be cut into bite-sized portions before the meal is served, so that the child can still eat independently.

Discomfort from edema may require creative interventions by the nurse. Distraction with toys or activities appropriate to the child's developmental level can be useful. Interventions to treat the underlying problem also reduce the edema and its accompanying discomfort. Interventions for edema should

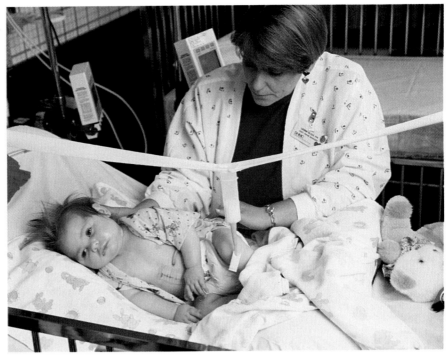

FIGURE 7–13 Edematous tissue is easily damaged. It must be kept clean and dry and free of pressure.

be added to the nursing management of the underlying condition that causes the edema. Administration of the prescribed medical therapy and observation for the complications of therapy are nursing responsibilities. Embarrassment regarding appearance can be addressed at the child's developmental level.

Principles of Electrolyte Homeostasis

All body fluids contain electrolytes, although the concentration of those electrolytes varies, depending on the type and location of the fluid. When a serum electrolyte value is reported from the laboratory, it provides information about the concentration of that electrolyte in the blood. It may not, however, give information about the concentration of the electrolyte in other body compartments.

A child develops an electrolyte imbalance when electrolyte homeostasis is altered. The simple bathtub analogy in Figure 7–14 illustrates electrolyte homeostasis (A), plasma electrolyte excess (B), and plasma electrolyte deficit (C).[10] In a healthy child there may be no loss of electrolyte through an abnormal route. Abnormal routes of electrolyte loss for children include emesis, wound drainage, and nasogastric suction.

Remember that serum sodium disorders are caused by concentration or dilution of body fluids. Thus, this bathtub analogy applies only to the homeostasis and imbalances of other electrolytes. The components of electrolyte homeostasis will be used in this chapter as the framework for discussion of potassium, calcium, and magnesium imbalances.

Potassium Imbalances

The concentration of potassium ions inside and outside muscle cells determines how well muscles will respond to a neural stimulus.

FIGURE 7-14 A bathtub provides a simple analogy for **(A)** electrolyte homeostasis, **(B)** plasma electrolyte excess, and **(C)** plasma electrolyte deficit.

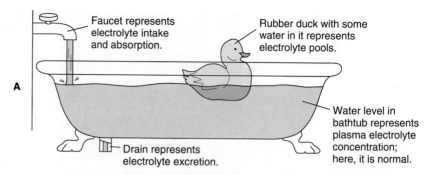

A, Electrolytes enter body through many routes (e.g., oral, intravenous). Oral electrolytes are then absorbed from gastrointestinal tract. *Electrolyte intake and absorption* are symbolized by partly open faucet on bathtub. *Electrolyte distribution* then carries electrolytes into extracellular fluid and into pools of electrolytes in other places in body (e.g., inside cells, in bones). Water level in bathtub symbolizes plasma concentration of electrolyte. Rubber duck (which also contains water) symbolizes electrolyte pools in other places in body. *Electrolyte excretion* occurs through normal routes of urine, feces, and sweat. In bathtub analogy, electrolyte excretion is symbolized by partially open drain. Clearly, water level in bathtub (plasma electrolyte concentration) varies, depending on faucet (intake and absorption), amount of water that leaks into duck (distribution to electrolyte pools), and drain (excretion). In this normal situation there is no electrolyte loss by an abnormal route.

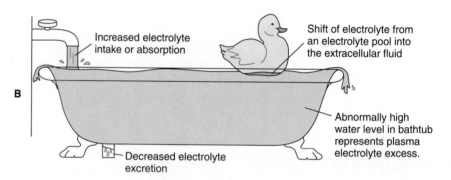

B, The three causes of a high plasma electrolyte concentration (too much water in bathtub) are *increased electrolyte intake or absorption* (faucet is wide open), *shift of electrolyte into an electrolyte pool* or physiologically unavailable form (rubber duck is swollen with water), and *decreased electrolyte excretion* (drain is closed).

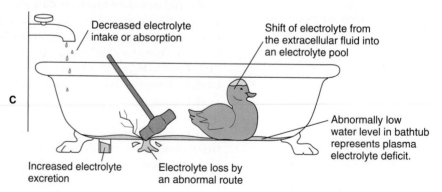

C, The four causes of a low plasma electrolyte concentration (not enough water in bathtub) are *decreased electrolyte intake or absorption* (faucet is closed), *shift of electrolyte out of an electrolyte pool* (rubber duck has given up most of its water), *increased electrolyte excretion* (drain is wide open), and *loss of electrolyte through abnormal routes* (jackhammer has made a hole in bathtub).

Potassium *intake* in healthy children comes from potassium-rich foods such as fruits and vegetables. Potassium is *absorbed* easily from the intestines. A normal potassium *distribution* is important for proper function. Most of the potassium ions in the body are inside the cells. The sodium-potassium pump in cell membranes moves potassium ions into cells to maintain the high intracellular potassium concentration. Potassium ions can be shifted into or out of cells by various physiologic factors (Fig. 7–15). Acidosis due to organic acids does not have the potassium-shifting effect of acidosis due to mineral acids. Potassium is *excreted* from the body through urine, feces, and sweat. The hormone aldosterone increases potassium excretion in the urine.

A potassium imbalance arises when the serum potassium concentration rises or falls outside the normal range. Potassium imbalances are caused by alterations in potassium intake, distribution, or excretion; by loss of potassium through an abnormal route; or by a combination of these factors.

FIGURE 7–15 Factors that shift potassium ions into or out of cells.

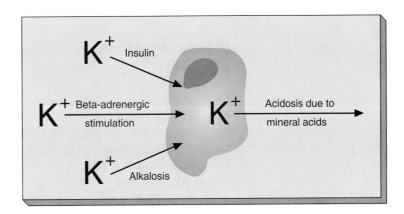

Hyperkalemia

Hyperkalemia is an excess of potassium ions in the blood. Although the plasma potassium concentration is elevated, whole body potassium content (including potassium inside the cells) may be elevated, normal, or decreased.

Clinical Manifestations

Serum potassium values above 5.0 mEq/L (5.9 mEq/L in infants) are diagnostic of hyperkalemia. The clinical manifestations of hyperkalemia are all related to muscle dysfunction. Dysfunction of gastrointestinal smooth muscle causes intestinal cramping and diarrhea in some children. The skeletal muscles become weak. The muscle weakness of hyperkalemia typically arises in the legs and ascends bilaterally. Weakness may progress to flaccid paralysis. Dysfunction of cardiac muscle in hyperkalemia causes cardiac arrhythmias and may result in cardiac arrest.

Etiology and Pathophysiology

Hyperkalemia is caused by conditions that involve increased potassium intake, shift of potassium from cells into the extracellular fluid, and decreased potassium excretion. *Increased potassium intake* that causes hyperkalemia is usually due to intravenous potassium overload. Excessive or too rapid intravenous administration of potassium chloride or other potassium-containing solutions may occur.

Blood transfusion is another source of potassium intake that may cause hyperkalemia. Potassium ions leak out of red blood cells that are stored in a blood bank. The longer blood is stored, the more potassium leaks out of the cells and accumulates in the fluid portion of the transfusion. Hyperkalemia from administration of stored blood arises when multiple units are transfused, as when infants receive exchange transfusions or children receive multiple blood transfusions after an automobile crash.

Shift of potassium from cells into the extracellular fluid occurs when there is massive cell death, as with a crush injury, in a sickle cell anemia hemolytic crisis, or when chemotherapy for a malignancy is rapidly effective. The dead cells release their high-potassium contents into the extracellular fluid. Potassium ions also shift out of cells in metabolic acidosis caused by diarrhea and in diabetes mellitus when insulin levels are low.

Decreased potassium excretion occurs with acute or chronic oliguric renal failure, severe hypovolemia, and conditions that decrease the secretion of aldosterone (Addison disease, hypoaldosteronism, and lead poisoning). Several medications can cause hyperkalemia.

Medical Management

Hyperkalemia is treated by management of the underlying condition that caused the imbalance. If the serum potassium concentration is very high or is causing dangerous cardiac arrhythmias, treatments to decrease the serum potassium level may be ordered. These treatments may remove potassium from the body or drive it from the extracellular fluid into the cells. Potassium is removed from the body by peritoneal dialysis or hemodialysis, by potassium-wasting diuretics, or with a cation exchange resin (Kayexalate) that is administered orally or rectally. Medical treatments that drive potassium ions into cells are intravenous bicarbonate or intravenous insulin and glucose.

Nursing Assessment

Monitor serum potassium levels. A child may report legs feeling "heavy" or be observed to have difficulty climbing stairs. A hyperkalemic infant will kick less vigorously and be more flaccid than usual. Ongoing assessment of muscle strength is important because the muscle weakness may progress to flaccid paralysis. This paralysis is reversible on correction of the potassium imbalance. An older child may complain of intestinal cramping. Monitoring for cardiac arrhythmias is vital in hyperkalemia because of the potentially fatal nature of the imbalance.

Nursing Diagnosis

Nursing diagnoses for a child who has hyperkalemia will depend on the severity of the clinical manifestations. The cause of the imbalance may also lead to useful diagnoses that will guide teaching for the child and the parents. The following nursing diagnoses may apply:

- High Risk for Decreased Cardiac Output related to cardiac arrhythmias
- High Risk for Injury related to muscle weakness
- Self-Care Deficit related to severe muscle weakness
- Anxiety related to decreased muscle function
- Knowledge Deficit (Parent) regarding management of potassium intake in chronic renal failure
- Noncompliance with dietary potassium restriction

Nursing Management

Any child who is receiving an intravenous infusion that contains potassium is at risk for hyperkalemia. Check that urine output is normal before administering intravenous potassium solutions. Intravenous containers to which potassium has been added should be turned end to end to mix the contents thoroughly before they are connected to the infusion tubing.[11]

The nurse's responsibilities when administering the prescribed medical therapy for hyperkalemia include monitoring for the complications of that therapy. Kayexalate is administered with sorbitol to prevent constipation. The glucose level must be noted frequently during infusion of insulin and glucose in case hypoglycemia develops. If bicarbonate infusion is used to treat hyperkalemia, transient ionized hypocalcemia may occur. Nursing assessment for this imbalance is discussed in the section on hypocalcemia in this chapter.

Medications that are high in potassium should be withheld. Intravenous solutions that contain potassium (including Ringer solution) should be discontinued, and potassium-free solutions should be substituted until the potassium concentration is decreasing toward normal. Request a change in the fluid orders if this has not been done. Several types of oral electrolyte solutions (e.g., Pedialyte) given to infants contain potassium; potassium-free oral solutions are needed for hyperkalemic infants.

The longer a unit of blood or packed red blood cells is stored in the blood bank, the more potassium is contained in the solution. To prevent hyperkalemia, be sure that fresh blood is obtained for a child who will receive multiple transfusions. This can be accomplished by reminding the physician who writes the blood order or, alternatively, by direct request to the blood bank.

For detection and management of hyperkalemia, a cardiac monitor should be applied during exchange transfusions, when a child will receive multiple units of blood or packed cells, and initially when hyperkalemia has been detected. Request an order for a cardiac monitor if one is not provided in these situations.

Adequate caloric intake is necessary to prevent tissue breakdown and the resultant potassium release from cells. Careful planning of snacks may be needed for a hyperkalemic child who has little appetite. Anxiety regarding muscle weakness or paralysis may be addressed directly in an older child. Explaining that the weakness is expected to go away as the potassium level decreases may reassure the child old enough to understand the idea.

If a child has chronic renal failure, parents and children (if old enough) need to be taught which foods are high in potassium and how to restrict them. Noncompliance in an older child will need to be addressed in the context of emotional and developmental needs and family dynamics. Potassium chloride (KCl) salt substitutes pose a danger to small children. To prevent hyperkalemia, all adults should be cautioned to keep KCl salt substitutes out of the reach of children.

Hypokalemia

Hypokalemia occurs when the serum potassium concentration is too low. Whole body potassium may be decreased, normal, or even increased when the serum level is low, depending on the cause of the imbalance.

Clinical Manifestations

Serum potassium levels below 3.5 mEq/L (3.9 mEq/L in infants) are diagnostic of hypokalemia. Since the ratio of intracellular to extracellular potas-

■ SAFETY PRECAUTIONS

A child who has the muscle weakness of hyperkalemia may need assistance with climbing into bed and other activities involving the leg muscles.

■ POTASSIUM-RICH FOODS

Apricots	Orange juice
Bananas	Peaches
Cantaloupe	Potatoes
Cherries	Prunes
Dates	Raisins
Figs	Strawberries
Molasses	Tomato juice

sium determines the responsiveness of muscle cells to neural stimuli, it is not surprising that the clinical manifestations of hypokalemia involve muscle dysfunction. Gastrointestinal smooth muscle in hypokalemia is lethargic, causing abdominal distention, constipation, or paralytic ileus. Skeletal muscles are weak and unresponsive to stimuli. As in hyperkalemia, this weakness is bilateral and ascending and may progress to flaccid paralysis. The respiratory muscles may become impaired. Cardiac arrhythmias also occur with hypokalemia. Polyuria results from changes in the kidney caused by hypokalemia.

Etiology and Pathophysiology

Hypokalemia is caused by conditions that involve decreased potassium intake, shift of potassium from the extracellular fluid into cells, increased potassium excretion, and loss of potassium by an abnormal route. *Decreased potassium intake* causes hypokalemia slowly or more rapidly if combined with increased excretion or loss of potassium. Hospitalized children may be placed on NPO status and receive prolonged intravenous therapy without potassium. Teenagers concerned about weight loss may embark on fad diets that are low in potassium. Teens with anorexia nervosa often consume little potassium.[12]

Shift of potassium from the extracellular fluid into cells occurs in alkalosis and hypothermia (unintentional or induced for surgery). Hyperalimentation often causes hypersecretion of insulin, which also shifts potassium into cells.

Increased potassium excretion is a major cause of hypokalemia. In addition to diuretics and other drugs, causes of increased urinary potassium excretion are osmotic diuresis (e.g., glucose in urine), hypomagnesemia, increased aldosterone (hyperaldosteronism, congestive heart failure, nephrotic syndrome, cirrhosis), and increased cortisol (Cushing disease and syndrome). Eating large amounts of black licorice increases renal excretion of potassium. Diarrhea causes greatly increased excretion of potassium in the feces. In the case study at the beginning of this chapter, Seth had increased potassium excretion through diarrhea.

Loss of potassium by an abnormal route occurs through emesis. Self-induced vomiting in bulimia falls into this category. Nasogastric suctioning (Fig. 7–16) and intestinal decompression also cause loss of potassium. Hypokalemia can be caused by several medications.

■ DRUGS THAT MAY CAUSE HYPOKALEMIA

Beta-adrenergic agonists
Insulin
Potassium-wasting diuretics
Parenteral penicillins
Glucocorticoids
Aminoglycoside antimicrobials
Systemic antifungals
Antineoplastics
Laxatives (if abused)

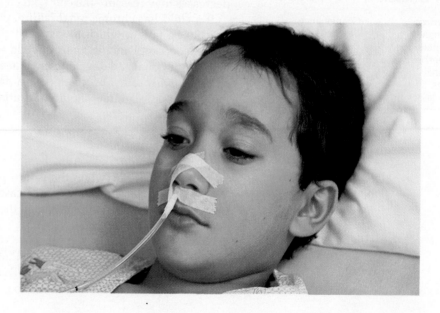

FIGURE 7–16 Because this child has a nasogastric tube in place that requires suctioning, it is important to monitor his potassium levels.

Medical Management

Medical management of hypokalemia focuses on replacement of potassium while treating the cause of the imbalance. Potassium replacement may be given intravenously or orally. If the hypokalemia is due to hypomagnesemia, the magnesium must be replaced before the potassium can be retained in the body.

Nursing Assessment

Monitor serum potassium levels. The muscle weakness of hypokalemia is frequently detected first in the legs, which feel "heavy" or weak. In the case study at the beginning of the chapter, Seth's skeletal muscle strength was difficult to assess because he was so lethargic. Muscle weakness may affect the respiratory muscles. The respirations of a hospitalized hypokalemic child should be assessed frequently to detect this problem and determine the need for mechanical ventilation.

Assessment of the gastrointestinal manifestations of hypokalemia should include listening for diminished bowel sounds. Cardiac monitoring is important for continued assessment of hypokalemia-associated arrhythmias. The polyuria of chronic hypokalemia may be identified by asking the parents if the child recently has been awakening to use the toilet in the night or has begun bedwetting after previously having been dry at night.

Nursing assessment of a child with hypokalemia should also include the child's ability to engage in active play, since muscle weakness may restrict activity and impair play interactions with peers.

Nursing Diagnosis

The most important nursing diagnoses in severe hypokalemia are related to cardiac arrhythmias and respiratory muscle weakness. The following nursing diagnoses may apply:

- High Risk for Decreased Cardiac Output related to cardiac arrhythmias
- Ineffective Breathing Pattern related to respiratory muscle weakness
- High Risk for Injury related to muscle weakness
- Self-Care Deficit related to severe muscle weakness
- Constipation related to decreased bowel function
- Anxiety related to decreased muscle function
- Knowledge Deficit (Parent) regarding management of potassium supplements or high-potassium diet
- Noncompliance with prescribed potassium therapy
- Knowledge Deficit (Adolescent) regarding safe weight loss diet

Nursing Management

Since potassium is excreted from the body every day, daily potassium intake is necessary to prevent hypokalemia. Some children who have no oral intake receive intravenous fluids that do not contain potassium. Unless a child is hyperkalemic, the nurse should ask for a potassium order to prevent hypokalemia.

The nursing diagnoses for a child with hypokalemia direct the nurse to use safety precautions appropriate to the child's developmental level and to provide frequent skin care if muscle weakness impairs movement.

Hypokalemia potentiates digitalis toxicity. A hypokalemic child who is receiving digitalis needs careful surveillance for digitalis toxicity, which is manifested as anorexia, nausea, vomiting, and bradycardia. Since the normal heart rate varies with age (see Chapter 12), definition of bradycardia varies with the age of the child.

Before potassium supplements are given, check the adequacy of urine output to prevent hyperkalemia. A nurse who administers potassium supplements to treat or prevent hypokalemia needs to watch for the complications of this therapy and report them if they develop.

Interventions to reduce constipation are discussed in Chapter 15. These interventions can be evaluated by monitoring bowel function.

A hypokalemic child who is able to eat needs a high-potassium diet. Teach parents (and the child if old enough) which foods are high in potassium and how to incorporate them in the daily diet.

Teenagers who want to lose weight need to be guided by a balanced weight-loss diet that contains low-calorie potassium-rich foods such as cantaloupe. When anorexia nervosa or bulimia is detected, the teenager needs professional help. The muscle weakness of hypokalemia may provide an opening for discussion of the problem and referral to a therapist.

If a child is discharged from the hospital with a prescription for potassium supplements, the parents need to be taught how to manage them at home. Liquid or powdered potassium supplements can be mixed with juice or with orange sherbet to improve the taste. The parent should call the mixture "medicine" so that the child does not learn to dislike all juices.

■ COMPLICATIONS OF POTASSIUM SUPPLEMENTS

Oral Potassium
Gastrointestinal distress
Occult blood in stool

Intravenous Potassium
Burning, redness, heat along vein
Elevated serum potassium level

■ Calcium Imbalances

A normal serum calcium concentration is important for many physiologic functions, including muscle and nerve function, secretion of hormones, and clotting of the blood.

Calcium intake in a traditional North American diet is primarily through dairy products. In other cultures it may be primarily through fishbones or dark green leafy vegetables after a child is weaned. *Calcium absorption* requires vitamin D for maximum efficiency and is greatest in the duodenum. *Calcium distribution* involves calcium entry into and exit from bones and the distribution of different forms of calcium in the plasma.

Calcium excretion occurs in urine, feces, and sweat. Parathyroid hormone is the major regulator of the plasma calcium concentration. It increases the plasma calcium concentration by increasing calcium absorption, increasing calcium withdrawal from bones, and decreasing calcium excretion in the urine.

Calcium imbalances are caused by alterations in calcium intake, absorption, distribution, or excretion; by loss of calcium through an abnormal route; or by a combination of these factors. The plasma calcium concentration has an important influence on cell membrane permeability and influences the threshold potential of excitable cells. For this reason calcium imbalances alter neuromuscular irritability.

■ NORMAL SERUM CALCIUM CONCENTRATION

9–11 mg/dL (4.5–5.5 mEq/L)

■ THE THREE FORMS OF CALCIUM IN PLASMA

Calcium bound to protein
Calcium bound to small organic ions (e.g., citrate)
Free ionized calcium (Ca^{++}), which is the only physiologically active form

Hypercalcemia

Hypercalcemia denotes a plasma excess of calcium. Because so much calcium is in the bones, the serum levels of calcium may not reflect body stores.

Clinical Manifestations

Serum calcium levels above 11 mg/dL are diagnostic of hypercalcemia. Many of the signs and symptoms of hypercalcemia are manifestations of *decreased neuromuscular excitability*. Constipation, anorexia, nausea, and perhaps vomiting occur. Fatigue and skeletal muscle weakness predominate. Hypercalcemia may also cause changes in personality and mood. Confusion and lethargy are common. Polyuria develops. Severe hypercalcemia may cause cardiac arrest. Neonates with hypercalcemia have flaccid muscles and exhibit failure to thrive.

Etiology and Pathophysiology

Hypercalcemia is caused by conditions that involve increased calcium intake or absorption, shift of calcium from bones into the extracellular fluid, and decreased calcium excretion. Hypercalcemia due to *increased calcium intake or absorption* may occur if an infant is fed large amounts of chicken liver (source of vitamin A) or is given megadoses of vitamin D or vitamin A or if a child or adolescent consumes large amounts of calcium-rich foods concurrently with antacids (milk-alkali syndrome).

In pediatric patients most hypercalcemia is due to *shift of calcium from bones into the extracellular fluid*. The excessive amounts of parathyroid hormone produced in hyperparathyroidism cause calcium withdrawal from bones. Hyperparathyroidism in infants and children may be congenital or hereditary. Prolonged immobilization also causes withdrawal of calcium from bones. Frequently the excess calcium ions are excreted in the urine. However, if calcium is withdrawn from bones faster than the kidneys can excrete it, hypercalcemia results. Hypercalcemia also occurs with many types of malignancies (e.g., leukemias). The malignant cells produce substances that circulate in the blood to the bones and cause bone resorption. The calcium from the bones then enters the extracellular fluid, causing hypercalcemia. Bone tumors destroy bone directly, leading to release of calcium.

Thiazide diuretics *decrease calcium excretion* in the urine and may contribute to development of hypercalcemia.

Medical Management

Hypercalcemia is treated by increasing urine excretion of calcium (increased fluids, the diuretic furosemide), decreasing intestinal absorption of calcium (glucocorticoids), and decreasing bone resorption (glucocorticoids, calcitonin). Phosphate is sometimes used to treat hypercalcemia but may cause dangerous precipitation of calcium phosphate salts in body tissues. Dialysis may be used if necessary.

Nursing Assessment

Nursing assessment of a child with hypercalcemia includes monitoring serum calcium levels, level of consciousness, gastrointestinal function, urine volume, specific gravity, cardiac rhythm, and pH. With chronic hypercalcemia, assessment of activity tolerance and developmental level becomes important.

Nursing Diagnosis

Many nursing diagnoses are appropriate for children who have hypercalcemia. Diagnoses that address cardiac and neuromuscular manifestations are especially important. The following nursing diagnoses may apply:

- High Risk for Decreased Cardiac Output related to cardiac arrest
- High Risk for Injury related to decreased level of consciousness
- High Risk for Injury related to muscle weakness
- High Risk for Injury related to risk of pathologic fractures
- Self-Care Deficit related to fatigue and muscle weakness
- Anxiety related to decreased muscle function
- Constipation related to decreased bowel function
- High Risk for Altered Nutrition: Less Than Body Requirements related to anorexia and nausea
- High Risk for Impaired Urinary Elimination related to renal calculi

Nursing Management

Children who have hypercalcemia need to decrease their calcium intake. Therefore calcium-rich foods and calcium antacids should not be used. Parents need this information to provide home care. Vitamin D supplementation should be avoided, because it increases calcium absorption from the gastrointestinal tract.

Increasing the fluid intake is an important nursing intervention for a child who has hypercalcemia or who is immobilized. A large fluid intake, appropriate to the child's age, is necessary to keep the urine dilute. An acidic urine helps to keep the calcium from forming stones. Many urinary tract infections cause the urine to be alkaline. Thus nursing interventions to prevent urinary tract infection are necessary in hypercalcemia. Thiazide diuretics (e.g., hydrochlorothiazide) decrease calcium excretion and should not be given to a hypercalcemic child.

Nursing interventions to avoid constipation are also important because hypercalcemia often causes constipation.

Increasing mobility through assisted weight-bearing helps to decrease the withdrawal of calcium from bones that is caused by immobility. If the hypercalcemia is caused by withdrawal of calcium from the bones, the child will be at risk for pathologic fractures and must be handled gently.

Hypocalcemia

Hypocalcemia denotes a plasma deficit of calcium. Serum calcium levels may not reflect body stores.

Clinical Manifestations

Serum calcium levels below 9 mg/dL are diagnostic of hypocalcemia. The signs and symptoms of hypocalcemia are manifestations of *increased neuromuscular excitability* (tetany). In children they include muscle twitching and cramping, tingling around the mouth or in the fingers (perioral or digital paresthesias), carpal spasm, and pedal spasm. Laryngospasm, seizures, and cardiac arrhythmias are more severe manifestations of hypocalcemia and may be fatal. Hypocalcemia in infants is more frequently manifested as tremors, muscle twitches, and brief tonic-clonic seizures. Hypocalcemia may cause congestive heart failure, especially in neonates.

Etiology and Pathophysiology

Hypocalcemia is caused by conditions that involve decreased calcium intake or absorption, shift of calcium to a physiologically unavailable form, increased calcium excretion, and loss of calcium by an abnormal route. *Decreased calcium intake or absorption* causes hypocalcemia in children with severe chronic malnutrition. Even with a normal calcium intake, hypocalcemia occurs if calcium is not absorbed. If a child does not have enough vitamin D, calcium is not absorbed efficiently from the duodenum. Sunlight speeds formation of vitamin D in the skin. Children who are institutionalized without access to sunlight (e.g., severely developmentally delayed children) may become hypocalcemic because of the lack of vitamin D. The uremic syndrome is another cause of vitamin D deficiency. It interferes with the kidney's ability to activate vitamin D. Chronic diarrhea and steatorrhea (fatty stools) also reduce calcium absorption from the gastrointestinal tract.

Shift of calcium into a physiologically unavailable form occurs when calcium shifts into bone or free ionized calcium in plasma binds to proteins or small organic ions in the plasma. Too much calcium shifts into bones in various types of hypoparathyroidism, including DiGeorge syndrome (congenital absence of the parathyroid glands). Hypomagnesemia impairs parathyroid hormone function and may cause hypocalcemia. Some types of neonatal hypocalcemia are associated with delayed parathyroid hormone function or hypomagnesemia. Calcium shifts rapidly into bone when rickets is treated (hungry bone syndrome). A high plasma phosphate concentration causes plasma calcium to decrease. Ionized hypocalcemia, which is due to increased binding of plasma ionized calcium, occurs very rapidly. The ionized hypocalcemia persists until the alkalosis resolves or the citrate is metabolized by the liver. Children who receive liver transplants are hypocalcemic for several days because of impaired citrate metabolism.[13]

Increased calcium excretion occurs in steatorrhea (fatty stools), when calcium secreted into the gastrointestinal fluids binds to the fecal fat in addition to the dietary calcium that is bound in the feces. A similar situation occurs in acute pancreatitis.

Loss of calcium by an abnormal route may contribute to hypocalcemia as calcium is lost from the body through burn or wound drainage or sequestered in acute pancreatitis. Many different medications can cause hypocalcemia.

Medical Management

Hypocalcemia is treated by oral or intravenous administration of calcium. The original cause of the imbalance is also treated. If the hypocalcemia is due to hypomagnesemia, the magnesium must be replenished before the calcium replacement can be successful.

Nursing Assessment

A child who develops hypocalcemia may give a subjective history of muscle cramps, stiffness, and clumsiness. Grimacing caused by spasms of facial muscles may be observed, as may twitching of the arm muscles. Many healthy newborns have a positive Chvostek sign, so this assessment should be reserved for children over several months of age. Laryngospasm may be recognized initially by the honking sound made by the child who is having difficulty breathing. In addition to monitoring serum calcium levels, cardiac monitoring is also important to detect cardiac arrhythmias.

Nursing Diagnosis

The effects of the increased neuromuscular excitability of hypocalcemia are the basis for several nursing diagnoses. These include:

CAUSES OF IONIZED HYPOCALCEMIA

Alkalosis, which causes more calcium to bind to plasma proteins
Citrate in transfused blood products, which binds calcium

DRUGS THAT MAY CAUSE HYPOCALCEMIA

Antacids (if overused)
Laxatives (if abused)
Oil-based bowel lubricants
Anticonvulsants
Phosphate-containing preparations
Protein-type plasma expanders (if rapid infusion)
Antineoplastics

COMPLICATIONS OF CALCIUM SUPPLEMENTS

Oral Calcium
Constipation

Intravenous Calcium
Infiltration, tissue sloughing
Elevated serum calcium level
Decreased serum phosphate level

◼ CLINICAL TIP

Increased neuromuscular excitability may be detected by testing for Trousseau sign. A blood pressure cuff is applied to the arm and left inflated for 3 minutes. If a carpal spasm occurs, Trousseau sign is positive. Another assessment for increased neuromuscular excitability is Chvostek sign. The skin is tapped lightly just in front of the ear (over the facial nerve). If the corner of the mouth draws up because of muscle contraction, Chvostek sign is positive.

- High Risk for Injury related to increased neuromuscular excitability
- High Risk for Ineffective Breathing Pattern related to laryngospasm
- High Risk for Decreased Cardiac Output related to cardiac arrhythmias
- Sensory/Perceptual Alteration (paresthesias) related to increased neuromuscular excitability
- Anxiety related to increased neuromuscular excitability
- Knowledge Deficit (Parent) regarding nondairy sources of calcium

Nursing Management

Safety is a prime consideration in hypocalcemia. Seizure precautions may be necessary. An older child may find some comfort in an explanation of the cause of the muscle cramps. A younger child may be less anxious when given a stuffed animal or familiar toy to hug.

Calcium is given orally or intravenously. A 10% calcium gluconate solution should be readily available for emergency intravenous use in severe hypocalcemia. Calcium is *never* given intramuscularly because that would cause tissue necrosis. A hypocalcemic child who is able to eat needs a calcium-rich diet. Parents and children need to be taught about calcium-rich foods and ways to use milk in the diet. For example, calcium in the diet can be increased by adding dried milk when baking. A child who has chronic diarrhea needs a long-term increase in calcium intake to prevent hypocalcemia.

A child who has lactose intolerance will be unable to tolerate milk and other dairy products. Teach nondairy calcium sources to parents of children with lactose intolerance. Large grocery stores carry milk that is treated with lactase so that it is digestible for these children. This milk is more expensive than untreated milk, so it is important to explore the family's financial situation when recommending this product. Inexpensive calcium carbonate tablets also are available.

■ NONDAIRY FOODS RICH IN CALCIUM

Almonds	Okra
Bok choy cabbage	Oranges
Broccoli	Salmon (canned)
Cactus (nopales)	Sardines (canned)
Chocolate	Spinach
Cream of Wheat	Tofu
Farina	

■ Magnesium Imbalances

The electrolyte magnesium is necessary for enzyme function, acetylcholine release, and bone formation. Cellular chemistry will be impaired in a child who has a magnesium imbalance.

Since magnesium is a component of chlorophyll, magnesium *intake* is aided by eating dark green leafy vegetables. Nuts and grains are also good sources of magnesium. Magnesium is *absorbed* primarily from the terminal ileum.

Magnesium is *distributed* among the extracellular fluid (small amounts), the cells (larger amounts), and the bones (large amounts). Magnesium *excretion* occurs in urine, feces, and sweat.

Magnesium imbalances are caused by alterations in magnesium intake, distribution, or excretion; by loss of magnesium through an abnormal route; or by a combination of these factors. The plasma magnesium concentration influences the release of acetylcholine at neuromuscular junctions. Thus magnesium imbalances are characterized by alterations in neuromuscular irritability.

■ NORMAL SERUM MAGNESIUM CONCENTRATION

1.5–2.5 mEq/L (0.75–1.25 mmol/L)

Hypermagnesemia

Hypermagnesemia occurs when the plasma magnesium concentration is too high. The serum levels measured in the laboratory may not reflect body magnesium stores because most of the magnesium in the body is in bones and inside the cells.

Clinical Manifestations

Serum magnesium levels above 2.5 mEq/L (1.25 mmol/L) are diagnostic of hypermagnesemia. Hypermagnesemia causes decreased neuromuscular irritability. The clinical manifestations include hypotension, bradycardia, drowsiness, lethargy, and weak or absent deep tendon reflexes. In severe hypermagnesemia, flaccid muscle paralysis, fatal respiratory depression, cardiac arrhythmias, and cardiac arrest may occur.

Etiology and Pathophysiology

Hypermagnesemia is caused by conditions that involve increased magnesium intake and decreased magnesium excretion. *Increased magnesium intake* through magnesium sulfate ($MgSO_4$) treatment of eclampsia shortly before delivery or $MgSO_4$ enemas given to infants have also caused hypermagnesemia. Aspiration of seawater, as in near-drowning, is an uncommon but potentially serious source of excessive magnesium intake.

Shift of magnesium from bones into the extracellular fluid does not usually cause hypermagnesemia in children.

Decreased magnesium excretion is an important cause of hypermagnesemia. In both oliguric renal failure and adrenal insufficiency, magnesium ions that cannot be excreted in the urine accumulate in the extracellular fluid. Medication containing magnesium may cause hypermagnesemia.

Medical Management

Hypermagnesemia is managed primarily by increasing the urinary excretion of magnesium. This is usually accomplished by increasing fluid intake (except in oliguric renal failure) and administering diuretics. Dialysis may be necessary.

Nursing Assessment

In addition to monitoring serum magnesium levels, nursing assessment in hypermagnesemia includes blood pressure (hypotension), heart rate and rhythm (bradycardia and cardiac arrhythmias), respiratory rate and depth (respiratory depression), muscle tone (deep tendon reflexes) and movement (weak deep tendon reflexes and flaccid paralysis) (Fig. 7–17), and level of consciousness (lethargy). If a serum magnesium level is not known for a child who has major risk factors and early manifestations of hypermagnesemia, request that magnesium be measured.

Nursing Diagnosis

The impaired physiologic functions of children who have hypermagnesemia are the basis for several nursing diagnoses. These include:

- High Risk for Decreased Cardiac Output related to cardiac arrhythmias
- Ineffective Breathing Pattern related to respiratory depression
- High Risk for Injury related to decreased level of consciousness and flaccid paralysis

■ **DRUGS THAT MAY CAUSE HYPERMAGNESEMIA**

Magnesium-containing cathartics (if overused)

Magnesium antacids (if overused)

FIGURE 7–17 The flaccid muscle tone of the infant could be due to hypermagnesemia.

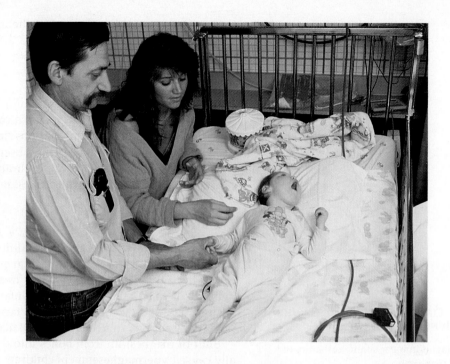

- Self-Care Deficit related to decreased level of consciousness and flaccid paralysis
- Anxiety related to decreased muscle function
- Knowledge Deficit (Parent) regarding sources of magnesium

Nursing Management

Since hypermagnesemia causes lethargy and muscle weakness, the side rails of the bed must be raised for safety. Any child who has hypermagnesemia should not be given magnesium-containing medications or sea salt. To prevent hypermagnesemia from developing, these preparations should also be withheld from any child who becomes oliguric.

Parents of children who have chronic renal failure need to understand that these children should never be given milk of magnesia, antacids that contain magnesium, or other sources of magnesium such as sea salt. Older children can be included in this teaching. If hypermagnesemia is being treated with diuretics, monitoring the serum potassium levels is important because the diuretics also increase potassium excretion.

Hypomagnesemia

Hypomagnesemia indicates that the plasma magnesium concentration is too low. The serum levels of magnesium may not reflect body stores, since much of the magnesium in the body is inside cells and in the bones.

Clinical Manifestations

Serum magnesium levels below 1.5 mEq/L (0.75 mmol/L) are diagnostic of hypomagnesemia. Hypomagnesemia is characterized by *increased neuromuscular excitability* (tetany). The clinical manifestations are hyperactive reflexes, skeletal muscle cramps, twitching, tremors, and cardiac arrhythmias. Seizures occur with severe hypomagnesemia.

■ CLINICAL TIP

Teaching for parents of a child with chronic renal failure should include practice reading labels to detect magnesium in antacids and cathartics.

Etiology and Pathophysiology

Hypomagnesemia is caused by conditions that involve decreased magnesium intake or absorption, shift of magnesium to a physiologically unavailable form, increased magnesium excretion, and loss of magnesium by an abnormal route. *Decreased magnesium intake or absorption* causes hypomagnesemia if a child who is not eating has prolonged intravenous therapy without magnesium. Chronic malnutrition is another cause of decreased magnesium intake. Magnesium absorption is decreased in chronic diarrhea, short bowel syndrome, malabsorption syndromes, and steatorrhea.

Shift of magnesium to a physiologically unavailable form occurs with massive transfusion of citrated blood products because magnesium bound to the citrate is not physiologically active. Such transfusions cause prolonged hypomagnesemia in liver transplant patients, who have impaired citrate metabolism. Magnesium shifts rapidly into bones in the hungry bone syndrome.

Increased magnesium excretion in the urine occurs with diuretic therapy, the diuretic phase of acute renal failure, diabetic ketoacidosis, and hyperaldosteronism. Chronic alcoholism, occasionally seen in adolescents, increases urinary magnesium excretion. Magnesium contained in gastrointestinal secretions is bound to fat and excreted fecally in steatorrhea.

Loss of magnesium by an abnormal route occurs with prolonged nasogastric suction and through sequestration of magnesium in acute pancreatitis. Several medications may cause hypomagnesemia.

■ DRUGS THAT MAY CAUSE HYPOMAGNESEMIA

Magnesium-wasting diuretics
Antineoplastics
Systemic antifungals
Aminoglycoside antimicrobials
Laxatives (if abused)

Medical Management

Hypomagnesemia is treated by administering magnesium and treating the underlying cause of the imbalance.

Nursing Assessment

In addition to monitoring serum magnesium levels, nursing assessment of hypomagnesemia includes monitoring deep tendon reflexes, testing Trousseau sign and Chvostek sign (unreliable in young infants), monitoring cardiac function, and observing for muscle twitching. Children who are able to talk report muscle cramping. Since magnesium levels are not routinely measured in many hospitals, it is very important to request a serum magnesium level for any child who has risk factors and early manifestations of hypomagnesemia.

■ COMPLICATIONS OF MAGNESIUM SUPPLEMENTS

Oral Magnesium
Diarrhea

Intramuscular Magnesium
Elevated serum magnesium level

Intravenous Magnesium
Flushing, feeling of warmth
Elevated serum magnesium level
Cardiac arrhythmias
Decreased deep tendon reflexes

Nursing Diagnosis

The increased neuromuscular excitability of hypomagnesemia provides the basis for several important nursing diagnoses. These include:

- High Risk for Injury related to increased neuromuscular excitability
- High Risk for Decreased Cardiac Output related to cardiac arrhythmias
- Sensory/Perceptual Alteration related to increased neuromuscular excitability
- Anxiety related to increased neuromuscular excitability
- Knowledge Deficit (Parent) regarding management of magnesium-rich diet for a child with chronic bowel problem

Nursing Management

Safety interventions, including seizure precautions in severe hypomagnesemia, are important. Explanations and a soft, familiar toy to hug may decrease a child's anxiety related to increased neuromuscular excitability.

Before administering magnesium replacements, verify that the child's urine output is adequate. Deep tendon reflexes should be monitored during intravenous infusion of magnesium. If reflexes diminish, the infusion should be stopped and a serum magnesium level obtained. Parents need to include magnesium-rich foods in the diet of a child who has hypomagnesemia or continuing risk factors (e.g., chronic diarrhea) for this imbalance.

■ Summary of Clinical Assessment of Fluid and Electrolyte Imbalances

■ **RISK FACTOR ASSESSMENT FOR FLUID IMBALANCES**

Isotonic Fluid (Extracellular Fluid Volume Imbalances)
Source of increased intake?
Aldosterone secretion increased or decreased?
Source of loss from the body?

Water (Osmolality Imbalances)
Source of increased intake?
Antidiuretic hormone secretion increased or decreased?
Source of unusual loss from the body?

■ **RISK FACTOR ASSESSMENT FOR ELECTROLYTE IMBALANCES**

(Think through separately for potassium, calcium, and magnesium)

Electrolyte Intake and Absorption
Increased? Decreased?

Electrolyte Shifts
From electrolyte pool into plasma?
From plasma into electrolyte pool?

Electrolyte Excretion
Decreased? Increased?

Electrolyte Loss by Abnormal Routes
Any abnormal routes present?

How can you assess children appropriately for fluid and electrolyte imbalances without thinking through the clinical manifestations of every possible disorder one after the other? First, performing a rapid *risk factor assessment* on each child is useful and efficient to see which (if any) fluid or electrolyte imbalances are in the high-risk category.

A risk factor assessment may be performed mentally during routine tasks. For a specific child a *fluid imbalance risk factor assessment* looks for factors that alter the intake, retention, and loss of isotonic fluid and water. This information is used to decide what fluid imbalance (if any) is most likely for the child. Similarly, an *electrolyte imbalance risk factor assessment* looks for factors, in a specific child, that alter electrolyte intake and absorption, distribution between plasma and other electrolyte pools, excretion, and abnormal routes of electrolyte loss. This information about factors that alter electrolyte homeostasis is used to decide which (if any) electrolyte imbalances are in the high-risk category for the child.

After deciding what the high-risk imbalances are for a specific child, the next step is the clinical assessment. Assessment of fluid imbalances is performed by assessing weight changes, vascular volume, interstitial volume, and cerebral function (Table 7–10). Assessment of electrolyte imbalances is performed by assessing serum electrolyte levels, skeletal muscle strength, neuromuscular excitability, gastrointestinal tract function, and cardiac rhythm (Table 7–11). After these assessments, check for other manifestations that are specific to a particular high-risk imbalance (e.g., polyuria in hypokalemia). This method of *risk factor assessment followed by clinical assessment* provides a rapid, yet thorough approach to assessment for fluid and electrolyte imbalances.

TABLE 7-10 Summary of Clinical Assessment of Fluid Imbalances

Assessment Category	Specific Assessments	Changes with Fluid Imbalances
Rapid changes in weight	Daily weights	Weight gain—extracellular volume excess Weight loss—extracellular volume deficit; clinical dehydration
Vascular volume	Small vein filling time	Increased—extracellular volume deficit; clinical dehydration
	Capillary refill time	Increased—extracellular volume deficit; clinical dehydration
	Character of pulse	Bounding—extracellular volume excess Thready—extracellular volume deficit; clinical dehydration
	Postural blood pressure measurements	Postural drop—extracellular volume deficit; clinical dehydration
	Lung sounds in dependent portions	Crackles—extracellular volume excess
	Central venous pressure	Increased—extracellular volume excess Decreased—extracellular volume deficit; clinical dehydration
	Tenseness of fontanel (infants)	Bulging—extracellular volume excess Sunken—extracellular volume deficit; clinical dehydration
	Neck vein filling (older children)	Full when upright—extracellular volume excess Flat when supine—extracellular volume deficit; clinical dehydration
Interstitial volume	Skin turgor	Skin tents—extracellular volume deficit; clinical dehydration
	Presence or absence of edema	Edema—extracellular volume excess
Cerebral function	Level of consciousness	Decreased—hyponatremia; hypernatremia; clinical dehydration

TABLE 7-11 Summary of Clinical Assessment of Electrolyte Imbalances

Assessment Category	Specific Assessments	Changes with Electrolyte Imbalances
Skeletal muscle function	Muscle strength	Weakness, flaccid paralysis—hyperkalemia; hypokalemia
Neuromuscular excitability	Deep tendon reflexes	Depressed—hypercalcemia; hypermagnesemia Hyperactive—hypocalcemia; hypomagnesemia
	Chvostek sign (not infants)	Positive—hypocalcemia; hypomagnesemia
	Trousseau sign	Positive—hypocalcemia; hypomagnesemia
	Paresthesias	Digital or perioral—hypocalcemia
	Muscle cramping or twitching	Present—hypocalcemia; hypomagnesemia
Gastrointestinal tract function	Bowel sounds	Decreased or absent—hypokalemia
	Elimination pattern	Constipation—hypokalemia; hypercalcemia Diarrhea—hyperkalemia
Cardiac rhythm	Regularity of pulse	Irregular—hyperkalemia; hypokalemia; hypercalcemia; hypocalcemia; hypermagnesemia; hypomagnesemia
	Electrocardiogram	Abnormal—hyperkalemia; hypokalemia; hypercalcemia; hypocalcemia; hypermagnesemia; hypomagnesemia

Fluid and Electrolyte Imbalances Caused by Selected Clinical Conditions

Although the fluid and electrolyte imbalances have been presented one at a time in this chapter, several imbalances may occur simultaneously in clinical situations. For these patients assessment and nursing management of the different imbalances can be combined into a comprehensive plan of care. Fluid and electrolyte imbalances commonly seen in children with vomiting, diarrhea, diabetic ketoacidosis, and oliguric renal failure are presented in Table 7–12.

TABLE 7-12 Fluid and Electrolyte Imbalances Associated with Selected Clinical Conditions

Condition	Imbalance	Major Cause
Vomiting	Extracellular fluid volume deficit	Loss of saline
	Hypernatremia	Loss of relatively more water than salt
	Hypokalemia	Loss of potassium by abnormal route; increased renal potassium excretion due to alkalosis
	Metabolic alkalosis	Loss of acid (see Chapter 8)
Diarrhea	Extracellular fluid volume deficit	Loss of saline
	Hypernatremia	Loss of relatively more water than salt
	Hypokalemia	Increased potassium excretion
	Hypocalcemia (chronic diarrhea)	Decreased calcium absorption; increased calcium excretion
	Hypomagnesemia (chronic diarrhea)	Decreased magnesium absorption; increased magnesium excretion
	Metabolic acidosis	Loss of bicarbonate (see Chapter 8)
Diabetic keto-acidosis	Extracellular fluid volume deficit	Osmotic diuresis
	Hyperkalemia (before treatment)	Shift of potassium from cells into extracellular fluid due to lack of insulin
	Hypokalemia (after treatment)	Increased potassium excretion in osmotic diuresis; insulin treatment causes remaining potassium to shift into cells
	Hyperphosphatemia (before treatment)	Ketoacids cause organic phosphates to decompose and release inorganic phosphates from cells into extracellular fluid
	Hypophosphatemia (after treatment)	Increased phosphate excretion in osmotic diuresis; insulin treatment causes remaining phosphates to shift into cells
	Metabolic acidosis	Production of ketoacids (see Chapter 8)
Oliguric renal failure	Extracellular fluid volume excess	Decreased saline excretion
	Hyperkalemia	Decreased potassium excretion
	Hypermagnesemia	Decreased magnesium excretion
	Hyperphosphatemia	Decreased phosphate excretion
	Hypocalcemia (chronic renal failure)	Decreased calcium absorption due to lack of active form of vitamin D; hyperphosphatemia
	or	
	Hypercalcemia (chronic renal failure)	Secondary hyperparathyroidism

REFERENCES

1 Skorecki, K., & Brenner, B. (1981). Body fluid homeostasis in man: A contemporary overview. *American Journal of Medicine, 70,* 77–88.

2 Pflaum, S. (1979). Investigation of intake-output as a means of assessing body fluid balance. *Heart and Lung, 8,* 495–498.

3 Reubi, F. (1980). Hemodynamic changes in isotonic dehydration. *Contributions to Nephrology, 21,* 55–61.

4 Abrams, C., Phillips, L., Berkowitz, C., Blackett, P., & Priebe, C. (1975). Hazards of overconcentrated milk formula. *Journal of the American Medical Association, 232,* 1136–1140.

5 Chesney, R., & Brusilow, S. (1981). Extreme hypernatremia as a presenting sign of child abuse and psychosocial dwarfism. *Johns Hopkins Medical Journal, 148,* 11–13.

6 Tucker, J., & Sussman-Karten, K. (1987). Treating acute diarrhea and dehydration with an oral rehydration solution. *Pediatric Nursing, 13,* 269–274.

7 Mortimer, J. (1980). Acute water intoxication as another unusual manifestation of child abuse. *Archives of Diseases of Childhood, 55,* 401–403.

8 Bennett, H., Wagner, T., & Fields, A. (1983). Acute hyponatremia and seizures in an infant after a swimming lesson. *Pediatrics, 72,* 125–127.

9 Nardone, D., & McAfee, J. (1987). Causes of peripheral edema. *Hospital Medicine, 23,* 162–182.

10 Felver, L., & Pendarvis, J. (1989). Electrolyte imbalances in operating room patients: Risk factors and survey of OR nurses. *AORN Journal, 49,* 992–998.

11 Williams, R. (1973). Potassium overdosage: A potential hazard of non-rigid parenteral fluid containers. *British Medical Journal, 1,* 714–715.

12 Felver, L., & Pendarvis, J. (1988). Perioperative risk factors for hypokalemia. *Today's OR Nurse, 10,* 26–32.

13 Sommerauer, J., Gayle, M., Frewen, T., Wall, W., Gamt, D., Girvan, D., Ghent, C., Jenner, M., & Stiller, C. (1988). Intensive care course following liver transplantation in children. *Journal of Pediatric Surgery, 23,* 705–708.

SUGGESTED READINGS

Cullen, L. (1992). Interventions related to fluid and electrolyte balance. *Nursing Clinics of North America, 27,* 569–597.

Drew, D., & Schumann, D. (1986). Homogeneity of potassium chloride in small volume intravenous containers. *Nursing Research, 35,* 325–329.

Felver, L. (1980). Electrolytes across the age continuum—implications for the practicing nurse. *Washington State Journal of Nursing, 52,* 19–32.

Ichikawa, I. (Ed.). (1990). *Pediatric textbook of fluids and electrolytes.* Baltimore: Williams & Wilkins.

McFadden, E., Zaloga, G., & Chernow, B. (1983). Hypocalcemia: A medical emergency. *American Journal of Nursing, 83,* 227–230.

Rose, B.D. (1989). *Clinical physiology of acid-base and electrolyte disorders* (3rd ed.). New York: McGraw-Hill.

Smith, L. (1988). Home treatment of mild, acute diarrhea and secondary dehydration of infants and small children: An educational program for parents in a shelter for the homeless. *Journal of Professional Nursing, 4,* 60–63.

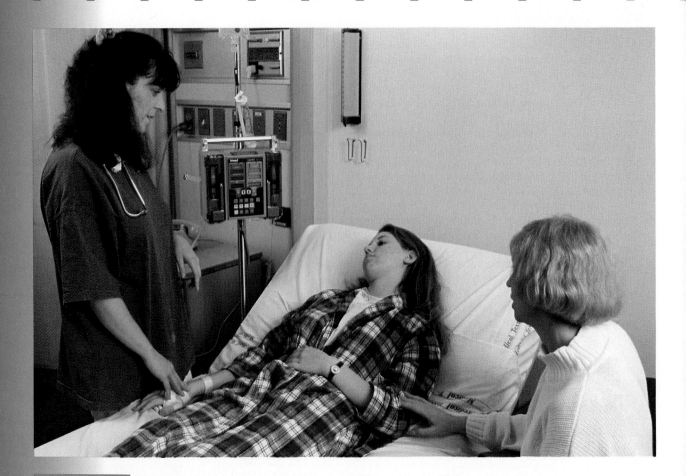

J ean, 15 years old, has been trying to lose weight. She has not eaten anything for 5 days; she is drinking nothing but bouillon. Her mother and younger brothers have the "flu." Two days ago, Jean's muscles began to ache and she developed diarrhea. This morning Jean did not come downstairs in time to catch the school bus. After her mother called to her and received no answer, she went to Jean's room and found her lying on the bed, breathing deeply. Although Jean opened her eyes, she responded slowly to questions and then with only one word at a time. With the help of a neighbor, her mother took Jean to the emergency department. Arterial blood drawn in the emergency room showed a pH of 7.20, PCO_2 to be 21 mm Hg, and bicarbonate to be 8 mEq/L. Jean has metabolic acidosis.

How did Jean get metabolic acidosis? What happens inside the body when metabolic acidosis occurs? Why was Jean breathing so deeply? What nursing management is important to help Jean recover? What teaching do she and her mother need to prevent metabolic acidosis in the future?

ALTERATIONS IN ACID-BASE BALANCE

8

TERMINOLOGY

acidemia   Decreased blood pH.

acidosis   Condition caused by too much acid in the blood.

alkalemia   Increased blood pH.

alkalosis   Condition caused by too little acid in the blood.

buffer   Related acid-base pair that gives up or takes up hydrogen ions as needed to prevent large changes in pH of a solution.

carbonic acid H_2CO_3; excreted by the lungs in the form of carbon dioxide and water.

compensation   Process that tends to restore blood pH to normal by making either the partial pressure of carbon dioxide (PCO_2) or the bicarbonate ion concentration abnormal. Compensation does not fix the cause of the acid-base imbalance.

correction   Process that tends to restore blood pH to normal by fixing the cause of the acid-base imbalance.

hyperventilation   Condition in which more air than normal is moved in and out of the lungs.

pH   Negative logarithm of the hydrogen ion concentration; used to monitor the acidity of body fluid.

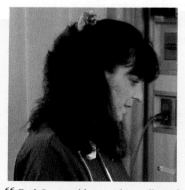

66 Both Jean and her mother will need teaching about how to prevent another episode of metabolic acidosis. While focusing on the importance of a reduced-calorie diet and exercise, I will emphasize that the starvation approach to weight loss that Jean tried can be very dangerous to her health. 99

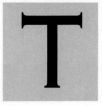

This chapter describes how the body regulates acid-base status and explains acid-base imbalances. It provides guidance for nursing management of children like Jean who have acid-base imbalances. Using information in this chapter, you will be able to assist with restoring normal acid-base balance and provide teaching to prevent similar problems in the future.

Regulation of Acid-Base Balance

A normal acid-base balance is necessary for the cells (and thus, the body) to work properly. The number of hydrogen ions (H^+) present in a fluid determines how acidic it is. Increasing the hydrogen ion concentration makes a solution more acidic. Because the hydrogen ion concentration in body fluids is very small, acidity is expressed as **pH** (the negative logarithm of the hydrogen ion concentration) rather than as the hydrogen ion concentration itself. The range of pH is 1 to 14. A pH of 7 is neutral. The lower the pH, the more acidic the solution. A pH above 7 is basic. The higher the pH, the more basic the solution. Body fluids are normally slightly basic.

The pH of body fluids is regulated carefully to provide a suitable environment for cell function. The pH of the blood influences the pH inside cells. In order for the enzymes inside cells to function optimally, the pH must be in the normal range. If the pH inside cells becomes too high or too low, then the speed of chemical reactions becomes inappropriate for proper cell function. Thus acid-base imbalances result in clinical signs and symptoms, and, in severe cases, they may cause death.

In the course of their normal function, all cells in the body produce acids. Cells produce two kinds of acids: **carbonic acid** (H_2CO_3) and metabolic (noncarbonic) acids. These acids are released into the extracellular fluid and must be neutralized or excreted from the body to prevent dangerous accumulation. They can be neutralized to some degree by the buffers in body fluids. Carbonic acid is excreted by the lungs in the form of carbon dioxide and water. Metabolic acids are excreted by the kidneys.

Buffers

All body fluids have buffers to provide initial protection against rapid changes in pH. A **buffer** is a related acid-base pair that works together to neutralize acids or bases. If too much base is present, the acid part of the buffer pair releases hydrogen ions to neutralize the base (Fig. 8–1). On the other hand, if too much acid is present, the base part of the buffer pair takes up excess hydrogen ions to neutralize the acid (Fig. 8–2).

Several different kinds of buffers are present in the body. Different body

FIGURE 8–1 How buffers respond to an excess of base. If the blood has too much base, the acid portion of a buffer pair (e.g., H_2CO_3 of the bicarbonate buffer system) releases hydrogen ions (H^+) to help return pH to normal.

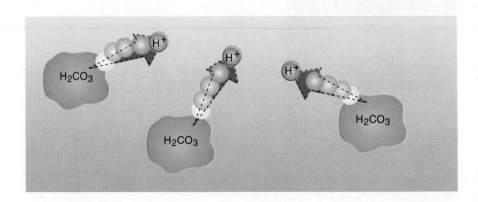

FIGURE 8-2 How buffers respond to an excess of acid. If the blood has too much acid, the base portion of a buffer pair (e.g., HCO_3^- of the bicarbonate buffer system) takes up hydrogen ions (H^+) to help return pH to normal.

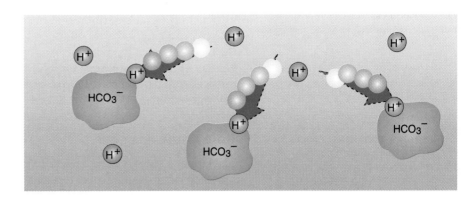

TABLE 8-1 Important Buffers

Buffer	Major Locations in the Body
Bicarbonate	Plasma; interstitial fluid
Protein	Plasma; inside cells
Hemoglobin	Inside red blood cells
Phosphate	Inside cells; urine

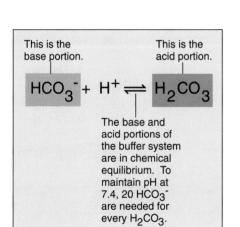

This is the base portion.   This is the acid portion.

$$HCO_3^- + H^+ \rightleftharpoons H_2CO_3$$

The base and acid portions of the buffer system are in chemical equilibrium. To maintain pH at 7.4, 20 HCO_3^- are needed for every H_2CO_3.

FIGURE 8-3 The bicarbonate buffer system.

Carbonic acid = carbon dioxide + water

$$H_2CO_3 = CO_2 + H_2O$$

▪ NORMAL VALUES OF ARTERIAL BLOOD PCO₂

Values may vary from laboratory to laboratory.
Infant: 30–34 mm Hg
School-age child: 35–41 mm Hg
Adolescent: 38–44 mm Hg

fluids have buffers to meet their special needs (Table 8–1). The bicarbonate buffer system neutralizes metabolic acids (Fig. 8–3). It cannot neutralize carbonic acid.

All buffer systems have limits. For example, if there are too many metabolic acids, the bicarbonate buffers become depleted. The acids then accumulate in the body until they are excreted by the kidneys. Clinically, this situation is seen as a decreased serum bicarbonate concentration (depleted bicarbonate buffers) and a decreased blood pH (accumulation of acid).

Role of the Lungs

The lungs are responsible for excreting carbonic acid from the body. A child breathes out carbon dioxide and water (carbonic acid) every time he or she exhales. The faster and deeper a child breathes, the more carbonic acid is excreted. A certain amount of carbonic acid is necessary in the body. Since carbonic acid is converted in the body to carbon dioxide and water by the enzyme carbonic anhydrase, an indirect laboratory measurement of carbonic acid is PCO_2.

Although a child can voluntarily increase or decrease the rate and depth of breathing, respiratory rate and depth are usually involuntarily controlled. The PCO_2 and pH of the blood are monitored by chemoreceptors in the brain (hypothalamus) and the periphery (aorta and carotid arteries). The peripheral chemoreceptors also monitor the PO_2 of the blood. The input from the chemoreceptors is combined with other neural input to modify ventilation according to the body's needs. If the PCO_2 begins to rise (carbonic acid accumulating) in a healthy child, the rate and depth of breathing increases and the excess carbonic acid is soon excreted. Then breathing returns to normal. If the PCO_2 begins to decrease (less carbonic acid present) in a healthy child, then breathing becomes a little more shallow so that less carbon dioxide is excreted and more carbonic acid is retained. Under normal conditions the lungs regulate the level of carbonic acid in the body effectively.

If a child has a condition that decreases the excretion of carbonic acid or causes breathing to be too slow and shallow, carbonic acid accumulates in the blood. Clinically, this is seen as an increased blood PCO_2. If, on the other hand, a child's breathing is too rapid and deep, too much carbon dioxide is excreted and carbonic acid is depleted in the blood. Clinically, this is seen as a decreased blood PCO_2.

Role of the Kidneys

The kidneys are responsible for excreting metabolic acids from the body. The blood bicarbonate ion concentration is an indicator of the amount of metabolic acids present, since bicarbonate is used in buffering these acids. A bicarbonate concentration within the normal range indicates that metabolic acids are present in the normal amount.

In the process of excreting some of the hydrogen ions from metabolic acids, the kidneys recycle bicarbonate ions (base). In this way, metabolic acids that are produced by cellular metabolism are eliminated from the body while the bicarbonate buffers are preserved. The recycling of bicarbonate with acid excretion occurs in the proximal tubules of the nephrons (Fig. 8–4). The ability to recycle bicarbonate (and thus secrete acid) matures after birth. Low-birth-weight infants are less efficient in recycling bicarbonate than are term infants. Even for term infants, this process requires several years to mature fully (Fig. 8–5).[1]

In the distal tubules and collecting ducts, hydrogen ions can be secreted from the blood into the renal tubular fluid by other mechanisms. Once the hydrogen ions enter the distal tubules, they are taken up by urinary buffers (primarily phosphate) or by ammonia (Fig. 8–6). The distal tubules can also

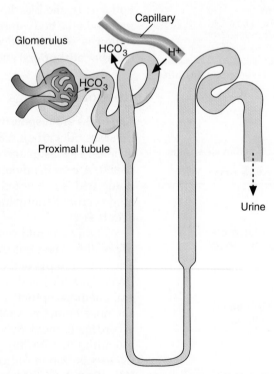

FIGURE 8–4 Recycling of bicarbonate by the kidneys. Bicarbonate ions that are in the blood are filtered into the renal tubules at the glomerulus. In the proximal tubules, bicarbonate ions are reabsorbed into the blood at the same time that hydrogen ions are transported from the blood into the renal tubular fluid.

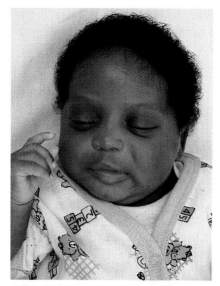

FIGURE 8–5 Developmental variation in the infant. An infant's kidneys are not efficient at recycling bicarbonate and thus excrete more bicarbonate in the urine. Thus, infants are at risk if they are given an acid load.

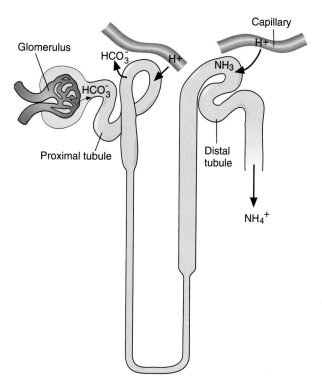

FIGURE 8–6 Secretion and buffering of H^+ in the kidneys. If the urine is too acidic, the cells that line the urinary tract could be damaged. To prevent this problem, hydrogen ions secreted into the distal tubules are neutralized by phosphate buffers or bound to ammonia and excreted in the form of ammonium ions.

■ GROWTH AND DEVELOPMENT CONSIDERATIONS

An infant is less effective in excreting acid through the kidneys than is an older child.

secrete bicarbonate ions into the renal tubular fluid or reabsorb them back into the blood. These distal processes allow the body to excrete more metabolic acids and to regenerate bicarbonate buffers.

In a healthy child the net result of these renal processes is excretion of metabolic acids and maintenance of blood bicarbonate concentration within normal limits. If the body needs to excrete more metabolic acids than usual, it can increase the production of ammonia by the cells that form the renal tubules. This mechanism allows more binding of hydrogen ions in the tubular fluid and thus more acid excretion. If too few metabolic acids are present in the blood, the kidneys can decrease their production of ammonia, excrete less acid, and excrete more bicarbonate to return the pH to normal. A child whose kidneys are not producing enough urine may be unable to excrete metabolic acids effectively. Accumulation of these acids uses up many of the bicarbonate buffers. Clinically, this accumulation of metabolic acids is detected as a decreased serum bicarbonate concentration.

Acid-Base Imbalances

There are four primary acid-base imbalances. Two of these imbalances are the result of processes that cause relatively too much acid in the body; each is called **acidosis**. The other two imbalances are the result of processes that cause relatively too little acid in the body; each is called **alkalosis**. An acid-base disorder caused by too much or too little carbonic acid is called a *respiratory* acid-base imbalance. A disorder caused by too much or too little metabolic acid is called a *metabolic* acid-base imbalance.

Acidosis: Relatively too much acid
  Respiratory acidosis: Relatively too
  much carbonic acid
  Metabolic acidosis: Relatively too
  much metabolic acid
Alkalosis: Relatively too little acid
  Respiratory alkalosis: Relatively too
  little carbonic acid
  Metabolic alkalosis: Relatively too lit-
  tle metabolic acid

Many conditions that result in acid-base disorders are discussed else-where in this book. The following discussion focuses on nursing care that ad-dresses only the acid-base aspects of these underlying conditions.

Respiratory Acidosis

Respiratory acidosis is caused by accumulation of carbon dioxide in the blood. Since carbon dioxide and water can be combined into carbonic acid, respiratory acidosis is sometimes called carbonic acid excess. This condition may be acute or chronic.

Clinical Manifestations

Carbon dioxide diffuses rapidly through cell membranes, and intracellular acidosis soon follows the **acidemia** (decreased blood pH) of respiratory aci-dosis. Acidosis in the brain cells causes central nervous system depression. Therefore, children who have acute respiratory acidosis may be disoriented, confused, lethargic, or even comatose. Acute respiratory acidosis may also be accompanied by headache (vasodilation of cerebral blood vessels), tachy-cardia (sympathetic nervous system stimulation), and cardiac arrhythmias (intracellular acidosis in myocardial cells). Children who have chronic respi-ratory acidosis are likely to be somewhat confused and sleepy.[2]

The child's arterial blood gases always show increased PCO_2, the labora-tory marker of increased carbonic acid. The pH is decreased or normal.

Etiology and Pathophysiology

Any factor that interferes with the ability of the lungs to excrete carbon diox-ide can cause respiratory acidosis. These factors may interfere with the gaseous exchange within the lungs, may impair the neuromuscular pump that moves air in and out of the lungs, or may depress the respiratory rate (Table 8–2, Fig. 8–7).

TABLE 8-2 Causes of Respiratory Acidosis

Factors Affecting the Lungs	Factors Affecting Central Control of Respiration
Aspiration	Drug overdose
Spasm of airways	General anesthesia
Epiglottitis	Head injury
Croup	Brain tumor
Pulmonary edema	Central sleep apnea
Atelectasis	
Cystic fibrosis	
Bronchopulmonary dysplasia	

Factors Affecting the Neuromuscular Pump

Flail chest
Pneumothorax or hemothorax
Mechanical underventilation
Hypokalemic muscle weakness
High cervical spinal cord injury
Botulism
Tetanus
Kyphoscoliosis
Poliomyelitis
Muscular dystrophy
Congenital diaphragmatic hernia

FIGURE 8-7 This child may develop respiratory acidosis or respiratory alkalosis. If the tidal volume is set too low during mechanical ventilation, carbon dioxide (carbonic acid) will accumulate in the body (respiratory acidosis) because it is not being excreted by the lungs. If the tidal volume is set too high, carbon dioxide will be depleted in the body (respiratory alkalosis) because it is being excreted in great quantities.

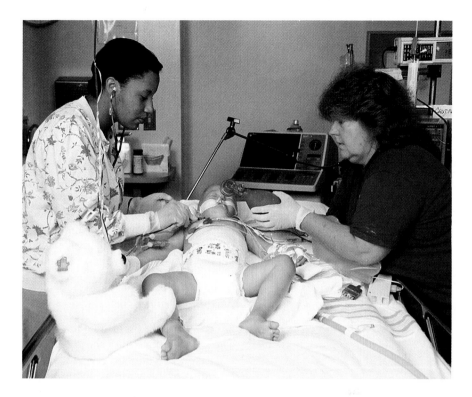

As the PCO_2 begins to increase, the pH of the blood begins to decrease. When the pH of the blood changes, two processes, correction and compensation, occur in the body. **Correction** tends to restore blood pH to normal by fixing the cause of the imbalance. **Compensation** does not fix the cause of the problem but tends to restore blood pH to normal by making either the PCO_2 or the plasma bicarbonate concentration abnormal. Both of these processes help protect the cells from the potentially fatal effects of acid-base imbalances.

Lung function must be restored in order to correct respiratory acidosis. If respiratory acidosis persists, compensation begins. Although the kidneys cannot excrete carbonic acid, they can excrete other acids. Excreting other acids from the body does not correct the problem, but it does help move the pH back toward the normal range and may prevent the severe clinical consequences of a very low pH.

Renal compensation takes several days to become fully effective and is likely to be less efficient in infants, since their ability to excrete acid is not as well developed as it is in older children. As the kidneys excrete more metabolic acids, the bicarbonate concentration of the blood rises because less bicarbonate is needed for buffering metabolic acids (Table 8–3).

TABLE 8-3 Laboratory Values in Uncompensated and Compensated Respiratory Acidosis

	PCO_2	pH	HCO_3^-
Uncompensated	Increased	Decreased	Normal
Partially compensated	Increased	Decreasing but moving toward normal	Increasing
Fully compensated	Increased	Normal	Increased

Medical Management

The main goal of medical management is treatment of the underlying cause of the respiratory acidosis. For example, treatment may include bronchodilators for bronchospasm or mechanical ventilation for neuromuscular defects.

Nursing Assessment

It is important to assess the child's level of consciousness. Adjust the assessment for the developmental level of the child. Observe an infant's general level of alertness and response to stimuli or assess an older child's ability to respond to questions. A child who is old enough to respond can be asked about headache. Assess the rate and depth of respirations. Count the child's apical pulse frequently, watching for tachycardia. If the pulse is irregular, a cardiac monitor should be applied. Serial arterial blood gas measurements should be taken to evaluate the child's changing status.

Nursing Diagnosis

Several nursing diagnoses may apply to the child with respiratory acidosis. The most important of these addresses the child's risk for injury. Other nursing diagnoses depend on the specific clinical manifestations and the particular cause of the acidosis. Examples include:

- High Risk for Injury related to decreased level of consciousness
- High Risk for Decreased Cardiac Output related to cardiac arrhythmias
- Ineffective Breathing Pattern (hypoventilation) related to (many possible etiologies)
- Pain related to cerebral vasodilation
- Noncompliance with previously prescribed bronchodilator therapy

Nursing Management

Protect the child who has a decreased level of consciousness from injury. Position the child so that the chest is not compressed or twisted to help increase ventilation to excrete the excess carbon dioxide (Fig. 8–8).

Use interventions to improve respiratory function. Depending on the cause of the respiratory acidosis, these may include encouraging the child to cough and take deep breaths, suctioning, or administering prescribed medications. Maintain sufficient fluid intake to produce a brisk flow of urine (unless contraindicated by the child's medical condition) to support renal compensation.

After the child is stabilized, teaching to prevent further episodes of respiratory acidosis becomes important. Use the cause of the respiratory acidosis to guide the teaching. Teach the parent (and child, if old enough) how to manage a chronic respiratory condition in order to prevent another episode of acidosis. If the respiratory acidosis occurred in an adolescent who has a chronic condition, then barriers to compliance with prescribed therapy need to be identified. Compliance must always be viewed in the context of the child's developmental needs and family dynamics.

Respiratory Alkalosis

Respiratory alkalosis occurs when the blood contains too little carbon dioxide. It is sometimes called carbonic acid deficit.

■ SAFETY PRECAUTIONS

Safety interventions for a child who has a decreased level of consciousness include keeping the bedrails up, making sure the child does not become tangled in the bedcovers, turning the child frequently, and positioning the child in good body alignment.

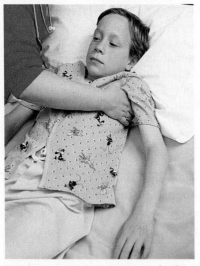

FIGURE 8–8 Positioning to facilitate chest expansion. If the child is positioned to avoid chest compression or slumping to the side, this will help correct respiratory acidosis.

Clinical Manifestations

Respiratory alkalosis results in cerebral vasoconstriction and leads to decreased oxygen perfusion of brain tissue. The **alkalemia** (increased blood pH) leads to intracellular alkalosis. Therefore, children with respiratory alkalosis are often lightheaded and confused. Diaphoresis may occur. The neuromuscular irritability caused by the alkalosis is manifested by digital and circumoral paresthesias. Muscle cramping and carpal or pedal spasms may also be seen. The arterial blood gases show a decreased PCO_2. The pH is elevated or normal.

Etiology and Pathophysiology

Respiratory alkalosis is caused by **hyperventilation**, the condition in which more air than normal is moved in and out of the lungs. The increased rate and depth of respirations result in excretion of more than the normal amount of carbon dioxide and water (carbonic acid). Common causes of hyperventilation are listed in Table 8–4.[2] It is critical to recognize that hypoxemia may cause hyperventilation.

Many cases of respiratory alkalosis last only several hours and renal compensation does not occur because the compensatory process takes several days. If respiratory alkalosis persists, the kidneys retain more acid and excrete more bicarbonate. Although this compensatory process does not correct the imbalance, it protects cellular function by returning the pH to normal. If full renal compensation occurs, the pH is normal and the bicarbonate concentration is decreased. The PCO_2 is decreased (Table 8–5).

Medical Management

Treatment focuses on correcting the condition causing the hyperventilation and the resultant alkalosis.

Nursing Assessment

Assess the child's level of consciousness and ask if the child feels lightheaded or has tingling sensations or numbness in the fingers, toes, or around the mouth. Increased neuromuscular irritability should be assessed by checking Chvostek sign or Trousseau sign (see Chapter 7). Assess rate and depth of respirations to monitor the effectiveness of the therapy to reduce the hyperventilation. Assess the child's level of oxygenation by monitoring the PO_2. Take serial arterial blood gas measurements to evaluate the changing status of the child's condition.

TABLE 8-4 Causes of Hyperventilation

Related to:

Hypoxemia
Anxiety
Pain
Fever
Salicylate poisoning
Meningitis
Encephalitis
Septicemia caused by Gram-negative bacteria
Mechanical overventilation

■ **NURSING ALERT**

The PO_2 must be checked before any therapy for respiratory alkalosis is started because it is dangerous to stop hyperventilation if oxygenation is poor.

TABLE 8-5 Laboratory Values in Uncompensated and Compensated Respiratory Alkalosis

	PCO_2	pH	HCO_3^-
Uncompensated	Decreased	Increased	Normal
Partially compensated	Decreased	Increased but moving toward normal	Decreasing
Fully compensated	Decreased	Normal	Decreased

Nursing Diagnosis

Several nursing diagnoses may apply to a child who has respiratory alkalosis. The most important of these address the child's hyperventilation and risk for injury. Examples include:

- Ineffective Breathing Pattern (hyperventilation) related to (many possible etiologies)
- High Risk for Injury related to confusion and lightheadedness
- Anxiety related to paresthesias and muscle cramps

Nursing Management

The cause of the respiratory alkalosis influences the nursing interventions. It is important to assist with improving oxygenation in a child who has respiratory alkalosis resulting from hypoxemia. Use appropriate pain control interventions (see Chapter 5) if the hyperventilation is due to pain.

If the hyperventilation is not caused by hypoxemia or chemical stimulation of the central nervous system, an older child may be able to decrease respirations if the nurse counts or breathes with the child. Breathing into a paper bag for a short time, which increases the carbon dioxide content of the inspired air, is frequently used with adolescents and adults but may be frightening for young children. Drawing a funny face or friendly animal on the bag may help.

Take precautions to ensure the child's safety. Make sure the bedrails are in the up position. Assist the child who is lightheaded when he or she is walking to the bathroom.

Reducing anxiety is also important, since the symptoms of respiratory alkalosis (paresthesias and lightheadedness) are alarming and may lead to additional hyperventilation. Nursing interventions should be based on the child's developmental level and modified according to the child's responses (Table 8–6).

Metabolic Acidosis

Metabolic acidosis is a condition in which there is an excess of any acid except carbonic acid. For this reason, it is sometimes called noncarbonic acid excess.

TABLE 8–6 Techniques for Reducing Anxiety in Children with Paresthesias

Infant
Calming touch, quiet voice, swaddling, holding quietly

Toddler or Preschooler
As above (omit swaddling), plus stuffed toy to hug, singing familiar quiet nursery songs, acknowledging the child's feelings

Young School-Age Child
As above, plus talking quietly about a happy event, telling a familiar story, reading a familiar book together, explaining that the tingling will go away, use of simple guided imagery, supportive listening

Older School-Age Child or Adolescent
Above interventions as appropriate, plus explaining the reason for the tingling and that it will go away, use of guided imagery, familiar music on tape or radio, asking what the child does when anxious or "scared," and talking about coping strategies

---

Clinical Manifestations

Like Jean in the case study at the beginning of this chapter, children with metabolic acidosis may be confused, drowsy, or lethargic. They may be stuporous or even comatose.[2] This decreased level of consciousness is caused by intracellular acidosis in cerebral neurons. Headache (resulting from cerebral vasodilation) and abdominal pain often occur. Cardiac arrhythmias result from intracellular acidosis of the myocardial cells. Respiratory compensation leads to an increased rate and depth of respiration (Kussmaul respirations). The blood bicarbonate ion concentration is decreased, and the pH may be decreased or normal.

Etiology and Pathophysiology

Metabolic acidosis can be caused by increased metabolic acids or by loss of bicarbonate. Both mechanisms cause a net increase in acid (Table 8–7).

Metabolic acids can accumulate in the body by three mechanisms. First, a child may eat or drink acids or substances that are converted to acid in the body. These substances include aspirin, boric acid, antifreeze, and methanol (automobile windshield cleaner). Second, a child's renal secretion of acid may be impaired, as in oliguric renal failure (Fig. 8–9). Third, a child may develop conditions that speed up cellular metabolism or cause cells to make unusual acids.[3] Ketoacidosis caused by diabetes mellitus or starvation is one such condition. In the case study, Jean had not eaten for 5 days, and her body had begun to break down fat to provide needed energy. When fat is metabolized in the absence of available glucose, metabolism is incomplete. The ketoacids resulting from the incomplete metabolism accumulate faster than the kidneys can excrete them, causing metabolic acidosis.

TABLE 8–7 Causes of Metabolic Acidosis

Gain of Metabolic Acid

Ingestion of acids (e.g., aspirin)
Ingestion of acid precursors (e.g., antifreeze)
Oliguria (e.g., renal failure)
Distal renal tubular acidosis
Diabetic ketoacidosis
Starvation ketoacidosis
Some inborn errors of metabolism (e.g., maple syrup urine disease)
Tissue hypoxia (lactic acidosis)

Loss of Bicarbonate

Diarrhea
Intestinal or pancreatic fistula
Proximal renal tubular acidosis

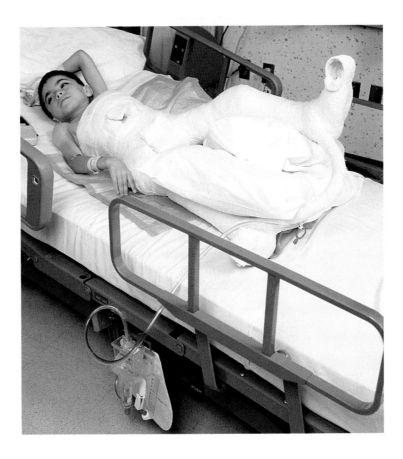

FIGURE 8–9 With any postoperative or immobilized child, it is important to monitor urine output to detect oliguria. If the kidneys do not produce very much urine, the metabolic acids accumulate in the body and cause metabolic acidosis. Inadequate fluid intake in the postoperative or immobilized child can lead to oliguria and, potentially, metabolic acidosis.

TABLE 8-8 Laboratory Values in Uncompensated and Compensated Metabolic Acidosis

	HCO_3^-	pH	PCO_2
Uncompensated	Decreased	Decreased	Normal
Partially compensated	Decreased	Decreased but moving toward normal	Decreasing
Fully compensated	Decreased	Normal	Decreased

Bicarbonate can be lost from the body through the urine or through excessive loss of bicarbonate-rich intestinal fluid.[4] Pancreatic secretions, which are released into the intestines, are rich in bicarbonate. In children who have diarrhea, like Jean, the bicarbonate-rich fluid leaves the body, causing metabolic acidosis. As illustrated in the case study, metabolic acidosis may develop from more than one cause in a particular child.

When the pH of the blood decreases below normal, the chemoreceptors in the brain and peripheral arteries are stimulated and respiratory compensation begins. The child's rate and depth of breathing increase and carbonic acid is removed from the body. Removing carbonic acid does not correct the problem, which is caused by a net increase of metabolic acids, but it makes the blood less acidic and shifts the pH toward the normal range. This compensation, which protects the cells from the potentially fatal effects of extreme acidemia, takes several hours to exert a major effect. Respiratory compensation can be seen as a decreased PCO_2 value.

Depending on how long metabolic acidosis has been present and the effectiveness of respiratory compensation, the pH may be decreased or in the normal range and the PCO_2 may be normal or decreased (Table 8–8).

Medical Management

The main goal of medical management is treatment of the underlying cause of the acidosis. In severe metabolic acidosis, intravenous sodium bicarbonate may be used to raise the pH to prevent the occurrence of fatal cardiac arrhythmias. The use of sodium bicarbonate is becoming less common, especially in the treatment of diabetic ketoacidosis.[5] However, it may still be given to some children to increase blood pH while treatment of the original cause takes effect.[6]

Nursing Assessment

Assess the child's level of consciousness frequently. Question the child who is able to talk about headache and abdominal pain. If the child has cardiac arrhythmias, a cardiac monitor should be applied. Assess the rate and depth of respirations to evaluate the child's ability to perform respiratory compensation (increased respiratory rate and depth). Take serial arterial blood gas measurements to evaluate the child's status.

Nursing Diagnosis

Several nursing diagnoses may apply to a child with metabolic acidosis. The most important nursing diagnosis addresses the child's risk for injury. Additional nursing diagnoses can be derived from the child's specific signs and symptoms and from teaching needs related to the specific cause of the imbalance. Examples include:

- High Risk for Injury related to altered level of consciousness
- High Risk for Decreased Cardiac Output related to cardiac arrhythmias
- High Risk for Altered Oral Mucous Membrane related to hyperventilation
- Pain related to cerebral vasodilation
- Anxiety related to pain and altered sensorium
- Knowledge Deficit (Parent and Child) regarding safe weight loss diet
- Noncompliance with previously prescribed insulin therapy

Nursing Management

Ensure the child's safety, taking into account the child's current level of consciousness and developmental stage. Turn the child who is stuporous or comatose frequently to prevent complications of immobility. Protect the child who has cardiac arrhythmias from increased oxygen demand by using interventions to reduce the child's activity.

Do not try to decrease the rate of the rapid, deep respirations because this respiratory compensation helps reverse the acidemia. Position the child to facilitate chest expansion to allow respiratory compensation. Provide frequent oral care so that the oral mucous membranes do not become dry and cracked. Narcotic analgesics should not be used routinely for headaches or abdominal pain associated with metabolic acidosis because they tend to depress respiration.

Reducing anxiety is also important. Suggested interventions for decreasing anxiety in children at different developmental stages are presented in the respiratory alkalosis section.

If intravenous sodium bicarbonate is used to raise blood pH, monitor for the electrolyte imbalance complications of this therapy: ionized hypocalcemia and hypokalemia. Rebound metabolic alkalosis occurs if too much sodium bicarbonate is given. To detect it, draw blood gases if the child's level of consciousness lessens after it has been improving or if the child develops paresthesias of fingers, toes, or around the mouth.

After the child's acid-base status is stabilized, nursing interventions to prevent further episodes of metabolic acidosis become important. For example, in the case study, Jean and her mother needed teaching regarding reduced-calorie diet, exercise, and appropriate weight loss goals. For children whose metabolic acidosis has other causes, teach what is needed to prevent this disorder. For example, teach parents how to keep acids away from a young child (Fig. 8–10) or explore the factors that make a diabetic adolescent noncompliant with previously prescribed insulin therapy.

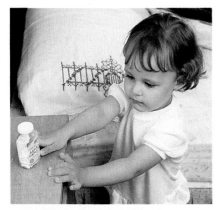

FIGURE 8–10 The parents of this child need teaching by a nurse! Teaching parents to use safety latches on cabinets to keep aspirin away from small children can help prevent metabolic acidosis.

Metabolic Alkalosis

Metabolic alkalosis occurs when there are too few metabolic acids. It is sometimes called noncarbonic acid deficit.

Clinical Manifestations

Increased neuromuscular irritability, with paresthesias, tetany, or seizures, may occur initially. Children may have nausea and vomiting. A period of belligerence and increased arousal (resulting from central nervous system excitation) may be followed by confusion, lethargy, and coma (resulting

TABLE 8–9 Causes of Metabolic Alkalosis

TABLE 8–9 Causes of Metabolic Alkalosis

Gain of Bicarbonate

Ingestion of baking soda
Ingestion of large quantities of bicarbonate antacids
Exchange transfusion or massive transfusion (citrate is metabolized to bicarbonate)

Loss of Metabolic Acid

Prolonged vomiting (e.g., pyloric stenosis)
Nasogastric suction
Cystic fibrosis
Hypokalemia
Diuretic therapy
Hyperaldosteronism
Adrenogenital syndrome
Cushing syndrome

from subsequent central nervous system depression). To compensate for metabolic alkalosis, respirations usually decrease in rate and depth. The blood bicarbonate concentration is elevated and the pH is increased.

Etiology and Pathophysiology

Metabolic alkalosis is caused by a gain of bicarbonate or by a loss of metabolic acid (any acid except carbonic acid) (Table 8–9). Bicarbonate is gained through ingestion of baking soda or bicarbonate antacids or through metabolism of bicarbonate precursors such as the citrate contained in blood transfusions. Acid can be lost from the body through the gastrointestinal tract, as in emesis; the kidneys, as in hyperaldosteronism; or shifted into cells, as in hypokalemia.[7]

When the blood bicarbonate concentration rises, the pH also rises, reflecting the increasing alkalinity of body fluids. The chemoreceptors in the brain and peripheral arteries detect the rising pH and the rate and depth of respiration decrease in response. This hypoventilation, a compensatory response to metabolic alkalosis, causes retention of carbonic acid in the body. The carbonic acid helps to neutralize the excess base and return the pH toward normal. Respiratory compensation for metabolic alkalosis usually does not normalize the pH completely, however, because the need for oxygen drives respiration and limits compensation. The PCO_2 is normal or increased (Table 8–10).

Medical Management

Medical treatment is directed at the underlying cause of the condition. Increasing the extracellular fluid volume with intravenous normal saline is used to facilitate renal excretion of bicarbonate.

Nursing Assessment

Assess the child's level of consciousness frequently. Level of consciousness may decrease after an initial excitation (belligerence, increased activity), so assessment should continue at regular intervals until the imbalance resolves. Monitor neuromuscular irritability. Question the child about nausea and vomiting. Assess rate and depth of respirations because respiratory compensation depresses respirations. Take serial arterial blood gas measurements.

Nursing Diagnosis

Several nursing diagnoses may apply to the child with metabolic alkalosis. The most important of these addresses the child's risk for injury. Other nurs-

TABLE 8–10 Laboratory Values in Uncompensated and Compensated Metabolic Alkalosis

	HCO_3^-	pH	PCO_2
Acute condition; uncompensated	Increased	Increased	Normal
Partially compensated	Increased	Increased but moving toward normal	Increasing
Fully compensated	The need for oxygen drives respirations and limits full compensation for metabolic alkalosis.		

ing diagnoses address safety issues, anxiety, and teaching needs. Examples include:

- High Risk for Injury related to altered level of consciousness
- High Risk for Aspiration related to nausea and decreased level of consciousness
- High Risk for Injury related to potential tetany and seizures
- Anxiety related to paresthesias and muscle cramps
- Knowledge Deficit (Parent and Child) regarding use of bicarbonate antacids

Nursing Management

■ NURSING ALERT

A child with metabolic alkalosis who is nauseous should be positioned on the side to avoid aspiration of vomitus.

The most important nursing interventions ensure the child's safety and should be modified as the child's condition changes. The bedrails may need to be padded initially. However, if the child's level of consciousness decreases, frequent turning may be more important. Use age-appropriate interventions to reduce anxiety.

To prevent metabolic alkalosis, make sure older children and adolescents understand that metabolic alkalosis may be caused by ingestion of baking soda or bicarbonate antacids. Tell parents not to apply baking soda over a large area of an infant's broken skin as a remedy for diaper rash. The sodium bicarbonate may be absorbed through the skin, causing metabolic alkalosis.

Mixed Acid-Base Imbalances

Although uncommon, it is possible for a child to develop two primary acid-base imbalances at the same time. For example, a child who has cystic fibrosis may develop respiratory acidosis from the lung problems and concurrent metabolic alkalosis from emesis and chloride loss in sweat. Similarly, chronic pulmonary insufficiency of the premature infant causes respiratory acidosis. Treatment with diuretics may cause concurrent metabolic alkalosis resulting from extracellular volume depletion and hypokalemia. Mixed acid-base imbalances are treated by correcting the underlying causes of the imbalance. Nursing management focuses on protecting the child from injury, reversing the physiologic processes that cause the disorders, and teaching to prevent these imbalances from occurring again. Since children who have mixed acid-base imbalances are generally seriously ill, frequent assessment and modification of care are essential.

■ How to Interpret Arterial Blood Gas Measurements

Arterial blood gas measurements (ABGs) provide a laboratory assessment of a child's current acid-base status. This discussion focuses on interpretation of the pH, PCO_2, and bicarbonate concentrations, which are the most important acid-base measures. The PO_2, a measure of oxygenation, is not discussed here. In some settings, end-tidal CO_2 measurements are available to provide a continuous noninvasive measurement that may parallel the arterial PCO_2 measure and allow for less frequent blood sampling for ABGs.

The key to understanding ABGs is remembering that the PCO_2 reflects the carbonic acid status (respiratory acid-base imbalances) and the bicarbonate concentration reflects the metabolic acid status (metabolic acid-base imbalances). Use an organized approach when looking at an arterial blood gas report.

1. *Look at the pH.* Is the pH above the normal range? If so, the child has alkalosis. Is it below normal? If so, the child has acidosis. If the pH is within

the normal range, either the child has no acid-base imbalance or has a fully compensated imbalance. A pH above 7.40 but still within the normal range might be fully compensated alkalosis. A pH below 7.40 but still within the normal range might be fully compensated acidosis. The other blood gas values will enable you to decide which is the situation.

2. *Look at the PCO₂.* Is the PCO_2 above the normal range? If so, the child has respiratory acidosis. This may be the primary disorder or it may be a compensatory response to metabolic alkalosis. Looking at the bicarbonate concentration later will enable you to decide. Is the PCO_2 below normal? If so, the child has respiratory alkalosis. This may be the primary disorder or it may be a compensatory response to metabolic acidosis. If the PCO_2 is within the normal range, the child does not have a respiratory acid-base imbalance.

3. *Look at the bicarbonate concentration.* Is the bicarbonate concentration above the normal range? If so, the child has metabolic alkalosis. This may be the primary disorder or it may be a compensatory response to respiratory acidosis. Is the bicarbonate concentration below normal? If so, the child has metabolic acidosis. This may be the primary disorder or it may be a compensatory response to respiratory alkalosis. If the bicarbonate concentration is within the normal range, the child does not have a metabolic acid-base imbalance.

4. *Interpret the results.* Now think about the three laboratory values together. If the pH is abnormal and either the PCO_2 or the bicarbonate concentration is normal, there is an uncompensated acid-base disorder. For example, if the pH is below normal and the PCO_2 is elevated, then the child has uncompensated respiratory acidosis. If all three values are abnormal, the child has a partially compensated disorder and the pH will provide the definitive answer. For example, in the case study, Jean's PCO_2 and bicarbonate concentration were both decreased. She might have had partially compensated metabolic acidosis or partially compensated respiratory alkalosis. Her decreased pH indicated partially compensated metabolic acidosis. The same reasoning applies if the PCO_2 and the bicarbonate concentration are abnormal but the pH is within the normal range. In this case, the child has a fully compensated acid-base disorder and the pH will indicate which one is present. For example, if both the PCO_2 and the bicarbonate concentration are elevated and the pH is within the normal range, the child might have fully compensated metabolic alkalosis or fully compensated respiratory acidosis. If the pH is normal but below 7.40, then the child has fully compensated metabolic acidosis.

5. *Think about the child.* Does your interpretation of the ABGs fit with the child's clinical situation? For example, if the blood gases indicate partially compensated metabolic acidosis, does the child have a factor that causes a relative increase of metabolic acids? In other words, does your interpretation of the ABGs make sense? In the case study, Jean had two such factors: diarrhea and production of ketoacids after not eating for 5 days. The interpretation of her ABGs did, indeed, make sense. This last step will help you integrate laboratory data with the clinical picture in order to strengthen your nursing care of the child who has an acid-base imbalance.

REFERENCES

1 Ichikawa, I., Narins, R., & Harris, H. (1990). Regulation of acid-base homeostasis. In I. Ichikawa (Ed.). *Pediatric textbook of fluids and electrolytes*. Baltimore: Williams & Wilkins.

2 Ichikawa, I., Narins, R., & Harris, H. (1990). Acid-base disorders. In I. Ichikawa (Ed.). *Pediatric textbook of fluids and electrolytes*. Baltimore: Williams & Wilkins.

3 Goldberg, G., & Greene, C. (1992). Update on inborn errors of metabolism: Primary lactic acidemia. *Journal of Pediatric Health Care, 6*, 176–181.

4 Santos, F., & Chan, J. (1986). Renal tubular acidosis in children: Diagnosis, treatment, and prognosis. *American Journal of Nephrology, 6*, 289–295.

5 Graf, H., & Arieff, A. (1986). The use of sodium bicarbonate in the therapy of organic acidosis. *Intensive Care Medicine, 12*, 285–288.

6 Narins, R., & Cohen, J. (1987). Bicarbonate therapy for organic acidosis: The case for its continued use. *Annals of Internal Medicine, 106*, 615–618.

7 Mathew, P., Hamdan, J., & Nazer, H. (1991). Cystic fibrosis presenting with recurrent vomiting and metabolic alkalosis. *European Journal of Pediatrics, 150*, 264–266.

SUGGESTED READINGS

Curley, M., & Thompson, J. (1990). End-tidal CO_2 monitoring in critically ill infants and children. *Pediatric Nursing, 16*, 397–403.

Ichikawa, I. (Ed.), (1990). *Pediatric textbook of fluids and electrolytes*. Baltimore: Williams & Wilkins.

Mims, B. (1991). Interpreting ABG's. *RN, 54*, 42–46.

Rose, B. (1989). *Clinical physiology of acid-base and electrolyte disorders* (3rd ed.). New York: McGraw-Hill.

Weizman, Z., Houri, S., & Gradus, D. (1992). Type of acidosis and clinical outcome in infantile gastroenteritis. *Journal of Pediatric Gastroenterology and Nutrition, 14*, 187–191.

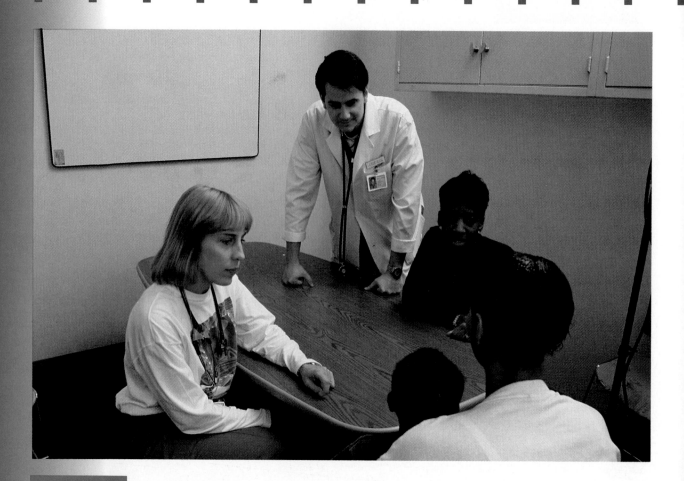

R aymond, a 2-year-old child, has had recurrent infections since he was born. In the last three months he has had bronchitis twice, otitis media three times, and several colds. Raymond has had a slight fever, vomiting, and diarrhea for several days. His grandmother brings him to a walk-in clinic to find out what is wrong.

Blood tests are performed to assess Raymond's immune function. On the basis of a thorough evaluation of Raymond's clinical symptoms and the results of the laboratory tests, he is diagnosed with acquired immunodeficiency syndrome (AIDS).

Raymond is admitted to a special unit of the hospital for children with AIDS where special precautions are taken to prevent infection. Like many of the other children, Raymond is often irritable and difficult to console. Because he vomits frequently, the nurses pay particular attention to Raymond's nutritional problems, giving him frequent small feedings.

Raymond is diagnosed as having failure to thrive, a common sequela of AIDS. Broad-spectrum antibiotics are given, and he is assessed frequently for the development of new infections. A multidisciplinary team, involving nurses, physicians, psychologists, nutritionists, and social services professionals, confer daily to ensure that Raymond receives the best care.

ALTERATIONS IN IMMUNE FUNCTION

9

▪ TERMINOLOGY

allergen An antigen capable of inducing hypersensitivity.

antibody A protein that is capable of reacting specifically to an antigen.

antigen A foreign substance that triggers an immune response.

graft-versus-host disease Series of immunologic responses mounted by the host of a transplanted organ with the purpose of destroying the transplant cells.

hypersensitivity response An overreaction of the immune system, responsible for allergic reactions.

immunodeficiency A state of the immune system in which it cannot cope effectively with foreign antigens.

immunoglobulins A protein that functions as an antibody. Immunoglobulins are responsible for humoral immunity.

opportunistic infection An infection that is often caused by normally nonpathogenic organisms in persons who lack normal immunity.

primary immune response The process in which B lymphocytes produce antibodies specific to a particular antigen on first exposure.

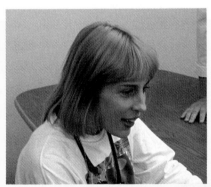

❝ Raymond's family is learning to deal with the reality of AIDS. All of us on the team are trying to give them the support they need now and to prepare them for the future. **❞**

W

hat are the signs and symptoms of immunologic disorders in children? Many times they are nonspecific. Raymond's admitting signs and symptoms, described in the opening scenario, are characteristic of several different immunodeficiency disorders.

The immune system is one of the few body systems that regulates, either directly or indirectly, all other body functions. Thus a problem with the immune system can have multisystem consequences and may be life-threatening. Allergic reactions to food or frequent episodes of otitis media may indicate a disorder of immune function. Congenital abnormalities sometimes signal a defect in cellular immunity (e.g., DiGeorge syndrome).

In this chapter, we will examine some of the more common disorders of immune function and discuss nursing care for children who have these diseases and their families.

Anatomy and Physiology of Pediatric Differences

The function of the immune system is to recognize any foreign material and to eliminate that foreign substance as efficiently as possible. Whenever the body recognizes the presence of a substance that it cannot identify as part of itself, the body protects itself through the immune response. Normally, the immune system responds to an invasion of foreign substances, or **antigens,** by producing antibodies and sensitized lymphocytes.

Immunity is either natural or acquired. Natural immune defenses are those the infant is born with, such as intact skin, body pH, natural antibodies from the mother, and inflammatory and phagocytic properties. Acquired immunity is composed of humoral (antibody-mediated) and cell-mediated immunity and is not fully developed until a child is about 6 years of age.

Humoral immunity is responsible for destroying bacterial antigens. B lymphocytes, produced in the bone marrow, develop into plasma cells that produce antibodies. An **antibody** is a class of proteins called **immunoglobu-**

FIGURE 9–1 Primary immune response.

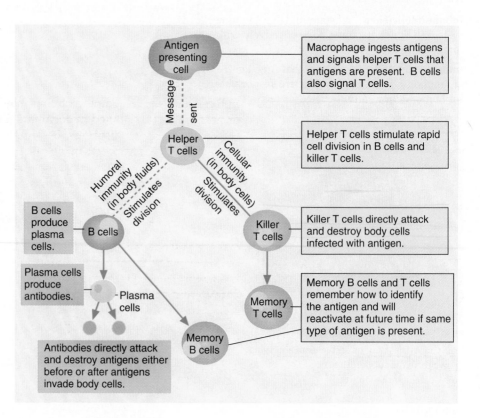

lins. Antibodies are found in serum, body fluids, and certain tissues. When a child is first exposed to an antigen, the B lymphocyte system begins to produce antibodies that react specifically to that antigen (Fig. 9–1). It takes approximately 3 days for this process, known as **primary immune response,** to occur. Subsequent encounters with the antigen trigger memory cells, resulting in an immune response within 24 hours. Children under the age of 6 years become ill so frequently because they have a limited supply of antibodies against commonly encountered bacteria.

In contrast, cell-mediated immunity achieves full function early in life. T lymphocytes, produced in the thymus, provide cellular immunity and protect against most viruses, fungi, and slowly developing bacterial infections such as tuberculosis. In addition, they control the timing of the response in delayed hypersensitivity reactions, such as the purified protein derivative (PPD) test, and they are responsible for the rejection of foreign grafts, such as transplants. Specialized types of T lymphocytes include killer T cells, suppressor T cells, and helper T cells. Suppressor T cells inhibit B lymphocytes from differentiating into plasma cells. Helper T cells aid this process.

Complement is a component of blood serum consisting of 11 protein compounds. It is an inactive enzyme that activates in response to antigen-antibody functions, resulting in a generalized inflammatory reaction that kills foreign cells.

Immunodeficiency Disorders

Immunodeficiency, a state of decreased responsiveness of the immune system, can occur to varying degrees in response to any number of events. Children with congenital immunodeficiency, or primary immune deficiency, are born with a failure of humoral antibody formation (B cell disorder), a deficient cellular immune system (T cell disorder), or a combination of both defects. This immune deficiency is not caused by another condition. Immunodeficiency may also be acquired, as in human immunodeficiency virus (HIV) infection.

B Cell and T Cell Disorders

In B cell disorders, immunoglobulins may be present in inadequate numbers or nearly absent. X-linked hypogammaglobulinemia and selective IgA deficiency are two such disorders. Because newborns are protected from infection by maternal antibodies in the first months after birth, symptoms of B cell disorders usually become apparent after 3 months of age. These infants have frequent recurrent bacterial infections and failure to thrive. With treatment, intravenous immunoglobulins and antibiotics, most children survive into adulthood. Prognosis depends on the degree of antibody deficiency.

T cell disorders are characterized by inadequate numbers of T lymphocytes or absence of T cell functions. Isolated T cell disorders are rare and may be associated with congenital abnormalities (as in DiGeorge syndrome) or of unknown cause. DiGeorge syndrome is characterized by the absence of parathyroid or thymus glands, cardiac and ear defects, tetany 48 hours after birth, and viral and fungal infections in the neonatal period (Fig. 9–2). Children with the disorder are treated with antibiotics, oral calcium, and thymus transplant. Without thymus transplant, few children survive beyond 5 years.

Refer to Table 9–1, which compares laboratory values for selected congenital immunodeficiency disorders.

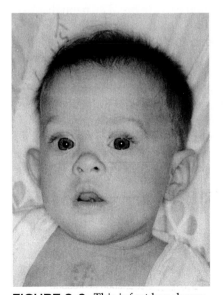

FIGURE 9–2 This infant has characteristic features of DiGeorge syndrome. Note the low-set and malformed ears.

From Stites, D.P., & Terr, A.I. (1991). *Basic & clinical immunology* (7th ed.) (p. 336). Norwalk, CT: Appleton & Lange.

TABLE 9-1 Congenital Immunodeficiency Disorders

Disorders	Laboratory Findings
B Cell	
X-linked hypogammaglobulinemia (inherited disorder)	Reduced IgG (<200 µL), absent IgM, IgA, IgD, IgE, absence of B cells in peripheral blood, normal T cells
Selective IgA deficiency	IgA <5 mg/dL
T Cell	
DiGeorge syndrome (birth defect)	Lymphopenia; absent T cell functions, decreased T cells, normal B cells
Combined	
Severe combined immunodeficiency syndrome (SCID)	Complete absence of both T and B cell immunity; severe reduction or absence of T and B cells
Wiskott-Aldrich syndrome	Thrombocytopenia, normal IgG, decreased IgM, increased IgA, increased IgE; inability to respond to polysaccharide antigens

Adapted from Griffin, J. (1986). *Hematology & immunology: Concepts of nursing.* Norwalk, CT: Appleton & Lange.

Severe Combined Immunodeficiency Disease

Severe combined immunodeficiency disease (SCID) is a congenital condition characterized by absence of both humoral and cellular immunity. SCID occurs in X-linked recessive, autosomal recessive, and sporadic forms. Without appropriate treatment, children born with SCID usually die within the first 2 years of life.

Clinical Manifestations

Symptoms in a child born with SCID develop early in life. The neonate often demonstrates a susceptibility to infection by 3 months of age. The disorder is characterized by chronic infection, failure to completely recover from infection, frequent reinfection, and infection with viruses such as cytomegalovirus and the bacterium *Pneumocystis carinii*. Often the first infection seen is a resistant oral candidiasis. Children are also highly susceptible to sepsis and pneumonia. Failure to thrive is a consequence of persistent illness.

Some infants experience **graft-versus-host disease** as a result of placental transfer of maternal T lymphocytes. If the child receives foreign tissue, for example, in a blood transfusion, signs such as skin rash, fever, hepatosplenomegaly, and diarrhea may occur.

Etiology and Pathophysiology

The exact cause of SCID is unknown. Defective stem cells, thymus dysfunction, and enzymatic disorder have been proposed as possible etiologies.

Diagnostic Tests and Medical Management

A marked reduction in lymphocyte counts indicates SCID. B and T lymphocytes are few in number or absent from the peripheral blood and lymphoid tissues. Immunoglobulin levels are significantly reduced. Refer to Table 9–1 for laboratory findings in SCID.

The goal of medical management is to restore immune function. Thymic hormones have been given to some children with limited success. Bone marrow transplantation offers hope for children with SCID (see Chapter 13). However, the donor must be a histocompatible donor, such as a sibling.

Prognosis is poor without aggressive therapy. Some children have survived 10 years after a successful bone marrow transplant.[1]

Nursing Assessment

Obtain a thorough history of infections, including age of onset, type of causal organism, frequency, and severity. Take a family history, and find out if the child has had any unusual reactions to vaccines, medications, or foods. Measure the child's height and weight accurately to determine failure to thrive. Look for any evidence of infections on the skin, subcutaneous tissues, and mucous membranes. Palpate the abdomen for hepatomegaly and the lymph nodes for lymphadenopathy.

Assess family support systems, and coping mechanisms.

Nursing Diagnosis

The primary nursing diagnosis for a child with SCID is High Risk for Infection related to immunodeficiency. Other nursing diagnoses may include:

- High Risk for Altered Nutrition: Less Than Body Requirements related to chronic diarrhea and infections
- High Risk for Impaired Skin Integrity related to chronic infections
- High Risk for Caregiver Role Strain related to chronic, life-threatening disease in child
- High Risk for Altered Growth and Development related to restricted activities and chronic illness

■ SAFETY PRECAUTIONS

Children with immune disorders, their siblings, or other household contacts should not be immunized with the oral polio vaccine, which contains a live virus, because of the risk of giving the virus to the immunodeficient child. Inactivated polio virus should be used instead.

Nursing Management

Nursing care of the immunodeficient child focuses on preventing infection. However, even with the use of environmental controls, such as keeping children inside bubbles to maintain a sterile environment, these children are prone to **opportunistic infections** (infections caused by normal flora that develop in immunocompromised or immunodeficient persons).

Prevent Systemic Infection. Frequent and thorough handwashing is important. Use aseptic technique when caring for all sites where catheters, central lines, endotracheal tubes, pressure monitoring lines, and peripheral intravenous lines enter the child's body.

Promote Skin Integrity. The skin is the only intact defense that many of these children have. Provide good skin care, and observe all possible pressure areas closely for signs of breakdown or infection. Turn the child frequently. Encourage range of motion exercises. Avoid any skin trauma.

Provide Emotional Support. SCID is a life-threatening and devastating disease. Even with aggressive therapy, the prognosis is poor. Evaluate the family's knowledge about the disease. The parents may be experiencing guilt because of the genetic nature of the disease and the difficulties of treatment. Listen closely to their concerns and encourage them to discuss their fears. Refer them to an appropriate support group or counselor if needed. Genetic counseling should be encouraged if the parents plan to have more children.

Wiskott-Aldrich Syndrome

This combined congenital immunodeficiency syndrome is an X-linked disorder, characterized by thrombocytopenia, eczema, hemorrhagic tendencies, and recurrent infections. Thrombocytopenia with bleeding tendencies appears during the neonatal period. Eczema appears by 1 year of age. Infections involve the middle ear and often lead to chronic otitis media. Children are particularly susceptible to infections from herpes viruses and lymphoreticular malignancies, especially of the lymphatic system.

The cause of the basic defect is unknown. The diagnosis is made in the early neonatal period on the basis of the thrombocytopenia (refer to Table 9–1). How and when Wiskott-Aldrich syndrome manifests itself varies, with some children maintaining normal lymphocyte levels for years. Treatment is symptomatic and includes antibiotic prophylaxis together with platelet infusions and intravenous immunoglobulin therapy. Without bone marrow transplantation, most children die within the first 5 years of life. Transplantation does not, however, reverse all of the defects of this disease and the ultimate impact on long-term survival is not known.[2]

Nursing Management

Nursing care is similar to that for the child with SCID. Refer the parents for genetic counseling to help them understand the transmission of the disease and the probability of having another child with the same disorder. Arrange for psychological support for those parents who may be overwhelmed with guilt from learning that the illness is inherited.

Help the parents and family cope with the knowledge that the child has a chronic and potentially fatal illness. Referral to family counseling may be appropriate.

Acquired Immunodeficiency Syndrome

Soon after acquired immunodeficiency syndrome (AIDS) was recognized in homosexual adults and intravenous drug abusers, cases of AIDS were seen in children. Increasing numbers of children infected with the human immunodeficiency virus (HIV) have been diagnosed, making HIV infection a leading cause of immune disease in infants and children. The virus affects multiple systems and eventually destroys the child's immune system. An understanding of the natural history of HIV disease is still evolving.

Clinical Manifestations

The interval from HIV infection to the onset of overt AIDS is shorter in children than in adults, and shorter in children infected perinatally than in those infected through transfusion.[3-5] Most children with AIDS have nonspecific findings, including lymphadenopathy, hepatosplenomegaly, oral candidiasis, failure to thrive and weight loss, diarrhea, chronic eczema, and fever. Raymond, described at the beginning of this chapter, had several of these findings, as well as a history of recurrent infections (bronchitis, otitis media, and colds). Bacterial and opportunistic infections, such as *Streptococcus, Haemophilus influenzae, Salmonella,* and *Pneumocystis carinii* pneumonia, as well as malignancies such as lymphomas frequently occur as the disease progresses. Lymphocytic interstitial pneumonitis is a common manifestation of pediatric AIDS. Frequently children develop encephalopathy resulting in developmental delay or a deterioration of motor skills and intellectual functioning.

Etiology and Pathophysiology

Acquired immunodeficiency syndrome is caused by the human immunodeficiency virus (HIV-1). Children may acquire HIV infection from their mothers transplacentally or during delivery. Perinatal transmission can occur during birth from blood, amniotic fluid, and exposure to genital tract secretions and through breast milk from HIV-positive mothers.

Thirteen percent of children with AIDS contracted the virus through transfusion of blood products.[6] Most of these children were infected during treatment of hemophilia. This occurred before mandatory screening of blood and blood products was instituted in 1985. Adolescents frequently acquire the virus through intravenous drug abuse and through homosexual or heterosexual activities.

The HIV virus selectively targets and destroys T cells, thereby decreasing and eventually eliminating cellular immunity. Humoral immunity is also affected. Thus, the child is left unprotected against a myriad of bacterial, viral, fungal, and opportunistic infections, which are ultimately fatal.

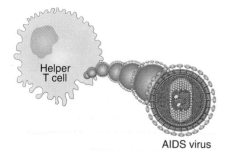

Helper T cell

AIDS virus

Diagnostic Tests and Medical Management

Fifty percent of children with AIDS are diagnosed during the first year of life, and 82 percent by the age of 3 years.[6] Serologic tests for detection of the virus are the enzyme-linked immunosorbent assay (ELISA) and the Western blot. Both tests detect antibodies to the virus. The Centers for Disease Control and Prevention (CDC) considers children under 13 years of age to be infected if their symptoms meet the CDC criteria for AIDS, if they have HIV in the blood or tissues, or if they have antibody to HIV (Table 9–2).

Medical management is supportive. There is no cure for AIDS. Intravenous gamma immunoglobulin has been used to prevent bacterial infec-

---

TABLE 9-2 CDC Definition of AIDS in Children

1. Children under 15 months of age whose mothers are not thought to have had HIV infection during the perinatal period; however, these infants and children are repeatedly reactive for HIV antibody by ELISA with a subsequent positive Western blot or immunofluorescence assay.

2. Children under 15 months of age whose mothers are thought to have had HIV infection during the perinatal period; the infant or child is repeatedly reactive for HIV antibody, has elevated serum immunoglobulin levels, has a positive Western blot or immunofluorescence assay, and has at least one of the following:
   a. Decreased absolute lymphocyte count
   b. Depressed T helper lymphocyte count
   c. Decreased T helper to T suppressor lymphocyte ratio

3. Children 15 months of age or older who are repeatedly reactive for HIV antibody by ELISA with subsequent positive results from Western blot or immunofluorescence assay.

4. Children less than 13 years of age who have multiple or recurrent serious bacterial infections, lymphoid interstitial pneumonia, or pulmonary lymphoid hyperplasia and laboratory evidence of HIV infection. A presumptive diagnosis may be made in the absence of a positive ELISA for lymphoid interstitial pneumonia or pulmonary lymphoid hyperplasia.

5. Children who have a progressive loss of behavioral or developmental milestones not related to any other known condition and laboratory evidence of HIV.

6. Children who fail to thrive and have laboratory evidence of HIV.

Adapted from Centers for Disease Control and Prevention. (1987). Classification system for human immunodeficiency virus infection in children under 13 years of age. *Morbidity & Mortality Weekly Report, 36,* 225–230; and Centers for Disease Control and Prevention. (1992). Revised classification system for HIV infection and expanded surveillance case definition for AIDS among adolescents and adults. *Morbidity & Morality Weekly Report, 41,* RR–17.

tions in children under the age of 2. Treatment involves prompt therapy for bacterial and opportunistic infections. Children between 3 months and 12 years of age have been receiving experimental therapy with antiretroviral drugs such as zidovudine (azidothymidine [AZT]). Zidovudine theoretically slows replication of the virus. The earlier the child develops AIDS, the poorer the prognosis.

Nursing Assessment

Assessment centers on observation and evaluation of potential sites of infection. Assess breath sounds, respiratory status, arterial blood gases, level of consciousness, and mental status. Any evidence of lymphocytic interstitial pneumonitis or neurologic abnormalities should be reported. Assess the child's height and weight frequently. Look for *Candida* infections in the mouth and the diaper area. Note any developmental delays in motor skills or intellectual functioning, which could result from encephalopathy.

Assess family support systems and coping mechanisms, as the stressors of caring for a child with AIDS may overwhelm parents. Assess the family's ability to care for the child. If the mother is infected, inquire about the extended family's ability to provide daily care as well as emotional support. When assessing an adolescent who has AIDS, evaluate the teen's understanding of how AIDS is transmitted.

Nursing Diagnosis

The accompanying Nursing Care Plan includes common nursing diagnoses that may apply to a child with AIDS. Other nursing diagnoses may include:

- Diarrhea related to gastrointestinal infection, malignancy, or drug reactions
- Impaired Gas Exchange related to pulmonary disease
- Altered Growth and Development related to HIV encephalopathy
- High Risk for Ineffective Family Coping: Compromised related to life-threatening illness

Nursing Management

Nursing care of the child with AIDS is primarily supportive and centers on preventing infection, promoting adequate nutritional intake, promoting respiratory function, providing mouth care, and providing emotional support to parents and child. The Nursing Care Plan summarizes nursing care for the child with acquired immunodeficiency syndrome.

Prevent Infection. Immunosuppressed children become infected with bacteria as well as other organisms that are common in the environment. Frequent handwashing and limiting exposure of the child to individuals with upper respiratory infections or other infections are a few of the interventions used to protect the child from infections. Teach sexually active adolescents the importance of practicing safe sex and the ramifications of high-risk sexual behaviors and intravenous drug abuse.

Promote Respiratory Function. Because many children with AIDS develop pneumonia, encourage the child to cough and deep breathe every 2 to 4 hours. Blowing cotton balls with a straw, blowing bubbles, or other games

■ SAFETY PRECAUTIONS

Health care workers who come in contact with blood or other body fluids of children infected with HIV are at risk for exposure to the virus. Universal precautions should be used at all times (see the Atlas of Pediatric Procedures).

may engage the interest of a younger child. Rest periods to conserve energy and lower the body's demand for oxygen are important.

Promote Adequate Nutritional Intake. Because many children with AIDS have failure to thrive, nutrition is an important part of their care. A nutritionist should be involved in planning an appropriate diet for the child. Adequate nutrition is sometimes provided by hyperalimentation.

Diarrhea resulting from gastrointestinal infection is a common finding in these children and complicates other nutritional disturbances. Antidiarrheal medications may be prescribed. Keep the child's lips and mouth moist and pay close attention to hydration status. Monitor the skin turgor and urine output, and provide careful perineal skin care to prevent infection.

Provide Mouth Care. The frequency of *Candida* infections leads to blisters, cracking, and discharge of the oral mucous membranes. Mouth care with a non-alcohol-based solution such as normal saline or lemon-glycerine swabs should be done every 2 to 4 hours.

Provide Emotional Support. The family of the child with AIDS is under great strain. Integrate social services and support groups into the care of the child as soon as the diagnosis is made. Spend time talking with the family about their fears and feelings. In many parts of the United States, AIDS still carries a tremendous stigma, and the family may not be able to discuss their feelings outside of the hospital environment.

Discharge Planning and Patient and Family Home Care Teaching. Home care needs should be identified and addressed well in advance of discharge. The diagnosis of AIDS is surrounded by strong emotions and fears. Be honest and direct. Education is essential. Explain that there is no evidence that casual contact among family members can spread the infection.

Make sure the child and family understand that AIDS is transmitted through blood, urine, stool, and other body secretions. Teach family members the importance of careful hygiene. Encourage careful handwashing and tell parents to avoid handling body fluids. Explain that they should wear gloves when changing diapers; disposing of urine, stool, and emesis; and when treating the child's cuts and scrapes. Instruct parents to use a bleach solution for disinfection of objects when necessary.

School attendance guidelines for children with AIDS have been published by the American Academy of Pediatrics and the Centers for Disease Control and Prevention. These guidelines recommend that children with AIDS or AIDS-related complex have unrestricted school attendance as long as their physician approves. Contraindications to school attendance include lack of control of body secretions, biting, and open wounds that cannot be covered.

Support groups, home health care nursing services, financial assistance, and psychological counseling are usually needed at some point during the child's illness, and the family should be aware of the availability of such services. Help the family deal with guilt feelings about the child's condition.

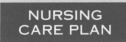
THE CHILD WITH ACQUIRED IMMUNODEFICIENCY SYNDROME

GOAL	INTERVENTION	RATIONALE	EXPECTED OUTCOME
1. High Risk for Infection related to immunosuppression			
Child will remain free of infection.	Assess child every 2 to 4 hours for fever; lesions in the mouth; redness, inflammation, soreness, and lesions on the skin or around intravenous lines.	Fever is one of the few signs of infection in the immunosuppressed child who does not have a sufficient number of white blood cells.	Child has no fever and shows no other signs of infection.
	Auscultate for changes in breath sounds every 2 hours. Perform pulmonary toilet (coughing, deep breathing, incentive spirometry) every 2 to 4 hours.	Pneumonia is a likely infection in the child with AIDS.	
	Enforce strict handwashing. Allow no fresh flowers, fruits, or vegetables in child's room. Screen visitors for colds or recent exposure to varicella. Use blood and body fluid precautions (see the Atlas of Pediatric Procedures). Practice strict asepsis for dressing changes and suctioning.	Control of environmental factors helps prevent infection.	
	Coordinate patient care assignments to avoid exposing child to individuals with recent infections or immunizations.	Planning minimizes chances for infection.	
	Organize patient care activities to allow for adequate periods of rest.	Rest periods allow child to regain energy.	
2. Altered Nutrition: Less Than Body Requirements related to decreased intake and absorption of nutrients			
Child will have adequate nutritional intake to meet metabolic needs.	Encourage frequent small meals to promote nutritional and fluid intake.	Additional nutrition is required to rebuild the immune system.	Child eats frequent meals of adequate nutritional content.
	Maintain nasogastric tube feeding, if ordered. Hyperalimentation may be necessary to ensure adequate nutrition.		
	Eliminate unpleasant stimuli and odors from the environment during meals.	Unpleasant stimuli decrease the desire for food.	
	Monitor skin turgor every shift.	Skin turgor reflects hydration status.	
	Involve nutritionist in planning a diet for the child that includes favorite foods.	Including favorite foods encourages intake.	

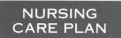
THE CHILD WITH ACQUIRED IMMUNODEFICIENCY SYNDROME—CONTINUED

GOAL	INTERVENTION	RATIONALE	EXPECTED OUTCOME
3. High Risk for Impaired Skin Integrity related to skin infection, immobility, or diarrhea			
Child will have minimal or no skin breakdown.	Observe all pressure areas closely for signs of infection or breakdown.	Skin care is important in the immunocompromised child. The skin may be the only intact defense the child has.	Child is free of preventable skin breakdown.
	Keep skin clean and dry. Provide perineal care to minimize irritation from diarrhea.	Prevents breaking or cracking of skin.	
4. High Risk for Altered Oral Mucous Membranes related to infection			
Child will have intact oral mucous membranes.	Inspect mouth for signs of blistering or lesions.	Candidal infection is frequently associated with immunodeficiency.	Child has intact oral mucous membranes.
	Provide mouth care with normal saline solution or lemon-glycerine swabs every 2 to 4 hours.	Provides comfort and promotes healing.	
5. Knowledge Deficit (Parent) related to home care of child with AIDS			
Parent will verbalize knowledge about home care, measures to prevent infection, and signs and symptoms to report to health care providers.	Explain the importance of optimizing the child's health status and reducing risk of complications through diet, rest, and meticulous personal hygiene. Be sure that parents and other family members understand how AIDS is spread and appropriate precautions.	Knowledge about the disorder and preventive measures are necessary in order to provide safe and effective home care for the child.	Parent describes appropriate home care and preventive measures for a child with AIDS.
	Discuss with parents and child reasons for protective measures.	Knowledge of rationale increases compliance.	
	Inform family about signs and symptoms of infection that should be reported promptly to the physician or nurse (fever, chills, cough, mild erythema).	Prompt treatment improves outcome.	
6. Caregiver Role Strain related to anxiety about child's condition and demands of providing care			
Parent will report decreased anxiety related to child's condition and care.	Encourage family members to express fears and concerns regarding the child's prognosis.	Expression of fears helps to decrease anxiety.	Parent states decreased anxiety.
	Advise family about support services or other resources available in the community.	Provides additional support to help family cope with the child's illness and the dying process, when needed.	

Autoimmune Disorders

In an immune system damaged by pathologic changes, an immune response may occur to some of the body's own proteins, resulting in the production of autoantibodies. These pathologic conditions in which the body directs the immune response against itself are called autoimmune disorders.

The primary feature of autoimmune disorders is tissue injury caused by a probable immunologic reaction of the host with its own tissues. Structural or functional changes occur as immune cells attack other cells in the body.

The autoimmune disorders are grouped into systemic and organ-specific diseases. Systemic diseases, which largely involve more than one organ, include systemic lupus erythematosus and juvenile rheumatoid arthritis. Organ-specific diseases, which primarily affect a single organ, include juvenile diabetes mellitus (see Chapter 19) and thyroiditis.

Systemic Lupus Erythematosus

Systemic lupus erythematosus (SLE), a generalized disorder seen mainly in females, is a chronic inflammatory disease of unknown origin that involves many organ systems. SLE affects approximately 1 in 100,000 people, and it is more common in blacks than whites. The majority of cases are diagnosed between the ages of 16 and 30 years.[7,8]

Clinical Manifestations

Symptoms depend on the organ involved and the amount of tissue damage that has occurred. Initial symptoms include fever, chills, fatigue, malaise, and weight loss. The most common symptoms are arthritis and skin rash. A butterfly rash on the face, consisting of a pink or red rash over the bridge of the nose extending to the cheeks, is a characteristic finding. Children with SLE may have hemolytic anemia, with a low white blood cell and platelet count; bleeding disorders; hypergammaglobulinemia; and vasculitis.

Etiology and Pathophysiology

The exact etiology of SLE is unknown. It is believed that an outside environmental agent causes the body to have a negative response to its own immune system. Damage to organs is believed to occur because the immune complexes (antigen-antibody complexes) are deposited in the vascular system, leading to widespread inflammation and tissue damage. The tissues most likely to be affected are the small blood vessels, glomeruli, joints, spleen, and heart valves. Because many systems can be affected at the same time, organ damage with subsequent system failure may occur.

Diagnostic Tests and Medical Management

Blood tests show anemia, elevated blood urea nitrogen, abnormal plasma proteins, and a positive LE (lupus erythematosus) cell reaction, which indicates nonspecific inflammation. Urinalysis may reveal proteinuria.

The goal of medical management is to prevent complications. Corticosteroids, such as prednisone, are prescribed to control inflammation. Antimalarial preparations, such as hydroxychloroquine and chloroquine, are used to treat symptoms associated with skin lesions and renal and arthritic problems. Although the exact action of these drugs on SLE is not known, they often permit continued remission with a lowered dose of steroids. Nonsteroidal anti-inflammatory drugs (aspirin) are used to relieve muscle and joint pains. Immunosuppressant drugs, such as cyclosporin and methotrexate, have been used to help control SLE. Diet may be restricted if the child has

■ NURSING ALERT

The side effects of steroids, immunosuppressant drugs, and antimalarial drugs are significant and include hair loss, susceptibility to infection, "moon face," retinal damage, and bone loss.

excessive weight gain or fluid retention from steroids and renal damage.

Prognosis depends on the severity of the disease. The 5-year survival rate now approaches 80% to 90% because of improved treatment measures.[1]

Nursing Assessment

A thorough assessment is needed as symptoms are widespread. Assess for rash, petechiae, cyanosis, skin ulcers, joint deformity, friction rub, edema, and splenomegaly. Assess family interactions, exploring stressful situations such as divorce or trauma.

Because SLE is a chronic disease that affects primarily adolescents, psychosocial assessment is indicated. Treatment-related restrictions and changes in appearance can lead to withdrawal, depression, and suicidal tendencies.

Nursing Diagnosis

Several nursing diagnoses may apply to the child with SLE. These include:

- High Risk for Ineffective Management of Therapeutic Regimen related to denial
- High Risk for Altered Renal Tissue Perfusion related to renal vasculitis
- High Risk for Impaired Skin Integrity related to rashes and photosensitivity
- High Risk for Activity Intolerance related to chronic disease
- High Risk for Body Image Disturbance related to side effects of medications
- Risk of Infection related to immunosuppressive medications

Nursing Management

The goal of nursing care is to assist the child to manage and cope with a chronic disease.

Maintain Fluid Balance. Since most children with SLE have renal involvement, it is important to monitor intake and output and frequently evaluate the child's fluid and electrolyte status. Renal dysfunction can manifest itself by edema, muscle cramps, diarrhea, tetany, and convulsions.

Promote Skin Integrity. Presence of the rash on mucous membranes can cause weakening of the tissues, placing the child at increased risk for infection. Encourage the use of good hygienic measures and a mild soap. Recommend that adolescents limit their use of cosmetics. Reinforce the importance of avoiding sunlight as much as possible and the use of sun protection factor (SPF) of 15 at all times when in the sun.

Promote Rest and Comfort. Because of fatigue and joint pain, the child has little energy reserve during acute episodes of the disease. Encourage frequent rest periods and a nutritious diet to maximize energy stores. A physical therapist can plan a program to encourage mobility and increase muscle strength.

Provide Emotional Support. Adolescents may have an altered body image as a result of rash, alopecia, arthritic changes in the joints, and chronic disease. Referral to a lupus support group, social services, or counseling may be helpful. The American Lupus Society and the Lupus Foundation of America can provide information to help parents and children adjust to the disease (see Appendix F). The Arthritis Foundation also publishes a useful pamphlet, *Meeting the Challenge: A Young Person's Guide to Living with Lupus.*

Juvenile Rheumatoid Arthritis

Juvenile rheumatoid arthritis (JRA) is an autoimmune inflammatory disease with no known cause. It occurs slightly more often in girls than in boys. JRA usually occurs in children between 2 and 5 or between 9 and 12 years of age, and it may disappear in adolescence.[1]

Clinical Manifestations

JRA may be restricted to a few joints or be systemic with involvement of multiple joints. Symptoms can include fever, rash, lymphadenopathy, splenomegaly, and hepatomegaly. The child may develop a limp or obviously favor one extremity over the other. Pain, stiffness, loss of motion and swelling occur in the large joints such as the knees. Older children may develop symmetrical involvement of the small joints of the hand.

Etiology and Pathophysiology

The cause of JRA is unknown, but it is thought to have an autoimmune basis. Inflammation begins in the joint and leads to pain and swelling. Scar tissue eventually develops, resulting in limited range of motion.

Diagnostic Tests and Medical Management

Diagnosis is made primarily on the basis of the history and assessment findings. There are no specific tests for the disease. In some children, rheumatoid factor and antinuclear antibody tests are positive.[1]

Medical management involves drug therapy, physical therapy, and, when necessary, surgery. The goals of treatment are to relieve pain and prevent contractures. Salicylates (aspirin) or nonsteroidal anti-inflammatory drugs (tolmetin sodium, naproxen, ibuprofen) are prescribed to reduce inflammation. Steroids may be used with children who have moderately active disease. Children who do not respond to aspirin or nonsteroidal anti-inflammatory drugs may be treated with intramuscular injections of gold salts.[9] Immunosuppressants, such as methotrexate or cyclophosphamide, may be given. Surgery may be performed to relieve pain and maintain or improve joint function in children with joint contractures.

Seventy percent of children with JRA experience a spontaneous and permanent remission of the disease by adulthood. Rarely, the disease is unresponsive to treatment. Children with early onset have a better prognosis.[1]

Nursing Assessment

A careful history is important, as it is sometimes the primary mode for diagnosis. Assess for joint swelling and deformities, fever, nodules under the skin, and enlarged lymph nodes.

Nursing Diagnosis

Several nursing diagnoses may apply to the child with JRA. They include:

- Activity Intolerance related to joint swelling and pain
- Impaired Physical Mobility related to joint inflammation
- Anxiety related to chronic illness and uncertain prognosis
- Pain related to joint inflammation

Nursing Management

Nursing care focuses on promoting mobility, encouraging adequate nutrition, and providing emotional support.

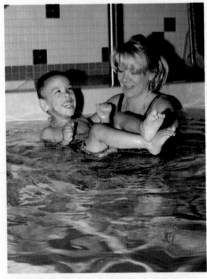

FIGURE 9–3 The physical therapist uses hydrotherapy to help maintain joint function in a child who has juvenile rheumatoid arthritis.

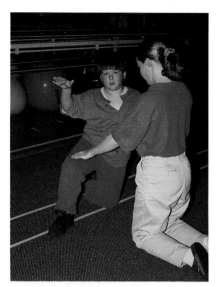

FIGURE 9–4 Stretching exercises are an important part of physical therapy for a child who has juvenile rheumatoid arthritis.

Allergic Reactions

Promote Improved Mobility. Physical therapists should be involved in the child's treatment. The goal of physical therapy is to maintain joint function, strengthen muscles, increase tone, maintain body alignment, and prevent permanent deformities such as contractures. Range of motion exercises, stretching, hydrotherapy, and swimming exercises help to prevent deformities (Figs. 9–3 and 9–4). Encourage the child to perform activities of daily living. Medications may be given to reduce joint swelling and inflammation. Warm compresses to the involved joints are soothing.

Encourage Adequate Nutrition. Promote general health by encouraging a well-balanced diet. Children with decreased mobility may have reduced metabolic needs, and excess weight causes additional muscle strain.

Discharge Planning and Patient and Family Home Care Teaching. Teach parents about the child's condition and prognosis, and answer their questions about the child's treatment. The child may need support to adjust to the diagnosis of a chronic illness. Encourage the child to maintain contact with peers and to attend school whenever possible. Explain to the child and parents that overexertion may lead to exacerbation of JRA. Inform parents about possible complications of the disease, such as altered growth related to early closure of epiphyseal plates, small joint contractures, and synovitis. Parents and children can be referred to the Arthritis Foundation and the American Juvenile Arthritis Foundation for further information and support (see Appendix F).

According to a 1985 National Institutes of Health (NIH) survey, 40 million Americans suffer from one or more allergic diseases.[9] Allergy is one of the major chronic illnesses of children today. Why are some children allergic to cats, for instance, while no one else in the family has allergies? In order to answer this question, the nurse needs to have a basic understanding of the mechanisms of allergy.

Allergy is an abnormal or altered reaction to an antigen. Antigens responsible for clinical manifestations of allergy are called **allergens.** Allergens can be ingested in food or drugs or injected or absorbed through contact with unbroken skin. An allergic reaction is an antigen-antibody reaction and can manifest itself as anaphylaxis, atopic disease, serum sickness, or contact der-

---

TABLE 9–3 Characteristic Findings in Children with Allergies

Respiratory System: Asthma, rhinitis (seasonal and perennial), serous otitis media, cough, pneumonia, croup, edema of glottis

Gastrointestinal System: Abdominal pain and colic, stomatitis, constipation, diarrhea, bloody stools, geographical tongue, vomiting

Skin: Angioedema, urticaria, eczema, atopic dermatitis, erythema multiforme, purpura, drug and food rashes, contact dermatitis

Nervous System: Headache, tension, fatigue, convulsions, Ménière syndrome, tremor

Eye: Conjunctivitis, cataract, ciliary spasm, iritis

Blood: Thrombocytopenia purpura, hemolytic anemia, leukopenia, agranulocytosis

Musculoskeletal System: Arthralgia, myalgia, rheumatoid arthritis, torticollis

Genitourinary System: Dysuria, vulvovaginitis, enuresis

Miscellaneous: Anaphylactic shock, serum sickness, autoimmune diseases

---

TABLE 9-4   Types of Hypersensitivity Reactions

Type	Mechanism of Action	Clinical Manifestations	Examples
Type I: Localized or systemic reactions (anaphylaxis)	Antibodies bind to certain cells, causing release of chemical substances that produce an inflammatory reaction	Hypotension, wheezing, gastrointestinal or uterine spasm, stridor, urticaria	Extrinsic asthma, hay fever
Type II: Tissue-specific reactions	Antibodies cause activation of complement system, which leads to tissue damage	Variable; may include dyspnea or fever	Transfusion reaction, ABO incompatibility, hemolytic disease of the newborn
Type III: Immune-complex reactions	Immune complexes are deposited in tissues where they activate complement, which results in a generalized inflammatory reaction	Urticaria, fever, and joint pain	Acute glomerulonephritis, serum sickness
Type IV: Delayed reactions	Antigens stimulate T cells that release lymphokines, which cause inflammation and tissue damage	Variable; may include fever, erythema, itching	Contact dermatitis, tuberculin skin test, graft-versus-host disease, allograft rejection

matitis. Characteristic findings in children with allergies are summarized in Table 9-3.

The **hypersensitivity response,** an overreaction of the immune system, is responsible for allergic reactions. Hypersensitivity reactions have been classified into four types (Table 9-4). Type I hypersensitivity reactions are immediate reactions that occur within seconds or minutes of exposure to the antigen. Symptoms can include a wheal and flare in the skin, edema, spasm of smooth muscle, wheezing, vomiting, diarrhea, or anaphylaxis. The release of chemical substances such as histamine is responsible for the signs and symptoms exhibited. The first time a child is exposed to the allergen, there is no reaction. With every exposure thereafter, however, the allergic child may have a reaction to the allergen.

Type IV reactions are delayed responses that do not appear until several hours after exposure and require 24 to 72 hours to develop fully. A type IV reaction, which is not confined to any specific tissue, is elicited by relatively complex antigens such as those of bacteria and viruses and by simple antigens such as drugs and metals. Symptoms include contact dermatitis, itching, and blistering.

Nursing Management

The child with allergies requires a thorough assessment, including a complete past medical history, family history, personal and social history, and review of symptoms. The history focuses on the following areas:

- What symptoms does the child experience? Encourage the child to describe the difficulty in his or her own words.
- Are the symptoms continuous or intermittent? What is the frequency and duration of episodes?
- When did the child first begin to experience symptoms? Did the child have eczema or a feeding problem in infancy or childhood? Did the infant have frequent bouts of colic or skin problems when new foods were introduced? Was there a change in symptoms at puberty? Are the symptoms becoming worse or spontaneously improving?

- What known agents in the environment cause difficulties?
- Are there seasonal variations in symptoms? At what time of the day or night do symptoms usually occur?

Assessment should also include a complete physical examination, laboratory studies, x-rays, pulmonary function studies, tests of nasal function, and skin testing.

Nursing care focuses on treating the symptoms, alleviating the anxiety of the child and parents, and identifying the allergens. Teaching the child and family how to minimize or avoid exposure to allergens is important. Parents of children who have had severe reactions to bee or wasp stings should be taught how to take precautions and how to provide emergency treatment if the child is stung.

Families may need instructions on allergy-proofing the home. Pets, dust, carpets, fabrics, feather pillows and bedding, and cigarette smoke can all cause allergic reactions. If families are reluctant to give up pets, frequent baths can reduce dander, which is the usual allergen.

Review any dietary restrictions for a child who has a food allergy with the child and family, and teach parents to read labels. Referral to a nutritionist is usually necessary.

■ SAFETY PRECAUTIONS

If the child has had a severe reaction in the past to a bee or wasp sting, ensure that the parents know how to handle an anaphylactic reaction if the child is stung again. Kits with syringes of premeasured adrenaline are available on a prescription basis. Instruct family members on how to use the kit.

REFERENCES

1 Stites, D.P., & Terr, A.T. (1991). *Basic & clinical immunology* (7th ed.). Norwalk, CT: Appleton & Lange.

2 Workman, L., Ellerhorst-Ryan, J., & Hargrave-Koertge, V. (1993). *Nursing care of the immunocompromised patient*. Philadelphia: W.B. Saunders.

3 Griffin, J. (1986). *Hematology & immunology: Concepts for nursing*. Norwalk, CT: Appleton & Lange.

4 Centers for Disease Control. (1987). Classification system for HIV infection in children under 13 years of age. *Morbidity & Mortality Weekly Report, 36*, 225–230.

5 Centers for Disease Control. (1992). Revised classification system for HIV infection and expanded surveillance case definition for AIDS among adolescents and adults. *Morbidity and Mortality Weekly Report, 41*, RR–17.

6 DeVita, V., Hellman, S., & Rosenberg, S. (1988). *AIDS: Etiology, diagnosis, treatment, and prevention*. Philadelphia: J.B. Lippincott.

7 Conderni, J.J. (1987). The autoimmune diseases. *JAMA, 258*, 2920–2929.

8 Long, B., Phipps, W., & Cassmeyer, V. (1992). *Medical surgical nursing: A nursing process approach* (3rd ed.). St. Louis: Mosby–Year Book.

9 Rudolph, A.M., Hoffman, J.I.E., & Rudolph, C.D. (1991). *Rudolph's pediatrics* (19th ed.). Norwalk, CT: Appleton & Lange.

SUGGESTED READINGS

Bellanti, J. (1985). *Immunology III*. Philadelphia: W.B. Saunders.

Buckley, R.H. (1987). Immunodeficiency diseases. *JAMA, 258*, 2841–2850.

Fritsch, D.F., & Fredrick Pilat, D.M. (1993). Exposing latex allergies. *Nursing, 23*(8), 46–48.

Griffin, J.P. (1986). Nursing care of the critically ill immunosuppressed patient. *Critical Care Nursing Quarterly, 9*(1), 25–34.

Ignatavicius, D. (1987). Meeting the psychosocial needs of patients with rheumatoid arthritis. *Orthopedic Nursing, 6*(3), 16–21.

Kluppel, J.H. (1990). SLE, treatment-related complications. *JAMA, 263*(13), 1811–1815.

Lyons, M. (1993). Immunosuppressive therapy after cardiac transplantation: Teaching pediatric patients and their families. *Critical Care Nurse, 13*(1), 39–45.

Parillo, J., & Masur, H. (1987). *The critically ill immunosuppressed patient*. Rockville, MD: Aspen Publications.

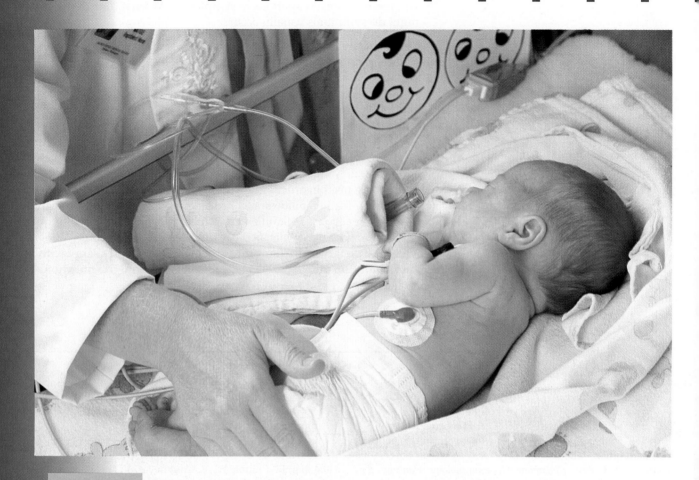

M ichael, 3 weeks old, is rushed to the local hospital when he suddenly stops breathing. Although Michael's mother had a healthy pregnancy, he was born prematurely at 35 weeks' gestation and weighed 5½ pounds when he left the hospital 2 days after birth. He has been eating well and gaining weight appropriately since going home.

Michael's mother had just finished giving him his morning bottle when he suddenly stopped breathing. Quickly she raised Michael's head and brought him to a sitting position. Michael then began to breathe again on his own. At the local emergency department, Michael's mother, visibly upset, tells staff that he had just dozed off to sleep when "he turned blue around his lips and seemed to go limp for a long time, maybe about 30 seconds!" Michael has experienced an episode of apnea of prematurity.

Although few children have such serious threats to health, all parents soon learn that infants and young children have numerous minor respiratory conditions. What accounts for the high incidence of respiratory conditions in infants and young children? What can you tell parents about their child's respiratory functioning that will help them promote healthy growth and development, prevent illness, and recognize danger signs of respiratory distress?

ALTERATIONS IN RESPIRATORY FUNCTION

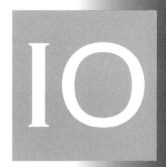

TERMINOLOGY

apnea Cessation of respiration lasting longer than 20 seconds.

airway resistance The effort or force needed to move oxygen through the trachea to the lungs.

alveolar hypoventilation The condition in which the volume of air entering the alveoli during gas exchange is inadequate to meet the body's metabolic needs.

dysphonia Muffled, hoarse, or absent voice sounds.

dyspnea Shortness of breath; difficulty in breathing.

hypercapnia Greater than normal amounts of carbon dioxide in the blood.

hypoxia Lower than normal amounts of oxygen in the blood.

laryngospasm Spasmodic vibrations of the larynx, which create sudden, violent, unpredictable, involuntary contraction of airway muscles.

periodic breathing Pauses in respiration lasting less than 20 seconds; a normal breathing pattern in infancy and childhood.

retractions A visible drawing in of the skin of the neck and chest, which occurs on inhalation in infants and young children in respiratory distress.

stridor An abnormal, high-pitched musical respiratory sound caused when air moves through a narrowed larynx or trachea.

tachypnea An abnormally rapid rate of respiration.

trigger A stimulus that initiates an asthmatic episode; a substance or condition, including exercise, infection, allergy, irritants, weather, or emotions.

❝ I can't tell you how terrified I was when my baby stopped breathing. I felt much better after the nursing staff explained what was going on, what to do if it happened again, and how to do it. **❞**

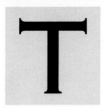

This chapter explores several special factors in the child's respiratory system that create ongoing threats to respiratory function and overall health. Most respiratory problems in children produce mild symptoms, last a short time, and can be managed at home. Nevertheless, acute respiratory problems are the most common cause of illness requiring hospitalization in infants and children under 15 years of age.[1]

Pediatric respiratory conditions may occur as a primary problem or as a complication of nonrespiratory conditions. Respiratory problems in children may be life threatening and may have long-term implications. For these reasons nurses must learn to assess the child's current respiratory status quickly, monitor progress, and anticipate potential complications (Table 10–1).

Respiratory problems may be a result of structural problems, functional problems, or a combination of both. Structural problems involve alterations in the size and shape of parts of the respiratory tract. Functional problems involve alterations in gas exchange and threats to this normal process from irritants (such as large particles and chemicals) or invaders (such as viruses or bacteria). Alterations in other organ systems, especially the immune and neurologic systems, may also threaten respiratory function. As you read the chapter, keep this distinction between structural and functional problems in mind to help you understand what is normal and what is abnormal about the child's maturing respiratory system.

TABLE 10–1 Assessment Guidelines for a Child in Respiratory Distress

Quality of Respirations
- Inspect the rate, depth, and ease of respirations.
- Identify signs of respiratory distress: tachypnea (abnormally rapid rate of respirations), retractions, nasal flaring, inspiratory stridor, expiratory grunting.
- Note lack of simultaneous chest and abdominal rise with inspiration (paradoxic breathing).
- Auscultate breath sounds: bilateral, diminished or absent, adventitious (wheezes, crackles, rhonchi).

Quality of Pulse
- Assess the rate and rhythm: tachycardia may indicate hypoxia.
- Compare pulse sites (apical to brachial) for strength and rate.

Color
- Observe overall color: with respiratory distress, color progresses from pallor to mottled to cyanosis; central cyanosis is a late sign of respiratory distress.
- Compare peripheral and central color: assess capillary refill and nailbed color and inspect mucous membranes; central cyanosis in mucous membranes is more ominous.
- Note whether crying improves or worsens color.

Cough
- Quality: note whether dry (nonproductive), wet (productive, mucousy), brassy (noisy, musical), croupy (barking, seal like).
- Effort: note whether forceful or weak; weak cough may indicate an airway obstruction or fatigue from prolonged respiratory effort (not valid in neonates).

Behavior Change
- Watch for abrupt behavior changes (restlessness, irritability) and lowered level of consciousness, which indicate increasing hypoxia.
- Note level of consciousness: alert or lethargic.
- Restlessness and irritability are associated with hypoxia.

Signs of Dehydration
- Inspect for dry mucous membranes, poor skin turgor, and decreased urine output, which indicate that fluid needs are not being met.

Anatomy and Physiology of Pediatric Differences

The child's respiratory tract constantly grows and changes until about 12 years of age. The young child's neck is shorter than an adult's, resulting in airway structures that are closer together.

Upper Airway Differences

The child's airway is shorter and narrower than an adult's. These differences create a greater potential for obstruction (Fig. 10–1 and Table 10–2). The infant's airway is approximately 4 mm in diameter, about the width of a drinking straw, in contrast to the adult's airway diameter of 20 mm. The upper airway primarily increases in length rather than diameter during the first 5 years of life.

The child's narrower airway causes an increase in **airway resistance,** the effort or force needed to move oxygen through the trachea to the lungs. As air moves from the child's nares down the trachea to the distal airways (alveoli), it must flow through a relatively small area. Friction and increasing resistance are generated as air passes through the airway. When edema and

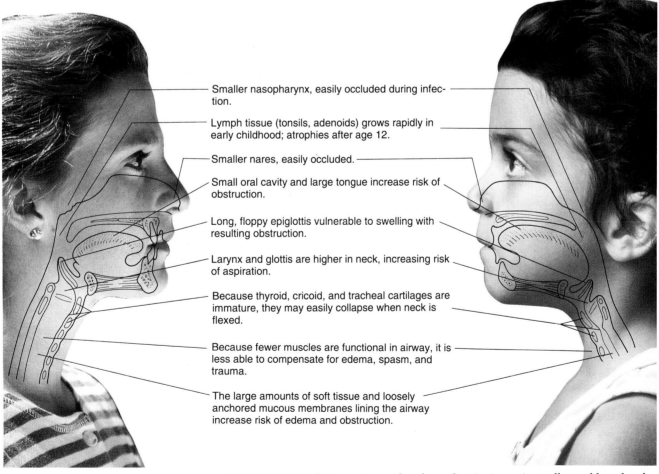

Smaller nasopharynx, easily occluded during infection.

Lymph tissue (tonsils, adenoids) grows rapidly in early childhood; atrophies after age 12.

Smaller nares, easily occluded.

Small oral cavity and large tongue increase risk of obstruction.

Long, floppy epiglottis vulnerable to swelling with resulting obstruction.

Larynx and glottis are higher in neck, increasing risk of aspiration.

Because thyroid, cricoid, and tracheal cartilages are immature, they may easily collapse when neck is flexed.

Because fewer muscles are functional in airway, it is less able to compensate for edema, spasm, and trauma.

The large amounts of soft tissue and loosely anchored mucous membranes lining the airway increase risk of edema and obstruction.

FIGURE 10–1 It is easy to see that the pediatric airway is smaller and less developed than the adult airway, but why is this important? Because things such as upper respiratory tract infections, allergic reactions, positioning of the head and neck during sleep, and the small objects children play with can have serious consequences in the child.

TABLE 10–2 Summary of Upper Airway Differences Between Children and Adults

Difference in Children	Significance
Small oral cavity and large tongue	Increases risk of obstruction; nasal patency is critical in infants
Rapid growth of lymph tissue (tonsils and adenoids) during early childhood, atrophy after age 12	Larger tissues in smaller pharyngeal structures; infection can easily cause obstruction of upper airway as lymph tissues swell in response
Larynx and glottis high in neck	Increases chance of aspiration
Thyroid, cricoid, and tracheal cartilages immature and incomplete	Easily collapse when neck is flexed, further narrowing airway; less protective of glottis
Large amount of soft tissue and loosely anchored mucous membranes lining length of airway	Increases likelihood of airway edema and obstruction
Long, floppy epiglottis	Vulnerable to swelling with resultant obstruction
Fewer functional muscles in the airways	Less able to compensate for edema, spasm and trauma; may swallow more mucus than able to sneeze or cough out

swelling occur in response to a virus, bacterium, or other irritant, the airway is further narrowed, increasing airway resistance even more. The trachea in a child is higher and at a different angle than the adult's (Fig. 10–2).

Physiologically the upper airway is the port for inspiration of oxygen and expiration of carbon dioxide. Older infants, children, and adults can breathe through either the nose or the mouth. Until about 6 months of age, infants are obligatory nose breathers. This is because coordination of mouth breathing is controlled by maturing neurologic pathways. Young infants do not automatically open the mouth to breathe when the nose is obstructed. The only time these infants breathe through the mouth is when they are crying. Nasal patency in young infants is therefore essential for such normal activities as breathing and eating.

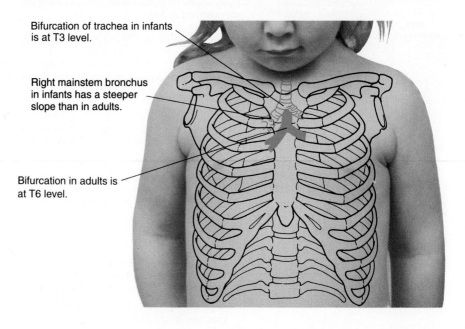

Bifurcation of trachea in infants is at T3 level.

Right mainstem bronchus in infants has a steeper slope than in adults.

Bifurcation in adults is at T6 level.

FIGURE 10–2 In children the trachea is shorter and the angle of the right bronchus at bifurcation is more acute than in the adult. When you are resuscitating or suctioning, you must allow for the differences. Do you think that this difference is significant in respiratory infection? Why?

Lower Airway Differences

The child's lower airway is also constantly growing. The developing alveoli change size and shape, and their numbers increase until respiratory maturity is attained at 12 years of age. This alveolar growth increases the area available for gas exchange. At birth the distal (peripheral) bronchioles that extend to the alveoli are narrow and fewer in number than in an adult. The child's overall growth can be correlated to the increased branching of the peripheral bronchioles as the alveoli continue to multiply. The taller the child, the greater the lung surface area.

The bronchi and bronchioles are lined with smooth muscle. The newborn does not have enough smooth muscle bundles to help trap airway invaders. By 5 months of age, however, sufficient muscles exist to react to irritants by bronchospasm and muscle contraction. Smooth muscle development is complete and comparable to that of an adult by 1 year of age.[2]

The lungs, which have no muscles of their own, rely on the diaphragm and intercostal muscles to power respiration. Children up to 6 years of age are primarily diaphragmatic breathers. The intercostal muscles are immature, and the ribs are primarily cartilage and very flexible. In cases of respiratory distress the extra effort of the diaphragm increases the negative pressure on the chest wall. **Retractions** occur as the flexible rib cage is pulled inward on inspiration. By 6 years of age the child begins to use the intercostal muscles more effectively for breathing.[2]

Urgent Respiratory Threats

From the moment a child is born, airway integrity is threatened because of immaturity of the respiratory muscles and neurologic system. Learn to recognize the early signs of respiratory compromise so that you will be able to intervene quickly to assist the infant in distress.

Apnea

Infants normally breathe with an irregular rhythm and may have pauses of up to 20 seconds between breaths. This **periodic breathing** should not be confused with apnea. **Apnea,** by definition, is cessation of respiration lasting longer than 20 seconds. Apnea may be the first major sign of respiratory dysfunction in the neonate.[1,3,4]

There are two types of apnea: apnea of prematurity (AOP) and an apparent life-threatening event (ALTE). AOP occurs in preterm infants, usually as a result of immaturity. This was the case with Michael, the infant who was described at the beginning of the chapter. ALTE (sometimes referred to as apnea of infancy) occurs in near-term or term infants. In the past, both AOP and ALTE were often called "near-miss sudden infant death" or "aborted crib death." These terms erroneously implied a close association between such episodes and sudden infant death syndrome (SIDS). SIDS should *not* be confused with apnea and is discussed separately later in this chapter.

Apnea of Prematurity

AOP may be caused by functional or structural problems. Functional problems involve neurologic and immunologic immaturity. Structural problems involve immature muscle development and coordination. Table 10–3 summarizes possible causes of AOP.

Apparent Life-Threatening Event

ALTE is defined as an episode of apnea accompanied by a color change (cyanosis, pallor, or occasionally ruddiness), limp muscle tone, choking, or gagging, occurring in a near-term or term infant who is greater than 37 weeks' gestation.[4,5] These episodes may occur during sleep, wakefulness, or feeding. A variety of identifiable diseases and conditions can cause ALTE (Table 10–3). In 50% of cases, however, no cause is ever identified.[4]

ALTE can frighten the parent or observer, who often fears the infant has died. Emergency resuscitation is usually required.

Nursing Management

After AOP or ALTE, infants are usually admitted to the hospital for 48 hours for evaluation and cardiorespiratory monitoring. Nursing care of infants with AOP and ALTE includes observing and monitoring cardiorespiratory

---

TABLE 10–3 Causes and Clinical Manifestations of Apnea of Prematurity and Apparent Life-Threatening Event

Cause	Clinical Manifestations	Diagnostic Tests
Functional or structural airway problem or immaturity	Apnea of 20 seconds or longer; bradycardia or cyanosis accompanying episode	Cardiorespiratory monitoring, sleep study, sepsis workup
Aspiration as a result of dysfunctional swallowing or gastroesophageal reflux	Choking, coughing, cyanosis, vomiting	Barium swallow, esophageal pH probe
Cardiac problems	Tachycardia, tachypnea, dyspnea (shortness of breath)	Cardiorespiratory monitoring, electrocardiogram, echocardiogram
Drug toxicity or poisoning	Central nervous system depression, hypotonia, maternal history or ingestion	Serum magnesium level, toxicity screen
Environmental	Lethargy, tachypnea, hypothermia or hyperthermia	Cardiorespiratory and temperature monitoring, environmental temperature level (ambient air temperature)
Impaired oxygenation, respiratory disease	Cyanosis, tachypnea, respiratory distress, anemia, choking, coughing	Oximetry, chest radiograph, arterial blood gases, complete blood count, upper airway evaluation, sleep study, serum electrolytes
Acute infection	Feeding intolerance, lethargy, temperature instability	Complete blood count, cultures when appropriate
Intracranial pathology	Abnormal neurologic examination, seizures	Cranial ultrasound, computed tomography scan, electroencephalogram, magnetic resonance imaging
Metabolic disorders	Jitteriness, poor feeding, lethargy, central nervous system depression or irritability	Serum electrolytes, glucose, calcium

Modified from Eichenwald, E., & Stark, A. (1992). Apnea of prematurity: Etiology and management. *Tufts University School of Medicine Reports on Neonatal Respiratory Diseases, 2*(1), 1-11.

status, providing supportive care to the infant and family, and anticipating the need for emergency resuscitation.

Monitor Cardiorespiratory Status. Cardiorespiratory monitoring records heart rate and respiratory rate while the infant is awake and asleep. Transcutaneous Po_2 (oxygen saturation or oximetry) monitoring provides continuous evaluation of the infant's oxygenation status.

Provide Emotional Support. Establishing rapport and open communication with the parents is essential for creating a sense of trust. To obtain further information about the episode, the nurse uses open-ended questions and active listening skills. The nurse should not give parents the impression that their parenting skills are being judged or questioned. Parents experience fear and anxiety about the infant's prognosis. Explanations of tests and treatment help to decrease their anxiety and increase their understanding of the situation.

During hospitalization the infant should be held and cuddled to provide a sense of security and well-being. Encouraging parents' participation in the infant's care helps to meet these needs and promotes family bonding. Often parents are afraid to touch the infant because they might disconnect the monitoring cable. Wrapping the cable inside the infant's blanket helps secure the wires, increasing parents' feelings of confidence in handling the infant.

Provide Tactile Stimulation. Tactile stimulation, such as rubbing the infant's back or feet, often is enough to halt an apneic episode. Continuous stimulation from an oscillating waterbed reduces the frequency of apneic episodes in some infants.[4] Both methods of stimulation remind the infant to take a breath.

Administer Medications. Methylxanthines (aminophylline, caffeine) or doxapram may be administered to stimulate the respiratory center in the brain. Infants have immature hepatic and renal systems, so the rate and efficiency of drug absorption and excretion are affected. Serum drug levels should be monitored frequently after drug therapy is begun because drug metabolism and distribution can be unpredictable.

Anticipate Emergency Resuscitation. Because the infant who has had AOP or ALTE continues to be at risk for cardiopulmonary arrest, emergency resuscitation equipment and drugs should be readily accessible at all times.

Discharge Planning and Patient/Family Home Care Teaching. Home care needs should be identified and addressed well in advance of discharge. The infant is sent home with an apnea monitor, and parents need to be taught how to operate the machine. Parents also need to learn what to do when the infant has an apneic episode (Table 10–4). They should be taught cardiopulmonary resuscitation (CPR) and choking prevention techniques (refer to the Atlas of Pediatric Procedures).

TABLE 10-4 Parent Teaching: Home Care Instructions for the Child Requiring Apnea Monitoring

Apnea Equipment
- Understand monitor type, lead wires, placement of skin electrodes or chest belt, battery power, manual for troubleshooting.

Emergency Preparation
- Notify telephone company, electric company, local rescue squad, local emergency department (establishes priority status).
- Post phone numbers of rescue squad, physician, equipment company, power company, emergency number, cardiopulmonary resuscitation (CPR) guidelines, other important numbers (neighbor, parents' work numbers) in at least two places in the home; have at least one added extension phone.

Safety Precautions
- Place monitor on firm surface; keep away from other appliances (television, microwave oven) and water.
- Ensure that alarms are audible from all locations.
- Double-check that monitor is *on* before going to bed.
- Thread cable and wires through lower end of child's clothes.
- Ensure integrity of leads, monitor cable, power cord (replace if frayed).

Routine Care
- Understand reasons for apnea monitor and frequency of use.
- Be able to attach and detach infant chest leads and belt.
- Evaluate skin for irritation or breakdown from electrode placement and give skin care (no oils or lotion; move patches correctly).

Emergency Care
- Develop plan for respiratory failure and power failure.
- Demonstrate CPR and Heimlich maneuver.
- Understand how to respond to alarms for apnea, bradycardia, or loose lead.

Apnea Alarm
- Observe infant's respiratory movement.
- If respiration is absent or infant is lethargic, stimulate by calling name and gentle touch, proceeding to vigorous touch if needed.
- If no response, proceed with CPR.

Bradycardia Alarm
- Stimulate infant; infant should respond quickly.

Loose Lead
- Check electrode patch. Is it loose? Dirty? Belt loose?
- Check wires from electrode or monitor cable.
- Check power supply. Is battery low? Power failure? Monitor malfunctioning?

Sudden Infant Death Syndrome

SIDS has been defined as the sudden death of an infant under 1 year of age that remains unexplained after a complete autopsy and review of the history. The deaths of one third to one half of infants who die between 1 month and 1 year of age are attributed to SIDS.[6] The peak incidence is between 2 and 3 months of age. SIDS occurs rarely in infants less than 2 weeks or older than 6 months of age.

SIDS is referred to as a "syndrome" because of the many and varied autopsy and clinical findings that characterize most infants who die of the disorder.[6,7] The autopsy typically does not identify a disease process that caused the death. Clinical findings include evidence of a struggle or change in position and the presence of frothy, blood-tinged secretions from the mouth and nares. SIDS occurs more often in the winter and between midnight and 9 AM.

TABLE 10-5 Risk Factors for Sudden Infant Death Syndrome

Infant

- Prematurity
- Low birth weight
- Twin or triplet birth
- Race (in decreasing order of frequency): most common in Native American infants, followed by black, Hispanic, white, and Asian infants
- Sex: more common in males than females
- Age: most common in infants between 2 and 3 months of age
- Time of year: more prevalent in winter months

Maternal and Familial

- Maternal age less than 20 years
- History of smoking and illicit drug use (increases incidence 10 times)
- Anemia
- Multiple pregnancies, with short intervals between births
- History of sibling with sudden infant death syndrome (increases incidence four to five times)
- Low socioeconomic status; crowding

Most deaths are unobserved and are thought to occur while the infant sleeps. Typically parents find the infant dead in the crib in the morning and report having heard no cries or disturbances during the night. A mild respiratory illness often precedes the death.

Although many reasons have been proposed for SIDS, including airway obstruction (as a result of anatomic, neuromuscular, and developmental factors), abnormal cardiorespiratory control, and hyperactive airway reflexes, the cause of the disorder remains unknown. Several infant, maternal, and familial factors appear to place infants at risk for SIDS (Table 10–5).

Nursing Management

The sudden, unexpected nature of the infant's death is confirmed in the emergency department. The nurse's role is to be empathetic and provide support during one of the greatest crises a family must face. The focus is on supporting the family during the acute grieving period (Table 10–6).

The nurse reassures the parents that they are not responsible for the infant's death and assists them in contacting other family members and mobilizing support. Older children may need reassurance that SIDS will not happen to them. They may also believe that bad thoughts or wishes about their baby brother or sister caused the death. Support groups can help parents, siblings, and other family members express these fears and work through their feelings about the infant's death. The SIDS Alliance (see Appendix F) is an organization that can help families to locate a support group in their geographic area.

Nurses can also play an important role in educating the public about the link between SIDS and infant positioning during sleep.

■ SAFETY PRECAUTIONS

Recent research shows a relationship between sudden infant death syndrome (SIDS) and sleeping on the abdomen. For this reason, the American Academy of Pediatrics now advises that infants be placed on their side or back for sleep.

Respiratory Failure

Respiratory failure occurs when the body can no longer maintain effective gas exchange because of functional or structural failure of the respiratory mechanism. Other body systems may also contribute directly or indirectly to increased workload and resultant failure of the respiratory system. The clinical manifestations of respiratory failure are signs of respiratory distress:

TABLE 10–6 Supportive Care for the Family of an Infant with Sudden Infant Death Syndrome (SIDS)

Nursing Interventions	Rationale
1. Provide parents with a private area and a support person who reinforces that the infant's death was not their fault.	1. Parents needs to be able to express their grief in their own way and know that they are not being blamed for the infant's death.
2. Prepare the family for the viewing of the infant. Describe how the infant will look and feel.	2. You can say "Paul's (use the infant's name) skin will feel cool. He will feel very still and his eyes are closed." They probably know this, but a gentle explanation demonstrates empathy. Advise that pooling of blood on the dependent areas will look like bruises.
3. Allow parents to hold, touch, and rock the infant if desired.	3. Viewing the infant allows parents a chance to say good-bye. Before bringing the infant to parents, wrap in a clean blanket, comb the hair, wash the face, swab the mouth clean, and apply Vaseline to lips.
4. Reinforce the physician's explanation about the need for an autopsy.	4. An autopsy is required for all unexplained deaths. You can say to parents, "It is the only way we can be absolutely sure of what caused your baby's death."
5. Answer parents' questions and provide them with sources for further information. Provide literature and a name of the local contact for a SIDS support group, as well as for the national foundation.	5. Parents may not be able to take in all of your answers. Many emergency departments and pediatric units have a social worker who provides ongoing contact with the family. Provide names of resource persons and phone numbers for SIDS support groups.
6. Advise parents that surviving siblings may benefit from psychologic support.	6. Siblings often require emotional support in the weeks and months after the death. Social workers can help the family obtain counseling and support for all members.
7. Provide parents with a lock of hair, footprints, and handprints.	7. Personal items can be placed in a memory book. This reaffirms the child's existence.

▨ LABORATORY VALUES: RESPIRATORY FAILURE

Arterial blood gas levels indicative of respiratory failure are PO_2 level less than 50 mm Hg and PCO_2 level greater than 50 mm Hg.

hypoxia (lower than normal blood oxygen level) and **hypercapnia** (an excess of carbon dioxide in the blood) (Table 10–7).

The physiologic process that ends in respiratory failure begins with **alveolar hypoventilation**. Alveolar hypoventilation occurs when one or any combination of these factors exist: (1) oxygen need exceeds actual oxygen intake, (2) the airway is partially occluded, or (3) transfer of oxygen and carbon dioxide in the alveoli is disrupted. This disruption may occur either because of a malfunction of respiratory center stimulation (the alveoli do not receive the message to diffuse) or because the alveolar membrane is defective (a structural problem).

Alveolar hypoventilation results in hypoxia and hypercapnia. When the blood levels of oxygen and carbon dioxide reach abnormal levels, respiratory failure begins. Signs of impending respiratory failure include irritability, lethargy, cyanosis, **dyspnea** (difficulty breathing), **tachypnea** (increased respiratory rate), nasal flaring, and intercostal retractions (Fig. 10–3). Any signs of respiratory failure should be reported immediately.[2,8,9]

TABLE 10-7 Clinical Manifestations of Respiratory Failure and Imminent Respiratory Arrest

Clinical Manifestations	Physiologic Cause
Respiratory failure	These signs occur because child is attempting to compensate for oxygen deficit and airway blockage
Initial Signs	Oxygen supply is inadequate; behavior and vital signs reflect compensation and beginning hypoxia
Restlessness	
Tachypnea	
Tachycardia	
Diaphoresis	
Early decompensation	Child attempts to use accessory muscles to assist oxygen intake; hypoxia persists and efforts now waste more oxygen than is obtained
Nasal flaring	
Retractions	
Grunting	
Wheezing	
Anxiety and irritability	
Headache	
Hypertension	
Confusion	
Imminent respiratory arrest	These signs occur because oxygen deficit is overwhelming and beyond spontaneous recovery
Severe hypoxia	Cerebral oxygenation is dramatically affected; central nervous system changes are ominous
Dyspnea	
Bradycardia	
Cyanosis	
Stupor and coma	

■ NURSING ALERT

The depth and location of retractions seen is associated with the severity of respiratory distress. Isolated intercostal retractions indicate mild distress. Subcostal, suprasternal, and supraclavicular retractions indicate moderate distress. These retractions accompanied by use of accessory muscles indicate severe distress.

Nursing Management

Early recognition of impending respiratory distress is the most important aspect of care for a child with any signs of respiratory compromise. The child who has even a slight degree of respiratory distress should immediately be placed in an upright position (by elevating the head of the bed). Next, respiratory quality and vital signs are assessed: respiratory rate, followed by apical pulse rate and then temperature. Oxygen administration equipment and

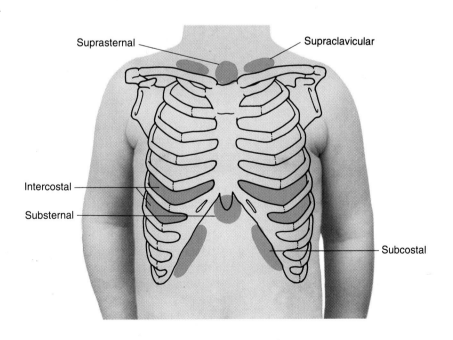

FIGURE 10-3 Retraction sites. Retractions may occur in the very young infant in the suprasternal area. In the older infant and child, retractions occur when the airway is severely obstructed, as in croup.

respiratory emergency equipment should be kept at the child's bedside. The nurse obtains an order for oxygen or ensures that oxygen is administered, monitors for changes in vital signs and level of consciousness, and is prepared to assist ventilations if respiratory status deteriorates.

Using Artificial Airways. Respiratory problems that do not respond to oxygen therapy, medications, or position change require the insertion of an artificial airway, such as an endotracheal tube or a tracheostomy tube. Endotracheal intubation is the placement of a tube in the trachea. This is considered an emergency or temporary measure to stabilize the airway. A tracheostomy is the creation of a surgical opening into the trachea through the anterior neck at the cricoid cartilage. Usually a skilled surgeon performs the procedure in the operating room. However, tracheostomy may also be performed in an emergency department or other setting when the situation dictates immediate intervention. (Refer to the Atlas of Pediatric Procedures for additional information on endotracheal and tracheostomy tubes.) These children usually require admission to the intensive care unit (ICU) for extensive and skilled monitoring.

Because endotracheal and tracheostomy tubes prevent vocal cord vibration, intubated children cannot cry or talk. Infants and young children often express initial frustration when they realize they cannot communicate verbally. They usually develop other noise-making behaviors, such as striking the mattress to gain attention. When time permits, the nurse should teach the parents and child what to expect before insertion of the endotracheal or tracheostomy tube.

A child may be discharged from the hospital and maintained at home for an extended period with a tracheostomy tube in place. Parent education about maintaining the airway, cleaning the tracheostomy site, and changing the tube is essential. Enrollment in a home care program may provide the best follow-up support for some families.

Reactive Airway Disorders

Reactive airway disorders occur when airway tissue reacts to invasion by a virus, bacterium, allergen, or irritant. These invaders cause airway tissue to respond with inflammation, edema, increased mucus production, and bronchospasm. Reactive airway disorders are reversible, usually self-limiting, and generally responsive to supportive therapies. They occur in either upper or lower airways and include croup syndromes, asthma, and bronchiolitis.

Croup Syndromes

Croup is a term applied to a broad classification of upper airway illnesses that result from swelling of the epiglottis and larynx. The swelling usually extends into the trachea and bronchi. Included under the classification of croup syndromes are viral syndromes, such as spasmodic laryngitis (spasmodic croup), laryngotracheitis, and laryngotracheobronchitis (LTB), and bacterial syndromes, such as bacterial tracheitis and epiglottitis (Fig. 10–4, Table 10–8).

LTB, epiglottitis, and bacterial tracheitis are referred to as the "big three" of pediatric respiratory illness because they affect the greatest number of children across all age groups in both sexes. The initial symptoms of all three conditions include inspiratory **stridor** (a high-pitched, musical sound that is created by narrowing of the airway), a "barking" cough, and hoarseness. LTB is the most common disorder, but epiglottitis and bacterial tracheitis are more serious.

FIGURE 10–4 There are two important changes in the upper airway in croup: the epiglottis swells, thereby occluding the airway, and the trachea swells against the cricoid cartilage, causing restriction.

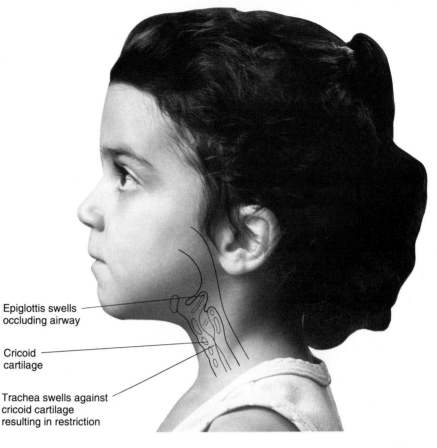

Epiglottis swells occluding airway

Cricoid cartilage

Trachea swells against cricoid cartilage resulting in restriction

TABLE 10–8 Summary of Croup Syndromes

	Viral Syndromes			Bacterial Syndromes	
	Acute Spasmodic Laryngitis (Spasmodic Croup)	**Laryngotracheitis**	**Laryngotracheobronchitis**	**Bacterial Tracheitis**	**Epiglottitis (Supraglottitis)**
Severity	Least serious	Most common*	Most serious; progresses if untreated	Guarded; requires close observation	Most life threatening (medical emergency)*
Age affected	3 months to 3 years	3 months to 8 years	3 months to 8 years	1 month to 6 years*	2 years to 8 years
Onset	Abrupt onset; peaks at night, resolves by morning (recurs)*	Gradual onset; starts as URI, progresses to moderate respiratory difficulty	Gradual onset; starts as URI, progresses to symptoms of respiratory distress	Progressive from URI (1–2 days)	Progresses rapidly (hours)*
Clinical manifestations	Afebrile; mild respiratory distress; barking-seal cough	*Early*: mild fever (<102.2° F); hoarseness; barking-seal, brassy, croupy cough; rhinorrhea; sore throat; stridor; apprehension (inspiratory) *Progressing to* labored respirations	*Early*: mild fever; (<102.2° F) barking-seal, brassy, croupy cough; rhinorrhea; sore throat; stridor (inspiratory); apprehension; restless/irritable *Progressing to* retractions (progressive); increasing stridor; cyanosis	High fever (>102.2° F); URI appears as viral croupy cough; croup initially; stridor (tracheal); purulent secretions	High fever (>102.2° F); URI; intense sore throat; dysphagia*; drooling*; increased pulse and respiratory rate; prefers upright position (tripod position with chin thrust)*
Etiology	Unknown; suspect viral with allergic/emotional influences	Parainfluenza, type 1 and other viruses	Parainfluenza, type 1 and other viruses	*Staphylococcus*	*Haemophilus influenzae*

*Classic parameter or key point (distinguishes condition).

Laryngitis and laryngotracheitis are mild illnesses that can be managed at home. Because LTB is the most serious type of viral croup, frequently necessitating hospitalization of infants and children under 6 years,[1] it is the focus of the following discussion.

Laryngotracheobronchitis

Although the term "croup" is applied to several viral and bacterial syndromes, it is most often used to refer to LTB, a viral invasion of the upper airway that extends throughout the larynx, trachea, and bronchi. Table 10–8 compares LTB and other croup syndromes.

Clinical Manifestations

A child who is brought to the hospital with LTB has usually been ill for several days with upper respiratory symptoms of increased respiratory rate, and a hoarse cough, especially at night. The cough has a seal-like, barking quality. The child has a runny nose, which appears red and irritated, a persistent low-grade fever (100.4° to 102.2°F), and a sore throat. Fluid status is usually altered because of an increased loss of fluid (fever) and decreased intake (sore throat). The child looks tired and ill and may say that he or she feels awful.

Etiology and Pathophysiology

Acute viral LTB is most common in children 3 months to 4 years of age but can occur up to 8 years of age. Boys are affected more often than girls. LTB is of greatest concern in infants and children under the age of 6 years, because of potential airway obstruction. The causative organism is usually one of the group of parainfluenzaviruses that appear during winter months in clustered outbreaks.[2,8]

Airway tissues respond to the invading virus by producing copious, tenacious secretions and swelling, which increase the child's respiratory distress. The laryngeal edema narrows the airway diameter in the subglottic area, the narrowest part of the airway. Even small amounts of mucus or edema can quickly obstruct the airway (Fig. 10–4). These secretions may cause further complications by allowing infection to take hold in other respiratory structures. The result may be pneumonia, bronchiolitis, or otitis media.

Diagnostic Tests and Medical Management

Some hospitals advocate anteroposterior (AP) and lateral x-ray studies of the neck to identify the area of airway narrowing.[2] The inner mouth and throat areas should *not* be probed. Selected blood studies (serum electrolytes and glucose) may be deemed appropriate once the potential for airway obstruction has decreased or been eliminated. White blood cell and differential counts may be used to distinguish between viral and bacterial illnesses.

Medical management consists of maintaining and improving respiratory effort by administering supplemental oxygen and creating a high-humidity environment. Cool humidified air with added oxygen helps to moisturize the irritated airway tissue and decrease mucosal swelling. The use of medications to treat LTB is controversial. The benefit of their use must be weighed against potential complications (Table 10–9).

Airway obstruction is a potential complication of LTB. The child may require intubation and transfer to the ICU to maintain airway patency if obstruction occurs. Most children, however, respond positively to the high humidity and oxygen therapy and are discharged within 48 to 72 hours.

■ NURSING ALERT

Throat cultures and visual inspection of the inner mouth and throat are *contraindicated* in children with LTB and epiglottitis. These procedures can cause laryngospasms (spasmodic vibrations that close the larynx) to occur as a result of the child's anxiety or of probing this reactive and already compromised area.

TABLE 10-9 Medications Used for Symptomatic Treatment of Laryngotracheobronchitis

Medication	Action/Indication	Nursing Considerations
Beta-agonists and beta-adrenergics (e.g., albuterol, racemic epinephrine): aerosolized through face mask	Rapid-acting bronchodilator, used to decrease symptoms of respiratory distress	Provides only temporary relief; child may develop tolerance quickly, increasing frequency with which drug is required; *child may experience tachycardia* (160–200 bpm) and hypertension; dizziness, headache, and nausea may necessitate stopping medication; watch for rebound edema up to 2 hours after discontinuing medication
Corticosteroids (e.g., methylprednisolone): systemic through IV route	Antiinflammatory, used to decrease edema	Child may experience cardiovascular symptoms (hypertension): requires close observation for individual response; relief of croup symptoms is questionable; may worsen infection by decreasing immune response
Sedatives (e.g., chloral hydrate)	Rapidly metabolized sedative with few side effects, used to promote rest and sleep	Very selective use; requires close observation of individual response

■ NURSING ALERT

Continually observe for inability to swallow, absence of voice sounds, increasing degree of respiratory distress, and acute onset of drooling (an ominous sign of supraglottic obstruction). If *any* of these signs occur, get medical assistance *immediately. The quieter the child, the greater the cause for concern.*

Nursing Assessment

PHYSIOLOGIC ASSESSMENT. The initial and ongoing physical assessment of the child focuses on adequacy of respiratory functioning. Close monitoring is required to identify changes in airway patency. The child should be observed every 20 minutes for the first hour (Tables 10–10 and 10–11) and then every 2 to 4 hours or more frequently for the first 24 hours as the child's condition warrants.

Particular attention should be paid to the child's respiratory effort and breath sounds. Physical exhaustion can diminish the intensity of retractions and stridor. As the child uses the remaining energy reserve to maintain ventilation, breath sounds may actually diminish. Noisy breathing (audible airway congestion, coarse breath sounds) in this situation verifies adequate energy stores.

TABLE 10-10 Nursing Assessment of Child with a Reactive Airway Disorder

Nursing Action	Rationale
Assess heart rate and respiratory rate	Tachypnea and tachycardia indicate increasing respiratory effort
Check position of child (sitting? prone? supine?)	Upright or semi-Fowler's promotes airway patency; child's change to one of these positions may signal increased distress
Assess overall quality of respiratory effort:	
Determine inspiratory and expiratory breath sounds, ability to speak, and presence of stridor, cough, retractions, nasal flaring, cyanosis	Reflects overall adequacy of airway and respiratory function
Initiate croup score (Table 10–11) and continue scoring every 2–4 hours or more frequently if distress increases; initiate nursing actions appropriate for croup score	Provides consistent and objective assessment data with quantitative score for future comparison
Attach cardiorespiratory monitor and pulse oximeter	Provides continuous assessment data as part of ongoing physiologic monitoring

TABLE 10-11 Croup Scale to Identify the Severity of Croup

Signs	Severity Score			
	0	1	2	3
Stridor	None	Mild	Moderate at rest	Severe, on inspiration + expiration
Retractions	None	Mild	Suprasternal, intercostal	Severe, may see sternal retractions
Color	Normal	Normal score = 0	Normal score = 0	Dusky or cyanotic
Breath sounds	Normal	Mildly decreased	Moderately decreased	Markedly decreased
Level of consciousness	Normal	Restless when disturbed	Anxious, agitated	Lethargic

Scoring: To quantify the severity of croup, add up the individual scores for each of the sign categories. A score between 0 to 15 is possible. The rating of mild, moderate, and severe is as follows: 4–5 is mild, 6–8 is moderate, > 8 or any sign in the severe category is severe.
Modified from Davis, H.W., et al (1981). *Pediatric Clinics of North America, 28*:4.

PSYCHOSOCIAL ASSESSMENT. The hospital environment and technical procedures create stress and anxiety for the child and parents. Observation of their initial behaviors helps direct nursing interventions during admission and throughout hospitalization (Table 10–12). Chapter 4 presents techniques for reducing the stress that is associated with hospitalization in children.

Nursing Diagnosis

The accompanying Nursing Care Plan lists common nursing diagnoses for the child with acute LTB. The following diagnoses might also be appropriate:

- Ineffective Breathing Pattern related to tracheobronchial obstruction, decreased energy, and fatigue
- Impaired Gas Exchange related to altered oxygen supply (narrowed air inlet)
- Altered Nutrition: Less than Body Requirements related to expenditure of glycogen stores and to inadequate food and fluid intake prior to admission

TABLE 10-12 Psychosocial Assessment for the Child with an Acute Respiratory Illness

Child

- Assess for indications of anxiety or fear that may have an impact on respiratory status.
- For young children, inquire about security objects (such as a blanket or doll), the child's reaction to strangers, and reaction to absence of parents.
- For older children, ask whether this is the first hospital stay and what previous illness and hospital experiences have meant to the child.

Parents

- Assess parents' reactions: Are they anxious? Fearful? Verbal or quiet? Asking appropriate questions?
- Observe for nonverbal cues. Often parents have financial worries (cost of hospital stay, lost work and wages) and personal worries (siblings at home who are ill) that they may not readily share with staff.

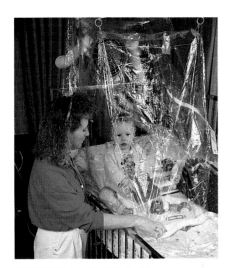

FIGURE 10–5 Washable, water-resistant toys provide the best mist tent "companions." Provide the child with favorite items and toys from home.

Nursing Management

Skillful nursing care can greatly assist children with LTB and their families to cope with the symptoms of the illness and effects of hospitalization. Nursing care focuses on maintaining airway patency, promoting fluid balance and nutrition, encouraging rest, reducing stress, and educating the child and family for discharge. The accompanying Nursing Care Plan summarizes nursing care for the child with LTB.

MAINTAIN AIRWAY PATENCY. A high-humidity mist tent provides a cool, moist, oxygen-rich environment. Children are often fearful and anxious because of the noise, confinement, and moisture inside the tent. Parents can be invaluable in keeping the child calm, quiet, and in the tent (Fig. 10–5). Tucking the loose tent edges under the mattress prevents oxygen loss and increases moisture within the tent. The mist tent should not, however, create such excess condensation that water droplets run down the tent sides.

An important developmental consideration is the child's ability to communicate reliably. The nurse must be immediately available to attend to the child's respiratory needs. The child should be roomed near the nurses' station and emergency resuscitation equipment kept at the bedside.

MEET FLUID AND NUTRITIONAL NEEDS. The illness preceding hospitalization may have compromised the child's fluid status. Recognizing fluid deficit and monitoring the child's hydration and nutritional status are essential. Fluids promote liquification of secretions and provide calories for energy and metabolism. Parents can be encouraged to participate in feeding to gain the child's cooperation in taking oral fluids. Parents can also identify food preferences, which can be incorporated into the daily diet. An intravenous infusion may be necessary to rehydrate the child, maintain fluid balance and provide emergency access if needed. The child should be observed closely for difficulty in swallowing, which may be an early sign of epiglottitis or bacterial tracheitis.

PROMOTE REST AND COMFORT. Care should be scheduled to give the child uninterrupted periods of rest. Drawing bed curtains, closing the room door, and posting a "SHHH! I'm sleeping" sign on the door also promote uninterrupted sleep.

The mist tent makes the child's hair, bedding, and pajamas very moist. Thus an important part of care is keeping the child dry and in a comfortable position.

DISCHARGE PLANNING AND PATIENT/FAMILY HOME CARE TEACHING. During the child's hospitalization nurses should take every opportunity to advise the family about what to expect as the child's respiratory system returns to normal. The nurse should assess the parents' knowledge of symptoms of LTB and discuss actions to take if symptoms recur (Table 10–13). If the parents require home care assistance, the nurse makes follow-up arrangements and initiates a referral for home care before the child's discharge.

Epiglottitis (Supraglottitis)

Epiglottitis (also known as supraglottitis) is an inflammation of the epiglottis, the long narrow structure that closes off the glottis during swallowing (Fig. 10–4). Because edema in this area can rapidly (within minutes or hours) obstruct the airway by occluding the trachea, epiglottitis is considered a potentially life-threatening condition. (Table 10–8 compares epiglottitis and other croup syndromes.)

Characteristically, a previously healthy child *suddenly* becomes very ill. The child initially develops a high fever (greater than 102.2° F) , with a sore throat, **dysphonia** (muffled, hoarse, or absent voice sounds), and dysphagia

FIGURE 10–6 The phrase "thumb sign" has been used to describe this enlargement of the epiglottis. Recall the trachea's usual "little finger" size. Do you see the stiff, enlarged "thumb" above it in this lateral neck x-ray?

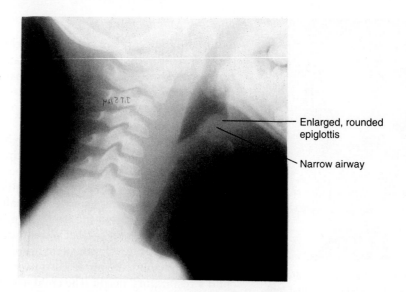

Enlarged, rounded epiglottis

Narrow airway

(difficulty in swallowing). As the larynx becomes obstructed, inspiratory stridor develops. The child resists normal swallowing of saliva because of intense throat pain and swelling, resulting in drooling. To fully open the airway and improve air intake, the child sits up and leans forward with the jaw thrust forward in the classic "sniffing" or tripod posture and refuses to lie down.

Epiglottitis is most often caused by bacterial invasion of the soft tissue of the larynx by *Haemophilus influenzae*, type B (HIB). The resulting inflammation and edema enlarge and stiffen the epiglottis. Fortunately, since use of the HIB vaccine has become widespread, the number of cases of epiglottitis has decreased significantly.

Diagnosis is based on a lateral neck x-ray (Fig. 10–6), which reveals an enlarged, rounded epiglottis, seen as a mass at the base of the tongue. A narrowed airway is also visible. **Laryngospasm** can occur as a result of the severe irritation and hypersensitivity of the airway muscles. For this reason, visual inspection of the mouth and throat is contraindicated in children with suspected epiglottitis unless carried out by a physican in an environment where immediate intubation can be performed.[8] Obstruction is almost certain if stress or physical manipulation further irritates the fragile airway.

Immediate medical therapy consists of interventions to maintain an open airway, usually by insertion of an endotracheal tube. Chloramphenicol and ampicillin are the antibiotics of choice and can be individually effective against HIB. They may be combined or given separately for a 7- to 10-day period.[8] Antipyretics (acetaminophen, ibuprofen) may be useful in managing fever and sore throat pain.

Nursing Management

Nursing management consists of airway management, drug therapy, hydration, and emotional and psychosocial support of the child and parents. Until the endotracheal tube is removed, the child is usually managed in the intensive care unit to ensure continual observation.

MAINTAIN AIRWAY PATENCY. Cool mist and supplemental oxygen promote better airway function. The child may be placed in a high-humidity tent to provide oxygen and cool moisture. The child should be observed closely and often. A quiet environment with as little stress as possible is essential. A quiet, undisturbed child will be less anxious and less inclined to cry. Crying

TABLE 10-13 Parent Teaching: Home Care Instructions for the Child with Laryngotracheobronchitis

When Symptoms Begin (or If They Recur):

- Provide a high-humidity (warm steam) environment to ease breathing by running hot water in both the sink and shower and closing the door. Hold the child and protect from hot water or splashing burns.
- Observe the child's response to warm steam for 10 minutes:
  - If breathing does not improve or distress increases, call 911 for assistance or take the child to the nearest emergency room.
  - If breathing improves, take the child to the phone with you while you call the physician for further instructions. While on the phone, use a cool mist vaporizer near the child or open a window to let in cool air. (Cool air can relieve symptoms during the breathing distress.)
- Ensure that the child is in an upright or seated position to ease breathing. Use distractions (television, music, or a story) to relax the child. Stay calm.
- Maintain high humidity in the bathroom. The child may require a return to the warm steam environment if breathing distress returns during the first hour of steam and cool air treatment (see section on contact physician or hospital [below] for further information).

Posthospital/Postsymptom Care (Once Child Is Breathing More Easily and Returns Home):

- Medication is usually not necessary (laryngotracheobronchitis is the most commonly viral and runs its own course). The child's physician will provide drugs for special needs only.
- Encourage the child to rest and run a cool mist vaporizer at the child's bedside for a few nights and at naptimes. Be sure that unit and cord are out of child's reach. Change water in the humidifier daily to prevent organism growth.
- Fluids are most important for energy and hydration (child may have little or no interest in food for a few days). Provide frequent, small amounts of water, noncitrus juice, or noncaffeinated tea or cola. Milk is not recommended because it is digested slowly and may create nausea and vomiting. Cool, flat soda pop causes less throat soreness and can be "de-fizzed" by adding a few granules of sugar and stirring to eliminate bubbles.

Contact Your Physician or the Nearest Hospital If:

- The child cannot swallow saliva or water, is drooling uncontrollably, and breathing is labored. *This is an emergency!* Call 911 or meet your physician at the nearest emergency room.
- The child's breathing is rapid while resting, breathing looks difficult, and the skin of the neck and chest draws in with each inhalation (retractions).
- Mild symptoms do *not* improve within 1 hour of humidity and cool air treatment.

stimulates the airway, increases oxygen consumption, and can precipitate laryngospasm; the calmer the child, the better the respiratory function.[8] A supine position is contraindicated because it can compromise the function of the diaphragm and make the child feel as if he or she is choking.

ADMINISTER MEDICATIONS AND FLUIDS. Antibiotics are administered to treat the infection and fluids to provide hydration. Because the child was febrile with a sore throat before admission, fluid intake may have been compromised. The nurse should be alert for signs of dehydration. Careful monitoring of intake and output and specific gravity provides valuable data about hydration status.

PROVIDE EMOTIONAL SUPPORT. The loss of voice, or even the inability to create sounds, can be frightening to a child. The unfamiliar hospital environment and strange equipment can create stress for child and parent alike. The nurse reassures the parents that the child's voice loss is temporary and explains the need for the various pieces of equipment. Twenty-four-hour visitation for parents or immediate family members is advisable. This provides

■ **NURSING ALERT**

A communication method is needed if the child will be left alone for even a brief period. Because infants and preverbal toddlers cannot alert the nurse if they have respiratory distress, they must not be left alone during the acute phase of the illness.

reassurance for the child and allows parents to take turns so that each can have a break.

DISCHARGE PLANNING AND PATIENT/FAMILY HOME CARE TEACHING. Most children show rapid improvement once cool mist and oxygen, antibiotics, and fluid therapy are started. Usually recovery occurs quickly and the endotracheal tube can be removed within 24 to 36 hours.[9] Home care may involve completing the course of antibiotics. Parents need instructions on proper administration and potential problems of drug therapy.

NURSING
CARE PLAN

THE CHILD WITH LARYNGOTRACHEOBRONCHITIS

GOAL	INTERVENTION	RATIONALE	EXPECTED OUTCOME
1. Ineffective Airway Clearance related to laryngeal edema, mucosal inflammation, and decreased energy (fatigue)			
Child will return to respiratory baseline. Child will not experience respiratory distress.	Assess respiratory status (Table 10–1) a minimum of every 2–4 hours or more often, as indicated. Cardiorespiratory monitor attached with alarms set, if ordered. Record and report changes promptly to physician.	Assessment and monitoring reveal rate and quality of air exchange. Frequent assessment and monitoring provides objective evidence of changes in the quality of respiratory effort, enabling prompt and effective intervention.	Child returns to respiratory baseline within 24–48 hours.
2. Altered Tissue Perfusion (cardiopulmonary) related to partially obstructed airway			
Child's oxygenation status will return to baseline.	Administer high humidity, cool mist, and oxygen via tent.	Cool, moist air with added oxygen acts locally to decrease swollen laryngeal tissue and provide needed extra oxygen and moisture.	Child's respiratory effort eases as evidenced by lack of stridor with breathing. Pulse oximetry reading remains >94% oxygen saturation during treatment.
	Note child's response to tent and ordered medications (nebulizer treatments, IV medications).	Medications act systemically and locally (on respiratory tissue) to open airways. However, side effects may necessitate their discontinuation.	Child tolerates therapeutic measures with no adverse effects.
	Position head of bed up or place child in postition of comfort on parent's lap, if crying or struggling in tent.	Position facilitates improved aeration and promotes decrease in anxiety (especially in toddlers) and energy expenditure.	Child rests quietly in position of comfort.
	Keep emergency oxygen, suction, and tracheostomy/intubation tray at bedside.	Laryngeal edema can lead to unpredictable and rapid airway obstruction.	Child has no further airway obstruction requiring emergency intervention.

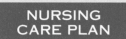

GOAL	INTERVENTION	RATIONALE	EXPECTED OUTCOME
3. High Risk for Fluid Volume Deficit related to inability to meet body requirements and increased metabolic demand			
Child will be adequately hydrated, be able to tolerate oral fluids, and progress to normal diet.	Maintain strict intake and output monitoring and evaluate specific gravity at least every 8 hours.	Monitoring provides objective evidence of fluid loss and ongoing hydration status.	Child takes adequate oral fluids after 24–48 hours to maintain hydration.
	Perform daily weight measurement on the same scale at the same time of day. Evaluate skin turgor.	Further evidence of improvement of hydration status.	Child's weight stabilizes after 24–48 hours; skin turgor is supple.
	Offer clear fluids and incorporate parent in care. Offer fluid choice.	Choice of fluid offered by parent gains child's cooperation.	Child accepts beverage of choice from parent or nursing staff.
Child's immediate fluid deficit is corrected.	Evaluate need for intravenous fluids. Maintain IV, if ordered.	Previous fluid loss may require immediate replacement.	Child's hydration status is maintained during acute phase of illness.
	Observe swallowing ability, mucous membranes, and presence of tears. Report changes promptly to physician.	Absence of swallowing is an early sign of epiglottitis or bacterial tracheitis. Moist mucous membranes and tears provide observable evidence of hydration.	Child evidences adequate swallowing and improved hydration.
4. Fear/Anxiety (Child and Parent) related to acute illness, hospitalization, and uncertain course of illness and treatment			
Child and parents will evidence behaviors that indicate decrease in anxiety.	Encourage parents to express fears and ask questions; provide direct answers and discuss care, procedures, and condition changes.	Provides opportunity to vent feelings and receive timely, relevant information. Helps reduce parents' anxiety and increase trust in nursing staff.	Parents and child show decreasing anxiety and decreasing fear as symptoms improve and as child and parents feel more secure in hospital environment. *Parent* freely asks questions and participates in child's care. *Child* cries less and allows staff to hold and/or touch him or her.
	Incorporate parents in child's care. Encourage parents to bring familiar objects from home (Fig. 10–5). Ask about and incorporate in care plan the home routines for feeding and sleeping.	Familiar people, routines, and objects decrease child's anxiety and increase parents' sense of control over unexpected, uncertain situation.	
5. Knowledge Deficit (Child or Parent) related to diagnosis, treatment, prognosis, and home care needs			
Parent will verbalize knowledge of croup symptoms and use of home care methods before the child's discharge from hospital.	Explain symptoms, treatment, and home care of croup (see Table 10–13).	Anticipate potential for recurrence. Assist family to be prepared should croup symptoms recur after discharge.	Parent accurately describes croup symptoms and says that a mist vaporizer is available in child's room at home.
	Provide written instructions for follow-up care arrangements, as needed.	Written, as well as oral, instructions reinforce knowledge. Parents may not "hear" and remember the particulars of home care if presented only orally.	Parents take instructions home when child is discharged.

Bacterial Tracheitis

Bacterial tracheitis is an infection of the upper trachea that is most often caused by *Staphylococcus aureus*. The disorder starts with croupy cough and stridor but progresses to include a high fever (greater than 102.2° F), which persists for several days.[10] (Table 10–8 compares bacterial tracheitis and other croup syndromes.)

Because of the similarity of symptoms, bacterial tracheitis is often misdiagnosed initially as LTB. Instead of improving with therapy, however, the child's condition becomes worse. Children generally prefer lying flat to sitting up. This seems to be a position of comfort that allows the child to conserve energy. Diagnosis is often made by blood cultures identifying the causative organism or by complete blood count values suggesting bacterial rather than viral illness.

Nursing Management

Nursing management involves the following:

- Administration of humidified oxygen
- Administration of antibiotics
- Careful airway assessment and support
- Airway maintenance (artificial airway assistance is often required because of the thick tracheal secretions that pool high in the upper airway)
- Suctioning as needed (mechanical suction enables easier removal of secretions and helps maintain a patent airway)

The section on epiglottitis discusses other nursing care interventions.

Asthma

Asthma (also called bronchial asthma) is a reactive airway disease that has been described in medical writings since ancient times. This common chronic illness occurs in infants, children, and adolescents and accounts for a large percentage of school absenteeism.[11] Most children with asthma experience their first symptoms before the age of 5 years.[8] Asthma occurs more frequently in boys than girls until the teen years, when the incidence equalizes.[10]

Asthma is a chronic condition with acute exacerbations. Children require continuous coordinated care to control sudden symptoms and minimize long-term airway changes. Although unusual in the past, untreatable asthma is more common now. Mortality from asthma in children rose 31% between 1980 and 1987.[11] How does this chronic condition pose a threat to children?

Clinical Manifestations

Asthma is characterized by airway obstruction or narrowing, airway inflammation, and airway hyperresponsiveness. The sudden appearance of breathing difficulty is often referred to as an asthma "attack" or "episode."

During an acute attack, respirations are rapid and labored and the child often appears tired because of the ongoing exertion of breathing. Nasal flaring and intercostal retractions may be visible. The child exhibits a productive cough and expiratory wheezing, use of accessory muscles, decreased air movement, and respiratory fatigue. The resulting hypoxia, as well as the cumulative effect of previously administered medications, contributes to behaviors ranging from wide-eyed agitation to lethargic irritability.

In children who have repeated acute exacerbations, a barrel chest and the use of accessory muscles of respiration are common findings. The child with chronic asthma is often small according to standard growth charts but usually catches up in adolescence.

Etiology and Pathophysiology

The respiratory difficulties that occur during an asthma attack are created because, for unknown reasons, the normal protective mechanisms of the lungs (mucus formation, mucosal swelling, and airway muscle contraction) react excessively in response to a stimulus.

The stimulus, more correctly termed a **trigger,** that initiates an asthmatic episode can be a substance or condition. Asthmatic triggers include exercise, infection, allergy (to mold, dust, or pollen), food additives, irritants, weather, and emotions. The role of emotions as a trigger is often misunderstood and misinterpreted. A common myth is that children with asthma have psychologic problems that precipitate acute attacks. Although some psychologic problems may be present, they do not account for the acute attack. The reactive airway responses to stimuli are present *before* the trigger initiates the physiologic sequence that results in an asthma attack.

Airway narrowing results from airway swelling and production of copious amounts of mucus. Mucus clogs small airways, trapping air below the plugs (Fig. 10–7). The airways swell, creating muscle spasms that often become uncontrolled in the large airways. With time, repeated episodes of bronchospasm, mucosal edema, and mucus plugging can damage the respiratory cells that line the airway. This process leaves the airway chronically irritated and scarred and results in air trapping, called hyperinflation.

The psychologic sequence of events during an asthmatic episode starts with moderate anxiety as the episode begins. The anxiety becomes severe as the episode intensifies. Severe anxiety, in turn, intensifies physical responses and symptoms, and a vicious cycle is established. Recognizing and address-

FIGURE 10–7 What can cause an asthma attack? Some asthma triggers are exercise, infection, and allergies. Shown is how asthma obstructs airflow through constriction and narrowing of the airway.

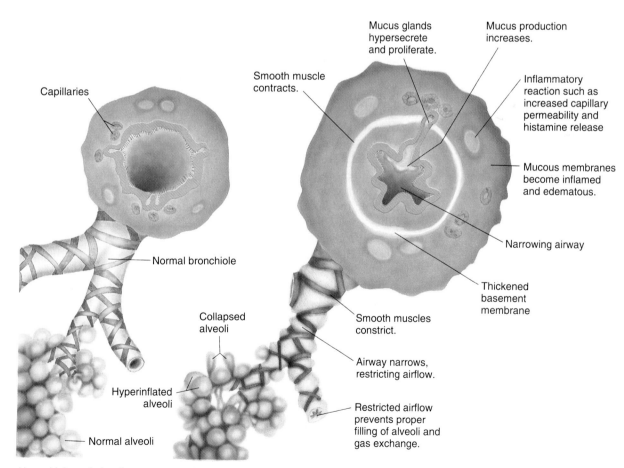

Mucus glands hypersecrete and proliferate.

Mucus production increases.

Smooth muscle contracts.

Inflammatory reaction such as increased capillary permeability and histamine release

Capillaries

Mucous membranes become inflamed and edematous.

Narrowing airway

Normal bronchiole

Thickened basement membrane

Collapsed alveoli

Smooth muscles constrict.

Airway narrows, restricting airflow.

Hyperinflated alveoli

Restricted airflow prevents proper filling of alveoli and gas exchange.

Normal alveoli

Normal bronchiole and alveoli

ing the child's fear and panic are essential for reestablishing normal respirations.

Diagnostic Tests and Medical Management

The diagnosis of asthma is confirmed through pulmonary function studies. A spirometer is used to measure the volume of air the lungs can move in and out. Because the test requires children to cooperate and follow instructions, it is usually administered to children over 5 years of age.[8] Findings determine the extent of airway restriction and assist in selecting the appropriate treatment. Skin testing may be used to identify allergens (asthma triggers).

Medical management includes medications, support of parents and child, and education. Pharmacologic treatment attempts to promote optimal respiratory function (Table 10–14). In children as young as 3 years, the use of a peak expiratory flow rate (PEFR) meter can assist in the management of asthma by helping to identify when obstruction occurs.[12] This device measures the child's ability to push air forcefully out of the lungs. Medication administration can be based on PEFR readings and the effectiveness of treatment confirmed by improved PEFR numbers. Support of the parents and child focuses on helping them to cope with and understand the diagnosis and the need for life-style changes. This includes teaching the family to recognize the child's triggers and modify the environment to eliminate or avoid them. The overall goal is to help the child achieve near-normal respiratory function while continuing normal growth and development.

Nursing Assessment

The nurse usually encounters the child and family in the emergency department or nursing unit. Acute care has become necessary because the child's level of respiratory compromise cannot be managed at home. What needs to be done first? What is the nurse's role during an acute asthmatic episode?

PHYSIOLOGIC ASSESSMENT. First the nurse identifies the child's current respiratory status by assessing the airway, breathing, and circulation. If the child is moving air or talking, the nurse assesses the quality of breathing. Is the child wheezing? Is stridor present? Are retractions visible (Fig. 10–3). What is the respiratory rate? What is the quality of breath sounds? Color and heart rate are assessed. Oxygen saturation is obtained via pulse oximeter. Only after no life-threatening respiratory distress is found should the assessment move on to other systems. The nurse assesses skin turgor, intake and output, and specific gravity. Because asthma can be a symptom of another illness, a head-to-toe assessment should be performed to identify other associated problems (Tables 10–1 and 10–10).

PSYCHOSOCIAL ASSESSMENT. Is the child anxious? Crying? In an older child whose asthma was previously diagnosed, have the asthmatic episode and hospitalization created guilt about doing something the child thinks he or she should have avoided or about forgetting to take medication? The nurse should look for clues to hidden stress and self-blaming.

Nursing Diagnosis

Common nursing diagnoses for the child experiencing an acute asthmatic episode include the following:

- Ineffective Airway Clearance related to airway compromise, copious mucus secretion, and coughing
- Ineffective Breathing Pattern related to airway obstruction, possible additional respiratory illness, and poor response to medication

TABLE 10-14 Medications Used to Treat Asthma

Medication	Action/Indication	Nursing Considerations
Bronchodilators		
Beta-agonists Albuterol, terbutaline: subcutaneous, inhaled, or by mouth	Relax smooth muscle in airway, resulting in rapid bronchodilation; *drugs of choice for acute or daily therapy (inhaled route)*	Have some side effects, but these are usually dose related; repetitive or excessive use can mask increasing airway inflammation and hyper-responsiveness
Methylxanthines Theophylline (related to caffeine): intravenous or by mouth	Relax muscle bundles that constrict airways; dilate airway; provide continuous airway relaxation	Continuous administration needed; work best when a specific amount is maintained in the bloodstream (therapeutic serum level); requires serum level checks and dose adjustment; have many and varied side effects (including tachycardia, restlessness, insomnia, hypotension, vomiting, and diarrhea)
Antiinflammatory Agents		
Cromolyn sodium: inhaled, only	*Preventive medication,* best taken daily to stop chemicals associated with producing asthma; controls seasonal, allergic, and exercise-induced asthma	Less effective in older children; once wheezing starts, this medication is ineffective
Corticosteroids: intravenous, by mouth, or inhaled	Effectively reduce mucosal edema in airways; best absorbed intravenously, but can be useful if inhaled; usually combined with other asthma medications	Side effects (such as abnormalities in glucose metabolism, increased appetite, fluid retention, weight gain, moon face, mood alteration, and hypertension) may be severe if used long term; if used on daily basis, lowest therapeutic dose should be given
Other		
Hyposensitization (allergy shots): subcutaneous	Series of injections that can reduce sensitivity to unavoidable allergens (e.g., environmental organisms—mold, pollen); gradual dose increase over time (called a "build-up") increases child's tolerance to allergic substances; has been of help in some children	Use is controversial; some question about actual effect

- Anxiety/Fear (Child or Parents) related to change in health status, difficulty breathing
- Knowledge Deficit related to medical management of chronic disease

Nursing Management

Pharmacologic and supportive therapies are used to reverse the airway obstruction and promote respiratory function. Nursing interventions center on maintaining airway patency, meeting fluid needs, promoting rest and stress reduction for child and parents, and providing the family with information to enable them to manage the child's acute asthmatic episodes and ongoing needs.

MAINTAIN AIRWAY PATENCY. If the child is exhibiting breathing difficulty, supplemental oxygen is required. Oxygen is best administered by nasal cannula or face mask (see Atlas of Pediatric Procedures). Humidified oxygen should be used to prevent drying and thickening of mucus secretion. The child should be placed in a sitting (semi-Fowler's) or upright position to promote and ease respiratory effort. The effectiveness of positioning and oxygen administration is evaluated by transcutaneous oxygen monitoring (pulse oximeter) and by observing for improved respiratory status.

The respiratory distress and need for supplemental oxygen can be stressful for parents and child alike. Encouraging the parents' presence can be reassuring for the child. The parents should be kept informed of procedures and results, and their input should be obtained in developing the treatment plan.

Many medications are given by the aerosol route (Fig. 10–8). The advantages of aerosol are that the medication acts quickly, enabling the pulmonary blood vessels to absorb the inhaled medication, systemic effects are minimized, and the inhaled droplets provide the added benefit of moisture. The disadvantage is that the medication is quickly absorbed; a child in severe distress may require aerosol administration as often as every hour.[11]

MEET FLUID NEEDS. Fluid therapy is often necessary to restore and maintain adequate fluid balance. Adequate hydration is essential to thin and break up trapped mucus plugs in the narrowed airways. An adequate oral intake may not be possible with the child's compromised respiratory status. An intravenous infusion may be needed, and this route also may be used for administering medications and providing glucose.

As respiratory difficulty diminishes, oral fluids can be offered slowly. Intake and output are monitored and specific gravity is assessed frequently to evaluate the child's hydration status. Involving parents in feeding can help

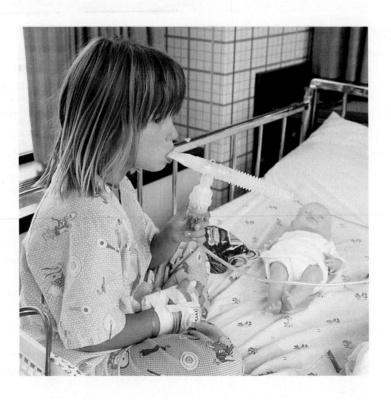

FIGURE 10–8 Medications given by aerosol therapy allow children the freedom to play and entertain themselves.

FIGURE 10–9 This educational piece from the American Lung Association explains what triggers an asthma attack. The required life-style changes for the child and family will be significant, so be sensitive to the family's situation and needs. Culture could be a significant influence.

From American Lung Association—The "Christmas Seal" People. Copyright © 1989 American Lung Association.

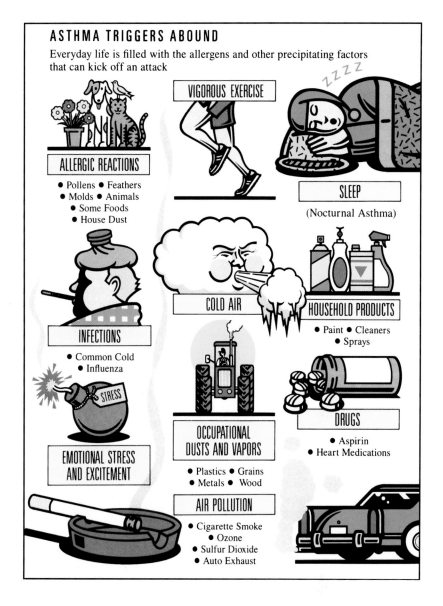

ASTHMA TRIGGERS ABOUND

Everyday life is filled with the allergens and other precipitating factors that can kick off an attack

ALLERGIC REACTIONS
- Pollens • Feathers
- Molds • Animals
- Some Foods
- House Dust

VIGOROUS EXERCISE

SLEEP
(Nocturnal Asthma)

INFECTIONS
- Common Cold
- Influenza

COLD AIR

HOUSEHOLD PRODUCTS
- Paint • Cleaners
- Sprays

EMOTIONAL STRESS AND EXCITEMENT

OCCUPATIONAL DUSTS AND VAPORS
- Plastics • Grains
- Metals • Wood

DRUGS
- Aspirin
- Heart Medications

AIR POLLUTION
- Cigarette Smoke
- Ozone
- Sulfur Dioxide
- Auto Exhaust

gain the child's cooperation in taking oral fluids. The child's fluid preferences should be determined and choices provided where possible.

PROMOTE REST AND STRESS REDUCTION. The child who has had an acute asthmatic episode is usually very tired when admitted to the nursing unit. Labored breathing and low oxygen status have left the child exhausted. The child should be placed in a quiet, private room if possible, to promote relaxation and allow the child to rest. By grouping tasks, nurses can avoid repeatedly disturbing the child. For example, vital signs can be taken when aerosol medications are administered. The parents also need rest and should be encouraged to take breaks as needed.

DISCHARGE PLANNING AND PATIENT/FAMILY HOME CARE TEACHING. Parents need a thorough understanding of asthma, how to prevent attacks and treatment to maintain the child's health and avoid unnecessary hospitalization. The American Lung Association is an excellent resource for parents (see Appendix F). Through printed educational materials and referral to a local support group, parents gain additional knowledge and confidence that enable them to help their child lead a normal life (Fig. 10–9).[12]

Length of hospitalization depends on the child's response to therapy. Any underlying or accompanying health problem, such as preexisting lung dis-

TABLE 10-15 Parent Teaching: Home Care Instructions for the Child with Asthma

1. Identify parents' knowledge about the condition:
   a. Review why asthma occurs and evaluate parents' understanding of the physiologic process. Ask:
      - Do you understand what happens in your child's lungs during an asthma attack?
      - Do you know the early warning signs of an asthma episode in your child?
      - What are your child's symptoms and how does he or she respond to them?
   b. Identify asthma triggers and evaluate parents' understanding of how to prevent, avoid, or minimize their effect in a timely manner. Ask:
      - Do you know your child's personal asthma triggers? (Suggest that parents and child keep a notebook to track episodes so they can learn more about these patterns.)
      - What steps can you take to minimize or eliminate your child's exposure? (quitting smoking etc.)
2. Set up a schedule for parents to learn asthma management. Ask:
   - Do you know when and where to seek emergency medical help?
   - What quick action can you take before seeking medical assistance?
3. Review parents' understanding of medication therapy:
   - Provide information about medications: name, type of drug, dose, method of administration, expected effect, possible side effects, use of peak expiratory flow rate meter.
4. Address associated issues:
   - Do parents know how to store and properly transport medications?
   - What are the financial considerations of medication cost and life-style changes?
   - Has the child's school or teacher been notified?
   - Has a MedicAlert bracelet or medallion been obtained for the child to facilitate assistance when away from home?
5. Identify need for follow-up care:
   - Do parents know when to see a physician? When drug levels need to be checked?
   - Does child need to see an allergist?
   - Do the child or parents have special emotional needs?
   - Would self-help group or camp experience be helpful for the child?

ease or pneumonia, can complicate and extend the child's hospital stay. The nurse should communicate with the family at least once a day about the child's condition.

Discharge planning for the asthmatic child focuses on increasing the family's knowledge about the disease, medication therapy, and the need for follow-up care (Table 10–15). The required life-style changes may be difficult for both child and parents. The need to modify the home by removing a loved pet, for example, may create stress. The nurse can play a role in keeping lines of communication open and can facilitate discussion and clarification of ways to prevent asthmatic episodes. The family should be reassured that most children with asthma can lead a normal life with some modifications. Parents should communicate with school personnel regarding the child's condition, need to take medications, and ability to participate in activities.[11]

Status Asthmaticus

Status asthmaticus is unrelenting, severe respiratory distress in an asthmatic child, which persists despite pharmacologic and supportive interventions. Without immediate intervention the child with status asthmaticus may die. The child is placed in an intensive care unit and may require endotracheal intubation with assisted ventilation. The section on respiratory failure earlier in the chapter gives additional information on the nurse's role in providing emergency respiratory care.

Lower Airway Disorders

The lower airway, or bronchial tree, lies below the trachea and includes the bronchi, bronchioles, and alveoli. Lower airway disorders occur because a structural or functional problem interferes with the lungs' ability to complete the respiratory cycle. Lower airway disorders include respiratory distress syndrome, bronchopulmonary dysplasia, bronchitis, bronchiolitis, pneumonia, tuberculosis, and cystic fibrosis.

Respiratory Distress Syndrome

Respiratory distress syndrome (RDS), also called hyaline membrane disease, manifests during the first 8 hours of life in newborn infants with severely compromised respiratory systems. RDS is the leading cause of death for preterm infants during the first 28 days of life and is best managed in an intensive care unit.[1]

Clinical manifestations include tachypnea (70 to 120 breaths per minute), retractions, grunting, rales, pallor, cyanosis, slow capillary refill, hypothermia, peripheral edema, flaccid muscle tone, gastrointestinal shutdown (paralytic ileus), jaundice, and acidosis.

RDS results from inadequate synthesis, secretion, or storage of pulmonary surfactant.[6] Surfactant is a substance that lowers the surface tension of the alveoli by keeping the alveoli inflated and preventing the interior walls from adhering. Without sufficient surfactant, the alveoli cannot reinflate and collapse.

This same process occurs when the infant takes its first breath after birth. In utero the fetal lungs are filled with fluid. At birth this fluid is expelled from the alveoli. If insufficient surfactant is present, the alveolar walls adhere together. As a result, oxygen and carbon dioxide cannot be exchanged, which creates a threat to life. The alveoli themselves become damaged and die, creating thick scar tissue (the hyaline membrane tissue) in the alveolar space. The alveoli are replaced with fibrous nonfunctional tissue that stiffens the lung.[1]

Diagnosis usually occurs in the newborn nursery. A chest radiograph showing air in the bronchial tree and decreased lung expansion confirms the diagnosis. Medical management focuses on mechanical ventilatory support to expand the alveoli and preserve respiratory function. Intravenous fluid therapy and medications (primarily theophylline) are administered to support function of the respiratory and other body systems.[1,6] A newer therapy is artificial surfactant, which is used to prevent atelectasis. Blood products may be administered to expand blood volume, increasing oxygen capacity.

Nursing Management

The respiratory status of the infant with RDS is closely monitored for at least the first 8 hours of life. Nursing assessment focuses on identifying changes in respiratory status, such as quality of respirations and pulse, overall color, signs of dehydration, changes in the infant's behavior, and vital sign trends.

Care of the infant is organized to eliminate any unnecessary physical stimulation, since this additional stress contributes to respiratory compromise. The infant is usually placed in a warmer to reduce metabolic demands. Parents need clear explanations about the infant's health status and planned interventions. By remaining available to parents and answering their questions, the nurse establishes a positive relationship and facilitates essential communication.

Survival after 72 hours usually results in discharge from the hospital after a long hospitalization.[1]

■ CLINICAL TIP

An alveolus can be thought of as a small balloon filled with water. When the balloon is emptied, the water droplets that remain inside the balloon cause the surface tension to increase. As a result the sides of the balloon stick together. The increased surface tension makes reinflation almost impossible.

Because of the potential for respiratory distress and ongoing respiratory problems after discharge, parents should be taught CPR. (Refer to Atlas of Pediatric Procedures.) The infant is also monitored at home for apnea, and medical follow-up should be continuous. Parents may benefit from referral to support groups.

Bronchopulmonary Dysplasia

Bronchopulmonary dysplasia (BPD) is an iatrogenic (treatment-induced) condition that results in chronic respiratory dysfunction. It is the most prevalent and serious chronic respiratory disorder that begins during infancy. Premature infants are affected more often than full-term infants, and morbidity is greater in males than in females.[6]

The infant with BPD has persistent signs of respiratory distress: tachypnea, hypoxia, irritability, nasal flaring, and retractions. Normal activities, such as feeding, can create increased oxygen demands that are difficult for the compromised infant to meet.

BPD is a direct result of the treatment provided to premature and term infants with such conditions as RDS, congenital heart disease, meconium aspiration, and tracheoesophageal fistula. Treating these conditions with high oxygen concentrations, intubation, and long-term, high-pressure ventilation contributes to BPD.

In BPD the alveoli and bronchioles are damaged and become scarred, thick, and fibrous, resulting in inefficient gas exchange and poor mucus clearing. Air trapping and small airway obstruction cause areas of overdistention and carbon dioxide retention. This, in turn, creates chronic low oxygenation (hypoxemia). The alveoli continue to develop, but the lungs never completely heal.

The chest radiograph is the best indicator of lung changes and is the key to medical diagnosis. It shows areas of hyperinflation (air trapping or emphysema) called "white out," a classic sign of BPD. The air trapping persists and in time causes the chest to assume a barrel shape. Medical management focuses on symptomatic treatment that supports respiratory function. Supplemental oxygen, chest physiotherapy, and medication therapy are used (Table 10–16).[6]

Nursing Management

Nursing management focuses on promoting respiratory function and preparing the family for home care needs. Nursing assessment includes close

TABLE 10–16 Medications Used to Treat Bronchopulmonary Dysplasia

Medication	Action/Indication
Bronchodilators (theophylline, beta-adrenergics, anticholinergics)	Open the airways by relaxing airway muscles; different drugs work together for best response
Antiinflammatory agents (corticosteroids, cromolyn)	Used in severe bronchopulmonary dysplasia; long-term therapy to prevent wheezing in combination with bronchodilators
Diuretics (furosemide, chlorothiazide, spironolactone)	Help remove excess fluid from lungs; may cause electrolyte imbalances
Antibiotics	Low-dose prophylactic therapy to prevent severe illness; specific treatment for identified organisms

monitoring of respirations, pulse, color, behavior changes, and vital sign trends. The infant with chronic BPD may become acutely ill at any time.

Once home, many infants need ventilation therapy, oxygen respiratory support, and drug therapy. Frequent rehospitalization may be necessary because, although the lungs may function adequately, they remain vulnerable throughout childhood to common respiratory illnesses. Infants with BPD do not have the same respiratory reserve as healthy infants, and they can become much more ill more quickly.

It is important to provide for the infant's normal development through rest, nutrition, stimulation, and family support. Including parents in the infant's care early on promotes bonding and prepares them for home care responsibilities. Some families require home nursing assistance. Referrals for needed respiratory supplies, medications, and follow-up care must be carefully planned and coordinated well in advance of the infant's discharge date.

Bronchitis

Bronchitis, inflammation of the bronchi, rarely occurs as an isolated problem. The bronchi can be affected simultaneously with adjacent respiratory structures during a respiratory illness. Bronchitis occurs most often in children under 4 years of age, usually following a mild upper respiratory tract problem.[10,13] Bronchitis is caused most often by a virus but may also result from invasion of bacteria or in response to an allergen or irritant.

The classic symptom of bronchitis is a coarse, hacking cough, which increases in severity at night. Children with bronchitis look tired and report that they feel awful. The chest and ribs may be sore because of the deep and frequent coughing. There is often a deep, rattling quality to breathing. Some children have audible wheezing that can be heard without a stethoscope.

Nursing Management

Nursing management includes supporting respiratory function through rest, humidification, hydration, and symptomatic treatment. The sections on asthma and pneumonia give detailed information on treatment measures.

Discharge planning should emphasize the self-limiting nature of the disorder. Because passive smoke and pollutant inhalation may contribute to its recurrence, eliminating or reducing the child's exposure to these irritants may improve overall respiratory function.[14] Parents who smoke should be advised that quitting or refraining from smoking in the child's presence may benefit the child.

Bronchiolitis

Bronchiolitis is one of the most frequent causes of hospitalization in infants[6] and poses one of the greatest threats to the respiratory system of infants and small children. Although some infants and children have mild symptoms that are easily managed at home, others become acutely ill with severe respiratory distress that can become a life-threatening emergency. What makes bronchiolitis such a potential threat?

Bronchiolitis is a lower respiratory tract illness that occurs when an infecting agent (virus or bacterium) causes inflammation and obstruction of the small airways, the bronchioles. Infection occurs most frequently in toddlers and preschoolers. Infection is most severe in infants under 6 months of age. Newborns and infants under 2 months of age are particularly vulnerable, and they are routinely hospitalized when bronchiolitis is diagnosed.

Clinical Manifestations

The infant or child with bronchiolitis may have been ill with upper respiratory symptoms such as nasal stuffiness, cough (not usually noted in infants), and fever (less than 102.2° F) for a few days. As the illness progresses, symptoms increase and include a deeper, more frequent cough and more stressful, labored breathing. Respirations are rapid, shallow, and accompanied by nasal flaring and retractions (signs of severe distress). Parents report that the infant or child is acting more ill—appearing sicker, less playful, and less interested in eating. Infants, especially, may refuse to feed or may spit up what they do eat along with thick, clear mucus, and thus alarm parents.

Etiology and Pathophysiology

Bacterial and viral organisms may cause bronchiolitis; however, infection with respiratory syncytial virus (RSV) is the most common cause. RSV is transmitted through direct or close contact with respiratory secretions of infected individuals.

Viruses, acting as parasites, are able to invade the mucosal cells that line the bronchioles. The invaded cells die when the virus bursts from inside the cell to invade adjacent cells. The resulting cell debris clogs and obstructs the bronchioles and irritates the airway. In response the airway lining swells and produces excessive mucus. Despite this protective effort by the bronchioles, the actual effect is partial airway obstruction and bronchospasms.

The cycle is repeated throughout both lungs as the airway cells are invaded by the virus. The partially obstructed airways allow air in, but the mucus and airway swelling block expulsion of the air. This creates the wheezing and crackles in the airways. Air trapped below the obstruction also interferes with normal gas exchange. The child with RSV is therefore at risk for respiratory failure as the oxygen level decreases and the carbon dioxide level increases.

As the airflow continues to decrease, breath sounds diminish. Thus the noisier the lungs, the better, since this indicates that the child is still able to move air in and out of the lungs. The first 24 to 72 hours is the most critical period.[6]

Diagnostic Tests and Medical Management

The history and physical examination provide the data needed to diagnose bronchiolitis.

Nasopharyngeal secretions are cultured to confirm the presence of RSV. Children who test positive for RSV are isolated, roomed together, or placed on the same ward to minimize the spread of the virus to other hospitalized children. Medical management is frequently supportive, especially when the causative agent is unknown (Table 10–17).

There is evidence that bronchiolitis in infancy may increase the chances of childhood wheezing and asthma. It also may be a major risk factor for chronic obstructive pulmonary disease later in life.[10]

Nursing Assessment

Physiologic Assessment. Airway and respiratory function are assessed carefully. Good observation skills are important to ensure timely interventions for worsening respiratory symptoms and prevention of respiratory distress (Tables 10–1 and 10–17).

◼ RESPIRATORY SYNCYTIAL VIRUS

Respiratory syncytial virus (RSV) occurs in annual epidemics from October to March. By the age of 3 years most children have been infected with RSV, and reinfection (via siblings or close family contacts) throughout life is common. Hospital personnel should follow principles of good handwashing, since the virus is easily transmitted.

TABLE 10-17 Medical Management for Bronchiolitis

Medical Therapy	Rationale
Full-Term Infant or Child	
Cardiorespiratory monitor and pulse oximetry	Enable provider to follow trends and assess need for specific therapies
Oxygen therapy via mask, nasal cannula, face tent, or high-humidity mist tent	Delivery method determined by desired concentration of oxygen, degree of moisture, and child's response; oxygen must be humidified
Hydration via intravenous or oral fluids	Provider must consider insensible fluid loss, decreased intake, and child's current electrolyte and hydration status
Inhaled medications and pulmonary hygiene (postural drainage and chest physiotherapy)	Nebulizer therapy (bronchodilators, steroids, and beta-antagonists) act directly on inflamed and obstructed airways; pulmonary hygiene helps to further loosen trapped mucus
Systemic medications	Symptomatic treatment may include antipyretics (acetaminophen preferred) or mild sedative (chloral hydrate selectively); no antibiotics are given unless evidence of secondary bacterial infection (e.g., otitis media) is present; no over-the-counter medications are given, especially not antihistamines, which dry and thicken airway secretions
High-Risk Infant or Child*	
Antiviral therapy (Ribavirin)	Ribavirin is an antiviral agent specific for respiratory syncytial virus

*Defined as an infant or child with congenital heart disease, bronchopulmonary dysplasia, chronic lung problems, or cystic fibrosis or who is premature or severely ill and less than 6 weeks old.

Psychosocial Assessment. Children and their parents should be observed for signs of fear and anxiety (Table 10–12). The unfamiliar hospital environment and procedures can increase stress. Parents' questions, as well as their non-verbal cues, help direct nursing interventions during admission and throughout hospitalization.

Developmental Assessment. The nurse should observe for signs of stranger and separation anxieties, which are common in the age group most often hospitalized for bronchiolitis (infants and small children). Involving parents in procedures and care, when appropriate, can promote emotional security.

Nursing Diagnosis

Common nursing diagnoses for the child with bronchiolitis include the following:
- Ineffective Airway Clearance related to increased airway secretions, fatigue from coughing and dyspnea, and air trapping
- Ineffective Breathing Pattern related to inflamed tracheobronchial tree and progression of bronchiolitis
- Fluid Volume Deficit related to inability to meet fluid needs and increased metabolic demands (insensible loss, fever, thickened or increased respiratory secretions)
- Fear/Anxiety (Parent or Child) related to uncertainty of prognosis, unfamiliar surroundings, and procedures
- Knowledge Deficit (Parent) related to medications, therapies, and follow-up care required after discharge

Nursing Management

Nursing management focuses on maintaining respiratory function, supporting overall physiologic function and hydration, reducing the child's and family's anxiety, and preparing the family for home care.

Maintain Respiratory Function. Close monitoring is essential to evaluate the child's improvement or to spot early signs of deterioration. Oxygen and pulmonary care therapies are administered. High humidity and supplemental oxygen may be provided with a mist tent if the child requires only moisture and minimal oxygen. If more concentrated oxygen is required, it can be given via nasal cannula or face mask or tent. Pulse oximetry is used to evaluate oxygenation.

Patent nares are important to promote oxygen intake. A bulb syringe is a helpful tool that can quickly and easily clear the nasal passages. The head of the bed should be elevated to ease the work of breathing and drain mucus from the upper airways. Pulmonary hygiene and nebulized medications are usually administered by a respiratory therapist.

Support Physiologic Function. Grouping nursing tasks promotes the child's physiologic function by decreasing stress and promoting rest. Rest is a key component in improving the child's breathing and overall health. Medications may be administered to control temperature and promote sleep as needed. An intravenous infusion may be ordered to rehydrate and maintain fluid balance until the child is capable of taking sufficient oral fluids.

Reduce Anxiety. The need for hospitalization and assistive therapies creates anxiety and fear in child and parents alike. An important part of nursing care is anticipating, recognizing, and acting to decrease the child's and parents' anxiety. The nurse provides parents with thorough explanations and daily updates and encourages their participation in the child's care.

The presence of parents and their ability to calm the infant or child can be helpful in the child's recovery. The parents may themselves be frightened by the child's continued respiratory difficulty and the presence of assistive equipment at the bedside. They should be reassured that holding or touching the child will not dislodge wires or tubing.

If the child has been ill for a few days before admission, the parents are likely to be tired. Acknowledging parents' physical and emotional needs facilitates a spirit of caring and enhances communication between staff and family. The parents should be encouraged to take turns at the child's bedside and to take breaks for meals and rest.

▧ DISCHARGE TEACHING: BRONCHIOLITIS

Advise parents to call the physician if:
- Respiratory symptoms interfere with sleep or eating
- Breathing is rapid or difficult
- Symptoms persist in a child who is less than 1 year old, has heart or lung disease, or was premature and had lung disease after birth
- The child acts sicker—appears tired, less playful, less interested in food (parents just "feel" the child is not improving)

Discharge Planning and Patient/Family Home Care Teaching. Children are discharged once they show sufficient stability in maintaining adequate oxygenation (as evidenced by easing of respiratory effort, decreased mucus production, and absence of coughing). In most children symptoms abate within 24 to 72 hours. The same supportive therapies implemented in the hospital may be needed at home:

- Use of the bulb syringe to suction the nares of an infant under 1 year of age
- Fluid intake to thin respiratory secretions (making them easier to clear) and provide glucose for energy (since the child's appetite may not return to normal for several days)
- Rest

Children are usually capable of recognizing their own activity limits. However, parents should encourage active toddlers to nap and take rest periods.

The nurse teaches the parents proper administration of medications. Acetaminophen may be prescribed for persistent low-grade fevers and general achiness. Parents need to know that RSV can recur, how to recognize symptoms, and when to call the physician.

Pneumonia

Pneumonia is an inflammation or infection of the bronchioles and alveolar spaces of the lungs. It occurs most often in infants and young children. Pneumonia in children often resolves much sooner than in adults. The key is early recognition, enabling the child to be managed at home rather than in the hospital.

Pneumonia is classified as typical or atypical, according to the invading causative organism or irritant. Typical pneumonia is bacterial in origin; atypical pneumonia is nonbacterial. Regardless of the causative agent, symptoms include elevated temperature, cough, dyspnea, tachypnea, abnormal breath sounds, and malaise that may progress to respiratory failure.[10,15]

What physiologic process occurs to precipitate the symptoms? Bacterial and viral invaders act differently within the lungs. Typical (bacterial) invaders circulate through the bloodstream to the lungs, where they damage cells. Bacteria tend to be distributed evenly throughout one or more lobes of a single lung, a pattern termed unilateral lobar pneumonia. Atypical (viral or mycoplasma) invaders, on the other hand, are parasites of cells. Viruses frequently enter from the upper respiratory tract, infiltrating the alveoli nearest the bronchi of one or both lungs. There they invade the cells, replicate, and burst out forcefully, killing the cells and sending out cell debris. They rapidly invade adjacent areas, distributing themselves in a scattered, patchy pattern referred to as bronchopneumonia.[15] The end result of bacterial, viral, or mycoplasma invasion is the presence of exudate resulting from cell death, which fills the alveolar spaces, pooling and clumping in dependent areas of the lung to create areas of consolidation.

In children, reliably differentiating typical from atypical pneumonias is often difficult. The child's age, severity of symptoms, and presence of an underlying lung, cardiac, or immunodeficiency disease can create varying responses. The important point is that inflammation and immune responses in the bronchioles and alveoli of a susceptible child invariably lead to pneumonia.[10]

Medical management for all types of pneumonia includes symptomatic therapy (pain and fever control) and supportive care through airway management, fluids, and rest. Mycoplasma and other bacterial pneumonias are treated with organism-sensitive antibiotics; viral pneumonias usually improve independent of antibiotics.

Nursing Management

Nursing care incorporates supportive measures and medical therapies as appropriate. Nursing measures used to manage the child with bronchiolitis are generally applicable to the child with pneumonia.

In addition to ongoing respiratory assessment and supportive therapies (pulmonary care, antibiotics, hydration), the child may need relief from pain when coughing and deep breathing. Pain medication (acetaminophen) can provide the added benefits of temperature control and may aid in sleep. Frequent chest radiographs may be necessary to follow the progress of the condition. Hospitalization may be as brief as 24 hours or as long as several weeks.

■ CLINICAL TIP

Teach the child and parent how to splint the chest, by hugging a small pillow, teddy bear, or doll, to make coughing less painful.

The goal of nursing care is to restore optimal respiratory function. Discharge planning should be addressed early in the hospital stay. Medications, especially antibiotics, must be taken at prescribed intervals and for the full course. Parents should be taught proper administration of drugs and any side effects. Follow-up may include monthly chest radiographs until the lungs are clear. Symptoms of pneumonia usually disappear long before the lungs are completely healed. Some children continue to have worsening reactive airway problems or abnormal results on pulmonary function tests. Most children, however, recover uneventfully.[10]

Preventive measures against pneumonia are limited. An immunization against pneumococcal bacteria is being used on a limited basis for children under 2 years of age and those who are immunosuppressed or otherwise at risk.[10]

Tuberculosis

Tuberculosis (TB) is caused by the organism *Mycobacterium tuberculosis*, which is transmitted through the air in infectious particles called droplet nuclei. Since 1985 the incidence of TB has been on the rise, particularly among blacks and Hispanics between the ages of 25 and 45 years. These individuals are of childbearing age and frequently have close contact with children and adolescents. Adults with active laryngeal or pulmonary TB place children at risk for contracting TB.[16]

Clinical manifestations of TB in children include a chronic cough, anorexia, weight loss or failure to gain weight, and fever.

By coughing, sneezing, speaking, or singing, a person with active TB sends out tiny droplets of moisture that remain in the air. If these droplets are inhaled, the bacillus may infect the new host. Frequently, however, the organism is trapped in the upper airway, preventing infection. Infection occurs *only* when the bacillus reaches the alveoli.[16]

Once the organism reaches the alveoli, an immune response is initiated to combat the invader. The immune system sends macrophages to surround and wall off the bacillus in small hard capsules, called tubercles. There the bacillus can remain dormant (inactive) indefinitely or can progress to active TB. If the tubercle extends into a blood vessel, the bacillus may spread through the bloodstream to affect the liver, spleen, bone marrow, or meninges (tubercular meningitis). This systemic form of TB (called miliary tuberculosis) may lead to serious illness or death. Miliary tuberculosis is *not*, however, transmissible; only active pulmonary TB has the potential to infect another individual.[10]

Several tests may be required to confirm the diagnosis (Table 10–18). Medical management focuses on diagnosis and treatment of active TB with antitubercular and corticosteroid drug therapy. Tuberculosis is a major public health problem and must be promptly reported to designated government agencies.

Nursing Management

Nursing care centers on administration of medications to treat the disease and supportive care measures. Parent education includes the disease process, prescribed medications, possible side effects, and long-term nature of therapy (for example, that drug therapy may last for 6 to 12 months). Most children with TB are able to lead essentially normal lives. The nurse should emphasize the importance of taking medications as prescribed, and ensuring proper nutrition and rest to promote normal growth and development.

The earlier discussion of pneumonia and the discussion of meningitis in Chapter 14 (regarding tubercular meningitis) give other nursing care measures appropriate for the child with TB.

TABLE 10-18 Diagnostic Tests for Tuberculosis

Test	Indication
Mantoux test (intradermal injection of purified protein derivative [PPD])	Confirms *infection* with the TB organism (2 to 10 weeks after exposure)
Chest x-ray examination (anterioposterior and lateral views)	Confirms presence of pulmonary tuberculosis (small, seedlike opacities may be visible)
Blood cultures for *Mycobacterium tuberculosis*	Proves diagnosis; defines specific drug sensitivity
Gastric washings (early morning after overnight fast; three consecutive days)	Confirms pulmonary tuberculosis (active form of tuberculosis)
Sputum cultures (expectorated or from bronchoscopic examination)	Confirms active pulmonary tuberculosis
Pleural biopsy for culture and tissue examination	Taken when pleural effusion is present
Lumbar puncture	Confirms meningeal tuberculosis (inactive form of tuberculosis)

Cystic Fibrosis

Cystic fibrosis is an inherited autosomal recessive disorder of the exocrine glands that results in physiologic alterations in the respiratory, gastrointestinal, integumentary, musculoskeletal, and reproductive systems (Fig. 10–10). The disorder occurs predominantly in white children. Sex is not a factor in incidence (Fig. 10–11).

Clinical Manifestations

The primary symptom of cystic fibrosis is the production of thick, sticky mucus. One of the earliest signs in the newborn is meconium ileus, a small bowel obstruction that occurs during the first few days of life. In infants and toddlers, fecal impaction and intussusception ("telescoping" of the bowel)

■ **THE FOUR F'S OF CYSTIC FIBROSIS**

Stools of a child with cystic fibrosis are characteristically:
- Frothy (bulky and large-quantity)
- Foul-smelling
- Fat-containing (greasy)
- Float

FIGURE 10–10 Pattern of inheritance in an autosomal recessive disorder such as cystic fibrosis. If both parents carry the gene, there is a 1 in 4 chance with each pregnancy of passing the disorder on to their child and a 1 in 2 chance that the child will be a carrier.

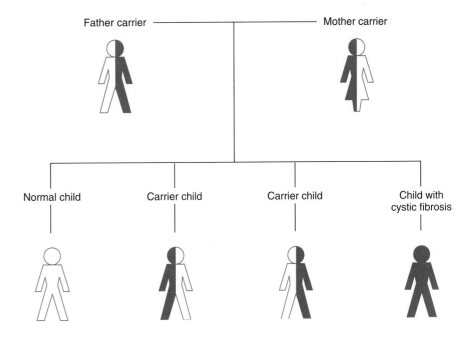

Father carrier — Mother carrier

Normal child — Carrier child — Carrier child — Child with cystic fibrosis

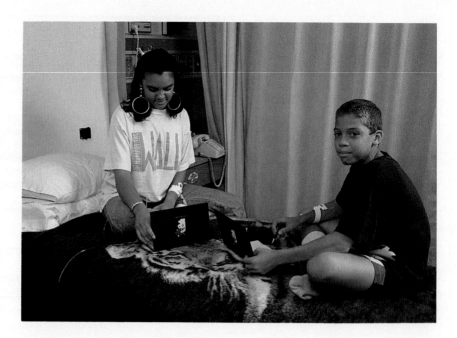

FIGURE 10–11 Cystic fibrosis is an inherited autosomal recessive disorder of the exocrine glands, so it is not uncommon to see siblings with it such as this brother and sister.

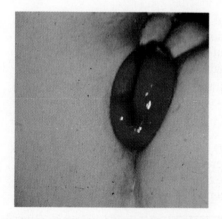

Rectal prolapse

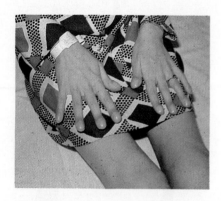

Digital clubbing

may be the first signs of the disorder.[10] Steatorrhea (fatty stool) is one of the characteristic signs of cystic fibrosis. The sticky, thick stool is thought to create the initial obstruction. Intestinal peristalsis (controlled by the autonomic nervous system) is also adversely affected. Rectal prolapse, resulting from the large, bulky, difficult-to-pass stools, is a common gastrointestinal problem in infants and children with cystic fibrosis.

Other signs and symptoms include a chronic moist, productive cough and frequent respiratory infections. Most children have difficulty maintaining and gaining weight despite a voracious appetite. Infants and children may have a delayed bone age, short stature, and delayed onset of puberty.[17] Clubbing of the tips of the fingers and toes occurs as the disease progresses.

Ralph Turner's Story

My name is Ralph Turner and I am a cystic.

One day I went to the store with my mother. It was winter and it was real cold outside and when I got in the store I started coughing. And my mother started pounding on me so I could get up the mucus and I wouldn't be coughing. But then this lady said, "Look at that mother beating on that kid who has a cold." And my mother told the lady to shut up and she told her what I had. And the lady didn't say nothing else.

I know some more things about cystic fibrosis. When I play baseball, I run to the bases and start coughing sometimes and I have to rest for a little while and then I am fine. And then I can play again. I can ride my bike and—ooh!—I ride my bike and that is good for us. It helps us bring up the mucus. That's right! When we go real fast we bring up the mucus!

The mucus is the stuff that I cough up. It is called phlegm. If I told you everything I did when I cough—you'd be amazed! Like when I jump and I land real hard on my feet—I cough! I want to be like Reggie Jackson and be on the Orioles. When people grow up they don't have that much trouble. They have to cough but not that much. Like I know this man who has cystic fibrosis and he is my father's friend and he doesn't have that much trouble.

My cousin has cystic fibrosis and his name is Ralph Paul Turner. He is 14 years old. Sometimes he has trouble like me. We were born with cystic fibrosis but they didn't know I had cystic fibrosis until I was 4 months old. Now I am 7.

I hope they find a cure for us kids soon.

by Ralph Dwayne Turner. Age, 7 years old
Died, 9 years old

Etiology and Pathophysiology

Metabolic function is altered as a result of the imbalances created by excessive electrolyte loss through perspiration, saliva, and mucus secretion. Enzyme abnormalities further disrupt metabolism by preventing nutrient absorption.

Because the blocked pancreatic ducts cannot secrete the natural enzymes necessary to digest fats and proteins, essential nutrients are excreted in the stool.

The classic cough occurs because the lungs are always filled with mucus, which the respiratory cilia cannot clear. This causes air to become trapped in the small airways, resulting in atelectasis (pulmonary collapse). Secondary respiratory infections occur because secretions provide an environment conducive to bacterial growth.

The "salty taste" of the skin is the result of sodium chloride that makes its way through skin pores to the skin surface.

Nearly all males who have cystic fibrosis are sterile because of blockage or absence of the vas deferens.[16] Females have difficulty conceiving because increased mucus secretions in the reproductive tract interfere with the passage of sperm.[18]

Diagnostic Tests and Medical Management

Cystic fibrosis is usually diagnosed in infancy or early childhood. Some children with a milder form of the disease, however, reach the teen or young adult years before symptoms appear.[10,18]

Cystic fibrosis is diagnosed definitively by two positive sweat tests and the presence of classic symptoms (Table 10–19).[6] The sweat test may be performed at the child's bedside or on an outpatient basis. The parents should be present to hold and reassure the infant or small child. They should be informed that the test will indicate whether the child has cystic fibrosis and that two tests may be ordered to confirm the diagnosis. This is especially important when the test is performed on adolescents, since girls who have monthly menses may have cyclically fluctuating sweat electrolyte levels. Pubertal boys may also show fluctuations.[19]

Medical management focuses on maintaining respiratory function, managing infection, promoting exercise and optimal nutrition, and preventing gastrointestinal blockage (Table 10–20). Improvements in medical management now enable many children with cystic fibrosis to survive into adulthood. The disease is ultimately terminal, however, because of the progressive multisystem changes and the difficulty of long-term infection management.[18]

Care of the child with previously diagnosed cystic fibrosis is the focus of the following discussion.

"I kissed my baby's cheek and tasted salt! Nothing would be the same after that."
—The mother of a 1-week-old infant with cystic fibrosis

▨ GENETIC CONSIDERATIONS

Recent advances in localization of the cystic fibrosis gene (on chromosome 7) by genetic linkage studies greatly enhance the likelihood that successful techniques for prenatal diagnosis will be developed. The possibility of gene therapy by transfer of the normal gene to airway epithelial cells is also being investigated.

TABLE 10–19 **Diagnostic Test for Cystic Fibrosis (Sweat Test)**

Test	Purpose	Normal Values	Diagnostic Values
Sweat test (pilocarpine iontophoresis)	Analysis of sodium and chloride content in sweat	Sodium: 10–30 mEq/L; chloride: 10–35 mEq/L	Chloride: 50–60 mEq/L—suspicious; >60 mEq/L—diagnostic with other clinical signs

TABLE 10-20 Medical Management for Cystic Fibrosis

Medical Therapy	Rationale
Respiratory Therapy	
Nebulization treatments with mucolytic and bronchodilating agents	Loosens, liquifies, and thins pulmonary secretions; opens large and small airways
Chest physiotherapy for all lung segments (bilateral percussion-vibration and forceful coughing)	Mobilizes secretions to bronchi for expectoration
Adjust medications given as prescribed (e.g., oral bronchodilators, steroids)	Promotes airway patency
Infection Management (Most Susceptible to H. influenzae, S. aureus, *and* P. aeruginosa *Bacteria and Viral Agents)*	
Antibiotics	Treatment based on sputum culture results
Nutritional Needs	
Pancreatic enzyme supplements (Cotazym-S, Pancrease, Viokase) taken with meals and snacks	Assists in digestion of nutrients and decreasing fat and bulk
Diet supplies well-balanced, nutritious food with all high caloric value and moderate fat; nutritional counseling necessary	Promotes essential nutrient balance for health, growth, and weight maintenance; considers child food preferences and cultural-socioeconomic issues
Multivitamins and vitamin E in water-soluble form; vitamins A, D, and K given when deficient	Cystic fibrosis interferes with vitamin production; supplements are required in water-soluble form for better absorption (vitamins A, D, E, and K are naturally fat soluble)

Nursing Assessment

Physiologic Assessment. Physical assessment of the child focuses on adequacy of respiratory function. The child with cystic fibrosis usually is admitted with symptoms of an upper respiratory infection (Table 10–1). A set of baseline vital signs, including temperature, pulse, respirations, and blood pressure, along with a weight measurement, should be obtained on admission. The nurse observes the child's physical appearance, noting overall body proportions and any changes characteristic of long-term cystic fibrosis.

Psychosocial Assessment. The emotional stress of this chronic disease may not be readily apparent on admission, particularly if the child's symptoms are mild and not imminently life threatening. Ongoing observation of the child's and parents' behavior helps direct nursing interventions throughout hospitalization (Table 10–12). The siblings may also show signs of difficulty in dealing with the illness.

The nurse should ask parents how the child's illness has affected day-to-day functioning. What have parents told the child and siblings about the disease? What kind of questions have the child and siblings asked about cystic fibrosis, and how have parents answered them? Has the child ever asked about his or her life expectancy? If not, what would parents say if asked?

Developmental Assessment. Growth and development may be altered by the chronic nature of the disease. The nurse compares the child's height and weight to age norms and observes the adolescent for the appearance of secondary sex characteristics, which are often delayed. School-age children and adolescents often are embarrassed at being viewed as different from playmates and peers. Ask how the child and adolescent feels about the need for special diet, medications, and limitations.

Nursing Diagnosis

Common nursing diagnoses for the child with cystic fibrosis include the following:

- Ineffective Airway Clearance related to thick mucus in lungs
- Ineffective Breathing Pattern related to thick tracheobronchial secretions and airway obstruction
- High Risk for Infection related to the presence of mucous secretions conducive to bacterial growth
- Altered Nutrition: Less than Body Requirements related to inability to digest nutrients
- Fear/Anxiety (Parent or Child) related to prognosis and effect of illness on growth and development
- Knowledge Deficit (Parent or Child) related to diet, therapies, and follow-up care

Nursing Management

Nursing management involves supporting the child and family initially, when the diagnosis is made, and during subsequent hospitalizations. The nurse's role begins with implementing specific medical therapies and providing nursing care to meet the child's physiologic and psychosocial needs. Respiratory therapy, medications, and diet must be coordinated to promote optimal body function. Psychosocial support and reinforcement of the child's daily care needs are important in preparation for home care.

Children with cystic fibrosis require periodic hospitalization when a severe infection occurs. Including parents in the child's routine care as much as possible helps them to maintain the child's home schedule while hospitalized. However, parents may view the hospital stay as a break from the rigorous daily pulmonary routine at home and need support in taking advantage of some "down" time. The family often becomes proficient at providing physical care to the child, but the nurse should take the opportunity provided during rehospitalization to review basic information about respiratory care, medications, and nutrition. Keeping lines of communication open and validating parents' understanding of their child's disease and care needs are important steps in preparing the family to cope with this chronic health challenge.[20]

Provide Respiratory Therapy. Chest physiotherapy is usually performed one to three times per day before meals to clear secretions from the lungs (Fig. 10–12). Parents and other family members can learn to help with these necessary treatments. (See Atlas of Pediatric Procedures.) Pulmonary care may involve aerosol treatments and antibiotics when indicated (Table 10–20).

Administer Medications and Meet Nutritional Needs. Digestive problems can be eased with special medications and dietary modification (Table 10–20). Pancreatic enzyme supplements come in powder sprinkles and capsule form and are taken orally with all meals and large snacks. The amount needed is individualized based on the child's nutritional needs and digestive response to these supplements. The goal is to achieve near-normal, well-formed stools and adequate weight gain.

Some fat-soluble vitamins (A, D, E, and K) are not completely absorbed

FIGURE 10–12 Postural drainage can be achieved by clapping with a cupped hand on the chest wall over the segment to be drained to create vibrations that are transmitted to the bronchi to dislodge secretions. **A,** If the obstruction is in the posterior apical segment of the lung, the nurse can do this with the patient sitting up. **B,** If the obstruction is in the left posterior segment, the patient should be lying on his or her right side. Several other positions can be used depending on the location of the obstruction.

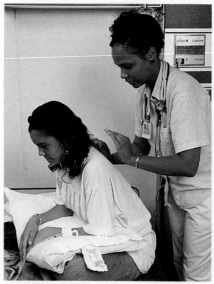
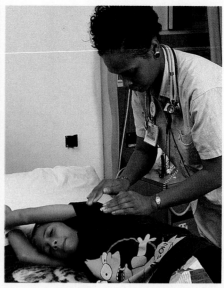

A   B

from food; therefore they must be taken in water-soluble form. Multivitamins taken once or twice daily usually are sufficient to prevent deficiency.

Diet should be well-balanced, with an emphasis on high caloric value. Respiratory complications necessitate additional energy expenditure, and some children require special nutritional supplements to gain and maintain weight.

Fats and salt are both necessary in the diet. Balanced with pancreatic enzyme supplements, moderate fat intake adds an important source of extra fuel. Children with cystic fibrosis lose more than normal amounts of salt in their sweat. This loss can become intensified during hot weather, strenuous exercise, and fever. Parents should allow the child to add extra salt to food and should permit some salty snacks (pretzels with salt, pickles, carbonated soda). During periods of increased sweat, the child should be encouraged to drink more fluids and increase salt intake. Parents need to recognize early symptoms of salt depletion, including fatigue, weakness, abdominal pain, and vomiting, and contact the child's health care provider.

Provide Anticipatory Guidance. The nurse should assist the parents and child to learn what they must do to maintain health after discharge. Emotional support is essential because the diagnosis of this invariably fatal disorder creates anxiety and fear in both parents and child. They need assistance with emotional and psychosocial issues relating to discipline, body image (stooling and odor), frequent rehospitalization, the fatal nature of the illness, the child's feeling of being different from friends, and overall financial, social, and family concerns. Because the disorder is inherited, families may have more than one child with cystic fibrosis. Parents may have unspoken feelings of anger and guilt, blaming themselves for their children's condition.

Discharge Planning and Patient/Family Home Care Teaching. The financial burden of medications, supplies, and medical follow-up may not be recognized immediately by a family already overwhelmed by the diagnosis. Because of the chronicity of cystic fibrosis, home care is as important as care of the child in the hospital. Initially, parents need assistance in obtaining necessary equipment. If the family needs financial assistance, they should be referred to the appropriate social services. Home care of the child with cystic fibrosis is expensive and can be draining on the family.

Parents need to learn chest physiotherapy, which the child will need as often as 3 to 4 times a day. Arranging for a visiting nurse and a respiratory therapist to visit the family frequently can provide reassurance and relief to the family. Managing the child's nutritional needs is important and takes time and energy.

Parents need to learn how to mix enzymes for young children, what vitamins need to be given daily, and what foods should be avoided or eliminated because of the child's digestive problems. Referral should be made to a dietician either before or at the time of discharge.

Cystic fibrosis affects all family members and disrupts activities of daily living for everyone. It is important to refer familes to family counseling and group therapy with familes of other children with cystic fibrosis if indicated. The Cystic Fibrosis Foundation (see Appendix F) is a source for information on current advances in cystic fibrosis. Local chapter activities also provide emotional support for parents and children.

Injuries of the Respiratory System

Airway compromise after an unintentional injury is a major cause of death in children.[21] Why are children so vulnerable to changes in respiratory function after accidental injury?

The small size of the child's airway makes it vulnerable to obstruction. The tongue, small amounts of blood, mucus, or foreign debris, or swelling in the respiratory tract or adjacent neck tissue may block the airway and lead to hypoxia and respiratory failure. If the child's neck is flexed or hyperextended, the soft laryngeal cartilage may compress and obstruct the airway.

Infants and young children rely on the diaphragm for air movement. They are abdominal (or "belly") breathers. Excessive crying and anxiety deplete metabolic reserves. External ventilatory support and vigorous crying may impede diaphragm function if the stomach becomes distended with air. Because the child's metabolic rate is about double that of an adult, the child has a greater need for oxygen. Respiratory distress, anxiety, and even fever can dramatically add to the child's oxygen demand.

■ **NURSING ALERT**

Never allow a child's neck to hyperextend (bend completely backward) or hyperflex (bend completely forward). Hyperextension flattens the trachea because there is no firm cartilage to provide structural support. Hyperflexion can kink and compress the trachea. Both maneuvers obstruct rather than open the airway.

Airway Obstruction

Airway obstruction exists when air passage in the respiratory tract and lungs is slowed or blocked. If the blockage occurs above the trachea, inhalation is more affected. If the blockage occurs below the trachea, exhalation is more affected. Earlier sections dealt with structural and functional problems that may lead to airway obstruction. This section addresses two common conditions of airway obstruction in children that result from unintentional injury: foreign body aspiration and near-drowning.

■ **GROWTH AND DEVELOPMENT CONSIDERATIONS**

Foreign body aspiration is a major health problem for infants and young toddlers because of their increasing mobility and tendency to place small objects in the mouth.

Foreign Body Aspiration

Foreign body aspiration is the inhalation of any object (solid or liquid, food or nonfood) into the respiratory tract. Aspiration occurs most often during feeding and reaching activities, while crawling, or during playtime in children aged 6 months to 4 years.[9] However, aspiration may occur in children of any age.

Clinical Manifestations

Children are usually brought to the hospital after a sudden episode of coughing. Discovery of an open container with small objects may prompt parents to seek medical assistance for the child. The child may have spasmodic coughing, respiratory distress, or gagging. Sudden respiratory distress in the absence of fever or other symptoms of illness strongly suggests foreign body aspiration.[9]

Etiology and Pathophysiology

In infants over 6 months and children, aspiration may be caused by any number of small objects that make their way into the child's mouth. Foods such as nuts, popcorn, or small pieces of raw vegetables or hot dog; small, loose toy parts such as small wheels and bells; or household objects and substances such as beads, safety pins, coins, buttons, latex balloon pieces, colorful liquids (mouthwash, perfume) in enticing packages (screw top bottles) are frequent causes of airway obstruction.

The severity of the obstruction depends on the size and composition of the object or substance and its location within the respiratory tract. The majority of aspirated foreign bodies (AFBs) usually cause bronchial, not tracheal, obstruction. An object lodged high in the airway above the vocal cords is frequently coughed out easily or with some assistance (such as use of chest and back thrusts or the Heimlich maneuver) (refer to Atlas of Pediatric Procedures). An object lodged in the trachea is a life-threatening situation.

Coughing, choking, gagging, and wheezing may be brief or may persist for several hours if the object drops below the trachea into one of the mainstem bronchi. The right lung is the most common site of lower airway aspiration because of the sloped angle of its bronchus (Fig. 10–2). Objects may migrate from higher to lower airway locations. An object may also move back up to the trachea, creating extreme respiratory difficulty.[6,8,10] If oxygen is depleted for an extended time, brain damage may occur.

Diagnostic Tests and Medical Management

Medical management focuses on taking a careful history to determine whether aspiration has indeed occurred. Choking associated with feeding or crawling on the floor is usually a confirming event. The physical examination often reveals decreased breath sounds and respiratory distress. A special radiograph, called a forced expiratory film, may be ordered. This shows local hyperinflation and mediastinal shift away from the affected side.[6,9] Sometimes, when the object aspirated is radiopaque, it can be seen on a radiograph. Fluoroscopy and fiberoptic bronchoscopy may be used to identify, locate, and extract the AFB.

The child with an AFB is usually stabilized in the emergency department and admitted for overnight observation. Mechanical ventilation may be needed temporarily. Depending on the type of object and degree of obstruction, surgical removal of the object may be required.

■ CLINICAL TIP

If the child cannot say the "P" in words like Pluto or Peter Pan, the expiratory effort is noticeably diminished as a result of the foreign body.

Nursing Assessment

PHYSIOLOGIC ASSESSMENT. If the object remains lodged, the child is observed for increasing signs of respiratory distress, especially vital signs and audible wheezing on auscultation. Changes in breath sounds, from noisy to decreasing to absent, on the affected side are noted. This can indicate that the object is moving and blocking a mainstem bronchus.

PSYCHOSOCIAL ASSESSMENT. The unexpected and acute nature of the hospitalization creates anxiety for both parents and child. The child and parents also may be experiencing a variety of other emotions—fear, anger, or guilt. The nurse should assess coping and level of stress. Providing a quiet environment and encouraging the presence of the parents help to reduce the child's fear and anxiety.

DEVELOPMENTAL ASSESSMENT. As the child's condition stabilizes, the nurse observes how well the child's abilities match the parents' understanding of age-appropriate behaviors. Providing anticipatory teaching or reinforcing information about developmental characteristics (see Chapter 2) helps parents to anticipate safety hazards in the future.

Nursing Diagnoses

Common nursing diagnoses for a child with an AFB include the following:

- Ineffective Airway Clearance related to foreign object trauma (previously removed or coughed out object)
- Ineffective Breathing Pattern related to inflamed tracheobronchial tree (object in place, or removed with traumatic edema)
- Fear/Anxiety (Parent or Child) related to uncertainty of prognosis, unfamiliar surroundings and procedures
- Knowledge Deficit (Parent) related to follow-up required after discharge, childproofing the home

Nursing Management

The first 12 hours after aspiration are critical, and subtle changes in the child's respiratory status during this period must be documented and reported promptly.[8] The child and family should be apprised of procedures and provided with emotional support.

DISCHARGE PLANNING AND PATIENT/FAMILY HOME CARE TEACHING. Discharge planning centers on anticipatory guidance about childproofing the home (see Chapter 2) and encouraging the parents to learn CPR, choking prevention techniques, and foreign body removal (Heimlich maneuver) (refer to the Atlas of Pediatric Procedures).

Near-Drowning

Near-drowning incidents and death by drowning are most prevalent in children under 5 years of age. In this age group, drowning is the single leading cause of death resulting from injury.[22] Groups at high risk include toddlers, teenage boys, and children with seizure disorders. Children with seizure disorders may experience sudden and uncontrollable loss of body position that places them at risk without warning.

Near-drowning has been called an accident of uncertainty. It is defined as survival for 24 hours following a submersion injury. Near-drowning may result in complete recovery, severe brain injury, or variable neurologic deficits.[23] A key feature influencing survival is initiation of spontaneous respiratory effort by the child within 5 minutes after removal from the water.[22] In the absence of spontaneous respirations, mouth-to-mouth ventilation should be started as quickly as possible. The mouth is cleaned of foreign matter, but time should not be wasted trying to remove water from the lungs. The sooner the child is ventilated, the better the chance of survival with normal neurologic potential. Emergency transport to a hospital should occur as soon as possible, even if spontaneous breathing is initiated.

Most drownings occur in the child's home pool or at the residence of a neighbor, friend, or relative. Usually the child is playing, is not wearing a swimsuit, and is briefly unsupervised before the immersion. Other common drowning sites for young children include bathtubs, hot tubs, toilets, and even large water-filled buckets. A child can drown in as little as 2 inches of water and an infant in 1 inch.[22] In most immersion cases, hypoxemia begins within seconds and irreversible nervous system cell changes begin within 4 to 6 minutes (refer to Chapter 14).[23]

Nursing Management

Nursing management focuses on observation and support of cardiopulmonary and central nervous system function (see Chapter 14). Frequent monitoring and assessment of vital signs provide valuable baseline information. The nurse should document any change in respiratory status and notify the physician promptly. A chest radiograph may be ordered to establish baseline information about lung expansion and pulmonary integrity. Pulse oximetry will be ordered to provide ongoing data about the child's oxygenation status.

The child and family need support to work through the feelings surrounding the near-drowning incident, the unexpected hospitalization, and an uncertain prognosis that may mean the child will not return to normal functioning. Prevention is the key to avoiding a similar mishap in the future.

Smoke Inhalation Injury

Exposure to fire conditions sets up dramatic responses in the respiratory tract of children. In every age group, inhalation injury significantly increases the child's chance of death.[24]

The severity of the smoke inhalation injury is influenced by the type of material burned. The composition of materials determines how easily they ignite, how fast they burn, and how much heat they release. These factors influence the production of smoke and toxic gases. Smoke, a product of the burning process that is composed of gases and particles, is generated in varying volumes and density. The type and concentration of toxic gases, which are usually invisible, affect the severity of pulmonary damage. Smoke particles are carried deep into the respiratory tract (sometimes as far as the alveoli), where they combine with water in the lungs. This can produce strong acids that burn the tissue, causing loss of cilia, loss of surfactant, and edema. Toxic gases, such as cyanide and ammonia, produce tissue destruction, edema, and loss of gas exchange capacity. The duration of exposure to the smoke produced and any toxic gases contribute significantly to the child's prognosis.

Exposure to extreme heat, common in house fires, leads to surface injury and upper airway damage. The upper airway normally removes heat from inhaled gases, sparing the lower airway from thermal damage. However, this action results in marked edema, placing the small child at particular risk for airway obstruction. Edema develops rapidly over a few hours and may create marked respiratory distress. Burns of the face and neck, singed nasal hairs, soot around the mouth or nose, and hoarseness with stridor or voice change all indicate inhalation injury.

Carbon monoxide (CO) is a clear, colorless, odorless gas that is present in all fire conditions. The CO molecule binds more firmly to hemoglobin than does oxygen. As a result, it replaces oxygen in circulation and rapidly produces hypoxia in the child. The longer the exposure to CO, the greater the hypoxia. The brain receives inadequate oxygen, resulting in confusion. This accounts for the inability of fire victims to escape as confusion progresses to loss of consciousness. The process can be rapidly reversed, however, by timely administration of 100% oxygen.[24]

Damage to the lower airway most often results from chemicals or toxic gas inhalation. Soot is carried deep into the lungs and deposits acid-producing chemicals on the lung tissue. Tissue destruction, edema, and gas exchange disruption produce the initial insult to the lungs. Days later, the damaged tissue sloughs off, obstructing the airways. Because the cilia that normally help in removing debris have been destroyed, the lungs become a breeding ground for microorganisms. Pneumonia becomes a major health concern. The damaged alveoli heal by scar tissue formation. This can greatly reduce the future functioning of the lungs.

Nursing Management

Most children who survive smoke inhalation injury are admitted for close observation and ventilatory support, if indicated. Respiratory assessment and pulmonary therapy are usually required to reestablish adequate oxygenation and respiratory function.

Blunt Chest Trauma

Blunt trauma is a common result of injury in children.[8] Chest injuries may not be obvious and can be extremely difficult to evaluate.

After sustaining blunt trauma, most children die from lack of oxygen caused by poor airway and ventilatory control. A child's elastic, pliable chest wall and thin abdominal muscles provide minimal protection to underlying organs. This elasticity often spares bone but not the underlying organs. The energy from blunt trauma is transferred directly from an external force to the internal organs, often causing a pulmonary contusion or pneumothorax.

Pulmonary Contusion

A pulmonary contusion is defined as bruising damage to the tissues of the lung. This causes bleeding into the alveoli, which may lead to capillary rupture in the air sacs. Edema develops in the lower airways as blood and fluid from damaged tissues accumulate. Lower airway obstruction and atelectasis may result.[25]

Pulmonary contusion occurs in up to 76% of children with nonpenetrating chest trauma. Initially the child may appear asymptomatic. Careful observation is required during the first 12 hours after the injury.

Nursing Management

Nursing care centers on providing necessary physiologic support. The child's level of consciousness is an excellent indicator of respiratory function. Agitation and lethargy can signal increasing hypoxia. The thorax should be inspected for symmetric chest wall movement and equal presence of breath sounds in both lungs. The child may initially appear well but requires careful and thorough monitoring to detect signs of deterioration. Children with significant injuries are cared for in the intensive care unit. Some children require ventilator support as the pulmonary tissues heal.

Pneumothorax

A pneumothorax occurs when air collects between the pleural layers, causing the lung to collapse. If blood collects in the pleural space, it is called a hemothorax, and if blood and air collect, it is called a pneumohemothorax. A pneumothorax is one of the more common thoracic injuries in pediatric trauma patients.

There are three types of pneumothorax: open, closed, and tension. Open pneumothorax, sometimes referred to as a sucking chest wound, results from any penetrating injury that exposes the pleural space to atmospheric pressure, thereby collapsing the lung.

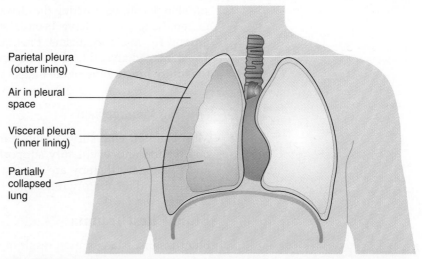

FIGURE 10–13 A pneumothorax is air in the pleural space that causes a lung to collapse. Whether the air results from an open injury or from bursting of alveoli due to a blunt injury, it is important to focus on airway management and maintain lung inflation.

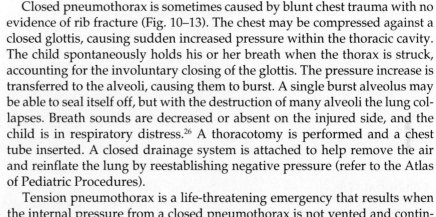

Closed pneumothorax is sometimes caused by blunt chest trauma with no evidence of rib fracture (Fig. 10–13). The chest may be compressed against a closed glottis, causing sudden increased pressure within the thoracic cavity. The child spontaneously holds his or her breath when the thorax is struck, accounting for the involuntary closing of the glottis. The pressure increase is transferred to the alveoli, causing them to burst. A single burst alveolus may be able to seal itself off, but with the destruction of many alveoli the lung collapses. Breath sounds are decreased or absent on the injured side, and the child is in respiratory distress.[26] A thoracotomy is performed and a chest tube inserted. A closed drainage system is attached to help remove the air and reinflate the lung by reestablishing negative pressure (refer to the Atlas of Pediatric Procedures).

Tension pneumothorax is a life-threatening emergency that results when the internal pressure from a closed pneumothorax is not vented and continues to build, compressing the chest contents and collapsing the lung. Air leaks into the chest cavity during inhalation but is trapped from escape during exhalation. Venous return to the heart is impaired as the trachea, heart, vena cava, and esophagus are compressed toward the unaffected lung when the mediastinum shifts. Signs of tension pneumothorax include increasing respiratory distress, decreased breath sounds, and paradoxic chest motion or "see-sawing" of the chest.

Nursing Management

Nursing management focuses on airway management and maintaining lung inflation. The child arrives on the nursing unit with a chest tube and drainage system in place. Continued close observation for respiratory distress is essential. Vital signs are carefully monitored. Complications include hemothorax (if the thoracotomy and chest tube are improperly placed), lung tissue injury, and scarring from poor tube placement (especially if the tube is placed too near the breast in girls).[27]

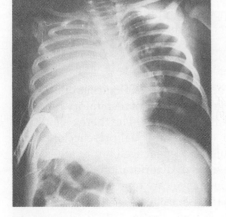

Pneumothorax

REFERENCES

1 U.S. Dept of Health and Human Services. (1986). *Pediatric respiratory disorders.* (NIH Publication No. 86-2107). Bethesda, MD: Division of Lung Diseases.

2 DeJong, S., & McCandless, S. (1983). *The respiratory system.* In Smith, J.B. (Ed.), Pediatric critical care. (pp. 21–87). New York: John Wiley & Sons.

3 National Institutes of Health Consensus Development Conference on Infantile Apnea and Home Monitoring. (1986). *Pediatrics, 79(2),* 292–299.

4 Eichenwald, E., & Stark, A. (1992). Apnea of prematurity: etiology and management. *Tufts University School of Medicine Reports on Neonatal Respiratory Diseases, 2(1),* 1–11.

5 Rosenstein, B.J., & Fosarelli, P.D. (1989). *Pediatric pearls.* St. Louis: Mosby.

6 Betz, C.L., & Poster, E.C. (1989). *Pediatric nursing reference.* St. Louis: Mosby.

7 Selekman, J. (1988). *Pediatric nursing: a study and learning tool.* Springhouse, PA: Springhouse.

8 Thompson, S.W. (1990). *Emergency care of children.* Boston: Jones & Bartlett.

9 Hazinski, M.F. (1992). *Nursing care of the critically ill child.* (2nd ed.). St. Louis: Mosby.

10 Hathaway, W.E., Hay, W.W., Groothuis, J.R., & Paisley, J.W. (Eds.). (1993). *Current pediatric diagnosis and treatment.* (11th ed.). Norwalk, CT: Appleton & Lange.

11 National Asthma Education Program, Expert Panel on the Management of Asthma. (1991). *Guidelines for the diagnosis and management of asthma* (DHHS Publication No. 91-3042A). Washington, D.C.: U.S. Government Printing Office.

12 Reinke, L.F., & Hoffman, L.A. (1992). How to teach asthma co-management. *American Journal of Nursing, 10,* 40–51.

13 Feeg, V.D., & Harbin, R.E. (Eds.). (1991). *Core curriculum and resource manual.* Pitman, NJ: Anthony J. Jannetti.

14 EPA to affirm passive smoke as cancer risk. (1993, January). *USA Today,* p. 1D.

15 Coleman, D.A. (1986). Pneumonia: where nursing care really counts. *RN, 2,* 22–29.

16 Boutotte, J. (1993). T.B. The second time around.... *Nursing, 5,* 42–50.

17 Landon, C., & Rosenfeld, R.G. (1984). Short stature and pubertal delay in male adolescents with cystic fibrosis. *American Journal of Diseases in Children, 138(4),* 388–391.

18 George, M.R. (1990). CF: not just a pediatric problem anymore. *RN, 9,* 60–65.

19 Nurses Reference Library. (1986). *Diagnostics* (2nd ed.). Springhouse, PA: Springhouse.

20 Canam, C. (1986). Talking about cystic fibrosis within the family—what parents need to know. *Issues in Comprehensive Pediatric Nursing, 9,* 167–178.

21 Campbell, L.S., & Thomas, D.O. (1991). Pediatric trauma: When kids get hurt. *RN, 8,* 32–39.

22 Wintemute, G.J. (1992). Drowning in early childhood. *Pediatric Annals, 21(7),* 417–421.

23 Coffman, S.P. (1992). Home care of the child and family after near-drowning. *Journal of Pediatric Health Care, 6,* 18–24.

24 Lybarger, P.M. (1987). Inhalation injury in children: Nursing care. *Issues in Comprehensive Pediatric Nursing, 10,* 33–50.

25 Jordan, K. (1990). Chest trauma. *Nursing, 9,* 34–42.

26 Eichelberger, M.R., Ball, J.W., Pratsch, G.S., & Runion, E. (1992). *Pediatric emergencies.* Englewood Cliffs, NJ: Brady.

27 Eichelberger, M.R., & Pratsch, G.L. (1988). *Pediatric trauma care.* Rockville, MD: Aspen.

SUGGESTED READINGS

American Lung Association. (1990). Childhood asthma—a matter of control (Publication No. 6012).

Back, K.J. (1991). Sudden, unexpected pediatric death: Caring for the parents. *Pediatric Nursing, 17(6),* 571–575.

Betz, C.L., & Poster, E.C. (1989). *Pediatric nursing reference.* St. Louis: Mosby.

Campbell, L.S., & Thomas, D.O. (1991). Pediatric trauma: When kids get hurt. *RN, 8,* 32–39.

Carlson, K.L. (1989). Assessing a child's chest. *RN, 11,* 26–32.

Cunningham, J.C., & Taussig, L.M. (1991). An introduction to cystic fibrosis for patients and families (Publication No. N8554A-4). Bethesda, MD: Cystic Fibrosis Foundation.

Clarke, P.H., & Deeds, N.C. (1988). The child in a mist tent. *Pediatric Nursing, 14(6),* 446–450.

Coffman, S.P. (1992). Home care of the child and family after near-drowning. *Journal of Pediatric Health Care, 6,* 18–24.

Dickison, A.E. (1990). Child with upper airway obstruction: Part I. *Choices in Respiratory Management, 20(2),* 29–34.

Dickison, A.E. (1990). Child with upper airway obstruction: Part II. *Choices in Respiratory Management, 20(3),* 66–68.

Fernbach, S.D., & Thomson, E.J. (1992) Molecular genetic technology in cystic fibrosis: Implications for nursing practice. *Journal of Pediatric Nursing, 7(1),* 20–25.

Griffith, H.W. (1989). *Complete guide to pediatric symptoms, illness & medications.* Los Angeles: The Body Press.

Hathaway, W.E., Hay, W.W., Groothuis, J.R., & Paisley, J.W. (Eds.). (1993). *Current pediatric diagnosis & treatment* (11th ed.). Norwalk, CT: Appleton & Lange.

Lybarger, P.M. (1987). Inhalation injury in children: Nursing care. *Issues in Comprehensive Pediatric Nursing, 10,* 33–50.

Manley, L.K. (1987). Pediatric trauma: Initial assessment and management. *Journal of Emergency Nursing, 13(2),* 77–87.

Nelson, N., & Beckel, J. (1987). *Nursing care plans for pediatric patients.* St. Louis: Mosby.

Polin, R.A., & Ditmar, M.F. (1989). *Pediatric secrets.* St. Louis: Mosby.

Smith, J. (1983). Pediatric critical care. New York: John Wiley & Sons.

Thompson, S.W. (1990). *Emergency care of children.* Boston: Jones & Bartlett.

Wintemute, G.J. (1992). Drowning in early childhood. *Pediatric Annals, 21(7),* 417–421.

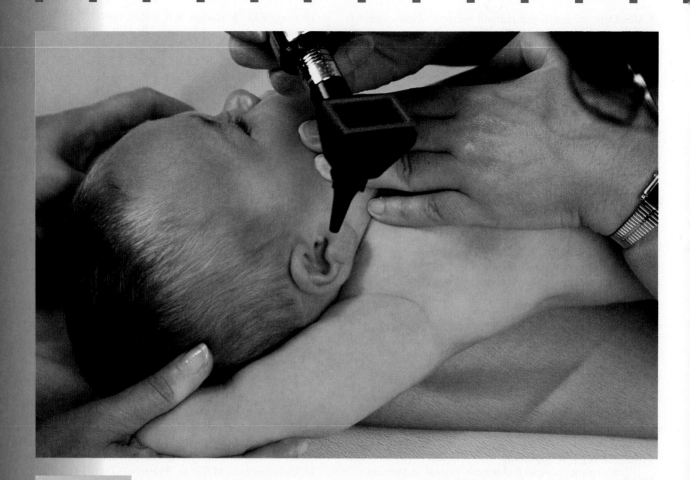

Tommy, a 12-month-old child, has been in the hospital 1 day for treatment of an acute upper respiratory infection. He has no appetite, has diarrhea, and is cranky. Tommy awoke several times last night and has been pulling at his ear. He has had two previous ear infections since the age of 5 months. Each one was cured by a 10-day course of antibiotics.

On assessment, Tommy's tympanic membrane shows signs of infection. He is diagnosed as having otitis media. The course of antibiotics being used to treat his respiratory infection will also treat his ear infection. However, long-term antibiotic therapy most likely will be necessary to prevent future ear infections.

Three months later Tommy is examined in his normal well-child care visit. A tympanogram shows that the mobility of the tympanic membrane has improved. Although this is a positive outcome, Tommy will need follow-up monitoring to ensure that his hearing and development are normal.

ALTERATIONS IN EYE, EAR, NOSE, AND THROAT FUNCTION

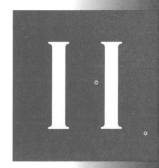

II

audiography   A test used to assess hearing in which sounds of various pitches and intensity are presented to children through earphones.

conductive hearing loss   Hearing loss caused by inadequate conduction of sound from the outer to the middle ear.

decibels   Units used to measure the loudness of sounds.

myringotomy   Making an incision in the tympanic membrane to drain fluid.

sensorineural hearing loss   Hearing loss caused by damage to the inner ear structures or the auditory nerve.

tympanostomy tubes   Small Teflon tubes inserted surgically into the tympanic membrane to promote fluid drainage and ventilate the middle ear.

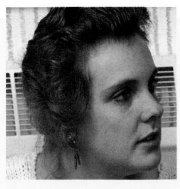

❝ I was very worried about Tommy's ear infections. I wondered if they would affect his hearing and maybe even his ability to talk. The nurse says the important thing is to try to prevent ear infections in the future. ❞

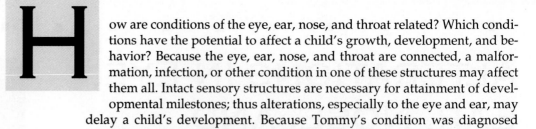

ow are conditions of the eye, ear, nose, and throat related? Which conditions have the potential to affect a child's growth, development, and behavior? Because the eye, ear, nose, and throat are connected, a malformation, infection, or other condition in one of these structures may affect them all. Intact sensory structures are necessary for attainment of developmental milestones; thus alterations, especially to the eye and ear, may delay a child's development. Because Tommy's condition was diagnosed and treated when he was very young, he should develop normally.

Most children with eye, ear, nose, and throat disorders are treated at home rather than in the hospital.

Anatomy and Physiology of Pediatric Differences

Eye

How are the eyes of children different from those of adults? Chapter 3 provides a detailed discussion of the assessment of the eyes and visual acuity. The eyes of neonates differ from the eyes of adults in several ways. Visual acuity in neonates ranges between 20/100 and 20/400. The lens is more spherical and cannot accommodate to both near and far objects, which means that the neonate sees best at a distance of about 8 inches. Since the optic nerve is not yet completely myelinated, the ability to distinguish color and other details is decreased. If the infant is preterm, especially less than 32 weeks' gestation, retinal vascularization, particularly in the periphery of the retina, may be incomplete. The rectus muscles that control binocular vision may be somewhat uncoordinated at birth. The eyes should be aligned and movement coordinated by the age of 3 months.

As infants grow, their eyes mature and their vision improves. By the age of 2 or 3 years most children have 20/50 vision, and by the age of 6 or 7 they have 20/20 vision.

The eyeball of the infant and young child occupies a larger portion of the orbit than in the adult. Since the eyeball is relatively unprotected laterally, it is more easily injured. The sclera of the neonate is thin and translucent with a bluish tinge. The iris of newborns is blue or gray. Eye color changes during the first 6 months of life.

Infants produce tears to nourish and oxygenate the outer layers of the cornea. Parents do not see tears when a young infant cries because the infant's lacrimal system efficiently drains tears into the nasal cavity.

Ear

Why do infants and young children have more ear problems than adults? The eustachian tube, which connects the nasopharynx to the middle ear, is proportionately shorter, wider, and straighter in infants than in older children or adults (Fig. 11–1). During sucking, yawning, and other movements the tube opens for milliseconds, allowing free passage of air between the nasopharynx and the middle ear.

The external ear canal is small at birth, although the internal ear and middle ear are relatively large. As a result the tympanic membrane is close to the surface and can be easily injured.

Nose and Throat

Up to the age of 6 months, infants can breathe only through the nose and not through the mouth. Edema and nasal discharge may interfere with adequate air intake and feeding. Mucosal swelling and exudate may block the small nasal passages of young children.

FIGURE 11-1 Of the three anatomic differences in the eustachian tube between adults and small children (shorter, wider, straighter), which do you think could cause more problems for the child and why? Answer: Straighter. Small children who are bottle-fed in a supine position have a greater probability of developing otitis media because the eustachian tube opens when the child sucks and the straight angle of the tube provides easy access to the middle ear. In older children the greater angle helps keep foreign substances and germs away from the middle ear.

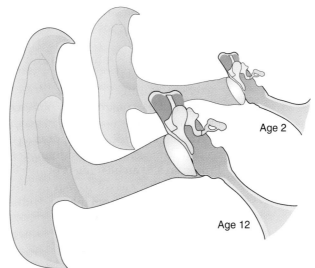

Position of eustachian tube is at a lesser angle in the young child, resulting in decreased drainage.

Age 2

End of eustachian tube in nasal pharynx opens during sucking.

Eustachian tube equalizes air pressure between the middle ear and the outside environment and allows for drainage of secretions from middle ear mucosa.

Age 12

The palatine tonsils, which are visible on oral examination, are located on each side of the oropharynx. The method for examining a child's throat is given in Chapter 3. Although tonsils vary in size considerably during childhood, they are normally large, especially in school-age children. The nasopharyngeal tonsils (adenoids) lie in the posterior wall of the nasopharynx, just above the oropharynx. In children the adenoids may become enlarged, harboring bacteria and interfering with breathing.

Disorders of the Eye

Infectious Conjunctivitis

Conjunctivitis is inflammation of the conjunctiva, the clear membrane that lines the inside of the lid and sclera. Bacteria, viruses, allergies, trauma, or irritants cause the conjunctiva to become swollen and red with a yellow or white discharge (Fig. 11-2). Organisms such as *Chlamydia trachomatis* and *Neisseria gonorrhoeae* are responsible for conjunctivitis in neonates but are less common or do not occur in older children.

In infants who have frequent tearing and "mattering" (eyelid discharge that has formed a crust) on awakening, a plugged lacrimal duct may mimic

FIGURE 11-2 Acute conjunctivitis. The major difference between bacterial and viral conjunctivitis is that bacterial conjunctivitis has a purulent discharge that may result in crusting whereas discharge from viral conjunctivitis is serous (watery). Allergic conjunctivitis produces watery to thick drainage and is characterized by itching.
Adapted from Newell, F.W. (1992). *Ophthalmology: Principles and concepts* (7th ed.). St. Louis: Mosby–Year Book.

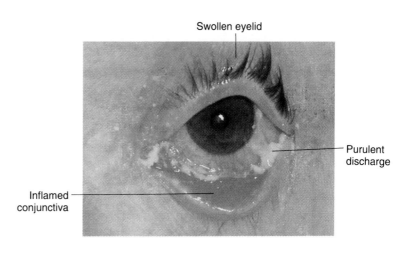

Swollen eyelid

Purulent discharge

Inflamed conjunctiva

conjunctivitis. Treatment involves massaging the tear duct every 4 hours when the infant is awake. Lacrimal ducts that remain plugged after the age of 1 year may have to be opened surgically.

Older children with conjunctivitis complain of itching or burning, mild photophobia, and a feeling of roughness under the lids. Parents may notice increased tearing or a mucoid or mucopurulent discharge, redness and swelling of the conjunctiva, a pink sclera, and crusty eyelids, especially in the morning. There is no change in vision.

Antibiotic eye drops are prescribed if a bacterial infection is suspected. Directions concerning their administration are given in the Atlas of Pediatric Procedures. If an allergen is believed to be the cause, antihistamines administered orally or as drops may be prescribed. Parents should be instructed to clean the exudate from the eye with a washcloth or cotton ball before instilling the medication.

Nursing Management

Since infectious conjunctivitis is extremely contagious, tell parents that children should not return to school until they have been taking an antibiotic for 24 hours. Instruct parents of the need for careful handwashing and avoidance of sharing towels. Tell parents that children should not rub their eyes. Mittens may help prevent infants from rubbing their eyes. Toddlers may be distracted by activities that keep their hands busy. Children should be kept in an upright position to reduce swelling.

Periorbital Cellulitis

Periorbital cellulitis is an infection of the eyelid and surrounding tissues (Fig. 11–3). It is usually caused by bacteria. Children present with swollen, tender, red or purple eyelids; restricted, painful movement of the area around the eye; and fever. Periorbital cellulitis should be treated promptly to prevent the spread of the infection to the optic nerve. Management includes hospitalization for intravenous administration of antibiotics and the application of hot packs. Children usually respond favorably within 48 to 72 hours.

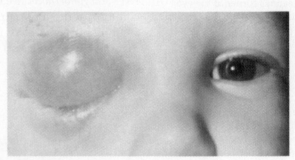

FIGURE 11–3 Periorbital cellulitis is an infection of the eyelid and surrounding tissue, not the eye itself. It is a serious bacterial infection that can spread to the optic nerve if not treated promptly with intravenous antibiotics.
From Malinow, I., & Powell, K.R. (1993). *Pediatric Annals, 22*(4), 244.

Visual Disorders

Visual disorders must be diagnosed and treated promptly to prevent impairment or loss of vision. The description and management of strabismus, amblyopia, cataracts, and glaucoma are presented in Table 11–1.

TABLE 11-1 Visual Disorders

Disorder	Treatment
Strabismus	
Eyes appear misaligned to observer. Most common types: Esotropia: inward deviation of eyes ("crossed eyes") Exotropia: outward deviation of eyes ("wall-eyes") May occur only when child is tired Symptoms include: squinting and frowning when reading; closing one eye to see; having trouble picking up objects; dizziness and headache Corneal light reflex and cover-uncover tests confirm diagnosis	**Occlusion therapy** (patching the fixating or good eye to force use of the weak eye) Corrective lenses Surgery of the rectus muscles to correct muscle imbalance; should be performed only after eye patching Eye drops to cause blurring of the good eye Prisms Eye exercises If treatment is begun before 24 months of age, amblyopia (reduced vision in one or both eyes) may be prevented
Amblyopia	
Reduced vision in one or both eyes Amblyopia can result from untreated strabismus, with the child "tuning out" the image in deviating eye Symptoms are the same as for strabismus Vision testing can be used to diagnose condition	Corrective lenses Occlusion therapy Treatment is discontinued when visual acuity no longer improves; 20/20 vision rarely attained
Cataracts	
Occur when all or part of lens of eye becomes opaque, which prevents refraction of light rays onto retina Can affect one or both eyes and may be congenital or acquired Clouding of lens indicates presence of cataract; however, cataracts are not always visible to naked eye Symptoms include: distorted red reflex; symptoms of vision loss (see strabismus)	Specific treatment depends on whether one or both eyes are affected, extent of clouding, and presence of other ocular abnormalities Surgical removal of lens and corrective lenses; contact lenses frequently used; results of surgery are good; surgery before the age of 2 months is associated with the best results; visual acuity in 55% of children is 20/40 or better Eye protectors and restraints are used postoperatively to prevent injury; antibiotic or steroid drops may be used for several weeks; treatment for amblyopia may be necessary
Glaucoma	
Increased intraocular pressure damages eye and impairs visual function; ciliary body of eye produces aqueous fluid that flows between iris and lens into anterior chamber; if enough fluid accumulates, blindness results May be congenital or acquired and affect one or both eyes Symptoms of congenital glaucoma include: tearing, corneal clouding, eyelid spasms, and progressive enlargement of eye; photophobia (extreme sensitivity to light) Symptoms of acquired glaucoma include: constant bumping into objects in child's periphery (painless visual field loss); seeing halos around objects Diagnosis is made using **tonometer**, which measures intraocular pressure	Surgery to reduce intraocular pressure is treatment of choice, since medications used to combat glaucoma in adults are not effective in children Corrective lenses used following surgery Treatment is not always successful, especially if the child has congenital glaucoma, so parents' feelings regarding care of a visually handicapped child should be explored

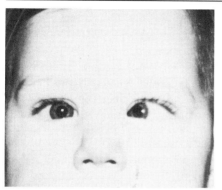

Strabismus.
From Newell, F.W. (1992). *Opthalmology: Principles and concepts* (7th ed.) (p. 409). St. Louis: Mosby–Year Book.

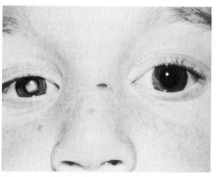

Congenital cataract.
From Vaughan, D., Asbury, T., & Riordan-Eva, P. (1992). *General opthalmology* (13th ed.) (p. 172). Norwalk, CT: Appleton & Lange.

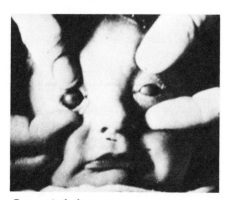

Congenital glaucoma.
From Vaughan, D., Asbury, T., & Riordan-Eva, P. (1992). *General opthalmology* (13th ed.) (p. 172). Norwalk, CT: Appleton & Lange.

Retinopathy of Prematurity

Retinopathy of prematurity (ROP) occurs when immature retinal blood vessels constrict and become necrotic. This condition, which may occur in infants of low birth weight or of short gestation, eventually leads to retinal detachment and impaired vision or blindness. Although excessive oxygen therapy is associated with the development of ROP, other factors such as apnea and infection may lead to this disorder.

Retinal changes become visible when infants with ROP are between 4 and 9 weeks of age. ROP spontaneously arrests in 75% to 90% of infants.[1]

Injuries of the Eye

In the United States eye injuries are most common in boys 11 to 15 years of age.[2] Foreign bodies, blunt and sharp objects, chemical and thermal burns, physical irritants, toys, and abuse may cause eye trauma. Some injuries can

TABLE 11–2 Emergency Treatment of Eye Injuries

Injury	Treatment
Subconjunctival hemorrhage (caused by coughing, mild trauma, or increased physical activity)	Usually heals spontaneously; child should see ophthalmologist if most of sclera is covered or if condition does not clear up in 1 to 2 weeks
Periorbital ecchymosis ("black eye")	Apply ice to eye area for 5 to 15 minutes every hour for the first 1 to 2 days after injury; then apply warm compresses; even if only one eye is affected, gravity may cause both eyes to discolor
Foreign body on conjunctiva	Do not let child rub eye; remove material on surface of eye by closing upper lid over lower lid, irrigating or everting upper lid, visualizing material, and removing it with slightly damp handkerchief; patch eye and transport child to emergency department if foreign body cannot be removed
Corneal abrasion	Superficial corneal abrasions are diagnosed by touching sterile fluorescein strip to lower conjunctiva; dye remains where corneal epithelial cells are disrupted; most corneal abrasions heal spontaneously or antibiotic ointment may be prescribed and eyes patched in some children
Burns (alkaline burns readily penetrate cornea and are more serious than acid burns)	For child with chemical burn, irrigate eye for 15 to 30 minutes; transport child to emergency department, where irrigation should continue (see Atlas of Pediatric Procedures); pupils are dilated to reduce pain and prevent adhesions; after irrigation is complete, eyes are patched and antibiotics are prescribed
Penetrating and perforating injuries	Obtain medical assistance immediately; *never* try to remove an object that has penetrated the child's eye; such objects should be removed by an ophthalmologist; prevent the child from rubbing injured eye; cover both eyes with shield before transportation to emergency department
Eye injuries caused by severe blows to head and eye (blunt trauma can seriously injure all eye structures, including orbit, which can be fractured)	Transport immediately to ophthalmologist's office or emergency department for evaluation and treatment

be treated at home, but many necessitate a trip to the emergency room or require hospitalization. Table 11–2 summarizes emergency treatment of common eye injuries.

Disorders of the Ear

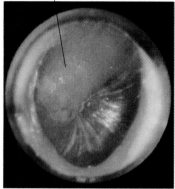

Bulging tympanic membrane

FIGURE 11–4 Acute otitis media is characterized by pain and a red, bulging, nonmobile tympanic membrane.

From Malasanos, L., Barkauskas, V., & Stoltenberg-Allen, K. (1990). *Health assessment* (4th ed.) (Plate 2). St. Louis: Mosby–Year Book. Courtesy Richard A. Buckingham, M.D., Clinical Professor, Otolaryngology, University of Illinois College of Medicine at Chicago, Chicago, IL.

Otitis Media

Otitis media, or inflammation of the middle ear, is sometimes accompanied by infection. This condition is one of the most common childhood illnesses. Between 76% and 95% of all children have at least one episode by 6 years of age,[3] and the greatest incidence is between 6 and 36 months of age.[3,4] Otitis media occurs more frequently among boys and in children who attend day care centers. It is most common during the winter months.

Clinical Manifestations

Otitis media is categorized according to symptoms and the length of time the condition has been present (Table 11–3). Pulling at the ear is a sign of ear pain. Diarrhea, vomiting, and fever are typical of otitis media. Irritability and "acting out" may be signs of a related hearing impairment. Since some children with otitis media are asymptomatic, an ear examination should be performed at every health care visit (see Chapter 3). A red, bulging, nonmobile tympanic membrane is a sign of otitis media (Fig. 11–4).

Etiology and Pathophysiology

The specific cause of otitis media is unknown, but it appears to be related to eustachian tube dysfunction. Often an upper respiratory infection precedes the development of otitis media, leading to a predictable sequence of events as was the case with Tommy. Infection causes the mucous membranes of the eustachian tube to become edematous. As a result air, which normally fills the middle ear, is reabsorbed into the bloodstream. Fluid is pulled from the

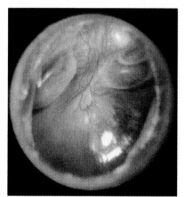

FIGURE 11–5 Otitis media with effusion is noted on otoscopy by fluid line or air bubbles.

From Malasanos, L., Barkauskas, V., & Stoltenberg-Allen, K. (1990). *Health assessment* (4th ed.) (Plate 2). St. Louis: Mosby–Year Book. Courtesy Richard A. Buckingham, M.D., Clinical Professor, Otolaryngology, University of Illinois College of Medicine at Chicago, Chicago, IL.

TABLE 11–3 Types of Otitis Media

Type	Duration	Clinical Manifestations
Acute otitis media (AOM)	Rapid onset; 1 to 3 weeks' duration	Tympanic membrane (TM) red, retracted or bulging, and painful; ear pulling; fever; hearing loss caused by presence of fluid; possible spontaneous TM rupture resulting in fluid drainage and reduction of pain
Recurrent otitis media (ROM)	Similar onset and duration to AOM, but repeated episodes in succession	Similar to those of AOM
Otitis media with effusion (OME) (Fig. 11–5)	May precede or follow any stage of OM	Ear popping; feeling of pressure in middle ear; pain; hearing loss; TM retracted; fluid line or bubbles via otoscopy
Chronic otitis media (COM)	Slow onset and persistence of 3 months or more	TM thick, immobile, retracted; if TM perforated, drainage from ear; tympanogram abnormal; hearing loss

Modified from Novak, J.C., & Novak, R.E. (1993). *Small Talk* 5(2), 1, 3-7.

mucosal lining into the former air space, providing a medium for the rapid growth of pathogens. The tympanic membrane and fluid behind it become infected. The most common causative organisms are *Streptococcus pneumoniae, Haemophilus influenzae,* and *Neisseria catarrhalis.*[3-6]

Other conditions, such as enlarged adenoids or edema from allergic rhinitis, can also obstruct the eustachian tube and lead to otitis media. Since children with certain facial malformations (cleft palate) and genetic conditions (Down syndrome) usually have compromised eustachian tubes, these children are more vulnerable to the development of otitis media.[3,6]

Diagnostic Tests and Medical Management

Diagnosis is based on otoscopic examination. A "flat" tympanogram is also suggestive of otitis media.

Acute and recurrent otitis media are treated with antibiotic therapy for 10 to 14 days. The choice of antibiotic depends on the probable organism, ease of administration, cost, previous effectiveness, and any history of allergies.[6,7] First-line drugs include amoxicillin, trimethoprim-sulfamethoxazole, erythromycin, and doxycycline.[8] Cephalosporins are commonly used for recurrent infections. Diarrhea and skin rash are the most common side effects of antibiotic therapy.[5,6,8] Treatment of recurrent or chronic otitis media may include a 6-month trial of prophylactic antibiotics.[6]

Neither decongestants nor antihistamines have been shown to be effective in the treatment of otitis media. The HIB vaccine routinely given to children, beginning at 2 months of age, may reduce the incidence of disease in children that is caused by *Haemophilus influenzae* type B. If infection recurs, **myringotomy** (surgical incision of the tympanic membrane) may be performed and **tympanostomy tubes** inserted to drain fluid from the middle ear. Although surgical treatment is believed to reduce recurrent infection and improve hearing, research has shown that this approach may be no more effective than waiting for the condition to resolve on its own.[6] Enlarged and infected adenoids may be removed at the same time.

Prolonged otitis media may result in sensorineural or conductive hearing loss and cochlear damage.

Nursing Assessment

The tympanic membrane is assessed for color, transparency, mobility, presence of landmarks, and light reflex.

Nursing Diagnosis

Several nursing diagnoses that may apply to the child with otitis media are included in the accompanying Nursing Care Plan.

Nursing Management

Since most children with otitis media are not hospitalized (unless myringotomy or adenoidectomy is being performed), nursing management centers on care of the child in the home. Occasionally, children admitted to the hospital for other problems have a concurrent ear infection that requires nursing care. The accompanying Nursing Care Plan summarizes nursing care for the hospitalized child with otitis media.

Chronic otitis media can create many problems for the family. The child's waking at night with ear pain results in lack of sleep and parental fatigue. Parents often become frustrated and disillusioned with the inability of the

■ **PARENT TEACHING: TYMPANOSTOMY TUBES**

- Water should not enter the ears. Children should use earplugs when bathing and swimming and should not put their head under water.
- Tympanostomy tubes do not have to be removed. They usually fall out spontaneously after 6 months.

■ **GROWTH AND DEVELOPMENT CONSIDERATIONS**

Fluid accumulation in the middle ear prevents the efficient transmission of sound and can result in hearing loss over a period of time, potentially delaying speech and language development. These delays may manifest as cognitive deficits or behavior problems.

health care system to cure the child and may fear a permanent hearing impairment. Reassure parents that as the child grows older, the recurrent infections eventually cease.

Injuries of the Ear

Ear injuries of many types commonly occur in children. Lacerations, infections, and hematomas may occur in the external ear structures, especially the pinna. Children may place foreign objects in the ear, and insects may enter the ear canal. Rupture of the tympanic membrane may result from head injuries, blows to the ear, or insertion of objects into the ear canal.

Table 11–4 presents information on the emergency treatment of ear injuries. Any injury resulting in earache, decreased hearing, persistent bleeding, or other discharge should be seen by a physician.

TABLE 11–4 Emergency Treatment of Ear Injuries

Injury	Treatment
Pinna	
Minor cuts or abrasions	Wash thoroughly with soap and water and rinse well; leave exposed to air if possible or apply adhesive bandage; monitor for infection
Hematomas	Needle aspiration should be performed and pressure dressing applied; undrained hematomas may become fibrotic; "cauliflower ear" deformity may develop
Cellulitis or abscesses	Apply moist heat intermittently; make sure that prescribed antibiotic is taken; minor surgery may be performed for an abscess
Deep lacerations	Apply pressure to stop bleeding; transport to physician's office or emergency department for suturing
Ear Canal	
Foreign bodies	Have child lie on back and turn head over edge of bed, with affected side down; wiggle earlobe and have child shake head; foreign object may fall out as result of gravity; if object remains in ear, call physician; do not try to remove foreign body with tweezers since this may push the object further into the ear
Insects	Shine flashlight into ear to try to attract insect; instilling a few drops of mineral oil, olive oil, or alcohol kills insect, and irrigating ear canal gently may remove dead insect (see Atlas of Pediatric Procedures)
Tympanic Membrane	
Ruptures	Call physician if child has persistent ear pain after blow, blast injury, or insertion of foreign object; cover external ear loosely with piece of sterile cotton or gauze; if tympanic membrane has been ruptured, systemic antibiotics are prescribed

THE CHILD WITH OTITIS MEDIA

GOAL	INTERVENTION	RATIONALE	EXPECTED OUTCOME
1. Pain related to inflammation and pressure on tympanic membrane			
Child or parent will indicate absence of pain.	Give analgesic such as acetaminophen. Use analgesic eardrops.	Analgesics alter perception or response to pain.	Verbal child states that pain is relieved. Nonverbal child has improved disposition and comfort.
	Have child sit up, raise head on pillows, or lie on unaffected ear.	Elevation decreases pressure from fluid.	
	Apply heating pad or warm hot water bottle.	Heat increases blood supply and reduces discomfort.	
	Ask an older child to pinch nose, close lips, and force air through eustachian tube. Have younger child chew gum or blow on balloon.	Clearing actions may help aerate middle ear.	
2. Infection related to presence of pathogens			
Child will be free of infection.	Instruct parents to administer antibiotics exactly as directed and to complete prescribed course of medication.	Blood level of antibiotic must remain constant for prescribed time period to kill pathogens.	Child's temperature is normal, symptoms have disappeared and tympanic membrane shows no signs of infection.
	Telephone parents 2 or 3 days after initiation of antibiotic therapy.	If symptoms have not improved in 36 hours, a new antibiotic may have to be prescribed.	
	Examine ear 3 or 4 days after completion of antibiotic treatment.	Check-up determines whether infection has cleared up and if effusion is present.	
3. High Risk for Caregiver Role Strain related to chronic disease			
Parents will manage child's condition with minimal stress.	Determine parent's ability to manage condition. Provide frequent information and feedback.	Many parents can treat children at home. Knowledge of condition allows parents to make informed decisions and to manage condition effectively.	Parents express confidence about treating the child and state that stress is reduced.
	Encourage parental input in managing care.	Active participation increases confidence and ability to manage condition.	
	Listen carefully to parental expressions of frustration and fatigue and try to understand parents' feelings.	Reacting empathetically encourages parents to communicate.	

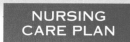

THE CHILD WITH OTITIS MEDIA—CONTINUED

GOAL	INTERVENTION	RATIONALE	EXPECTED OUTCOME

4. Knowledge Deficit related to common recurrence of infection in children resulting from anatomic differences in young children and frequent exposure to infectious agents

GOAL	INTERVENTION	RATIONALE	EXPECTED OUTCOME
Parents will state understanding of preventive measures.	Teach family members to cover mouths and noses when sneezing or coughing and to wash hands frequently. Have parents isolate sick children.	Good hygiene prevents spread of pathogens.	Child has fewer recurrences or reinfections.
	Encourage optimal nutrition, rest, and exercise.	Physical well-being helps body fight disease.	
	Position bottle-fed infants upright when feeding. Do not prop bottles.	Elevated position prevents injection of milk and pathogens into eustachian tube.	
	Eliminate allergens and upper respiratory irritants such as tobacco, smoke, and dust.	Fewer irritants and allergens may decrease susceptibility to respiratory infections. Secondhand smoke contributes to higher incidence of otitis media.	

5. High Risk for Altered Growth and Development related to hearing loss

GOAL	INTERVENTION	RATIONALE	EXPECTED OUTCOME
Child will have normal hearing.	Assess hearing ability frequently.	Monitoring detects hearing loss early.	Child's general health and hearing improve, and incidence of condition decreases.

Disorders of the Nose and Throat

Epistaxis

Epistaxis, or nosebleed, is common in school-age children, especially boys. Kiesselbach's plexus, an area of plentiful veins located in the anterior nares, is the most common source of bleeding. The most common cause is irritation from nosepicking, foreign bodies, or low humidity. Other causes include forceful coughing, allergies, or infections resulting in congestion of the nasal mucosa. Bleeding from the posterior septum is more serious and may be life threatening. Hospitalization may be necessary. Posterior nosebleeds have a variety of causes, some of which may indicate systemic disease (i.e., bleeding disorder) or injury.

Children with nosebleeds are sometimes brought to the emergency department by a parent who has been unable to stop the flow of blood in a few minutes. Both parent and child may be frightened. The parent should be questioned briefly about any history of nosebleeds and other contributing factors, including medications. The child's pulse and blood pressure should be taken to assess for excessive blood loss. The nasal mucosa should be carefully examined by asking the child to blow any clots out gently, if possible. Suctioning may be necessary.

Observing the flow may help determine whether the blood comes from an anterior or a posterior location. A nosebleed confined to one side of the nose is almost always anterior, but posterior bleeding can flow on one or both sides. If blood cannot be observed, the child may be swallowing it and may become nauseous. Suspect posterior bleeding in children with blunt trauma or in other children at high risk.

The child with anterior bleeding should sit upright quietly. The head should be tilted forward to prevent trickling of blood down the throat, which may lead to vomiting. The nares should be squeezed just below the nasal bone and held for 10 minutes while the child breathes through the mouth. If the bleeding does not stop, a cotton ball or swab soaked with Neo-Synephrine, epinephrine, thrombin, or lidocaine may be inserted into the affected nostril to promote topical vasoconstriction or anesthesia. Once the bleeding has ceased, the nostril may have to be cauterized by means of silver nitrate or electrocautery. If the bleeding cannot be stopped, the child should be sedated and one or both nostrils packed with gauze impregnated with petroleum jelly. The packing should remain in place between 1 and 7 days.[9]

Posterior bleeding must also be stopped by packing, and the child must be monitored carefully in the hospital.

Nursing Management

The child's hematocrit or hemoglobin should be assessed if significant bleeding has occurred. Children with frequent epistaxis should have a complete history taken and physical examination performed to rule out systemic disease.

After the nosebleed has stopped, the child is more vulnerable to rebleeding and should avoid bending over, stooping, strenuous exercise, hot drinks, and hot baths or showers for the next 3 to 4 days. Sleeping with the head elevated on two or three pillows and humidifying the air may also prevent relapse. Provide parents with general suggestions for prevention and home management of epistaxis (Table 11–5).

TABLE 11–5 Discharge Teaching: Prevention and Home Management of Epistaxis

Prevention

- Humidify the child's room, especially during the winter.
- Discourage the child from picking or rubbing the nose or inserting foreign objects into the nose.
- Moisten the nasal mucosa by applying normal saline nose drops.
- Instruct the child to blow the nose gently and release sneezes through the mouth.
- Apply a thin layer of petroleum jelly twice a day to the septum to relieve dryness and irritation.

Home Management

- Keep the child calm.
- Sit the child upright with head tilted slightly forward so blood does not run down the throat.
- Insert a cotton ball with hydrogen peroxide, nasal decongestant, petroleum jelly, or plain water into the affected nostril. The cotton ball should be moist.
- Apply steady pressure to both nostrils just below the nasal bone with the thumb and forefinger for 10 to 15 minutes. Time by the clock.
- Apply an ice pack or cold compress to the bridge of the nose or the back of the neck.
- Gently remove the cotton ball after the time is up.
- Call physician if the bleeding does not stop.

Modified from Wolff, R. (1982). *Nurse Practitioner*, 7(10), 16. Reprinted with permission of Elsevier Science Publishing. Copyright © 1982.

■ CULTURAL CONSIDERATIONS

Many Hispanic and Asian cultural groups believe in the "hot and cold theory" of disease, in which health and disease are viewed as the result of a balance or imbalance. For example, Mexican-Americans traditionally treat a cold disease, such as an earache or common cold, with hot substances. Nurses should be aware of such culturally influenced beliefs about health and illness.

Nasopharyngitis

Nasopharyngitis, also known as the "common cold," causes inflammation and infection of the nose and throat and is probably the most common illness of infancy and childhood. More than 200 viruses and numerous bacteria cause this condition. The most common viruses include rhinovirus and coronavirus, and the most frequently occurring bacterium is group A Streptococcus. The organisms incubate in 1 to 3 days, and the infection is communicable several hours before symptoms develop and for 1 to 2 days after they begin.[10] Symptoms may last 4 to 10 days or longer. The pathogens are believed to spread when the infected person touches the hand of an uninfected individual, who then touches his or her mouth or nose, resulting in self-inoculation.

A red nasal mucosa with clear nasal discharge and an infected throat with enlarged tonsils may be apparent in children with nasopharyngitis. Vesicles may be present on the soft palate and in the pharynx. Clinical manifestations may vary, depending on the child's age (Table 11–6).

Between episodes of nasopharyngitis, children should be asymptomatic. If children have continual upper respiratory infections, the presence of underlying conditions such as allergy, asthma, or polyps should be ruled out.

Nursing Management

For infants who cannot breathe through the mouth, normal saline nose drops can be administered every 3 to 4 hours, especially before feeding. (Refer to the Atlas of Pediatric Procedures for instructions on how to administer nose drops.) For infants over 9 months of age, nasal stuffiness can be treated with either normal saline nose drops or a decongestant such as phenylephrine (0.125% to 0.25%, depending on the child's age). Older children can use nasal sprays.

Although nose drops and sprays are more effective than systemic decongestants, they should not be used for more than 4 or 5 days. Antihistamines may be helpful for children with allergic rhinitis or profuse nasal drainage. Long-acting nasal sprays and medications with several ingredients are not recommended.

Room humidification may help prevent drying of nasal secretions. Antipyretics such as acetaminophen reduce fever and make the child more comfortable. Aspirin is not recommended because of its association with Reye syndrome (refer to Chapter 14).

Children should avoid strenuous physical activity and engage in quiet play that includes reading, listening to music or stories, or watching television or videotapes. Children should not be forced to eat, but the intake of favorite fluids to liquify secretions should be encouraged. Parents should be told that no medicine or vaccine can prevent the common cold, but eliminating contact with infected persons can reduce the spread of infection. Good handwashing and proper disposal of tissues also discourage spread of the infection.

Pharyngitis

Acute pharyngitis is an infection that primarily affects the pharynx, including the tonsils (Fig. 11–6). It is seen most frequently in children 4 to 7 years of age and is rare in children less than 1 year of age.[10] Approximately 80% of these infections are caused by viruses; the rest are caused by bacteria. Bacterial infection, commonly known as "strep throat," results from infection by group A beta-hemolytic *Streptococcus* (GABHS).

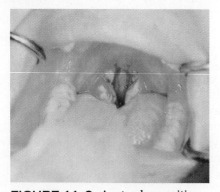

FIGURE 11-6 Acute pharyngitis primarily affects the pharynx but often involves the tonsils, as in this child.

From Malasanos, L., Barkauskas, V., & Stoltenberg-Allen, K. (1990). *Health assessment*. (4th ed.) (Plate 4). St. Louis: Mosby–Year Book. Courtesy Edward L. Applebaum, M.D., Chicago.

TABLE 11-7 Clinical Manifestations of Viral Pharyngitis and Strep Throat (Group A Beta-Hemolytic *Streptococcus* [GABHS])*

Viral Pharyngitis	Strep Throat
Nasal congestion	Tonsillar exudate†
Mild sore throat	Painful cervical lymphadenopathy†
Conjunctivitis	Abdominal pain
Cough	Vomiting
Hoarseness	Severe sore throat
Mild pharyngeal redness	Headache
Minimal tonsillar exudate	Fever >101° F
Mildly tender anterior cervical lymphadenopathy	Petechial mottling of soft palate
Fever <101° F	

*Children 6 months to 3 years of age may have streptococcosis with symptoms that resemble those of viral pharyngitis. Children with scarlet fever have the symptoms of strep throat plus a sandpaper-textured erythematous generalized rash and pallor around the lips.
†Classic signs of strep throat.

The major complaint is a sore throat. Table 11–7 contrasts clinical manifestations of viral pharyngitis and strep throat. Children who have symptoms of strep throat; who have minimal throat redness and pain, exudate, mild lymphadenopathy, and low fever; and who have been exposed to someone who has pharyngitis should have a throat culture. A child who finds swallowing difficult or extremely painful, who drools, or who exhibits respiratory distress or dehydration should be seen by a physician immediately. These could be symptoms of serious conditions such as epiglottitis, peritonsillar or retropharyngeal abscess, or diphtheria.

The diagnosis of strep throat is made by throat culture. Early signs of strep throat should be treated with oral penicillin for 10 days or given in one injection immediately, even before the result of the culture is available.[9,11,12] If the child is allergic to penicillin, erythromycin is also effective. Acute symptoms should resolve within 24 hours of therapy, at which time the child is no longer contagious.[10-13]

Nursing Management

Nursing care focuses on symptomatic relief. Acetaminophen reduces throat pain and generalized fever. Cool, nonacidic fluids and soft foods, ice chips, or frozen juice pops given frequently in small amounts facilitate swallowing and prevent dehydration. Humidification, sucking on hard candy, and gargling with warm salt water (1 teaspoon salt to 8 ounces water) soothe irritated throats. Commercial throat sprays or throat lozenges are no more effective than hard candy and contain ingredients that can lead to allergies.[12] Encourage the child to rest, to conserve energy and promote recovery.

Teach parents the importance of completing the 10-day course of antibiotics. Untreated streptococcal infections may lead to rheumatic fever, cervical adenitis, sinusitis, or meningitis. Other possible complications of streptococcal infections include peritonsillar abscess and retropharyngeal abscess.

Tonsillitis

Tonsillitis is an infection or inflammation (hypertrophy) of the palatine tonsils. Although most children with pharyngitis may have infected tonsils, they do not necessarily have tonsillitis.

■ **CLINICAL TIP**

Throat cultures must be properly performed for accurate diagnosis. A sterile cotton- or Dacron-tipped applicator is swabbed across the tonsils, posterior edge of the soft palate, and uvula.
- Cooperative children can be asked to put their hands under their buttocks, open their mouth, and laugh or pant like a dog. The throat is quickly swabbed.
- Uncooperative and younger children are placed on their back with their hands next to their head and held by parent or other person. The tongue is gently depressed with a tongue blade and the throat is swabbed.

■ **CLINICAL TIP**

Children may be more willing to gargle with salt water if the mixture is placed in a spray bottle and sprayed gently toward the throat.

Clinical Manifestations

Symptoms suggestive of tonsillitis include frequent throat infections with breathing and swallowing difficulties; persistent redness of the anterior pillars; and enlargement of the cervical lymph nodes. If children breathe through their mouths continuously, the mucous membranes may become dry and irritated.

Etiology and Pathophysiology

Like pharyngitis, tonsillitis may be caused by viruses or bacteria. The primary site of infection is the tonsils.

Diagnostic Tests and Medical Management

Diagnosis is made on the basis of visual inspection and clinical manifestations. Symptomatic treatment for tonsillitis is the same as for pharyngitis. Surgical removal of tonsils is controversial and does not always eliminate the symptoms.[10] However, children who have chronically hypertrophied tonsils that obstruct breathing and swallowing or who have repeated infections with cervical adenitis are candidates for tonsillectomy.[10,14] If the child is under 3 years of age, the surgery is postponed if possible because it may stimulate growth of other lymphoid tissue in the nasopharynx. If the pharyngeal tonsils (adenoids) are enlarged, as suggested by mouth breathing, cough, impaired taste and smell, a muffled quality to the voice, and chronic otitis media, they may be removed at the same time.

Nursing Assessment

If surgery is indicated, take a complete history of the child preoperatively. Monitor vital signs and observe for hemorrhage and dehydration postoperatively.

Nursing Diagnosis

Several nursing diagnoses may apply to the child with tonsillitis. They include:

- Pain related to inflammation of the pharynx
- High Risk for Fluid Volume Deficit related to throat pain and reluctance to swallow
- High Risk for Ineffective Breathing Pattern related to obstruction by enlarged tonsils

Nursing diagnoses for the child who is having a tonsillectomy are found in the accompanying Nursing Care Plan.

Nursing Management

The nurse provides general supportive care and, if medication is prescribed, encourages completion of the full course of treatment. The nursing management of children with tonsillitis is similar to that of children with pharyngitis (see earlier discussion).

If surgery is indicated, the parents are helped to prepare their child for a short-term surgical procedure with an overnight stay in the hospital. Children should be free of sore throat, fever, or upper respiratory infection for at least 1 week before surgery. They should not be given aspirin or ibuprofen for 2 weeks before surgery, since these medications can increase bleeding.

Postoperative care of the child is described in the accompanying Nursing Care Plan. The child usually remains overnight in the hospital.

Discharge Planning and Patient and Family Home Care Teaching. Discharge planning includes teaching parents about pain management, fluid and nutrition intake, activity restrictions, and possible complications in the postoperative period. Most children will have a sore throat for 7 to 10 days after tonsillectomy. After an adenoidectomy, the sore throat will be mild, lasting only 1 to 2 days. Advise parents that to relieve the child's throat pain, they should:

- Have the child drink adequate fluids or chew gum, since this reduces spasms in the muscles surrounding the throat.
- Give acetaminophen elixir, as ordered.
- Apply an ice collar around the child's neck.
- Have the child gargle with a solution of ½ teaspoon each of baking soda and salt in a glass of water.
- Have the child rinse the mouth well with viscous lidocaine and then swallow the solution.

Children may experience ear pain, especially when swallowing, between 4 and 8 days after tonsillectomy. Advise parents that this is the result of pain referred from the tonsillar area and does not indicate ear infection.

Emphasize to parents the importance of adequate fluid intake. Children should be given any liquid they prefer for the first week, except citrus juices, which may produce a burning sensation in the throat. Soft foods such as gelatin and mashed potatoes can be added as tolerated.

Children do not need to be confined to bed, but vigorous exercise should be avoided for the first week after surgery. Advise parents that the child may return to school approximately 10 days after tonsillectomy or 3 to 4 days after adenoidectomy.

Any surgery carries with it the risk of postoperative complications. Teach parents the normal signs of healing in the postoperative period, as well as signs of complications (Table 11–8).

TABLE 11–8 Discharge Teaching: Complications of Tonsillectomy and Adenoidectomy

Bleeding
- To prevent bleeding, aspirin should not be given for pain for the first postoperative week. Use acetaminophen instead.
- Bleeding is most likely to occur within the first 24 hours or 7 to 10 days after the tonsillectomy, when the scar is forming. Report any trickle of bright red blood to the physician immediately.

Infection
- The back of the throat will look white and have an odor for the first 7 to 8 days after the surgery. The child also may have a low-grade fever. These are not signs of infection.
- For temperatures over 101° F, acetaminophen may be used.
- Call the physician if the child develops a fever above 102° F.

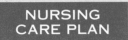
THE CHILD UNDERGOING A TONSILLECTOMY

GOAL	INTERVENTION	RATIONALE	EXPECTED OUTCOME
1. Pain related to surgical procedure			
Child and parents will indicate that pain is controlled.	Assess pain by: Asking child or parent about pain Observing for signs of discomfort such as restlessness Pain scale Give pain medication every 3 to 4 hours (acetaminophen or acetaminophen with codeine) Use nonpharmacologic pain strategies such as ice collar or distraction (playing, reading, watching television)	Adequate pain management promotes faster healing. Nonpharmacologic methods can be an effective adjunct to pain medications.	Child and parents indicate that pain is controlled.
2. High Risk for Fluid Volume Deficit related to reluctance to swallow due to pain			
Child will be hydrated.	Maintain intravenous line until child is taking oral fluids. Encourage the child to take cold or cool foods or liquids such as ice chips, ice pops (no red or brown), or ice cream. Do not give the child citrus juice or carbonated beverages.	Intravenous fluids can maintain adequate fluid balance. Throat pain can lead to spasm and reduce the desire to swallow. Cool liquids provide an anesthetic effect to the throat. Red or brown liquids can be confused with blood if they are vomited. Citrus juices and carbonated beverages may cause more pain.	Child shows signs of hydration (moist mucous membranes, good skin turgor, adequate urinary output).
3. High Risk for Injury related to postoperative complications			
Child will have no symptoms of fresh bleeding.	Avoid irritating the surgical site with hot liquids, irritating foods or straws. Instruct the child to avoid clearing throat or coughing vigorously. Observe for signs of hemorrhage, including frequent swallowing, large amounts of bright red bloody emesis or coffee-ground emesis, restlessness, pallor, elevated pulse and respiratory rate. Report signs of bleeding to physician immediately.	Surgical site can be irritated by hot or rough-textured foods. Straws have the potential to create a vacuum and initiate bleeding. The force of coughing can initiate bleeding. Bleeding is the most common immediate postoperative complication of tonsillectomy. The child needs to be returned to surgery for ligation or cautery of bleeding vessel before life-threatening shock develops. Hemorrhage may result in hypovolemic shock if not detected early.	Child has no symptoms of fresh bleeding. If bleeding is discovered, child does not develop hypovolemic shock.

Continued.

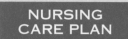
THE CHILD UNDERGOING A TONSILLECTOMY—CONTINUED

GOAL	INTERVENTION	RATIONALE	EXPECTED OUTCOME
4. Impaired Swallowing related to inflammation and pain			
Child will not aspirate secretions.	Place child in flat, side-lying, or prone position immediately after surgery.	Proper positioning facilitates drainage of secretions.	Child aspirates neither secretions nor fluids.
	Do not give liquids until the child is completely awake.	Swallowing when conscious prevents aspiration.	
	Have parents or nurse stay with child.	Assistance and vigilance by continuous presence may prevent aspiration of secretions.	
	Use bulb syringe to suction. Have suction machine available for anterior oral suction only.	Bulb syringe or suction machine ensures prompt removal of secretions.	
5. Knowledge Deficit related to discharge care			
Parents will state understanding of postoperative instructions and restrictions.	Assess parents' anxiety about caring for child at home. Discuss discharge instructions and potential complications with parents (Table 11–8).	Information helps to reduce parental anxiety.	Parents describe appropriate monitoring and care of child at home. Parents describe actions to take if complications occur.

Child with a Sensory Impairment

Visual Impairment

Children whose vision cannot be corrected by prescription lenses are considered to be visually impaired. Approximately 2 of every 500 schoolchildren in the United States do not have corrected 20/20 vision.[15] Children who see no better than 20/70 in their best eye, when corrected, are said to have poor vision. Legal blindness is defined as 20/200 or worse in the corrected eye; about 1 child in 2500 is legally blind.[15]

The manifestations of visual impairment depend on the cause and degree of the problem and the age of the child (Table 11–9). The child's eyes may appear crossed or watery, and the lids may be crusty. Verbal children may complain of itching, dizziness, headache, blurred vision, seeing double, or poor vision.

Many conditions discussed in the section on alterations in eye function lead to temporary or permanent visual impairment. Infants who are premature, whose mothers were infected prenatally with rubella, toxoplasmosis, or other viruses, and who have certain congenital and hereditary conditions have a high risk of visual problems (Table 11–10).[15]

Medical management depends on the child's condition and may include surgery, medication, and supportive aids. In the case of a disorder that results in permanent visual impairment, an interdisciplinary team of specialists works with the child and family.

TABLE 11–9 Clinical Manifestations of Visual Impairment

Infants

May be unable to follow lights or objects
Do not make eye contact
Have a dull, vacant stare
Do not imitate facial expressions

Toddlers and Older Children

May rub, shut, or cover eyes
Tilt or thrust head forward
Blink frequently
Hold objects close
Bump into objects
Squint

TABLE 11-10 Common Causes of Visual Impairment in Children

Congenital or Hereditary

Cataracts
Glaucoma
Tay-Sachs disease
Marfan syndrome
Prenatal infections (maternal infection)
    Rubella
    Toxoplasmosis
    Herpes simplex
Retinoblastoma

Acquired

Injury to eye or head
Infections
    Rubella
    Measles
    Chickenpox
Brain tumor
Retinopathy of prematurity

■ GROWTH AND DEVELOPMENT CONSIDERATIONS

Vision affects both fine and gross motor skills, so skills such as hand-to-mouth coordination and walking may be delayed in children who are visually impaired. Children who have vision problems may also take longer to master self-help skills such as feeding and dressing.

Nursing Assessment

Vision screening facilitates early detection and treatment of conditions that can lead to vision loss.

Visual testing can be done at any age, including immediately after birth. Developmental milestones that require vision, such as following bright lights, reaching for objects, or looking at pictures in a book, can be used to assess vision. For children over the age of 3 years, visual acuity is most frequently measured by means of an age-appropriate Snellen chart (see Chapter 3 and the Atlas of Pediatric Procedures). Visual fields and ability to discriminate colors are not tested until school age, when children can cooperate.

Children who are visually impaired lag in development of cognitive and other skills. Sighted children learn the word "cup" using four senses—sight, touch, hearing, and taste—to obtain the information necessary to connect words with the objects they represent. In contrast, children with vision impairment rely on only three senses—touch, hearing, and taste. They learn concepts through differences in sounds, textures, and shapes. Children with vision problems are highly verbal and imitative, with good memories. However, they may use words and phrases out of context.

Nursing Diagnosis

Common nursing diagnoses for the child with impaired vision include:

- Sensory/Perceptual Alteration (Visual) related to specific condition
- High Risk for Injury related to poor vision
- High Risk for Altered Growth and Development related to visual impairment
- High Risk for Ineffective Family Coping related to a child with a sensory impairment

Nursing Management

Nursing care focuses on encouraging the child's use of all senses, promoting socialization, helping parents to meet the child's schooling needs, and providing emotional support to parents.

Encourage Use of All Senses. Children who are partially sighted or blind use other senses to a great extent. Encouraging the use of the eyes as much as possible is important even if a child has poor vision.

- Encourage a toddler or preschooler who is visually impaired to look at pictures in well-lit settings. Have a school-age child read large-print books. Computers with large letters are also available.
- Expose the infant and child to everyday sounds.
- Suggest that the parents encourage the infant to use the sense of touch to explore people and objects. Have the parents purchase toys with sound and texture in mind. Directional concepts can be taught using games. Responding to the infant's and child's vocalizations encourages the use of speech.
- Teach specific techniques for toileting, dressing, bathing, eating, and safety. When the child becomes mobile, furniture and other objects in the environment should be kept in the same positions so the child can safely move around independently.
- Emphasize the child's abilities. Adolescents can use seeing-eye dogs to function independently.

- If the child is in a hospital or another strange environment, orient the child to the placement of objects and do not rearrange them. Always announce your presence to the child when approaching. When walking with a blind child, walk slightly ahead of the child so the child can sense your movements, and let the child hold your arm rather than the reverse. Identify the contents of meal trays. Encourage the child to function independently within normal developmental parameters.

Promote Socialization. The child's interactions and socializations should be as normal as possible (similar to those of sighted children of the same age and development).

- Stroke, rock, and hug infants and children who are visually impaired. Sing and talk to them. These infants do not make eye contact and have rather blank expressions.
- Teach parents to read body language and vocalization as expressions of emotion. Facial expressions give a great deal of information, but infants and children with poor vision do not have the ability to learn by visual imitation. Show parents how to use tactile means to teach appropriate facial expressions.
- Explain to parents that discipline and rewards for children with poor vision should be the same as those for other children in the family. The child should be given age-appropriate tasks.
- Encourage contact with peers as the child grows older. Teach the child to look directly at persons who are talking to him or her. Play, sports, and other activities can be modified to give the visually impaired child the same social experiences as a sighted child.

Help Parents to Meet Child's Schooling Needs. Public laws require that each state provide educational and related services for impaired children (see Chapter 1). Parents and professionals should develop an individual education plan that maximizes the child's learning ability. If possible, the child with a vision problem should attend day care and preschool with children who are not impaired.

- Provide parents with information about educational options before their child reaches school age. Education should take place in a setting that allows the child to have contact with other children and to participate in social activities. The child may be mainstreamed with a tutor, be partially mainstreamed in a resource room, attend special classes, or be tutored at home. If the child is to attend public school, suggest to parents that they contact the school well before enrollment to ensure that the personnel understand the child's disability.
- Make sure that equipment such as large-print books, braille materials, audio equipment, or an Optacon (a device that raises print so it can be felt by the child) is available.
- Familiarize the child with the environment.

Provide Emotional Support. The family often needs help to understand the child's abilities and disabilities.

- Encourage habilitation as soon as realistically possible. Make the adjustment easier by providing information about the child's specific type of visual impairment, available community services, and groups or associations for children with similar vision conditions. Refer to Appendix F for a list of resources for families of children with vision disorders.

- Be supportive and listen to the family's concerns regarding the child's visual deficit.
- Make sure the parents meet their own physical and emotional needs so that they are better able to care for and provide support to their child.

Hearing Impairment

Approximately 1 million children in the United States have some form of hearing impairment. Hearing impairment is expressed in terms of **decibels** (dB), which are units of loudness, and is rated according to severity (Table 11–11). Children who have only a mild hearing loss (35 to 40 dB) may miss 50% of everyday conversation and are considered at high risk for school failure. Children with more than a 90 dB hearing loss are considered legally deaf.

Infants and children at risk for hearing loss include those with recurrent otitis media, congenital perinatal infections such as rubella or herpes, anatomic malformations involving the head or neck, low birth weight (less than 1500 g), hyperbilirubinemia, bacterial meningitis, and severe asphyxia at birth.[16] Parents should be aware of excessive noise at home and at school. Teenagers who use earphones at high volumes or attend many rock concerts are at risk for hearing loss.

Hearing disorders can be classified according to the location of the deficit. **Conductive hearing loss** occurs when conditions in the external auditory canal or tympanic membrane prevent sound from reaching the middle ear. Common causes include impacted cerumen, the most frequent reason for conductive loss; outer ear infection ("swimmer's ear"); trauma; or a foreign body. Conductive loss also occurs if the tympanic membrane does not fully vibrate, as in otitis media. The loss of acuity may be gradual or rapid and results in diminished hearing in all ranges.

Sensorineural hearing loss occurs when the hair cells in the cochlea or along the auditory nerve (cranial nerve VIII) are damaged. This leads to permanent hearing loss. Conditions leading to this type of hearing loss may be congenital (maternal rubella), genetic (Tay-Sachs disease), or acquired (from ototoxic drugs or loud noise).[16] In sensorineural hearing loss, high-frequency sounds are most affected. Mixed hearing loss is a combination of conductive and sensorineural loss.

Hearing is both an innate and a learned behavior. Infants and children who are hearing impaired exhibit a range of behaviors depending on the child's age and the severity of the deficit. Infants who hear normally respond to sound in both obvious and subtle ways that do not occur in those who are hearing impaired (Table 11–12). As children with hearing impairments mature, language skills are affected. Hearing loss is often manifest as a cognitive deficit, a behavioral problem, or both.

■ GROWTH AND DEVELOPMENT CONSIDERATIONS

Infants and children first respond automatically with a blink or the startle reflex to unexpected or loud sounds. As they mature, they localize the sound source, then understand speech, and then communicate verbally.

TABLE 11-11 Severity of Hearing Loss

Type of Loss	Hearing Ability
Slight/mild	Some speech sounds are difficult to percieve, particularly unvoiced consonant sounds
Moderate	Most normal conversational speech sounds are missed
Severe	Speech sounds cannot be heard at normal conversational level
Profound	No speech sounds can be heard; considered legally deaf
Deaf	No sound at all can be heard

TABLE 11-12 Behaviors Suggestive of Hearing Impairment

Age	Behavior
Infant	Has a diminished or absent startle reflex to loud sound Does not awaken when environment is very noisy Awakens only to touch Does not turn head to sound at 3 to 4 months Does not localize sound at 6 to 10 months Babbles little or not at all
Toddler and preschooler	Speaks unintelligibly, in a monotone, or not at all Communicates needs through gestures Appears developmentally delayed Appears emotionally immature, yells inappropriately Does not respond to doorbell or telephone Appears more interested in objects than people and prefers to play alone Focuses on facial expressions rather than verbal communications
School-age child and adolescent	Asks to have statements repeated Answers questions inappropriately, except when able to view speaker's face Daydreams and is inattentive Performs poorly at school or is truant Has speech abnormalities or speaks in a monotone Sits close to or turns television or radio up loudly Prefers to play alone

Nursing Assessment

The child's hearing should be assessed at every well child visit. The best judges of hearing are parents; they should be asked if they have any concerns about their child's hearing. An infant's reaction to rattles, bells, or handclapping (about 12 inches from the ear) is an important observation. Language milestones should be evaluated when the older infant and child are examined. Deaf infants begin to babble at about 5 to 6 months of age, the same age as hearing infants. This babbling ceases several months later.

An otoscopic examination with a tympanogram can be performed on an older infant to determine conductive hearing. A "flat" tympanogram suggests conductive hearing loss. **Audiography** can be used with cooperative children over 3 years of age. Sounds of various frequencies and intensities are presented to the child through earphones, and the child is instructed to raise his or her hand when the sound is heard. Audiography cannot detect loss caused by middle ear effusion but can indicate sensorineural loss.

The hearing of preschool and school-age children is tested by asking them to repeat whispered words or to indicate whether or not they hear a ticking watch. Hearing of school-age children and adolescents also is assessed with the Weber and Rinne tests (see Chapter 3).

If a hearing loss is uncorrectable, a team composed of a physician, audiologist, speech-language pathologist, psychologist, nurse, teacher, and social worker should work with the child and family. A hearing aid may be prescribed for a conductive loss. A sensorineural loss is more difficult to treat, but cochlear implants and bone conduction hearing aids have been used in some children. For children with both types of hearing loss, several approaches are used to enhance communication (Table 11–13). Children with hearing impairment may receive speech therapy and instructions in lipreading, signing, cuing, and fingerspelling.

TABLE 11–13 Communication Techniques for Children Who Are Hearing Impaired

Technique	Description
Cued speech	Supplement to lipreading; eight hand shapes represent groups of consonant sounds and four positions about the face represent groups of vowel sounds; based on the sounds the letters make, not the letters themselves; child can "see-hear" every spoken syllable a hearing person hears
Oral approach	Uses only spoken language for face-to-face communication; avoids use of formal signs; uses hearing aids and residual hearing
Total communication	Uses speech and sign, fingerspelling, lipreading, and residual hearing simultaneously; child selects communication technique depending on the situation

From Schwartz, S. (1987). *Choices in deafness: A parent's guide.* Rockville, MD: Woodbine House. Reprinted with permission.
For publications related to hearing-impaired children, contact Woodbine House (see Appendix F).

Nursing Diagnosis

Common nursing diagnoses for the child with impaired hearing include:

- Sensory/Perceptual Alteration (Auditory) related to a specific condition
- High Risk for Impaired Verbal Communication related to hearing loss
- High Risk for Altered Growth and Development related to communication impairment
- High Risk for Ineffective Family Coping related to a child with a hearing impairment

Nursing Management

Nursing care focuses on facilitating the child's ability to receive spoken language and to send information, helping parents to meet the child's schooling needs, and providing emotional support to parents.

Facilitate Ability to Receive Spoken Language. Be aware of how the child compensates for hearing loss and use these strategies in communication.

- If hearing loss is mild or temporary or if the child reads lips, first obtain the child's visual attention by lightly touching the child or saying the child's name. Position your face 3 to 6 feet from the child's face and make sure that the child's eyes are focused on your face and lips. Make sure lighting is good, with no backlighting. Speak at a normal rate and tone, and use facial expressions that show caring or concern. If the child does not understand, rephrase the information in shorter, simpler sentences. Use specific, concrete explanations, and give the child time to comprehend. Watch for subtle signs of misinterpretations and give consistent and immediate feedback. Only 30% of the English language is visible on the lips.[17,18]
- Be familiar with the different types of hearing aids. Hearing aids, which are microphones that amplify all sounds, can be worn in or behind the ear, in the frame of glasses, or on the body with a wire attached to the ear. When talking to a child with a hearing aid, speak slowly within 6 to 18 inches from the microphone using a normal conversational tone. Talk to the child even if the child is not looking at

you. Make sure the batteries are fresh for the best reception. Since all sound is amplified, reduce background noise as much as possible.

Acoustic feedback, an audible whistling sound that cannot always be heard by the child, is one of the most common problems with hearing aids. To eliminate this sound, readjust the hearing aid to make sure that it is inserted properly and that no hair or ear wax is caught between the ear mold and canal. Turning down the volume may also help.

A remote microphone system is another type of device designed to improve hearing. This is often used in the classroom situation because background noise is eliminated. The speaker wears a transmitter that picks up the voice and transmits it to a receiver worn by the child.

Facilitate Ability to Send Information. Many children with impaired hearing communicate using speech, which is enhanced through speech therapy. In addition, they are taught to sign, fingerspell, or use cued speech. Articulation may be difficult, and understanding what the child is trying to say may be frustrating for both the nurse and the child. Taking time to listen carefully is important.

- Ask the parents to explain the child's communication techniques and to help interpret words. Have younger children point to pictures. Use assisted technologies such as a picture board or drawings or gestures if necessary. This is especially helpful for communicating feelings of pain and hunger during hospitalization. If the child signs or fingerspells, make sure that you understand the signs for important functions.
- Give older children a pad of paper and pencil to write requests. People other than parents should be able to understand what the child is trying to communicate.

Help Parents to Meet Child's Schooling Needs. Public laws apply to the education of children who are hearing impaired (see Chapter 1). After diagnosis, the parents and professionals together agree on an individualized educational plan. Day care and preschool are recommended for children with hearing problems.

- Provide parents with information about adjustments that may have to be made for the hearing-impaired child who attends public school. By sitting at the front of the classroom, the child can hear and see more clearly. The teacher should always face the child when speaking, and background noise should be reduced.
- Tell parents that children who are hearing impaired have the same intelligence quotient distribution as children without hearing impairment. However, most deaf high school graduates read at about the fourth-grade level because communication and learning are difficult.[18] Children with hearing impairment should reach their intellectual potential, although development in certain areas may take place more slowly than it does in non-hearing-impaired children.

Provide Emotional Support. By recognizing the effects of the diagnosis on the family, the nurse can help the family deal with their reaction to the child's hearing loss. Supporting healthy coping is an important intervention to help the parents carry on with their lives.

- Help the parents understand the child's disability and its effect on speech and language development. Provide accurate information about their concerns. Work jointly with other health care professionals and social service workers if necessary.

- Tell the family about the community services available for medical, nursing, psychologic, and financial assistance. Refer to Appendix F for a list of resources for families of children with hearing disorders.

REFERENCES

1 Hunter, D.G., & Mukai, S. (1992). Retinopathy of prematurity: Nursing interventions. *International Ophthalmologic Clinics: Pediatric Ophthalmology, 32*(1), 163–181.

2 Catalano, R. (1992). Special considerations in the pediatric patient. In *Ocular emergencies* (pp. 91–105). Philadelphia: Saunders.

3 Novak, J.C., & Novak, R.E. (1993). Impact of otitis media on hearing and communication. *Small Talk, 5*(2), 1, 3–7.

4 Facione, N. (1990). Otitis media: An overview of acute and chronic disease. *Nurse Practitioner, 15*(10), 11–19.

5 Zenk, K.E., & Ma, H. (1990). Pharmacologic treatment of otitis media and sinusitis in pediatrics. *Journal of Pediatric Health Care, 4*(6), 297–303.

6 Kempthorne, J., & Giebink, G.S. (1991). Pediatric approach to diagnosis and management of otitis media. *Otolaryngologic Clinics of North America, 24*(2), 905–929.

7 Murph, J.R. (1989). Ear infections in young children. *Small Talk, 1*(2), 1, 3–6.

8 Harrison, C.J., & Belhorn, T.H. (1992). Acute otitis media. *Clinical Reviews, 2*(4), 53–65.

9 Wolff, R. (1982). Pediatric epistaxis. *Nurse Practitioner, 17*(10), 12–14, 16.

10 Arnold, J.E. (1992). The respiratory system: Upper respiratory tract. In R.E. Behrman (Ed.), *Nelson's textbook of pediatrics* (pp. 1054–1061). Philadelphia: Saunders.

11 Kenna, M.A. (1990). Sore throat in children. In Bluestone, C.D., & Stool, S. (Eds.), *Pediatric otolaryngology.* (2nd ed.). (Vol. II, pp 837–842.) Philadelphia: Saunders.

12 Schmitt, B.S. (1980). Sore throat. In *Pediatric telephone advice* (pp. 60–64.) Boston: Little, Brown.

13 Wald, E.R. (1990). Rhinitis and acute and chronic sinusitis. In Bluestone, C.D., & Stool, S. (Eds.), *Pediatric otolaryngology.* (2nd ed.). (Vol. II, pp. 729–744.) Philadelphia: Saunders.

14 Paradise, J.L. (1990). Tonsillectomy and adenoidectomy. In Bluestone, C.D., & Stool, S. (Eds.), *Pediatric otolaryngology.* (2nd ed.). (Vol. II, pp. 915–926.) Philadelphia: Saunders.

15 Kovalesky, A. (1985). The child with a visual impairment. In *Nurses' guide to children's eyes* (pp. 272–273). Orlando, FL: Grune & Stratton.

16 Letko, M.D. (1992). Detecting and preventing infant hearing loss. *Neonatal Network, 11*(5) 33–37.

17 Northcott, W.H. (1978). *Curriculum guide: Hearing impaired children and their parents.* Washington, DC: Alexander Graham Bell Association for the Deaf.

18 Bergh-Jackson, C. (1990). Primary health care for deaf children, Part II. *Journal of Pediatric Health Care, 4*(1), 39–40.

SUGGESTED READINGS

Futcher, J.A. (1988). Chronic illness and family dynamics. *Pediatric Nursing, 14*(5), 381–385.

Gardner, S.L., & Hagedorn, M.I. (1990). Physiologic sequelae of prematurity: The nurse practitioner's role. Part II. Retinopathy of prematurity. *Journal of Pediatric Health Care, 4*(2), 72–76.

George, D., Stephens, S., Fellows, R.R., & Bremer, D.L. (1988). The latest on retinopathy of prematurity. *MCN, 32*(4), 254–258.

Jackson, C.B. (1989). Primary health care for deaf children. Part I. *Journal of Pediatric Health Care, 3*(6), 316–318.

Kaye, B. (1990). The cure for lazy eye. *Journal of Ophthalmic Nursing and Technology, 9*(3), 90–93.

Long, C.A. (1989). Cryotherapy: A new treatment for retinopathy of prematurity. *Pediatric Nursing, 15*(3), 269–272.

Neumann, E., Friedman, Z., & Able-Peleg, B. (1987). Prevention of strabismic amblyopia of early onset. *Journal of Ophthalmic Nursing & Technology, 6*(6), 242–237.

Riley, M.A. (1987). *Nursing care of clients with ear, nose and throat disorders* (pp. 179–184). New York: Springer.

Tumulty, G., & Resler, M.M. (1984). Eye trauma. *American Journal of Nursing, 84*(6), 740–744.

White, G.L., Liss, R.P., & Crandall, A.S. (1991). Congenital glaucoma. *Physician Assistant, 15*(1), 45–46, 48–49, 69–71.

Wurst, J., & Stern, P.N. (1990). Childhood otitis media: The family's endless quest for relief. *Issues in Comprehensive Pediatric Nursing, 13*(1), 25–39.

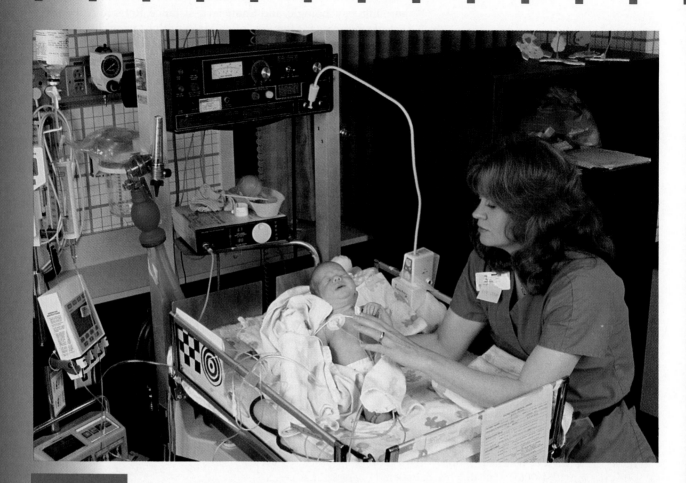

H elena, who is 1 month old, had a ventricular septal defect (VSD) at birth. Her parents are just beginning to accept that Helena has a congenital heart defect that may need surgical repair. Helena's cardiologist has advised them to watch their daughter for signs of respiratory distress and difficulty in feeding that could indicate the development of complications.

Helena's mother has become concerned because her daughter has been more difficult to feed and has been crying frequently for 2 days. Today she seems short of breath. On physical examination, Helena is lethargic and pale. Her heart rate is 166 beats per minute, her respiratory rate is 62 breaths per minute, and her liver is enlarged. She has gained 0.5 kg (1 pound) since her well-child visit 2 weeks ago.

Helena is immediately hospitalized with a diagnosis of congestive heart failure. She is treated with digoxin, furosemide (Lasix), and potassium. Over the next 2 days she loses the fluid weight she had gained. She feeds more actively, completes feedings, and smiles more often. Helena's parents take her home with instructions for daily administration of digoxin and furosemide and a description of the signs of congestive heart failure.

What are the causes of congestive heart failure? How is this condition treated? Will Helena need surgery sooner now that complications have occurred? What teaching and support do Helena's parents need?

ALTERATIONS IN CARDIOVASCULAR FUNCTION

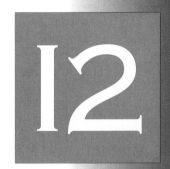

TERMINOLOGY

compliance Amount of distention or expansion that ventricles can achieve to increase stroke volume.

desaturated blood Blood with a lower than normal oxygen level resulting when a heart defect causes oxygenated and unoxygenated blood to mix.

digitalization Process of giving a higher than normal dose of digoxin initially to speed response to the drug.

hemodynamics Pressures generated by blood and passage of blood through the heart and pulmonary system.

hypoxemia Abnormally decreased arterial blood oxygen concentration.

palliative procedure Intervention used to preserve life in children with potentially lethal heart defects.

polycythemia Overproduction of red blood cells to increase the amount of hemoglobin available to carry oxygen.

preload Volume of blood in the ventricle at the end of diastole that stretches the heart muscle before contraction.

pulmonary hypertension Condition resulting from a chronic blood volume overload through the pulmonary arteries. It is often irreversible and leads to a life-threatening increase in pulmonary vascular resistance.

shunt Movement of blood between heart chambers through an abnormal anatomic or surgically created opening.

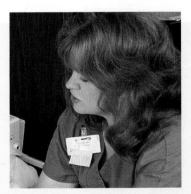

❝ Helena's parents should do fine caring for her at home. But they have already experienced a lot of stress and the next few weeks will be difficult. I am recommending that they attend support group sessions so they can talk over their concerns with other parents in similar situations. ❞

Alterations in cardiovascular function may be a result of a congenital defect, acquired infection, or injury. Heart disease is the fifth leading cause of death in children in the United States.[1] Congenital heart defects, like Helena's ventricular septal defect, occur in approximately 1% of all live births[2] and often require surgical correction. Rapid advances in the treatment of congenital heart defects have resulted in children having surgery at younger ages. As a result, nursing care required to identify and manage responses of infants and children with heart disease has become more challenging.

Anatomy and Physiology of Pediatric Differences

Transition from Fetal to Pulmonary Circulation

After the umbilical cord has been cut, the newborn must quickly adapt to receiving oxygen from the lungs. The transition from fetal to pulmonary circulation occurs in just a few hours. During fetal circulation the constricted pulmonary vessels limit blood flow to the lungs (high pulmonary vascular resistance). Blood, however, flows easily to the extremities because systemic vascular resistance is low. The foramen ovale, an opening between the atria in the fetal heart, allows blood to flow from the right to the left atrium. Systemic vascular resistance increases after the umbilical cord is cut, causing a backup of blood flow. The pressure in the left side of the heart increases, stimulating closure of the foramen ovale. Once breathing has been initiated, the lungs expand and pulmonary vascular resistance falls. Blood that was previously shunted from the lungs through the ductus arteriosus to the aorta flows to the lungs. Figure 12–1 compares fetal and pulmonary circulation.

The ductus arteriosus, responding to higher oxygen saturation, normally constricts and closes within 10 to 15 hours after birth. Permanent closure occurs by 10 to 21 days after birth, unless oxygen saturation remains low. Fetal tissues are accustomed to low oxygen saturation. This may explain why newborns with cyanotic heart disease appear relatively comfortable even

FIGURE 12–1 Normal circulation of the heart. **A,** Fetal (prenatal) circulation. **B,** Pulmonary (postnatal) circulation. *LA,* left atrium; *LV,* left ventricle; *RA,* right atrium; *RV,* right ventricle.

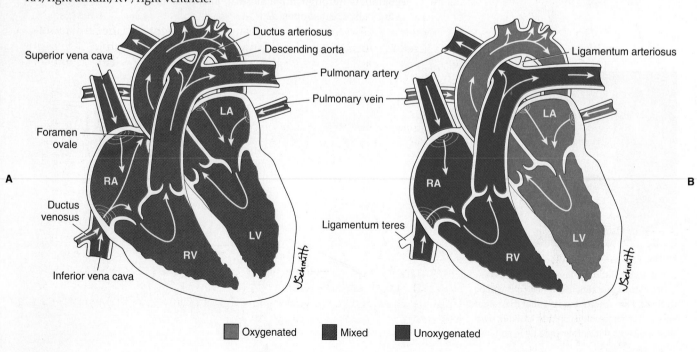

Superior vena cava
Foramen ovale
Ductus venosus
Inferior vena cava

Ductus arteriosus
Descending aorta
Pulmonary artery
Pulmonary vein

Ligamentum arteriosus
Ligamentum teres

☐ Oxygenated ■ Mixed ■ Unoxygenated

when the arterial partial pressure of oxygen (PaO_2) is 20 to 25 mm Hg. Acidosis, cerebral anoxia, and death would occur in minutes in older children and adults with a comparable PaO_2.[3]

The ventricles are equal in size at birth, but by 2 months of age the left ventricle is twice as large as the right ventricle. The higher systemic vascular pressures force the left ventricle to develop quickly.

Infants have a greater risk of heart failure than older children because the immature heart is more sensitive to volume or pressure overload. During infancy the muscle fibers of the heart are less developed and less organized, resulting in limited functional capacity. Less **compliance** (amount of distention or expansion the ventricles can achieve to increase stroke volume) of the heart muscle means that stroke volume cannot increase substantially. The heart muscle fibers develop during early childhood so that heart function is comparable to a healthy adult's by 5 years of age.[4]

Oxygenation

Oxygen bound to hemoglobin is transported to the tissues by the systemic circulation. Hematocrit and hemoglobin concentrations appropriate for the child's age are necessary for adequate oxygen transport (see Chapter 13). The oxygen arterial saturation is the amount of oxygen that can potentially be delivered to the tissues. **Desaturated blood** results when oxygenated and unoxygenated blood mix because of a congenital heart defect.

Cyanosis, which indicates **hypoxemia** (an abnormally decreased arterial blood oxygen concentration), results from the presence of 5 or more grams of unoxygenated hemoglobin per 100 mL of blood.[5]

The child's bone marrow responds to chronic hypoxemia by producing more red blood cells to increase the amount of hemoglobin available for oxygenation. This increase is known as **polycythemia**. A hematocrit value of 50% or higher is common in children with cyanotic heart defects.

Cardiac Functioning

Oxygen requirements are high for the first 8 weeks of life. Normally the newborn's heart rate increases to provide adequate oxygen transport. The infant has little cardiac output reserve capacity until oxygen requirements begin to decrease.[6] Cardiac output depends almost completely on heart rate until the heart muscle is fully developed at 5 years of age. Weight-specific cardiac output decreases during childhood. However, total cardiac output increases with growth.[7] During stress, exercise, fever, or respiratory distress, infants and children have tachycardia, which increases their cardiac output.

Children respond to severe hypoxemia with bradycardia. Cardiac arrest in children generally results from prolonged hypoxemia related to respiratory failure or shock rather than from a primary cardiac insult as in adults. Bradycardia is therefore a significant warning sign of cardiac arrest. Appropriate management of hypoxemia reverses bradycardia and prevents cardiac arrest.

Congestive Heart Failure

Congestive heart failure is a condition in which cardiac output is inadequate to support the body's metabolic needs. It may result from a congenital heart defect that causes an obstruction or fluid overload in the heart, from problems with heart contractility, or from pathologic conditions that require high cardiac output, such as severe anemia.

Clinical Manifestations

Congestive heart failure often develops subtly, and symptoms may not be recognized at first. The infant tires easily, especially during feeding. Weight loss or lack of normal weight gain, diaphoresis, irritability, and frequent infections may be evident.

As the disease progresses, symptoms such as tachypnea, tachycardia, nasal flaring, grunting, retractions, cough, or crackles may occur. Generalized fluid volume overload is seen more commonly in toddlers and older children. Periorbital and facial edema, jugular vein distention, and hepatomegaly are signs of fluid volume excess. Cyanosis, weak peripheral pulses, cool extremities, hypotension, and heart murmur are precursors of cardiogenic shock. (Cardiogenic shock is discussed later in this chapter.)

Etiology and Pathophysiology

Congenital heart defects are the most common cause of congestive heart failure in children.[6] Some defects allow blood to flow from the left side of the heart to the right so that extra blood must be pumped to the pulmonary system rather than through the aorta when the left ventricle contracts. Even though the heart rate increases to manage the extra blood volume, the pulmonary system becomes overloaded. Helena, described at the beginning of this chapter, had a ventricular septal defect that led to the development of congestive heart failure. Other congenital defects restrict the flow of blood so that normal pressures in the heart are disrupted. For example, if the aorta or pulmonary vessels are abnormally small, the heart must work harder to force blood through these structures. As a result the heart muscle hypertrophies, which increases cardiac output initially, but eventually the hypertrophied muscle becomes ineffective and dies.[9] Initially the right or left side of the heart may fail, but eventually failure is bilateral.

When cardiac output remains insufficient, the body's sympathetic response is activated. Peripheral vasoconstriction and decreased blood flow to internal organs such as the brain and kidneys lead to fatigue and dizziness. The kidneys respond to the lowered volume by activating the renin-angiotensin mechanism, which temporarily corrects the problem. Renal vasoconstriction results when aldosterone is secreted, and salt and water are retained. This protective measure eventually fails, leading to systemic edema or pulmonary congestion.

Diagnostic Tests and Medical Management

Diagnosis is based primarily on clinical manifestations such as tachycardia, respiratory distress, and crackles. A chest x-ray study may reveal cardiac enlargement and increased pulmonary vascular markings. Echocardiography may be performed to diagnose cardiac dysfunction. An electrocardiogram rarely shows abnormalities but may rule out cardiac dysrhythmias.

The goals of medical management are to make the heart work more efficiently and to remove excess fluid, thus improving peripheral circulation.[10] Digoxin is the drug most commonly used to improve the heart's ability to contract and therefore increase its output. Occasionally a higher than normal dose is given initially, followed by a lower maintenance dose. This process, called **digitalization**, speeds the child's response to the drug.

Diuretics, such as furosemide, chlorothiazide, ethacrynic acid, and spironolactone, are given to promote fluid excretion. Furosemide is the most commonly used. Since most diuretics (except for spironolactone) cause potassium loss, serum potassium levels are monitored and potassium sup-

FIGURE 12-2 Jooti is receiving intravenous fluids and oxygen. Her condition is being continuously monitored for congestive heart failure.

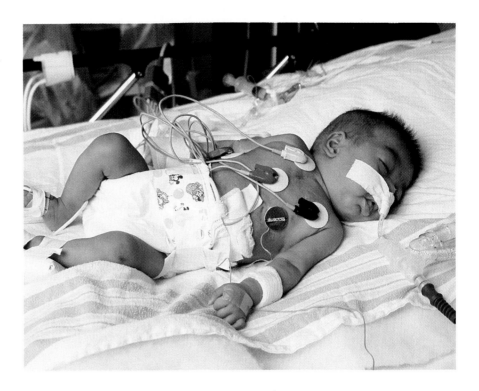

plements may be ordered. Vasodilating drugs may be given to reduce pulmonary and systemic vasoconstriction and to decrease the work of the heart.[11]

Other medical therapy is supportive. Oxygen therapy, rest, and fluid and dietary management are also part of the treatment plan (Fig. 12–2).

Most children improve rapidly after medication is administered. When congestive heart failure develops in a child with a correctable heart defect, surgery may be scheduled sooner than had been planned to prevent further deterioration and damage to the heart.

Nursing Assessment

Physiologic Assessment. Since diagnosis of congestive heart failure depends primarily on physical symptoms, nursing observations are important. Assess the child's behavioral patterns, cardiac function, respiratory function, and fluid status (Table 12–1). Obtain a detailed history of the onset of symptoms from the parents, since congestive heart failure often develops slowly.

Psychosocial Assessment. Take a history of the child's previous hospitalizations and assess the family's knowledge about the child's condition. Families of children with congestive heart failure are anxious and fear the potential serious outcome of the problem and the need for providing ongoing care.[6,12] Assess the family's anxiety level and coping strategies. Evaluate the family's economic status. Medication is crucial to treatment, and a family's inability to afford the necessary medicines jeopardizes the child's outcome.

The family is often overprotective and reluctant to leave the child with other caregivers. Find out if a knowledgeable person who can safely administer medications and watch the child is available for respite care.

TABLE 12-1 Physical Assessment of a Child in Congestive Heart Failure

Behavioral Manifestations

Lethargy
Listlessness
Tiring on feeding (infant)
Tiring with play (child)
Irritability

Cardiac Function and Fluid Status

Tachycardia
Cyanosis (late sign unless a cyanotic defect)
Cool extremities
Peripheral edema
Slow capillary refill time
Hypotension (rare; late sign)
Jugular vein distention (children)
Heart murmur

Respiratory Function

Tachypnea
Nasal flaring
Retractions
Crackles
Orthopnea
Cough
Grunting

Nonspecific Signs

Poor weight gain (infant)
Ascites
Hepatomegaly
Diaphoresis
Frequent infections (e.g., otitis media, respiratory)
Oliguria

Developmental Assessment. Since fatigue limits the activities of the child with congestive heart failure, the child does not have the opportunity to practice the skills needed to attain normal developmental milestones. Perform developmental assessment with a tool such as the Denver II (see Chapter 3). In addition, ask parents about the attainment of expected developmental milestones such as sitting, manipulating objects, standing, or walking. When congestive heart failure is well controlled, the child's energy level increases and developmental skills often improve. In infants and toddlers assessments every 2 to 3 months are useful to observe development and evaluate disease management.

Parents may limit the child's contact with other children because of frequent infections and exercise intolerance. Ask parents about contact and play with other children and a typical day's activity schedule.

Nursing Diagnosis

Several nursing diagnoses that may apply to the child with congestive heart failure are given in the accompanying Nursing Care Plan. The primary nursing diagnosis is Decreased Cardiac Output related to cardiac defect.

Nursing Management

Nursing care for the child with congestive heart failure focuses on administering and monitoring effects of medications, maintaining adequate oxygenation and myocardial function, promoting rest, fostering development, providing adequate nutrition, and providing emotional support to the child and family. The accompanying Nursing Care Plan summarizes nursing care for the child with congestive heart failure.

Administer and Monitor Prescribed Medications. Children with congestive heart failure usually receive digoxin and furosemide. These medications are potent and must be administered correctly. Digoxin is given intravenously or orally in extremely small doses. Carefully measure and verify the doses. If

■ CLINICAL TIP

Take an apical pulse with a stethoscope for 1 full minute before every dose of digoxin. If bradycardia is detected (<100 beats/min for infants and toddlers, <80 beats/min in older children, or <60 beats/min in adolescents), call for a physician's advice before administering the drug.

a child taking digoxin orally is NPO or vomiting, seek a physician's order for course of action; the drug must not be omitted. On the other hand, vomiting can be a signal that digoxin is at a toxic level. It is important to observe the child carefully for digoxin toxicity. Blood is drawn 6 to 8 hours after digoxin is given to monitor serum levels. A therapeutic serum level ranges from 1.1 to 1.7 ng/mL. Levels below 0.5 ng/mL are ineffective, and those over 2 ng/mL can lead to toxicity. Digoxin overdose is more common when potassium levels are low, so check serum potassium levels when a potassium-depleting diuretic is given.

Measure intake and output carefully. Weigh the infant's diapers before and after changing (1 g = 30 ounces urine). Observe for changes in peripheral edema and circulation. Weigh the child at the same time each day because fluid volume varies throughout the day. If ascites is present, take serial abdominal measurements to monitor changes (see Fig. 7–12). Turn the child frequently, and provide skin care when edema is present (see Fig. 7–13).

Maintain Oxygenation and Myocardial Function. Oxygen therapy may be ordered. Make sure that tubing is patent, the oxygen flow rate is correct, the oxygen delivery device is working properly, and humidification is provided. Keep the child calm and quiet. Position the child in a semi-Fowler or 45-degree angle position to promote maximum oxygenation. Infants are generally most comfortable eating at a 45-degree angle, which facilitates breathing while eating.

Promote Rest. Group assessments and interventions together to ensure that the child has some uninterrupted rest each hour. Feedings should last no more than 20 to 30 minutes. Frequent small feedings generally work best, with burping after every half ounce of intake to minimize vomiting.[12] Rocking is restful for infants. Encourage older children to engage in quiet activities such as playing board games or watching television.

Foster Development. Encourage parents to play with the child, using toys to stimulate eye-hand coordination and fine motor movements. Such toys include rattles, blocks, and stuffed animals for infants and books, paper and pencil, and dolls for older children. Encourage sitting, standing, or walking for short periods with adequate rest afterward to promote the development of large muscles. Singing, talking, and playing music facilitate cognitive and language skills.

Provide Adequate Nutrition. Teach parents about feeding techniques. The mother who chooses to breast feed the infant should not be discouraged. The antibodies contained in breast milk reduce infections, and the milk is naturally low in sodium. However, the sucking involved in feeding may cause dyspnea that forces the infant to rest frequently during feeding. Infants should be burped frequently to permit rest and prevent vomiting. They may need small frequent feedings and longer feeding periods. Make sure that parents understand that changes in feeding habits (decreased intake, vomiting, sleeping through feedings, increased perspiration with feedings) may indicate deteriorating cardiac status.[13] The American Heart Association publishes the booklet *Feeding Infants with Congenital Heart Disease* for parents (see Appendix F).

Adequate nutrition is needed to support the infant's growth. When infants have significant dyspnea with feeding, special feeding techniques are needed. Some infants need a higher caloric formula (24 calories per ounce or higher) to obtain adequate nutrition. Other infants require nutrition supplementation by nasogastric or gastrostomy tube. Parents are often advised to give the infant a chance to feed normally for a specific period. The remainder of the formula is then given by nasogastric or gastrostomy tube.

Provide Emotional Support. When a child is hospitalized with congestive heart failure, the family is often anxious about his or her condition. Give parents an opportunity to express concerns about their child's heart condition. Explain the child's treatment regimen, and make sure family members understand the child's need for nutrition and rest. Answer any questions about the child's prognosis and the ultimate outcome. Provide family members with information, and relay questions to the physician. Talking to other parents of children with cardiac conditions may be a source of emotional support. Refer parents to the appropriate support groups.

Discharge Planning and Patient and Family Home Care Teaching. Home care needs should be identified and addressed well in advance of discharge. While the child is hospitalized, teach the family about the administration of medications and signs of worsening condition.

Demonstrate administration of drugs, and then supervise while the parents show how to measure and administer medications. Emphasize that a calibrated dropper must be used to administer digoxin elixir. Teach parents about the toxic effects of digoxin. Advise them to notify the physician immediately if any of these side effects occur.

Tell parents to watch for symptoms such as increased feeding difficulty, irritability, lethargy, breathing difficulty, and puffiness around the eyes or extremities that indicate congestive heart failure is worsening. Parents are frequently taught to take the child's pulse and to report any significant change to the physician. An increase in pulse rate can signal congestive failure, and a decrease in pulse rate can indicate digoxin toxicity.

Evaluate family resources so that adequate child or respite care can be arranged if needed. The caregiver must understand the importance of proper medication administration and report any feeding difficulties.

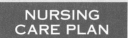

THE CHILD WITH CONGESTIVE HEART FAILURE

GOAL	INTERVENTION	RATIONALE	EXPECTED OUTCOME
1. Decreased Cardiac Output related to congenital heart defect			
Child's cardiac output will be sufficient to meet body's metabolic demands.	Administer digoxin as ordered.	Digoxin increases contractility of heart and force of contraction.	Child's cardiac output is sufficient as indicated by increased energy, adequate feeding intake, and decreased edema.
	Take apical pulse and listen to heart sounds regularly, especially before each dose of digoxin. Record apical pulse with each recorded dose of digoxin.	Digoxin may cause bradycardia. Pulse and heart sounds provide information about heart functioning.	
	Use cardiac monitor if ordered.	Monitor notes tachycardia and dysrhythmias.	
	Prevent injury by monitoring for digoxin side effects. Monitor serum level of digoxin and serum potassium level.	Digoxin is a potent drug with serious side effects. Hypokalemia increases risk of digoxin toxicity.	Child maintains normal serum levels of potassium and therapeutic levels of digoxin.
	Provide for rest periods each hour.	Rest decreases need for high cardiac output.	Child rests hourly and has adequate energy to eat and play.
2. Altered Tissue Perfusion related to sympathetic response to congestive heart failure			
Child's peripheral and central edema will decrease.	Provide skin care for edematous body parts and elevate extremities.	Edematous skin breaks down easily. Elevation promotes return of fluid from extremities.	Child shows no edema.
	Weigh daily. Measure abdominal girth daily if ascites is present. Observe for peripheral edema.	Evaluations demonstrate effectiveness of therapy.	
Child's urinary output will remain within normal levels.	Measure intake and output carefully.	Adequate output is a good indicator of renal perfusion.	Child's intake and output are proportional, and electrolyte levels remain within normal ranges.
	Maintain fluid restricted diet if ordered.	Fluid restriction is sometimes used to decrease cardiac fluid load.	
	Administer diuretics as ordered.	Diuretics mobilize fluids and facilitate excretion.	
	Monitor electrolytes.	Electrolyte imbalance is common when fluids are restricted and diuretics are given.	
3. Impaired Gas Exchange related to pulmonary congestion			
Child will manifest adequate oxygenation.	Place child in semi-Fowler's position.	Position facilitates lung expansion.	Child has normal respiratory rate for age with no evidence of adventitious sounds or diaphoresis.
	Evaluate respiratory rate and sounds. Take pulse oximetry readings to determine oxygen saturation.	Absence of tachypnea and adventitious sounds and oxygen saturation above 95% indicate ease of respiration.	
	Provide oxygen and humidification if ordered.	Supplemental oxygen decreases tachypnea, and humidification moistens secretions to keep airway clear.	
	Observe for diaphoresis, a sign of increased respiratory effort.		

Continued.

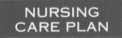
THE CHILD WITH CONGESTIVE HEART FAILURE— CONTINUED

GOAL	INTERVENTION	RATIONALE	EXPECTED OUTCOME
4. Altered Nutrition: Less Than Body Requirements related to rapid tiring while feeding			
Infant or child will demonstrate normal weight gain for age.	Hold infant at 45-degree angle for feeding. Record intake carefully. Weigh child daily. Give frequent small meals with rest periods in between. Give high-calorie snacks. Use soothing approaches such as holding infants for feeding and having parents eat with older child.	Position facilitates breathing while eating. Evaluation of intake indicates whether caloric and other nutritional needs are met. Weight gain indicates growth (in absence of edematous symptoms of congestive heart failure). Digesting small meals requires less energy. High-calorie snacks provide calories efficiently. Restful approach facilitates intake with minimal cardiac work.	Infant or child gains recommended weight according to growth grids. All dietary requirements are met, and meal times are pleasant.
5. Altered Growth and Development related to low energy level			
Child will meet developmental milestones for age group.	Plan for short play periods after rest. Introduce age-appropriate toys and activities such as rattles and blocks for infants and art projects for older children. Perform baseline developmental assessment.	Short play periods maintain energy and facilitate play. Play activities facilitate learning and mastery of developmental tasks. Assessment provides comparison for later assessments and basis for planning specific games, toys, and activities.	Child displays normal language, fine motor, and gross motor activity.
6. Knowledge Deficit (Parent) related to treatment regimen			
Parents will demonstrate correct administration of medications. Parents will state side effects of medications and symptoms of congestive heart failure.	Demonstrate administration of digoxin, diuretics, and other medications. Have parents administer them under supervision of nurse. Describe side effects of medications. Give parents handouts with telephone number to call to ask questions or report side effects. Describe subtle onset of congestive heart failure and its symptoms (increasing weakness, exhaustion, irritability, difficulty feeding, cough or difficult respirations, edema).	Demonstration with return demonstration is an excellent method of learning psychomotor skills. If side effects are understood, serious complications can be avoided. Parents can evaluate child regularly and note subtle changes requiring medical management.	Parents report that child continues to demonstrate improvement and adequate cardiac output with absence of congestive failure episodes.

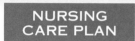
THE CHILD WITH CONGESTIVE HEART FAILURE— CONTINUED

GOAL	INTERVENTION	RATIONALE	EXPECTED OUTCOME
7. Anxiety (Parent) related to unknown nature of child's disease			
Parent will express lessened anxiety as hospitalization proceeds.	Encourage parents to room in or stay with child. Explain procedures and treatment. Involve parents in care as much as possible. Have parents plan child's play periods.	Involvement in child's care lessens parental anxiety and fear of unknown.	Parents demonstrate comfort in providing care for child.
	At discharge, provide clear instructions and information about whom and where to call with questions.	Having resources available provides feeling of security.	
	Allow parents to verbalize questions, concerns, and feelings. Refer parents to support groups or other resources as needed.	Emotional support is needed to lessen anxiety.	

Congenital Heart Disease

Congenital heart disease is a defect in the heart or great vessels, or persistence of a fetal structure after birth.[6] Congenital heart defects are estimated to occur in 1% of all live births. In spontaneously aborted and stillborn fetuses the incidence is much higher.[2]

The occurrence of congenital heart defects is influenced by the following factors:

- Fetal exposure to drugs such as phenytoin and lithium
- Maternal viral infections such as rubella
- Maternal metabolic disorders such as phenylketonuria and diabetes mellitus
- Maternal complications of pregnancy such as increased age and antepartal bleeding
- Genetic factors (family recurrence patterns)
- Chromosomal abnormalities such as Turner syndrome, Down syndrome, and trisomy syndromes 13 and 18[7]

The occurrence of a congenital heart defect is usually the result of a combined or interactive effect of genetic and environmental factors. A child often has more than one defect at the same time. Depending on the type of defect, signs and symptoms may be present at birth or develop later.

Congenital heart defects are generally divided into two categories, cyanotic and acyanotic, based on the hallmark sign of cyanosis. However, a child with an acyanotic defect may show clinical signs of cyanosis. The pathophysiology of a heart defect is related to **hemodynamics,** which refers to the pressures generated by blood and the pathways blood takes through the heart and pulmonary system.

Acyanotic Defects

The majority of children with congenital heart defects have acyanotic conditions. There are two types of acyanotic defects: nonobstructive lesions, which do not interfere with the flow of blood, and obstructive lesions, which block the outflow of blood from the heart. Nonobstructive defects include patent ductus arteriosus (PDA), atrial septal defect (ASD), atrioventricular canal (endocardial cushion defect), and ventricular septal defect (VSD). Obstructive defects include pulmonic stenosis (PS), aortic stenosis (AS), and coarctation of the aorta. Table 12–2 summarizes clinical manifestations, diagnostic tests, and medical management for these defects.

TABLE 12–2   Acyanotic Heart Defects

Condition

NONOBSTRUCTIVE LESIONS
Patent Ductus Arteriosus (PDA)

Common congenital defect caused by persistent fetal circulation. When pulmonary circulation is established and systemic vascular resistance increases at birth, pressures in aorta become greater than in the pulmonary arteries. Blood is then shunted from aorta to pulmonary arteries, increasing circulation to pulmonary system.

Clinical Manifestations

Dyspnea; tachypnea; full, bounding pulses; and poor development occur. Infant is at risk for frequent respiratory infections and subacute endocarditis. When a large PDA exists, congestive heart failure, intercostal retractions, hepatomegaly, and growth failure are also seen. A continuous systolic murmur is auscultated, and a thrill may be palpated in pulmonic area.

Diagnostic Tests

When murmur is detected, diagnosis is confirmed by chest x-ray study, electrocardiogram (ECG), and echocardiogram. Chest x-ray film and ECG show left ventricular hypertrophy. PDA can be visualized, and left-to-right shunt can be measured on echocardiogram.

Medical Management

Surgical ligation of PDA is the treatment of choice. Intravenous indomethacin often stimulates closure of the ductus arteriosus in premature infants. Transcatheter closure by obstructive device is sometimes attempted in children over 18 months of age.

PROGNOSIS: If PDA is not treated, child's life span is shortened because pulmonary hypertension and vascular obstructive disease develop.

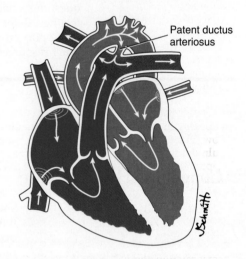

Patent ductus arteriosus

Atrial Septal Defect (ASD)

An opening at any point in atrial septum that permits left-to-right shunting of blood. Opening may be small, as when the foramen ovale fails to close, or septum may be completely absent.

Clinical Manifestations

Infants and young children usually have no symptoms, since small and moderate-sized ASDs are usually not diagnosed until preschool years or later. Congestive heart failure, easy fatigue, and poor growth occur with a large ASD. Soft systolic murmur is usually heard in pulmonic area with wide splitting of S_2.

Diagnostic Tests

Diagnosis is made by echocardiogram that identifies right ventricular overload and shunt size. Chest x-ray film and ECG reveal little information unless ASD is large and excessive shunting is present.

Medical Management

Surgery to close or patch ASD is performed to prevent pulmonary vascular obstructive disease. Some ASDs may be closed by transcatheter device during cardiac catheterization.

PROGNOSIS: Many persons with uncorrected small and moderate-sized ASDs have lived to middle age without symptoms. Atrial dysrhythmias are common late complications.

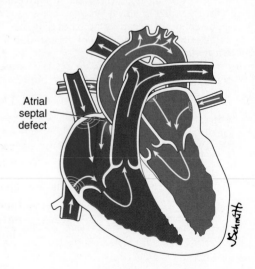

Atrial septal defect

TABLE 12-2 Acyanotic Heart Defects *Continued*

Condition

Atrioventricular Canal (Endocardial Cushion Defect)

Atrioventricular (AV) canal refers to a combination of defects in atrial and ventricular septa and portions of tricuspid and mitral valves. This defect is associated with Down syndrome. Endocardial cushions are fetal growth centers for mitral and tricuspid valves and AV septum. The most complex AV canal malformation results in one AV valve and large septal defects between both atria and ventricles.

Clinical Manifestations

Severity of symptoms depends on amount of mitral regurgitation. Infants have congestive heart failure, poor growth, and repeated respiratory failure, as well as systolic murmur, which is loudest at left lower sternal border.

Diagnostic Tests

On chest x-ray film, heart appears large and pulmonary vascular markings are present. Echocardiogram reveals presence of septal defects and details of valvular malformation. Cardiac catheterization is performed to evaluate pulmonary hypertension and pulmonary resistance.

Medical Management

Surgery is performed during infancy to prevent pulmonary vascular disease. Patches are placed over septal defects, and valve tissue is used to form functioning valves. Oxygen may be required until surgery.

PROGNOSIS: Information on long-term survival following successful surgery is lacking. There is no difference in short-term survival rates between infants with and without Down syndrome.

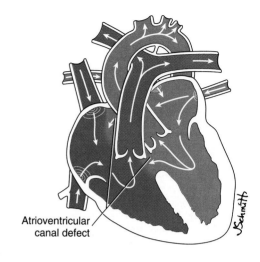

Atrioventricular canal defect

Ventricular Septal Defect (VSD)

An opening in the ventricular septum results in increased pulmonary blood flow. Blood is shunted from left ventricle directly across open septum into pulmonary artery. The most common congenital heart defect, occurring in approximately 30% to 40% of all children with congenital heart disease.*

Clinical Manifestations

Only 15% of VSDs are large enough to cause symptoms, such as tachypnea, dyspnea, poor growth, reduced fluid intake, congestive heart failure, and pulmonary hypertension. Systolic murmur is auscultated in lower left sternal border.

Diagnostic Tests

Chest x-ray film and ECG reveal few findings in cases of small VSDs. Larger VSDs with shunting are associated with enlarged heart and pulmonary vascular markings on chest x-ray film and left ventricular hypertrophy on ECG. Echocardiogram establishes diagnosis if shunting is present. Cardiac catheterization is used only in preparation for surgery.

Medical Management

Most small VSDs close spontaneously. Treatment is conservative when no signs of congestive heart disease or pulmonary hypertension are present. Surgical patching of VSD during infancy is performed when poor growth is evident. Closure of VSD by transcatheter device during cardiac catheterization may be attempted for some defects. Prophylaxis for infective endocarditis is required.

PROGNOSIS: Highest risk associated with surgical repair is in the first few months of life. Children respond well to surgery and experience substantial "catch-up" growth. A dysrhythmia, complete right bundle branch block, is complication found in more than 30% of patients.†

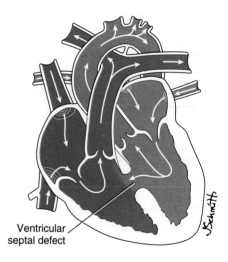

Ventricular septal defect

---

*Information from Hoffman, J.I.E. (1990). Congenital heart disease: Incidence and inheritance. *Pediatric Clinics of North America, 37,* 25–43.
†Information from Fyler, D.C. (1992). Ventricular septal defect. In *Nadas' pediatric cardiology* (pp. 453–457). Philadelphia: Hanley & Belfus.

Continued

TABLE 12-2 Acyanotic Heart Defects *Continued*

Condition

OBSTRUCTIVE LESIONS   *All this have ↓ Cardiac Output.*
Pulmonic Stenosis

Stenosis (narrowing of valve or valve area) can be above valve, below valve, or at valve. Stenosis obstructs blood flow into pulmonary artery. This increases preload. Right ventricular hypertrophy occurs. Pulmonic stenosis is second most frequent congenital heart defect.

Clinical Manifestations

Children with mild stenosis may have no symptoms and grow normally. In moderate stenosis, dyspnea and fatigue occur on exertion. Signs of heart failure are rare but may result from chronic pressure overload. Systolic murmur with a fixed split S_2 and thrill may be found in pulmonic listening area.

Diagnostic Tests

Diagnosis is usually made at birth after auscultation of murmur. The chest x-ray film may show heart enlargement, and the ECG may demonstrate right ventricular hypertrophy. Echocardiogram provides information about pressure gradient across valve and size of valve ring.

Medical Management

Dilation by balloon valvuloplasty, performed during cardiac catheterization, has been widely successful for treatment of simple pulmonic stenosis. Surgical valvotomy is still used, especially when other defects such as ASD are present. Pulmonary regurgitation may result, but is not significant problem.

PROGNOSIS: Pulmonic stenosis does not typically increase in severity. Lifelong infective endocarditis prophylaxis is necessary.

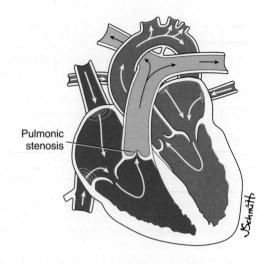

Pulmonic stenosis

Aortic Stenosis

Narrowing of the aortic valve obstructs blood flow to systemic circulation. This defect is often associated with bicuspid rather than normal tricuspid valve. Stenosis is usually progressive during childhood. Approximately 75% of affected children are boys.

Clinical Manifestations

Majority of infants and young children are asymptomatic and grow and develop normally. Occasionally child complains of chest pain after exercise, but exercise intolerance is uncommon. Peripheral pulses may be weak. Fainting and dizziness are serious signs that require intervention. Congestive heart failure develops in symptomatic infants. Systolic heart murmur and thrill in the aortic listening area is usually detected in routine physical examination in school-aged child or adolescent.

Diagnostic Tests

Chest x-ray film and ECG are usually normal in mild cases. Echocardiogram reveals number of valve cusps, pressure gradient across valve, and size of aorta. Stress testing may be used in asymptomatic children to determine amount of obstruction present with exercise.

Medical Management

Aortic valve may be successfully dilated by balloon valvuloplasty during cardiac catheterization. Surgical valvuloplasty is still performed. Aortic valve replacement is performed when stenosis is severe or if significant regurgitation results from other interventions. Surgical treatment is palliative rather than curative.

PROGNOSIS: Sudden death can occur in symptomatic children, particularly during vigorous exercise. Stenosis is usually progressive during childhood. Valve replacement may ultimately be necessary. Lifelong infective endocarditis prophylaxis is required.

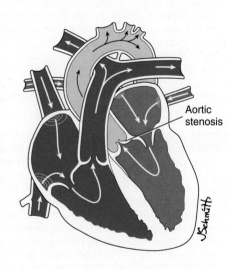

Aortic stenosis

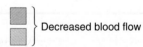

Decreased blood flow

TABLE 12–2 Acyanotic Heart Defects *Continued*

Condition

Coarctation of the Aorta

Narrowing or constriction in the descending aorta, often near ductus arteriosus, obstructs systemic blood outflow. This defect is common, occurring in 9% of all children with congenital heart disease.

Clinical Manifestations

Many children are asymptomatic and grow normally, but constriction is progressive. Reduction in blood flow through descending aorta causes lower blood pressure in legs and higher blood pressure in arms, neck, and head. Brachial and radial pulses are full, but femoral pulses are weak or absent. Infants with constriction between aorta and the ductus arteriosus may have signs of congestive heart failure and cyanosis in lower half of body.

Diagnostic Tests

ECG shows left ventricular hypertrophy. Chest x-ray film may reveal indentation of descending aorta, but rib notching is rarely seen before 10 years of age. Magnetic resonance imaging shows coarctation.

Medical Management

Balloon dilation during cardiac catheterization may provide initial relief. Surgical resection and anastomosis are palliative, since the coarctation usually recurs. The subclavian artery can be used as a patch in the infant.

PROGNOSIS: Persistent hypertension is common.

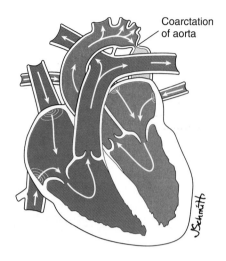

Coarctation of aorta

Clinical Manifestations

The child with a nonobstructive acyanotic heart defect may be asymptomatic except for a heart murmur. Congestive heart failure may develop if the amount of blood passing from the left to the right side of the heart overloads the pulmonary system. If this occurs, the child has hepatomegaly, dyspnea, tachypnea, intercostal retractions, poor growth, and frequent respiratory infections.

The child with an obstructive acyanotic heart defect also has a heart murmur. Although some children have fatigue and exercise intolerance because of their inability to increase cardiac output, many children are asymptomatic and grow normally.

Etiology and Pathophysiology

Beginning at birth the left side of the heart normally generates higher pressures than the right side in response to increasing systemic vascular resistance and decreasing pulmonary vascular resistance. In children who have nonobstructive defects such as openings in the septal wall, a left-to-right **shunt** (movement of blood between heart chambers through an abnormal opening) occurs. Oxygenated blood mixes with unoxygenated blood. The extra blood volume overloads the pulmonary system and causes congestive heart failure. **Pulmonary hypertension,** an often irreversible condition leading to life-threatening pulmonary vascular resistance, occurs if chronic volume overload of the pulmonary arteries is not corrected.

Diagnostic Tests and Medical Management

The presence of a heart murmur is often the first indication of an acyanotic defect. A loud murmur indicates higher pressures of blood flowing across

The following tests are used in the diagnosis of congenital heart disease:

Chest x-ray study: size of the heart and characteristics of pulmonary vascular markings

Electrocardiogram (ECG): quality of major electrical activity in the heart

Echocardiogram: heart's structures, the pattern of movement, and the presence of defects

Cardiac catheterization: precise measurement of oxygen saturation and pressures in each chamber and heart vessel; also identifies anatomic alterations

the shunt or through the narrowed valve or vessel. Once the heart murmur is discovered, a chest x-ray examination, electrocardiography, and echocardiography are performed. The echocardiogram usually clearly shows the defect, shunt, and heart pressures.

The selection of treatment for acyanotic defects depends on the severity of symptoms and whether the condition is imminently life threatening. Surgical correction is the treatment of choice for most acyanotic defects. Table 12–3 lists the types of surgical procedures performed on children with congenital heart defects. Conservative treatment, such as waiting until the child is asymptomatic, may be selected initially. For example, a ventricular septal defect may close spontaneously or growth of the child may increase the probability of success of surgery. Surgical correction of defects that cause pulmonary hypertension is performed in infancy to prevent irreversible pulmonary vascular disease.

Surgery often results in complete repair of the acyanotic defect. Unless complications develop before surgery, the child should make a complete recovery without limitations. The major complication of acyanotic heart defects is pulmonary hypertension.

Cardiac catheterization, an invasive procedure previously used exclusively for diagnosis of some congenital heart defects, is now more often performed as a therapeutic procedure. Recently developed techniques using balloons and other transcatheter devices permit treatment of many acyanotic heart defects during cardiac catheterization.

TABLE 12–3 Surgical Procedures for Congenital Heart Defects

Procedure	Purpose	Therapeutic Use
Arterial switch	Reattachment of great arteries with correct ventricle for transposition of great vessels	Corrective
Fontan	Creation of conduit between right atrium and pulmonary artery to increase pulmonary blood flow	Corrective
Modified Blalock-Taussig	Creation of conduit to increase pulmonary blood flow	Palliative
Mustard or Senning	Baffling blood in the atria to re-establish a proper blood flow in transposition of the great vessels	Corrective
Norwood	Creation of conduit between aorta and pulmonary artery to increase blood flow to aorta	Palliative or corrective
Patent ductus arteriosus ligation	Closure of ductus arteriosus	Corrective
Pulmonary artery banding	Placement of constricting band around pulmonary artery to reduce pulmonary blood flow	Palliative
Rashkind	Creation of larger defect between atria to increase blood mixing	Palliative
Transcatheter closure	Closure of septal defect by umbrella device during cardiac catheterization	Corrective
Transplant	Replacement of diseased heart with donor heart	Corrective
Valvuloplasty	Repair of valve to relieve stenosis by balloon dilation during cardiac catheterization or surgery	Palliative or corrective

Potential complications of cardiac catheterization include perforation of the pulmonary artery, allergic reaction to the contrast media, dysrhythmias, hypotension, stroke, vascular compromise in the leg, and bleeding.

Nursing Care of the Child Undergoing a Cardiac Catheterization

Prepare the child for cardiac catheterization with age-appropriate information. A tour of the catheterization laboratory may reduce the child's fears about the large equipment. Since the child will be sedated but arousable for the procedure, explain the sensations that the child will experience.

Diagnostic cardiac catheterization is an outpatient procedure. Therapeutic catheterization with dilation usually requires that the child be admitted for observation. The child is NPO after midnight, except for medications, and arrives at the catheterization laboratory the morning of the procedure. Before entering the laboratory, the child is asked to void and is given an oral sedative.

Nursing Assessment

Before the procedure, assess the child's vital signs, hematocrit and hemoglobin concentrations, and strength of pedal pulses for comparison with post-catheterization assessments.

For several hours after the procedure, monitor the child for potential complications such as dysrhythmia, bleeding, hematoma development, thrombus formation, and infection. No bleeding should occur at the catheterization site. Assess vital signs, neurovascular status of the lower extremities, and pressure dressing over the catheterization site every 15 minutes for 1 hour and then every 30 minutes for 1 hour. The child's temperature, heart rate, respiratory rate, and blood pressure should remain stable. Monitor intake and output because the contrast medium may cause diuresis. The child's intake and output should be balanced. Pedal pulses, capillary refill, sensation, warmth, and color of the lower extremities should match the precatheterization assessment.

Nursing Diagnosis

The following nursing diagnoses may apply to the child who undergoes cardiac catheterization:

- Knowledge Deficit (Child and Parent) related to cardiac catheterization procedure
- High Risk for Infection related to invasive procedure
- High Risk for Fluid Volume Deficit related to blood loss, period of time NPO, and diuretic effect of contrast medium
- Altered Tissue Perfusion (Cardiopulmonary) related to potential thrombus formation and hemorrhage
- High Risk for Decreased Cardiac Output related to obstruction by balloon catheter

Nursing Management

Nursing care during a cardiac catheterization focuses on monitoring the child's vital signs, reassuring the child, and providing emergency care if necessary. After the catheters and guidewires are removed at the end of the procedure, direct pressure must be applied for 15 minutes. A pressure dressing is then placed over the site for 6 hours.

The child is kept on bed rest for 6 hours. Activity is then limited for 24 hours. Provide quiet diversional activities to keep the child occupied.

Encourage the intake of small amounts of clear liquids initially, and then progress to other fluids and food as the child tolerates them. Maintaining hydration is important because the contrast medium used during the procedure has a diuretic effect. Monitor intake and output.

DISCHARGE PLANNING AND PATIENT AND FAMILY HOME CARE TEACHING. Routinely children are discharged several hours after the cardiac catheterization. Teach the parents to watch the child for signs of complications and make sure they know when to notify the physician. An elevated temperature may indicate infection. It is essential that parents specifically check the catheterization site for bleeding or a hematoma for 24 hours. Emphasize that quiet play *only* is allowed for 24 hours.

Children whose heart defect is corrected by cardiac catheterization have the same risks for infective endocarditis as children with surgical correction. Use the information provided in Table 12–6 to teach parents about antibiotic prophylaxis.

Nursing Care of the Child Undergoing Surgery for an Acyanotic Defect

Children with acyanotic heart defects are hospitalized either because of complications, such as congestive heart failure, or for surgery. Refer to the earlier discussion of nursing management in congestive heart failure for care of children with this condition.

Nursing Assessment

Assess the ability of the parents to cope with the diagnosis of their child's congenital heart defect. Initially parents may be in shock and feel guilty and anxious. The child often looks healthy and has few symptoms.

Parents need an opportunity to express their feelings and learn to cope. They need special support if their infant has a life-threatening heart defect. Members of the cardiology team, including nurses, must provide counseling for the family. Counseling information may include the following:

- General information about the congenital heart disease, including a description of the heart's anatomy and physiology and the defect
- Specific information about the multiple interactive factors associated with congenital heart disease, which helps reduce parents' guilt about the child's defect
- Sample case histories with good and poor prognoses
- Overview of the child's prognosis and timing of medical and surgical interventions

Parents may need genetic counseling if planning a future pregnancy. Fetal echocardiography can identify structural heart defects as early as 18 to 20 weeks of gestation (Table 12–4).

The American Heart Association publishes the booklet *If Your Child Has a Congenital Heart Defect*. A copy can be obtained from the local chapter of the association. See Appendix F for information about contacting the national headquarters.

Following surgical correction of the heart defect, the child is usually cared for in an intensive care unit until stable. The child may be intubated and ven-

TABLE 12-4 Fetal Development of Specific Heart Defects

Defect	Critical Time (Weeks of Gestation)
Patent ductus arteriosus	3–8
Coarctation of the aorta	4–28
Ventricular septal defect	4–7
Transposition of the great vessels	3–4
Tricuspid or mitral atresia	3–6
Truncus arteriosus	6–7
Total anomalous pulmonary venous return	3–8

From Keith, J.D., Rowe, R.D., & Vlad, P., (Eds.). (1978). *Heart disease in infancy and childhood* (3rd ed). New York: Macmillan.

tilated for a few hours. In the immediate postoperative period, assess the child's vital signs, level of consciousness, heart functioning, and dysrhythmias. Monitor intake and output. Check for hemorrhage, adequate ventilation and tissue perfusion, and acid-base and electrolyte imbalances.[14]

After the child's return to the general nursing unit, nursing assessment focuses on signs of surgical complications such as infection, dysrhythmias, and impaired tissue perfusion. Monitor the child's temperature, and inspect the surgical incision site. Fever, excessive incisional pain, spreading erythema around the incision, and wound drainage beginning 3 to 4 days postoperatively may be early signs of infection. Assess the respiratory system for breath sounds, respiratory effort, and signs of distress that may indicate pneumonia or fluid in the pleural space.

Since the child may no longer be on a cardiac monitor, auscultation of the apical pulse to detect an irregular heart rate or bradycardia is essential. Either condition is an indication of reduced cardiac output that requires intervention. To assess for impaired tissue perfusion, check capillary refill, extremity warmth, pedal pulses, level of consciousness, and urine output. Reduced urine output is a sign of decreased cardiac output. Assess the child's pain.

Nursing Diagnosis

Several nursing diagnoses may be associated with acyanotic heart defects and their complications. They include:

- Fluid Volume Excess related to pulmonary vasculature overload
- Decreased Cardiac Output related to an obstructed outflow tract
- Ineffective Breathing Pattern related to pulmonary vasculature overload
- Altered Nutrition: Less Than Body Requirements related to ineffective feeding pattern
- Ineffective Infant Feeding Pattern related to shortness of breath and fatigue
- High Risk for Infection related to altered immune function, surgery, or pulmonary overload
- High Risk for Activity Intolerance related to chronic pulmonary vasculature overload
- Altered Family Processes related to guilt and grieving over lack of perfect infant
- High Risk for Caregiver Role Strain related to chronic health condition
- Knowledge Deficit (Parents) related to special care for chronic condition

Nursing Management

Children are often managed at home until surgery is scheduled. See Table 12–5 for parent education guidelines.

TABLE 12–5 Home Care of Children with Congenital Heart Defects Before Surgery

Routine Health Care

Provide well-child care and all immunizations, including pneumovaccine and influenza vaccine.

Provide preventive dental care with fluoride treatment beginning at 2 years of age.

Administration of Medications

Give medications safely with a dosage schedule that fits the family's routine.

Signs of Illness

Notify physician if the child has the following signs: fever, vomiting, diarrhea, or is feeding poorly.

Activity

Allow the child to set his or her own activity level. Children with congenital heart defects usually do not overexert themselves.

Nursing care following surgery focuses on promoting the child's recuperation. Pain management should be provided for several days postoperatively. Follow the guidelines given in Chapter 5.

Encourage the child to perform spirometry exercises regularly to promote full lung expansion. Chest physiotherapy may be performed in children under 3 years of age. Inspect the child's incision regularly and cleanse it with hydrogen peroxide if ordered (Fig. 12–3).

Administer antibiotics as ordered. Intravenous lines are often converted to heparin locks to continue antibiotic administration once the child's oral intake is normal. Although oral fluids are rarely limited, intake and output should be assessed carefully.

Encourage the child to increase activity gradually with longer periods out of bed every day. Provide opportunities for therapeutic play so the child can better manage the stresses associated with pain and frightening procedures.

DISCHARGE PLANNING AND PATIENT AND FAMILY HOME CARE TEACHING. Infants and children may be discharged from the hospital 1 week after surgery. Parents need discharge teaching in preparation for continuing care of the child at home. Instructions should include the following:

- Allow the child to increase activity gradually as tolerated. Report any changes in activity level to the physician.
- Observe for signs of wound infection, fever, flulike symptoms, or an increased respiratory rate or respiratory distress.[15] Report these signs to the physician.
- Allow the child to return to school in approximately 3 weeks. Physical activities such as rough play, bike riding, or climbing should be postponed for 6 weeks until the incision has healed completely.

Reassure parents by telling them that the child with a repaired cardiac defect should have no further cardiovascular problems. Encourage them to allow the child to live a normal and active life.

Children are at risk for infective endocarditis, especially within the first 6 months after surgery. The child should receive prophylactic antibiotics according to the American Heart Association recommendations (Table 12–6). Any unexplained fever or malaise seen in the 2 months following repair or after dental work may be a sign of infection. The child should be examined for petechiae and splenomegaly. Blood cultures, blood cell count, and urinalysis should be performed.[16]

FIGURE 12–3 A child with atrial septal defect repair. Surgery is performed with this type of defect to prevent pulmonary vascular obstructive disease.

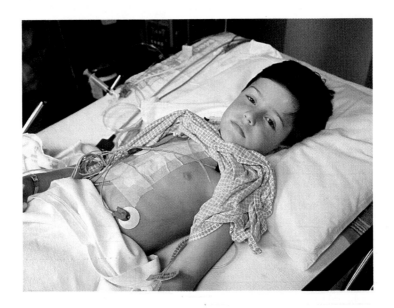

TABLE 12–6 **Antibiotic Recommendations for Endocarditis Prophylaxis in Children***

For Dental, Oral, or Upper Respiratory Tract Procedures
Amoxicillin

For Children Allergic to Penicillin
Erythromycin or clindamycin

For Genitourinary and Gastrointestinal Procedures
Ampicillin, gentamicin, amoxicillin

For Children Allergic to Penicillin
Vancomycin

Modified from Committee on Rheumatic Fever, Endocarditis, and Kawasaki Disease (1990). Prevention of bacterial endocarditis: Recommendations of the American Heart Association. *Journal of the American Medical Association, 264*, 2919–2922.
Routine dosage: Large dose is given 1 hour before procedure. Smaller dose is given 6 hours after procedure.

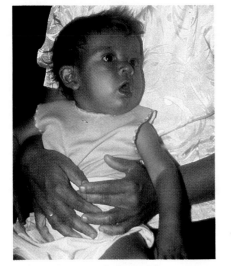

FIGURE 12–4 Infant with a cyanotic heart defect. What is the prognosis for an infant who has either of the most common malformations—tetralogy of Fallot or transposition of the great vessels?

Cyanotic Defects

Cyanotic heart disease is generally caused by a valvular or vascular malformation. The most common malformations are tetralogy of Fallot and transposition of the great vessels (Fig. 12–4). Table 12–7 summarizes clinical manifestations, diagnostic tests, and medical management for these defects.

Other less common congenital heart defects include hypoplastic left heart syndrome, tricuspid atresia, pulmonary atresia, truncus arteriosus, and total anomalous pulmonary venous return (Table 12–8). Not all of these defects cause cyanosis.

Clinical Manifestations

Cyanosis often occurs when the ductus arteriosus closes, causing chronic hypoxemia, fatigue, clubbing of the fingers and toes, exertional dyspnea, and delayed developmental milestones. Because infants tire easily with feeding, they receive fewer calories, and do not grow normally. Congestive heart failure develops in some children.

TABLE 12–7 Cyanotic Heart Defects

Condition

Tetralogy of Fallot

Combination of four defects: pulmonic stenosis, right ventricular hypertrophy, ventricular septal defect (VSD), and overriding of aorta. Some children have fifth defect: open foramen ovale or atrial septal defect (ASD). Between 4% and 8% of children with congenital heart defects have tetralogy of Fallot. This defect is characterized by elevated pressures in right side of heart, causing right-to-left shunt.

Clinical Manifestations

As ductus arteriosus closes, infant becomes hypoxic and cyanotic. Degree of pulmonary stenosis determines severity of symptoms. Polycythemia, hypoxic spells, metabolic acidosis, poor growth, clubbing, and exercise intolerance may develop. Infants have systolic murmur heard in pulmonic area that is transmitted to suprasternal notch.

Diagnostic Tests

Chest x-ray film shows a boot-shaped heart due to the large right ventricle with decreased pulmonary vascular markings. Electrocardiogram (ECG) shows right ventricular hypertrophy. Echocardiogram demonstrates VSD, obstruction of pulmonary outflow, and overriding aorta. Cardiac catheterization is required before surgical correction to completely identify the location of all anatomic structures and any additional defects.

Medical Management

Cyanotic spells are managed according to guidelines given in section on nursing management of cyanotic defects. Monitoring child for metabolic acidosis or prolonged unconsciousness is critical. Palliative surgery may be performed before corrective surgery. Corrective surgery may be attempted in symptomatic children by 6 months of age.

PROGNOSIS: Dysrhythmias and myocardial dysfunction are believed to be related to surgical intervention. Sudden death from ventricular dysrhythmias occurs in 2%–7% of patients several years after surgery.* Lifelong infective endocarditis prophylaxis is required.

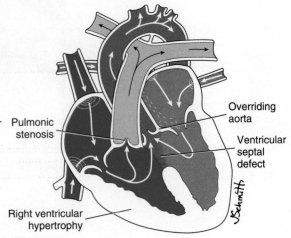

Pulmonic stenosis

Overriding aorta

Ventricular septal defect

Right ventricular hypertrophy

Transposition of the Great Vessels (TGV)

Pulmonary artery is outflow for left ventricle, and aorta is outflow for right ventricle. This condition is life threatening at birth, and survival initially depends on open ductus arteriosus and foramen ovale. This condition occurs in about 10% of children with cyanotic congenital heart disease. ASD or VSD may also be present with TGV.

Clinical Manifestations

Cyanosis, apparent soon after birth, progresses to hypoxia and acidosis. Cyanosis does not improve with oxygen administration. However, cyanosis may be less apparent when large VSD is also present, and congestive heart failure may develop over days or weeks. Tachypnea (60 respirations/min) is often present without retractions or other signs of dyspnea. Infants take long time to feed and need frequent rest periods because of rapid respiratory rate and fatigue. Growth failure may be evident as early as 2 weeks of age if corrective surgery is not performed.

Diagnostic Tests

Diagnosis is made by echocardiogram when position of arteries arising from ventricles is visible.

Medical Management

Prostaglandin E_1 is initially ordered to maintain patent ductus arteriosus until palliative procedure can be performed. Corrective surgery is usually performed before 1 week of age. Large opening between atria is created with balloon during cardiac catheterization in newborns. This may also be corrected surgically.

PROGNOSIS: Survival without surgery is impossible. Infective endocarditis prophylaxis may be necessary.

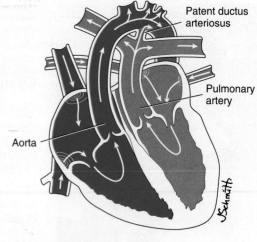

Patent ductus arteriosus

Pulmonary artery

Aorta

☐ Decreased blood flow

---

*Fyler, D.C. (1992). Tetralogy of Fallot. In *Nadas' pediatric cardiology* (pp. 471–491). Philadelphia: Hanley & Belfus.

TABLE 12-8 Less Common Congenital Heart Defects

Condition	Clinical Manifestations	Diagnostic Tests	Medical Management
Hypoplastic Left Heart Syndrome			
Absence or stenosis of mitral and aortic values associated with an abnormally small left ventricle and aortic arch. Signs are initiated with closure of ductus arteriosus.	Signs include tachypnea, retractions, decreased peripheral pulses, poor peripheral perfusion, pulmonary edema, and increased right ventricular impulse, eventually leading to shock and death.	Echocardiogram is used for initial diagnosis.	Prostaglandin E_1 is given to maintain patent ductus arteriosus. Palliative Norwood procedure, and then a modified Fontan procedure or transplantation may be performed. Survival rate is low.
Tricuspid Atresia/Pulmonary Atresia			
This defect is absence of tricuspid or pulmonary valve. Ventricular septal defect (VSD) is also often present.	Early cyanosis, dyspnea, congestive heart failure, hepatomegaly, acidosis, hypoxic spells, clubbing, polycythemia, and growth delays occur. Continuous murmur is heard in aortic area.	Chest x-ray study and echocardiogram are used for initial diagnosis.	Prostaglandin E_1 is given to maintain patent ductus arteriosus. Digoxin and diuretics are also used. Palliative surgery increases pulmonary blood flow. Modified Fontan procedure results in improved survival for tricuspid atresia. The Rashkind procedure is used for pulmonary atresia.
Truncus Arteriosus			
A single large vessel empties both ventricles. VSD is usually present.	Cyanosis develops soon after birth, severe congestive heart failure, dyspnea, retractions, fatigue, poor feeding, polycythemia, clubbing, increased pulse pressure, bounding peripheral pulses, increased respiratory infections, and cardiomegaly also occur.	Chest x-ray and echocardiogram give initial diagnosis. Cardiac catheterization is used before surgery.	Surgery is performed to close VSD and create passage to pulmonary arteries. Digoxin and diuretics are given. Repeated surgery is necessary to enlarge pulmonary artery conduit. Survival is improved, but long-term prognosis is unknown.
Total Anomalous Pulmonary Venous Return			
Pulmonary veins empty into right atrium or systemic veins.	Mild cyanosis and increased right ventricular impulse may occur. With severe pulmonary overload, tachycardia, dyspnea, pulmonary edema, retractions, cyanosis, hepatomegaly, poor feedings, irritability, and failure to thrive are seen.	Chest x-ray study, echocardiogram, and cardiac catheterization are used for diagnosis.	Surgery to reconnect or baffle the pulmonary veins to left atrium is performed. Survivors have lived more than 20 years after correction.

The skin may have a ruddy or mottled appearance before cyanosis is observed. When pulmonary circulation is impaired, hemoglobin may not become reoxygenated. Cyanosis may not be apparent in children who have anemia because there is not enough unoxygenated red blood cells to produce the cyanosis.

Cyanotic (hypoxic) spells, the most significant problem to develop in infants and toddlers with heart defects, usually appear between 2 months and 2 years of age. Cyanotic spells can develop suddenly. Signs include:

- Increased rate and depth of respirations
- Increased cyanosis
- Increased heart rate
- Pallor and poor tissue perfusion
- Agitation or irritability

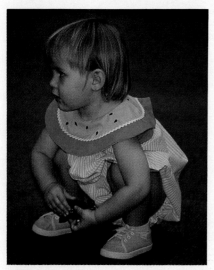

FIGURE 12-5 A child with a cyanotic heart defect squats (assumes a knee-chest position) to relieve cyanotic spells.

Children with uncorrected cyanotic heart disease often squat to relieve dyspnea (Fig. 12–5). The knee-chest position reduces the cardiac output by decreasing the venous return from the lower extremities and by increasing the systemic vascular resistance.

Etiology and Pathophysiology

Cyanotic defects are generally caused by a malformation or combination of defects that prevents adequate oxygenation of the blood. When the defect is associated with decreased pulmonary blood flow, pressures from obstructed blood in the right side of the heart exceed those in the left. Unoxygenated blood is shunted to the left side of the heart. Oxygenated blood destined for the systemic circulation is diluted, resulting in chronic hypoxemia and cyanosis.

When children with cyanosis rise in the morning, they may experience an abrupt decrease in pulmonary blood flow. A cyanotic spell may be triggered by this decrease when combined with a sudden increase in cardiac output and venous return caused by crying, feeding, exercise, and straining with defecation. The partial pressure of oxygen (PO_2) is lowered, and the partial pressure of carbon dioxide (PCO_2) rises. The hypoxemia becomes progressively worse as the respiratory center in the brain overreacts, increasing the respiratory effort. The additional respiratory effort further increases the cardiac output and contributes to a life-threatening decline unless rapid intervention is successful.

Children with cyanotic defects are at increased risk for thromboembolism. The chronic hypoxemia leads to polycythemia in an attempt to increase the hemoglobin available to carry oxygen. Brain abscesses are more common in children with cyanotic heart disease. Bacteria in the blood returning from the systemic circulation are usually filtered out by the capillaries in the lungs. When unoxygenated blood enters the systemic circulation through the right-to-left shunt, bacteria can travel directly to the brain.

Diagnostic Tests and Medical Management

A systolic heart murmur may be apparent after cyanosis develops. A chest x-ray study, electrocardiogram, and echocardiogram are obtained. Usually the echocardiogram clearly shows the defect, shunt, and heart pressures. Cardiac catheterization is often used to obtain detailed anatomic information before surgery.

Early management of cyanotic heart defects is important to prevent secondary damage to the heart, lungs, and brain, including the adverse effects of hypoxemia on the child's cognitive and psychomotor development.[17] For this reason, corrective surgery is being performed at younger ages, often in infancy. A **palliative procedure** may be performed to preserve life in children with potentially lethal heart defects and complications (see Table 12–4). With many defects the success of corrective surgery is better after the infant has had an opportunity to grow.

If closure of the ductus arteriosus causes life-threatening cyanosis in newborns, prostaglandin E_1 (PGE_1) is prescribed to reopen the ductus arteriosus. These infants depend on a patent ductus arteriosus for survival or improvement in pulmonary or systemic blood flow. Treatment with PGE_1 provides time for the newborn to be transferred to a cardiac center for surgical intervention. Response time to PGE_1 varies depending on the type of defect. Cyanotic infants respond within 30 minutes, but infants with acyanotic lesions such as coarctation of the aorta may take up to 3 hours to respond.[18]

The child's hemoglobin level and hematocrit values must be monitored to ensure that the blood does not become too viscous. Polycythemia may be managed by red blood cell pheresis if the blood viscosity becomes too high.

Cyanotic spells are treated aggressively. The initial treatment is placing the child in the knee-chest position, calming the child, and giving oxygen. Morphine is administered. All unpleasant procedures must be postponed. If the spell continues, treatment involves intravenous fluid volume expansion, sodium bicarbonate for acidosis, and drugs to increase vascular resistance. Once a cyanotic spell has occurred, immediate palliative or corrective surgery is often scheduled.[19]

Antibiotic prophylaxis for infective endocarditis is needed before and after surgical correction for all cyanotic conditions. See Table 12–6 for a list of recommended antibiotics.

Nursing Assessment

Frequently monitor the cardiovascular status of infants receiving PGE_1 therapy. Assess vital signs, heart rhythm, skin color, peripheral pulses, and capillary refill time. Observe for signs of improvement in vital signs and color as the oxygen saturation increases and acidosis decreases following the initial treatment. In addition, watch for tachycardia, tachypnea, crackles, frothy secretions, low urine output, and edema because these infants are at risk for congestive heart failure.

Observe the child carefully for signs of increased cyanosis in the morning or at other high risk times. Watch for neurologic signs of thromboembolitic complications from polycythemia such as headache, dizziness, excessive irritability, and paralysis. Older children with cyanotic defects may have clubbing (Fig. 12–6).

Nursing Diagnosis

Common nursing diagnoses for the child with cyanotic heart disease include:

- Altered Cardiopulmonary Tissue Perfusion related to reduced pulmonary blood flow
- Decreased Cardiac Output related to developing congestive heart failure
- High Risk for Infection related to unfiltered bacteria in the blood and sites of blood shunting that promote bacterial growth
- Altered Nutrition: Less Than Body Requirements related to dyspnea and fatigue with feeding
- Ineffective Infant Feeding Pattern related to dyspnea and fatigue
- High Risk for Caregiver Role Strain related to care of a child with chronic illness
- Activity Intolerance related to cyanosis and dyspnea on exertion
- Altered Growth and Development related to hypoxemia
- High Risk for Ineffective Management of Therapeutic Regimen related to prophylactic antibiotics for dental care procedures
- Knowledge Deficit (Parents) related to assessment and management of cyanotic spells, which are unpredictable events

Nursing Management

Children with tetralogy of Fallot are often managed at home until surgery is scheduled. Home care involves reducing parental anxiety, providing adequate nutrition, helping parents recognize signs of illness, and formulating a plan for emergency treatment. Nursing care of the hospitalized child focuses on monitoring PGE_1 therapy (for newborn only, used until palliative surgery is performed), treating cyanotic spells, and providing postsurgical care.

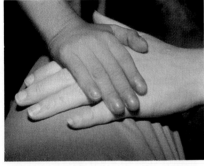

FIGURE 12–6 Clubbing of the fingers is one manifestation of a cyanotic defect in an older child. What neurologic signs may be associated with such a defect?

HOME CARE OF THE CHILD BEFORE SURGERY. Parents are usually anxious because of the need to wait before surgery can be performed. They often fear that the infant will not survive until surgery or that they will be unable to manage any problems the infant may have. Provide parents with information and teach them how to care for the child at home. Some infants have such special home care needs that home health nursing and other community resources are needed. Many of these children require supplemental oxygen and nutrition, either for emergencies or for regular use.

Cyanosis with or without congestive heart failure often results in delayed gross motor skills. Developmental specialists can help parents set realistic developmental goals for the child. Make referrals to community-based Zero to Three Early Intervention Programs to promote the child's development.

Encourage parents to treat the infant as normally as possible. The child should be able to tolerate crying for a few minutes without difficulty. Prolonged crying should not be permitted because it causes fatigue and further hypoxia.

Vomiting and diarrhea may lead to dehydration, and parents must notify the physician whenever the infant or child has these symptoms. Dehydration is a particular risk in children with polycythemia because the blood can become even more viscous. Fever and dehydration may increase cyanosis. The systemic vascular resistance is decreased, resulting in a further decrease in blood flow to the pulmonary system. Aggressive management with antipyretic medication and fluid volume replacement is necessary.[20]

Teach parents to observe the child for signs of infective endocarditis, including low-grade fever, fatigue, and malaise. They need to notify the physician if these symptoms occur within 2 months of surgery or a high-risk procedure. Parents must learn to request antibiotic prophylaxis for the child (Table 12–6). Children also need preventive dental care to reduce the risk of endocarditis.

Parents may want to formulate an emergency plan in case the infant develops acute problems such as a cyanotic spell or respiratory distress. Cardiopulmonary resuscitation should be taught to the parents. Ask parents to notify the local rescue squad about the infant's problem. Prepare a card or brief history form with information about the child's condition, medications, and necessary emergency care and the physician's name for parents to keep at home. When an acute problem occurs, this card gives important information to the emergency medical technicians and emergency department staff.

Although parents may travel with cyanotic children, they should not take these children to areas of high altitude without consulting with the physician first. Arrangements for supplemental oxygen when traveling on an airplane may be necessary.

CARE OF THE INFANT AND CHILD UNDERGOING SURGERY. Monitor and carefully maintain the central, umbilical, or peripheral intravenous lines in the infant receiving continuous infusion of PGE_1. Observe the infant for side effects of prostaglandin treatment. Have intubation equipment and a bag and mask at the bedside in case apnea occurs. Have intravenous fluids available to control hypotension.

If a cyanotic spell occurs, immediately place the child in the knee-chest position and administer oxygen. Administer morphine as ordered. Immediately notify the physician for further orders if these procedures are ineffective and the spell continues. Avoid any unpleasant or anxiety-provoking procedures.

Children are admitted to the intensive care unit following surgery. Refer to the section on nursing assessment in nursing care of the child undergoing

■ NURSING ALERT

Common side effects of PGE_1 therapy include cutaneous vasodilation, bradycardia, tachycardia, hypotension, seizure activity, fever, and apnea.

surgery (see Chapter 4). Postoperative bleeding is a potential risk in children with polycythemia because bleeding times are prolonged and platelet counts are low. Chest tube output is monitored carefully for bright red blood or excessive volume. Bright red blood in the chest tube is a significant sign of hemorrhage. Fluids and diuretics are used to maintain **preload** (the volume of blood in the ventricle at the end of diastole that stretches the heart muscle before contraction) in the right ventricle while inotropic drugs are used to support cardiac output. Children are transferred to the general nursing unit once heart function has stabilized.

Monitor the heart functioning of children following surgery. Assess vital signs, skin color, perfusion of the skin by capillary refill, and distal pulses. A sudden sustained increase in pulse and respirations and a decrease in peripheral perfusion may be early signs of hemorrhage. Monitoring fluid intake and output following surgery is critical. Note any signs of respiratory distress that may indicate the development of a pneumothorax or congestive heart failure.

Acquired Heart Diseases

Rheumatic Fever

Rheumatic fever is an inflammatory disease that follows an initial infection by some strains of group A beta-hemolytic streptococci. This disorder causes changes in the heart, joints, skin, and, less often, the central nervous system. As a result of effective treatment of streptococcal infections, the incidence of rheumatic fever reached a low in the United States in the 1970s. The disease has occurred more frequently in recent years, probably because of an increase in number and severity of group A streptococcal infections.[21] The exact cause of the disease is unknown. Possible causes include a bacterial toxin or an altered immune response.

Several weeks after an untreated streptococcal infection, the hallmark signs of rheumatic fever may occur. Aschoff bodies (hemorrhagic bullous lesions) develop in the connective tissue of the heart. Endocarditis may lead to permanent heart valve damage. The child's joints become inflamed and painful (migratory polyarthritis), although this condition improves in several weeks. Subcutaneous nodules may be palpable near joints. A skin rash called erythema marginatum, with pink macules and blanching in the middle of the lesions, is frequently seen. Spiking fever often occurs. A condition known as Sydenham chorea (St. Vitus dance), which is characterized by aimless movements of the extremities and facial grimacing, may be seen if the central nervous system is involved. Mild anemia may also occur.

Diagnosis is based on clinical signs (Jones criteria) (Table 12–9) and laboratory testing for antistreptolysin-O. An elevated antistreptolysin-O (ASO) antibody titer indicates a recent streptococcal infection.

Medical treatment includes antibiotics (penicillin or erythromycin) to eradicate the streptococcal infection. Aspirin may be given to control joint inflammation and reduce fever. Children should be monitored carefully for potential heart involvement. Most children recover fully.

Nursing Management

The most important role of the nurse is prevention of rheumatic fever. All children with possible streptococcal infections should have a throat culture.

TABLE 12–9 Guidelines for Diagnosis of Initial Attack of Rheumatic Fever (Jones Criteria, updated 1992)*

Major Manifestations	Minor Manifestations
Carditis	*Clinical findings*
Polyarthritis	Arthralgia
Chorea	Fever
Erythema marginatum	*Laboratory findings*
	Elevated acute-phase reactants
Subcutaneous nodules	Erythrocyte sedimentation rate
	C-reactive protein
	Prolonged PR interval

Supporting evidence of antecedent group A streptococcal infection: (1) positive throat culture or rapid streptococcal antigen test; (2) elevated or rising streptococcal antibody titer.

*If supported by evidence of preceding group A streptococcal infection, the presence of two major manifestations or of one major and two minor manifestations indicates a high probability of acute rheumatic fever.
Data from Special Writing Group of the Committee on Rheumatic Fever, Endocarditis, and Kawasaki Disease of the Council on Cardiovascular Disease in the Young (1992). Dallas, TX: American Heart Association.

It is important that a child with a positive culture complete the 10-day course of antibiotics.

When the child with rheumatic fever is hospitalized, nursing care focuses on assessing the child's condition, promoting recovery, and ensuring compliance with the treatment regimen.

During the acute inflammatory phase, take the child's temperature at least every 4 hours and monitor vital signs. Auscultate the child's heart and note any unusual sounds. Observe the child for changes in skin, joints, or behavior. Family members should have throat cultures done to identify possible asymptomatic streptococcal carriers.

Administer penicillin and aspirin as ordered. The child is usually lethargic and often has joint pain. Position the child's joints and handle them carefully. Use tepid sponges and cool compresses to control spiking fevers. Provide quiet activities, since the child is often confined to bed. The child is usually placed in isolation. Encourage visits or telephone calls from family members and friends. For the child with chorea, provide emotional support because the purposeless involuntary movements can be disturbing. Encourage the family to participate in the child's hospital care.

During the recovery phase the child's activities may be limited, especially if heart damage is suspected. Help parents plan quiet activities, such as playing board games, working with computers, or reading, and arrange rest periods after the child returns to school. Reassure the child and parents that the effects of chorea will eventually subside.

On discharge a daily oral low-dose antibiotic is prescribed or monthly long-acting antibiotic injection is given. Make sure the child and parents understand the importance of taking prescribed medication indefinitely to prevent future infection and possible heart damage from recurrent rheumatic fever. Stress the importance of telling future health care providers, including dentists and surgeons, about the child's rheumatic fever history so prophylactic antibiotics can be given to prevent infective endocarditis during invasive procedures.

Make sure the parents understand that their child's future sore throats may be streptococcal and that a throat culture should be taken even when the child is taking daily antibiotics. Emphasize the importance of follow-up care to prevent new infection and to monitor heart function.

Infective Endocarditis

Endocarditis is an inflammation of the heart lining and valves. Infective endocarditis, also known as subacute bacterial endocarditis, is the most common type of this infection.

Symptoms can be mild and develop slowly, or they can be severe and develop rapidly. Common symptoms are fever (often with elevations in the afternoon), fatigue, joint and muscle aches, headache, and gastrointestinal discomfort.[22] Other signs include chest pain, dyspnea, weight loss, splenomegaly, and dysrhythmias or murmurs.

Most infections are caused by *Streptococcus* or *Staphylococcus*. Children who have a congenital heart defect, rheumatic heart disease, or a central venous catheter or who have had heart surgery are at risk for infective endocarditis. Infections frequently occur after the causal organism enters the bloodstream during dental work or surgery.

Infective endocarditis is diagnosed primarily by blood culture; however, urine and cerebrospinal fluid also may be cultured. Elevated erythrocyte sedimentation rate, anemia, elevated C-reactive protein level, increased white blood cell count, alterations in electrocardiogram, and changes in heart sounds and murmurs are indicators of the diagnosis. Echocardiography may be used to identify the presence of infective lesions in the heart.

Treatment consists of administering antibiotics such as penicillin G, ampicillin, vancomycin, nafcillin, or gentamicin. Intravenous administration is preferred, with therapy continuing for 2 to 8 weeks. Serum levels of antibiotics are monitored to maintain a therapeutic range. Occasionally surgery is necessary to drain an abscess or because of heart valve failure. If congestive heart failure occurs, bed rest and medications such as digoxin and furosemide are given. Although treatment is effective in the majority of children, 20% to 25% die because of heart damage.[22]

Nursing Management

Nursing care focuses on assessing the child's condition, administering medications, and teaching the parents about the child's care. Take the child's vital signs and assess gastrointestinal discomfort. Administer medications as ordered and monitor serum antibiotic levels. Monitor for side effects of antibiotics and for infiltration or extravasation at the infusion site. Keep invasive procedures to a minimum. Use careful aseptic technique in performing venipunctures, urinary catheterizations, and other procedures.

The child is often lethargic and on bed rest. Encourage parents to assist with the child's care and plan quiet age-appropriate activities. At discharge, instruct parents about administration of oral antibiotics at home and reinforce the need for follow-up visits. Explain the importance of informing physicians and dentists about the child's history of endocarditis so that care is taken to prevent infection before invasive procedures.

Cardiac Dysrhythmias

Cardiac dysrhythmias (abnormal rhythms) are not uncommon in children. Most are not harmful and do not require intervention.[23] These include tachydysrhythmias (sinus tachycardia) and bradydysrhythmias (sinus bradycardia) that occur with acute conditions and resolve once the condition is treated. Other abnormal rates and rhythms should be evaluated by a cardiologist. Supraventricular tachycardia is the most common abnormal dysrhythmia. Other dysrhythmias, which are usually associated with congenital heart disease, include atrial fibrillation, atrial flutter, ventricular fibrillation, and heart block.

Supraventricular tachycardia is a sudden, rapid, but regular heart rate, often too fast to count. Neonates and young children may be predisposed to the condition because of a congenital heart defect or Wolff-Parkinson-White syndrome. Short periods of dysrhythmia (several seconds), which may be caused by paroxysmal atrial tachycardia, are rarely dangerous. However, prolonged episodes may lead to congestive heart failure or death. Recurrent attacks are common. Electrocardiography is used to confirm the diagnosis.

The condition is life threatening and quickly progresses to congestive heart failure or cardiogenic shock if untreated. Cardiac output is affected because diastolic filling cannot occur with such a rapid heart rate.

Vagal stimulation such as application of ice or iced saline solution to the face may reduce the heart rate. An older child can perform the Valsalva maneuver to increase intrathoracic and venous pressures and thus slow the heart rate. Adenosine is the recommended emergency medication. Cardioversion may be used for life-threatening episodes if other treatments are not effective. Digoxin and propranolol may be given to reduce the frequency of episodes.[22,24]

Nursing Management

Nursing care focuses on assessing the child's condition, administering medications, and providing emotional support to the child and parents. Children are treated in the emergency department or intensive care unit. The child is placed on a cardiac monitor, and frequent assessment is critical. Report continued abnormal rates or rhythms to the physician. Carefully observe and record changes in level of consciousness, color, weakness, irritability, and feeding pattern. Administer medications as ordered. Have emergency drugs and resuscitation equipment available at the bedside. Provide for rest and adequate nutrition.

Episodes of dysrhythmia are frightening for both the child and parents. Carefully explain the treatment plan and home care. Teach parents to take the child's apical pulse. Provide telephone numbers of emergency medical facilities and help parents plan how to seek emergency care. Emphasize that the prognosis after extended treatment with digoxin is favorable.

Vascular Diseases

Kawasaki Disease

Kawasaki disease, also known as mucocutaneous lymph node syndrome, is an acute systemic inflammatory illness. Although this disorder is most commonly found in Japanese children, it is seen in all races. It occurs primarily in toddlers. In the United States, Kawasaki disease is the most common cause of acquired heart disease in children, and its incidence is increasing.[25]

The acute stage of the disease is characterized by fever, conjunctival hyperemia, red throat, swollen hands and feet, rash, and enlargement of the cervical lymph nodes. The subacute stage is characterized by cracking lips and fissures, desquamation of the skin on the tips of the fingers and toes, joint pain, cardiac disease, and thrombocytosis. In the convalescent stage the child appears normal but lingering signs of inflammation may be present.

The etiology of Kawasaki disease is unknown, but the primary cause is infection with an organism or toxin. The disease occurs most often in late summer and early spring. It is not spread by person-to-person contact.

Diagnosis is based on clinical signs using the criteria given in Table 12–10. Blood studies show some abnormalities such as elevated erythrocyte sedimentation rate, elevated white blood cell count, mild anemia, elevated platelet count, and elevated C-reactive protein level. Echocardiogram may reveal some heart changes.

Medical management of Kawasaki disease involves the use of aspirin and gamma globulin. High doses of aspirin (80 to 100 mg/kg/day) are given while the fever is high. The dose is decreased to 10 mg/kg/day or less once the fever has dropped. Aspirin is taken until the platelet count is normal and may be continued on a long-term basis if cardiac abnormalities occur.

TABLE 12–10 Diagnostic Criteria for Kawasaki Disease

Kawasaki disease is diagnosed when fever lasts for 5 days and four of the following five criteria are present:
- Bilateral conjunctivitis without exudate
- Mucous membrane changes such as erythema of lips and tongue
- Skin changes of extremities such as edema, erythema, or desquamation
- Polymorphous rash with absence of vesicles or crusts
- Cervical lymphadenopathy with at least one node over 1.5 cm in diameter

From Plauth, W.H. (1985). *Critical Care Quarterly, 8,* 39–47.

Gamma globulin given early in the disease has been shown to reduce the incidence of coronary artery lesions and aneurysms, although the mechanism is unknown.[26]

Children are usually hospitalized as long as fever persists. Most children recover fully. Careful monitoring for cardiac disease continues for several weeks or months. Cardiac involvement is the most serious complication. Aneurysms and other vessel changes lead to dysrhythmias, congestive heart failure, myocardial infarction, and, potentially, death.

Nursing Management

Nursing care focuses on promoting comfort, monitoring for early signs of complications or disease progression, and supporting the family.

Assessment is important in identifying signs of Kawasaki disease, since the acute phase of this disorder is commonly confused with other diseases. Take the child's temperature every 4 hours and before each dose of aspirin. Carefully assess the extremities for edema, redness, and desquamation every 8 hours. Examine the eyes for conjunctivitis and the mucous membranes for inflammation. Monitor the child's dietary and fluid intake and weigh the child daily. Carefully assess heart sounds and rhythm.

Administer aspirin and gamma globulin as ordered. Monitor for side effects of aspirin such as bleeding and gastrointestinal upset. Administer intravenous gamma globulin as a blood product, carefully regulating the rate to run slowly according to the physician's orders, and watching for any reactions to the infusion. If symptoms of reaction are noted, *stop* the infusion immediately (see the Atlas of Pediatric Procedures).

Promote the child's comfort. Keep the child's skin clean and dry, and lubricate the lips. Use cool compresses and tepid sponges to keep the feverish child more comfortable. Change the child's clothes and bed linens frequently. Give the child frequent small feedings of soft foods and liquids that are neither too hot nor too cold. Use passive range of motion exercises to facilitate joint movement.

Since the child is frequently lethargic and irritable, plan rest periods and quiet age-appropriate activities. Encourage the parents to participate in their child's care. This comforts and reassures the child. Provide the parents with information about the disease and the child's treatment.

Before the child is discharged, teach the parents to administer aspirin as ordered and watch for side effects. Have them take the child's temperature daily and report any fever above 100° F (37.8° C) to the physician. Emphasize the need for follow-up care to monitor for cardiac complications.

Hyperlipidemia

Hyperlipidemia is excessive fat in the blood that may eventually lead to atherosclerosis. Although children do not usually die of atherosclerotic heart disease, coronary heart disease, the major cause of death in the United States, begins in childhood and progresses through the adult years.[28] It is important to identify children who have a genetic history or life-style that makes them more susceptible to future coronary heart disease (Table 12–11).

As the excessive fat circulates, it causes changes in blood vessels. The fatty streaks that appear in childhood become fibrous plaques in adolescence. These atherosclerotic plaques continue to grow in adulthood and may cause hemorrhage, thrombi, and occlusion of vessels.[29]

Hyperlipidemia is identified by a blood test. Cholesterol, including total cholesterol (TC), high-density lipoprotein cholesterol (HDL), very low-density lipoprotein cholesterol (VLDL), and triglycerides are measured. The

TABLE 12–11 Risk Factors for Hyperlipidemia

Family history of coronary heart disease before age 55
Cigarette smoking
Hypertension
Diabetes
Lack of exercise
High fat intake
Obesity

low-density lipoprotein cholesterol (LDL) level is calculated using an equation based on the triglyceride, VLDL, HDL, and total cholesterol levels. It has been recommended that all children who have a family history of cardiovascular disease before age 55 years (parents or grandparents) or who have a parent with elevated total serum cholesterol (≥240 mg/dL) be screened.[28] Some clinicians choose to screen all children, especially those with an unknown family history, during childhood or sometime after the age of 2 years. Based on total cholesterol value, children are placed in a low-, moderate-, or high-risk category. The LDL cholesterol level is examined carefully in children with elevated total cholesterol (≥200 mg/dL). LDL cholesterol should be less than 110 mg/dL. High HDL and low LDL cholesterol levels provide protection against heart disease.

Some children have hereditary disorders of lipid metabolism characterized by high levels of cholesterol, triglycerides, or both.[30] Children with hypercholesterolemia, for example, have cholesterol levels of 600 to 1000 mg/dL, resulting in lipid deposits in their corneas and tendons. These uncommon conditions require treatment by a lipid specialist.

Hyperlipidemia in most children can be managed by dietary modifications and other changes in life-style. The child's diet is carefully analyzed, and changes are made to satisfy the dietary guidelines given in Table 12–12. If the child continues to have high serum lipid levels, a lipid specialist should be consulted. Cholestyramine or colestipol, which bind bile acid in the intestine, are occasionally prescribed for children over 10 years of age.

Long-term studies of the effect of childhood lipid levels on life span are not yet concluded. It is hoped that careful monitoring and management of lipid levels in childhood will decrease the incidence of cardiovascular disease.

Nursing Management

Nursing care focuses on identifying children at risk for hyperlipidemia, providing education about diet and exercise, and monitoring eating patterns. The child's history of exercise patterns, weight percentile, and dietary intake provides important information. Obtain information on familial heart disease, hypertension, diabetes, and smoking to determine risk factors. Tell parents that the child will need to fast for 12 hours before blood is drawn to evaluate serum lipid levels.

Work with nutritionists to provide dietary teaching and monitor family eating patterns. Emphasize the importance of exercise in keeping the heart and blood vessels free from atherosclerotic changes. Help the child select an aerobic activity and encourage participation at least three times weekly.

Smoking by the child or the parents should be discouraged. Secondhand smoke may affect blood pressure and increase the risk for the development of cardiovascular disease.[31]

■ AEROBIC ACTIVITIES

Running	Biking
Jogging	Soccer
Fast walking	Aerobic dancing
Hiking	Rollerblading
Swimming	

TABLE 12–12 Recommended Nutrient Intake in Children and Adolescents with Hyperlipidemia

Nutrient	Recommended Intake
Saturated fatty acid	Less than 10% of calories
Total fat	Average no more than 30% of calories
Polyunsaturated	Up to 10% of calories
Monounsaturated	10%–15% of calories
Cholesterol	Less than 300 mg/day

Modified from National Cholesterol Education Program Coordinating Committee. (1991). *Report of the Expert Panel on Blood Cholesterol Levels in Children and Adolescents.* Washington, DC: U.S. Department of Health and Human Services.

Include the entire family in the treatment plan, since changing eating and exercise patterns is difficult for a single family member.[32] The family of a child with hyperlipidemia requires continual teaching and reinforcement. Nutrition assessments and evaluation of family diet should be performed periodically.

Hypertension

Hypertension is uncommon in children. Most cases are caused by underlying conditions such as kidney disease or heart defects. However, a genetic predisposition to hypertension may be manifested in some children by high normal or slightly elevated blood pressures. All children with blood pressures in the 90th percentile for age are significantly more likely to develop hypertension as adults.[33]

Take a complete history for the child with borderline hypertension and no other associated diseases. Are parents or siblings hypertensive? Is the child obese? What is the child's daily salt intake? What are the child's daily exercise routines? Serum lipid studies should be performed to determine whether hyperlipidemia exists.

Teach both the child and the parents how to improve the diet and develop exercise routines. Teaching that involves the entire family is usually the most effective. Take the child's blood pressure regularly to monitor changes.

Persistent Pulmonary Hypertension

Persistent pulmonary hypertension is a disease of newborns, especially premature infants, resulting from pulmonary artery constriction. The increased pressure leads to a right-to-left shunt. In some children with congenital heart defects, excessive pulmonary blood flow leads to pulmonary vascular resistance.

Hypoxemia results from pulmonary hypertension, and the infant displays tachypnea, cyanosis, retractions, and fatigue. Feeding is difficult, and weight loss with fluid and electrolyte imbalance is likely.

The pulmonary hypertension may be caused by hyaline membrane disease, polycythemia, meconium aspiration, a respiratory infection, or a congenital heart defect.[22] After the cause is determined, the infant is treated with oxygen, ventilation, and medications.

Nursing care focuses on promoting rest for oxygen conservation, monitoring fluid intake and output carefully, and administering medications and oxygen. Newborns often require mechanical ventilation. Give parents needed support and information about their infant. Encourage them to visit but to avoid any stimulation of the newborn.

Injuries of the Cardiovascular System

Shock

Shock is an acute complex state of circulatory dysfunction resulting in failure to deliver sufficient oxygen and other nutrients to meet tissue demands. It can be caused by a variety of conditions.

Hypovolemic Shock

Hypovolemic shock is a clinical state of inadequate tissue and organ perfusion resulting from the movement of blood or plasma out of the intravascular compartment.[34] The blood or plasma in the vascular space may be decreased because of hemorrhage or fluid movement into the interstitial spaces. Hypovolemia is the most common cause of shock in infants and children.[35]

Clinical Manifestations

Signs of early hypovolemic shock in children are nonspecific but need to be recognized before hypotension occurs. Signs indicating that the child is compensating for a decreased blood volume are tachycardia, usually sustained at a rate greater than 130 beats per minute, increased respiratory effort, delayed capillary refill (>2 seconds), weak peripheral pulses, pallor, and cold extremities (signs of decreased perfusion). Although the child's body attempts to compensate by preserving circulation to vital organs, a decreased level of consciousness ultimately results from reduced cerebral blood flow. Urine output decreases when renal blood flow drops.

If treatment is not initiated in the early stages of hypovolemic shock, the condition progresses until the child can no longer compensate. At that time the systolic blood pressure drops and the pulse pressure decreases. In cases of dehydration, dry mucous membranes and poor skin turgor are also present. Table 12–13 compares the signs associated with early, uncompensated, and profound shock.

Etiology and Pathophysiology

Major causes of decreased intravascular blood volume include:

- Hemorrhage from significant injury
- Plasma loss from burns, nephrotic syndrome, and sepsis
- Fluid and electrolyte loss associated with dehydration, diabetic ketoacidosis, and diabetes insipidus
- Vasodilating drugs

Shock results in inadequate delivery of oxygen and nutrients to cells and accumulation of toxic wastes in the capillaries. This reduction in circulating

TABLE 12-13 Signs of Hypovolemic Shock

System	Early Shock	Uncompensated Shock	Profound Shock
Cardiac	Tachycardia, weak distal pulses	Tachycardia, absent distal pulses, decreasing systolic blood pressure	Frank hypotension, bradycardia, weak central pulses
Neurologic	Normal, anxious, irritable, or combative behavior	Confusion, lethargy, decreased pain response	Comatose state
Skin	Mottled appearance; capillary refill time ≥ 2 seconds; cool, clammy extremities	Cyanosis, capillary refill time > 3 seconds, cold extremities	Pale, cold skin
Renal	Decreased urine output, increased specific gravity	Oliguria, increased specific gravity	No urine output

Modified from Waisman, H., Eichelberger, M.R. (1993). Hypovolemic shock. In Eichelberger, M.R. (Ed.), *Pediatric trauma: Prevention, acute care, rehabilitation* (p. 182). St. Louis: Mosby–Year Book.

blood volume causes a decrease in cardiac output and mean arterial pressure. Cellular hypoxia and acidosis develop simultaneously. The accumulation of toxins and inadequate tissue oxygenation cause cellular damage.

The child's body attempts to compensate by the following:

- The heart rate and myocardial contractility increase to improve cardiac output.
- The respiratory rate increases to improve oxygenation and decrease waste accumulation in the cells.
- The hydrostatic pressure falls, permitting fluid to shift into the vascular space and increasing the circulating blood volume.
- The peripheral vasculature constricts to maintain the systemic vascular resistance as long as possible.

The child is able to compensate until 20% to 25% of volume loss occurs, and then life-threatening hypotension results.

Diagnostic Tests and Medical Management

No laboratory values can be used to evaluate the volume deficit rapidly and diagnose hypovolemic shock. The child is examined for characteristic signs to confirm the diagnosis.

Laboratory tests commonly performed after hypovolemic shock is diagnosed include hematocrit and hemoglobin, arterial blood gases, serum electrolytes, glucose, osmolality, blood urea nitrogen, and urinalysis.

Emergency care focuses on improving tissue perfusion. An open airway is established, oxygen is administered, and ventilation is assisted if necessary. Bleeding is controlled, and an IV is started to provide large volumes of crystalloid fluids (Ringer's lactate).

Ringer's lactate solution is the preferred fluid for initial resuscitation. A fluid volume of 20 mL/kg is administered rapidly over 5 minutes. The same amount of fluid is given in 5 minutes if the child's physiologic condition does not improve after fluid is first administered. If no improvement is seen after the second fluid bolus, blood or albumin is usually ordered.

Once the child's physiologic condition is stabilized, the cause of the hypovolemic shock becomes the focus of examination and treatment.

Nursing Assessment

Ask the parent (or child, if appropriate) about possible injuries or the duration and severity of acute illnesses. If no external bleeding is evident, determine whether an injury may be causing internal bleeding. For example, the liver and spleen are highly vascular organs that have little protection from direct blunt forces. Significant bleeding from injury to one of these organs can cause hypovolemic shock without evidence of bleeding. An acute illness such as gastroenteritis with prolonged vomiting and diarrhea can also result in dehydration and hypovolemic shock.

If external bleeding is apparent, determine the amount of blood lost. Although children lose the same amount of blood from a laceration as adults, the total volume of blood lost is proportional to their weight.

When an injured child is admitted to the hospital for a problem such as a liver or spleen laceration, assess the child's circulatory status frequently. Current medical treatment for these injuries is conservative. Surgeons give the liver or spleen a chance to heal spontaneously rather than perform immediate surgery to control bleeding and repair the laceration. Even if the child's circulatory condition was stabilized during emergency care, shock can develop again if bleeding continues.

■ GROWTH AND DEVELOPMENT
CONSIDERATIONS

The child's total blood volume varies by weight. The child has approximately 80 mL of blood for every kilogram of body weight.[36]

Newborn: 3 kg × 80 mL = 240 mL (1 cup)

5-year-old child: 25 kg × 80 mL = 2000 mL (2 quarts)

13-year-old child: 50 kg × 80 mL = 4000 mL (1 gallon)

Frequently assess the child's heart rate, respiratory rate, blood pressure, capillary refill time, level of consciousness (with the Glasgow Coma Scale) (see Chapter 14), color, and skin temperature to identify any changes that indicate improvement or deterioration in the child's condition. Monitor urine output and specific gravity hourly. Signs of the child's improved status include:

- A decrease in heart rate, respiratory rate, and capillary refill time
- An increase in systolic blood pressure and urine output
- Improved color, level of consciousness, and skin temperature
- Regaining of lost weight

Nursing Diagnosis

Several nursing diagnoses may apply to the child with hypovolemic shock. They include:

- Decreased Cardiac Output related to blood loss or dehydration
- Fluid Volume Deficit related to dehydration
- Altered Cardiopulmonary, Renal, and Cerebral Tissue Perfusion related to decreased circulating blood volume
- Ineffective Airway Clearance related to altered level of consciousness
- Ineffective Family Coping: Compromised related to life-threatening condition of the child
- Anxiety related to unexpected hospitalization for an emergency condition

Nursing Management

Nurses in the emergency department and intensive care unit participate in the resuscitation of the child in hypovolemic shock. Assist with the child's assessment and the establishment of intravenous access. Calculate and prepare the amount of intravenous fluid needed for administration according to the child's weight (20 mL/kg). Ensure rapid fluid administration by intravenous push or pressure bag. Monitor the child's physiologic response to the fluid bolus within 5 minutes. Prepare a second and third fluid bolus.

Use warmed intravenous fluids for resuscitation because hypothermia may interfere with the child's response to treatment. Keep the child covered or use heat lamps to reduce body heat loss.

When packed red blood cells are administered, verify that the correct blood has been obtained for the child. Change the intravenous fluid to normal saline solution to prevent clotting during blood administration. Assess the child carefully for a transfusion reaction (see Chapter 13). Monitor the child's physiologic circulatory responses for improvement or deterioration in status. Notify the physician of any deterioration.

Provide support to the child and family during the acute phase of treatment. Parents and children with hypovolemic shock resulting from injury are usually apprehensive. The child may be fearful because of the sudden hospitalization or agitated because of an altered level of consciousness. Determine the causes of the child's anxiety. The parents often fear for the child's life in cases of injury. Update the parents about the child's condition frequently. Explain the care being provided and how it helps the child. Listen to their concerns and correct any misconceptions.

Distributive Shock

Distributive (septic) shock is an abnormal pooling of blood in the extremities that may be caused by anaphylaxis, sepsis, or spinal cord injury. Immunodeficient children are at high risk for septic shock. The blood accumulates in the extremities because of vasodilation. Less blood is returned to the heart, so preload drops and cardiac output falls.

Septic shock has two phases, warm (hyperdynamic) and cold (hypodynamic). During the hyperdynamic phase, perfusion appears adequate. The child has a fever and tachycardia, tachypnea, warm extremities, bounding pulses, and brisk capillary refill.

Cardiac output is high but systemic vascular resistance is low, leading to an uneven flow and pooling in the extremities. Blood moves sluggishly, and anaerobic metabolism and lactic acidosis occur in tissue beds where oxygen no longer circulates. As the syndrome progresses, the hypodynamic phase develops. Cardiac output is low, and systemic vascular resistance is high. Blood has already pooled in the extremities. During the hypodynamic phase the child is cool, hypotensive, pale, and oliguric. Blood is shunted away from the kidneys, muscles, and skin to the heart and brain. Multisystem organ failure occurs if treatment does not improve regional perfusion.

Treatment for septic shock is initiated even before the diagnosis is confirmed. Fluid resuscitation is used in early septic shock to stabilize the circulation and ensure adequate tissue perfusion. Antibiotics effective against the suspected organism are given. Vasopressors are given during the hypodynamic phase. Morbidity and mortality are high even when treatment is initiated early. Complications include disseminated intravascular coagulation and adult respiratory distress syndrome.

Obstructive Shock

Obstructive shock occurs when a blockage of the main bloodstream interferes with tissue perfusion. Causes in children include compression of the vena cava, pericardial tamponade, pulmonary embolism, tension pneumothorax, pleural effusion, and congenital heart defects with outflow obstruction (for example, coarctation of the aorta). Management is focused on treatment of the underlying condition.

Cardiogenic Shock

Cardiogenic shock is an abnormality of myocardial function leading to low cardiac output and inadequate tissue perfusion. Causes of cardiogenic shock in children may include congestive heart failure, congenital heart disease, and dysrhythmias such as bradycardia and supraventricular tachycardia. Cardiogenic shock may also be an end stage for other acute and chronic conditions such as sepsis, prolonged shock, hypoglycemia, and muscular dystrophy. Heart failure may result from obstructed outflow in congenital heart defects such as coarctation of the aorta.

Clinically, cardiogenic shock resembles hypovolemic shock. Tachycardia, hypotension, cool extremities, depressed level of consciousness, acidosis, and oliguria are common signs. Increased systemic vascular resistance puts more stress on the failing heart.

The goal of medical treatment is restoration of myocardial function with adequate ventilation, correction of dysrhythmias, fluid management, and administration of diuretics and inotropic drugs.

Myocardial Contusion

Myocardial contusion, a rare injury in children, results from a strong, blunt force against the chest wall that injures the heart muscle. Blood flow to areas of the heart muscle is disrupted, or myocardial cells are directly destroyed. This potentially life-threatening condition is often associated with a motor vehicle–related injury. It most often occurs in adolescents who have struck the steering wheel of a motor vehicle during a crash.

A myocardial contusion should be suspected in cases of injury to the anterior chest. This condition is often overlooked during the initial emergency assessment. The child has chest discomfort because of fractured ribs or chest wall contusion. An electrocardiogram reveals dysrhythmias or signs of myocardial infarct. An echocardiogram may show an abnormality in heart wall movement. Cardiac isoenzyme concentrations are elevated. Because of the risk of sudden dysrhythmias, the child is admitted to the intensive care unit for cardiac monitoring.

REFERENCES

1 National Center for Health Statistics. (1993). *National vital statistics system*, unpublished data.

2 Hoffman, J.I.E. (1990). Congenital heart disease: Incidence and inheritance. *Pediatric Clinics of North America, 37*, 25–43.

3 Freed, M.D. (1992). Fetal and transitional circulation. In Fyler, D.C. (Ed.), *Nadas' pediatric cardiology* (p. 59). Philadelphia: Hanley & Belfus.

4 Ludwig, S., & Loiselle, J. (1993). Anatomy, growth, and development: Impact on injury. In Eichelberger, M.R. (Ed.), *Pediatric trauma: Prevention, acute care, rehabilitation* (pp. 39–58). St. Louis: Mosby–Year Book.

5 Carroll, P.L.F. (1988). Cyanosis: The sign you can't count on. *Nursing 88, 18*, 50.

6 Hazinski, M.F. (1992). *Nursing care of the critically ill child* (2nd ed.). St. Louis: Mosby–Year Book.

7 Sims, S.L. (1990). Alterations in cardiovascular function in children. In McCance, K.L., & Huether, S.E. (Eds.), *Pathophysiology: The biologic basis for disease in adults and children*. St. Louis: Mosby–Year Book.

8 Eichelberger, M.R., Ball, J.W., Pratsch, G.S., & Runion, E.F. (1992). *Pediatric emergencies*. Englewood Cliffs, NJ: Brady.

9 Katz, A. (1990). Cardiomyopathy of overload. *New England Journal of Medicine, 322*(2), 100–110.

10 Slota, M. (1982). Congestive heart failure. *Critical Care Nurse, 2*(6), 58–61.

11 Zimmerman, S., & Gildea, J. (1985). *Critical care pediatrics*. Philadelphia: W.B. Saunders.

12 Higgins, S., & Kashani, I. (1984). Congestive heart failure: Parent support and teaching. *Critical Care Nurse, 4*(4), 21–24.

13 O'Brien, P., & Boisvert, J.T. (1989). Discharge planning for children with heart disease. *Critical Care Nursing Clinics of North America, 1*, 297–305.

14 Callow, L.B. (1987). Postoperative nursing care of the patient who has undergone the Fontan procedure. *Focus on Critical Care, 14*(4), 24–31.

15 Higgins, S.S., & Kashani, I.A. (1986). The cyanotic child: Heart defects and parental learning needs. *Maternal Child Nursing, 11*, 259–262.

16 Engle, M.A., & O'Loughlin, J.E. (1987). Complications of cardiac surgery in children. *Pediatrics in Review, 9*, 147–154.

17 Castaneda, A.R. (1990). Classical repair of tetralogy of Fallot: Timing, technique, and results. *Seminars in Thoracic and Cardiovascular Surgery, 2*, 70–75.

18 Rikard, D.H. (1993). Nursing care of the neonate receiving prostaglandin E_1 therapy. *Neonatal Network, 12*, 17–22.

19 Driscoll, D.J. (1990). Evaluation of the cyanotic newborn. *Pediatric Clinics of North America, 37*, 1–23.

20 Flynn, P.A., Engle, M.A., & Ehlers, K.H. (1992). Cardiac issues in the pediatric emergency room. *Pediatric Clinics of North America, 39*, 955–986.

21 Denny, F. (1993). New developments: Group A streptococcal infections, 1993. *Current Problems in Pediatrics, 23*(5), 179–185.

22 Behrman, R. (1992). *Nelson's textbook of pediatrics*. Philadelphia: W.B. Saunders.

23 Strong, W., & Alpert, B. (1982). The child with heart disease: Play, recreation, and sports. *Current Problems in Pediatrics, 13*(2), 6–34.

24 Ros, S., Fisher, E., & Bell, T. (1991). Adenosine in the emergency management of supraventricular tachycardia. *Pediatric Emergency Care, 7*(4), 222–223.

25 Lux, K. (1991). New hope for children with Kawasaki disease. *Journal of Pediatric Nursing, 6*(3), 159–165.

26 Newburger, J.W., et al. (1986). The treatment of Kawasaki syndrome with intravenous gamma globulin. *New England Journal of Medicine, 315*, 341–347.

27 McEnhill, M., & Vitale, K. (1989). Kawasaki disease: New challenges in care. *Maternal Child Nursing, 14*(6), 406–410.

28 National Cholesterol Education Program. (1991). *Report of the Expert Panel on Blood Cholesterol Levels in Children and Adolescents*. Washington, DC: U.S. Department of Health & Human Services.

29 Gates, D., & McClure, M.J. (1989). Forestalling the progress of heart disease. *Maternal Child Nursing, 14*(3), 174–178.

30 Kwiterovich, P.O. (1989). *Beyond cholesterol*. Baltimore: Johns Hopkins University Press.

31 Howard, J., Bindler, R., Dimico, G., et al. (1991). Cardiovascular risk factors in children: A Bloomsday research report. *Journal of Pediatric Nursing, 6*(4), 222–229.

32 McCabe, E. (1993). Monitoring the fat and cholesterol intake of children and adolescents. *Journal of Pediatric Health Care, 7*(2), 61–70.

33 Lauer, R., Clarke, W., Mahoney, L., & Witt, J. (1993). Childhood predictors for high adult blood pressure: The Muscatine study. *Pediatric Clinics of North America, 40*(1), 23–40.

34 Waisman, Y., & Eichelberger, M.R. (1993). Hypovolemic shock. In Eichelberger, M.R. (Ed.), *Pediatric trauma: Prevention, acute care, rehabilitation* (pp. 178–185). St. Louis: Mosby–Year Book.

35 Rimar, J.M. (1988). Recognizing shock syndromes in infants and children. *Maternal Child Nursing, 13*, 32–37.

36 DiMaio, A.M., & Singh, J. (1992)) The infant with cyanosis in the emergency room. *Pediatric Clinics of North America, 39*, 987–1006.

SUGGESTED READINGS

Beaver, B.L., & Laschinger, J.C. (1992). Pediatric thoracic trauma. *Seminars in Thoracic and Cardiovascular Surgery, 4*, 255–262.

Berro, E.A., & Bechler-Karsch, A. (1993). A closer look at septic shock. *Pediatric Nursing, 19*, 289–297, 314.

Caire, J.B., & Erickson, S. (1986). Reducing distress in pediatric patients undergoing cardiac catheterization. *Children's Health Care, 14*, 146–152.

Cowell, J., Montgomery, A., & Talashek, M. (1992). Cardiovascular risk stability: From grade school to high school. *Journal of Pediatric Health Care, 6*(6), 349–354.

DeBruin, W.J., Greenwald, B.M., & Notterman, A. (1992). Fluid resuscitation in pediatrics. *Critical Care Clinics, 8*, 423–438.

Grimes, D., & Woolbert, L. (1990). Facts and fallacies about streptococcal infection and rheumatic fever. *Journal of Pediatric Health Care, 4*(4), 186–192.

Hayden, R.A. (1992). What keeps oxygen on track? *American Journal of Nursing, 92*, 32–40.

Jensen, C.A. (1992). Nursing care of a child following an arterial switch procedure for transposition of the great arteries. *Critical Care Nurse, 12*, 51–57.

Kashani, I.A., & Higgins, S.S. (1986). Counseling strategies for families of children with heart disease. *Pediatric Nursing, 12*, 38–40.

Klein, D.M. (1991). Shock: Physiology, signs, and symptoms. *Nursing 91, 21*, 74–76.

McCubbin, H., Thompson, E., Thompson, A., McCubbin, M., & Kaston, A. (1993). Culture, ethnicity, and the family: Critical factors in childhood chronic illnesses and disabilities. *Pediatrics, 91*(5), 1063–1070.

Mistretta, E., & Strond, S. (1990). Hypercholesterolemia in children: Risk and management. *Pediatric Nursing, 16*(2), 152–154.

Nicklaus, T., Farris, R., Srinivasan, S., Webber, L., & Berenson, G. (1989). Nutritional studies in children and implications for change: The Bogalusa heart study. *Journal of Advancement in Medicine, 2*(3), 451–473.

Ohler, L., Fleagle, D.J., & Lee, B.I. (1989). Aortic valvuloplasty: Medical and critical care nursing perspectives. *Focus on Critical Care, 16*, 275–287.

Page, G.G. (1986). Tetralogy of Fallot. *Reviews in Critical Care, 15*, 390–399.

Perkin, R.M. (1992). Shock states. In Fuhrmann, B.P., & Zimmerman, J.J., *Pediatric critical care* (pp. 287–298). St. Louis: Mosby–Year Book.

Pryor, R.W., Kline, M.W., & Matson, J.R. (1989). Septic shock: Principles of management in the emergency department. *Pediatric Emergency Care, 5*, 193–197.

Radtke, W., & Lock, J. (1990). Balloon dilation. *Pediatric Clinics of North America, 37*, 193–209.

Rimar, J.M. (1988). Shock in infants and children: Assessment and treatment. *Maternal Child Nursing, 13*, 98–105.

Rowley, A., & Gonzalez-Crussi, F. (1991). Kawasaki syndrome. *Current Problems in Pediatrics, 21*(9), 380–405.

Sade, R.M., & Fyfe, D.A. (1990). Tricuspid atresia: Current concepts in diagnosis and treatment. *Pediatric Clinics of North America, 37*, 151–169.

Stradtman, J.C., & Ballenger, M.J. (1989). Nursing implications in sternal and mediastinal infections after open heart surgery. *Focus on Critical Care, 16*, 178–183.

Uzark, K., Messiter, E., & Rosenthal, A. (1986). Promoting dental health care in children with congenital heart disease. *Pediatric Nursing, 12*, 96–99.

Uzark, K., VonBargen-Mazza, P., & Messiter, E. (1989). Health education needs of adolescents with congenital heart disease. *Journal of Pediatric Health Care, 3*, 137–143.

Warshaw, M.P., & Winn, C.W. (1988). Pulmonary valvuloplasty as an alternative to surgery in the pediatric patient: Implications for nursing. *Heart & Lung, 15*, 521–527.

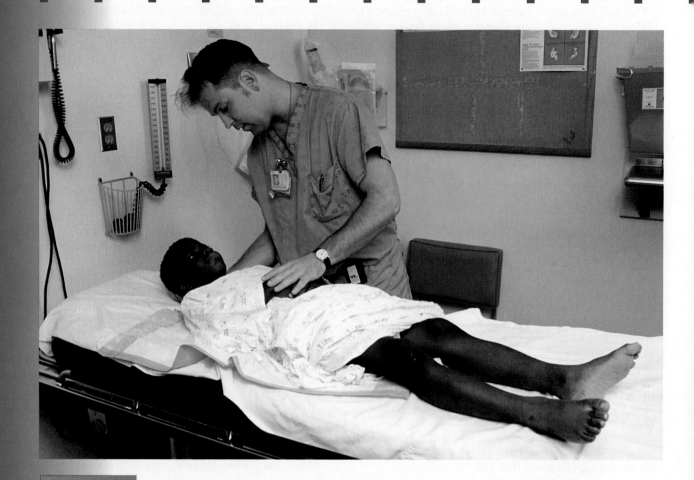

M ark is a 12-year-old black child who, following a viral illness, has been brought to the emergency department for severe abdominal pain. Although his parents are with him, Mark is extremely anxious and frightened. On assessment, you note that he is thin for his age. Mark has two ulcers on his shin and three others that are partially healed. His parents report that he has complained of blood in his urine (hematuria).

Mark is in sickle cell crisis, a severe hematologic disorder that occurs in children with sickle cell anemia. The increased blood viscosity and destruction of red blood cells associated with this disorder result in a wide range of symptoms, including the chronic leg ulcers experienced by Mark. Although sickle cell anemia may be identified during screening in the neonatal period, many children are not diagnosed with the disorder until they begin to develop symptoms or are in sickle cell crisis in early childhood.

What immediate and long-term care will Mark require? What should you tell Mark and his parents about sickle cell anemia? How can you help them cope with the implications of this chronic disease?

ALTERATIONS IN HEMATOLOGIC FUNCTION

13

▓ TERMINOLOGY

anemia Reduction in the number of red blood cells, the quantity of hemoglobin, and the volume of packed red cells per 100 mL of blood to below-normal levels.

ecchymosis A bruise.

erythropoiesis Formation of red blood cells.

hemarthrosis Bleeding into joint cavities.

hematopoiesis Blood cell production.

hemoglobinopathy Disease characterized by abnormal hemoglobin.

hemosiderosis Increased deposition of iron in body tissues associated with diseases involving destruction of red blood cells.

leukopenia A low white blood cell count.

pancytopenia A decreased number of blood cell components.

petechiae Pinpoint red lesions, usually indicative of a bleeding disorder.

polycythemia Above-normal increase in the number of red cells in the blood.

purpura Condition characterized by bleeding into the tissues, particularly beneath the skin and mucous membranes, and lesions that vary from red to purple.

thrombocytopenia A low platelet count.

vaso-occlusion Blockage of a blood vessel.

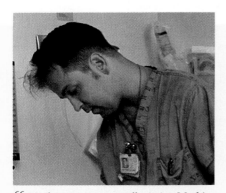

❝ My first concern was alleviating Mark's pain. The first analgesic given to him was not effective. Mark obviously needed to have a stronger analgesic to prevent his pain from recurring. Dealing with Mark's fear was as important as controlling his pain. ❞

he hematologic system is one of a few body systems that regulate, directly or indirectly, all other body functions. Because blood is involved in the function of all tissues and organs, changes in the blood may result in altered functioning of many body organs and structures. Are you aware that a tendency toward easy bruising is a characteristic sign of many bleeding disorders? Other signs include nosebleeds, pallor, frequent infections, and lethargy. This chapter discusses the most common disorders of the blood and blood-forming organs in children. (See Chapter 16 for a discussion of leukemia.)

Anatomy and Physiology of Pediatric Differences

Blood has two components: a fluid portion called plasma and a cellular portion known as the formed elements of the blood. The cellular elements are red blood cells (erythrocytes), white blood cells (leukocytes), and platelets (thrombocytes) (Fig. 13–1). Table 13–1 gives normal values for these blood components in children.

FIGURE 13–1 Types of blood cells.

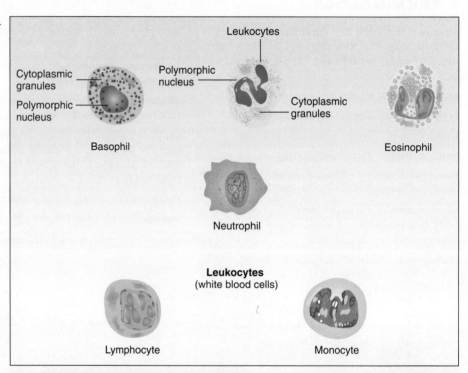

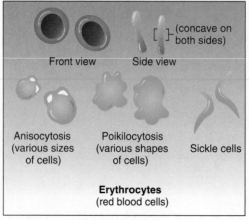

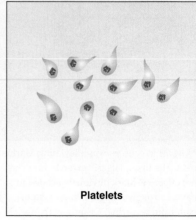

TABLE 13–1 Normal Blood Values in Children

	Newborn	1 Year	5 Years	8–12 Years
Red blood cells (RBCs) (millions/μL)	5.9 (4.1–7.5)	4.6 (4.1–5.1)	4.7 (4.2–5.2)	5 (4.5–5.4)
Hemoglobin (Hgb) (g/dL)	19 (14–24)	12 (11–15)	13.5 (12.5–15)	14 (13–15.5)
White blood cells (WBCs) (per μL)	17,000 (8–38)	10,000 (5–15)	8,000 (5–13)	8,000 (5–12)
Platelets (per μL)	350,000			260,000
Hematocrit (Hct) (%)	54 + 10	36	38	40

Adapted from Merenstein, G.B., Kaplan, D.W., & Rosenberg, A.A. (1994). *Silver, Kempe, Bruyn & Fulginiti's handbook of pediatrics* (17th ed.). Norwalk, CT: Appleton & Lange, pp. 1032–1035.

■ CULTURAL CONSIDERATIONS

According to traditional Chinese beliefs, a person who does not feel well is lacking in *chi* (inner energy) and blood. Chinese-Americans who follow traditional practices may be hesitant to have blood drawn for laboratory studies for fear of causing bodily weakness.

TABLE 13–2 White Blood Cells and Their Functions

Type	Function
Neutrophils	Phagocytosis
Eosinophils	Allergic reactions
Basophils	Inflammatory reactions
Monocytes (macrophages)	Phagocytosis, antigen processing
Lymphocytes	Humoral immunity (B cell), cellular immunity (T cell)
Plasma cells	Antibody production

At birth, **hematopoiesis,** or blood cell production, occurs in almost every bone. The flat bones, such as the sternum, ribs, pelvic and shoulder girdles, vertebrae, and hips, retain most of their hematopoietic activity throughout life.[1]

Red Blood Cells

Red blood cells, or erythrocytes, are the most abundant of the cellular elements of blood. They are formed through a process called **erythropoiesis.** The primary function of red blood cells is to transport oxygen from the lungs to the tissues. These cells also help to carry carbon dioxide back to the lungs. Hemoglobin, a red pigment composed of protein and iron, is essential to this function. Any condition that causes the quantity of oxygen transported to the tissues to decrease ordinarily increases the rate of red blood cell production. When a child becomes anemic secondary to hemorrhage, for instance, the bone marrow immediately begins to produce large quantities of red cells. **Polycythemia** is an above-normal increase in the number of red cells in the blood.

White Blood Cells

White blood cells, or leukocytes, are the mobile units of the body's protective system. They are formed in bone marrow and lymph tissue. There are five types of white blood cells, each with a distinct function (Table 13–2).

Platelets

Platelets, or thrombocytes, are cell fragments that can form hemostatic plugs and stop bleeding. They are synthesized from components in the red bone marrow and are stored in the spleen.

Anemias

■ TYPES OF ANEMIA

- Iron deficiency
- β-Thalassemia
- Aplastic
- Pernicious
- Sickle cell

Anemia is defined as a reduction in the number of red blood cells, the quantity of hemoglobin, and the volume of packed red cells to below-normal levels. This condition can be caused by loss or destruction of existing red blood cells or by an impaired or decreased rate of red cell production. Anemia also can be a clinical manifestation of an underlying disorder, such as lead poisoning or hypersplenism.

TABLE 13-3 Sickle Cell Disorders

Sickle Cell Trait (Hgb SA)

Most common form of sickle cell disease in the United States
Heterozygous condition (child has one sickle cell hemoglobin gene and one normal hemoglobin gene)
Child is carrier of sickle cell anemia and rarely has symptoms of the disease

Sickle Cell Anemia (Hgb SS)

Homozygous condition (child has two sickle hemoglobin genes)
Child is subject to sickle cell crises

Sickle Cell Syndromes
Sickle cell–Hgb C disease (Hgb SC)

Second most frequent form of sickle cell disease in blacks
Different from sickle cell anemia only in that the sickle cell assumes a C shape instead of an S shape

Sickle Cell–β-Thalassemia Disease (Hgb SB)

Rarely occurs
Combination of sickle cell trait and thalassemia trait most often seen in people of Mediterranean descent

Sickle Cell Anemia*

Sickle cell anemia is a hereditary **hemoglobinopathy,** characterized by the partial or complete replacement of normal hemoglobin with abnormal sickle-shaped hemoglobin (Hgb S) (Table 13–3). Although sickle cell anemia occurs primarily in blacks, occasionally it affects people of Mediterranean descent. Sickle cell anemia occurs in about 1 in 500 black infants born in the United States.

Clinical Manifestations

Affected children are usually asymptomatic until 4 to 6 months of age because sickling is inhibited by high levels of fetal hemoglobin. Clinical manifestations are directly related to the shortened life span of blood cells (hemolytic anemia) and tissue destruction resulting from **vaso-occlusion.**[2] Pathologic changes occur in most body systems and result in multiple signs and symptoms (Table 13–4).

Illness results from recurrent vaso-occlusive events that involve painful crises and chronic organ damage.[3, 4] Sickle cell crises are acute exacerbations of the disease that vary markedly in severity and frequency (Table 13–5). Mark, the child described at the beginning of this chapter, was in sickle cell crisis.

Etiology and Pathophysiology

Sickle cell anemia is an autosomal recessive disorder. In the United States, 1 in 12 black individuals carries the trait.[3] If both parents have the trait, with each pregnancy the risk of having a child with the disease is 25%.

In sickle cell anemia, the hemoglobin in the red blood cell acquires an elongated crescent or sickle shape (Fig. 13–2). Sickling may be triggered by fever and emotional or physical stress. Precipitating factors for sickle cell crisis include increased blood viscosity (such as from a low fluid intake or

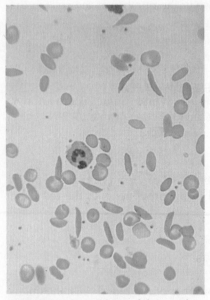

FIGURE 13-2 Many of these red blood cells show elongated crescent shape characteristic of sickle cell anemia.
Courtesy of the American Society of Hematology, Brookline, MA.

*Material for the discussion of sickle cell anemia was provided by Sara Zimmerman, R.N., M.Ed., Children's National Medical Center, Washington, DC.

TABLE 13-4 Clinical Manifestations of Sickle Cell Anemia

Area Affected	Clinical Manifestations	Cause
Liver	Hepatomegaly, cirrhosis	Impaired blood flow from capillary obstruction leads to enlargement and scarring
Spleen	Nonfunctioning spleen, increased number of infections	Infarct in spleen leads to fibrosis
Kidneys	Enuresis, hematuria, inability to concentrate urine	Ischemia of kidneys
Bones	Osteoporosis, osteomyelitis, spinal deformities, aseptic necrosis of femoral head	Chronic ischemia of bones leads to susceptibility to infection and bone degeneration
Skin	Leg ulcers	Decreased peripheral circulation
Brain	Headache, aphasia, convulsions, visual disturbances	Cerebrovascular infarction
Eyes	Diminished vision	Retinopathy, retinal detachment
Penis	Priapism	Microcirculatory obstruction and engorgement of penis
Extremities	Peripheral neuropathy, weakness, arthralgia	Vaso-occlusion and chronic ischemia

TABLE 13-5 Sickle Cell Crises

Vaso-occlusive Crises (Thrombotic)

Most common type of crisis; painful
Caused by stasis of blood with clumping of cells in the microcirculation, ischemia, and infarction
Signs include fever, pain, tissue engorgement

Splenic Sequestration

Life-threatening crisis; death can occur within hours
Caused by pooling of blood in the spleen
Signs include profound anemia, hypovolemia, and shock

Aplastic Crises

Diminished production and increased destruction of red blood cells
Triggered by viral infection or depletion of folic acid
Signs include profound anemia, pallor

fever) and hypoxia or low oxygen tension. Potential causes of hypoxia or low oxygen tension include high altitudes, poorly pressurized airplanes, hypoventilation, vasoconstriction when cold, or an emotionally stressful event. Any condition that increases the body's need for oxygen or alters the transport of oxygen (such as infection, trauma, or dehydration) may result in sickle cell crisis. Sickled cells are rigid and obstruct capillary blood flow. Microscopic obstructions lead to engorgement and tissue ischemia. This local tissue hypoxia causes further sickling and ultimately large infarctions. Damaged tissues in organs become scarred, resulting in impaired function. For example, children with sickle cell anemia have severely compromised immunity because the spleen is rarely functional after 5 years of age.

Sickled cells can resume a normal shape when rehydrated and reoxygenated. The membrane of these cells becomes more fragile, however, and cell life is shortened to 10 to 20 days rather than the usual 120 days. Bone marrow spaces enlarge to produce more red blood cells. Continuous formation and destruction of the child's red blood cells contributes to the severe hemolytic anemia that is characteristic of sickle cell anemia.

Diagnostic Tests and Medical Management

The initial diagnosis of sickle cell anemia in black newborns is often made by testing cord blood using hemoglobin electrophoresis. The sickle-turbidity test (Sickledex) may be used for quick screening purposes in children over 6 months of age, once the fetal hemoglobin levels have fallen. Hemoglobin electrophoresis is performed to verify positive Sickledex test results.

No cure for sickle cell anemia exists. Supportive care is aimed at the prevention and treatment of sickling episodes. Preventing exposure to infections and maintaining normal hydration are important in avoiding crises. The reticulocyte count is monitored regularly to make sure that the bone marrow is still functioning.

Treatment of crises involves hydration, oxygen, pain management, and bed rest to reduce energy expenditure. Cultures (blood, urine, and throat) are taken to identify sources of infection. Other therapeutic measures include blood transfusions to treat the anemia and to make the sickled blood less viscous. If given early in the crisis, blood transfusions may sometimes relieve the ischemia in major organs and body parts (spleen, lung, kidney, brain, and penis) caused by the vaso-occlusion. Antibiotics are administered for infection control.

Prognosis depends on the severity of the child's disease. The major cause of death is from infection because the nonfunctional spleen results in an immunocompromised state. Neonatal screening, early intervention, prophylactic antibiotics, and parent education have allowed children with sickle cell disease to live into adulthood.

Nursing Assessment

A comprehensive physical assessment is essential because the disease can affect any body system. In children who are known to have sickle cell anemia, obtain a detailed history from the child or parents about past crises, precipitating events, medical treatment, and home management. Measure the child's height and weight accurately and compare to past measurements, since failure to thrive is common.

When the child is in crisis, assess pain and note the presence of any signs of inflammation or infection. Carefully monitor the child for signs of shock (see Chapter 12).

Nursing Diagnosis

Common nursing diagnoses are presented in the Nursing Care Plan for the Child with Sickle Cell Anemia.

Nursing Management

The accompanying Nursing Care Plan summarizes nursing care for the child with sickle cell anemia. Nursing management for the child in crisis focuses on increasing tissue perfusion, promoting hydration, controlling pain, preventing infection, ensuring adequate nutrition, and preventing complications.

Increase Tissue Perfusion. Administer blood transfusions and oxygen as ordered. Never give cold blood; use a blood warming coil before infusing. The

---

■ **SAFETY CONSIDERATIONS**

When administering blood, carefully cross-check the information on the unit with the child's blood type and patient record number. Most hospitals require two nurses to check the blood unit before starting a transfusion.

■ **NURSING ALERT**

Blood reactions can occur as soon as the blood transfusion begins. Administer the first 20 mL of blood slowly and observe the child carefully for a reaction. Repeatedly assess the child according to hospital policy.

TABLE 13–6 Nursing Considerations for Blood Transfusion Reactions

Type of Reaction	Cause	Clinical Manifestations	Nursing Interventions
Allergic reaction	Immune response	Urticaria, itching, respiratory distress	Stop the transfusion; call physician; give antihistamines as ordered; monitor vital signs; change IV to normal saline; keep IV line open; check urine for hematuria
Hemolytic reaction	Mismatched blood, history of multiple trans-fusions	Fever, chills, hematuria, headache, chest pain; can progress to shock	

■ CLINICAL TIP

To encourage fluid intake in a small child:
- Use a special cup or glass
- Use straws
- Take advantage of times when the child is thirsty, such as on awakening or after play
- Leave a cup within easy reach of the child
- Offer frozen juice pops, crushed ice drinks, and flavored ice chips

■ NURSING ALERT

Neither heat nor cold compresses should be used for pain management in the child who has sickle cell anemia. Ischemic tissue is fragile and has reduced sensation, increasing the risk of burn injury. Cold compresses promote sickling.

■ COMPLICATIONS OF SICKLE CELL ANEMIA

Poor growth
Delayed maturation
Nonfunctional spleen
Infection
Crisis

IV fluid used before and after a blood transfusion must be saline rather than D_5W to prevent hemolysis. In small children, the blood is usually infused without saline because the child cannot manage the extra volume. Monitor for transfusion reactions (Table 13–6). Encourage the child to rest. Work with the child and family to avoid emotional stress. Any activities that increase cellular metabolism also result in tissue hypoxia. Schedule caregiving activities and play to allow for optimal rest.

Promote Hydration. The child with sickle cell anemia is adversely affected by dehydration. Calculate the child's fluid maintenance requirements (minimum daily fluid intake) (see Chapter 7) and monitor the child's oral fluid intake. Administer IV fluids as ordered. Adjust oral intake as necessary to keep the child well hydrated.

Control Pain. Give prescribed analgesics around the clock during crises. Allow the child to assume a position of comfort. Do not put stress on painful joints.

Prevent Infection. Infection makes the child more susceptible to a crisis, and the crisis makes the child more susceptible to infection. Watch for evidence of infection and report any signs to the physician immediately.

Ensure Adequate Nutrition. Emphasize the importance of adequate nutrition to promote growth. Encourage the child to eat a high-protein, high-calorie diet. Emphasize the importance of folic acid supplements as ordered.

Prevent Complications of Crises. Observe the child for signs of increasing anemia and shock (mental status change, pallor, vital sign changes). Assess the child's neurologic status for evidence of altered cerebral function. If ordered, assess for an enlarged spleen by gentle palpation. Administer blood transfusions and watch the child for any adverse reaction.

Discharge Planning and Patient and Family Home Care Teaching. Home care needs should be identified and addressed well in advance of discharge. Provide parents with information about sickle cell disease and their child's treatment. Explain the basic effect of tissue hypoxia and the effects of sickling on circulation. Refer parents to support groups such as the National Association of Sickle Cell Disease if they wish to obtain more information about the disorder (see Appendix F).

Teach parents to look for signs of dehydration, such as dry mucous membranes, weight loss, and sunken fontanels in infants. Give specific instructions about how many ounces of liquid the child needs to drink each day.

THE CHILD WITH SICKLE CELL ANEMIA

GOAL	INTERVENTION	RATIONALE	EXPECTED OUTCOME
1. High Risk for Altered Tissue Perfusion related to sickle cell crises			
Child will show few signs and symptoms of tissue hypoxia.	Instruct child to avoid physical exertion, emotional stress, low-oxygen environments (e.g., airplanes, high altitudes), and known sources of infection.	Decreased activity and exposure reduce body's need for oxygen.	Child has no shortness of breath and shows no signs of hypoxia.
	Administer blood transfusions as ordered.	Packed cells increase number of red blood cells available to carry oxygen to tissue cells. Transfusions promote circulation.	
	Perform several caregiving activities together whenever possible.	Grouping activities allows for optimum rest.	
	Give oxygen as ordered.	High concentration of oxygen in alveoli increases diffusion of gas across membranes.	
2. High Risk for Fluid Volume Deficit related to sickle cell crises			
Child will maintain or be restored to adequate hydration.	Calculate child's daily fluid requirements. Monitor the child's usual fluid consumption and make necessary adjustments. Encourage child to take fluids. Observe for signs of dehydration.	Optimizing fluid intake ensures that child gets needed fluid. Dehydration exacerbates crises.	Child shows signs of adequate hydration.
	Record intake and output.	Recording enables nurse to monitor daily fluid intake and spacing throughout the day.	
3. Pain related to sickle cell crises			
Child will verbalize that pain is controlled.	Apply heat to affected area. Avoid cold compresses.	Heat is soothing. Cold may promote sickling.	Child is pain-free or pain control is significantly improved.
	Administer analgesics, such as morphine or hydromorphine (Dilaudid), as ordered. Continuous intravenous infusion is used for the duration of a painful crisis.	Pain of sickle cell crises is excruciating.	
	Position carefully.	Joints and extremities can be extremely painful.	

Emphasize that increased fluid intake is needed to replace the fluids lost from overheating or exposure to hot weather.

Make sure both the child and family understand the triggers and precipitating factors for sickle cell crises. Encourage them to avoid situations that cause crises. Instruct the child and parents about early signs and symptoms of crises that should be reported to their health care provider (see Table 13–5).

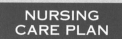

THE CHILD WITH SICKLE CELL ANEMIA—CONTINUED

GOAL	INTERVENTION	RATIONALE	EXPECTED OUTCOME
4. High Risk for Infection related to chronic disease and splenic malfunction			
Child will not develop infection.	Ensure adequate nutrition by providing high-calorie, high-protein diet. Make sure that child's immunizations are up to date. Report any signs of infection to physician immediately.	Chronically ill children are at greater risk of infection.	Child is free of infection.
	Isolate child from possible sources of infection. Instruct parents about signs of infection.	Restriction of persons with infection decreases child's contact with infectious agents.	
5. Knowledge Deficit (Child and Parents) related to cause and treatment of sickle cell anemia			
Child and family will verbalize understanding of risk factors for sickle cell crises and how to minimize them.	Review basics of sickle cell disease. Teach child and family about signs and symptoms of crises.	Knowledge of disease helps ensure compliance with medical regimen and adherence to preventive measures.	Child and parent can verbalize precipitating events of crises.
	Arrange for genetic counseling and testing for sickle cell trait for family members if desired.	Questions and concerns regarding future pregnancies can be allayed through knowledge of disease and transmission.	

Advise parents to inform all treating physicians and dentists of their child's medical condition. The child should also wear some type of medical identification (e.g., Medic Alert bracelet). Special precautions are necessary when the child undergoes surgery of any kind, since hypoxia that results from anesthesia is a major surgical risk.

Encourage older children with sickle cell anemia to participate in activities with other children between crises but to avoid strenuous physical exertion and contact sports. Play and social interactions that promote learning and development are important.

Genetic counseling should be made available to parents who plan to have more children and to adolescents with sickle cell trait or disease.

Iron Deficiency Anemia

Iron deficiency anemia is the most common type of anemia in children. It can occur secondary to blood loss or as a result of increased internal demands (rapid growth) for blood production or poor nutritional intake.

Clinical manifestations depend on the severity of the anemia. Pallor, fatigue, and irritability are characteristic findings in infants. Rapidly growing adolescents whose diets are high in fat and low in vitamins and minerals are particularly susceptible to this form of anemia. Infants who are breast-fed exclusively after 6 months of age are also at risk because neonatal iron stores have been depleted by this time and their iron needs are not being met

Diagnosis is made on the basis of laboratory studies, including hemoglobin level, mean corpuscular volume, microscopic analysis (Fig. 13–3), and serum iron-binding capacity. Treatment involves correction of the iron deficiency with oral elemental iron preparations and a diet high in iron.

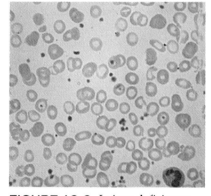

FIGURE 13-3 In iron deficiency anemia, red blood cells appear hypochromic as a result of decreased hemoglobin synthesis.
Courtesy of Department of Hematology/Oncology, Children's National Medical Center, Washington, DC.

Nursing Management

Nursing care focuses on educating the parents and child about the causes of iron deficiency anemia, dietary management, and the importance of complying with the medication regimen. Dietary management is the preferred treatment. Teach the child and family about foods that are rich in iron. Oral iron preparations are given when the anemia is severe. Teach the child and family that the iron preparation should be taken through a straw because it stains the teeth. Instruct about side effects such as black stools, constipation, and a foul aftertaste. Emphasize the importance of maintaining adequate hydration to minimize side effects.

β-Thalassemia

The thalassemias are a group of inherited blood disorders of hemoglobin synthesis characterized by anemia that can be mild or severe. β-Thalassemia, also known as Cooley anemia, is the most common type. These disorders most often occur in people of Mediterranean descent but also are found among Middle Eastern, Asian, and African populations.[5] If both parents carry the abnormal gene, with each pregnancy there is a 25% chance of passing the disorder on to their child.

There are three types of β-thalassemia: thalassemia minor, or thalassemia trait (produces mild anemia); thalassemia intermedia (produces severe anemia); and thalassemia major (produces anemia requiring transfusion). The clinical manifestations listed in Table 13–7 are caused by the defective syn-

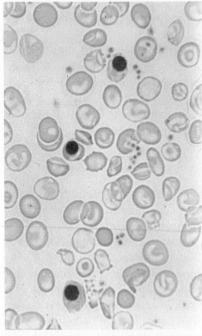

FIGURE 13-4 Red blood cell appearance in β-thalassemia. What characteristic abnormalities can be seen on this microscopic view?
Copyright © MEDCOM, Inc., Garden Grove, CA.

TABLE 13-7 Clinical Manifestations of β-Thalassemia

Anemia

Hypochromic and microcytic changes
Folic acid deficiency
Frequent epistaxis

Skeletal Changes

Osteoporosis
Delayed growth
Susceptibility to pathologic fractures
Facial deformities: enlarged head, prominent forehead due to frontal and parietal bossing, prominent cheek bones, broadened and depressed bridge of nose, enlarged maxilla with protruding front teeth, eyes with mongoloid slant and epicanthal fold

Heart

Chronic congestive heart failure
Myocardial fibrosis
Murmurs

Liver/Gallbladder

Hepatomegaly
Hepatic insufficiency

Spleen

Splenomegaly

Endocrine System

Delayed sexual maturation
Fibrotic pancreas, resulting in diabetes mellitus

Skin

Darkening of skin

thesis of hemoglobin, structurally impaired red blood cells (Fig. 13–4), and the shortened life span of the red blood cells.

β-Thalassemia can be detected early in infancy. The infant with β-thalassemia manifests pallor, failure to thrive, hepatosplenomegaly, and severe anemia (hemoglobin <6 g/dL).[5] Diagnosis is made by hemoglobin electrophoresis, which shows a decreased production of one of the globin chains in hemoglobin. Characteristic erythrocyte cell changes often can be recognized in infants by 6 weeks of age.

Treatment is supportive. The goal of medical management is to maintain normal hemoglobin levels. Blood transfusion is the conventional therapy used to treat children with severe disease. However, frequent transfusions may result in an overload of iron in the body. The iron is stored in tissues and organs (**hemosiderosis**) because the body has no way of excreting it. For this reason an iron-chelating drug such as deferoxamine is given along with vitamin C to promote iron excretion. Other potential complications of long-term transfusion therapy are transfusion reactions and alloimmunization (antibody formation).[5] Bone marrow transplantation may be offered as an alternative therapy for children newly diagnosed with the disorder.[5]

Nursing Management

Nursing care focuses on observing for complications of transfusion therapy, providing emotional support, and referring for genetic counseling. Transfusions of packed cells are often given. Watch for blood transfusion reactions (see Table 13–6).

Provide parents with information about thalassemia and its treatment. Genetic counseling should be provided. Provide emotional support and encourage parents to take an active role in the child's treatment regimen.

Compliance with transfusion therapy often becomes an issue as children reach adolescence. Offering the adolescent treatment options, such as when to undergo transfusion, can help to improve compliance.[5] Adolescents with β-thalassemia and parents of newly diagnosed children can be referred to the Thalassemia Action Group, a national organization for patients, or to the Cooley's Anemia Foundation (see Appendix F).

Aplastic Anemia

Aplastic anemia is a deficiency of the formed elements of the blood that results from failure of the bone marrow to produce adequate numbers of circulating blood cells. The condition may be congenital or acquired.

Congenital aplastic anemia (Fanconi anemia) is a rare autosomal recessive syndrome consisting of multiple congenital anomalies. Symptoms can include **purpura** (bleeding into the tissues) (Fig. 13–5), **petechiae** (pinpoint lesions), bleeding, fatigue, and pallor. Laboratory findings include neutropenia or anemia and **thrombocytopenia** (low platelet count) that progresses to **pancytopenia** (decreased number of blood cell components). Children are at risk for developing malignancies such as acute nonlymphocytic leukemia.[2] The treatment of choice is bone marrow transplantation. The prognosis is poor, and death usually results from overwhelming infection, hemorrhage, or malignancy.

Acquired aplastic anemia in children is either idiopathic or occurs from a drug reaction. It can develop after exposure to ionizing radiation or insecticides or after ingestion of drugs such as sulfonamides, chloramphenicol, quinacrine, benzene solvents in model airplane glue, or lead.[6] This type of anemia can also be a result of an infectious process such as viral hepatitis or mononucleosis.

Symptoms are related to the degree of bone marrow failure and can include petechiae, purpura, bleeding, pallor, weakness, and fatigue.[5] Diagno-

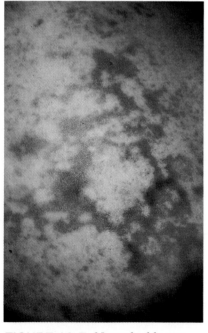

FIGURE 13–5 Nonpalpable purpura with bleeding into the tissues below the skin.

Courtesy of the Department of Hematology/Oncology, Children's National Medical Center, Washington, DC.

sis is made by blood studies (which reveal **leukopenia** [decreased white blood cell count] with marked neutropenia, thrombocytopenia, and pancytopenia) and bone marrow aspiration (which reveals yellow, fatty bone marrow instead of red bone marrow).

Treatment is supportive and includes transfusions of packed cells and/or platelets. The treatment of choice is bone marrow transplantation from a compatible sibling or family member donor or immunosuppressive therapy.

Nursing Management

Nursing care is similar to care provided for the child with leukemia (see Chapter 16). Nursing care focuses on preventing bleeding, administering and monitoring blood transfusions, preventing infection, encouraging mobility as tolerated, educating the parents and child about the disorder, and providing emotional support. Families need support in dealing with a child who has a life-threatening disease. Refer them to support groups for counseling, if indicated, and to social services.

Clotting Disorders

Hemophilia

Hemophilia refers to a group of hereditary bleeding disorders that result from a deficiency in specific clotting factors. Hemophilia A, or classic hemophilia, is caused by a deficiency of factor VIII in the blood and accounts for 80% of persons with hemophilia. Hemophilia B, known as Christmas disease, is a deficiency of factor IX. Fifteen percent of persons with hemophilia have hemophilia B.

Clinical Manifestations

Spontaneous bleeding, **hemarthrosis** (bleeding into a joint space), and deep tissue hemorrhage occur with factor levels of less than 1%.[7] Affected children frequently experience bleeding into the joint spaces of the knees, ankles, and elbows. Bleeding into joint spaces or bursae causes the child to have limited motion because of pain, tenderness, and swelling.[6] Bone changes, contractures, and disabling deformities can result from immobility and from the effects of blood on the joint structures.

Children may have easy bruising **(ecchymosis)**, nosebleeds, hematuria, and bleeding after tooth extraction, minor trauma, or minor surgical procedures. Large subcutaneous and intramuscular hemorrhages sometimes occur. Bleeding into the tissues of the neck, mouth, or chest is particularly serious because of the potential for airway obstruction. Retroperitoneal and intracranial bleeding may also occur and can be life-threatening.

Etiology and Pathophysiology

Hemophilia is a sex-linked recessive trait seen almost exclusively in males. The gene is transmitted from father to daughter and from mother to son. Daughters also may acquire the trait from mothers who are carriers of the gene. A daughter who inherits the trait from her father has a 50% chance of transmitting it to her sons. However, as many as one third of hemophiliacs have no family members with a history of clotting disorders. In these cases the disorder is caused by a new mutation.

The degree of bleeding is related to the amount of clotting factor and the severity of the injury.

Diagnostic Tests and Medical Management

Diagnosis is made on the basis of the history, physical examination, and laboratory data. Prothrombin time, fibrinogen concentration, and platelet count as well as specific assays for factors VIII and IX are evaluated.

The goal of medical management is to control bleeding by replacing the missing clotting factor. Replacement therapy is indicated when the child experiences a mild or major hemorrhage or faces a life-threatening situation. Intravenous infusions consisting of plasma, fresh frozen plasma, cryoprecipitates, or factor concentrates are administered. The promptness and adequacy of treatment greatly affect the child's response to therapy.

The outlook for children with hemophilia has been greatly improved by the availability of transfusion therapy. Transfusions started at home and early interventions prevent many disease complications. In the past many children with factor VIII deficiency died in the first 5 years of life. Today children with moderate or mild hemophilia can lead normal lives.

A synthetic drug that is effective against mild hemophilia is desmopressin acetate (DDAVP). An analog of vasopressin and an antidiuretic hormone, DDAVP is administered intravenously and causes a two- to threefold increase in factor VIII activity.[6]

Nursing Assessment

Obtain a complete medical history from the child or parents. In particular, ask about previous episodes of prolonged bleeding and the occurrence of hemophilia or any other bleeding disorders in family members. The history of bleeding will vary, depending on the severity of the disease.

Assess the child for any joint pain, swelling, or permanent deformity, particularly around the knees, elbows, ankles, and shoulders. Note the presence of hematuria and mild flank pain. A neurologic assessment should be conducted, since risk for intracranial hemorrhage and bleeding can lead to peripheral neuropathies.

Nursing Diagnosis

The most important nursing diagnosis for the child with hemophilia is High Risk for Injury related to bleeding disorder. Other common nursing diagnoses include:

- Pain related to bleeding episodes
- Impaired Physical Mobility related to hemarthrosis
- Knowledge Deficit (Child and Parent) related to treatment plan

■ CLINICAL TIPS

Take the following precautions when caring for children with bleeding disorders.
- Avoid taking temperatures rectally or giving suppositories.
- Check blood pressure by cuff as infrequently as possible.
- Avoid any intramuscular or subcutaneous injections.
- Use only paper or silk tape for dressings.
- When indicated, perform mouth care every 3 hours with a glycerine swab.
- Except for factor replacement therapy, avoid all venipuncture.
- Use a peripheral fingerstick to obtain blood samples.
- Do not give aspirin.

Nursing Management

Nursing care focuses on preventing and controlling bleeding, limiting joint involvement and managing pain, and providing emotional support. Both short-term interventions and long-term management are necessary.

Prevent and Control Bleeding Episodes. Bleeding problems are rare in infants with hemophilia. As children learn to walk and develop other motor skills, however, they often fall and suffer cuts and bruises. The risk of injury can be reduced by emphasizing to parents the need for close supervision and a safe environment. Parents should encourage children to play with toys that are safe and age appropriate.

If dental surgery or tooth extraction is necessary, it should be performed in a controlled environment by experienced staff. Use of a dental irrigation device is often recommended if the child has excess bleeding from gums. Advise adolescents to shave only with an electric razor.

Control any superficial bleeding by applying pressure to the area for at least 15 minutes. Immobilize and elevate the affected area, and apply ice packs to promote vasoconstriction.

If significant bleeding does occur, offer supportive measures and assist with factor replacement therapy. Carefully monitor the child's condition for any side effects when factor replacement therapy is administered.

Limit Joint Involvement and Manage Pain. During bleeding episodes hemarthrosis is managed by elevating and immobilizing the joint and applying ice packs. Administer analgesics as ordered. Once bleeding has been controlled, range of motion exercises are performed to strengthen muscles and joints and to prevent flexion contractures. Because excessive weight can place an added stress on joints, encourage the child to maintain an appropriate weight.

Provide Emotional Support. The needs of families with hemophiliac children are best met through a comprehensive team approach. Refer the parents for genetic counseling as soon as possible after diagnosis.

Encourage the parents to verbalize their feelings. Be understanding and sensitive to their needs. Teach the parents about hemophilia and explain how the disorder affects both the child and other family members. Explain the cause of bleeding using simple terms so both child and parents understand the disease process. Explain what to expect during the child's hospitalization.

Discharge Planning and Patient and Family Home Care Teaching. Home care needs should be identified and addressed well in advance of discharge. Advise parents to have the child wear a Medic-Alert bracelet. Teach the child and family how to identify internal bleeding. Signs and symptoms such as joint pain, abdominal pain, and obvious bleeding are indicators for immediate factor infusion. Make sure the child and parents know what situations could cause bleeding to occur. Teach parents to give acetaminophen instead of aspirin to relieve pain.

Instruct the parents and the child, when appropriate, in the preparation and administration of factor concentrates. If infusion of the missing factor is scheduled on a regular basis, bleeding episodes can be controlled or avoided. Have the parents demonstrate the procedure and make sure they can administer the product correctly. The parents need to be familiar with properties of the factor concentrate to prepare the mixture correctly.

Help the family and school to plan an appropriate schedule of activities without overprotecting the child. Children with hemophilia should not engage in contact sports such as football and soccer, which may result in injury and trauma. Instead, sports such as swimming, hiking, and bicycling should be encouraged.

Hemophilia is not only a debilitating disorder for the child. It also can be financially draining for the family. Frequent outpatient visits, emergency room visits, hospital admissions, and the cost of factor concentrate can exhaust a family's resources. If indicated, referral should be made to appropriate social services (e.g., the state's maternal and child health program for children with special health care needs).

Put parents in contact with appropriate resource groups such as the National Hemophilia Foundation (see Appendix F). Sharing experiences with other families of children with hemophilia can provide support.

Von Willebrand Disease

Like hemophilia, von Willebrand disease is a hereditary bleeding disorder. It is caused by reduced levels of factor VIII and von Willebrand factor and by

■ GROWTH AND DEVELOPMENT CONSIDERATIONS

Encourage adolescents with hemophilia to participate in leisure activities such as computer games, reading clubs, and crafts. Knee pads, elbow pads, and helmets should be used for any physical sports. Coaches or teachers should be familiar with early signs of bleeding. The school nurse should be able to administer factor replacement therapy.

platelet dysfunction. The disorder is transmitted as an autosomal dominant trait, and it can occur in both males and females.

The characteristic manifestations are easy bruising and epistaxis. Children with von Willebrand disease frequently have gingival bleeding and increased bleeding with lacerations or during surgery. Affected teenage girls may have menorrhagia (increased menstrual bleeding).

Nursing management and treatment are similar to those for the child with hemophilia. Treatment options include fresh frozen plasma, cryoprecipitate, and certain factor VIII concentrates. However, because of the risk of transmission of the AIDS virus (even with adequate screening), cryoprecipitates are used as a last resort. Children are usually treated with desmopressin (DDAVP), given intravenously, which temporarily corrects the bleeding defect. DDAVP is not effective in treating all types of von Willebrand disease.

Teach parents not to give the child any aspirin or drugs that can cause bleeding or inhibit platelet function. During surgery and bleeding episodes, the child will need to have additional von Willebrand factor administered as well as antifibrinolytic drugs to assist in clotting. The prognosis is good, and children usually have a normal life expectancy.

Disseminated Intravascular Coagulation

Disseminated intravascular coagulation (DIC) is an acquired pathologic process in which the clotting system is abnormally activated, resulting in widespread clot formation in the small vessels throughout the body. This condition results in tissue hypoxia with eventual tissue necrosis.

Symptoms can include diffuse bleeding manifested by hematuria, petechiae, or purpura; an injection site that continues to ooze; circulatory collapse; and major vessel thrombosis.[2] DIC is seen as a complication of other serious illnesses in infants and children, such as hypoxia, shock, cancer, and viruses.

Medical management is supportive and includes identification and treatment of the underlying disorder; replacement of depleted coagulation factors, fibrinogen, and platelets; and anticoagulant therapy (heparin).[2]

Nursing Management

Nursing care focuses on assessing the bleeding, preventing further injury, and administering prescribed therapies. Every 1 to 2 hours observe for petechiae, ecchymoses, and oozing. Be sure to check dependent areas, since blood will pool in these areas. Intravenous sites are particularly prone to oozing and should be assessed every 15 minutes. Examine stool for the presence of blood, and measure blood loss as accurately as possible. Measure intake and output. Institute bleeding control precautions, as outlined in the section on nursing management for hemophilia.[8] Monitor prescribed therapy (transfusion, anticoagulant therapy) and report any signs of complications.

Idiopathic Thrombocytopenic Purpura

Idiopathic thrombocytopenic purpura (ITP), also known as autoimmune thrombocytopenic purpura, is a disorder characterized by increased destruction of platelets, even though platelet production in the bone marrow is normal. When the rate of platelet destruction exceeds the rate of platelet production, the number of circulating platelets decreases and blood clotting slows.

ITP is the most common bleeding disorder in children. It occurs most frequently in children 2 to 5 years of age and usually follows a viral infection such as measles, chickenpox, or rubella. Symptoms include multiple ecchymoses and petechiae.

Diagnosis is made by history and through physical and laboratory findings, which show a decreased platelet count and antiplatelet antibodies in the peripheral blood. Treatment includes administering corticosteroids and intravenous immunoglobulins. For those children who do not respond to drug therapy over a period of 6 months to 1 year, splenectomy may be the treatment of choice. Spontaneous remission is seen in 90% of children with ITP.[2]

Nursing Management

Nursing care focuses on controlling and reducing the number of bleeding episodes. Preventive measures are similar to those discussed earlier in this chapter for the child with hemophilia. Teach parents to use acetaminophen, rather than aspirin, to control pain. Provide emotional support.

Bone Marrow Transplantation

Bone marrow transplantation is a treatment that is used for immune diseases such as severe combined immunodeficiency disease, severe and unresponsive aplastic anemia, and leukemia (see Chapter 16). The transplantation procedure begins with chemotherapy directed at destroying the diseased bone marrow. The transplanted marrow, given via intravenous infusion, then plants itself in the bone and begins to grow. If the transplantation is successful, healthy bone marrow, capable of making blood cells, is the result.

There are three types of bone marrow transplant: autologous, isogeneic (or syngeneic), and allogeneic. In autologous transplantation, the child's own marrow is taken, stored, and reinfused after the child has received chemotherapy. In isogeneic transplantation, the marrow is taken from an identical twin. In allogeneic transplantation, the donor, usually a sibling, has a compatible human leukocyte antigen (HLA).

The child is without any immunity for a minimum of 10 days after transplantation. It takes 10 to 20 days before the donor cells begin to proliferate and mature.[9] This period is most critical, and the child should be kept in strict isolation in a special unit. However, once the bone marrow begins to produce new cells, graft-versus-host disease (rejection) may occur. Supportive care focuses on preventing infection, controlling bleeding, maintaining adequate nutrition and hydration, monitoring for signs of rejection, and providing psychosocial support. The nurse should encourage parents to discuss their feelings with other parents of children receiving bone marrow transplantation.

NATIONAL BONE MARROW REGISTRY

With the development of the National Bone Marrow Registry, bone marrow transplantation from HLA-matched unrelated donors has become an option for some children with immune disorders.

REFERENCES

1 Guyton, A. (1990). *Textbook of medical physiology* (8th ed.). Philadelphia: W.B. Saunders.
2 Hathaway, W.E., Way, W.W., Jr., Groothuis, J.R., & Paisley, J.W. (1993). *Current pediatric diagnosis & treatment* (11th ed.). Norwalk, CT: Appleton & Lange.
3 Baum, K., et al. (1987). The painful crises of homozygous sickle cell disease. *Archives in Internal Medicine, 147,* 1231–1234.
4 Lamb, C. (1985). Managing sickle cell emergencies. *Patient Care, 19*(1), 92–95.
5 Martin, M.B., & Butler, R.B. (1993). Understanding the basics of β thalassemia major. *Pediatric Nursing, 19*(2), 143–145.
6 Rudolph, A.M., Hoffman, J.I.E., & Rudolph, C.D. (Eds.). (1991). *Rudolph's pediatrics* (19th ed.). Norwalk, CT: Appleton & Lange.
7 Griffin, J. (1986). *Hematology & immunology: Concepts for nursing.* Norwalk, CT: Appleton-Century-Crofts.
8 Griffin, J. (1991). Interventions for clients with hematologic disorders. In D. Ignatavicus & M. Bayne (Eds.), *Medical surgical nursing.* Philadelphia: W.B. Saunders.
9 Brain, M., & Carbone, P. (1991). *Current therapy in hematology-oncology* (4th ed.). St. Louis: Mosby–Year Book.

SUGGESTED READINGS

Cerrato, P. (1986). Could you spot the other anemia? *RN, 49*(10), 63–64.
Griffin, J. (1986). Be prepared for the bleeding patient. *Nursing, 16*(6), 34–42.
Williams, W., Beutler, E., Ersley, A., & Lichtman, M. (1990). *Hematology* (4th ed.). New York: McGraw-Hill.
Yasko, J., & Green, P. (1987). Coping with problems relating to cancer and cancer treatment. *CA—A Cancer Journal for Clinicians, 37*(2), 106–125.

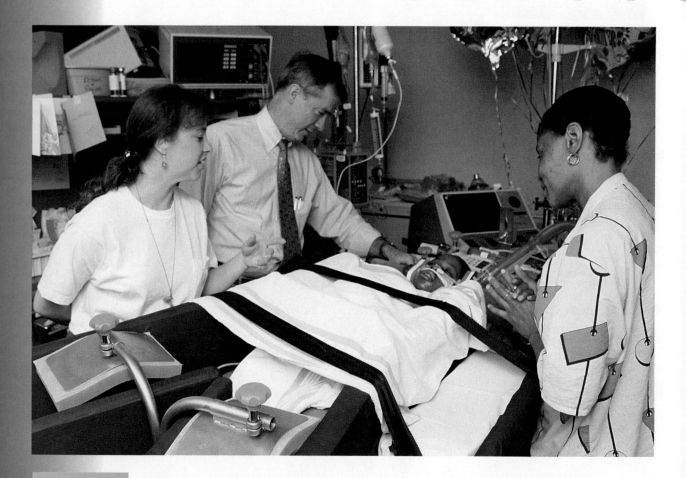

A ntwan, 10 years old, was injured when he was ejected from a motor vehicle that rolled over his lower spine. He was treated for shock in the emergency department, where his neurologic status and vital signs were frequently assessed. Initially Antwan's level of consciousness was good, although he displayed some motor deficits and decreased sensation in his legs. His level of consciousness gradually diminished, however, until he showed little response to stimuli. He was then intubated and medicated.

When Antwan's condition stabilized, he was taken to the radiology department for spinal films and computed tomography (CT) of the head and spine. Nurses monitored his vital signs closely, watching for further signs of deterioration. Radiologic findings revealed L-3 and L-4 spine fractures and a contusion to the frontotemporal lobe with a subarachnoid hemorrhage.

Surgery was performed to stabilize the spine and evacuate the hemorrhage. Postoperatively, Antwan's neurologic status and vital signs were closely monitored in the pediatric intensive care unit for increased intracranial pressure and poor perfusion. He was placed on a continuously rotating bed to maintain the spinal alignment and to reduce pressure points on his back. He remains intubated and sedated because of his decreased level of consciousness. It is likely that Antwan will have permanent damage to his spinal cord and need rehabilitation.

Alterations in Neurologic Function

TERMINOLOGY

areflexic No reflex response to verbal, sensory, or pain stimulation.

aura Subjective sensation, often olfactory or visual in nature, that is an early sign of a seizure.

clonic Alternating muscular contraction and relaxation; often used to describe seizure activity.

coma State of unconsciousness in which the child cannot be aroused, even with powerful stimuli.

confusion Disorientation to time, place, or person.

Cushing triad Reflex response associated with increased intracranial pressure or compromised blood flow to the brainstem; characterized by hypertension, increased systolic pressure with wide pulse pressure, bradycardia, and irregular respirations.

delirium State characterized by confusion, fear, agitation, hyperactivity, or anxiety.

focal Specific area of the brain; often used to describe seizures or neurologic deficits.

intracranial pressure Force exerted by brain tissue, cerebrospinal fluid, and blood within the cranial vault.

level of consciousness General description of cognitive, sensory, and motor response to stimuli.

obtunded Diminished level of consciousness with minimal response to stimuli.

postictal period Period after seizure activity during which the level of consciousness is decreased.

posturing Abnormal position assumed after injury or damage to the brain that may be seen as extreme flexion or extension of the limbs.

stupor Diminished level of consciousness with response only to vigorous stimulation.

tonic Continuous muscular contraction; often used to describe seizure activity.

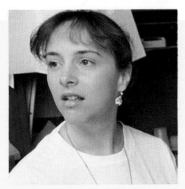

❝ Antwan has such a long course of rehabilitation ahead. I wish we knew the extent of his brain injury so we could better plan his long-term care. ❞

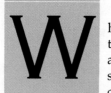

hy do certain neurologic disorders occur more often in children than in adults? What effect do these disorders have on a child's growth and development? Why are some neurologic injuries more likely to be seen in children and why do children recover from these injuries more completely than adults? What role do nurses play in ensuring early diagnosis and treatment of neurologic disorders? This chapter will enable you to answer these questions by examining some of the more common disorders of neurologic function in children.

Anatomy and Physiology of Pediatric Differences

Knowledge of the anatomy of the nervous system makes neurologic symptoms easier to understand. The brain, spinal cord, and nerves are the major structures of the nervous system (Fig. 14–1). The spinal cord transmits impulses to and from the brain, conveying sensory information and relaying impulses that stimulate motor responses. Because the nervous system helps to control and coordinate many body functions, alterations in neurologic function can have widespread effects on the normal operations of the body.

At birth, the nervous system is complete but immature. Although the infant is born with all of the nerve cells that will exist throughout life, the number of glial cells and dendrites continues to increase until approximately 4 years of age. Myelination, which increases the speed and accuracy of nerve impulses, is also incomplete at birth. This process continues throughout childhood, proceeding in a cephalocaudal direction.

The anatomic and physiologic differences between the nervous systems of children and adults help explain why children have different neurologic

FIGURE 14–1 Transverse section of the brain and spinal cord. Knowledge of the anatomy of the brain is helpful in understanding the symptoms of neurologic dysfunction.

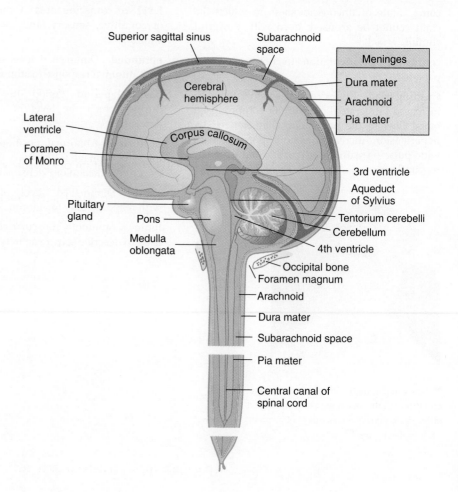

TABLE 14-1 Summary of Anatomic and Physiologic Differences Between Children and Adults

Difference	Significance
Top heavy; head is large in proportion to body; neck muscles not well developed	Prone to head injuries with falls; neck may not be able to support large head
Cranial bones thin and not well developed; unfused sutures	Prone to fracture
Brain highly vascular; subarachnoid space small; dura firmly attached but can strip away from pericranium	Brain prone to hemorrhage; there is less cerebrospinal fluid to cushion brain
Excessive spinal mobility; muscles, joint capsules, and ligaments of cervical spine immature	Greater risk for high cervical spine injury at C-1 to C-2 level
Wedge-shaped, cartilaginous vertebral bodies; ossification of vertebral bodies incomplete	Greater risk for compression fractures of vertebrae with falls

■ GROWTH AND DEVELOPMENT CONSIDERATIONS

Infants who have fontanels that are not yet closed have an elastic skull and room for brain expansion.

problems (Table 14–1). For example, the brain and spinal cord are protected by the skeletal structures of the skull and vertebrae. In infants, however, the cranial bones and vertebrae are not completely ossified. The infant's brain and spinal cord are thus at greater risk for injury resulting from trauma.

Altered States of Consciousness

Level of consciousness is perhaps the most important indicator of neurologic dysfunction. Consciousness, the responsiveness of the mind to sensory stimuli, has two components: alertness, or the ability to react to stimuli, and cognitive power, or the ability to process the data and respond either verbally or physically. Unconsciousness, on the other hand, is depressed cerebral function, or the inability of the brain to respond to stimuli.

Levels of deterioration can be further categorized as:

- **Confusion:** disorientation to time, place, or person. The child may seem alert. Answers to simple questions may be correct, but responses to complex ones may be inaccurate.
- **Delirium:** state characterized by confusion, fear, agitation, hyperactivity, or anxiety.
- **Stupor:** response to vigorous stimulation only; the child returns to the unresponsive state when the stimulus is removed. For example, the child may react to a needle stick but not respond to a milder stimulus such as touching the skin.
- **Coma:** state characterized by severely diminished response; the child cannot be aroused even by painful stimuli.

Clinical Manifestations

Declines in level of consciousness in children often follow a sequential pattern of deterioration. This was true in the case of Antwan, described at the beginning of the chapter. Children may initially appear awake and alert, responding appropriately to their environment. The first sign of change may

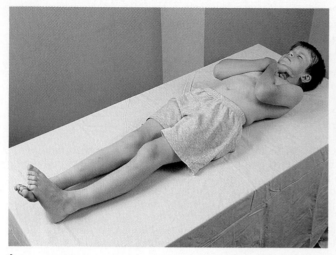 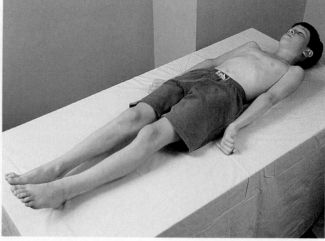

A   B

FIGURE 14-2 A, Decorticate posturing, characterized by rigid flexion, is associated with lesions above the brain stem in the corticospinal tracts. **B,** Decerebrate posturing, distinguished by rigid extension, is associated with lesions of the brain stem.

TABLE 14-2 Causes of Decreased Level of Consciousness

Trauma
Infection
Poisoning
Seizures
Endocrine or metabolic disturbance
Electrolyte or biochemical imbalance
Acid-base imbalance
Cerebrovascular pathology
Structural defects

---

be subtle, a slight disorientation to time, place, and person. Children may become restless or fussy, and actions that normally calm or soothe them only increase their irritability. Children may become drowsy, but they may still respond to loud verbal commands and withdraw from painful stimuli. Keeping them awake is sometimes difficult. Children's response to pain progresses from purposeful to nonpurposeful. Decorticate or decerebrate **posturing,** the abnormal positions assumed after injury or damage to the brain, may occur (Fig. 14-2).

Etiology and Pathophysiology

Trauma, infection, poisoning, seizures, or any other process that affects the central nervous system may alter the level of consciousness (Table 14-2). Discovering the cause of the decreased level of consciousness is important so that immediate treatment can begin to prevent possible secondary effects of the illness or injury.

Increased **intracranial pressure** (force exerted by brain tissue, cerebrospinal fluid, and blood within the cranial vault) may be noted in the comatose child. If this increased pressure level is marked and results from the accumulation of cerebrospinal fluid because of obstruction, a ventricular tap can be performed to decrease the pressure, thus relieving a life-threatening condition that can lead to coma.

Diagnostic Tests and Medical Management

Medical management focuses on early diagnosis, intervention, and prevention of complications.

A thorough history is one of the most important assessment tools. It is important to assess whether the child has had recent head trauma, infection, or ingested toxins. It is also important to determine if the child has a shunt, a tumor, or a condition that could affect his or her level of consciousness.

Laboratory tests include complete blood cell count, blood chemistry, clotting factors, and blood culture; toxicology assessments of both blood and urine; and urinalysis with culture.

TABLE 14–3 Glasgow Coma Scale for Assessment of Coma in Infants and Children

Category	Score	Infant and Young Child Criteria	Older Child and Adult Criteria
Eye opening	4	Spontaneous opening	Spontaneous
	3	To loud noise	To verbal stimuli
	2	To pain	To pain
	1	No response	No response
Verbal response	5	Smiles, coos, cries to appropriate stimuli	Oriented to time, place, and person; uses appropriate words and phrases
	4	Irritable; cries	Confused
	3	Inappropriate crying	Inappropriate words or verbal response
	2	Grunts, moans	Incomprehensible words
	1	No response	No response
Motor response	6	Spontaneous movement	Obeys commands
	5	Withdraws to touch	Localizes to pain
	4	Withdraws to pain	Withdraws to pain
	3	Abnormal flexion (decorticate)	Flexion to pain (decorticate)
	2	Abnormal extension (decerebrate)	Extension to pain (decerebrate)
	1	No response	No response

Add the score from each category to get the total. The maximum score is 15, indicating the best level of neurologic functioning. The minimum is 3, indicating total neurologic unresponsiveness.
From Teasdale, G., & Jennett, B. (1974). *Lancet 2*, 81–84; and James, H.E. (1986). *Pediatric Annals, 15*(1), 17.

A lumbar puncture may be performed to assess cerebrospinal fluid for protein, glucose, or blood cells. An electroencephalogram (EEG) identifies damaged or nonfunctioning areas of the brain.

Radiologic examination is an essential part of the diagnostic workup. Computed tomography (CT) or magnetic resonance imaging (MRI) is used to detect any lesions, structural abnormalities, vascular malformations, or edema. Skull x-ray studies are used to detect fractures or bony malformations.

The pediatric Glasgow Coma Scale is used to assess eye opening, verbal response, and motor response in infants and children (Table 14–3). The child's developmental age has to be taken into account when evaluating his or her responses to each category of the test.

- Eye opening. Note whether eye opening is spontaneous or occurs in response to a command. A dilated but reactive pupil may indicate an intracranial mass. A fixed and dilated pupil may be a sign of impending herniation resulting from increased intracranial pressure.
- Verbal response. Crying in an infant is a positive response. The 2-year-old child who says "no" to each command is also responding in an age-appropriate way.
- Motor response. Motor score is probably the most critical aspect of this test, since the child cannot control reflexes. A fearful toddler may refuse to open his or her eyes or talk to strangers, but the child's reflexes should automatically respond to appropriate stimuli.

Nursing Assessment

Initially assess the child's physiologic status, using the ABCs as described in Table 14–4. Assess the child's level of consciousness, vital signs, and breathing patterns frequently, since they can be indicators of neurologic deterioration.

TABLE 14-4 Physiologic Assessment Based on the ABCs

Assessment Area	Questions
Airway	Is the child's airway patent?
	Is it maintainable (for example, with a jaw thrust)?
	Is intubation necessary?
Breathing	What is the child's ventilatory status?
	Is the child's color normal? Does the child appear pale or cyanotic?
	What are the heart and respiratory rates?
	Is the child's breathing more labored? Does the child have nasal flaring, retractions, or grunting?
	What are the breath sounds?
	What is the pulse oximetry or arterial blood gas measurement?
Circulation	What are the heart rate and blood pressure?
	Is the capillary refill time greater than or less than 2 seconds?
Disability	What is the level of consciousness? How does the child respond to interventions or the environment?
	What is the pediatric Glasgow Coma Score?
Exposure	Is the body temperature normal, above or below normal?
	Are there any signs of injury or trauma?

TABLE 14-5 Assessment of Cranial Nerves in the Unconscious Child

Cranial Nerves	Reflex	Assessment
II, III	Pupillary	Shine light source in eye. Rapid, concentrally constricting pupils indicate intact cranial nerves II, III.
II, IV, VI	Oculocephalic (doll's eyes)	Should be performed with eyes held open and head turned from side to side. Eyes gazing straight up or lagging slightly behind head motion indicate intact cranial nerves. *Precaution:* C-spine must be cleared before this assessment is performed.
III, VIII	Oculovestibular	Place the head in a midline and slightly elevated position. Inject ice water into ear canal. Eyes deviating *toward* the irrigated ear indicate intact cranial nerves III, VIII. *Precautions:* C-spine must be cleared before this assessment is performed. Tympanic membrane must be intact; otherwise brain may be filled with bacteria-laden fluid. NOTE: This assessment is usually performed by a physician.
V, VII	Corneal	Cornea is gently swabbed with sterile cotton swab. A blink indicates intact cranial nerves V, VII.
IX, X	Gag	Pharynx is irritated with tongue depressor or cotton swab. Gagging response indicates intact cranial nerves IX, X.

■ CLINICAL TIP

When assessing the motor skills of a toddler, ask the child to reach for a finger puppet or doll rather than your hand. This makes the child feel less threatened. The toy is a reward.

A child's responses may differ significantly when stress and anxiety are reduced. Encourage the parents to take part in the examination to reduce the child's anxiety.

Assess the child's cranial nerves (Table 14–5). This is not difficult to perform in the conscious child (see Table 3–22), but the inability of an unconscious child to cooperate makes assessment difficult.

Assess the child's respiratory effort and color. Monitor pulse oximetry or arterial blood gas measurements. The child must be able to maintain adequate air exchange to keep oxygen and carbon dioxide levels within normal ranges; otherwise there is a risk of increased intracranial pressure. If the child cannot maintain an adequate tidal volume, mechanical ventilation will be necessary.

Nursing Diagnosis

Common nursing diagnoses for the child with an altered level of consciousness include:

- Ineffective Breathing Pattern related to decreased level of consciousness or increased intracranial pressure
- High Risk for Aspiration related to decreased level of consciousness
- Impaired Physical Mobility related to decreased level of consciousness
- Impaired Social Interaction related to diminished response to environment
- High Risk for Altered Family Processes related to care of child with disability

Nursing Management

Nursing care focuses on maintaining airway patency, monitoring neurologic status, performing routine care, providing sensory stimulation, and providing emotional support to parents.

Maintain Airway Patency. Make sure that the child's airway is clear at all times. Intubation, tracheostomy, and/or mechanical ventilation may be required. Pulse oximetry or arterial blood gas analysis is performed at regular intervals to ensure that gas exchange is adequate. If the child is having difficulty swallowing secretions or does not have a gag reflex, intubation is required. If long-term airway management is anticipated, a tracheostomy may be performed.

Monitor Neurologic Status. Perform routine neurologic checks. Evaluate pupil size and reactivity, eye movements, and motor function. Monitor vital signs. Increased systolic blood pressure, a wide pulse pressure, and bradycardia indicate increased intracranial pressure. Look for other signs of increased intracranial pressure listed in Table 14–6.

Be sure that adequate cerebral perfusion pressure (i.e., the amount of pressure needed to ensure that adequate oxygen and nutrients will be delivered to the brain) is maintained. If the child is hypovolemic (see Chapter 7) or has poor perfusion, give fluids. If the child has signs of fluid overload and is still poorly perfused, dopamine or dobutamine may be administered.

Keep suction apparatus with catheters, oxygen, resuscitation bag and mask, and extra tracheostomy tubes (if applicable) at the bedside in case of seizures. The siderails should be padded to protect the child from injury.

Perform Routine Care. If the corneal reflex is absent, place artificial tears in the eyes, pad the eyes with gauze, and tape the eyes so they remain closed. Perform routine mouth care by brushing the teeth and using glycerine swabs.

Provide adequate nutrition. Initially nutrients may be supplied intravenously. A gastrostomy tube may be inserted if the child remains unconscious or is not alert enough to take food by mouth.

TABLE 14–6 Signs of Increased Intracranial Pressure

Early Signs

Headache
Nausea and vomiting
Dizziness or vertigo
Slight change in vital signs
Pupils not as reactive or equal
Sunsetting eyes
Seizures
Slight change in level of consciousness
Infant has above signs plus:
    Bulging fontanel
    Wide sutures
    Dilated scalp veins
    High-pitched, catlike cry

Late Signs

Significant decrease in level of consciousness
Cushing triad
    Increased systolic blood pressure
    Wide pulse pressure
    Brachycardia
Irregular respirations
Fixed and dilated pupils

TABLE 14–7 Care of the Immobile Child

- Help keep body in proper alignment with splints or rolls made of towels or blankets.
- Change position every 2 hours.
- Perform passive or gentle range of motion exercises three or four times per day according to physician's orders.
- Maintain skin integrity.
- Place child on foam or egg-crate mattress or sheepskin covering.
- Massage child gently using lotion.

Prevent complications associated with immobility (muscle atrophy, contractures, and skin breakdown) as described in Table 14–7.

Provide Stimulation. Explain all procedures and actions. Because the child with a severely altered level of consciousness may still be able to hear, talking to him or her may be beneficial.

When the child becomes more alert, orient the child to time, place, and person, depending on age and level of understanding. Encourage parents to bring objects or toys from home to make the environment more familiar and promote a feeling of security.

Provide Emotional Support. Explain the child's condition in simple terms. Encourage parents to take part in their child's care and therapy as much as possible. If the child's condition is the result of trauma, infection, or tumor and he or she may never function normally, the family needs emotional support and referral to appropriate psychologic and social services (see Chapter 6 for more information about helping families cope with a child's life-threatening illness). Allow family members to express their feelings.

Discharge Planning and Patient and Family Home Care Teaching. Home care needs should be identified and addressed well in advance of discharge. Arrangements should be made for long-term care of the child who is **obtunded** (has a minimal response to stimuli). Possibilities include a long-term care facility, a rehabilitation facility, or home care. If the child will be managed at home, teach family members how to care for the child. Make sure they understand and can perform routine care activities, such as proper feeding, positioning, exercise, and skin care. Tell parents to watch for signs of respiratory distress. Parents should learn cardiopulmonary resuscitation (CPR) techniques.

Put parents in contact with social workers who can help arrange for financial assistance and the purchase of special equipment. Home care nurses play a vital role in the care of the child with a neurologic dysfunction. They coordinate care and services for the child and provide the family with needed emotional support. A knowledgeable person who can care for the child should be available for respite care.

■ Seizure Disorders

Seizures are periods of involuntary muscle contraction and relaxation. They are a common neurologic disorder in children. An estimated 3% to 5% of children have seizures during their early years.[1,2] Epilepsy is a chronic disorder characterized by recurrent seizures. It is secondary to underlying brain dysfunction and is often a sign of a central nervous system disorder.

Clinical Manifestations

The symptoms of a seizure depend on the type and duration of the seizure. Seizures are classified into two types: partial and generalized. The specific characteristics of the various types of partial and generalized seizures are presented in Table 14–8. The initial manifestations of the **tonic** phase of a generalized seizure are unconsciousness and continuous muscular contraction. The tonic phase is followed by the **clonic** phase, characterized by alternating muscular contraction and relaxation. In the **postictal period**, following seizure activity, the level of consciousness is decreased.

Febrile seizures are generalized seizures that occur in children and usually accompany such infections as otitis media, upper respiratory infections, and meningitis. These seizures usually occur with rapid temperature rise above 39° C (102° F) and rarely occur before 6 months or after 5 years of age. Febrile seizures involve generalized tonic-clonic movements that last less than 15 minutes. The length of the postictal period varies from child to child.

Etiology and Pathophysiology

Seizures are believed to be the result of spontaneous electrical discharge of hyperexcited cells in the brain. These cells can be triggered by either environmental or physiologic stimuli such as emotional stress, anxiety, fatigue, infection, or metabolic disturbances.

TABLE 14–8 Clinical Manifestations of Seizures

Type of Seizure	Clinical Manifestations
Partial Seizures	
Complex partial seizures (psychomotor seizures) *Onset:* 3 years of age to adolescence	Consciousness not completely lost, although level of consciousness decreases
	Aura frequently present
	Feelings of anxiety, fear, or déjà vu (sensation that an event has occurred before)
	Abdominal pain
	Unusual taste or odor
	Staring into space
	Mental confusion
	Posturing
	Performing repeated purposeless activities (automatisms)
	Lip smacking, lip chewing, or sucking
Simple partial seizures (focal seizures) *Onset:* any age	Consciousness generally not lost unless the seizure becomes generalized
	No aura
	Motor responses may involve one extremity, part of that extremity, or ipsilateral extremities with eyes and head turning in opposite direction
	Sensory responses involve paresthesias (decreased sensation or tingling) as well as auditory or visual sensations
	Motor and sensory involvement may be combined
	Jacksonian march (rare in young children):
	Tonic contractions of either fingers of one hand, toes of one foot, or one side of the face become clonic or tonic-clonic movements
	Activity then "marches" up to adjacent muscles of either affected extremity or same side of body (such as face)

Continued.

TABLE 14–8 Clinical Manifestations of Seizures—Continued

Type of Seizure	Clinical Manifestations
Generalized Seizures	
Tonic/clonic seizures (grand mal seizures) *Onset:* any age	Abrupt onset seizure in which there may not be aura
	Tonic phase of seizure lasts 10 to 30 seconds; clonic phase may persist from 30 seconds to 30 minutes
	Falling to ground during initial tonic phase when loss of consciousness occurs
	Intense muscular contractions
	Eyes rolling upward or deviating to one side with pupils dilated
	Abdominal and chest muscle rigidity with leg, head, and neck extended and arms flexed or contracted
	Pallor or cyanosis
	Cry or grunt as air is forced through rigid diaphragm
	Urinary or bowel incontinence
	Postictal phase of variable duration (few minutes to several hours). Characterized by:
	Sleepiness, difficulty in arousal
	Hypertension
	Diaphoresis
	Headache, nausea, vomiting
	Poor coordination, decreased muscle tone
	Confusion, amnesia
	Slurred speech
	Visual disturbances
	Combativeness
Primary generalized seizures (petit mal, pure absence, lapse seizures) *Onset:* age 4 years with remission in adolescence More prevalent in females	Brief loss of consciousness; usually last 5 to 10 seconds, rarely exceeding 30 seconds
	Attacks occur frequently (as often as 20 or more times daily)
	No aura
	Abrupt cessation of current activity
	Rolling of eyes
	Ptosis or fluttering of eyelids
	Staring
	Slight loss in muscle tone (head may droop, hand-held objects may be dropped)
	Amnesia
	Episodes may often be confused with inattentiveness or daydreaming
Myoclonic seizures *Onset:* as early as 2 years, but more prevalent in school-age child and adolescent	No loss of consciousness; child recovers in seconds
	Attacks occur most often upon falling asleep or awakening
	Head, extremity, or body contractions
	No postictal period
Infantile spasms (myoclonic epilepsy of infancy, salaam seizures) *Onset:* begin at age 3 months and resolve by 2 years	Possible loss of consciousness
	Episodes usually occur when infant is sleepy or drowsy
	Several seizures can occur throughout day
	Dropping of head, flexion of neck, extension of arms, and flexion of legs
	Rolling of eyes either upward or downward
	Crying, pallor, or cyanosis
	Children who display these seizures with positive history of gestational difficulties, developmental delays, or other neurologic abnormalities most likely have mental retardation and other types of seizures
Akinetic or atonic seizures (drop attacks) *Onset:* first seen at age 2 years and disappear by age 6	Momentary loss of consciousness
	Loss of muscle tone after which child falls to ground
	Inability to break fall

Some seizures are idiopathic. Genetic factors may lower the seizure threshold by making brain cells more vulnerable to abnormal electrical discharges. Acquired seizures may be caused by underlying pathologic conditions such as trauma, infection, hypoglycemia, endocrine dysfunction, toxins, tumors, or lesions that may be manifested at any time. Table 14–9 lists some of the causes of the different types of seizures.

Partial, or **focal**, seizures are caused by abnormal electrical activity in a specific area of the cerebral cortex, most often the temporal, frontal, or parietal lobes. The symptoms that are displayed depend on the region of the cortex affected.

In contrast, generalized seizures are the result of diffuse electrical activity that begins in one area of the brain and spreads throughout the cortex into the brainstem. Movements and spasms displayed by the child are bilateral and symmetric, since both hemispheres are affected.

The length of a seizure, especially that of a generalized seizure, is important because the airway may be compromised during the tonic phase. The basal metabolic rate rises during the peak of seizure activity. This change, in turn, increases the demand for oxygen and glucose. During a seizure the child may become pale or cyanotic as a result of hypoxia or hypoglycemia.

TABLE 14–9 Common Causes of Seizures

Type of Seizure	Cause
Partial	
Complex partial seizure	Lesions, cysts, or tumors
	Perinatal trauma
	Prolonged febrile seizures that may cause scarring of mediotemporal lobe
	Hamartomatous lesions
	Arteriovenous malformations
	Trauma
Simple partial seizure	Focal damage (e.g., with cerebral palsy)
	Tumors or lesions
	Arteriovenous malformations
	Brain abscesses
Generalized	
Grand mal seizure	Cerebral damage from birth injury, trauma, tumors, lesions, and metabolic and neuromuscular degenerative disorders; many are idiopathic
Petit mal seizure	Possible genetic link
Infantile spasm	Prenatal and perinatal encephalopathy
	Tuberous sclerosis
	Microcephaly
Akinetic/myoclonic seizures	Gray matter degenerative diseases and subacute sclerosing panencephalitis; many are idiopathic
Febrile seizure	Rapid rise in temperature, reaching 39° C (102° F)
	Associated with infections:
	Upper respiratory
	Urinary tract
	Otitis media
	Pharyngitis
	Roseola

Diagnostic Tests and Medical Management

After the child's first seizure, it is essential that a thorough history be taken from the parent, primary caretaker, or witnesses to the event. Table 14–10 lists the questions that should be asked. Details such as the description and length of the seizure, presence or absence of an **aura** (an early sign or warning of an impending seizure, most often olfactory or visual in nature), and whether the child lost consciousness or not should be noted.

A complete physical and neurologic examination is performed. Based on the physical findings and history, diagnostic tests are ordered. Laboratory tests include a complete blood cell count and blood chemistry. If the child is taking any anticonvulsants, blood levels of the medication should be monitored. Lumbar puncture and EEG may be performed. Radiologic tests include CT scanning or MRI and angiography.

Many convulsions are self-limiting and require no emergency intervention, but status epilepticus is considered a medical emergency. Status epilepticus is a continuous seizure that lasts more than 30 minutes or a series of seizures during which consciousness is not regained. Management of the

---

TABLE 14-10 Questions to Ask About Seizures

- Did the child complain of not feeling well or feeling "funny" just before the seizure?
- Did the child complain of headache, nausea, muscle pain? Did the child vomit?
- Did the child suffer any trauma before the seizure?
- Did the child get into any medications or poisons before the seizure?
- Was the child sick or feverish before the seizure?
- Were the child's movements tonic-clonic (periods of muscle rigidity followed by relaxation)?
- Was the child's vision normal?
- Were the pupils dilated or the eyes deviated to one side?
- Was the child incontinent of urine or stool?
- How long did the episode last?
- When did the child begin to wake up?
- Was the child lethargic, weak, or uncoordinated upon arousal?
- Did the child's movements involve one side of the body or one arm or leg?
- Did the child injure himself or herself during the convulsion?
- Did the child become pale or did the skin change color (e.g., red or blue)?
- Did the child lose consciousness?

TABLE 14-11 Management of Status Epilepticus

- A patent airway should be maintained. Muscle rigidity may compromise it.
- If the airway is obstructed, a jaw thrust maneuver should be performed.
- Suction equipment should be at the bedside in case of excessive secretions.
- Oxygen is given by mask as increased metabolic demands can deplete oxygen stores.
- The physical stress of the seizure may result in declining glucose levels. If the child is hypoglycemic, glucose should be administered.
- An intravenous line should be established to administer any necessary fluids or medications.
- Benzodiazepines such as diazepam, lorazepam, or midazolam are administered. If there is no response, the dose may be repeated.
- Phenytoin or phenobarbital may be necessary if seizure activity continues.

■ SAFETY PRECAUTIONS

Do not force a bite block between the teeth of a child during a seizure. Loose teeth may be knocked out and aspirated.

■ CLINICAL TIP

Children under the age of 5 years with specific types of seizures may be put on a ketogenic diet, which includes a ratio of 3 to 1 of fat versus carbohydrate and protein intake.[1] This high-fat diet is believed to slow the electrical impulses that cause seizures. Medium-chain triglycerides may be given as a supplement to increase the acidosis.

■ SAFETY PRECAUTIONS

Children who have frequent, recurrent seizures should wear helmets to protect their heads in case they fall. All children with seizure disorders should wear some form of medical identification (for example, a Medic-Alert bracelet).

child in status epilepticus is described in Table 14–11. The postictal period ranges from 30 minutes to 2 hours.

Most seizure disorders are treated with anticonvulsants (Table 14–12). Serum drug levels are monitored to maintain therapeutic levels. Maintaining a balance between seizure control and medication toxicity is difficult in children because increases in dosage may be needed as children grow.

A ketogenic diet may be advised for treatment of some seizure disorders in children.[1] Surgery may be necessary to remove tumors, lesions, or parts of the brain that have been identified as causing the seizures.

Nursing Assessment

Assess the child's status based on the ABCs (Table 14–4). Once the child is stable, a more definitive assessment can be made. Level of consciousness is one of the most important indicators of neurologic function. It is important to remember that lack of response in a child may be a result of the postictal state.

Nursing Diagnosis

Common nursing diagnoses for the child with a seizure disorder include:

- Ineffective Breathing Pattern related to decreased respiratory effort during the tonic phase of a seizure
- Ineffective Airway Clearance related to seizure activity
- High Risk for Aspiration related to decreased level of consciousness
- High Risk for Injury related to seizure activity
- Body Image Disturbance related to loss of body control during seizure activity
- High Risk for Anxiety related to distressing aspects of seizure disorder
- Altered Family Processes related to a chronic disorder

Nursing Management

Nursing care focuses on maintaining airway patency, ensuring safety, administering medications, and providing emotional support. Both acute care and long-term management are involved.

Maintain Airway Patency. Be sure that nothing is placed in the child's mouth during a seizure. Monitor the child to ensure adequate oxygenation: the child's color should be pink, the heart rate at a normal or slightly above normal rate for age, and the pulse oximetry reading greater than 95%. Administer oxygen at levels below this per physician's orders.

Ensure Safety. Protect the child from self-harm during violent convulsions. If the child is in bed, the siderails should be padded to prevent injury. A child who has a seizure when standing should be gently assisted to the floor and placed in a side-lying position. Clear the area of any objects that might harm the child.

Administer Medications. Take special precautions when administering intravenous drugs for the acute management of seizures. These drugs should be given very slowly to minimize the risk of respiratory or circulatory collapse.

Medications for management of chronic seizures are given by mouth. Crushing pills and mixing them in a teaspoonful of applesauce, pudding, or other soft food make them more palatable and easier for the child to swallow.

Educate the child and parents about medication regimens. Explain the purpose of each drug, its schedule for administration, and the importance of not skipping any doses. Teaching the older child to take medications without parental intervention gives the child a feeling of control. Provide information about the side effects of medications ordered, and alert parents to the signs of toxic reactions or the need to change the dosage. Help arrange for the school nurse to give the medication during school hours if necessary. Encourage follow-up care to monitor drug levels.

Parents and teachers should know what actions to take if the child has a seizure. They should also be aware of activities that are not recommended, such as contact sports. Swimming should only be permitted with close supervision. Generally, adolescents can drive after they have been seizure free for at least 2 years, depending on state laws. Tell parents to boost the child's self-image by emphasizing what the child can do.

Provide Emotional Support. The loss of control of body movements and possible loss of consciousness make seizures frightening and difficult to accept for the child, parents, and other family members. The child may be afraid of having a seizure in front of friends. Reassure the child and family that taking medications regularly should control seizures.

Discharge Planning and Patient and Family Home Care Teaching. Encourage parents to express their fears and anxieties. Answer their questions honestly, and refer them to organizations such as the Epilepsy Foundation of America where they can obtain more information about the disorder (Appendix F).

Parents often feel guilty about their child's seizure disorder, and to compensate for this, they do not discipline or restrict the child adequately. Stress the need to treat the child as normally as possible. Refer the child and family to support groups and counseling services if indicated.

Infectious Diseases

Bacterial Meningitis

Meningitis, an inflammation of the meninges, can be caused by either bacterial or viral agents. Bacterial meningitis is more virulent than viral meningitis and is sometimes fatal.[3] The child who is less than 1 year of age is at greatest risk for acquiring bacterial meningitis. Ninety percent of all cases appear before 5 years of age.[4]

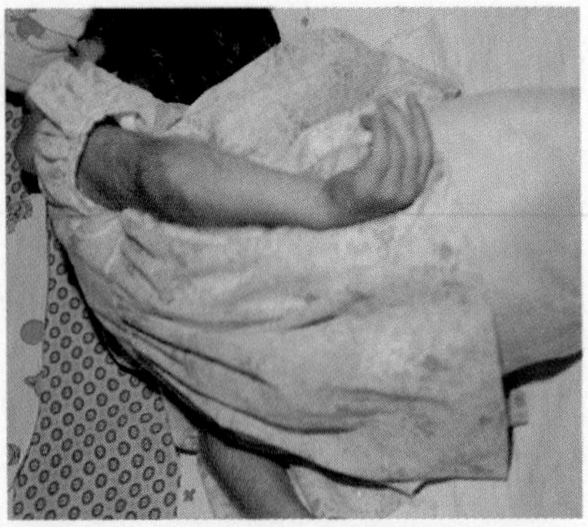

Clinical Manifestations

Symptoms are variable and depend on the child's age, the pathogen, and the length of the illness before diagnosis. Symptoms in the young infant may include fever, change in feeding pattern, vomiting, or diarrhea. The anterior fontanel may be bulging or flat. The infant may be alert, restless, lethargic, or irritable. Rocking or cuddling, which normally calms a fussy infant, only irritates the infant.

Older children are usually febrile, can be irritable or lethargic, and complain of muscle or joint pain. A hemorrhagic rash, first appearing as petechiae and changing to purpura or large necrotic patches, may be seen in

FIGURE 14-3 This child, who has bacterial meningitis, is hyperextending the head and neck (opisthotonic position) to relieve discomfort.

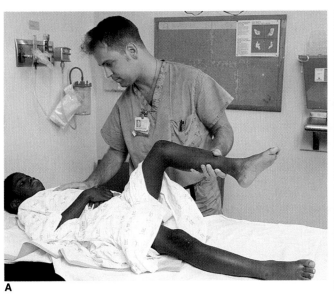
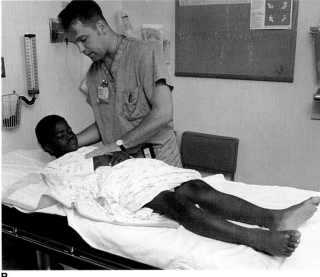

FIGURE 14–4 A child who has viral meningitis may have a positive Kernig sign (**A**) or Brudzinski sign (**B**), or both, on physical examination.

▮ KERNIG SIGN

Extend the child's leg at the knee. If any resistance is noted or any pain is felt, this result is a positive Kernig sign.

▮ BRUDZINSKI SIGN

With the child in a supine position, flex the child's head. If this action causes or makes the knees or hips flex involuntarily, this result is a positive Brudzinski sign.

meningococcal meningitis. The child displays other symptoms consistent with meningeal irritation: headache (most often frontal), photophobia, and nuchal (nape) rigidity.[4] The child is comfortable only in an opisthotonic position (hyperextension of the head and neck to relieve discomfort) (Fig. 14–3). The child may have a positive Kernig or Brudzinski sign, or both, on examination (Fig. 14–4).

Symptoms can progress to include seizures, apnea, cerebral edema, subdural effusion, hydrocephalus, disseminated intravascular coagulation (DIC), shock, and increased intracranial pressure. The bacteria may also colonize a joint and cause septic arthritis.

Etiology and Pathophysiology

Meningitis may occur secondary to other infections such as otitis media, sinusitis, pharyngitis, cellulitis, pneumonia, or septic arthritis; head trauma; or a neurosurgical procedure. The three most common causal agents in children more than 1 month of age are *Haemophilus influenzae* type b, *Neisseria meningitidis*, and *Streptococcus pneumoniae* (Table 14–13). Once the bacteria have spread to the meninges, they enter the cerebrospinal fluid and infect the subarachnoid space.[5] An inflammatory response follows. White blood cells accumulate, covering the surface of the brain with a thick, white, purulent exudate. The brain then becomes hyperemic and edematous. If the infection spreads to the ventricles, they can become obstructed and impede the flow of the cerebrospinal fluid, causing hydrocephalus.

Diagnostic Tests and Medical Management

Diagnosis is based on the history, clinical presentation, and laboratory findings. A thorough history should be taken and physical examination performed.

Laboratory tests include a complete blood count, cultures, serum electrolytes and osmolality, and clotting factors. A lumbar puncture is performed to evaluate the cerebrospinal fluid for number of white blood cells and protein and glucose levels. A Gram stain and culture are done.

TABLE 14-13 Common Organisms That Cause Bacterial and Viral Meningitis

Age	Bacterial Agents	Viral Agents
Neonates (age: less than 1 to 2 months)	*Escherichia coli;* group B *Streptococcus; Listeria monocytogenes; Haemophilus influenzae* type B; *Neisseria meningitidis; Streptococcus pneumoniae*	Herpes
Beyond neonatal period to early adolescence (age: 2 months to 12 years)	*Haemophilus influenzae* type B (in those not immunized); *Neisseria meningitidis; Streptococcus pneumoniae*	Enterovirus, mumps, adenovirus
Adolescence (age: more than 12 years)	*Neisseria meningitidis; Streptococcus pneumoniae*	Herpes, arbovirus, adenovirus

TABLE 14-14 Antibiotics Used in the Treatment of Bacterial Meningitis

Age Group	Organism	Antibiotic
4 to 12 weeks	Group B *Streptococcus; Escherichia coli; Listeria monocytogenes; Haemophilus influenzae; Streptococcus pneumoniae; Neisseria meningitidis*	Ampicillin plus gentamicin or cefotaxime
More than 12 weeks	*Haemophilis influenzae Streptococcus pneumoniae* or *Neisseria meningitidis*	Ceftriaxone, cefotaxime, ampicillin Penicillin G, ampicillin

Based on material from McCracken, G. (1992). *Pediatric Infectious Disease Journal, 11*(2), 169–174; and Roos, K. (1992). *Seminars in Neurology, 12*(3), 155–164, reprinted with permission by Thieme Medical Publishers, Inc.

TABLE 14-15 Complications of Bacterial Meningitis

Syndrome of inappropriate antidiuretic hormone secretion (SIADH)
Disseminated intravascular coagulopathy (DIC)
Subdural effusion
Sepsis
Septic arthritis
Seizures
Hearing loss

Medical management consists primarily of treating the child with appropriate antibiotics. Antibiotics are administered as soon as diagnostic tests are obtained (Table 14–14). These drugs are administered intravenously for 7 to 10 days, depending on the organism and the child's clinical response. Steroids are given as an adjunct to children over 6 weeks of age.[6,7] An adrenocorticosteroid (dexamethasone is the drug of choice) is given with the first dose of antibiotics and continued over several days.[4,8]

Many infants and children who have had bacterial meningitis suffer neurologic damage despite early, aggressive management. The most common sequelae involve cranial nerves, especially the eighth, resulting in hearing loss. In addition, attention deficits, seizures, developmental delay, septic arthritis, or other focal signs may occur (Table 14–15).

Nursing Assessment

Assess the child's physiologic status, including vital signs and level of consciousness. Assess for any sensory deficits.

Nursing Diagnosis

Several nursing diagnoses that may apply to the child with bacterial meningitis are given in the accompanying Nursing Care Plan.

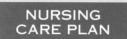

THE CHILD WITH BACTERIAL MENINGITIS

GOAL	INTERVENTION	RATIONALE	EXPECTED OUTCOME

1. Inability to Sustain Spontaneous Ventilation related to decreased level of consciousness

Child will not have respiratory arrest from apneic spells.	Place the child on either an apnea monitor or respiratory monitor with a 20-second alarm.	The alarm on the monitor alerts staff that the child is having an apneic spell.	Child's respiratory failure is easily managed with prompt assessment and treatment.
	Have resuscitation equipment, including oxygen, resuscitation bag with mask, and suction apparatus at the bedside.	Equipment should be at the bedside in case of respiratory arrest. Mouth-to-mouth resuscitation is not advised because the child's respiratory secretions contain bacteria.	
	Stimulate the child if apneic; if no response, begin manual ventilations and call for emergency resuscitation.	Stimulation may encourage spontaneous respirations; if not, ventilation is necessary. Calling for emergency resuscitation ensures help in managing the child in a timely manner.	
	Monitor heart rate and perform compressions if necessary.	The apneic child may have bradycardia resulting from cardiac hypoxia.	

2. Infection related to pathogens in cerebrospinal fluid

Child will be free of infection as quickly as possible.	Administer prescribed antibiotics and steroids as scheduled.	Antibiotics and steroids help eradicate the pathogen and prevent cerebral edema.	Child responds to the medication within 72 hours.
	Monitor vital signs, assess for signs of increased intracranial pressure, check head circumference for swelling, note changes in level of consciousness.	Watching for common sequelae such as subdural effusions or septic arthritis ensures prompt treatment.	
Caretakers or family members will have no apparent evidence of infection.	Explain rationale and dose and schedule for taking rifampin.	Rifampin provides prophylaxis for many bacterial pathogens responsible for meningitis.	Family members and other close contacts verbalize schedule of rifampin therapy.

3. High Risk for Ineffective Thermoregulation related to infection

| Child's thermoregulation will return to normal. | Administer antipyretics such as acetaminophen as ordered (aspirin is not advised because of risk of Reye syndrome). May give tepid bath. May use hypothermia blanket. | Administration of antipyretics and use of other techniques safely reduce fever. | Body temperature decreases or returns to normal. |

Continued.

GOAL	INTERVENTION	RATIONALE	EXPECTED OUTCOME
4. High Risk for Injury related to infection of cerebrospinal fluid and potential sequelae			
Child will suffer minimal central nervous system injury secondary to infection.	Give antibiotics and steroids as soon as possible. Note return of fever, nuchal rigidity, or irritability. Be alert for signs and symptoms of effusion, cerebrospinal fluid obstruction, or cerebral edema, and notify the physician immediately if they occur.	Prompt administration of antibiotics enhances eradication of the pathogen. Administration of steroids diminishes inflammatory response and reduces the chance of neurologic sequelae.	Child's condition significantly improves within 48 to 72 hours (fever decreases, photophobia becomes less severe).
	Measure head circumference once or twice daily.	Increasing head circumference may indicate subdural effusion or hydrocephalus.	
Child will not develop cerebral edema as result of water retention.	Monitor for syndrome of inappropriate antidiuretic hormone secretion (SIADH) and watch for signs of increased intracranial pressure (ICP).	SIADH can be either avoided or quickly managed if early recognition is achieved.	Cerebral edema does not develop. If SIADH or increased ICP occurs the condition is treated promptly so there will be minimal effects on the child.
	Perform strict intake and output measurements. Determine urine specific gravity. Check electrolytes and osmolality of both serum and urine. Weigh child daily. Administer fluids at two thirds of maintenance requirements.	Low urine output with a high specific gravity is a sign of fluid retention and SIADH. The child is maintained with lower fluids to reduced the possibility for cerebral edema.	
Child will be free of injury resulting from disseminated intravascular coagulopathy (DIC).	Be aware of needle sticks that continue to bleed and lesions that continue to ooze. Monitor clotting times.	Prompt recognition leads to management of the coagulopathy.	Child does not sustain injury from DIC.
	Administer blood products, vitamin K, or heparin as ordered.	Prompt recognition allows for early initial treatment of DIC. Child may bleed to death if treatment is delayed.	
	Maintain a safe environment. Protect child from injury.	Additional injury can be prevented.	
Child will be free of injury secondary to shock.	Monitor vital signs including pulse, respirations, and blood pressure. Note perfusion (capillary refill, central versus proximal pulses). Check level of consciousness. Note urine output.	Monitoring allows for prompt diagnosis of shock based on clinical signs.	Child recovers from shock quickly with no complications. Prompt management of shock can enhance the child's recovery, since it prevents complications associated with poor perfusion (tissue acidosis and ischemia).

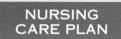
GOAL	INTERVENTION	RATIONALE	EXPECTED OUTCOME
	Begin fluid resuscitation as ordered.	Intravenous fluid bolus may improve perfusion.	
	Administer inotropes if ordered.	Inotropes enhance perfusion when response to fluid challenge is minimal.	
Child will have any hearing loss identified.	Arrange for hearing assessment prior to discharge.	Hearing loss is a common complication. Early intervention is needed to promote growth and development.	Children with identified hearing loss will be referred to appropriate specialist or program for intervention

5. Impaired Social Interaction related to decreased level of consciousness, hospitalization, and isolation

GOAL	INTERVENTION	RATIONALE	EXPECTED OUTCOME
Child's social interactions will be near normal despite isolation.	Educate parents and other visitors to use proper infection control techniques. Encourage parents to help with daily activities such as feeding and bathing.	Family members help fulfill the emotional and social needs of the ill and contagious child. Parental involvement in the child's care provides the child with a sense of security and emotional well-being. Parents have a sense of control and a feeling that they are doing something to enhance the child's recovery.	Child's social and developmental needs are met by family members despite child's illness and hospitalization.
	Have age-appropriate games and toys in the room. Play with the child. When the child is feeling better, encourage watching television or a videotape or listening to the radio or an audio tape.	Providing the child with toys and games as well as sensory stimulation helps the child achieve a sense of well-being.	Child engages in age-appropriate play.

6. Pain related to meningeal irritation

GOAL	INTERVENTION	RATIONALE	EXPECTED OUTCOME
Child will be as comfortable as possible.	Minimize tactile stimulation. Allow the child to assume a position of comfort. Keep the lights dim. Maintain a quiet environment. Keep doors closed.	Sensory stimulation increases discomfort. Child determines the most comfortable position. Opisthotonic position, with the head and neck hyperextended, may be the most comfortable. Dim lights reduce the discomfort from photophobia. Noise can disturb the child.	Child is calm and expresses increased comfort.

Nursing Management

Nursing care begins with emergency treatment and continues as the child's condition stabilizes. Monitor respiratory status, maintain hydration, administer medications, prevent complications, and promote social interaction. Monitor the child's response to antibiotic therapy. The accompanying Nursing Care Plan summarizes nursing care for the child with bacterial meningitis.

Discharge Planning and Patient and Family Home Care Teaching. Home care needs should be identified and addressed well in advance of discharge. Follow-up visits are important to monitor for complications and sequelae. Help parents deal with any physical requirements resulting from the child's illness and any emotional, social, and financial repercussions of the child's condition. Teach parents what to do if the child has a seizure.

Infants and toddlers with neurologic sequelae should be referred to an early intervention program. If the child has had a hearing loss, referral to an otolaryngologist and speech and language specialist should be made.

Children with learning or attention disorders need individualized educational plans, and parents may need assistance in planning for the child's special educational needs. Parents should be referred to the appropriate social service agencies for support and assistance.

Viral (Aseptic) Meningitis

Viral meningitis is an inflammatory response of the meninges characterized by an increased number of blood cells and protein in the cerebrospinal fluid.[5,9] An enterovirus is most often the cause of aseptic meningitis in the United States.[5]

Generally, the child with aseptic meningitis does not appear to be as ill as the child with bacterial meningitis. The child may be irritable or lethargic and usually has a fever. Other symptoms include general malaise, headache, photophobia, gastrointestinal distress, upper respiratory symptoms, and a maculopapular rash. The child may also show signs of meningeal irritation such as stiff neck, back pain, and positive Kernig and Brudzinski signs (Fig. 14–4). The infant may have a tense anterior fontanel. Seizures secondary to the fever may occur.[9] Symptoms usually resolve spontaneously within 3 to 10 days.

The child with fever and meningeal signs is hospitalized. Blood, urine, and cerebrospinal fluid analyses are performed. Until the diagnosis of aseptic meningitis is confirmed, the child is treated as if he or she has bacterial meningitis.

Nursing Management

Nursing care focuses on providing supportive care and teaching the child and family about the disease.

Give acetaminophen as ordered to reduce fever, headache, and muscle or joint pain. Keep the room dark and quiet (to decrease stimuli and meningeal irritation), give fluids either intravenously or orally, and promote comfort with proper positioning.

Explain medical and nursing procedures in terms that the child and family can understand. Encourage parents to bring toys and games to the hospital for the child.

Keep parents informed about the child's progress. Explain that complete recovery may take several weeks and that complications such as learning deficits or altered language development can occur.[2,9] Stress the importance of follow-up care.

Reye Syndrome

Reye syndrome is an acute metabolic encephalopathy of childhood that also affects the liver, causing hepatic dysfunction. It is characterized by cerebral edema and an enlarged, fatty, poorly functioning liver.

The clinical manifestations of Reye syndrome have been divided into five stages, as described in Table 14–16. The child is recovering from a viral illness when repeated vomiting begins (stage I). Within 24 to 48 hours after the vomiting, behavioral changes such as confusion, anxiety, fear, or detachment are observed. The child may be combative and use inappropriate language but soon slips into a coma, which may be interrupted by periods of screaming and ranting (stage II). The majority of children gradually recover, but the state of frenzy may deteriorate within another 24 hours into deeper coma with decorticate posturing (stage III). Decerebrate posturing then occurs, with many brainstem reflexes lost (stage IV). Seizures and respiratory arrest follow (stage V). Death usually follows within 2 to 3 days of onset. Thirty percent of these children die despite treatment.[10]

The etiology of Reye syndrome is unclear. The disorder usually develops after a mild viral illness, such as varicella, an upper respiratory infection, or gastroenteritis. It has also been associated with aspirin use.[10] The link between aspirin and Reye syndrome is not conclusive.[11] However, since more and more parents have begun giving children acetaminophen rather than aspirin, the incidence of Reye disorder has declined.

The diagnosis of Reye syndrome is based on an abrupt change in the child's level of consciousness and diagnostic laboratory tests. Liver enzyme levels (aspartate aminotransferase [AST] or alanine aminotransferase [ALT]) are elevated to twice their normal levels, ammonia levels are elevated, blood sugar levels are below normal, and clotting time is prolonged.[11] Liver biopsy is the only test that truly confirms the diagnosis.

Children with Reye syndrome should be placed in pediatric intensive care units because their condition may deteriorate rapidly. The goal of medical management is to provide supportive treatment and to prevent the secondary effects of cerebral edema and metabolic injury. Children should be checked for signs of increased intracranial pressure, which can be secondary to cerebral edema. Hypoglycemia should be treated with intravenous glucose. Electrolytes, blood chemistry, and blood pH should be monitored as well.

Nursing Management

Nursing care focuses on monitoring the child's physical status, providing emotional support, and teaching parents about disease prevention.

TABLE 14-16 Stages of Reye Syndrome

Stage	Clinical Manifestations
I	Vomiting; lethargy; appropriate responses to verbal commands; purposeful responses to pain; brisk pupillary reaction
II	Combativeness; stupor; inappropriate language; purposeful and nonpurposeful responses to pain; sluggish pupillary reaction; conjugate deviation with oculocephalic reflex; hyperactive reflexes
III	Coma; decorticate rigidity; conjugate deviation with diminished oculocephalic reflex; sluggish pupillary reaction
IV	Coma with brainstem dysfunction; decerebrate rigidity; inconsistent or absent oculocephalic reflex; loss of corneal reflex; sluggish pupillary reaction
V	Coma with seizures; flaccidity; loss of deep tendon reflexes; respiratory arrest

Check the child's respiratory and neurologic status frequently, and note any signs of improvement or deterioration. Orient the child who awakens from coma. See nursing management of altered states of consciousness for specific nursing interventions. Look for changes in laboratory values that indicate acidosis, an elevation of ammonia levels, or hypoglycemia. Monitor the child's intake and output. Correct imbalances by administering fluids, electrolytes, or medications as ordered. Prevent complications associated with immobility (Table 14–7).

Provide emotional support to the parents, who may feel guilty because they did not seek medical attention sooner. Keep them informed about their child's condition, and prepare them for the potentially deteriorating course of the disease. Explaining treatments reduces anxiety. Encourage the parents to participate in their child's care whenever possible.

Make sure parents understand the possible link between aspirin and Reye syndrome. Instruct them to check all over-the-counter medicines for the presence of aspirin compounds. Emphasize the importance of obtaining health care whenever a child's condition worsens at the end of a viral illness.

Guillain-Barré Syndrome (Postinfectious Polyneuritis)

Guillain-Barré syndrome is an acute demyelinating disease of the nervous system. This condition, which may lead to deteriorating motor function and paralysis, affects persons of all ages but is most commonly seen in children between the ages of 4 and 9 years.

Pain or paresthesias initially develop in the lower extremities and are followed by symmetric weakness or hypotonia. This weakness spreads to the upper extremities, trunk, chest, neck, face, and head. Respiratory effort may be inadequate to ensure proper ventilation. Facial paresis and difficulty swallowing follow. Cranial nerves may be affected. A dysfunctional autonomic nervous system may cause such symptoms as hypertension, postural hypotension, sinus tachycardia or bradycardia, excessive diaphoresis, urinary and bowel incontinence, and facial flushing.[12]

The etiology of Guillain-Barré syndrome is unknown. The disorder has been associated with viral illnesses and noninfectious factors such as surgery, trauma, drugs, immunizations, and heredity. Many children have nonspecific viral illnesses or infections several days or weeks before the occurrence of neurologic symptoms.

Two tests are used to diagnose Guillain-Barré syndrome. Lumbar puncture is performed to obtain cerebrospinal fluid; increased protein levels with fewer than 10 lymphocytes per cubic millimeter are a positive indicator of the condition.[13] Electroconduction tests such as electromyography are also used. An abnormal pattern of nerve conduction is indicative of Guillain-Barré syndrome.

Treatment for Guillain-Barré syndrome is supportive. In most cases the progression of weakness and paralysis ceases in 2 to 4 weeks, and children usually recover completely.

Nursing Management

Nursing care focuses on monitoring respiratory status, meeting nutritional needs, preventing complications associated with immobility, providing emotional support, and teaching the parents how to care for the child after discharge.

Monitor Respiratory Status. Monitor the child's respiratory status closely, especially in the early phase of illness. Look for such signs as fatigue, inadequate effort, color changes, and PaO$_2$ less than 70 mm Hg, which indicate the need for endotracheal intubation and mechanical ventilation.[13]

Meet Nutritional Needs. Assess whether the child is having difficulty swallowing. If the child has no gag reflex, nutritional needs are maintained with intravenous supplements or nasogastric tube feedings.

Prevent Complications. Prevent complications associated with immobility (Table 14–7). Ensure good postural alignment, and turn the child every 2 hours. Maintaining skin integrity is also important.

Evaluate the child's muscle tone, strength, and symmetry. When the child's condition begins to improve, recovery of lost strength is the priority. Active exercise is emphasized in physical therapy. Help the child practice exercises learned in physical therapy sessions, and encourage the child to perform activities of daily living, such as brushing teeth or combing hair.

Provide Emotional Support. Explain the progression of Guillain-Barré syndrome to the parents during the initial stages. Witnessing a rapid deterioration in their child's physical status can be frightening; therefore preparation is essential to reduce their anxieties. Be honest when discussing recovery and prognosis for the child.

Help the child adjust to any residual effects of Guillain-Barré syndrome. To promote a positive self-image, praise any effort the child makes to be self-sufficient. The child may have feelings of frustration and anger. Allow the child to express these feelings in an appropriate way, either during play or in conversation.

Encourage the family members to participate in the child's care, especially during the recovery phase. They can help with the activities of daily living and reinforce what the child has learned in physical therapy. Have them bring in favorite toys, dolls, or books to make the child feel more secure. Playing with the child or reading to the child is comforting.

Discharge Planning and Patient and Family Home Care Teaching. Home care needs should be identified and addressed well in advance of discharge. Support the parents as they prepare for the child's return home. Provide referral to home care nurses who can manage all treatment and follow-up. Refer the parents to social workers, who can help with financial arrangements and school considerations.

Encephalitis

Encephalitis is an inflammation of the brain usually caused by a viral infection. This condition affects more than 12,000 children each year in the United States.[5]

Signs and symptoms depend on the causative organism and the location of the infection within the brain. An acute onset of a febrile illness with neurologic signs is the classic manifestation of encephalitis. Initially the child may have a severe headache, signs of an upper respiratory infection, and nausea or vomiting. There may be signs of meningeal irritation such as nuchal rigidity, photophobia, and positive Kernig and Brudzinski signs (Fig. 14–4). Other neurologic signs vary. The child may be disoriented or confused, with behavior or personality changes. There may be speech disturbances; motor dysfunction such as hemiparesis, ataxia, or weakness; cranial

TABLE 14-17 Causative Viruses of Encephalitis

Enteroviruses
  Poliovirus
  Echovirus
  Coxsackievirus
Adenoviruses and herpesviruses
Arboviruses
Measles
Mumps
Rubella
Rabies
Hepatitis B

---

nerve deficits; or alterations in reflex response. Focal or generalized seizures may occur, alternating with periods of screaming, hallucinating, and moving in a bizarre fashion. The child's level of consciousness may deteriorate from stupor to coma.

Viruses are believed to cause most cases of encephalitis (Table 14-17). Herpes simplex type I is the most common cause after the newborn period.

Diagnosis is based on history and laboratory analyses. Information concerning recent immunizations, insect bites, or travel to areas where vectors are present should be obtained. Cerebrospinal fluid analysis, blood serologic tests, and nasopharyngeal and stool specimens should be evaluated to identify viral pathogens. A CT scan, MRI, and EEG may also be performed. The only positive means of identifying herpes simplex is to perform a brain biopsy.

The child with encephalitis is at risk for seizures, respiratory failure, and increased intracranial pressure and should be cared for in an intensive care unit. Treatment is both pharmacologic and supportive. The child with suspected bacterial disease should be treated with antibiotics until bacterial pathogens have been ruled out.[14] A child with herpes simplex virus should receive acyclovir or other antiviral agents.[15]

Children with encephalitis have many neurologic sequelae. Although some children recover completely, many more are left with intellectual, motor, visual, or auditory deficits. The cardiovascular system, lungs, or liver may also be affected. Generally, the younger the child, the more serious the illness and the more severe the residual effects.

Nursing Management

Nursing care focuses on monitoring cardiorespiratory function, preventing complications resulting from immobility, reorienting the child, and teaching the parents about the child's condition.

Monitor the child's cardiorespiratory function. Check the child's airway and ability to handle secretions. Monitor respiratory status by observing color, pulse oximetry reading, and arterial blood gas values. Observe cardiopulmonary status by monitoring heart rate, blood pressure, capillary refill time, and urine output. Provide seizure precautions, and have appropriate equipment for managing seizures at the bedside.

Prevent complications resulting from immobility as described in Table 14-7. Maintain skin integrity. Proper positioning with frequent turning is important. Perform chest physiotherapy to prevent pneumonia when indicated by the physician.

The child whose level of consciousness begins to improve may at first be confused and disoriented and may have residual effects of the disease. Orient the child to the hospital environment. Have the family help to reorient the child by bringing favorite stuffed animals or music from home. Engage in therapeutic play (refer to Chapter 4 for techniques). Give the child age-appropriate toys to encourage a return to normal behavior.

Provide the parents with information about their child's condition and prognosis. If the child receives physical, occupational, or speech therapy, explain the treatment regimen to the parents. Encourage the parents to learn specific therapies so they can work with their child both in the hospital and at home.

Discharge Planning and Patient and Family Home Care Teaching. Encourage parents to take an active role in the child's physical and emotional care in the hospital, and give them written instructions concerning care for their child at home. Refer parents to social services, family counseling, and support groups.

Tetanus

Tetanus, or lockjaw, is an acute but preventable disease. Fatality rates range from 45% to 55%. The incubation period varies from 1 day to several weeks. The more distant the wound from the central nervous system, the longer the incubation time and the more severe the illness.

Tetanus is caused by exotoxins produced by *Clostridium tetani,* an anaerobic, gram-positive bacterium that is found in soil and feces. The wound is usually insignificant, although burns, deep punctures, splinters, or compound fractures may be ports of entry. The earliest symptoms include hypertonicity of the jaw and neck muscles. Trismus, the inability to open the mouth because of muscle spasm, is present in more than 50% of cases.

Children whose immunizations are up to date are given tetanus toxoid prophylactically for clean, minor wounds if they have not been vaccinated in 10 years, or for contaminated wounds if they have not been vaccinated in 5 years. The child whose immunizations are not up to date should receive human tetanus immune globulin for protection from the exposure, as well as tetanus toxoid for activation of the immune system.

The child with tetanus should be cared for in the intensive care unit, with appropriate resuscitation equipment at the bedside. Attention must be paid to the airway, which may become obstructed, especially during seizure activity. Intubation may be needed prophylactically to keep the airway patent. Prescribed medications, such as sedatives or paralytics, should be administered to promote safety and comfort and to prevent seizures. A tracheostomy may be performed as an emergency procedure during seizure activity.

The environment should be kept as quiet and calm as possible, since the child with tetanus is hypersensitive to sensory stimuli. Lights should be dim, and doors should be closed. Contact with the child should be kept to a minimum because touch may precipitate seizure activity.

Parents are anxious about their child, and they also may feel guilty about the inadequate status of the child's immunizations. Keep them informed about their child's condition, and be compassionate and sympathetic. Reinforce the importance of having their other children immunized. Assist other members of the health care team with discharge planning. Arrange for home care nursing if indicated.

▪ Structural Defects

Hydrocephalus

Hydrocephalus is the body's response to an imbalance between the production and absorption of cerebrospinal fluid. Hydrocephalus in infancy is considered to be congenital or related to prematurity. The incidence is 4 per 1000 births. In older children it is usually a complication of illness or trauma.[12]

Clinical Manifestations

The signs and symptoms of hydrocephalus, which vary depending on the age of the child, are listed in Table 14–18. The predominant manifestation of the condition in infants is rapid head growth. Older children show signs of increased intracranial pressure (see Table 14–6).

TABLE 14-18 Clinical Manifestations of Hydrocephalus

Congenital Hydrocephalus in Infant

Rapid head growth (cranial sutures may separate)
Bossing (protrusion) of frontal area
Prominent scalp veins
Translucent skin
Sunsetting eyes (sclera visible above iris)
Tense or bulging anterior fontanel
Irritability or lethargy
Decline in level of consciousness
Late stages:
   Shrill, high-pitched cry
   Difficulty swallowing or feeding
   Cardiopulmonary depression (severe cases)

Acquired Hydrocephalus in Older Child

No head enlargement
Headache upon arising with nausea or vomiting
Fussiness, sleepiness, confusion, or apathy
Poor judgment or verbal incoherence
Ataxia or spasticity
Visual defects secondary to pressure on optic nerve
Signs of increased intracranial pressure

Etiology and Pathophysiology

Hydrocephalus may be either communicating or obstructive. Communicating hydrocephalus involves reduced absorption of cerebrospinal fluid in the subarachnoid space at the arachnoid villi (Fig. 14–5). It can be acquired, such as from postinfectious meningitis or subarachnoid hemorrhage; congenital; or of unknown etiology.

Obstructive hydrocephalus, which is responsible for 99% of all occurrences in children,[16] results from a blockage in the ventricular system that prevents cerebrospinal fluid from entering the subarachnoid space (Fig. 14–6). This obstruction can be caused by infection, hemorrhage, tumor, or structural deformity.

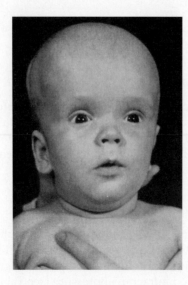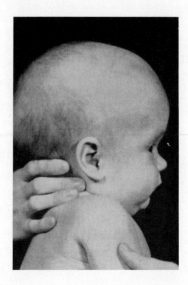

FIGURE 14-5 In communicating hydrocephalus, an excessive amount of cerebrospinal fluid accumulates in the subarachnoid space and produces the characteristic head enlargement seen here.

From Ingraham, F.D., & Matson, D.D. (1969). *Neurosurgery of infancy and childhood* (2nd ed.) (p. 226). Springfield, IL: Charles C Thomas, Publishers.

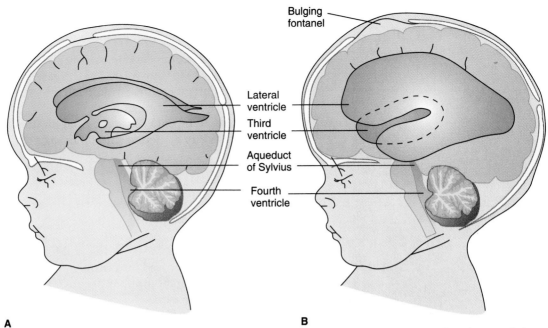

Lateral ventricle

Third ventricle

Aqueduct of Sylvius

Fourth ventricle

Bulging fontanel

A

B

FIGURE 14–6 **A,** Normal size of ventricle. **B,** Enlarged ventricles, characteristic of hydrocephalus.

Diagnostic Tests and Medical Management

Diagnosis of hydrocephalus is based on clinical manifestations. In the infant, rapid enlargement of the head is the first indication of hydrocephalus. Daily measurements of head circumference are critical.

CT scanning and MRI definitively identify hydrocephalus. In the infant whose fontanel is still open, ultrasonography or echoencephalography may be used to confirm the diagnosis.

Medical management of hydrocephalus occurs in three phases: identifying the cause, treating the cause (which may involve surgical removal of a lesion), and managing the hydrocephalus with placement of a shunting device.[16] Ventriculoperitoneal shunts (Fig. 14–7) are commonly used. Shunt systems consist of four parts: a ventricular catheter, a pumping chamber, a unidirectional pressure valve, and a distal catheter. Initial shunt placement usually occurs at 3 to 4 months of age, with replacement two to four times as the child grows.

Mechanical complications may include blockage at either the proximal or the distal end of the catheter, kinking of the tubing, or valve breakdown. Infants or children with shunt failure show signs and symptoms of recurrent hydrocephalus. Shunt failure is confirmed by CT scanning or MRI.

The most serious complication is shunt infection, which may occur at any time but is most prevalent in the first 2 months after placement. Symptoms include ventriculitis, low-grade fever, malaise, headache, and nausea. Antibiotics are usually prescribed, but if the infection is overwhelming, the shunt is removed and an external drainage device is placed. A new shunt is inserted when the infection resolves.

Nursing Assessment

It is important for nurses to become familiar with the clinical manifestations of hydrocephalus. Assess the child with a ventriculoperitoneal shunt for signs and symptoms of shunt failure and infection. Report any abnormalities to the physician immediately.

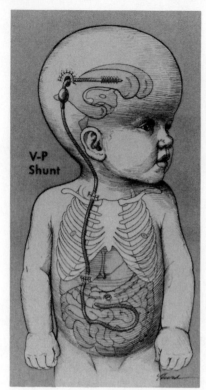

FIGURE 14-7 A ventriculoperitoneal shunt, commonly used to treat children with hydrocephalus, is usually placed at 3 to 4 months of age.

From McCullough, D.D. (1986). In Hoffman, H.J., & Epstein, F. *Disorders of the developing nervous system: Diagnosis and treatment* (p. 577). Cambridge, MA: Blackwell Scientific Publications.

Nursing Diagnosis

Common nursing diagnoses for the child with hydrocephalus include:

- High Risk for Infection related to presence of shunt
- Impaired Physical Mobility related to increased weight of head
- High Risk for Caregiver Role Strain related to care of child with chronic condition or life-threatening illness
- Anxiety related to repeated surgeries and life-threatening illness
- High Risk for Injury related to shunt blockage

Nursing Management

Nursing care focuses on providing both preoperative and postoperative care and providing emotional support.

Provide Preoperative Care. Measure the child's head circumference daily and watch for signs of increased intracranial pressure (Table 14–6).

Measure fluid intake and output as ordered. Carefully assess respiratory status. Provide good skin care.

Position the child carefully; do not stretch or strain the neck muscles, since they must support the large head. Holding the child may be difficult because of the additional weight of the head. Reduce the chances for skin breakdown by placing sheepskin or a lamb's wool blanket under the head. Prevent any other complications associated with immobility (Table 14–7).

Attend to the child's special nutritional needs. Since the child is prone to vomiting, frequent small feedings with frequent burping are beneficial.

Provide Postoperative Care. The child is usually placed in a flat position to prevent rapid cerebrospinal fluid drainage. The head of the bed is elevated gradually.

Take vital signs every 2 to 4 hours. Monitor the child carefully for any signs of shunt malfunction, increased intracranial pressure (Table 14–6), or infection.

Provide Emotional Support. Provide parents with explanations about the child's condition and all procedures to be performed. Encourage parents and family to help with the child's care in the hospital when appropriate. This gives them a sense of control. Be sympathetic and understanding, and allow parents to express their concerns. If hydrocephalus occurs in the neonatal period or early infancy, the parents are faced with anxiety about the initial blockage and subsequent surgical procedures. If hydrocephalus is secondary to neoplasm, however, the parents' anxieties are compounded by their child's life-threatening illness.

Assure parents that most children with shunts lead normal lives, attend school, and interact with their peers. Encourage parents not to be overprotective and to allow children to develop normally. Discourage participation in contact sports.

Discharge Planning and Patient and Family Home Care Teaching. Home care needs should be identified and addressed well in advance of discharge. Parents need to be taught how to care for a child with a shunt. Parents and other family members should be made aware of the signs and symptoms of both shunt failure (signs of increased intracranial pressure) and infection. Give them the telephone numbers of the pediatrician and the neurosurgeon, and make sure that they understand that they should contact a physician immediately if they suspect a problem. Inform them that a new shunt may need to be placed at one or more times in childhood as the child grows. Appropriate home care referrals should be arranged. Refer families to the appropriate psychologic and social services, such as the National Hydrocephalus Foundation (see Appendix F).

Spina Bifida

Spina bifida, a congenital neural tube defect that affects the head and spinal column, is the most common developmental disorder of the central nervous system. It is a malformation of the neural tube that can occur anywhere along the spine. The condition occurs in 0.4 to 1 per 1000 births in the United States each year.[17]

A saclike protrusion on the infant's back indicates spina bifida at birth (Fig. 14–8). There are several different types of spina bifida (Table 14–19). The clinical manifestations seen depend on the location of the defect: the higher the defect, the greater the neurologic dysfunction. The lower extremities may be completely paralyzed. Bowel and bladder sphincters may be affected. Renal involvement may occur secondary to neurologic impairment and urinary retention. Hydrocephalus may be present.

The cause of spina bifida is unknown, although environmental factors such as chemicals, medications, and poor maternal nutrition (especially low levels of folic acid) have been implicated. The increased incidence of the condition in families indicates a possible genetic influence.

Diagnosis is made by examination of the lesion and evaluation of neurologic status. Radiologic studies are also performed. CT scan, MRI, and flat films of the spinal column can pinpoint the bony defect. Surgery is usually performed to close and repair the lesion when the neonate is a few days old.

Children with spina bifida can have orthopedic problems with varying degrees of immobility. A team of physicians, nurses, and therapists from the neurosurgery, orthopedic, and physical medicine departments should work together to develop a plan of care and rehabilitation. Casting, splinting, brac-

FIGURE 14–8 Lumbosacral myelomeningocele is caused by a neural tube defect that results in incomplete closure of the vertebral column. As shown here, the meninges (and sometimes the spinal cord) protrude as a saclike structure.

From Ingraham, F.D., & Matson, D.D. (1969). *Neurosurgery of infancy and childhood* (2nd ed.) (p. 26). Springfield, IL: Charles C Thomas, Publishers.

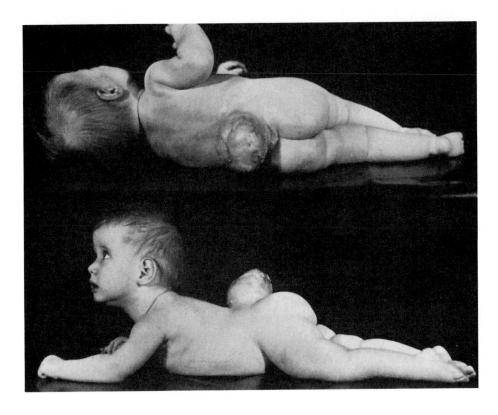

TABLE 14-19 Types of Spina Bifida

Spina bifida occulta	Failure of posterior vertebral arches to fuse, most commonly at fifth lumbar or first sacral vertebrae; no herniation of spinal cord or meninges; condition usually not visible externally
Spina bifida cystica	Defect in closure of posterior vertebral arch with protrusion through bony spine
Meningocele	Saclike protrusion through bony defect containing meninges and cerebrospinal fluid; sac covering defect may be translucent or membranous
Myelomeningocele	Saclike herniation through bony defect holding meninges, cerebrospinal fluid, as well as a portion of spinal cord or nerve roots; fluid leakage may also occur; lesion poorly covered with imperfect tissue

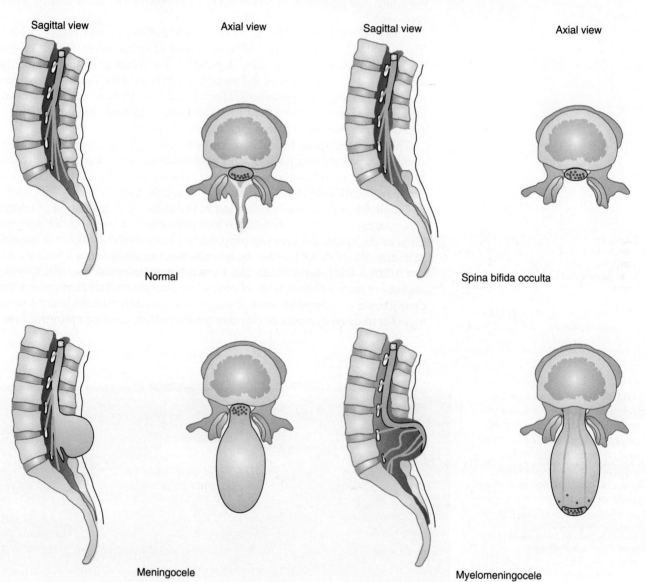

Sagittal view Axial view Sagittal view Axial view

Normal Spina bifida occulta

Meningocele Myelomeningocele

ing, traction, and surgical interventions are used to promote the child's chances for independent mobility. Children with lower spinal lesions may use walkers, crutches, and canes. Custom-designed wheelchairs are available for children with deformities higher in the spinal column.

Children with spina bifida often have neurogenic bladders and are subject to frequent urinary tract infections. Intermittent catheterization and medications to improve bladder capacity and continence are used to manage this condition. Stool softeners and high-fiber diets are used to regulate bowel function.

Prognosis depends on the type of defect, the level of the lesion, and the presence of other complicating factors.

Nursing Management

Nursing care focuses on providing preoperative and postoperative care, promoting mobility, and providing emotional support.

Provide Preoperative Care. Cover the sac with a sterile saline dressing to protect its integrity. Place the infant in a prone position with hips slightly flexed and legs abducted to minimize tension on the sac. Maintain this position using towel rolls placed between the knees.

Neurologic monitoring for motor deficits as well as bladder and bowel involvement should be performed regularly.

The infant is difficult to handle before surgery. Feed the infant with the head turned to one side until surgery has been performed. Comfort the infant before surgery with tactile stimulation such as touching, patting, and cuddling.

Provide Postoperative Care. Monitor the infant's vital signs carefully. Watch closely for symptoms of infection, especially meningitis. If a shunt was placed, watch for hydrocephalus, increased intracranial pressure, or infection. Inspect the surgical site for cerebrospinal fluid leakage. The infant should be placed in the prone or side-lying position; he or she may be held upright in some cases.

Promote Mobility. Begin performing gentle range of motion exercises as soon as possible to prevent muscle contractures and atrophy. Care must be taken because these children have brittle bones and are subject to idiopathic fractures that they may not be able to feel.

Provide Emotional Support. Keep parents informed about their child's status. Allow them to express their frustrations and anger. Parents who are faced with long-term management of their child will be concerned about the physical and financial issues of caring for the child at home. Parents may need assistance from social workers, members of the clergy, family members, and support groups.

Discharge Planning and Patient and Family Home Care Teaching. Home care needs should be identified and addressed well in advance of discharge. As soon as parents are able to cope with the child's condition, encourage them to become involved in the child's care in the hospital. Teach them about positioning, handling, feeding, and exercise. Parents may need to learn how to catheterize the child. Make sure family members understand how to care for the child at home. They may need to obtain special devices such as splints, wedges, and rolls to prevent complications. Special braces, walkers, or wheelchairs may need to be purchased later.

Make sure that the parents know the signs and symptoms of increased intracranial pressure, hydrocephalus, shunt infection or malfunction, and urinary tract infection. Safety issues should be emphasized as well. Children with spina bifida are prone to pressure sores, burns, or fractures of the lower extremities, resulting from lack of sensation and immobility, and brittle bones.

Home care nursing should be arranged, if necessary. The home care nurse reinforces the skills learned in the hospital setting and coordinates the numerous health care professionals who will be working with the child and family. Refer parents to resource groups such as the Spina Bifida Association of America (see Appendix F).

Craniosynostosis

Craniosynostosis is the premature closing of the cranial sutures. This condition occurs in up to 1 in 1900 births. Most children have no family history of the condition, although 10% to 20% have other inherited syndromes.[19]

Closure of the sutures usually takes place at predetermined times during the child's development. Problems arise if closure is premature. Bone growth continues in a direction parallel to the suture line, which leads to compensatory overgrowth at normal suture lines and the classic skull deformities associated with craniosynostosis.[19]

The cause of craniosynostosis is unknown. Diagnosis is made by clinical appearance, skull x-ray films, CT scan, and MRI.

Reconstructive surgery is the most common form of treatment. After surgery it is important for the incision to remain dry and intact. The nurse should also observe the child for symptoms of increased intracranial pressure (Table 14–6).

Explain to parents that surgery will improve the child's appearance. Assure them that most children with craniosynostosis who are otherwise healthy and without complications will develop normally. Provide emotional support, and be compassionate and understanding.

Drug-Addicted Infant (Neonatal Abstinence Syndrome)

Repeated use of narcotics leads to tolerance and physical dependence. All narcotics, regardless of their mode of administration, readily cross the placenta, enter the fetal circulation, and have the same effects on the fetus that they do in the mother. When administration of drugs stops during gestation, the mother and fetus both have withdrawal symptoms. If the infant is born to a mother who is still actively using drugs, the neonate goes into withdrawal shortly after birth. Heroin remains the leading street drug, although cocaine, meperidine, methadone, propoxyphene, amphetamines, alcohol, and marijuana are also used with great frequency.

In the newborn, irritability and jitteriness are the most common symptoms of drug withdrawal. Infants may have excoriated skin, especially on the heels, toes, hands, elbows, nose, or chin, as a result of their continuous movements on the crib sheets. Infants may also have a high-pitched, shrill cry; hyperreflexia; poor temperature control; episodes of tachypnea; abnormal sleep-wake patterns; flushing of the skin; and excessive diaphoresis. Additional symptoms can include poor feeding and poor coordination between sucking and swallowing, which can lead to aspiration and inadequate nutritional intake. Vomiting and diarrhea may occur as a result of a hyperactive bowel. These infants also have an increased risk of seizures.

TABLE 14-20 Signs of Narcotic Withdrawal in Neonates

W = wakefulness
I = irritability
T = tremulousness, temperature variation, tachypnea
H = hyperactivity, high-pitched cry, hyperreflexia, hypertonia, hiccups
D = diarrhea, diaphoresis, disorganized suck
R = rub marks (excoriations on knees and face), regurgitation (vomiting)
A = apneic spells, autonomic dysfunction
W = weight loss (or failure to gain weight)
A = alkalosis (respiratory)
L = lacrimation
S = stuffy nose, sneezing, seizures

From Rudolph, A.M., Hoffman, J.I.E., & Rudolph, C.D. (Eds.). (1991). *Rudolph's pediatrics* (19th ed.) (p. 811). Norwalk, CT: Appleton & Lange.

Between 50% and 90% of infants of drug-addicted mothers suffer withdrawal. Withdrawal symptoms usually appear 12 to 28 hours after birth. However, it is not uncommon for these symptoms to appear between 7 and 14 days after birth if the mother was taking heroin or methadone. The onset of symptoms may be attributed to the type and amount of drug taken by the mother and how soon before birth it was taken.[20] Signs of narcotic withdrawal in neonates are given in Table 14–20.

Treatment is generally supportive. Medications such as phenobarbitol, chlorpromazine, and paregoric may be prescribed to alleviate symptoms. The most serious and prevalent complication with drug abuse is AIDS, since the HIV virus readily crosses the placenta and is transmitted to the fetus.

Nursing Management

Nursing care focuses on monitoring withdrawal symptoms, administering prescribed medications, and satisfying emotional needs.

The drug-addicted infant should be monitored closely, since many of the symptoms of withdrawal are identical to those seen in infection, bowel obstruction, hydrocephalus, and intracranial anomaly. Administer prescribed medications. Provide frequent, small, high-calorie feedings, which are more readily tolerated. Keep the infant in a quiet environment with subdued lighting and minimal stimulation.

Satisfy the emotional needs of the neonate by swaddling, rocking, holding, and cuddling. Volunteers or hospital-based foster grandparents, if available, may help fulfill these needs.

Long-term and follow-up care should be planned to ensure regular developmental testing, assessment for fetal alcohol syndrome, and interventions as needed.

Cerebral Palsy

Cerebral palsy is motor dysfunction that occurs secondary to damage in the motor centers of the brain. The categories of this dysfunction are presented in Table 14–21. Cerebral palsy is the most common chronic disorder of childhood, occurring in an estimated 1 in 1000 children. Many children have some degree of mental retardation as well as physical disability.[1]

TABLE 14–21 Categories of Cerebral Palsy

Categories	Characteristics
Physiologic	
Hypotonia	Floppiness, increased range of motion of joints, diminished reflex response
Hypertonia	
Rigidity	Tense, tight muscles
Spasticity	Uncoordinated, awkward, stiff movements; scissoring or crossing of the legs; exaggerated reflex reactions
Athetosis	Constant involuntary writhing motions that are more severe distally
Ataxia	Irregularity in muscle coordination or action
Topographic	
Hemiplegia	Involvement of one side of the body with the upper extremities being more dysfunctional than the lower extremities
Diplegia	Involvement of the lower extremities, usually spastic
Quadriplegia	Involvement of all extremities with the arms in flexion and legs in extension

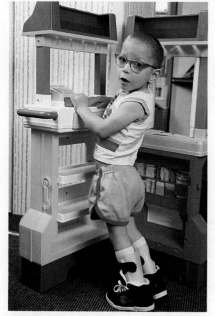

FIGURE 14–9 A child with cerebral palsy has abnormal muscle tone and lack of physical coordination.

Clinical Manifestations

Cerebral palsy is characterized by abnormal muscle tone and lack of coordination (Fig. 14–9). Children have a variety of symptoms depending on their age, as listed in Table 14–22. Usually they are delayed in meeting their developmental milestones. Children frequently have accompanying problems, including visual defects such as strabismus, nystagmus, or refractory errors; hearing loss; speech or language delay; speech impediment; seizures; or mental retardation.

Etiology and Pathophysiology

Cerebral palsy may be due to prenatal, antenatal, or postnatal trauma or to infection or lesion. During gestation, insufficient nutrients and oxygen can cause damage to the developing brain of the fetus. Premature infants are at especially high risk because of their immature central nervous systems. Injury at birth may be due to direct trauma to the brain or to asphyxia resulting from cord collapse or strangulation. As children grow older, head trauma becomes the major source of acquired brain injury and subsequent motor involvement.

Neonatal infections such as meningitis and infantile bilirubin encephalopathy (kernicterus) may also lead to the development of cerebral palsy.

Diagnostic Tests and Medical Management

Diagnosis is usually based on clinical findings. Generally cerebral palsy is not diagnosed until the child is 2 years of age. It is not uncommon for children who are delayed in meeting developmental milestones or have neuromuscular abnormalities at 1 year of age to show gradual improvement with signs of dysfunction disappearing entirely with physical maturation.

Medical management focuses on assisting the child to develop to his or her maximum potential. Appropriate referrals for physical, occupational, and speech therapy and special education are necessary. Surgical interventions may be required. The Achilles' tendon may be lengthened to increase

TABLE 14-22 Early Signs of Cerebral Palsy

Birth to 1 Month

Weak or absent sucking or swallowing
Episodes of bradycardia or apnea
High-pitched cry
Jitteriness
Hypotonia
Seizures
Difficulty in eliciting primitive reflex responses

Infants: 3 Months

Feeding difficulties
Tongue thrust
Irritability
Hypotonia but with advanced head control while prone
One or both hands fisted
Brisk tendon reflexes
Strabismus
Persistence of primitive reflexes

Infants: 6 Months

Delayed developmental milestones
Handedness (one hand dominant); continued fisting
Hypertonia; difficult to dress
Little spontaneous movement
Arching; tendency to stand
Persistence of primitive reflexes

Infants: 9 Months

Delayed motor milestones
    Abnormal crawl: may be asymmetric, using only arms for movement
    Abnormal reach: splaying of fingers with wrist extended; tremor
Abnormal movements
Keeping arms flexed

Infants: 12 Months

Scissoring
Toe walking
Athetoid (writhing) motions
Handedness

■ **CLINICAL TIP**

All infants who show symptoms of developmental delays, feeding difficulties caused by poor sucking, or abnormalities of muscle tone should be evaluated. Two simple screening assessments are:

- Place a clean diaper on the infant's face. The normal child will use two hands to remove it, but the infant with cerebral palsy will either use one hand or not remove the cloth at all.
- Turn the infant's head to one side. A persistent asymmetric tonic neck reflex (beyond 6 months of age) is an indicator of a pathologic condition.[1] Cerebral palsy should be suspected in any infant who has persistent primitive reflexes.

range of motion in the ankle, which allows the heel to touch the floor and thus improves ambulation. The hamstrings may be released to correct knee flexion contractures. Other procedures may be performed to improve hip adduction or correct the natural position of the foot.

Prognosis for infants and children with cerebral palsy depends on the level of physical involvement and on the presence of intellectual, visual, or hearing deficits. Many children with hemiplegia or ataxia show some improvement with maturation and are able to ambulate. However, a child who does not sit up independently by 2 years of age is unlikely to walk.[21]

Nursing Assessment

Assess the child for developmental delays. Any orthopedic, visual, auditory, or intellectual deficits should be noted. Assess for the presence of newborn reflexes, which may persist in a child with cerebral palsy.

Nursing Diagnosis

Common nursing diagnoses for the child with cerebral palsy include:

- Altered Nutrition: Less Than Body Requirements related to poor sucking and impaired swallowing and chewing
- Impaired Physical Mobility related to delayed neuromuscular development
- Self-Care Deficit (feeding, bathing/hygiene, dressing/grooming, toileting) related to physical disability
- High Risk for Injury related to neuromuscular impairment
- High Risk for Impaired Skin Integrity related to decreased mobility
- High Risk for Altered Parenting related to child with chronic disability
- Body Image Disturbance related to physical disability
- Chronic Low Self-Esteem related to dependence on others
- Altered Growth and Development related to hearing, vision, and speech abnormalities

Nursing Management

Nursing care focuses on providing adequate nutrition, maintaining skin integrity, promoting physical mobility, promoting growth and development, and providing emotional support.

Provide Adequate Nutrition. Children with cerebral palsy require high-calorie diets because of increased muscle tone due to spasticity. Many children have difficulty chewing and swallowing, which makes feeding difficult. Give the child small amounts of soft foods at a time. Feeding utensils with large, padded handles may be easier for the child to use.

Maintain Skin Integrity. Take special care to protect the bony prominences from skin breakdown. See Table 14–7 for specific nursing interventions.

Proper body alignment should be maintained whenever possible. Support the child with pillows, towels, and bolsters whether the child is in bed or in a chair. Support the head and body of a floppy infant. A spastic child with scissored, extended legs or an athetoid child who writhes constantly is difficult to carry and transport.

Promote Physical Mobility. Range of motion exercises are essential to prevent contractures and maintain joint flexibility. Consult with physical therapists who work with the child and assist with recommended exercises. Encourage parents to bring the child's adaptive appliances (customized wheelchairs, braces) to the hospital to prevent deterioration during hospitalizations.

Promote Growth and Development. Remember that many children with cerebral palsy are physically but not intellectually disabled. Use terminology appropriate for the child's developmental level. Help the child develop a positive self-image to ensure emotional health and social growth.

Provide Emotional Support. Refer parents to individual and family counseling if appropriate. Listen to the parents' concerns and encourage them to ask questions. Let them know what to expect regarding future treatment. Work with other health care professionals to help families adjust to this chronic disease.

Discharge Planning and Patient and Family Home Care Teaching. Home care needs should be identified and addressed well in advance of discharge.

■ CLINICAL TIP

Provide audio and visual activities for the child who is quadriplegic. Television, videotapes, and music are good diversions. Encourage the child who is paraplegic to use his or her arms and hands in interactive games. Children can use special hand controls or pointers to play video games or other adaptive devices to manipulate the television or radio.

Teach parents of a child with newly diagnosed cerebral palsy how to position, support, feed, and dress their child. Encourage them to promote their child's well-being and self-esteem.

Refer parents to developmental centers, support groups, and organizations such as the United Cerebral Palsy Association (see Appendix F) and Shriners hospitals. Other parents of children with cerebral palsy can provide needed support. Developmental centers can help parents learn how to meet their child's special needs, including physical, occupational, and speech therapy, as well as educational needs. Parents may need financial assistance to provide the care that the child needs and to obtain appliances such as braces, wheelchairs, or adaptive utensils.

Injuries of the Neurologic System

Head Injury

A head injury can be defined as any trauma involving the scalp, cranial bones, or structures within the skull resulting from force or penetration. Head injuries are the leading cause of mental retardation, physical disability, and seizures in children.[22] These injuries may also result in sensory deficiencies, attention deficits, and a variety of focal neurologic symptoms.

Children are prone to skull fractures, often resulting in hematomas and brain injury. They may suffer from secondary effects of trauma, such as diffuse cerebral edema, malignant brain edema, and increased intracranial pressure.

Children under the age of 10 years have the best chance of recovering from head injuries. Because of their anatomic immaturity and compensatory abilities (see Table 14–1), many of these children continue to improve and recuperate for up to 5 years after their injury.

Clinical Manifestations

The signs and symptoms of head injuries in children depend on the pathologic features and severity of the injury. The child with a mild head injury may remain conscious or lose consciousness for less than 5 minutes. The child with a moderate head injury loses consciousness for 5 to 10 minutes. Following mild and moderate head injuries, children may have amnesia about the event, headache, nausea, and vomiting. A child with a severe head injury is usually unconscious for more than 10 minutes and may show signs of increased intracranial pressure.

Unconsciousness may result from increased intracranial pressure, edema, hemorrhage, or parenchymal damage to both cerebral cortices or the brainstem.

Vital signs are important indicators of head injury. Changes in respiratory effort or periods of apnea can occur secondary to shock, injury to the spinal cord above C-4, or damage to or pressure on the medulla. Heart rate and blood pressure are indices of brainstem function. Tachycardia can be a sign of blood loss, shock, hypoxia, anxiety, or pain. **Cushing triad,** associated with increased intracranial pressure or compromised flow to the brainstem, is characterized by hypertension, increased systolic pressure with wide pulse pressure, bradycardia, and irregular respirations. Refer to the discussion of altered states of consciousness for more information about increased intracranial pressure.

Reflexes may be hyporesponsive, hyperresponsive, or nonexistent. The child may assume a decorticate, decerebrate, or flaccid **areflexive** posture (Fig. 14–2).

The younger the child, the greater the risk of head injuries. Fatalities from head injuries occur in children less than 1 year of age twice as often as they do in children aged 1 to 6 years, and three times as often as in children aged 6 to 12 years.[22]

Any infant who arrives in the emergency
department with seizures, failure to
thrive, vomiting, lethargy, respiratory irregularities, or coma should be evaluated
for child abuse, particularly "shaken
child syndrome."

Etiology and Pathophysiology

Falls are a major cause of unintentional head injuries in young children. Infants fall from dressing tables, beds, and sofas and also tumble down stairs,
especially in walkers. Child abuse accounts for a large number of head injuries in the child less than 1 year old. Toddlers and preschool age children
lack good judgment, and they may run out into the street without looking
where they are going or may lean out of windows and fall. School-age children may be injured in motor vehicle crashes, either as passengers or as
pedestrians, and they may be injured in bicycle or skateboard mishaps. Adolescents are frequently the drivers in motor vehicle crashes; often alcohol or
drugs are involved. Teenagers may also be injured in sports-related accidents.

Head injuries can be categorized as either primary or secondary. Primary
injuries occur at the time of the insult when the initial cellular damage takes
place. These injuries result from either a direct blow to the head (coup injury)
or acceleration-deceleration movement of the brain within the skull (contrecoup injury) (Fig. 14–10). At the time of impact, arterial and intracranial pressures increase and apnea and loss of consciousness occur.

The secondary phase of head trauma, which involves both the brain and
the body's response to the initial injury, can be manifested immediately or
several hours, days, or weeks later. Damage usually results from destruction
of brain tissue secondary to hypoxia, hypotension, edema, change in the
blood-brain barrier, or hemorrhage.[23] Whatever the underlying cause, however, the result is increased intracranial pressure. Irreversible brain damage
may result if the condition is left untreated.

Diagnostic Tests and Medical Management

Identifying the pathologic results of a head injury involves history, observation, examination, and diagnostic testing. The questions in Table 14–23 can
be used to determine what happened.

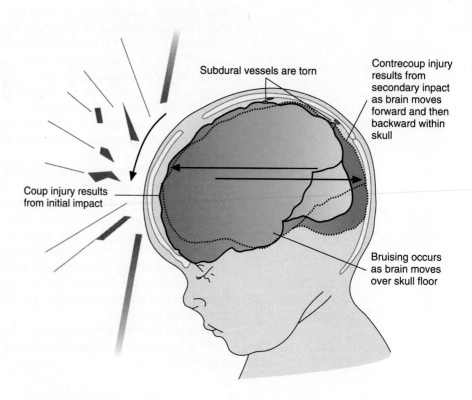

FIGURE 14–10 Head trauma can
result from a direct blow to the head
(coup injury) or the acceleration-deceleration movement of the brain (contrecoup injury).

Subdural vessels are torn

Contrecoup injury
results from
secondary inpact
as brain moves
forward and then
backward within
skull

Coup injury results
from initial impact

Bruising occurs
as brain moves
over skull floor

Neurologic evaluation with the pediatric Glasgow Coma Scale is performed frequently to evaluate whether the child's condition is improving, remaining constant, or deteriorating. Cranial nerves are assessed (see Table 14–5). See Chapter 3 and the discussion of altered states of consciousness for further details.

Laboratory tests include a complete blood cell count, blood chemistry, toxicology screening, and urinalysis.

Radiologic examination is performed to determine specific injury. Skull films are used to detect fractures. Structural injuries, such as fractures, hematomas, lacerations, or contusions, usually appear clearly on CT scan. Although a hemorrhage may not be evident on a CT scan taken shortly after the trauma, a repeat scan should be performed if the child shows clinical signs of injury. MRI may be performed in order to visualize subtle damage or injury.

The initial medical management of a child with a head injury is based on findings from assessment of the child's physiologic status (the ABCs) (see Table 14–4). The airway must be clear and stable. Hypoxia and hypercapnia have disastrous effects on cerebral function, since they can cause vasodilation and increase intracranial pressure. If indicated, the child is intubated, sedated, and chemically paralyzed.

Perfusion must be maintained to ensure adequate cerebral perfusion pressure. All sources of internal bleeding must be identified. Shock is treated aggressively with fluid boluses. Until adequate cerebral perfusion pressure is ensured, the head of the bed should be kept flat.[24] Inotropes may be used to ensure perfusion if cerebral edema is present.

Increased intracranial pressure must be controlled. Hyperventilation is the initial treatment of choice. After it has been determined that no cervical spine injury is present, the head of the bed is elevated to 30 degrees. The child's head is kept in the midline to promote venous (jugular) drainage. Hip flexion is avoided. Acetaminophen can be given for pain. The child's body temperature is kept within normal limits. The environment is kept as quiet as possible. Fluids may be restricted only after the child is hemodynamically stable.

Medications may be used to manage increased intracranial pressure. Diuretics such as mannitol or furosemide may be given to shrink brain volume. A urinary catheter is inserted to monitor output, and electrolytes should be checked frequently.

Invasive procedures may be necessary to reduce increased intracranial pressure. Burr holes may be made or more extensive surgery may be performed as a method of evacuating lesions or hematomas. A ventricular catheter may be placed to drain cerebrospinal fluid and to monitor pressure.

Nursing Assessment

The child's neurologic status is compared to his or her previous state, with improvement, stability, or deterioration noted. The cause of deterioration must be quickly determined and appropriate interventions taken.

Assess the child's neurologic status frequently. Evaluate the child's level of consciousness continually using the pediatric Glasgow Coma Scale (Table 14–3). A child who has a decreased level of consciousness shortly after a head injury may have had a posttraumatic seizure and may still be in the postictal state. Monitor vital signs closely. Changes in these signs may indicate hypoxia, decreased perfusion, shock, or increased intracranial pressure.

Nursing Diagnosis

Common nursing diagnoses for the child with a head injury include:

- Altered Cerebral Tissue Perfusion related to poor respiratory effort, hypovolemia and/or increased intracranial pressure
- High Risk for Fluid Volume Deficit related to hypovolemia
- Impaired Gas Exchange related to poor respiratory effort
- Ineffective Airway Clearance related to decreased level of consciousness
- Ineffective Breathing Pattern related to decreased level of consciousness
- High Risk for Caregiver Role Strain related to long-term care of child with neurologic complications
- High Risk for Altered Family Processes related to child's development of a disability
- Altered Growth and Development related to motor, cognitive, and perceptual deficits

Nursing Management

Nursing care focuses on maintaining cardiopulmonary function, preventing complications, promoting recovery, and providing emotional support. Nursing management is based on prevention of secondary injury and return to optimal level of function.

Maintain Cardiopulmonary Function. In the moderately injured child, observe breathing patterns and check color and level of consciousness. Check the pulse oximeter. If there is any indication of decreased oxygenation, notify the physician immediately.

Make sure that the siderails of the bed are padded to protect the child if a seizure occurs. Equipment for suction and ventilation should be at the bedside.

Prevent Complications. Position the child properly, maintain a quiet environment, and control body temperature. Administer medications as ordered. Check intracranial monitors or surgical sites if invasive measures have been taken. If any signs and symptoms of increased intracranial pressure are apparent (Table 14–6), alert the physician immediately so treatment can begin promptly.

Promote Recovery. Physical, occupational, and speech therapy should begin in the hospital. Work with physical, occupational, and speech therapists to reinforce these exercises and help teach parents the techniques so they can work with the child in the hospital and at home. The nurse can reinforce what has been done during these sessions, noting positive changes. In addition, if hospitalization is long term, visiting teachers may provide intellectual stimulation and contribute to the child's self-esteem. Using toys, books, music, or games, provide stimulation based on the child's age and ability. Encourage parents to bring in favorite toys, stuffed animals, and tape recordings of the child's favorite music or of family members talking.

Provide Emotional Support. Nurses, social workers, physicians, psychologists, rehabilitation therapists, and members of the clergy can support and help parents accept a child with a new disability. The child, for example, an adolescent facing long-term rehabilitation, will also need ongoing support.

Discharge Planning and Patient and Family Home Care Teaching. Home care needs should be identified and addressed well in advance of discharge. Give parents information about caring for children with head injuries at home. Refer parents to the National Head Injury Foundation for further information (see Appendix F).

Ask parents if it will be necessary for them to make adaptations to their home in order to care for their child. If the child has gross motor disabilities, the home may need to accommodate a wheelchair, walker, braces, or a special bed. Social work and home health agencies can often help the parents make special arrangements.

Inquire tactfully if parents need financial assistance. Many children with head injuries are disabled enough to qualify for Social Security SSI benefits or the state program for children with special health care needs. Put the parents in contact with a social worker if indicated.

Arrange for home care nursing and follow-up care, if necessary. The home care nurse can take over the case management of the child, make sure the environment is safe, and help the family plan any clinical appointments or hospitalizations. The home care nurse is available at all times for questions, concerns, or emergencies.

Some children require inpatient or outpatient rehabilitation. If the child returns to school, help prepare the other children for how their classmate is "different." Such sensitivity training makes reintegrating the child into the classroom easier.

Specific Head Injuries

Scalp Injuries. Injuries to the scalp, which can be caused by falls, blunt trauma, or penetration of a foreign body, are usually benign. Although bleeding may be extensive, hypovolemia or shock is uncommon unless the child is an infant.

Lacerations should be irrigated with copious amounts of sterile normal saline solution and inspected for bony fragments or depressions, cerebrospinal fluid leakage with a dural tear, or debris. If the injury is simple, the laceration can be sutured and the child discharged from the emergency department. If not, a neurosurgeon should be consulted.

Concussion. A concussion can involve transient impairment of consciousness (less than 5 minutes) that usually results from blunt head trauma. It is secondary to stretching, compression, or shearing of nerve fibers.[23] There is usually no gross structural damage or focal injury. The child may have amnesia of the event, headache, nausea with or without vomiting, or dizziness.

Treatment is supportive. Children are observed in the emergency department for several hours before being sent home with instructions to the parents to watch them closely. Any child who is unconscious for more than 5 minutes or has amnesia of the event should be admitted to the hospital to rule out other injury.

Pediatric concussive syndrome, which is believed to be caused by an injury to the brainstem, is seen in children who are less than 3 years old. Toddlers seem stunned at the time of injury, but they do not lose consciousness. Later, however, these children become pale, clammy, and lethargic, and they may vomit. They are usually brought to the hospital for treatment when these symptoms appear. These children are admitted overnight for observation and usually recover within 24 hours.

Postconcussive syndrome, which is common in both children and adults, may occur anytime after the initial head injury. Signs and symptoms can include headache, dizziness or vertigo, photophobia, subtle changes in personality, difficulty concentrating, and poor memory. Treatment is supportive. Symptoms usually disappear within several weeks. Parents and teachers should be informed to expect altered behavior in the child. They should be encouraged to help the child maintain self-esteem.

Skull Fractures. A fracture to any of the eight cranial bones is caused by a considerable force to the head. Any area of the skull with swelling or a hematoma should be evaluated for possible fracture. Diagnosis is made by visual inspection, palpation, x-ray study, or CT scan. Treatment should always include neurosurgical consultation.

Management of skull fractures depends on the type and extent of the injury (Table 14–24).

TABLE 14–24 Skull Fractures

Injury	Diagnosis and Management
Linear Fracture	
Results from impact to large area of the skull; usually no symptoms unless fracture cuts across suture lines near middle meningeal artery, in which case epidural hematoma may form	On x-ray study, fracture appears as a thin, clear line; child is hospitalized overnight for observation; fracture heals within 6 months A growing skull fracture may appear if the dura mater has been torn; management is surgical
Depressed Fracture	
Break in skull itself, which usually shatters it into many fragments; pieces of broken bone can be depressed into brain tissue, with hematoma forming on top; most common sites for injury are frontal or parietal areas	Diagnosis confirmed by x-ray study or CT scan, although fracture usually palpable; treatment may be surgical; any depressed area greater than thickness of skull or 5 mm must be elevated in operating room to prevent damage to underlying brain tissue; if this is not done within 24 hours, brain contusion or laceration may ensue; tetanus prophylaxis and antibiotics are given to prevent infection; seizures are common sequelae
Compound Fracture	
Combination of scalp laceration and depressed skull fracture	Diagnosis made visually, by x-ray study, or by CT scan; treatment involves surgical debridement and elevation of bony fragments, tetanus prophylaxis and antibiotics
Basilar Fracture	
Occurs in the inferior, posterior portion of skull; can involve frontal, ethmoid, sphenoid, temporal, or occipital bones; may have dural tear; classic signs are blood behind tympanic membrane with cerebrospinal fluid leaking from nose or ears; child also has periorbital ecchymosis (raccoon's eyes) and bruising of mastoid (Battle sign)	Diagnosis confirmed by CT scan; treatment includes hospitalization with observation; often dural tear heals in 1 week; however, if cerebrospinal fluid leakage persists, leak should be surgically repaired; possible damage to cranial nerves I, II, III, VII, and VIII

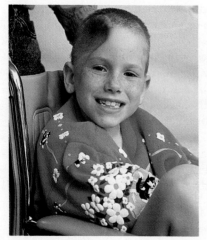

Depressed fracture

Data from Flint, N. (1988). Head trauma and spinal cord injuries. In Kelly, S. (Ed.). *Pediatric emergency nursing.* Norwalk, CT: Appleton & Lange.

Cerebral Contusion. A cerebral contusion, or the bruising of brain tissue, is secondary to blunt trauma and can occur with either coup or contrecoup injuries (Fig. 14–10). Such injuries are rare in children less than 1 year of age. The temporal or frontal sections of the skull are the most common sites of this injury, which involves damage to the parenchyma with tears in vessels or tissue, pulping, and subsequent areas of necrosis or infarction.

The child may have focal symptoms depending on the area of injury. Altered levels of consciousness range from confusion and disorientation to being totally obtunded. A CT scan is used for diagnosis.

Treatment involves hospitalization for observation and to rule out other injuries. Surgical treatment is rarely necessary.

Sequelae are focal and specific to the area of the brain that was injured. For example, an injury to the left temporal area may affect speech.

Intracranial Hematomas. Intracranial hematomas are space-occupying lesions that expand rapidly or slowly, depending on whether they are arterial or venous in origin. They must be located quickly. Some lesions require evacuation as soon as possible to minimize the secondary effects of the injury. Table 14–25 describes types of intracranial hematomas and their treatment.

Subarachnoid hemorrhages, associated with severe head injuries such as intracranial hematomas or contusions, result from laceration of arteries or veins in the subarachnoid space. Symptoms include decreased level of consciousness, ipsilateral pupil dilation, diplopia, hemiparesis, nausea and vomiting, nuchal rigidity, and headache.

Diagnosis is confirmed by CT scan. There is no specific treatment, and the clinical course depends on associated injuries.

Cerebral Edema. Cerebral edema is an increase in intracellular and extracellular fluid in the brain. This condition, which may not be seen until 24 to 48 hours after the head injury, results from anoxia, vasodilation, or vascular stasis. *Malignant brain edema* (cerebral hyperemia), which is more prevalent in children, is a vascular response to brain injury, resulting from a disruption in the blood-brain barrier. In both cases the child displays the signs and symptoms of increased intracranial pressure.

CT scan is used to diagnose these conditions. Management is similar to that of increased intracranial pressure and includes oxygen, hyperventilation, proper head positioning, and administration of diuretics.

It is estimated that up to 50% of children with these types of edema will die or have serious neurologic sequelae.

Penetrating Injuries. Gunshot wounds to the head can damage tissue, bone, and vessels. Low-velocity bullets enter but do not exit the skull; instead they ricochet within the cranial vault, destroying brain tissue and vessels. Although the child may be conscious just after the injury, the level of consciousness quickly deteriorates because of the edema surrounding the penetration tract. High-velocity bullets, on the other hand, cause immediate, severe damage on impact.

CT is used to evaluate gunshot trauma and pinpoint the location of bullet and bone fragments as well as parenchymal damage. Treatment involves surgical debridement of the tract, evacuation of any hematomas, and removal of accessible bone or bullet particles.

Approximately 50% of children with gunshot wounds to the head die. Those who survive may suffer multiple focal deficits and seizures.

TABLE 14-25 Intracranial Hematomas

Type of Hematoma	Diagnosis and Management
Subdural Hematoma	

Result of severe head injuries such as falls, assaults, motor vehicle crashes, or shaken child syndrome
Occurs most frequently in children less than 1 year old
Caused by laceration of the bridging veins; clot forms and presses directly on brain, leading to damage from two sources: original contusion and hematoma
Symptoms (may not appear until 48 to 72 hours after the injury) include:
   Change in level of consciousness (confusion, agitation, or lethargy)
   Nausea or vomiting
   Headache
   Retinal hemorrhages in both eyes
   Pupil on side of injury may be fixed and dilated
   Seizures
   Fever
	Diagnosis confirmed by CT scan
	Treatment is usually surgical; subdural taps may be necessary after surgery to give the brain room to expand
	More than half of children with subdural hematomas die; those who survive have 75% chance of developing seizures
	
	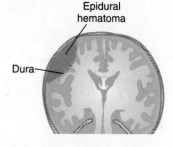
	
	Bleeding occurs between dura and brain

Epidural Hematoma	

Rare in children and almost never occurs in children less than 4 years of age
Results from blunt trauma (most often falls), motor vehicle crashes, or assaults
Temporal and parietal areas are most common sites
May be associated with linear skull fracture
May be fatal if bleeding is arterial
Symptoms include:
   Sleepiness or lethargy
   Headache
   Full fontanel
   Paresis of cranial nerves III and VI
   Papilledema
   Fixed and dilated pupil
   Signs of increased intracranial pressure
	Diagnosis confirmed by CT scan
	Treatment involves immediate surgical intervention; craniotomy is performed followed by evacuation of the hematoma
	Prognosis is good, although 25% of children have seizures
	
	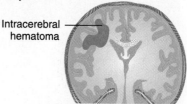
	
	Bleeding occurs between dura and skull

Intracerebral Hematoma	
Result of deep contusion or intra-cerebral laceration (secondary to foreign body or bony penetration or impalement) Causes diffuse bleeding in paren-chyma; there may be a hematoma with associated small areas of bleeding	Diagnosis confirmed by CT scan Surgical treatment not indicated Neurologic effects depend on size and location of lesion and whether bleeding can be controlled; hemiplegia or visual loss may result Bleeding occurs within cerebrum

Impalement Injuries. Impalement injuries frequently occur in children in association with lawn darts or dog bites. All objects *must* be left in place and removed in the operating room by a neurosurgeon.

The child with an impalement injury is at high risk for focal injury and infection.

After surgery children with this type of injury are managed as with other postoperative head injuries, with attention focused on level of consciousness, increased intracranial pressure, and infection control.

Spinal Cord Injury

Less than 10% of spinal injuries occur in children.[25] Yet over half of children with such injuries die within the first hour of trauma, and approximately 20% die during the first 3 months after trauma.[26]

Almost half of all spinal cord injuries are the result of motor vehicle crashes. In young children they are pedestrian-vehicular, bicycle-vehicular, or passenger-related. By adolescence the incidence of passenger-related injuries increases significantly, with alcohol and drugs contributing to about 25% of crashes.[26] Other causes of spinal injuries, especially in toddlers and young children, include falls and child abuse. Recreation-related trauma accounts for more injuries as children grow older. Penetrating injuries such as stab wounds and gunshots are becoming more prevalent.

The mechanism of injury determines the type of lesion that occurs (Fig. 14–11). Hyperflexion injuries produce tears or avulsions and fractures of ver-

FIGURE 14-11 Mechanics of injury to the spinal cord. **A,** Hyperflexion. **B,** Lateral flexion, **C,** Extension. **D,** Compression.

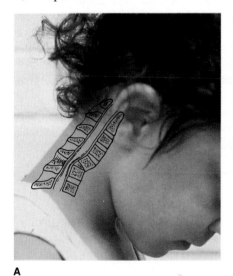
A

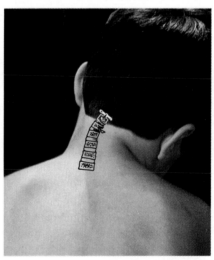
B

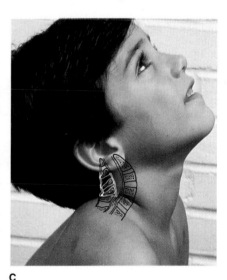
C

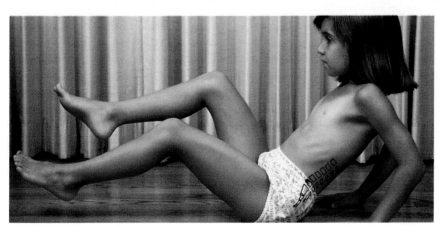
D

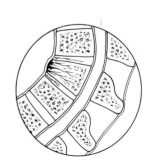

TABLE 14-26 Spinal Cord Injuries in Children

Cervical Region

- Site of 75% of spinal injuries in children through age 8 years and 60% between 8 and 14 years
- Highest incidence above C-3 segment
- Many of these injuries are fatal

Thoracolumbar Region

- Second most common area of injury; probably a result of improperly placed lap belts*

Thoracic Region

- Site of 20% of spinal injuries usually between ages 8 and 14 years

*Data from Luerssen, T. (1993). General characteristics of the neurological injury. In Eichelberger, (M., Ed.). *Pediatric trauma: Prevention, acute care, rehabilitation.* St. Louis: Mosby–Year Book.

■ SCIWORA

Spinal cord injury without radiographic abnormality (SCIWORA) accounts for 15% to 25% of all pediatric spinal cord trauma. SCIWORA occurs when initial films or CT scans show no bony deformity and the child is believed to be free of injury. The young child's spinal column can withstand up to 2 inches of stretch without disruption, while the cord itself ruptures with an elongation of only ¼ inch. This incongruity may account for the normal radiograph despite cord injury.[26]

tebral bodies, as well as subluxation and dislocation. Lateral flexion (rotation) may cause joint dislocations or unstable spinal fractures. Extension may result in the so-called hangman's fracture, ligament tears, avulsion fractures of vertebral bodies, as well as central or posterior spinal cord syndrome. Compression injuries cause anterior cord syndrome.

Spinal cord injuries are classified as complete or incomplete. Complete lesions are irreversible and involve a loss of sensory, motor, and autonomic function below the level of the injury. Incomplete lesions involve varying degrees of sensory, motor, and autonomic function below the level of injury.

Children are prone to specific kinds of spinal cord injuries because of the extreme mobility and flexibility of their spinal column. Table 14–26 describes the spinal cord injuries most common in children.

The higher the level of spinal cord injury, the more severe the neurologic damage. The child is often a victim of multiple trauma and may display signs of hypovolemic shock resulting from other injuries, increased intracranial pressure, or respiratory depression. Children can also experience neurogenic or spinal shock (see Chapter 12).

At the time of injury the child is flaccid and areflexic below the lesion and responds only to stimuli above the level of the injury. Priapism may be present. Muscle spasticity below the lesion occurs later.

Diagnosis is made by observation, neurologic examination, and x-ray studies. X-ray studies include lateral cervical spine and anteroposterior and lateral views of the thoracic and lumbosacral spine. In addition, CT scanning, MRI, fluoroscopy, or myelography may be performed. Many children have spinal cord injury without radiographic abnormality (SCIWORA).[27]

Spinal injuries are managed aggressively. The child with a spinal cord injury may be placed in skeletal traction or a halo device. Further surgical management of the injury may be necessary. Debridement and decompression should be accomplished within the first 8 hours after penetrating injury. A fusion using bone from another part of the body may be performed to stabilize the spinal cord. If more drastic measures are necessary, an internal fixation device may be required.

To further decrease neurologic sequelae, methylprednisolone is administered in high doses to children with motor deficits. Administration must be started within 8 hours of the injury.

Nursing Management

Nursing care focuses on monitoring vital signs, ensuring adequate nutrition, maintaining skin integrity, promoting independent functioning, encouraging therapeutic play, and providing emotional support.

Monitor Vital Signs. Be alert for any changes in vital signs, especially those that may signify increased intracranial pressure (Table 14–6). Monitor the child's respiratory status. Some children with cervical lesions have tracheostomies performed to help maintain airway patency; others with very high lesions are dependent on ventilators. Proper equipment should be at the bedside at all times.

Meet Nutritional Needs. Ensure adequate nutrition. A child with complete paralysis may require a gastrostomy tube.

Maintain Skin Integrity. Prevent skin breakdown (Table 14–7). Observe surgical sites for signs of infection or inflammation. Good skin care should be performed at the insertion site or the site of the external fixation device. (See Table 17–12.)

Promote Independent Functioning. Reinforce the exercises and skills learned in physical and occupational therapy. Use supports, boots, footboards, splints, and braces as recommended by the therapists. Encourage the child to be as independent as possible in a wheelchair.

Bowel and bladder control may be hard to achieve. Intermittent catheterizations may be necessary. Bowel training involves a diet high in fiber and the use of stool softeners.

Encourage Therapeutic Play. Therapeutic play appropriate for the child's developmental level is an important part of the healing process. Provide as many normal activities for the child as possible, but do not give the child tasks that he or she will have difficulty completing. Child life teachers or tutors can help the child keep up with schoolwork.

Television, videotapes, and music can offer diversion for prolonged hospitalization. Paraplegic children can learn to use their arms and hands to play interactive games. Devices can also be adapted so that the child can play video games or manipulate the television or radio.

Provide Emotional Support. Support the child emotionally. Avoid being overly solicitous or overprotective, but encourage the child to meet small, short-term goals, including those that involve self-care. Encourage the child to express fears and frustrations.

Be compassionate and understanding. Encourage siblings to visit, answer their questions honestly, and help them to discuss their feelings. Involve the parents and siblings in the care of the child as much as possible. When appropriate, encourage them to help with activities of daily living.

Discharge Planning and Patient and Family Home Care Teaching. Home care needs and safety issues should be identified and addressed well in advance of discharge. Assist with arrangements for the child's discharge from the hospital. Work closely with the child, parents, and other members of the health care team concerning placement. Many children go on to rehabilitation facilities. Refer families to social services, family counseling, and support groups if indicated.

Hypoxic-Ischemic Brain Injury (Drowning and Near-Drowning)

Drowning is defined as death within 24 hours of a submersion incident. Over 90% of drownings occur in fresh water. Fifty percent of these incidents occur in swimming pools, and 90% of these children drown in residential pools.[28]

Drowning is the second most common cause of injury-related deaths in children. The majority of pediatric victims are very young (under age 4 years) or in their teen years. Boys are five times more likely than girls to die from drowning.

There are two types of drowning. Wet drowning, which occurs more frequently, is the result of aspiration of fluid into the lungs. Dry drowning, which is seen in 10% to 15% of cases, is due to hypoxemia resulting from laryngospasm, with small or insignificant amounts of liquid aspirated.

The events preceding drowning follow a sequential pattern. The child trapped in water panics, struggles, attempts to move using swimming motions, and holds his or her breath. Then the child swallows a small amount of fluid, vomits, and aspirates the vomitus. This leads to a brief period of laryngospasm, which lasts no more than 2 minutes. Because of the increasing panic and hypoxia, the child swallows more liquid. Then either the child

■ GROWTH AND DEVELOPMENT CONSIDERATIONS

Between 40% and 50% of children who are injured in drowning incidents are under 4 years of age, with peak incidence between ages 1 and 2 years.

goes into profound laryngospasm, becomes severely hypoxic, has a seizure, and dies (dry drowning), or the child becomes unconscious, the laryngospasm relaxes as reflexes are lost, and the child passively aspirates even greater amounts of water into the airway and stomach (wet drowning).

Hypoxemia is the major insult associated with drowning. Aspiration leads to impaired gas exchange and ultimately affects pulmonary, cardiac, cerebral, and possibly renal functions. See Chapter 10 for a brief discussion of the effects of drowning on the respiratory system.

Prognosis and outcome are highly individual. The length of time submerged and the immediacy of intervention and treatment, especially cardiopulmonary resuscitation, affect the child's chances for survival.[29,30]

The child who has been immersed exhibits a wide variety of signs and symptoms depending on the length of time underwater, the temperature of the water, the response to the episode, and the initial treatment performed at the scene. Children who are immersed for short periods have few symptoms and recover without complication. The child with a longer immersion can experience the following symptoms: decreased level of consciousness ranging from stupor to total unresponsiveness, cerebral edema, increased intracranial pressure, seizures, respiratory acidosis, irregular respirations, apnea, and gastric distention.

Medical intervention begins at the scene of the drowning with immediate ventilation and compressions, when indicated. The sooner the treatment is started, the better is the prognosis.

Nursing Management

Nursing care of the child who survives the submersion incident focuses on monitoring the child's cardiopulmonary status and providing emotional support.

Monitor the child's respiratory status, cardiopulmonary function, and neurologic state. Administer prescribed medications and position the child properly. Other nursing interventions, especially for the obtunded child, are similar to those for any child in coma (see the discussion of altered states of consciousness).

Provide emotional support to the family. Be nonjudgmental and provide a forum for parents to express their feelings. Reassure parents who exhibit guilt reactions that their child is receiving all possible medical treatment. Parents may be faced with an unknown prognosis. Encourage parents to seek assistance from social workers, members of the clergy, close friends, and relatives. Arrange for appropriate referrals.

Home care needs should be identified and addressed well in advance of discharge. Assist with arrangements for the child with minor deficits. Help the parents decide whether the comatose child will go home or to a long-term facility.

■ NURSING ALERT

All near-drowning victims should be admitted to the hospital for at least 24 hours even when asymptomatic. Many life-threatening complications, including respiratory distress and cerebral edema, may not become evident for at least 12 hours after the incident.

■ SAFETY PRECAUTIONS

Drowning can be prevented by education. The nurse should emphasize the importance of closely supervising children when near or in water, whether at pools, at the beach, or in bathtubs; keeping residential pools inaccessible to toddlers; and emptying pails of liquid.

REFERENCES

1 Scipien, G., Chard, M., Howe, J., et al. (1990). *Pediatric nursing care*. St. Louis: Mosby–Year Book.

2 Barkin, R., & Rosen, P. (1990). *Emergency pediatrics—A guide to ambulatory care* (3rd ed.). St. Louis: Mosby–Year Book.

3 Lorens, X., & McCracken, G. (1990). Bacterial meningitis in neonates and children. In *Infectious Disease Clinics of North America* (Vol. 4, pp. 623–641). Philadelphia: W.B. Saunders.

4 Roos K. (1992). Management of bacterial meningitis in children and adults. *Seminars in Neurology, 12*(3), 155–164.

5 Ikeda, M., & Young, R. (1992). Meningoencephalitis. In R. Hoekelman (Ed.-in-chief), *Primary pediatric care* (2nd ed.). St. Louis: Mosby–Year Book.

6 Barker, E. (1990). Avoiding increased intracranial pressure. *Nursing 90, 90*(5), 64Q–64RR.

7 Jafari, H., & McCracken, G. (1993). Update on steroids for bacterial meningitis. *The Report on Pediatric Infectious Diseases, 3*(2), 1–2.

8 McCracken, G. (1992). Current management of bacterial meningitis in infants and children. *Pediatric Infectious Disease Journal, 11*(2), 169–174.

9 Cherry, J. (1992). Aseptic meningitis and viral meningitis. In R. Feigin & J. Cherry (Eds.), *Textbook of pediatric infectious diseases* (3rd ed.). Philadelphia: W.B. Saunders.

10 Keating, J. (1992). Reye syndrome. In R. Feigin & J. Cherry (Eds.), *Textbook of pediatric infectious diseases* (3rd ed.). Philadelphia: W.B. Saunders.

11 Maheady, C. (1989). Reye's syndrome: Review and update. *Journal of Pediatric Health Care, 3*(5), 246–250.

12 Thompson, J., McFarland, G., Hirsch, J., et al. (1989). *Mosby's manual of clinical nursing* (2nd ed.). St. Louis: Mosby–Year Book.

13 Glaze, D. (1992). Guillain-Barré syndrome. In R. Feigin & J. Cherry (Eds.), *Textbook of pediatric infectious diseases* (3rd ed.). Philadelphia: W.B. Saunders.

14 Cherry, J., & Shields, W. (1992). Encephalitis and meningoencephalitis. In R. Feigin & J. Cherry (Eds.), *Textbook of pediatric infectious diseases* (3rd ed.). Philadelphia: W.B. Saunders.

15 Whitley, R. (1990). Viral encephalitis. *The New England Journal of Medicine, 323*(4), 242–247.

16 Page, R. (1992). Hydrocephalus. In R. Hoekelman (Ed.-in-chief), *Primary pediatric care* (2nd ed.). St. Louis: Mosby–Year Book.

17 Peterson, P. (1992). Spina bifida—Nursing challenge. *RN, 55*(3), 40–47.

18 Slater, J., Mostello, L., & Shaer, C. (1991). Rubber-specific IgE in children with spina bifida. *The Journal of Urology, 146*(578), 578–579.

19 Simpson, D., & David, D. (1986). Craniosynostosis. In H. Hoffman & F. Epstein (Eds.), *Disorders of the developing nervous system: Diagnosis and treatment*. Cambridge, MA: Blackwell Scientific Publishers.

20 Davis, J., & Mercier, C. (1992). Infants of narcotic-addicted mothers. In R. Hoekelman (Ed.-in-chief), *Primary pediatric care* (2nd ed.). St. Louis: Mosby–Year Book.

21 Miller, G., & Couch, S. (1992). Cerebral palsy. In R. Hoekelman (Ed.-in-chief), *Primary pediatric care* (2nd ed.). St. Louis: Mosby–Year Book.

22 Reynolds, E. (1992). Controversies in caring for the child with a head injury. *Maternal Child Nursing, 17*(5), 246–251.

23 Bruce, D. (1993). Head trauma. In M. Eichelberger (Ed.), *Pediatric trauma: Prevention, acute care, rehabilitation*. St. Louis: Mosby–Year Book.

24 Pilmer, S., Duhaime, A., & Raphaely, R. (1993). Intracranial pressure control. In M. Eichelberger (Ed.), *Pediatric trauma: Prevention, acute care, rehabilitation*. St. Louis: Mosby–Year Book.

25 Luerssen, T. (1993). General characteristics of neurological injury. In M. Eichelberger (Ed.), *Pediatric trauma: Prevention, acute care, rehabilitation*. St. Louis: Mosby–Year Book.

26 Dickman, C., & Rekate, H. (1993). Spinal trauma. In M. Eichelberger (Ed.), *Pediatric trauma: Prevention, acute care, rehabilitation*. St. Louis: Mosby–Year Book.

27 Athey, R. (1991). A 3-year-old with spinal cord injury without radiologic abnormality (SCIWORA). *Journal of Emergency Nursing, 17*(6), 380–385.

28 Ochsenschlager, D. (1992). Drowning and near drowning. In R. Barkin (Ed.), *Pediatric emergency medicine: Concepts and clinical practice*. St Louis: Mosby–Year Book.

29 Orlowski, J. (1987). Drowning, near-drowning, and ice-water submersions. *Pediatric Clinics of North America, 34*(1), 75–92.

30 Fields, A. (1993). Near-drowning. In M. Eichelberger (Ed.), *Pediatric trauma: Prevention, acute care, rehabilitation*. St. Louis: Mosby–Year Book.

SUGGESTED READINGS

American Heart Association & American Academy of Pediatrics (1992). Guidelines for cardiopulmonary resuscitation and emergency care. *Journal of the American Medical Association, 162*(68), 2131–2334.

Bracken, M., Shepard, M., Collins, W., et al. (1990). A randomized, controlled trial of methylprednisolone or naloxone in the treatment of acute spinal cord injury. *The New England Journal of Medicine, 322*(20), 1406–1411.

Currier, R., & Crowell, R. (1992). *The yearbook of neurology and neurosurgery*. St. Louis: Mosby–Year Book.

Kelly, S. (1988). *Pediatric emergency nursing*. Norwalk, CT: Appleton & Lange.

McLaurin, R., Schut, L., Venes, J., & Epstein, F. (Eds.). (1989). *Pediatric neurosurgery* (2nd ed.). Philadelphia: W.B. Saunders.

Menkes, J. (1990). *Textbook of child neurology* (4th ed.). Philadelphia: Lea & Febiger.

Nichols, D., Yaster, M., Lappe, D., et al. (1991). *Golden hour: The handbook of advanced pediatric life support*. St. Louis: Mosby–Year Book.

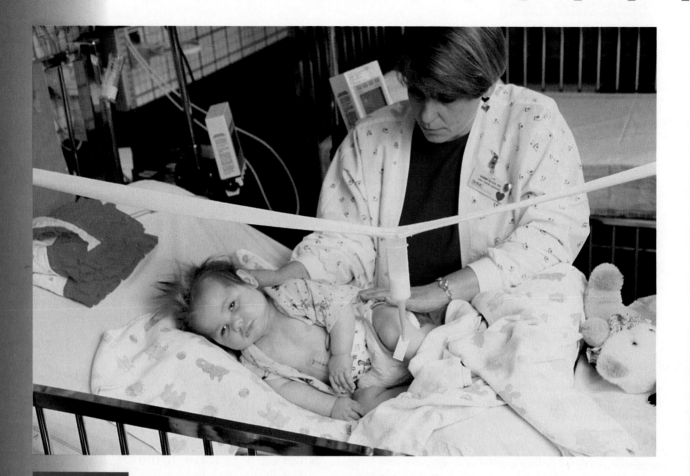

Jenny was born full term after a spontaneous vaginal birth. She had excessive oral and pharyngeal secretions and was slightly cyanotic in the delivery room. After suctioning of secretions, Jenny showed some improvement but quickly became cyanotic again. When the nurse attempted to insert a nasogastric tube through the esophagus into the stomach, resistance was felt. Esophageal atresia was suspected.

Jenny was kept NPO. An umbilical artery catheter was inserted. Diagnostic x-ray films revealed that Jenny's esophagus ended in a blind pouch, with the trachea connected to the stomach. A catheter was placed in the upper esophageal pouch and attached to continuous suction. Jenny was scheduled for immediate surgery.

Jenny underwent a staged operation for repair of the defect. The initial surgery was done to separate the trachea from the stomach. Jenny, who is now 9 months old, is receiving all of her nutritional intake through gastrostomy tube feedings. In the second stage of surgery, to be performed at 18 to 24 months of age, the two ends of the esophagus will be reconnected.

ALTERATIONS IN GASTROINTESTINAL FUNCTION

TERMINOLOGY

constipation Difficult and infrequent defecation with passage of hard, dry stool.

diarrhea Frequent passage of abnormally watery stool.

hernia Protrusion or projection of a body part or structure through the muscle wall of the cavity that normally contains it.

occult blood Blood that is present in minute quantities and can be seen only on microscopic examination or through chemical testing.

ostomy An artificial opening into the urinary or gastrointestinal canal that diverts urine or fecal matter to provide an outlet for it.

peristalsis A progressive, wavelike movement that occurs involuntarily throughout the gastrointestinal tract.

projectile vomiting Vomiting in which the stomach contents are ejected with great force.

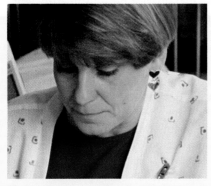

❝ After Jenny's initial surgery, I encouraged her parents to spend time with her—stroking her and talking to her. Sometimes they helped with her feedings too. The closeness that developed during that time helped Jenny's parents adjust to home care. ❞

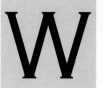hat causes structural defects like esophageal atresia? What care will Jenny require during the period before complete repair of her esophageal defect? This chapter discusses the care of infants, like Jenny, who have structural defects and those with other common disorders of gastrointestinal functioning.

Through the gastrointestinal (GI) tract, a child obtains the foods and fluids necessary to sustain life and promote growth. In most GI disturbances, symptoms are short term and interfere with nutrition and fluid balance for only a brief period. Some disorders or severe defects lead to complications that prevent optimal nutrition and adequate growth. This chapter explores some of the common GI disorders in children. (See Chapter 7 for a discussion of specific fluid imbalances that may accompany GI disorders.)

GI disorders can result from a congenital defect, acquired disease, infection, or injury. Structural problems may occur when development is altered or ceases in the first trimester of gestation. Infections can cause an increase or decrease in motility and prevent proper absorption of nutrients. Interruption or destruction of the GI system can also result from trauma or ingestion of caustic substances. As you read the chapter, remember that any interruption or alteration in the GI system will decrease the body's ability to obtain nutrients, thus impairing growth.

Anatomy and Physiology of Pediatric Differences

Although the fetus makes sucking and swallowing movements in utero and ingests amniotic fluid, the GI system is immature at birth. The processes of absorption and excretion do not begin until after birth because the placenta is responsible for providing nutrients and removing waste. Sucking is a primitive reflex that occurs whenever the lips or cheeks are stroked. The infant does not have voluntary control over swallowing until about 6 weeks of age.

The stomach capacity of the newborn is quite small, and intestinal motility (**peristalsis**) is greater than in older children. Those characteristics explain the newborn's need for small, frequent feedings and the increased frequency and liquid consistency of bowel movements. Because of the relaxed cardiac sphincter, infants frequently regurgitate small amounts of feedings.

Digestion takes place in the duodenum. Infants have a deficiency of several enzymes: amylase (which digests carbohydrates), lipase (which enhances fat absorption), and trypsin (which catabolizes protein into polypeptides and some amino acids). Enzymes are usually not present in sufficient quantity to aid digestion until 4 to 6 months of age. Thus abdominal distention from gas and flatus are common.

Liver functions are also immature. After the first few weeks of life the liver is able to conjugate bilirubin and excrete bile. The processes of gluconeogenesis (formation of glycogen from noncarbohydrates), plasma protein and ketone formation, vitamin storage, and deamination (removal of amino group from amino compound) remain immature during the first year of life.

By the second year of life, digestive processes are fairly complete. Stomach capacity increases to accommodate a three-meal-per-day feeding schedule. At about the same time, myelination of the spinal cord becomes complete and voluntary control over excretory functions is achieved.

■ GROWTH AND DEVELOPMENT CONSIDERATIONS

Stomach capacity increases throughout early childhood:

Age	Capacity (mL)
Newborn	10–20
1 week	30–90
2–3 weeks	75–100
1 month	90–150
3 months	150–200
1 year	210–360
2 years	500

Structural Defects

Structural defects can involve one or more areas of the GI tract. These defects occur when growth and development of fetal structures are interrupted during the first trimester. This can leave the structure incomplete, resulting in atresia (absence or closure of a normal body orifice), malposition, nonclosure, or other abnormalities.

Cleft Lip and Cleft Palate

Cleft lip and cleft palate are two distinct facial defects that can occur singly or in combination (Fig. 15–1). Incomplete fusion of the lip occurs in approximately 1 in 1000 births and is more common in boys. Incomplete fusion of the palate occurs in approximately 1 in 2500 births and is more common in girls.[1] There are various degrees of severity with each defect.

Clinical Manifestations

A cleft that involves the lip is apparent at birth. It may be a simple dimple in the vermilion border of the lip or a complete separation extending to the floor of the nose. The defect may be unilateral or bilateral and may occur alone or in combination with a cleft palate defect. Varying degrees of nasal deformity may also be present.

Cleft palate defects are less obvious when they occur without a cleft lip and may not be detected at birth. Clefts of the hard palate form a continuous opening between the mouth and nasal cavity and may be unilateral or bilateral.

Etiology and Pathophysiology

Cleft lip with or without cleft palate results from a failure of the maxillary processes to fuse with the elevations on the frontal prominence during the sixth week of gestation. Normally union of the upper lip is complete by the seventh week. Fusion of the secondary palate occurs between 7 and 12 weeks of gestation. Failure of the tongue to move downward at the correct time will prevent the palatine processes from fusing.

The intrauterine development of the hard and soft palates is completed in the first trimester. It is during this time that other major organ systems develop. Other congenital defects, such as tracheoesophageal fistulas and omphaloceles, are commonly associated with cleft lip and palate defects.

FIGURE 15-1 Cleft lip and cleft palate defects. **A,** Unilateral cleft lip. **B,** Bilateral cleft lip and cleft palate.

A from Rudolph, A.M., Hoffman, J.I.E., & Rudolph, C.D. (1991). *Rudolph's pediatrics* (19th ed.) (p. 964). Norwalk, CT: Appleton & Lange. B from Zitelli, B.J., & Davis, H.W. (Eds.) (1987). *Atlas of pediatric physical diagnosis* (p. 2.10). New York: Mosby–Year Book Europe Ltd.

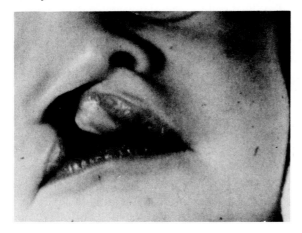

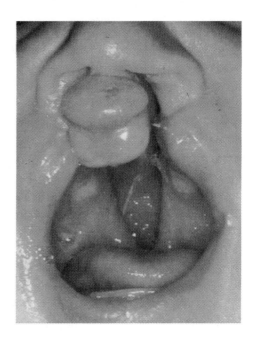

Diagnostic Tests and Medical Management

Cleft lip and palate are usually diagnosed at birth or during the newborn assessment. Medical management requires the combined efforts of a multidisciplinary team. Because speech, hearing, and dentition may be affected, coordinated care by specialists in plastic surgery, hearing, speech, and dentistry is necessary.[1] The cleft lip is usually repaired shortly after birth. The lip is sutured together, and a Logan bow or other stabilizing device or dressing is put in place to prevent tension on the suture line. After surgery the infant's elbows should be restrained to prevent flexion (see Atlas of Pediatric Procedures) and crying should be minimized to prevent injury.

Early closure of the lip enables the infant to form a better seal around the nipple for feeding. The sucking motion strengthens the muscles necessary for speech. Special feeding devices such as longer nipples with enlarged holes are available to help meet the infant's short-term nutritional needs before surgical correction.

Timing of the cleft palate repair is controversial and depends on the size and severity of the cleft. Most surgeons perform closure operations when the infant is 6 to 12 months old. This allows the infant to develop more normal speech patterns.

Infants with cleft lip and cleft palate are prone to recurrent otitis media, which can lead to tympanic membrane scarring and hearing loss. Antibiotic therapy is prescribed to treat any infections that might lead to an ear infection. Because infants with chronic otitis media often have difficulty hearing, speech patterns may be altered. These infants require early and continuous intervention to prevent complications. (Refer to Chapter 11 for care of the child with chronic otitis media.) The child who has had cleft palate repair will require orthodontic care. Early visits will permit assessment of tooth eruption and need for future orthodontic work.

Nursing Assessment

Physiologic Assessment. A cleft lip defect is observable at birth. A cleft palate defect is usually noted during the newborn assessment by palpation of the hard palate with the finger. A description of the location and extent of the defect will assist the nurse in determining the correct method of feeding.

Psychosocial Assessment. Assessment of the family's reactions is an integral part of the overall nursing assessment. Physical deformities, especially of the face, can devastate the parents. A delay in correction of the defect can impede the bonding process between the infant and parents. A poorly corrected defect can lead to the development of low self-esteem in the older child.

Nursing Diagnosis

The accompanying Nursing Care Plan lists common nursing diagnoses for the infant with a cleft lip and/or palate. Other diagnoses that might be appropriate include:

- Anxiety (Parent) related to surgical correction of cleft lip within the first few days of life, long-term management, and financial concerns
- Ineffective Feeding Pattern related to ineffective suck and anatomic abnormality
- High Risk for Caregiver Role Strain related to child with a chronic condition

- High Risk for Impaired Home Maintenance Management related to infant's defect(s) and inadequate family support

Nursing Management

Nursing care involves providing emotional support, performing postsurgical care, helping parents to coordinate care and maintain a healthy home environment, and making appropriate referrals. The accompanying Nursing Care Plan summarizes nursing care for the infant with a cleft lip and/or cleft palate.

Provide Emotional Support. Parents may need assistance to view their infant as a whole person, rather than focusing solely on the physical defect.[2,3] Nurses can promote parent-infant bonding by explaining the cause of the structural defect and the procedure for correction. Self-blame is common among parents. Parents can also be referred to the American Cleft Palate Association for information about the disorder (see Appendix F).

Parental anxiety is usual when children undergo surgery. This anxiety is heightened when the surgery involves an infant. To minimize anxiety, explanations to parents should be clear and concise. Allow sufficient time for parents to ask questions. Encourage parents to hold and cuddle the infant before surgery.

Provide Postoperative Care. Provide general postoperative care for the infant. (See the accompanying Nursing Care Plan for the Infant with Cleft Lip and/or Palate and the Nursing Care Plan for the Child Undergoing Surgery in Chapter 4.) Assess vital signs frequently and maintain the infant's airway. Measure intake and output. When oral fluids are started, they are usually given through a dropper or an Asepto syringe. Position the infant in a sitting position for the feedings to avoid aspiration. The infant then progresses to half-strength formula or breast milk. After each feeding clean the suture line with water or normal saline to avoid accumulation of feedings.

It is important to maintain the suture line to ensure healing. Position the infant in a supine or a side-lying position to avoid rubbing the suture line on bedding. Keep elbows in soft restraints. Maintain the metal bar or Steri-strips placed over the incision. Place antibiotic cream on the incision site. Medicate for pain regularly to minimize crying and stress on the suture line. After cleft palate surgery, avoid the use of metal utensils or straws, since they may disrupt the surgical site.

Discharge Planning and Patient and Family Home Care Teaching. Home care needs should be identified and addressed well in advance of discharge. Discuss all aspects of the infant's care with the parents throughout hospitalization and after surgery. Involve parents in the infant's care to increase their comfort level before discharge and to promote bonding. Teach them feeding techniques, how to recognize signs of infection, how to position the infant, and how to care for the suture line. Management, especially in the first few months of life, involves many different health care professionals. The parents are the best coordinators of the child's care. Encourage them to keep a diary listing the professionals with whom they talk and the content of the discussions.

Discuss with the parents the financial implications of long-term care. Private insurance does not always cover all the costs of care necessary for the child. Refer parents to appropriate social services familiar with programs and financial aid for which the parents and child may be eligible. Relief of financial worries enables parents to concentrate on caring for the child.

■ GROWTH AND DEVELOPMENT CONSIDERATIONS

The infant who has had a cleft lip repair needs stimulation to provide distraction. This approach will minimize crying, which can damage the suture line. Since the infant is positioned on the back or side, soft, colorful toys, mobiles, and other visual objects are helpful. Music also can be used to soothe the infant.

Discuss with parents how to care for the child after discharge. If the child has siblings, emphasize that they will need preparation to accept the child. Sibling rivalry can be heightened when one child receives more attention within the home. Remind parents of the importance of setting limits with all children and of spending time individually with them. Determine whether additional family supports are necessary. Provide parents with information on support groups, physicians, social workers, and local services that can help maintain family continuity.

Discuss ways to prevent the infant from touching the suture line. Teach parents how to bundle an infant in a blanket with arms tucked inside the blanket. A front-sling baby carrier may also be used to immobilize the arms. Carriers provide the additional benefits of comforting the infant through contact with the parent and of holding the infant upright, which aids in positioning during feeding.

After surgical repair, parents need to be taught how to feed the infant and how to identify signs of complications (fever, emesis, respiratory distress). Referral to a home health agency for home support may be helpful.

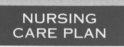
NURSING CARE PLAN

THE INFANT WITH A CLEFT LIP AND/OR PALATE

GOAL	INTERVENTION	RATIONALE	EXPECTED OUTCOME

Preoperative Care

1. High Risk for Aspiration (Breast Milk, Formula, or Mucus) related to anatomic defect

GOAL	INTERVENTION	RATIONALE	EXPECTED OUTCOME
Infant has no episodes of gagging or aspiration.	Assess respiratory status and monitor vital signs at least every 2 hours.	Allows for early identification of problems.	Infant exhibits no signs of respiratory distress.
	Position on side after feedings.	Prevents aspiration of feedings.	
	Feed slowly and use adaptive equipment as needed.	Facilitates intake while minimizing risk of aspiration.	
	Burp frequently (after every 15–30 mL of fluid).	Helps to prevent regurgitation and aspiration.	
	Position upright for feedings.	Minimizes passage of feedings through cleft.	
	Keep suction equipment and bulb syringe at bedside.	Suctioning may be necessary to remove milk or mucus.	

2. Ineffective Family Coping related to birth of child with visible and/or structural defect

GOAL	INTERVENTION	RATIONALE	EXPECTED OUTCOME
Parents will begin bonding process with infant.	Help parents to hold infant and facilitate feeding process.	Contact is essential for bonding.	Parents hold, comfort, and show concern for infant.
	Point out positive attributes of infant (hair, eyes, alertness, etc.).	Helps parents see child as a whole, rather than concentrating on the defect.	
	Explain surgical procedure and expected outcome. Show pictures of other children's cleft lip repair.	Eliminating unknown factors helps to decrease anxiety.	

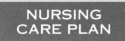
THE INFANT WITH A CLEFT LIP AND/OR PALATE—CONTINUED

GOAL	INTERVENTION	RATIONALE	EXPECTED OUTCOME
2. Ineffective Family Coping related to birth of child with visible and/or structural defect—Continued			
The family's coping ability will be maximized. Parents will verbalize the nature and sequelae of the defect.	Assess parents' knowledge of the defect, their degree of anxiety and level of discomfort, and the interpersonal relationships among family members.	Helps to determine the appropriate timing and amount of information to be given regarding the child's defect.	The family demonstrates improved coping ability before discharge.
	Explore reaction of extended family.	Extended family is an important source of support for most parents of a newborn. Family members can often help promote acceptance and compliance with the treatment plan.	
	Support open visitation.	Allows parents to begin the bonding process.	
	Encourage parents to participate in caretaking activities (holding, diapering, feeding).	Participation in infant care decreases anxiety and provides parents with a sense of purpose.	
	Provide information about the etiology of cleft lip and palate defects and the special needs of these infants. Encourage questions.	Concrete information allows parents time to understand the defect and reduces guilt.	
	Refer to parent support groups.	Support groups allow parents to express their feelings and concerns, to find people with concerns similar to their own, and to seek additional information.	
3. Altered Nutrition: Less Than Body Requirements related to infant's inability to form an adequate seal for sucking			
Infant will gain weight steadily.	Assess fluid and calorie intake daily. Assess weight daily (same scale, same time, with infant completely undressed).	Provides an objective measurement of whether the infant is receiving sufficient caloric intake to promote growth. Using the same scale and procedure when weighing the infant provides for consistent daily weights.	Infant maintains adequate nutritional intake and gains weight appropriately.
	Observe for any respiratory impairment.	Any symptoms of respiratory compromise will interfere with the infant's ability to suck. Feedings should be initiated only if there are no signs of respiratory distress.	

Continued

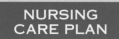

THE INFANT WITH A CLEFT LIP AND/OR PALATE—
CONTINUED

GOAL	INTERVENTION	RATIONALE	EXPECTED OUTCOME

3. Altered Nutrition: Less Than Body Requirements related to infant's inability to form an adequate seal for sucking—Continued

GOAL	INTERVENTION	RATIONALE	EXPECTED OUTCOME
	Provide 100–150 cal/kg/day and 100–130 mL/kg/day of feedings and fluid. If the infant needs an increased number of calories to grow, referral to a nutritionist should be made. Formulas with higher calorie concentrations per ounce are available without increasing total fluids.	Provides optimal calories and fluids for growth and hydration.	
	Facilitate breast-feeding.	Breast milk is recommended as the best food for an infant. The process of breast-feeding helps to promote bonding between mother and infant.	
	• Hold the infant in a semi-sitting position.	• Makes swallowing easier and reduces the amount of fluid return from the nose.	
	• Give the mother information on breast-feeding the infant with a cleft lip and/or palate such as plugging the cleft lip and eliciting a let-down reflex before nursing.	• Information and specific suggestions may encourage the mother to persist with breastfeeding.	
	• Contact the LaLeche League for the name of a support person (see Appendix F).	• The LaLeche League promotes breast-feeding for all infants. It can provide support people with experience who will aid the mother.	
	If the mother is unable to breast-feed (or prefers not to), initiate bottle feeding:		
	• Hold infant in an upright or semisitting position for feeding.	• Facilitates swallowing and minimizes the amount of return from the nose.	
	• Place nipple against the inside cheek toward the back of the tongue. May need to use a premature nipple (slightly longer and softer than regular nipple with a larger opening) or a Brecht feeder (an oval bottle with a long, soft nipple).	• Use of longer, softer nipples makes it easier for the infant to suck. A Brecht feeder decreases the amount of pressure in the bottle and makes the formula flow more easily.	

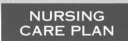
GOAL	INTERVENTION	RATIONALE	EXPECTED OUTCOME

3. Altered Nutrition: Less Than Body Requirements related to infant's inability to form an adequate seal for sucking—Continued

	• Feed small amounts slowly.	• Small amounts and slow feeding do not tire the infant as quickly as do larger amounts given at faster rate. They also decrease the calories used during feeding.	
	• Burp frequently, after 15–30 mL of formula has been given.	• Frequent burping prevents the accumulation of air in stomach, which can cause regurgitation or vomiting.	
	• Initiate nasogastric feedings if infant is unable to ingest sufficient calories by mouth.	• Adequate nutrition must be maintained. Use of a feeding tube allows the infant who has difficulty with oral feeding to receive adequate nutrition for growth.	

Postoperative Care

1. High Risk for Infection related to surgical procedure and accumulation of formula and secretions in the oral cavity

Infant's mucosal tissue will heal without infection.	Assess vital signs every 2 hours.	Elevated temperature may indicate infection.	Infant remains free of infection in the oral cavity. Tissues remain intact and pink.
	Assess oral cavity every 2 hours or as needed for tenderness, reddened areas, lesions, or presence of secretions.	Aids in identifying infection.	
	Cleanse suture line with normal saline or sterile water if ordered.	Helps decrease presence of bacteria.	
	Cleanse the cleft areas by giving 5–15 mL of water after each feeding.	Prevents accumulation of carbohydrates, which encourage bacterial growth.	
	If a crust has formed, use a cotton swab to apply a half-strength peroxide solution.	Helps loosen crust, aiding in removal.	
	Apply antibiotic cream to suture line as ordered.	Counteracts growth of bacteria.	
	Use careful handwashing and sterile technique when working with suture line.	Prevents spread of microorganisms from other sources.	

Continued

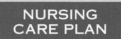

NURSING CARE PLAN

THE INFANT WITH A CLEFT LIP AND/OR PALATE—CONTINUED

GOAL	INTERVENTION	RATIONALE	EXPECTED OUTCOME
2. Ineffective Breathing Pattern related to anesthesia and increased secretions			
Infant will maintain effective breathing pattern.	Assess respiratory status and monitor vital signs at least every 2 hours.	Allows for early identification of problems.	Infant shows no signs of respiratory infection or compromise.
	Apply a cardiorespiratory monitor.	Enables early detection of abnormal respirations, facilitating prompt intervention.	
	Keep suction equipment and bulb syringe at bedside. Gently suction oropharynx and nasopharynx as needed.	Gentle suctioning will keep the airway clear. Suctioning that is too vigorous can irritate the mucosa.	
	Provide cool mist for first 24 hours postoperatively if ordered.	Moisturizes secretions to reduce pooling in lungs. Moisturizes oral cavity.	
	Reposition every 2 hours.	Ensures expansion of all lung fields.	
3. Impaired Tissue Integrity related to surgical correction of cleft			
Lip and/or palate will heal with minimal scarring or disruption.	Position infant with cleft lip repair on side or back only.	Prone position could cause rubbing on suture line.	Lip/palate heals without complications.
	Use soft elbow restraints. Remove every 2 hours and replace. Do not leave infant unattended when restraints are removed	Prevents infant's hands from rubbing surgical site. Regular removal allows for skin and neurovascular checks.	
	Maintain metal bar (Logan bow) or Steri-Strips placed over cleft lip repair.	Maintaining suture line will minimize scarring.	
	Avoid metal utensils or straws after cleft palate repair.	These devices may disrupt suture line.	
	Keep infant well medicated for pain in initial postoperative period. Have parents hold and comfort infant.	Good pain management minimizes crying, which can cause stress on suture line. Increases bonding and soothes child to decrease crying.	
	Provide developmentally appropriate activities (i.e., mobiles, music).	Soothes and keeps infant calm.	

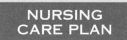
GOAL	INTERVENTION	RATIONALE	EXPECTED OUTCOME
4. Knowledge Deficit (Parent) related to diagnosis, treatment, prognosis, and home care needs			
Before discharge, parents will verbalize home care methods for care of infant with cleft lip and palate defect.	Explain care and treatment (both short-term and long-term). Discuss potential complications. Demonstrate feeding techniques and alternatives. Allow parents to redemonstrate before discharge. Provide written instructions for follow-up care arrangements. Introduce the parents (if possible) to a primary caregiver in the setting where the infant will receive follow-up care after discharge.	Assists the family to deal with the physical and psychosocial aspects of a child with a congenital defect. Provides visual instructions. Redemonstration confirms learning. Written instructions reinforce verbal instruction and provide a reference after discharge. Continuity of care is important. Since the infant will require long-term follow-up; a contact in the new environment is helpful.	Parents accurately describe and demonstrate feeding techniques to facilitate optimal growth of infant; describe interventions if respiratory distress occurs; and take the written instructions home with them on discharge.
5. Altered Nutrition: Less Than Body Requirements related to surgery and feeding difficulties			
Infant will receive adequate nutritional intake.	Maintain intravenous infusion as ordered. Begin with clear liquids, then give half-strength formula or breast milk as ordered. Use Asepto syringe or dropper in side of mouth. Do not allow pacifiers. Give high-calorie soft foods after cleft palate repair.	Provides fluid when NPO. Ensures adequate fluids and nutrients. Avoids suture line and resultant accumulation of formula in that area. Sucking can disrupt suture line. Rough foods, utensils, and straws could disrupt surgical site.	Infant receives adequate nutritional intake. Infant resumes usual feeding patterns and gains weight appropriately.

Esophageal Atresia and Tracheoesophageal Fistula

Esophageal atresia is a rare malformation that results from failure of the esophagus to develop as a continuous tube during the fourth and fifth weeks of gestation.

Symptoms in the newborn include excessive salivation and drooling, often accompanied by choking, coughing, and sneezing. During feeding, the infant returns fluid through the nose and mouth. Aspiration places the infant at risk for pneumonia. Depending on the type of defect, the abdomen may become distended because of air trapping.

In esophageal atresia the foregut fails to lengthen, separate, and fuse into two parallel tubes (the esophagus and trachea) during fetal development. Instead the esophagus may end in a blind pouch or develop as a pouch connected to the trachea by a fistula (tracheoesophageal fistula) (Fig. 15–2). Esophageal atresia often is associated with a maternal history of polyhydramnios.

Diagnosis is usually confirmed by attempting to pass a nasogastric tube into the stomach. In most cases the tube meets resistance and can be advanced only minimally. Specific defects are determined by x-ray examination. A delay in diagnosis can be fatal because ingested fluid or secretions may enter the lungs.

Surgical correction may be accomplished in several stages. The first stage usually involves ligation of the fistula and insertion of a gastrostomy tube. This was the case with Jenny, who was described in the vignette at the beginning of this chapter. In the second stage the two ends of the esophagus are reconnected, if possible. Potential postoperative complications include gastroesophageal reflux, aspiration, and stricture formation.[1] The prognosis is usually good with surgery.

Nursing Management

Esophageal atresia is a surgical emergency. Preoperatively the infant requires close observation and intervention to maintain a patent airway. Suction should be readily available to remove any secretions that accumulate in the nasopharyngeal airway. Place the infant with the head of the bed slightly lowered to drain secretions from the blind pouch and to minimize aspiration of secretions into the trachea. Continuous or low intermittent suction may be

■ CLINICAL TIP

When using a small-bore nasogastric tube, gurgling can occur when the tube is in the esophagus or lung. To confirm placement, aspiration of stomach contents and pH testing are required.

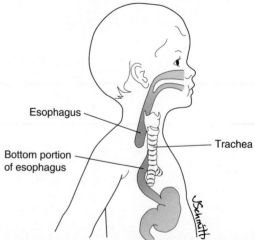

FIGURE 15–2 In the most common type of esophageal atresia and tracheoesophageal fistula, the upper segment of the esophagus ends in a blind pouch connected to the trachea; a fistula connects the lower segment to the trachea.

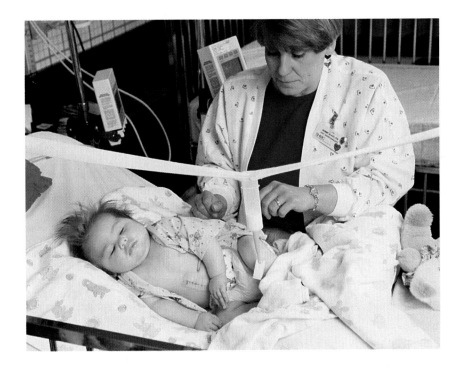

FIGURE 15–3 A gastrostomy tube is used for feeding of the child with a gastrointestinal disorder such as esophageal atresia.

used to remove secretions from the blind pouch. Oral fluids are withheld, and the infant is maintained with intravenous fluids administered through an umbilical artery catheter.

The parents require emotional support throughout the infant's hospitalization. All procedures should be clearly explained. Encourage parents to bond with the infant by stroking and talking to the infant. Eliciting questions and allowing parents to participate in the infant's care, especially feeding (when permitted), can facilitate bonding and help to prepare parents for postdischarge care.

Once enteral feedings have been established, the infant may be discharged from the hospital with a gastrostomy tube in place (Fig. 15–3). (See the Atlas of Pediatric Procedures for care of the child with a gastrostomy tube.) Parents require instruction about gastrostomy tube care and feeding, signs of infection, and prevention of postoperative complications (Table 15–1).

Pyloric Stenosis

Pyloric stenosis is a hypertrophic obstruction of the circular muscle of the pyloric canal. It is a common problem that most often affects first-born male infants.

Clinical Manifestations

Symptoms usually become evident 2 to 4 weeks after birth, although onset may vary.[4] Initially the infant appears well or regurgitates slightly after feedings. The parents may describe the infant as a "good eater" who vomits occasionally. As the obstruction progresses, the vomiting becomes projectile. In **projectile vomiting** the contents of the stomach may be ejected up to 3 feet from the infant. The vomitus is nonbilious and may become blood tinged because of repeated irritation to the esophagus. The infant is always hungry, appears irritable, fails to gain weight, and has a decreased number and volume of stools.

TABLE 15–1 Parent Teaching: Home Care Instructions for the Child Requiring Gastrostomy Tube Feedings and Care

Equipment

Prepared, prescribed feeding; enteral feeding pump; long-nosed syringe

Procedure

1. Wash hands.
2. Warm prescribed formula to room temperature.
3. Pour formula to run through the feeding bag.
4. Allow formula to run through the tubing to remove air. Close clamp.
5. Attach syringe to the end of the gastrostomy tube. Unclamp the gastrostomy tube.
6. Pull plunger back until resistance is felt. Check amount of formula in syringe. If more than half of the prescribed amount is withdrawn, refer to the section on problem solving (below). If less than the prescribed amount is withdrawn, push the formula gently back through the syringe.
7. Instill water through the tube.
8. Attach the feeding bag to the gastrostomy tube. Infuse at the prescribed rate.
9. Burp or bubble the infant throughout the feeding.
10. After feeding, flush the gastrostomy tube with water and clamp the tube.
11. Position the infant prone or side lying for ½ to 1 hour after feedings.

Psychosocial Needs

Hold and rock the infant or child during feedings.
Give a pacifier to an infant or a bottle or cup to a child to meet developmental needs.

Medication Administration

Use liquid medication whenever possible.
Crush only uncoated tablets.
Crush tablets to a fine powder and mix with water or juice.
Flush tubing before and after medication administration.

Stoma Care

Wash the area around the stoma twice a day with soap and water.
Use half-strength hydrogen peroxide to remove any crusting.
Look for signs of infection, such as redness, swelling, and discharge.
Notify the physician if any signs of infection or leakage are present.

Problem Solving

Problem	Cause	Action
Formula will not flow	Blocked tube (clamping, foreign material)	Check clamp. Reposition. Pull back on syringe. Instill water. Notify physician.
	Viscous formula	
	Pump malfunction	Check plug. Call company. Give feeding by gravity.
Large volume of un-digested formula removed before feeding	Delayed absorption	Reinfuse remaining formula. If more than half of feeding, subtract from the next feeding. Do not discard the residual.
	Constipation	Check for last bowel movement. Notify physician.
Constipation	Decreased free fluids	Give water and juice between feedings as tolerated. Report bowel problems or hard stools to physician.
Diarrhea	Hyperosmolar formula	Dilute formula.
	Rapid rate of flow	Feed at a slower rate.
	Cold formula	Warm formula to room temperature before feeding.
	Bacterial contamination	Treat with antibiotics.

Data from Gulanick, M., Knoll-Puzas, M., & Wilson, C. (Eds.) (1992). *Nursing care plans for newborns and children: Acute and critical care.* St. Louis: Mosby–Year Book; Skale, N. (1992). *Manual of pediatric nursing procedures.* Philadelphia: J.B. Lippincott; and Young, C., & White, S. (1992). Preparing patients for tube feeding at home. *American Journal of Nursing, 92,* 46–53.

Etiology and Pathophysiology

The exact cause of pyloric stenosis is unknown, although frequently there is a family history of the disorder. Hypertrophy of the circular pylorus muscle results in stenosis of the passage between the stomach and the duodenum, partially obstructing the lumen of the stomach. The lumen becomes inflamed and edematous, which narrows the opening until the obstruction becomes complete. At this time vomiting becomes more projectile. As the obstruction progresses, the infant becomes dehydrated and electrolytes are depleted, resulting in metabolic imbalances.

Diagnostic Tests and Medical Management

An upper GI series is performed to confirm the diagnosis, showing a delay in gastric emptying. Blood tests are used to determine the degree of dehydration and anemia (see Chapter 7).

Surgical correction is the treatment of choice. Preoperatively the infant's condition is stabilized with intravenous fluids and electrolytes. A nasogastric tube is inserted to decompress the stomach. Surgery is performed as soon as possible after the infant's condition is stabilized. During surgery the circular muscle fibers are released to allow the passage of food and fluid (Fredet-Ramstedt procedure). The prognosis is good, and the infant is usually discharged within 72 hours of surgery.

Nursing Assessment

During the physical examination of the infant, peristaltic waves may be observed. Bowel sounds are hyperactive on auscultation. Palpation reveals an olive-shaped mass in the right upper quadrant of the abdomen.

Assess skin turgor, fontanels, and orbital regions to determine whether hydration is adequate. Measure vomitus and describe vomiting episodes.

Nursing Diagnosis

Common nursing diagnoses for the child with pyloric stenosis include:

- Fluid Volume Deficit related to frequent vomiting
- Altered Nutrition: Less Than Body Requirements related to vomiting and lack of absorption of nutrients
- Sleep Pattern Disturbance related to constant hunger, vomiting, and esophageal irritation or pain
- High Risk for Infection related to surgical incision
- Altered Family Processes related to seriously ill infant requiring hospitalization and surgery

Nursing Management

Nursing care centers on meeting the infant's fluid needs, minimizing weight loss, promoting rest and comfort, preventing infection, and providing supportive care for parents.

Meet Fluid Needs. Because projectile vomiting will continue until the obstruction is relieved surgically, oral feedings are withheld. Intravenous fluid therapy is administered to correct fluid and electrolyte imbalances and to maintain adequate hydration. Monitor intake and output (including vomitus) and urine specific gravity. Inform parents that all diapers will be weighed to measure the infant's output of urine and stool.

Minimize Weight Loss. The infant loses weight because of frequent vomiting. Monitor weight daily both preoperatively and postoperatively. Small, frequent feedings consisting of clear liquids are begun within 4 to 6 hours postoperatively. If clear liquids are tolerated, the infant is advanced to formula feedings.

Promote Rest and Comfort. During the preoperative period the infant is hungry and cries often. The infant is swaddled to maintain warmth and provide comfort. Encourage the parents to hold and cuddle the infant. Provide a pacifier to meet the infant's need to suck.

Postoperatively the infant is uncomfortable because of the surgical incision. Instruct parents to avoid pressure on the incision. When diapering the infant, slide the diaper gently under the buttocks rather than lifting the legs. Swaddling, rocking, and use of a pacifier help to relax the infant. Acetaminophen or other analgesics can be administered to relieve discomfort as ordered. (See Chapter 5 for a discussion of pain management.)

Prevent Infection. Postoperatively the incision is covered with collodion or Steri-Strips and should be kept clean and dry. Check the incision site for redness, swelling, or discharge. Monitor the infant's temperature every 4 hours.

Provide Supportive Care. The need for hospitalization and surgery creates anxiety for parents. Encourage them to participate in the infant's care and to discuss their fears and concerns. Provide simple and clear explanations about the infant's condition and care. Advise parents that occasional vomiting after surgery may occur.

Discharge Planning and Patient and Family Home Care Teaching. Instruct parents to observe the incision for redness, swelling, or discharge and to notify the physician immediately if these occur or if the infant's temperature is higher than 101° F (38.5° C). To reduce the possibility of infection, advise parents to fold the infant's diaper so that it does not touch the incision.

Gastroesophageal Reflux

Gastroesophageal reflux, the return of gastric contents into the esophagus, is the result of an immature cardiac sphincter. It may occur at any time and is not necessarily related to having a full stomach.

Children with gastroesophageal reflux are frequently hungry and irritable. They eat often but still lose weight. They have a history of vomiting and frequent upper respiratory infections. Reflux of stomach contents can lead to aspiration, resulting in frequent bouts of pneumonia, reactive airway disease, or apnea.

Some "spitting up" after feedings is considered normal in newborn infants. However, regurgitation that continues and increases in frequency, resulting in delayed growth, requires further investigation. The disorder is more common in premature infants and in children with neurologic impairments. It often resolves without surgical intervention.[1,4]

Diagnosis is confirmed by a thorough history of the child's feeding patterns and by diagnostic evaluation using barium swallow, pH probe monitoring (insertion of a small catheter into the esophagus through the nose that is left in place for 18 to 24 hours to measure pH and thus determine number of reflux episodes), or gastroesophageal scintigraphy (radionuclide scanning to evaluate gastric emptying).

Treatment depends on the severity of the condition. Mild cases may require only a modification of feeding habits. The use of rice cereal in the infant's bottle to thicken feedings is controversial.[5] Some authorities believe that this decreases gastric motility and delays gastric emptying, adding material to be refluxed. Others say thickened feedings help to push the formula through the sphincter. Medications (cholinergics, antacids, and histamine antagonists) may be prescribed to reduce the amount of stomach acid and lessen the child's discomfort. The child should be positioned with the upper body raised after feedings.

Treatment for severe cases may include surgery to create a valve mechanism by wrapping the greater curvature of the stomach (fundus) around the distal esophagus (Nissen fundoplication). A gastrostomy tube is usually inserted during surgery.

The prognosis is good, both for infants with mild conditions and those undergoing surgical correction.

Nursing Management

Nursing management focuses on obtaining a thorough history of the child's feeding patterns. Observe vomiting episodes and document amount, color, and consistency of emesis.

Monitor the infant's weight daily and plot on a growth chart to note progress. Observe for any signs of respiratory distress, and keep the infant's nose and mouth clear of vomitus.

Adequate nutrition must be maintained. Infants receiving oral feedings should be given small, frequent feedings. Place the infant in a prone position with the head of the bed elevated to prevent aspiration if vomiting should occur. If the child has difficulty maintaining this position, a Tracy harness or reflux board may be used. The harness, which is pinned to the mattress, supports the infant in an upright position. If the child has a gastrostomy tube, it is important to maintain skin integrity around the stoma site.[6]

Discharge planning focuses on instructing parents in how to feed and position the infant (e.g., avoid use of infant seat[7]), as well as providing comfort and emotional support. Encourage parents to hold and cuddle the infant during all feedings. Providing the infant with a pacifier helps to meet nonnutritive sucking needs. Teach parents how to suction the nose and mouth if vomiting occurs.

■ NURSING ALERT

Do not place an infant with gastroesophageal reflux in an infant seat. The infant's position in this type of seat increases intraabdominal pressure and will actually worsen the condition.

Omphalocele

Omphaloceles are congenital malformations in which intraabdominal contents herniate through the umbilical cord (Fig. 15–4). They result from failure of the abdominal contents to return to the abdomen when the abdominal wall begins to close by the tenth week of gestation. The protrusion is covered by a translucent sac into which the umbilical cord inserts. Omphalocele is often associated with other congenital anomalies such as cardiac defects, genitourinary anomalies, tracheoesophageal fistula, and imperforate anus.[1]

The size of the sac varies depending on the extent of the protrusion. Rupture of the sac results in evisceration of the abdominal contents. Treatment involves immediate surgical repair to replace the abdominal contents and close the abdominal wall.[1] If the defect is severe, surgical correction may be performed in two steps. If an omphalocele occurs without associated defects, the prognosis is good.

FIGURE 15-4 In omphalocele, the size of the sac depends on the extent of the protrusion of abdominal contents through the umbilical cord.

From Rudolph, A.M., Hoffman, J.I.E., & Rudolph, C.D. (1991). *Rudolph's pediatrics* (19th ed.) (p. 1040). Norwalk, CT: Appleton & Lange.

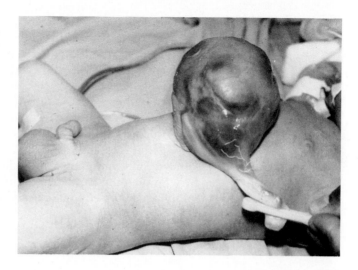

Nursing Management

Immediately after birth, the sac is covered with sterile gauze soaked in normal saline solution to prevent drying of the abdominal contents. A layer of plastic wrap is placed over the gauze to provide additional protection against heat and moisture loss. Monitor vital signs every 2 to 4 hours, and inspect the area for signs of infection.

Because the infant is NPO preoperatively, fluid and electrolyte balance is maintained by administering intravenous fluids. Postoperative care includes measures to control pain, prevent infection, maintain fluid and electrolyte balance, and ensure adequate nutritional intake.

Throughout the infant's hospitalization, parents need clear, accurate explanations about the infant's condition. To help the parents deal with the crisis of an acutely ill newborn, provide emotional support and encourage them to express their feelings.

Intussusception

Intussusception occurs when one portion of the intestine invaginates or telescopes into another. It is one of the most frequent causes of intestinal obstruction during infancy and most often occurs in boys between the ages of 3 months and 3 years.

The onset is usually abrupt. A previously healthy infant suddenly experiences acute abdominal pain with vomiting and passage of brown stool. As the condition worsens, the stools become red and resemble currant jelly because of the mix of blood and mucus. A palpable mass may be present in the upper right quadrant of the abdomen.

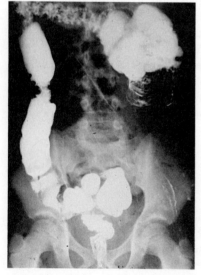

FIGURE 15-5 In infants, intussusception is commonly associated with measles, viral diseases, and gastroenteritis syndromes.

Copyright © MEDCOM, Inc., Garden Grove, CA.

The most common site of intussusception is the ileocecal valve (Fig. 15-5). Telescoping of the intestine obstructs the passage of stool. The walls of the intestine rub together, causing inflammation, edema, and decreased blood flow. This can lead to necrosis, perforation, hemorrhage, and peritonitis.

Diagnosis may be made on the basis of the history and confirmed by a barium enema. In some cases the hydrostatic pressure from the barium moves the bowel back into place. If this does not occur, surgical intervention to reduce the invaginated bowel and remove any necrotic tissue is necessary. The prognosis is good with early intervention.

Nursing Management

Nursing management focuses on maintaining or restoring fluid and electrolyte balance. Intravenous fluids are started immediately. Serum electrolyte monitoring is essential to correct imbalances.

Postoperative care focuses on monitoring for early signs of infection, managing the child's pain, and maintaining nasogastric tube patency. Assess vital signs, check for abdominal distention, and listen for bowel sounds every 4 hours. After normal bowel function returns, clear liquid feedings are begun. Feedings are advanced as the infant progresses.

Discharge usually occurs shortly after the infant begins taking full feedings. Instruct parents to watch for infection and to call the physician if symptoms recur, a fever develops, or appetite decreases.

Hirschsprung Disease

Hirschsprung disease, also known as congenital aganglionic megacolon, is a congenital anomaly in which inadequate motility causes mechanical obstruction of the intestine. The absence of autonomic parasympathetic ganglion cells in the colon prevents peristalsis at that portion of the intestine, resulting in accumulation of intestinal contents and abdominal distention. Hirschsprung disease is more common in boys and in children with Down syndrome. It can be acute or chronic.

Clinical manifestations vary depending on the child's age at onset. In newborns symptoms include failure to pass meconium, refusal to suck, abdominal distention, and bile-stained emesis. If Hirschsprung disease is not treated, the condition can lead to complete obstruction, respiratory distress, and shock.

In the older child symptoms may include failure to gain weight and delayed growth. The child may have a history of abdominal distention, severe constipation alternating with diarrhea, and vomiting.

Diagnosis is made on the basis of the history, bowel patterns, and radiographic contrast studies. Treatment in infancy involves surgical removal of the aganglionic bowel. A temporary colostomy is created to rest the bowel. Closure of the colostomy and reanastomosis are performed when the child reaches a weight of approximately 10 kg. For the child with a milder defect, management may involve dietary modification, stool softeners, and isotonic irrigations to prevent impaction until the child is toilet trained.

The prognosis is usually good. The return of normal bowel function depends on the amount of bowel involved. Some fecal incontinence and constipation may persist following closure of the colostomy.

NURSING ALERT

Because newborns are often discharged within 24 hours of birth, it is important to describe to parents the characteristics of infants' first bowel movements. Parents should be instructed to notify the physician if no stool is passed or if the abdomen becomes distended.

Nursing Management

Nursing assessment in the newborn period includes careful observation for the passage of meconium. When the disease is diagnosed later in infancy or in childhood, obtain a thorough history of weight gain, nutritional intake, and bowel habits.

Nursing management consists of carefully monitoring fluid and electrolyte balance and maintaining nutrition. Teach parents how to ensure regular bowel movements. Daily rectal irrigations with normal saline solution are necessary to promote adequate elimination and prevent obstruction. Teach parents how to prevent skin breakdown in the rectal area. Instruct parents to change diapers frequently, to cleanse the area carefully, and to apply protective ointment at each diaper change.

If surgical correction is necessary, nursing care will include monitoring for infection, managing pain, maintaining hydration, measuring abdominal circumference to detect any distention, and providing support to the child and family. Parents will need instruction in ostomy care (refer to the discussion later in this chapter). Provide appropriate referrals to an ostomy support group and enterostomal nurse specialist.

Anorectal Malformations

Malformations of the anus and rectum are common congenital anomalies. Minor anomalies occur as frequently as 1 in 500 births. More severe anomalies occur once in every 5000 births, usually in association with anomalies of the urinary tract, esophagus, and duodenum.[1] Table 15–2 describes the most common anorectal anomalies.

Diagnosis is usually made at birth or during the newborn assessment of anorectal structures and rectal patency. Failure to pass meconium may indicate a malformation higher in the colon. Stool in the urine is indicative of a fistula between the colon and urinary tract. Ultrasound and lower GI x-ray studies are used to confirm the diagnosis and demonstrate the extent of the anomaly.

Medical management depends on the extent of the malformation. An imperforate anal membrane (Fig. 15–6) is excised surgically, followed by daily manual dilations. More severe defects require reconstructive surgery. A temporary colostomy is sometimes performed to rest the bowel after reconstruction. Closure of the colostomy is generally performed between the age of 6 months and 1 year.

Nursing Management

During the initial newborn assessment, the perineal area is inspected for a poorly developed anal dimple or sacral anomalies. A rectal thermometer is lubricated and inserted a short distance into the rectum to determine patency. Observation and recording of passage of meconium are essential.

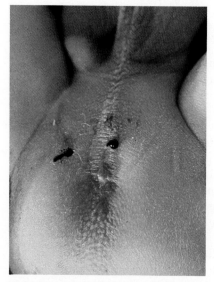

FIGURE 15–6 Imperforate anus, which is usually obvious at birth, can range from mild stenosis to a complex syndrome that includes associated congenital anomalies.

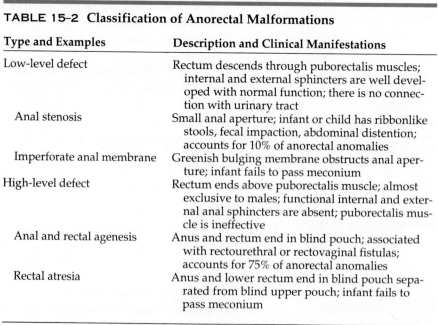

TABLE 15–2 Classification of Anorectal Malformations

Type and Examples	Description and Clinical Manifestations
Low-level defect	Rectum descends through puborectalis muscles; internal and external sphincters are well developed with normal function; there is no connection with urinary tract
Anal stenosis	Small anal aperture; infant or child has ribbonlike stools, fecal impaction, abdominal distention; accounts for 10% of anorectal anomalies
Imperforate anal membrane	Greenish bulging membrane obstructs anal aperture; infant fails to pass meconium
High-level defect	Rectum ends above puborectalis muscle; almost exclusive to males; functional internal and external anal sphincters are absent; puborectalis muscle is ineffective
Anal and rectal agenesis	Anus and rectum end in blind pouch; associated with rectourethral or rectovaginal fistulas; accounts for 75% of anorectal anomalies
Rectal atresia	Anus and lower rectum end in blind pouch separated from blind upper pouch; infant fails to pass meconium

Compiled from Hathaway W.E., Hay, W.W. Jr., Groothuis, J.R., & Paisley, J.W. (1991). *Current pediatric diagnosis and treatment* (7th ed.). Norwalk, CT: Appleton & Lange.

Once the diagnosis has been made, intravenous fluids are initiated and a nasogastric tube is inserted to decompress the stomach. Provide emotional support to the parents.

Postoperative care centers on preventing infection and other complications and maintaining hydration. Observe the incision for signs of infection, and provide careful wound care. Assess temperature every 4 hours.

Discharge Planning and Patient and Family Home Care Teaching. Teach parents how to take the infant's temperature using the axillary route. Have them demonstrate the proper technique before discharge. Explain signs and symptoms of infection. Discuss feeding regimens and bowel habits necessary to maintain adequate nutrition for growth and development. Advise parents that children with anorectal malformations often have difficulty achieving bowel control. Patience in toilet training is important.

If a colostomy is performed, teach parents how to care for the ostomy site (see discussion of ostomies later in this chapter). Discuss follow-up care and long-term management.

Hernias

A **hernia** is the protrusion or projection of an organ or a part of an organ through the muscle wall of the cavity that normally contains it. This protrusion may result from the failure of normal openings to close during fetal development or from weakness in the supporting musculature. When intraabdominal pressure increases (as when the infant cries or strains to pass stool), the weakened area separates, causing a protrusion of underlying organs. Inguinal hernias are the most common type of hernia occurring in children (see Chapter 18). Other hernias that occur frequently in children are diaphragmatic and umbilical.[8]

Diaphragmatic Hernia

In a diaphragmatic hernia, abdominal contents protrude into the thoracic cavity through an opening. Most often herniation occurs through the foramen of Bochdalek. This type of hernia usually results from failure of the pleuroperitoneal canal to close completely during embryonic development.

Diaphragmatic hernia is a life-threatening condition. Severe respiratory distress occurs shortly after birth. As the infant cries, abdominal organs expand, decreasing the size of the thoracic cavity. The infant becomes dyspneic and cyanotic. Characteristic findings include a barrel-shaped chest and sunken abdomen.

Diagnosis is confirmed by chest x-ray examination. Immediate respiratory support is essential. The infant is positioned with the head and thorax higher than the abdomen to facilitate downward movement of abdominal organs. A nasogastric tube is inserted to decompress the stomach. Ventilator support is necessary to manage respiratory compromise. Intravenous fluids are administered through an umbilical artery catheter. Once the infant's condition is stabilized, surgery is performed to correct the defect.

The prognosis is poor. The survival rate is 50%, with death usually resulting from pulmonary hydroplasia.[4]

Nursing Management

The infant with a diaphragmatic hernia requires continuous monitoring and is usually admitted to the NICU. Preoperative management centers on providing supportive care to the infant and parents. Note the infant's vital signs every 30 minutes on the cardiorespiratory monitor. Observe for worsening of respiratory compromise. Maintain intravenous fluid administration. Promote decreased stimulation to keep the infant calm and thus maintain low abdominal pressure. Keep parents informed about the infant's condition, and provide emotional support both before and after surgery.

Postoperative care includes positioning the infant on the affected side to facilitate expansion of the lung on the unaffected side, observing closely for signs of infection, and carefully monitoring fluid and electrolyte balance.

Before discharge, instruct parents in wound care, prevention of infection, and feeding techniques.

Umbilical Hernia

An umbilical hernia results from imperfect closure or weakness of the umbilical ring (Fig. 15–7). The condition is often associated with diastasis recti (lateral separation of the abdominal muscles). It is common in black children in the first year of life.[4]

The hernia appears as a soft swelling covered by skin. The herniated area protrudes with coughing, crying, or straining during a bowel movement. It is easily reduced by pushing the bowel back through the fibrous ring. The size of the defect may vary among individuals. Contents of the hernia include omentum or portions of the small intestine.

Most defects resolve spontaneously by 2 years of age. Surgery is indicated in cases of strangulation (closure of the umbilical ring around a portion of the bowel, preventing it from moving back into the abdomen), increased protrusion of the hernia after the age of 2 years, or little or no improvement in a large defect after the age of 4 years.[4]

Nursing management is generally supportive. Instruct parents not to use tapes, straps, or coins to reduce the hernia. This can cause strangulation of the hernia, necessitating immediate surgery. If surgery is required, it is usually performed in a short-stay unit. Postoperatively, teach parents how to care for the surgical site, to watch for bleeding, and to recognize signs of infection. Reinforce the importance of returning for follow-up.

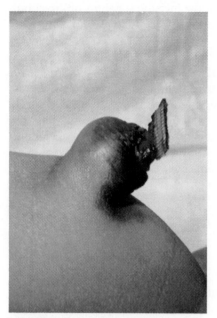

FIGURE 15-7 The umbilical hernia of the newborn usually closes as the muscles grow in later infancy and childhood.

From Zitelli, B.J., & Davis, H.W. (Eds.) (1987). *Atlas of pediatric physical diagnosis* (p. 2.10). New York: Mosby–Year Book Europe Ltd.

Inflammatory Disorders

Inflammatory disorders are reactions of specific tissues of the GI tract to trauma caused by injuries, foreign bodies, chemicals, microorganisms, or surgery. These disorders may be acute or chronic and may involve various segments of the GI tract.

Appendicitis

Appendicitis is an inflammation of the vermiform appendix, the small sac near the end of the cecum. Appendicitis occurs most often in adolescent boys (10 to 15 years of age). It is rarely seen before 5 years of age.

Clinical Manifestations

At onset, symptoms include midabdominal cramps, abdominal tenderness, and fever. In adolescent and young adult females, symptoms must be differentiated from those associated with ovulation (mittelschmerz), ruptured ectopic pregnancy, and pelvic inflammatory disease.[1] As the inflammation progresses, the pain in the right lower abdomen becomes constant. Pain is most intense at the McBurney point (halfway between the anterior superior iliac crest and the umbilicus). Symptoms progress to include rigidity and rebound tenderness following palpation over the right lower quadrant.

Vomiting, diarrhea, or constipation may be present. As the appendicitis progresses, the child remains motionless, usually in a side-lying position with knees flexed.

Etiology and Pathophysiology

Appendicitis almost always results from an obstruction in the appendiceal lumen. It can be caused by a fecalith (hard fecal mass), parasitic infestations, stenosis, hyperplasia of lymphoid tissue, or a tumor. Continued secretion of mucus following acute obstruction of the lumen increases pressure, causing ischemia, cellular death, and ulceration. Perforation or rupture of the appendix may occur, resulting in fecal and bacterial contamination of the peritoneum. Peritonitis spreads quickly and if untreated can result in small bowel obstruction, electrolyte imbalances, septicemia, and hypovolemic shock.[1]

Diagnostic Tests and Medical Management

An elevated white blood cell count (between 15,000 and 20,000/mm^3), in combination with a history of abdominal pain, is indicative of appendicitis. X-ray studies may identify the presence of a fecalith. An abdominal ultrasound may be helpful in locating an abscess.

Treatment involves immediate surgical removal (appendectomy). Preoperatively the child is kept NPO. Intravenous fluids, electrolytes, and antibiotics are administered. A nasogastric tube may be inserted before or after surgery. Postoperatively the child has an abdominal incision, and intravenous antibiotics are administered to prevent infection. If the appendix has ruptured before surgery, a Penrose drain is inserted and the wound may not be completely sutured. Wound irrigations may be needed to assist with cleansing of the peritoneum. The prognosis is good following uncomplicated removal of the appendix.

Nursing Assessment

Physiologic Assessment. A detailed pain assessment is necessary to differentiate appendicitis from other less serious illnesses (see Chapter 5). Ask the child to point to the painful area and to describe the pain. Note onset, location, and intensity of pain, precipitating factors, and relief measures tried. During abdominal assessment, perform light palpation last to avoid causing additional pain. Assess vital signs to determine baseline values, and monitor every 4 hours thereafter.

Psychosocial Assessment. Because appendicitis usually occurs in school-age children and adolescents, assessment of the child's coping skills is important. Adolescents, because of their preoccupation with body image, may be concerned about the surgical scar. Assess the parents' and child's anxiety about the sudden hospitalization and need for emergency surgery.

Nursing Diagnosis

Common nursing diagnoses for the child with appendicitis before surgery include:

- Pain related to inflammatory process

■ NURSING ALERT

Signs and symptoms of a ruptured appendix include:
- Fever
- Sudden relief from abdominal pain
- Guarding
- Abdominal distention
- Rapid shallow breathing
- Pallor
- Chills
- Irritability or restlessness

- High Risk for Fluid Volume Deficit related to vomiting
- Anxiety/Fear related to hospitalization, multiple painful procedures, and potential surgery

Postoperative nursing diagnoses might include:

- Pain related to abdominal incision
- High Risk for Infection related to incision, compromised skin integrity, and bowel manipulation
- High Risk for Ineffective Airway Clearance related to general anesthesia and incisional pain
- Anxiety (Parent and Child) related to child's sudden hospitalization and surgery

Nursing Management

Nursing management focuses on promoting comfort, maintaining hydration, providing emotional support, supporting respiratory function, providing care of the surgical site, and monitoring for symptoms of infection.

Promote Comfort. A side-lying position with knees bent is usually the most comfortable. Administer analgesics (preferably intravenously), and note relief from pain. Postoperative pain is managed in a similar manner. The child should be placed in a semi-Fowler or side-lying position on the right side. If the appendix has ruptured, lying on the right side facilitates drainage from the peritoneal cavity. Encourage the child to ask for pain medication when needed. Reassure the child that pain medication does not need to be given via intramuscular injection but can be administered through the existing intravenous line.

Maintain Hydration. Assess fluid volume status every 4 hours. Assess skin turgor, eyes, and mucous membranes for signs of dehydration. Monitor intake and output, and assess vital signs. An intravenous infusion is initiated preoperatively and continued until bowel function returns after surgery. Once bowel sounds return, offer water in small amounts and then other clear fluids.

Provide Emotional Support. For many children, this may be their first hospitalization and their first experience with health care personnel beyond their pediatrician's office. The nurse must elicit a history, perform a physical examination, coordinate diagnostic tests, and prepare the child for surgery in a short period of time. Emotional support is essential for both child and parents. Good preoperative education can reduce anxiety. Answer any questions the child or parents may have.

Support Respiratory Function. General anesthesia during surgery compromises respiratory function. It is important for the child to turn, cough, and breathe deeply to prevent atelectasis. Encourage the child to splint the incision area with a pillow during coughing to decrease pain.

Recognize Symptoms of Infection. Assess vital signs and observe the abdominal incision every 4 hours for erythema, edema, or drainage. If a drain is present, assess drainage for color, consistency, and amount. After the initial dressing has been changed, change dressings frequently and keep the incision area clean and dry. Administer antibiotics as prescribed.

Discharge Planning and Patient and Family Home Care Teaching. The child is discharged once bowel function returns and the child has a bowel move-

■ **NURSING ALERT**

Use of a heating pad is contraindicated in children with appendicitis. Heat will only increase the inflammation and may contribute to rupture of the bowel.

ment. Give parents instructions on reestablishing a nutritious diet slowly and as tolerated. Teach parents to recognize signs and symptoms of infection and to seek early treatment. Normal activities can be resumed fairly quickly, but strenuous activities and contact sports should be avoided in the immediate postoperative period. Parents should check with the child's physician before allowing the child to resume sports activities. Home tutoring may be needed for a short time so the child can keep up with schoolwork.

Necrotizing Enterocolitis

Necrotizing enterocolitis is a potentially life-threatening inflammatory disease of the intestinal tract that occurs primarily in premature infants.[1,9,10] It can be caused by several factors, including intestinal ischemia, bacterial or viral infection, and immaturity of the gut.

The infant may initially show signs of feeding intolerance (increased gastric residuals, vomiting, irritability, and abdominal distention). These signs are caused by inflammation and dilation of the bowel and accumulation of gas in the intestine. Bloody diarrhea may be present because of the hemorrhagic bowel. Signs of sepsis usually follow, and the infant's condition rapidly deteriorates.

Diagnosis is made on the basis of characteristic clinical findings and the presence of free peritoneal gas seen on abdominal x-rays. Necrotizing enterocolitis requires prompt intervention. Management begins with discontinuation of all enteral feedings. A nasogastric tube is inserted to prevent gastric distention, and intravenous fluids are started. Antibiotics are administered prophylactically or to treat sepsis. Perforation or necrosis of the bowel necessitates surgical resection of the bowel. An ileostomy or colostomy may be performed. Complications of necrotizing enterocolitis following intestinal resection include short bowel syndrome, infection or blockage of the central venous catheter, and cholestatic jaundice.[1]

Nursing Management

Nursing care centers on early detection of necrotizing enterocolitis to minimize bowel loss and providing postoperative care. Measure abdominal circumference in the premature or high-risk infant every 4 to 8 hours (see Fig. 7–12). Even minimal changes in circumference can indicate necrotizing enterocolitis and should be reported to the physician. Watch for feeding intolerance by aspirating gastric residual (if the infant is receiving enteral feedings).

Maintaining fluid and electrolyte balance is essential. Provide comfort by holding and cuddling an infant who is NPO, and offer a pacifier to meet non-nutritive sucking needs. Careful assessment for infection and maintenance of skin integrity are essential. Feedings are gradually reestablished once bowel function returns.

Parents need emotional support and reassurance and help in bonding with their infant. They are coping with the birth of an infant who is critically ill. Since the symptoms of necrotizing enterocolitis do not appear until approximately 5 to 7 days after feedings are begun, parents may not be prepared for the infant's decline. The recovery of a premature infant is slow and can be complicated. Give clear explanations and encourage parents to ask questions and express their fears and concerns.

Meckel Diverticulum

Meckel diverticulum results when the omphalomesenteric duct, which connects the midgut to the yolk sac during embryonic development, fails to atrophy. Instead, an outpouching of the ileum remains, usually located near the ileocecal valve. The pouch contains gastric or pancreatic tissue, which secretes acid, causing irritation and ulceration. Meckel diverticulum is the most common gastrointestinal malformation and occurs in 1% to 3% of the population. It is more common in males.[1,4,10]

Clinical manifestations usually appear by 2 years of age. The most common sign is painless dark or bright red rectal bleeding, which results from the obstruction or ulceration. Often blood is passed without stool. Abdominal pain is uncommon, but when it occurs, it may resemble the pain of appendicitis. The child may have symptoms of intussusception, incarcerated hernia, volvulus, or intestinal obstruction. If untreated, diverticulitis may progress to perforation and peritonitis.

Diagnosis is based on the history. Contrast studies are usually not helpful because the diverticulum is often too small to visualize and may not fill with barium. Radionuclide imaging and scanning can usually detect the gastric tissue, confirming the diagnosis. Treatment is surgical excision of the diverticulum and removal of any involved bowel. The prognosis is good following surgical excision.

Nursing Management

Preoperatively an intravenous infusion is initiated to correct fluid and electrolyte imbalances. Monitor intake and output. Observe for rectal bleeding, and test stools for occult blood. The child should be kept on bed rest. Assess vital signs every 2 to 4 hours, and monitor for signs of shock. Postoperative care is similar to that for an infant or child undergoing abdominal surgery. (See the earlier discussion of postsurgical nursing management of appendicitis and the Nursing Care Plan for the Child Undergoing Surgery in Chapter 4.)

At the time of discharge, parents need instructions on caring for the surgical site, preventing infection, providing an adequate diet, and administering prescribed medications.

Inflammatory Bowel Disease

Inflammatory bowel disease encompasses two distinct chronic disorders, Crohn disease and ulcerative colitis, that have similar symptoms and treatment.

Crohn disease is a chronic, inflammatory process. It may occur randomly throughout the GI tract, but in 90% of cases involves mainly the small intestine.[4,8,11] A distinct feature of Crohn disease is the development of enteric fistulas between loops of bowel or nearby organs. The etiology is unknown. There is strong evidence to support a genetic association.[4] Crohn disease is more common in whites and three to six times more prevalent in individuals of Jewish descent. It most often develops between 15 and 25 years of age.[4,8]

The onset of Crohn disease is subtle. Crampy abdominal pain is usually reported first, followed by diarrhea. Other symptoms include fever, anorexia, growth failure, general malaise, and joint pain. Diagnosis is based on laboratory evaluation and radiologic and biopsy examinations.

Ulcerative colitis is a chronic recurrent disease of the colon and rectal mucosa of unknown etiology. Inflammation is limited to the mucosa and can involve the entire length of the bowel with varying degrees of ulceration, hemorrhage, and edema. Emotional and other psychosocial factors may influence the presentation and course of the disease.[4] It is more prevalent among persons of Jewish heritage. The disease develops before 20 years of age with peak onset in adolescence.[11]

TABLE 15-3 Comparison of Ulcerative Colitis and Crohn Disease

	Ulcerative Colitis	Crohn Disease
Type of lesions	Continuous, superficial involvement	Segmental, transmural (through the wall) involvement
Clinical manifestations		
Anal or perianal lesions	Rare	Common
Anorexia	Mild to moderate	Can be severe
Diarrhea	Often severe	Moderate
Growth retardation	Mild	Significant
Pain	Present	Common
Rectal bleeding	Present	Absent
Weight loss	Moderate	Severe
Risk of cancer	Slightly increased	Greatly increased

The first symptom of ulcerative colitis usually is diarrhea. Lower abdominal pain and cramping are present before and during a bowel movement and are relieved by the passage of stool and flatus. The stool is often mixed with blood and mucus.

Diagnosis centers on evaluating the cause and identifying the extent of involved bowel and differentiating an infectious process (organisms such as *Shigella* and *Salmonella*) from ulcerative colitis. Endoscopy with biopsy is helpful to determine the extent and severity of the inflammatory process.[1,11]

Table 15–3 presents a comparison of the features of Crohn disease and ulcerative colitis. Both diseases have periods of remission and exacerbation. Treatment for both diseases includes pharmacologic interventions (administration of antibiotic, antiinflammatory, and antidiarrheal medications), nutrition therapy, and surgery. Corticosteroids are given orally and in the form of enemas to children with more severe disease. For children with milder disease, sulfasalazine has been shown to decrease the number of relapses.

The goal of nutrition therapy is to provide adequate caloric intake and nutrients necessary for growth. Vitamin, iron, zinc, and folic acid replacement is frequently required. Total parenteral nutrition (TPN) is often given to treat nutritional deficiencies and malnutrition, which accompany inflammatory bowel disease. A high-protein, high-carbohydrate, low-fiber diet with normal amounts of fat is recommended.

If other treatment measures fail to reduce inflammation, surgery is indicated. A temporary colostomy or ileostomy is performed to allow the bowel to rest. In Crohn disease, however, ulcerations tend to recur elsewhere in the GI tract. In ulcerative colitis, removal of the diseased bowel provides a permanent cure.

■ **NURSING ALERT**

Corticosteroids can decrease a child's immune response and alter growth. Immunizations (especially for polio) are contraindicated when steroids are being administered.

Nursing Management

Nursing management focuses on helping the child and family adjust to the emotional impact of a chronic disease, administering medications and diet therapy, and providing appropriate referrals. Provide emotional support and counseling to help the child adjust to feeling "different" from peers. Inability to compete with peers and frequent absences from school can affect the child's self-esteem. Encourage the hospitalized child to maintain contact with friends through telephone calls, cards, and visits.

If the child is unable to eat or the intake of calories is insufficient to meet

■ CLINICAL TIP

Instruct parents to continue to provide frequent small meals and avoid a three-meal-a-day pattern when the child returns home.

basic nutritional and metabolic needs, TPN will be ordered. If the child is able to eat, offer small, frequent, high-calorie meals or snacks. High-fiber foods should be avoided because they irritate the already inflamed bowel. Refer the parents and child to a nutritionist.

Body image is a major concern for children and adolescents with inflammatory bowel disease. Steroid therapy causes growth retardation and delayed sexual maturation. Encourage the child to discuss feelings about these side effects. If a permanent colostomy or ileostomy is required, the nurse can assist the child and family to understand the need for surgical treatment. (See the discussion of ostomies that follows.) Introduce the child and family to other children who have stomas.

Discharge planning is essential for children with ulcerative colitis and Crohn disease. Teach parents about medication administration and diet therapy. Reinforce to both the parents and child the importance of adhering to a strict medication regimen. Emphasize that medications should be continued even when the child is asymptomatic. Discuss the side effects of the drugs and what to do if any of these symptoms occur.

Parents also will need instructions for TPN and care of a central venous catheter, including dressing changes, sterile and nonsterile techniques, signs of infection, how to handle infusion pumps and tubing, and how to measure the child's intake and output. Assist parents in obtaining equipment and supplies necessary for the child's care. Be sure that parents demonstrate their mastery of care for the central venous catheter and understand TPN techniques before discharge.

Refer parents to social services, the visiting nurse association, and home health care agencies. For information about inflammatory bowel disease, refer families to the Crohn's Colitis Foundation (see Appendix F). Have the parents contact the school district to arrange for tutoring in case extended absences from school become necessary.

Peptic Ulcer

A peptic ulcer is an erosion of the mucosal tissue in the lower end of the esophagus, in the stomach (usually along the lesser curvature), or in the duodenum. Boys are more likely to have peptic ulcers than girls. Children with type O blood or a family history of peptic ulcer disease also have an increased incidence.[12,13]

Clinical manifestations vary according to the age of the child and location of the ulcer. The most common symptom is abdominal pain (burning) associated with an empty stomach, which may awaken the child at night. Vomiting after meals, anemia, **occult blood** in stools, and abdominal distention may also be present.

Ulcers are classified as primary or secondary, depending on their etiology. Primary peptic ulcers occur in healthy children. Secondary (stress) ulcers occur in children with a preexisting illness or injury (often a burn) and in children receiving medications such as salicylates, corticosteroids, and nonsteroidal antiinflammatory drugs.[4] Diet usually is not a major factor in the development of peptic ulcers in children, although caffeine and alcohol consumption in adolescents may exacerbate the disease.[1]

Diagnosis is based on the history and radiologic studies. The goals of medical management are to relieve discomfort and promote healing. A combination of antacids in liquid form (Maalox, Mylanta) and histamine antagonists (ranitidine, cimetidine, and famotidine) is used. Sucralfate may also be given. The prognosis is usually good with early intervention.

Nursing Management

Nursing care centers on interventions to promote adequate nutritional intake, promote healing, and prevent recurrences. A nutritionally sound, age-appropriate diet is developed. Foods should be omitted only if they exacerbate the disorder.

Emphasize the importance of continuing drug therapy after discharge. Children who attend school may prefer antacids in the form of tablets, which are easier to carry than liquid preparations. Parents should check with the child's physician before giving any additional medication. Caution parents to avoid aspirin products, which irritate the gastric mucosa. If an antipyretic or pain medication is needed, acetaminophen should be given. Advise parents to read medication labels if they are unsure of product contents.

Because psychologic stress can contribute to peptic ulcer disease, parents and child should be assisted to identify sources of stress in the child's life. Assess coping mechanisms and provide referral for psychologic counseling, if appropriate.

Ostomies

An **ostomy** is an opening into the small or large intestine that diverts fecal matter to provide an outlet for stool when a distal surgical anastomosis, obstruction, or nonfunctioning bowel prevents normal bowel elimination. Depending on the integrity and function of anatomic structures, the ostomy may be temporary or permanent.[14] Infants and small children with necrotizing enterocolitis, Hirschsprung disease, volvulus, or intussusception may require a temporary colostomy or ileostomy. Ostomies may also be indicated for children with inflammatory bowel disease, intestinal tumors, or abdominal trauma.

An ostomy may be elective or a surgical emergency. In all cases it affects a child's life-style, alters body image, causes anxiety, and increases the risk for alterations in physiologic processes (electrolyte imbalance, increased nutritional requirements). For adolescents, it may also result in dependence at a time when autonomy is a major developmental need.

In assessing the family and child approaching ostomy surgery, it is important to determine their ability to understand and accept the physical changes that will occur. Parents may feel guilt and anger about the ostomy surgery when the child has a genetically transmitted disease, has sustained an injury, or has developed an obstruction from necrosis of the bowel. Encourage the parents and child to express their feelings, and correct any misunderstandings. Parents and older children may be referred for counseling and to support groups to help them deal with their feelings. Adolescents often benefit from a visit with an adolescent ostomate (someone who has an ostomy) who can answer questions about living with an ostomy.

Preoperative Care

Preoperative education focuses on educating the child and family and preparing them for postoperative management. Discuss how the appliance will look, and explain the purpose of the pouch in developmentally appropriate terms. Encourage the parents and child to touch and manipulate all equipment. A younger child can be shown how to place a pouch on a doll. Older children can practice placing a pouch on their skin. These measures help relieve anxiety by providing information and increasing familiarity with the appliance.

In addition to discussion of the appliance, preoperative education should include discussion of pain control and measures that will be used to prevent postoperative complications (turning, coughing, and breathing deeply). Instructions should be geared to the child's developmental level. Encourage parental participation to promote compliance.

Postoperative Care

Postoperative care of a child with an ostomy is similar to that for any child who undergoes abdominal surgery. (See the earlier discussion of nursing management for appendicitis and the Nursing Care Plan for the Child Undergoing Surgery in Chapter 4.) Home care needs should be identified and addressed well in advance of discharge. Instructions include skin care, care of the stoma, appliance removal and application, and frequency of appliance changes. Teaching should begin immediately after surgery with responsibility for care transferred gradually to the parents and child as they are ready. (For information on caring for an ostomy, refer to the section on elimination in the Atlas of Pediatric Procedures.) Discuss diet, activity level, hygiene, clothing, equipment, and financial considerations.

Parents and children can be referred to the United Ostomy Association (see Appendix F) or a local ostomy group for information and support. Referrals should be made to social service, counseling, and a home health agency if appropriate.

Disorders of Motility

Fluids are produced in large quantities as part of normal GI functioning. As food passes through the intestines, fluids are reabsorbed and moderately soft stool is formed and evacuated. In disorders such as diarrhea and constipation, fluid production is altered, causing either more or less fluid to be reabsorbed. This can severely alter the characteristics of the stool. Reabsorption of too little water produces watery stools (**diarrhea**) and can lead to fluid and electrolyte alterations. Reabsorption of too much fluid can cause **constipation,** which if untreated can lead to bowel obstruction.

Gastroenteritis (Acute Diarrhea)

Gastroenteritis is an inflammation of the stomach and intestines that may be accompanied by vomiting and diarrhea. It can affect any part of the GI tract. Diarrhea is a common problem in children. It may be an acute problem, caused by viral, bacterial, or parasitic infections, or a chronic problem. Infants and small children with gastroenteritis or diarrhea can quickly become dehydrated and are at risk for hypovolemic shock if fluid and electrolyte losses are not replaced (see Chapter 7).

Clinical Manifestations

Diarrhea may be mild, moderate, or severe. In mild diarrhea, stools are slightly increased in number and have a more liquid consistency. In moderate diarrhea the child has several loose or watery stools. Other symptoms include irritability, anorexia, nausea, and vomiting. Moderate diarrhea is usually self-limiting, resolving without treatment within 1 or 2 days. In severe diarrhea, watery stools are continuous. The child exhibits symptoms of fluid and electrolyte imbalance, has cramping, and is extremely irritable and difficult to console.

TABLE 15–4 Causes of Diarrhea in Children

Causative Factor	Effect on Bowel Function
Emotional stress (anxiety, fatigue)	Increased motility
Intestinal infection (bacteria [*E. coli, Salmonella, Shigella*], viral [human rotavirus, enteric adenovirus] fungal overgrowth)	Inflammation of mucosa; increased mucus secretion in colon
Food sensitivity (gluten, cow's milk)	Decreased digestion of food
Food intolerance (lactose, introduction of new foods, overfeeding)	Increased motility; increased mucus secretion in colon
Medications (iron, antibiotics)	Irritation and suprainfection
Colon disease (colitis, necrotizing enterocolitis, enterocolitis)	Inflammation and ulceration of intestinal walls; reduced absorption of fluid; increased intestinal motility
Surgical alterations (short bowel syndrome)	Reduced size of colon; decreased absorption surface

Etiology and Pathophysiology

Diarrhea in children can have many different causes (Table 15–4).[15] The specific etiology is not always identified. The common mechanism is a decrease in the absorptive capacity of the bowel through inflammation, decrease in surface area for absorption, or alteration of parasympathetic innervation.

Diagnostic Tests and Medical Management

Diagnosis is based on the history, physical examination, and laboratory findings. A thorough history may help in identifying the causative factor. Ask parents about recent exposure to illnesses, use of antibiotics, travel, food and formula preparation, food sensitivities or allergies, and whether the child attends day care. Physical examination provides a guide to the severity of dehydration (see Chapter 7). The stool is examined for the presence of ova, parasites, infectious organisms, viruses, fat, and undigested sugars. Laboratory evaluation of serum and urine helps in recognizing electrolyte imbalances and other deficiencies.

Medical management depends on the severity of the diarrhea and fluid and electrolyte imbalances. The goal of treatment is to correct the fluid and electrolyte imbalances. For mild to moderate dehydration the child is rehydrated by means of oral replacement therapy. Commercially available solutions such as Pedialyte, Ricelyte, or Lytren are used for infants and young children; Gatorade is given to older children. Carbonated beverages and those containing sugar should not be given. Fermentation of sugar in the GI tract causes increased gas, abdominal distention, and increased frequency of diarrhea.

For severe dehydration, rehydration is accomplished by intravenous infusion with a solution chosen to correct the specific imbalances (see Chapter 7). The child is kept NPO to allow the bowel to rest. Once the dehydration has been corrected and the diarrhea has resolved, clear liquids are introduced. The child gradually progresses to a regular diet.

If the diarrhea is caused by bacteria or parasites, antimicrobial therapy may be prescribed. Absorbents such as Donnagel and Kaopectate will alter the appearance of stool but will not reduce the amount of fluid loss.

Nursing Assessment

The nurse usually encounters the child and family in the emergency department. If the child is hospitalized, it is important to assess onset, frequency, color, amount, and consistency of stools. If the child is also vomiting, monitor the amount and type of vomitus. Initial and ongoing physical assessment of the child focuses on observing for signs and symptoms of dehydration, which reflect underlying fluid and electrolyte status. Weigh the infant or child on admission and daily thereafter. Monitor vital signs every 2 to 4 hours. If the child is febrile, water loss will be increased, contributing to the dehydration. Assess skin integrity, especially in the perineal and rectal areas, and note any breakdown or rashes.

■ CLINICAL TIP

Avoid using commercial baby wipes when changing the diaper of an infant with diarrhea. Chemicals in the wipes may cause additional irritation and skin breakdown.

Nursing Diagnosis

The accompanying Nursing Care Plan lists common nursing diagnoses for a child with gastroenteritis. Other diagnoses that might also be appropriate include:

- Anxiety (Child and Parent) related to hospitalization
- Sleep Pattern Disturbance related to abdominal cramping and frequent bowel movements
- Altered Nutrition: Less Than Body Requirements related to inability to ingest sufficient nutrients and increased intestinal motility

Nursing Management

Nursing care focuses on relieving anxiety, promoting rest and comfort, and ensuring adequate nutrition. The accompanying Nursing Care Plan summarizes nursing care for the child with gastroenteritis.

Provide Emotional Support. The child may have been ill for several days or become suddenly ill a short time before admission. The child and parents are usually anxious, so it is important to allow them to talk and ask questions. The child may require frequent blood tests to help direct rehydration therapy. Using therapeutic play techniques, such as allowing the child to manipulate equipment, can reduce anxiety (see Chapter 4).[16] To promote a trusting relationship, be honest if a procedure will hurt. Encourage the child to express anger, fear, and pain.

Promote Rest and Comfort. Most children with gastroenteritis are quite ill and awaken frequently with periods of vomiting and diarrhea. Provide a quiet, restful environment. Darken the room and keep interruptions to a minimum. To reduce the child's anxiety, encourage parents to room-in. Place the child's favorite toys and comfort objects within reach. Keep the child's mouth moistened with a glycerine swab, a wet washcloth, or an occasional ice chip.

Ensure Adequate Nutrition. Once the dehydration has been corrected, clear liquids are offered. If tolerated, a lactose-free bland diet, such as the BRATS diet (bananas, rice cereal, applesauce, toast, and salted crackers), can be started. Infants are breast fed or given a lactose-free formula (Isomil, Nursoy, Prosobee) for a 1-week period. For older children a milk-free diet is recommended for 48 hours after symptoms have resolved. Oral feedings are started in the hospital and the child progresses to full feedings at home as tolerated.

Discharge Planning and Patient and Family Home Care Teaching. Discharge teaching should begin on admission. Instruct parents on what to expect as the child's GI system returns to normal function. Teach the parents about the symptoms of dehydration and what to do if diarrhea recurs. Be sure that parents understand the recommended diet progression. Refer them to a nutritionist, if necessary. Emphasize the necessity of good hygiene practices to prevent the spread of microorganisms that can cause gastroenteritis.

NURSING CARE PLAN — THE CHILD WITH GASTROENTERITIS

GOAL	INTERVENTION	RATIONALE	EXPECTED OUTCOME
1. Diarrhea related to altered gastrointestinal motility			
Child's bowel function will be restored to normal.	Obtain baseline vital signs and monitor every 2 to 4 hours.	Fluid and electrolyte imbalances can alter vital body functions.	Child's bowel function returns to normal.
	Observe stools for amount, color, consistency, odor, and frequency.	Aids in the diagnosis and in monitoring child's status.	
	Test stools for occult blood.	Frequent defecation and some infectious organisms can cause bleeding.	
	Monitor results of stool culture and sample for ova and parasites.	Rapid notification of the physician will facilitate treatment.	
	Wash hands well before and after contact with child.	Helps prevent transmission of microorganisms.	
	Isolate the child until the cause of the diarrhea is determined.	Prevents exposure of other patients and staff.	
	Assist child with toileting and hygiene.	Child may be weak, incontinent, physically impaired, or anxious and require assistance to use the bathroom.	
	Administer prescribed oral rehydration and intravenous solutions. Limit solid food intake.	Provides necessary fluids and nutrients while allowing the bowel to rest.	
	Notify the physician if diarrhea persists or characteristics change.	Ensures early intervention.	

Continued

GOAL	INTERVENTION	RATIONALE	EXPECTED OUTCOME

2. Fluid Volume Deficit related to diarrhea and vomiting

Child will remain hydrated and will begin to drink fluids within 24 hours of admission.	Monitor intake and output. Be sure to document time of each voiding.	Will determine if output exceeds input. Long periods of time without urine output can be an early indicator of poor renal function. A child should produce 1 mL of urine per kg per hour.	Child has normal fluid and electrolyte balance as indicated by laboratory evaluation and physical examination.
	Compare admission weight to preadmission weight. Assess weight daily.	The degree of dehydration can be determined by the percentage of weight loss. Daily weights aid in determining progress toward rehydration.	
	Assess level of consciousness, skin turgor, mucous membranes, skin color and temperature, capillary refill, eyes, and fontanels every 4 hours.	Will determine degree of hydration and adequacy of interventions.	
	Assess for vomiting.	Vomiting frequently accompanies diarrhea and contributes to child's fluid loss.	
	Provide oral fluid and electrolyte replacement solution if able to tolerate.	Less invasive than IV fluids. Provides for replacement of essential fluids and electrolytes.	
	Provide and maintain IV replacement therapy, as ordered.	Use of IV replacement is based on the degree of dehydration, ongoing losses, insensible water losses and electrolyte results.	

3. High Risk for Impaired Skin Integrity related to contact of skin with feces and frequent cleansing of skin

Child remains free of skin breakdown and rashes.	Assess skin of perineum and rectum for signs of skin breakdown or irritation.	Early assessment and intervention can prevent worsening of the condition.	Child's perianal and rectal tissue remains pink and intact.
	Provide prevention or restorative care for infants as follows:		
	Preventive care:		
	■ Change diapers every 2 hours or as needed.	■ Minimizes skin contact with chemical irritants from stool and urine.	
	■ Use cloth diapers rather than disposable.	■ Minimizes the mechanical and chemical irritation from disposables.	
	■ Wash diaper area after each soiling.	■ Removes traces of stool if present.	
	■ Apply A & D ointment.	■ Provides a barrier and protects intact or reddened skin from becoming excoriated.	

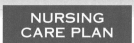

THE CHILD WITH GASTROENTERITIS—CONTINUED

GOAL	INTERVENTION	RATIONALE	EXPECTED OUTCOME

3. High Risk for Impaired Skin Integrity related to contact of skin with feces and frequent cleansing of skin—Continued

Restorative care:
- Place the infant prone and leave the buttocks open to air.
- Notify the physician if the skin is severely broken or peeling or if a rash is present.

For toddlers and older children:
- Tub bathe at least daily (if condition allows) in tepid water. Pat the area dry.
- Discourage the wearing of underwear if possible.

- Apply A & D ointment at least four times daily.

- Promotes air circulation to the area.

- Helps loosen any fecal matter without scrubbing, which can cause additional irritation to the skin.
- Allows air to circulate and prevents accumulation of moisture.
- Provides a barrier and protects intact or reddened skin from becoming excoriated.

Constipation

Constipation is characterized by a decrease in the frequency or passage of stools; the formation of hard, dry stools; or the oozing of liquid stool past a collection of hard, dry stool. Because stooling patterns vary among children, identification of an abnormal pattern is sometimes difficult. Infants usually have several bowel movements a day. For a young child, one bowel movement a day may be normal. As the child grows, however, three to four bowel movements a week may be a normal pattern.[17]

Constipation may be caused by an underlying disease, diet, or psychologic factor. It may result from defects in filling, or more commonly emptying, of the rectum. Pathologic causes of defective filling include ineffective colonic propulsive activity, caused by hypothyroidism or use of medication, and obstruction, caused by a structural anomaly (stricture or stenosis) or by an aganglionic segment (Hirschsprung disease). If the rectum fails to fill, stasis leads to excessive drying of the stools. Emptying of the rectum depends on the defecation reflex. Lesions of the spinal cord, weakness of the abdominal muscles, and local lesions blocking sphincter relaxation all may impede attempts to defecate.

Constipation during infancy is rare and is most often caused by mismanagement of diet. The transition from formula to cow's milk may cause a transient constipation because the bowel must adjust to the increased protein content of cow's milk. Constipation in young infants can usually be corrected by increasing the amount of fluids and juices given or by adding corn syrup to the formula. In older infants, increasing the intake of cereals, fruits, and vegetables in the diet should correct the problem.

Constipation occurs most frequently in the toddler and preschool age groups.[17] This increased incidence is often associated with learning to control bodily functions. Many children do not like the sensations of a bowel movement and may begin withholding stool, which accumulates in the rectum until the next urge to defecate. The increasingly painful bowel movement reinforces the child's behavior, and a self-perpetuating pattern develops.[1,4,17] Removing milk and milk products and constipating foods (bananas, rice, and cheese) from the child's diet often decreases the constipation. Increasing the child's intake of high-fiber foods (whole grain breads, raw fruits and vegetables) and increasing fluids also promote defecation.

In the school-age child, constipation may occur because time for toileting is limited. Busy school-age children may delay going to the bathroom. Children may also be hesitant to use an unfamiliar bathroom. Encouragement from parents and relaxation of bathroom privileges at school promote regularity and return of usual bowel patterns within a short time.

Diagnosis is based on a thorough history and physical examination. When constipation occurs along with growth failure, vomiting, or abdominal pain, further investigation is necessary to rule out other disorders. Dietary management is the treatment of choice for constipation that has no underlying pathologic cause.

Constipation may follow surgery, especially in children who are immobilized, such as by traction or a body cast. Stool softeners and a diet high in roughage and fluid are instituted to prevent and treat this problem.

Nursing Management

Take a diet history and obtain a description of bowel patterns from parents. Assessment of the child's food likes and dislikes may provide a clue to the cause of constipation. Nursing care focuses on teaching parents what constitutes normal bowel patterns in children and the importance of diet in maintaining normal bowel patterns. Regular bowel habits are encouraged by placing the child on the toilet 30 minutes after a meal or around the time defecation usually occurs. Providing positive reinforcement during toilet training helps to prevent a withholding pattern.

Teach parents dietary measures to promote regularity of bowel movements. Children can be given a high-fiber diet that includes fruits and vegetables. Cut up fresh fruits, dried fruits, and fruit juice can be offered as snacks. A glycerine suppository can be used periodically. This is a natural stimulant and lubricant of the bowel. Caution parents to avoid frequent use of laxatives, stool softeners, and enemas, since overuse can cause bowel dependency.

▓ Intestinal Parasitic Disorders

Intestinal parasitic disorders occur most frequently in tropical regions. Outbreaks take place in areas where water is not treated, food is incorrectly prepared, or people live in crowded conditions with poor sanitation. In the United States, outbreaks of diseases caused by protozoa or helminths (worms) are increasing. Young children, especially those in day care, are most at risk of infection. Young children often lack good hygiene practices and are apt to put objects and their hands in their mouths. The most common intestinal parasitic disorders are summarized in Table 15–5.

TABLE 15–5 Common Intestinal Parasitic Infections

Parasitic Infection	Transmission, Life Cycle, Pathogenesis	Clinical Manifestations	Treatment	Comments
Giardiasis				
Organism: protozoan *Giardia lamblia*	Transmission is through person-to-person contact, unfiltered water, improperly prepared infected food, and contact with animals. Cysts are ingested and passed into duodenum and proximal jejunum, where they begin actively feeding. Excreted in stool.	May be asymptomatic. *Infants:* diarrhea, vomiting, anorexia, failure to thrive *Older children:* abdominal cramps; intermittent loose, foul-smelling, watery, pale, and greasy stools	Available medications include furazolidone and quinacrine. Furazolidone has fewer side effects than quinacrine but is more expensive. Metronidazole is also effective but is not licensed in the United States for treatment of giardiasis.	Most common intestinal parasitic organism in United States. Infection may resolve spontaneously in 4 to 6 weeks without treatment. Parents or caregivers should wear gloves when handling diapers or stool of parasite-infected infant or child.
Enterobiasis (Pinworm)				
Organism: nematode *Enterobius vermicularis*	Transmission is from discharged eggs inhaled or carried from hand to mouth. Eggs hatch in upper intestine and mature in 15 to 28 days. Larvae then migrate to cecum. After mating, the female migrates out of the anus and lays up to 17,000 eggs. Movement of worms causes intense itching. Scratching deposits eggs on hands and under nails.	Intense perianal itching, irritability, restlessness, and short attention span; in females, can migrate to vagina and urethra to cause infection. Itching intensifies at night when female comes to anal opening to lay eggs.	Available medications include mebendazole, pyrantel pamoate, and piperazine citrate. The child and all household members should be treated at the same time. Treatment may be repeated in 2 to 3 weeks.	Most common helminthic infection in United States. Transmission is increased in crowded conditions such as housing developments, schools, and day care centers.

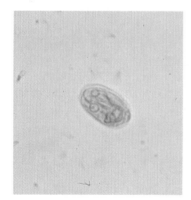

Giardia lamblia

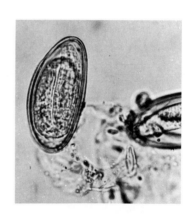

Pinworm

Giardia lamblia courtesy of the Centers for Disease Control and Prevention, Atlanta, GA; *pinworm* (p. 721), *roundworm* (p. 718), *hookworm* (p. 723), and *threadworm* (p. 724) from Rudolph, A.M., Hoffman, J.I.E., & Rudolph, C.D. (1991). *Rudolph's pediatrics* (19th ed.). Norwalk, CT: Appleton & Lange.

Continued

TABLE 15-5 Common Intestinal Parasitic Infections—Continued

Parasitic Infection	Transmission, Life Cycle, Pathogenesis	Clinical Manifestations	Treatment	Comments
Ascariasis (Roundworm)				
Organism: nematode *Ascaris lumbricoides*	Transmission is from discharged eggs carried from hand to mouth. Adult lays eggs in small intestine. Eggs are excreted in stool, where they incubate for 2 to 3 weeks. Swallowed eggs hatch in small intestine. Larvae may penetrate intestinal villi, entering portal vein and liver, then moving to lung. Larvae that ascend to upper respiratory tract are swallowed and proceed to small intestine, where they repeat cycle.	Mild infection may be asymptomatic. Severe infection may result in intestinal obstruction, peritonitis, obstructive jaundice, and lung involvement.	Available antihelmintic medications include mebendazole, pyrantel pamoate, or piperazine citrate. Stools should be examined 2 weeks after treatment and monthly for 3 months. Family members and contacts of child should be treated if indicated. If the child has intestinal obstruction, treatment can include administering piperazine through a nasogastric tube and duodenal suction. Obstructing worms sometimes have to be surgically removed.[1]	Most common in warm climates. Primarily affects children 1 to 4 years of age.
Hookworm disease				
Organism: nematode *Necator americanus*	Transmission is through direct contact with infected soil containing larvae. Worms live in small intestine and feed on villi, causing bleeding. Eggs are deposited in bowel and excreted in feces. Eggs hatch in damp shaded soil. Larvae attach to and penetrate skin then enter bloodstream migrating to lungs. Larvae then migrate to upper respiratory passages and are swallowed.	In healthy individuals mild infection seldom causes problems. More severe infection may result in anemia and malnutrition. Presence of larvae on skin may cause burning and itching, followed by redness and papular eruption.	Available medications include mebendazole and pyrantel pamoate. Stools should be examined 2 weeks after treatment and monthly for 3 months. Family members and contacts of child should be treated if indicated.	Children should wear shoes when outdoors, although other unprotected areas of skin may still come in contact with larvae.

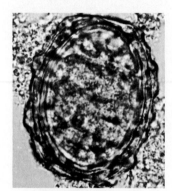

Roundworm

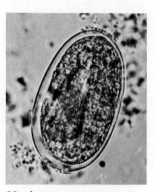

Hookworm

TABLE 15-5 Common Intestinal Parasitic Infections—Continued

Parasitic Infection	Transmission, Life Cycle, Pathogenesis	Clinical Manifestations	Treatment	Comments
Strongyloidiasis (Threadworm)				
Organism: nematode *Strongyloides stercoralis*	Transmission is from ingestion of discharged larvae in soil. Life cycle is similar to that of hookworm, except threadworm does not attach to intestinal mucosa and feeding larvae (rather than eggs) may be deposited in soil.	Light infection may be asymptomatic. Severe infection may result in abdominal pain and distention, nausea, vomiting, and diarrhea. Stools may be large and pale, with mucus. Severe infection may lead to nutritional deficiency.	Available medications include thiabendazole or mebendazole. Treatment may need to be repeated if symptoms recur after treatment. Family members and contacts of child should be examined and treated if indicated.	Most common in older children and adolescents.

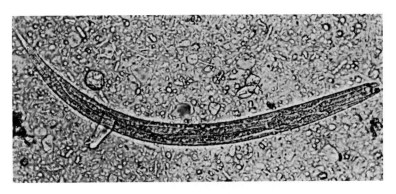

Threadworm

Parasitic Infection	Transmission, Life Cycle, Pathogenesis	Clinical Manifestations	Treatment	Comments
Visceral larva migrans (Toxocariasis)				
Organism: nematode *Toxocara canis* or *T. catis,* commonly found in dogs and cats	Transmission is through ingestion of eggs in soil. Ingested eggs hatch in intestine. Mobile larvae then migrate to liver and eventually to all major organs (including brain). Once migration is complete, they encapsulate in dense fibrous tissue.	Most cases are asymptomatic. Affected children may have low-grade fever and recurrent upper airway diseases. Severe symptoms include hepatomegaly, pulmonary infiltration, and neurologic disturbances. In all cases there is hypereosinophilia of blood.	There is no specific treatment. Corticosteroids have been used in severe cases. Thiabendazole has been recommended but efficacy is not established (infection usually resolves spontaneously).	Most common in toddlers. Deworm household pets monthly if indicated. Keep children away from areas contaminated with animal droppings.

     Laboratory examination of stool specimens identifies the causative organism (protozoa, worms, larvae, or ova). Treatment usually involves an anthelmintic. Nursing care centers on preventive teaching. Emphasize the importance of good hygiene practices, especially careful handwashing, after toileting and when handling food. Instruct parents to give prescribed medications as directed even if the child's condition seems to be improved.

Feeding Disorders

Feeding problems that interfere with a child's ability to ingest or tolerate formulas and foods usually become apparent during the first year of life. To prevent complications of poor nutrition, feeding methods or diet may need to be altered. The following discussion focuses on three common disorders: colic, food sensitivity and allergy, and rumination.

Colic

Colic is a feeding disorder characterized by paroxysmal abdominal pain of intestinal origin and severe crying. It usually occurs in infants under 3 months of age.

Characteristically the infant cries loudly and continuously, often for several hours. The infant's face may become flushed. The abdomen is distended and tense. Often the infant draws up the legs and clenches the hands. Episodes occur at the same time each day, usually in the late afternoon or early evening. Crying may stop only when the child is completely exhausted or after passage of flatus or stool. Carrying the child in the upright position is often helpful.

The etiology of colic is unknown. Proposed causes include feeding too rapidly and swallowing large amounts of air. Symptoms initially may resemble intestinal obstruction or peritoneal infection. These conditions must be ruled out along with sensitivity to formula. Treatment is supportive. Usually by 3 months of age the severity and frequency of symptoms decrease.

Nursing Management

Nursing care requires a thorough history of the infant's diet, daily schedule, and the events surrounding episodes of colicky behavior. Assessment of the infant's feeding patterns and diet includes type, frequency, and amount of feeding (if breast-feeding, maternal diet history) and frequency of burping. Episodes of colic are assessed for onset, duration, and characteristics of cry. Which family members are usually present during attacks? What are the activities of the caretaker before the episode (e.g., smoking, rushing to meet family demands)? What measures are used to relieve crying? How effective are they? When possible, the feeding method should be observed.

Parents of infants with colic are often tired and frustrated. They require frequent reassurance that they are not to blame for the infant's condition. Suggest ways of alleviating some of the infant's symptoms and discomfort (Table 15–6).

Food Sensitivity and Allergy

Food sensitivity encompasses any adverse reaction to foods or substances ingested in foods. The foods that most commonly cause a reaction are fish, shellfish, nuts, eggs, soy, wheat, corn, strawberries, and cow's milk products. Food antigens, chemical additives, antibiotics, preservatives, and food colorings also can cause food sensitivity reactions.

Allergic (IgE-mediated) reactions, on the other hand, are potentially systemic, characteristically rapid in onset, and may be manifest as swelling of the lips, mouth, uvula, or glottis, generalized urticaria, and, in severe reactions, shock.

Food allergies are more prevalent in children with a family history of allergic reactions to foods (atopy). Caution parents to be aware of "hidden"

TABLE 15-6 Parent Teaching: Suggestions for Alleviating Colic

Provide Rhythmic Movement

- Front-carrying sling carriers
- Infant swing (battery-operated swing provides continuous motion)
- Car ride

Alternate Positions

- Swaddle infant in a soft, stretchy blanket with knees flexed up against abdomen or with legs straight.
- Place infant prone on parent's arm, supporting the body with one hand under the abdomen and cradling the head in the crook of the other arm.

Reduce Environmental Stimuli

- Provide quiet, soothing music.
- Prevent sudden loud noises.
- Avoid smoking.

Provide Various Tactile Stimuli

- Offer a pacifier.
- Provide a warm bath.
- Massage abdomen.

Alter Intake

- Feed smaller amount and burp frequently.
- Use a bottle with a collapsible bag to prevent sucking air.
- Breast-feeding mothers: eliminate milk products and spicy or gas-producing foods.
- Hold upright for ½ hour after feeding

Above All, Respond Immediately to Crying

---

substances in prepared foods. For example, the child who is allergic to nuts will experience a reaction to a food if nut extracts are used in its preparation.

Delayed hypersensitivity reactions are attributed to digestive products of food and require a thorough diet history over several days to identify the offending food. These reactions are more difficult to diagnose, since the reaction can occur up to 24 hours after ingestion of the food.

Cow's milk may cause an allergy or a sensitivity reaction. In allergy, an IgE-mediated systemic reaction occurs. In sensitivity reaction, there is a gastrointestinal response to milk proteins (diarrhea, vomiting, abdominal pain). Infants often have vomiting and watery, blood-streaked, mucoid diarrhea.

Diagnostic tests to identify suspected food allergies include measurement of serum IgE levels, scratch tests, and the radioallergosorbent test (RAST), in which radioimmunoassay is used to measure IgE antibodies to specific allergens. A diet diary is kept, noting date, type of foods eaten, and reaction, if any. Foods should be eaten singly for several days to determine whether they cause a reaction.

Treatment consists of eliminating the offending foods from the child's diet. Children frequently outgrow food sensitivities. Careful reintroduction of the food after a 1- to 2-year absence may elicit no reaction in the previously sensitive child. Allergies are more commonly life-long. The foods involved should *always* be avoided.

Nursing Management

Prevention is the first step. Instruct parents of infants to introduce new foods at a rate of not more than one new food every 5 days. If a sensitivity is noted, the causative food can be easily identified. Discuss any changes in diet or preparation of formula. Reassure parents that the child's symptoms will disappear when the offending foods are removed from the diet.

Nursing care of a child with food allergies is primarily supportive. Help the family identify the offending foods. Explain to parents all tests, use of a food diary, and care of the child should a reaction occur. Emphasize the importance of reading food labels for hidden foods that can trigger an allergic reaction.

Rumination

Rumination is a rare and serious form of chronic regurgitation that may lead to malnutrition and growth failure in infancy. Chewing movements and mouthing of fingers often precede or accompany regurgitation. Close observation may reveal the infant actively initiating gagging with the tongue and fingers.

Rumination is most often associated with poor maternal-infant bonding. This kind of behavior is seen in infants who are deprived of tactile, visual, or auditory stimuli for long periods. The infant substitutes repetitive self-stimulation for the lack of appropriate external stimulation. (See the discussion of failure to thrive in Chapter 21.)

Diagnostic evaluation focuses on ruling out an organic cause and determining the degree and type of nutritional deficiencies. Treatment involves correcting the nutritional deficits and developing normal feeding patterns. Medical and nursing staff and social services are often involved in helping parents meet the infant's nutritional and psychologic needs (see Chapter 21).

Nursing Management

Nursing care focuses on establishing a warm, caring relationship with the infant and the parents. Making eye contact with the infant, providing food regularly, and stimulating the infant through all the senses are ways to break the pattern of rumination.

Parents need to be included in the infant's care. Discuss proper nutrition and demonstrate feeding techniques and interactions that promote development. Determine the parents' support needs and make a referral to social service agencies as appropriate. A parent who is preoccupied with financial or other problems is less likely to attend to an infant's needs, resulting in continuation or recurrence of the pattern of rumination.

Disorders of Malabsorption

Malabsorption occurs when a child is unable to digest or absorb nutrients in the diet. Disorders of malnutrition include celiac disease, lactose intolerance, and short bowel syndrome.

Celiac Disease

Celiac disease is a chronic malabsorption syndrome that is more common in Europe and is uncommon in black or Asian children. It is characterized by an intolerance for gluten, a protein found in wheat, barley, rye, and oats. Inability to digest glutenin and gliadin (protein fractions) results in the accumulation of the amino acid glutamine, which is toxic to mucosal cells in the intestine.[4] Damage to the villi ultimately impairs the absorptive process in the small intestine.

In the early stages celiac disease affects fat absorption, resulting in excretion of large quantities of fat in the stools (steatorrhea). Stools are greasy, foul smelling, frothy, and excessive. As changes in the villi continue, the absorption of protein, carbohydrates, calcium, iron, folic acid, and vitamins D, K, and B_{12} becomes impaired.

Symptoms usually occur when solid foods containing gluten are introduced to the child's diet (in the first 2 years of life). The child exhibits chronic diarrhea, vomiting, irritability, and failure to grow. If diagnosis is delayed, the child begins to show evidence of protein deficiency (wasted musculature, abdominal distention), delayed dentition, and changes in bone density.[4,8]

Diagnosis is confirmed through jejunal biopsy and removal of gluten products from the diet. Symptoms usually lessen within a week.[1] Growth should improve steadily, and height and weight should reach normal range within 1 year.

Nursing Management

Nursing care focuses on supporting the parents in maintaining a gluten-free diet for the child. The parents should receive a thorough explanation of the disease process. Emphasize the necessity of following a gluten-free diet. Help parents to understand that celiac disease requires lifelong dietary modifications that should not be discontinued when the child is symptom free. Discontinuation of the diet places the child at risk for growth retardation and the development of malignant lymphoma of the small intestine, esophageal cancer, and GI cancers in adulthood.

The diet of an infant or toddler is easily monitored at home. When the child enters school, however, ensuring adherence to dietary restrictions becomes more difficult. In addition to easily identified gluten-based foods, such as bread, cake, doughnuts, cookies, and crackers, the child must also avoid processed foods that contain gluten as a filler. School-age children and adolescents are often tempted to eat these foods, especially when among peers. Emphasize the need for compliance while meeting the child's developmental needs.

The child's special dietary needs can place a financial burden on the family. Parents will need to purchase prepared rice or corn flour products or make their own bread and bakery products. Advise parents that obtaining a dietary prescription will enable them to deduct the cost of these ingredients and commercially prepared products as a medical expense.

For information and support, parents and children can be referred to several organizations, including the American Celiac Society and the Celiac Sprue Association/United States of America. Written materials are also available from Children's Memorial Hospital in Chicago (see Appendix F).

Lactose Intolerance

Lactose intolerance is the inability to digest lactose, a disaccharide found in milk and other dairy products. It results from a congenital or acquired deficiency of the enzyme lactase. Congenital lactase deficiency of infancy is a rare disorder. Abdominal pain, flatulence, and diarrhea occur shortly after birth when the infant is unable to hydrolyze lactose. The prevalence of secondary (acquired) lactase deficiency is highest (approximately 100%) among Asian and Native American children and affects approximately 70% of North American blacks after the age of 3 years. Diarrhea develops rapidly after the child ingests milk and milk products.

Diagnosis is based on a thorough history and a hydrogen breath test,

■ NURSING ALERT

Many prepared foods contain hidden gluten. Examples include certain types of chocolate candy, some prepared hamburgers, hot dogs, luncheon meats, milk preparations such as malts and processed ice cream, and prepared soups.

which measures the amount of hydrogen left after fermentation of unabsorbed carbohydrates. Implementing a lactose-free diet for a period of time may eliminate the symptoms, confirming the diagnosis. Treatment for infants includes switching to a soy-based formula. For older children, eliminating lactose-containing foods is recommended. Enzyme tablets such as LactAid can be added to milk or sprinkled on foods to aid digestion.

Nursing Management

Nursing care is primarily supportive. Carefully explain dietary modifications to parents and include alternate sources of calcium (see Chapter 7). Discuss the need for supplementation of calcium and vitamin D to prevent deficiencies. Caution parents to read food labels carefully to identify hidden sources of lactose. For example, milk solids are found in breads, cakes, some candies (e.g., milk chocolate, caramels, and toffee), some salad dressings, margarine and various processed foods.

Short Bowel Syndrome

Short bowel syndrome is a decreased ability to digest and absorb a regular diet because of a shortened intestine. Loss of intestine may result from extensive bowel resection for treatment of necrotizing enterocolitis or inflammatory disorders or from a congenital bowel anomaly such as intestinal malrotation, gastroschisis, or atresia.[4]

The extent and location of the involved bowel determine the severity of the disorder. Complications arise when more than 25% of the intestine is removed or congenitally absent.[4] Over time the remaining bowel usually compensates for the absent intestine. However, the infant or young child requires nutritional support initially to provide sufficient nutrients for adequate growth and development. A combination of intravenous total parenteral nutrition and oral fluids may be required.

Nursing Management

Nursing care focuses on meeting the child's nutritional and fluid needs and teaching parents how to care for the child at home. Establishing an adequate nutritional intake and bowel pattern is a lengthy process. Total parenteral nutrition is provided initially until a feeding regimen can be established. Oral and enteral feedings are instituted gradually to allow the bowel time to compensate. Provide support to the family and child throughout this period. Discharge teaching for parents should include how to prepare and administer total parenteral feedings, ensure regular bowel function, and maintain skin integrity.

Hepatic Disorders

The liver is one of the most vital organs in the body. Among its essential functions are blood storage and filtration; secretion of bile and bilirubin; metabolism of fat, protein, and carbohydrates; synthesis of blood-clotting components; detoxification of hormones, drugs, and other substances; and storage of glycogen, iron, fat-soluble vitamins, and vitamin B_{12}.[1,8] Thus any inflammatory, obstructive, or degenerative disorder that affects liver function can be life threatening. The following discussion focuses on three common liver disorders in children: biliary atresia, acute hepatitis, and cirrhosis.

Biliary Atresia

Biliary atresia is the pathologic closure or absence of bile ducts outside the liver.[1] It is the most common pediatric liver disease necessitating transplantation.[18]

Initially the newborn is asymptomatic. Jaundice may not be detected until 2 to 3 weeks after birth. At that point bilirubin levels increase, accompanied by abdominal distention and hepatomegaly. As the disease progresses, splenomegaly occurs. The infant experiences easy bruising, prolonged bleeding time, and intense itching. Stools are puttylike in consistency and white or clay colored because of the absence of bile pigments. Excretion of bilirubin and bile salts results in tea-colored urine. Failure to thrive and malnutrition occur as the destructive changes of the disease progress.

The cause of biliary atresia is unknown. Absence or blockage of the extrahepatic bile ducts results in altered bile flow from the liver to the duodenum. This altered bile flow soon causes inflammation and fibrotic changes in the liver. Lack of bile acids also interferes with digestion of fat and absorption of fat-soluble vitamins A, D, E, and K, resulting in steatorrhea and nutritional deficiencies. Without treatment the disease is invariably fatal.

Diagnosis is based on the history, physical examination, and laboratory evaluation. Laboratory findings reveal elevated bilirubin levels, elevated serum transaminase and alkaline phosphatase values, prolonged prothrombin time, and increased ammonia levels. Because liver damage develops rapidly in infants with biliary atresia, early diagnosis is essential.

Treatment involves surgery to attempt correction of the obstruction (Kasai procedure) and supportive care. In the Kasai procedure (hepatoportoenterostomy) a segment of the intestine is anastomosed to the porta hepatis.[5] In most children this is a palliative treatment to maintain as much hepatic function as possible and prevent the complications of liver failure. Supportive treatment is directed at managing the bleeding tendencies by administering oral vitamin K; preventing rickets through vitamin D supplementation; controlling itching and irritability with cholestyramine and antihistamines; and promoting adequate nutrition.

Although the Kasai procedure improves the prognosis, complications of liver disease continue to develop and eventually necessitate liver transplantation. Advances in transplantation surgery now make it possible to perform partial liver transplants from living donor resections. This enables transplantation to be performed when the child is in optimal health, rather than waiting until an appropriate-size cadaver liver is available. These advances, along with the development of cyclosporine and other immunosuppressants, have improved the first-year survival rate for children receiving liver transplantation to between 30% and 75%.[18]

Nursing Management

Nursing care in the initial stages of biliary atresia is the same as that for any healthy newborn. As symptoms develop, the focus of nursing care becomes long-term management and support.

Diagnosis of this potentially fatal disorder can be devastating to parents. Provide emotional support and offer frequent explanations of tests during the initial diagnostic evaluation. As the disease progresses, the infant becomes irritable because of intense itching and the accumulation of toxins. Tepid baths may help to relieve itching and provide comfort. Promote rest by grouping nursing activities while the infant is awake. Care following the Kasai procedure is similar to that for a child undergoing abdominal surgery. (See the earlier discussion of postsurgical nursing management for appen-

■ CLINICAL TIP

When drying the skin, pat the towel against the skin rather than rubbing and massaging. Rubbing and massaging promote vasodilation, which worsens the infant's itching and irritation.

dicitis and the Nursing Care Plan for the Child Undergoing Surgery in Chapter 4.) Posttransplant care includes immunosuppressant drugs and close monitoring for vascular complications.

Discharge planning focuses on teaching parents how to care for the child's skin, provide for nutritional needs, administer medications, and, for children receiving transplants, how to identify signs of rejection (nausea, vomiting, fever, and jaundice). Refer parents to support groups, clergy, or social services if indicated.

Acute Hepatitis

Hepatitis is an inflammation of the liver caused by a viral infection. It may occur as an acute or chronic disease. Acute hepatitis is rapid in onset and if untreated may develop into chronic hepatitis. The most frequently diagnosed causative organisms are hepatitis A virus (HAV), hepatitis B virus (HBV), and non-A, non-B (NANB) virus. Hepatitis may also be caused by cytomegalovirus, herpesvirus, and Epstein-Barr virus.[19]

Clinical Manifestations

Acute hepatitis infection is characterized by two phases, the anicteric (absence of jaundice) phase and the icteric (jaundice) phase. The anicteric phase usually lasts 5 to 7 days. Signs and symptoms include nausea, vomiting, anorexia, malaise, fatigue, and fever (Table 15–7). The child becomes irritable, looks ill, and requires rest. In the icteric phase, signs and symptoms include darkening of urine, clay-colored stools, and the characteristic yellowing of the skin and sclera. As the jaundice worsens, the child begins to feel better. This phase lasts approximately 4 weeks. Complete recovery with return of normal liver function and laboratory values may take 1 to 3 months.

Not all children exhibit symptoms of the disease. Development of symptoms represents the body's ability to fight the disease. If the body is unable to develop an adequate defense against the viral antigen, the child may still harbor the virus as a chronic carrier.[19]

Etiology and Pathophysiology

Hepatitis A is the most common form of acute viral hepatitis. It is highly contagious and traditionally has been referred to as infectious hepatitis. Infection occurs primarily through the fecal-oral route. Transmission is by direct person-to-person spread or through ingestion of contaminated water or food (particularly shellfish). Hepatitis A frequently occurs in children in day care

TABLE 15–7 Comparison of Hepatitis A and Hepatitis B

	Hepatitis A	Hepatitis B
Incubation period	15–45 days	50–180 days
Onset	Acute	Insidious
Clinical manifestations		
Fever	Common	Less common
Nausea and vomiting	Common	Less common
Anorexia	Common	Mild to moderate
Jaundice	Present	Present
Urticaria	Rare	May be present
Arthralgia	Not present	May be present
Hepatosplenomegaly	Common	Common

settings where hygiene practices are poor. Because the virus is transmitted in the early stages of the disease when children are often asymptomatic or only mildly ill, large numbers of people may be exposed before the diagnosis is confirmed.

Hepatitis B, which has been known traditionally as serum hepatitis, is a serious disease. Transmission is usually by the parenteral route through the exchange of blood or any bodily secretion or fluid. Adolescents who use intravenous drugs and have unprotected sexual intercourse with multiple partners are at risk for contracting hepatitis B. Major sources for the spread of HBV are healthy chronic carriers. Maternal-infant transmission can occur in utero when maternal antibodies cross the placenta or the fetus ingests amniotic fluid or maternal blood, or through breast-feeding if the mother's nipples are cracked.[19] HBV may also be transmitted indirectly through cuts, burns, or abrasions. Onset is insidious, and the course of the disease parallels that of HIV infection.[19]

Non-A, non-B hepatitis represents a composite of undefined infections probably caused by two different viruses. In the United States over 90% of NANB hepatitis cases are associated with blood transfusions.[1,4,19] With the development of better screening techniques for blood and blood products the risk of transmission of NANB has been significantly reduced.

The liver's response to injury by the viruses that cause hepatitis is similar. Initially invasion of the parenchymal cells by the virus results in degeneration and necrosis. Subsequent infiltration of the parenchyma by lymphocytes, macrophages, plasma cells, eosinophils, and neutrophils causes inflammation. Structural changes of the hepatocyte account for altered liver functions, such as impaired bile excretion, elevated serum glutamate pyruvate transaminase (SGPT) and alkaline phosphatase levels, and decreased albumin synthesis. Regeneration of parenchymal cells occurs within 3 months, and most children recover completely.

In some children, however, a progressive and total destruction of the hepatic parenchyma known as acute fulminating hepatitis develops. Children with this form of the disease usually die of liver failure within 2 weeks of onset unless they receive a liver transplant. Another complication, chronic active hepatitis, may lead to scarring of the liver and progressive deterioration of liver function. The prognosis depends on the degree of liver involvement.

Diagnostic Tests and Medical Management

Diagnosis is often made on the basis of a thorough history and physical examination. A history of exposure to persons with the disease is significant. Physical examination reveals a tender, enlarged liver, abdominal pain, and flulike symptoms. Laboratory evaluation includes serologic testing (to detect the presence of antigens and antibodies to HAV or HBV) and liver function studies.

The three goals of medical management are early detection to prevent complications, support and monitoring during the acute phase of the disease, and prevention of disease spread. Early diagnosis is essential to follow the course of the illness and identify potential complications. Management of the illness includes bed rest during the flulike phase. If prothrombin times are increased, vitamin K is administered.

The spread of viral infections can be interrupted by elimination of the virus from the infected population, institution of proper hygiene, and passive or active immunization. To date, no antiviral agent has been developed to combat the hepatitis viruses. However, the antibiotic rifampin has been shown to be effective in preventing hepatitis A in exposed persons. For this reason it may be given for prophylactic management to children and staff at

---

■ **NURSING ALERT**

When hepatitis A is present, drug metabolism is altered and the liver's ability to detoxify drugs is decreased. As with all liver disorders, medications need to be administered carefully and the child's condition must be monitored for possible side effects.

■ **NURSING ALERT**

Health care workers who come in contact with blood or other body fluids of children infected with hepatitis B are at risk for contracting the virus. Universal precautions should be used at all times (see the Atlas of Pediatric Procedures). Hepatitis B immunization (three doses) is recommended for nurses and other persons at high risk for exposure as well as all infants (see the Atlas of Infectious and Communicable Diseases).

the day care center or school attended by an infected child. Prevention depends on breaking the cycle of infection.

Passive immunity to HAV can be achieved with standard pooled immune globulin. It must be administered within 2 weeks of exposure. Passive immunity to HBV can be achieved with hepatitis immune serum globulin (HBIG). It is used for one-time exposure and for infants of infected mothers. Heptavax B vaccine, developed in 1982, provides active immunity. This vaccine is now recommended for a three-dose administration for all infants and other individuals at risk. (Refer to the Atlas of Infectious and Communicable Diseases.)

Nursing Assessment

The nurse usually encounters the child and family in an outpatient setting. In addition to being observed for characteristic signs of hepatitis (jaundiced skin and sclera), the child is assessed for the presence of abdominal pain, anorexia, nausea and vomiting, malaise, and arthralgia. A history of the child's contacts over the past 45 days for HAV and up to 180 days for HBV is also obtained. This is especially important for children in day care centers.

Nursing Diagnosis

Common nursing diagnoses for the child with acute hepatitis include:

- High Risk for Altered Nutrition: Less Than Body Requirements related to anorexia, nausea, and vomiting
- Fatigue related to flulike symptoms and general feelings of malaise
- High Risk for Diversional Activity Deficit related to change in usual daily activities
- High Risk for Body Image Disturbance (Older Child) related to temporary jaundice
- Anxiety (Parent and Child) related to diagnosis and treatment measures

Nursing Management

Nursing care is mainly supportive, since children with hepatitis are seldom admitted to the hospital. The hospitalized child is placed in isolation. Educating parents about necessary precautions and infection control measures is a priority. In addition, teach parents the importance of maintaining adequate nutrition, promoting rest and comfort, and providing diversional activities.

Prevent Spread of Infection. Teach the parents and the child infection control measures to help prevent transmission of the virus. Good hygiene practices, such as washing hands before and after toileting and proper disposal of soiled diapers, should be reinforced to parents. Day care centers should be evaluated for diapering and toileting practices as well as food preparation and storage methods. Siblings of a child with hepatitis B who have not already been immunized with hepatitis B vaccine should be vaccinated immediately.

Maintain Adequate Nutrition. Initially the child is allowed to eat favorite foods. Once the anorexia and nausea have passed, a high-protein, high-carbohydrate, low-fat diet is recommended. Increased protein helps to maintain protein stores and prevent muscle wasting. Increased carbohydrates ensure adequate caloric intake and prevent protein depletion. The use of low-fat foods lessens stomach distention. Offer the child small, frequent feedings.

■ SAFETY PRECAUTIONS

Extreme care should be exercised when handling stool of a child infected with hepatitis A. The virus may continue to be excreted in the stool for up to 1 month after the appearance of jaundice. Children who attend day care should remain at home until 2 weeks after the onset of symptoms.

Promote Rest and Comfort. Bed rest is necessary only if the child has severe fatigue and malaise. However, most children voluntarily limit their activities during the initial phase of the disease. Keep the child quiet and comfortable. Offer comfort items such as favorite toys, blankets, and pillows.

Provide Diversional Activities. Hospitalized children with hepatitis are kept in isolation. Nonhospitalized children with hepatitis do not need to be isolated, but they should be kept at home for 2 weeks following the onset of symptoms. Parents who cannot arrange to take time off from work may need to arrange home sitters to stay with the child. Offer suggestions for diversional activities during this period. Young children can be provided with a new toy or favorite activities. Older children and adolescents can be provided with board games, puzzles, books or magazines, movies, or video games. Phone calls and short visits from friends help school-age children and adolescents maintain contact with peers.

Cirrhosis

Cirrhosis is a degenerative disease process that results in fibrotic changes and fatty infiltration in the liver. It can occur in children of any age as the end stage of several disorders. The diffuse destruction and regeneration of the hepatic parenchymal cells result in an increase in fibrous connective tissue and disorganization of the liver structure. The balance between destruction and regeneration determines the specific clinical presentation.

Clinical manifestations of cirrhosis vary. When the disease process results from obstruction, as in biliary atresia, jaundice is an initial sign that intensifies with progression of the disease. In other diseases that cause cirrhosis, jaundice may be a late sign, intermittent, or absent. Steatorrhea is frequently present and can lead to rickets, hemorrhage, and failure to gain weight. Anemia can occur as a result of chronic blood loss from the GI tract. Pruritus is common, particularly in children with biliary malformations. Clubbing of the digits and cyanosis are other common findings. Severe end-stage complications signaling hepatic failure can occur at any time and with little warning.

Diagnostic evaluation is based on the child's history of infection or disease with liver involvement. Physical examination may reveal jaundice, skin changes, ascites, and hemodynamic changes. Laboratory evaluation reveals abnormal liver function tests. A liver biopsy may help to determine the extent of the parenchymal damage.

Medical management focuses on treating the child's symptoms and achieving optimal nutritional status and growth. Table 15–8 summarizes

TABLE 15–8 Treatment for Complications of Cirrhosis

Complication	Treatment
Ascites	Restrict sodium, protein, and fluids. Administer diuretics (e.g., Lasix). Administer intravenous albumin.
Hepatic encephalopathy	Restrict protein. Administer lactulose (to control increased ammonia levels). Administer antibiotics. Correct any imbalances that can enhance coma (fluid and electrolyte imbalance).
Hemorrhage caused by esophageal varices	Administer blood and blood products. Replace fluid and electrolytes. Administer vitamin B complex and vitamin K. Insert Sengstaken-Blakemore tube in cases of severe bleeding.

treatment for complications of cirrhosis. Liver transplantation is the most common treatment for biliary atresia and metabolic disorders and is the only treatment for end-stage liver disease.

Nursing Management

Nursing care focuses on monitoring physiologic and psychosocial changes to identify early signs of end-stage hepatic failure. Monitor vital signs every 2 to 4 hours. Daily weight measurement is performed to assess for fluid retention. Close monitoring of electrolytes and liver function test results helps determine the need for fluid replacement therapy.

Careful administration of medications and monitoring for side effects are necessary because drug metabolism is altered in liver disorders. If ascites is present, provide a low-sodium, low-protein diet and restrict fluids. Remove all water pitchers, glasses, and straws to minimize the child's desire to drink.

Parents of a child with cirrhosis are coping with a life-threatening disorder, and their anxiety and stress are high. The child may be awaiting liver transplantation that represents the only hope for recovery. Provide support to parents and encourage them to verbalize their fears and concerns. Encourage parents to participate in the child's care. Referral to a support group or counseling may be beneficial.

Injuries to the Gastrointestinal System

Abdominal Trauma

Abdominal injuries may be caused by blunt or penetrating trauma. The kind of injury determines the extent of organ damage. Low-velocity trauma, which may occur when a child strikes the handlebars of a bicycle, usually results in single-organ injury. High-velocity blunt trauma, which may occur in motor vehicle crashes, usually results in multiple-organ involvement. Solid organs such as the liver and spleen are more vulnerable to injury than hollow organs such as the stomach, intestines, and bladder.

Motor vehicle crashes are the most common and also the most preventable unintentional injury in children.[20] On impact, small children who are held on a parent's lap or improperly restrained in a safety seat can easily become airborne, striking objects or being thrown from the car. When lap belts only are worn by older children involved in severe crashes, injury to the hollow organs may result.[21] Bicycles are another cause of abdominal injuries in children. Such injuries commonly occur when the child strikes the handlebars during a fall or sudden stop or is struck by a car. Child abuse is another major cause of abdominal trauma.

Suspected abdominal trauma in a child necessitates a thorough history and physical examination. The description of the event should be compared with the child's signs and symptoms. Clinical manifestations of abdominal injury include pain, abdominal distention, muscle guarding, decreased or absent bowel sounds, nausea and vomiting, hypotension, and shock.

■ PERITONEAL LAVAGE

In peritoneal lavage a dialysis catheter is inserted into the abdominal cavity and normal saline or lactated Ringer solution is instilled. The fluid is then drained and analyzed for the presence of red blood cells, amylase, and bacteria, which could indicate organ damage.

A sonogram or a CT scan is performed to assess for internal bleeding and air in the abdomen. CT scans are also used to locate areas of internal trauma. Peritoneal lavage may be performed. Baseline laboratory studies, including blood type and cross-match, are done. A Foley catheter may be inserted to check for the presence of blood and bladder rupture.

Treatment of a liver or spleen injury takes place in the ICU and focuses on preventing or managing hemorrhage and monitoring for signs of shock. An intravenous infusion is started for fluid maintenance and to provide access for blood products. The child will be kept NPO. A nasogastric tube is inserted. Blood transfusions and pharmacologic management are used to treat blood loss. Use of analgesics is minimized to avoid masking symptoms. Serial hematocrit levels are monitored during this period. Healing of the liver and spleen usually occurs without further intervention.

Exploratory laparatomy is performed to resect hollow organ injuries or to repair liver or spleen lacerations when bleeding is not controlled. The spleen is salvaged to help maintain immune function. The child is usually discharged within 5 to 7 days. No strenuous activity is allowed for 6 to 8 weeks. The prognosis is generally good.

Nursing Management

Nursing care includes initial and ongoing assessments of the child's condition. Monitor vital signs every hour as warranted. Measurement of abdominal circumference, intake and output monitoring, serial hematocrits, and auscultation of bowel sounds are also performed hourly. Notify the physician of any changes.

The child and parents are usually fearful and anxious when the child is admitted to the hospital. If the injury was preventable, parents may have feelings of guilt or anger. Provide emotional support and avoid judgmental comments or statements that assign blame.

Once the child's condition is stabilized, the focus of nursing care shifts to preventive teaching. Parents should be taught safety measures to prevent future injuries and given written materials, when available, to use as a reference when they return home.

Discuss the use of car safety restraint devices and rules for riding in an automobile (see Chapter 2). If the child's injury was the result of a bicycle fall or crash, discuss the importance of the proper bicycle size[22] and teach bike safety measures such as use of a helmet and knowledge and proper use of hand signals (see Chapter 2). Have the child practice safe biking habits at a bike rodeo sponsored by a local affiliate of the National SAFE KIDS Campaign (see Appendix F).

Poisoning

Poisoning is one of the most common causes of death in children between 1 and 4 years of age.[23] Young children are at risk for poisoning because of their characteristic behaviors, which involve exploration of the environment (see Chapter 2). Infants and toddlers commonly place objects in their mouths. Some household items are nontoxic and cause little harm. However, items that contain caustic agents or toxic chemicals can cause irreversible damage or death.

The Poison Prevention Packaging Act of 1970 mandates child protective devices for all potentially toxic substances, such as household cleansers and medications. Many other items commonly found in the home are less obvious sources of toxins. The leaves, stems, or flowers of many common household and garden plants are poisonous. Examples include Boston ivy, poinsettia, philodendron, lily-of-the-valley, daffodil (bulbs), azalea, and rhododendron. Table 15–9 summarizes clinical manifestations and treatment for several commonly ingested household toxins.

Most poisonings occur in the home (see Chapter 2). Parents who suspect that their child has ingested a poison should immediately call the Poison Control Center (PCC). The PCC will advise parents whether to begin treatment at home or to bring the child to the emergency department. If the child has vomited, the vomitus should be brought to the emergency department. With older children, the possibility of intentional ingestion needs to be considered.

TABLE 15-9 Commonly Ingested Toxic Agents

Type	Sources	Clinical manifestations	Treatment
Corrosives (strong acids and alkaline products that cause chemical burns of mucosal surfaces)	Batteries, household cleaners, Clinitest tablets, denture cleaners, bleach, toilet bowl cleaners	Severe burning pain in mouth, throat, or stomach; swelling of mucous membranes; edema of lips, tongue, and pharynx (respiratory obstruction); violent vomiting; hemoptysis; drooling; inability to clear secretions; signs of shock, anxiety, and agitation	*Do not induce vomiting!* Dilute toxin with water to prevent further damage. Give activated charcoal.
Hydrocarbons (organic compounds that contain carbon and hydrogen; most are distillates of petroleum)	Gasoline, kerosene, furniture polish, lighter fluid, paint thinners	Gagging, choking, coughing, nausea, vomiting, alteration in sensorium (lethargy), weakness, respiratory symptoms of pulmonary involvement, tachypnea, cyanosis, retractions, grunting	*Do not induce vomiting!* (Aspiration of hydrocarbons places child at high risk for pneumonia.) Use gastric lavage if severe central nervous system and respiratory impairment are present. Use of activated charcoal is controversial. Provide supportive care. Decontaminate skin by removing clothing and cleansing skin.
Acetaminophen	Many over-the-counter products	Nausea, vomiting, sweating, pallor, hepatic involvement (pain in upper right quadrant, jaundice, confusion, stupor, coagulation abnormalities)	Induce vomiting or perform gastric lavage, depending on amount ingested. Administer charcoal or NAC (concentrated form of Mucomyst), which binds with the metabolite, preventing absorption and protecting liver.
Salicylate	Products containing aspirin	Nausea, disorientation, vomiting, dehydration, diaphoresis, hyperpnea, hyperpyrexia, bleeding tendencies, oliguria, tinnitus, convulsions, coma	Depends on amount ingested. Induce vomiting. Administer intravenous sodium bicarbonate, fluids, and vitamin K.
Mercury	Broken thermometers, chemicals, paints, pesticides, fungicides	Tremors, memory loss, insomnia, weight loss, diarrhea, anorexia, gingivitis	Similar to that for lead poisoning (see below).
Iron	Multiple vitamin supplements	Vomiting, hematemesis, diarrhea, bloody stools, abdominal pain, metabolic acidosis, shock, seizures, coma	Induce vomiting. Administer intravenous fluids and sodium bicarbonate. Desferoxamine chelation therapy.

In the emergency department the child's vital signs and level of consciousness are assessed and specific information about the poison is obtained from the parent. The goal of treatment is to prevent further absorption of the poison and to reverse or eliminate its effects. Table 15–10 summarizes emergency management for poisoning.

Nursing Management

Once immediate care has been provided, the focus of nursing care shifts to providing emotional support and preventing recurrence.

Provide Emotional Support. Wait until the child is out of immediate danger before questioning parents in detail about the incident. Encourage parents to express feelings of anger, guilt, or fear about the incident.

The acronym SIRES is a useful mnemonic device for recalling the essentials of care in cases of poisoning:
   Stabilize the child's condition
   Identify the toxic substance
   Reverse its effect
   Eliminate the substance from the child's body
   Support the child physically and psychologically

TABLE 15–10 Emergency Management for Poisoning

1. Stabilize the child. Assess ABCs (airway, breathing, circulation). Provide ventilatory and oxygen support.
2. Perform a rapid physical examination, start an IV infusion, draw blood for toxicology screen, and apply a cardiac monitor.
3. Obtain a history of the ingestion, including substance ingested, where child was found, by whom, position, when, how long unsupervised, history of depression or suicide, allergies, and any other medical problems.
4. Reverse or eliminate the toxic substance using the appropriate method:

*Syrup of ipecac**

- Assess level of consciousness before administering. Recommended doses are:
  6–12 months: 10 mL; do not repeat
  1–12 years: 15 mL; may repeat one time if vomiting does not occur
  Over 12 years: 30 mL; may repeat one time if vomiting does not occur
- Administer clear fluids, 10–20 mL/kg, after giving ipecac.

Apomorphine

- Assess level of consciousness before administering.
- Given IM or SQ; has rapid onset
- Give plenty of oral fluids.

Gastric lavage

- Insert a gastric tube through the mouth (use the largest size possible for the size of the child).
- Instill normal saline solution until the return is clear. Considered a less effective method of removing ingested substances from the stomach than emesis. Reserved for children with central nervous system depression, diminished or absent gag reflex, or unwillingness to cooperate with other measures.
- *Contraindicated* in children who have ingested alkaline corrosive substances, since insertion of the tube might cause esophageal perforation. Used in children who have ingested acids to decrease continued damage and potential perforation of stomach and intestines.

Activated charcoal

- Given to absorb and remove any remaining particles of toxic substances.
- Mix activated charcoal powder with water and Sorbitol (to make it more palatable) and give orally or through a gastric tube. Activated charcoal also comes in a ready-to-drink solution in an opaque container. Use a covered cup and straw when giving orally, to prevent the child from seeing the black liquid and to minimize spillage. Give activated charcoal only after the child has stopped vomiting, since aspiration of charcoal is damaging to lung tissue.

Cathartics

- Hasten excretion of a toxic substance and minimize absorption. The most commonly used cathartic is magnesium sulfate.

Antidotes and antagonists

There are very few of these agents. The most common is Narcan, for opiate ingestion.

5. Other measures will depend on the child's condition, the nature of the ingested substance, and the time since ingestion. May include diuresis, fluid loading, cooling or warming measures, anticonvulsive measures, antiarrhythmic therapy, hemodialysis, or exchange transfusions.
6. Remember always to treat the child first, not the poison. Maintain airway, breathing, and circulation.

---

* The use of ipecac is no longer widely promoted, especially in the emergency department. Activated charcoal is considered by many to be more effective in the treatment of poisoning.

Prevent Recurrence. Discuss with parents the need to supervise infants and young children at all times. Ask parents how medicines and cleansing agents are stored and whether the house contains any plants. Teach parents proper methods of childproofing the home. Instruct parents to keep 2 bottles of syrup of ipecac available for each child in the home and to be familiar with its use and proper dosage. Suggest the following measures for preventing recurrence:

- Place household cleansers, medications, vitamins, and other potentially poisonous substances out of the reach of children or in locked cabinets. Use warning stickers such as Mr. Yuk on all containers.
- Buy products with childproof caps.
- Store products in their original containers. *Never* place household cleansers or other products in food or beverage containers.
- Remove all house plants from the child's play areas.
- Use caution when visiting other settings that are not childproofed (e.g., grandparents' homes).

■ SAFETY PRECAUTIONS

Since 1977 the content of lead in household paint has been regulated. However, chipping, peeling, or flaking paint in older buildings is a major source of harmful exposure to lead. Lead used in exterior paint may have contaminated the soil surrounding a home, becoming a source of long-term exposure. It is estimated that lead-based paint is present in 74% of privately owned homes built before 1980.[26]

Lead Poisoning

Lead poisoning is one of the most common pediatric health problems in the United States today, affecting millions of children from all socioeconomic levels.[24] Lead in paint is the most common source of lead exposure for preschool children.[25] Children are also exposed to lead when they ingest contaminated food, water, and soil or when they inhale dust contaminated with lead. Table 15–11 summarizes several sources of lead exposure.

Children are at greater risk for lead poisoning because they absorb and retain more lead in proportion to their weight than adults do. Lead is particularly harmful to children under the age of 7 years.[27]

Lead interferes with normal cell function, primarily of the nervous system, blood cells, and kidneys, and adversely affects the metabolism of vitamin D and calcium. Clinical manifestations depend on the degree of toxicity (Table 15–12). Neurologic effects include decreased IQ scores, cognitive deficits, impaired hearing, and growth delays. Impaired mental function can occur with blood levels as low as 10 μg/dL. Lead ingestion by a woman during pregnancy can result in fetal malformations, reduced birth weight, and premature birth. Severe lead poisoning, which can result in encephalopathy, coma, and death, is now rare.

Once in the body, lead accumulates in the blood, soft tissues (kidney, bone marrow, liver, and brain), bones, and teeth. Lead that is absorbed by the bones and teeth is released slowly. Thus exposure to even small doses, over time, can result in dangerously high levels of lead in the body.

The U.S. Department of Health and Human Services recommends universal screening for lead poisoning unless it can be demonstrated that the community does not have a lead poisoning problem.[24] A blood lead (Pb-B) level is the most useful screening and diagnostic test for lead exposure.

A Pb-B below 10 μg/dL is not indicative of lead poisoning. An environ-

---

TABLE 15-11 Sources of Lead Exposure

Lead-based paint
Soil and dust
Drinking water from coolers with lead-soldered or lead-lined tanks, from lead-soldered teapots, or from lead pipes or lead-soldered pipes
Food grown in contaminated soil, stored in lead-soldered cans or leaded crystal, or prepared in improperly fired pottery
Parental occupations and hobbies that involve exposure to lead (e.g., plumbing, battery manufacture, highway construction, furniture refinishing, stained glass work, pottery-making)
Airborne lead in areas surrounding smelters and battery-manufacturing plants

---

TABLE 15-12   Clinical Manifestations of Lead Poisoning

Mild Toxicity	Moderate Toxicity	Severe Toxicity
Myalgia or paresthesia	Arthralgia	Paresis or paralysis
Mild fatigue	General fatigue	Encephalopathy (may lead abruptly
Irritabiliity	Difficulty concen-	to seizures, changes in conscious-
Lethargy	trating	ness, coma, and death)
Occasional abdominal	Muscular exhaust-	Lead line (blue-black) on gingival
discomfort	ibility	tissue
	Tremor	Colic (intermittent, severe abdomi-
	Headache	nal cramps)
	Diffuse abdominal	
	pain	
	Vomiting	
	Weight loss	
	Constipation	
	Anemia	

From Agency for Toxic Substances and Disease Registry (1990). Lead toxicity. *Case studies in environmental medicine* (p. 11). Atlanta: Author.

mental history should be obtained for children with Pb-B levels between 10 and 19 μg/dL to identify removable sources of lead. Follow-up testing is required. Children with Pb-B levels between 20 and 69 μg/dL require a full medical evaluation, including a detailed environmental and behavioral history, physical examination, and tests for iron deficiency. Interventions to remove sources of lead from the child's environment are necessary. Depending on the child's Pb-B level, chelation therapy may also be administered. Children with Pb-B levels greater than 70 μg/dL are critically ill from lead poisoning and require immediate chelation therapy and interventions to provide a lead-free environment.

Chelation therapy involves the administration of an agent that binds with lead, increasing its rate of excretion from the body. Calcium disodium ethylenediamine tetraacetate (CaNa$_2$ EDTA), dimercaprol (BAL), D-penicillamine, or succimer (DMSA) may be used. Children with Pb-B levels between 45 and 69 μg/dL receive CaNa$_2$ EDTA for 5 to 7 days, followed by a rest period and then a second chelation treatment. Children with Pb-B levels greater than 70 μg/dL are given both BAL and CaNa$_2$ EDTA, followed by a rest period and a second chelation treatment using CaNa$_2$ EDTA alone. Long-term follow-up of children receiving chelation therapy is essential. The child should never be discharged unless a lead-free home environment has been ensured.

■ CULTURAL CONSIDERATIONS

Traditional medicines and cosmetics may contain large amounts of lead. Examples include *azarcon* and *greta*, preparations that are used by Mexican-Americans to treat *empacho*, a colic-like illness; *chifong tokuwan, pay-loo-ah, ghasard, bali goli*, and *kandu*, used by some Asian communities; and *alkohl, kohl, surma, saoott*, and *cebagin*, used by some Middle Eastern communities.[27]

Nursing Management

Nursing care centers on screening, education, and follow-up. Ask parents about the child's development, eating habits, and risk for lead exposure. Educate parents about sources of lead in the environment and techniques to reduce exposure. Emphasize the importance of housekeeping interventions to reduce exposure to lead dust. These interventions include damp mopping of hard surfaces, floors, window sills, and baseboards; washing the child's hands and face before meals; and frequent washing of toys and pacifiers.

Teach parents the importance of including foods high in iron and calcium in the child's diet to counteract losses of these minerals associated with lead exposure. The child should eat meals at regular intervals, since lead is absorbed more readily on an empty stomach.

Be sure that parents understand the importance of follow-up testing of lead levels. If the child is developmentally delayed, refer the family to an infant stimulation or child development program. Referral to social services and either a visiting nurse or home health care nurse may also be appropriate.

REFERENCES

1 Behrman, R., & Vaughan, V. (Eds.) (1992). *Nelson's textbook of pediatrics* (14th ed.). Philadelphia: W.B. Saunders.

2 Olds, S., London, M., & Ladewig, P. (1992). *Maternal newborn nursing: A family-centered approach* (4th ed.). Redwood City, CA: Addison-Wesley Nursing.

3 Bobak, I., & Jensen, M. (1993). *Maternity and gynecologic care: The nurse and the family* (5th ed.). St. Louis: Mosby–Year Book.

4 Lebenthal, E. (1989). *Textbook of gastroenterology and nutrition in infancy.* New York: Raven Press.

5 Orenstein, S., Magill, H., & Brooks, P. (1986). Thickening of infant feedings for therapy of gastroesophageal reflux. *Journal of Pediatrics, 1*(2), 181–186.

6 Sterling, C., Schaffer, S., & Jolley, S. (1991). Home management related to medical treatment for childhood gastroesophageal reflux. *Pediatric Nursing, 19*(2), 167–173.

7 Orenstein, S., Whittington, P., & Orenstein, D. (1983). The infant seat as treatment for esophageal reflux. *New England Journal of Medicine, 309,* 760–763.

8 Walker, W., Durie, P., Hamilton, J., Walker-Smith, J., & Watkins, J. (1991). *Pediatric gastrointestinal disease.* Philadelphia: B.C. Decker.

9 Korones, S., & Bada-Ellzey, H. (1993). *Neonatal decision making.* St. Louis: Mosby–Year Book.

10 Don, S., & Faix, R. (1991). *Neonatal emergencies.* Mount Kisco, NY: Futura.

11 Kirschener, B. (1988). Inflammatory bowel disease. *Pediatric Clinics of North America, 32*(1), 189–208.

12 Rogers, A. (1990). Medical treatment and prevention of peptic ulcer disease. *Postgraduate Medicine, 88*(5), 57–60.

13 Nord, K. (1988). Peptic ulcer disease in the pediatric population. *Nursing Clinics of North America, 35*(1), 117–140.

14 Klopp, A. (1992). In M. Gulanick, M. Knoll-Puzas, & C. Wilson (Eds.). *Nursing care plans for newborns and children.* St. Louis: Mosby–Year Book.

15 Rossi, T. (1988). Endoscopic examination of the colon in infancy and childhood. *Nursing Clinics of North America, 35*(2), 331–356.

16 Heiney, S. (1991). Helping children through painful procedures. *American Journal of Nursing, 93*(11), 20–24.

17 Hatch, T. (1988). Encopresis and constipation in children. *Pediatric Clinics of North America, 35*(2), 257–280.

18 Paradis, K., Freese, D., & Sharp, H. (1988). A pediatric perspective on liver transplantation. *Pediatric Clinics of North America, 35*(2), 409–433.

19 Balistreri, W. (1988). Viral hepatitis. *Pediatric Clinics of North America, 35,* 663–669.

20 Killam, P., & Smith, K. (1988). Getting kids into car seats. *Maternal Child Nursing, 13*(2), 124–126.

21 Eichelberger, M.R. (1993). *Pediatric trauma: Prevention, acute care, rehabilitation.* St. Louis: Mosby–Year Book.

22 American Academy of Pediatrics. (1978). *Child safety suggestions: Choosing the right size bicycle for your child.* Evanston, IL: Author.

23 American Academy of Pediatrics Committee on Accident and Poison Prevention. (1987). *Injury control for children and youth.* Elk Grove Village, IL: Author.

24 U.S. Department of Health and Human Services (1991). *Strategic plan for the elimination of childhood lead poisoning.* Washington, D.C.: Author.

25 Centers for Disease Control and Prevention (1991). *Preventing lead poisoning in young children.* Atlanta: Author.

26 U.S. Department of Housing and Urban Development (1990). *HUD interim guidelines on lead-based paint.* Washington, D.C.: Author.

27 Agency for Toxic Substances and Disease Registry (1990). Lead toxicity. *Case studies in environmental medicine.* Atlanta: Author.

SUGGESTED READINGS

Bazyk, S. (1990). Factors associated with the transition to oral feeding in infants fed by nasogastric tubes. *American Journal of Occupational Therapy, 44*(12), 1070–1078.

Campbell, L., & Thomas, D. (1991). Pediatric trauma: When kids get hurt. *RN, 8,* 32–39.

Curtin, G. (1990). The infant with cleft lip or palate: More than a surgical problem. *Journal of Perinatal/Neonatal Nursing, 3*(3), 80–89.

Ellett, M., & Schibler, K. (1988). Adolescent psychosocial adaptation to inflammatory bowel disease. *Journal of Pediatric Health Care, 2,* 57–66.

Gulanick, M., Knoll-Puzas, M., & Wilson, C. (Eds.) (1992). *Nursing care plans for newborns and children: Acute and critical care.* St. Louis: Mosby–Year Book.

Huddleston, K., & Ferraro, A. (1991). Preparing families of children with gastrostomies. *Pediatric Nursing, 17*(2), 153–158.

Huddleston, K., Vitarelli, R., Goodmundson, J., & Kok, S. (1989). MIC or Foley: Comparing gastrostomy tubes. *Maternal Child Nursing, 14,* 20–23.

Huth, M., & O'Brien, M. (1987). The gastrostomy feeding button. *Pediatric Nursing, 13,* 241–245.

Katzman, E. (1989). What's the most common helminth infection in the U.S.? *Maternal Child Nursing, 14*(3), 193–195.

Lehmann, S., & Barber, J.R. (1991). Giving medications by feeding tube: How to avoid problems. *Nursing '91, 21*(11), 58–61.

Lobo, M., Barnard, K., & Coombs, J. (1992). Failure to thrive: A parent-infant interaction perspective. *Journal of Pediatric Nursing, 7*(4), 251–260.

Lynch, M. (1989). Congenital defects: Parental issues and nursing supports. *Journal of Perinatal/Neonatal Nursing, 2*(4), 53–59.

McNichol, J. (1989). When eating doesn't come naturally. *Maternal Child Nursing, 14,* 23–26.

Milla, P. (1989). Small intestine and colon: Pathophysiology and therapeutics. *Current Opinions in Pediatrics, 1,* 358–362.

Neal, J., & Slayton, D. (1992). Neonatal and pediatric PEG tubes. *Maternal Child Nursing, 17,* 184–191.

Orenstein, S., & Orenstein, D. (1988). Gastroesophageal reflux and respiratory disease in children. *Journal of Pediatrics, 112*(6), 847–854.

Shannon, R. (1993). Gastroesophageal reflux in infancy: Review and update. *Journal of Pediatric Health Care, 7*(2), 71–76.

Skale, N. (1992). *Manual of pediatric nursing procedures.* Philadelphia: J.B. Lippincott.

Smith, C. (1988). Assessing bowel sounds. *Nursing '88, 18*(2), 42–43.

Soll, A. (1990). Pathogenesis of peptic ulcer and implications for therapy. *New England Journal of Medicine, 322,* 909–916.

Thompson, S. (1990). *Emergency care of children.* Boston: Jones & Bartlett.

Young, C., & White, S. (1992). Preparing patients for tube feeding at home. *American Journal of Nursing, 92,* 46–53.

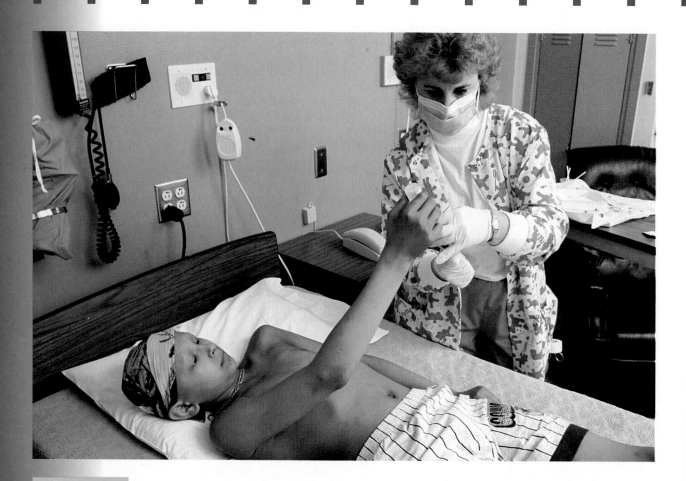

Danny is only 12 years old, but he is quick to understand that his disease is serious. His tests confirm that he has acute myelogenous leukemia. His parents try to be strong, but they are very worried about him.

Chemotherapy is begun immediately. With the treatment comes hope. Danny's parents visibly gain emotional strength each day. Danny tells everyone that he is strong and will beat the leukemia. He is discharged and continues treatment in the outpatient clinic.

Seven months later Danny is admitted with enterocolitis, an invasive infection of the small intestine and colon. Every day his condition worsens and his anxiety grows. His mother is unable to take time away from work to be with him, having taken a 6-month leave during the early phases of his treatment. At last, with aggressive antibiotic therapy and supportive nursing care, Danny conquers the complication and goes home.

Danny returns to school. His grades are high, and he loves the new computer that the Make-a-Wish organization has given him. He receives a letter from the president of the United States praising him for his bravery during his cancer treatments.

ALTERATIONS IN CELLULAR GROWTH

16

▇ TERMINOLOGY

benign A growth that does not endanger life or health.

bone marrow suppression Reduction in the activity of the bone marrow stem cells, which leads to a reduction in the number of blood cells produced by the bone marrow.

bone marrow transplantation The receipt of own (treated) or matched bone marrow by intravenous route following destruction of own bone marrow by chemotherapy and radiation.

carcinogens Chemicals or processes that, when combined with genetic traits and in interaction with one another, cause cancer.

chemotherapy Treatment that involves substances taken orally, intravenously, intrathecally, or by injection to combat cancer.

extravasation Damage that occurs when a chemotherapeutic drug leaks into soft tissue surrounding the infusion site.

immune therapy Cancer treatment that uses immune system modifiers to influence the response of the body.

leukocytosis Higher than normal leukocyte count.

leukopenia Lower than normal leukocyte count.

malignant The progressive growth of a tumor that will, if not checked by treatment, result in death.

metastasis Movement of cancer cells to additional sites in the body.

neoplasms Cancerous growths.

oncogene A portion of the DNA that is altered and, when duplicated, causes uncontrolled cellular division.

protooncogene A gene with the latent ability to change normal cells into cancer cells.

radiation Cancer treatment using unstable isotopes that release varying levels of energy to destroy cells.

tumor suppressor genes Genetic material that controls the growth of cells.

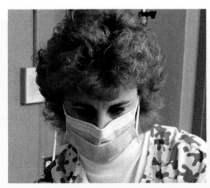

❝ The news that Danny had enterocolitis was a blow to him and his family, but that setback seemed to make Danny even more determined to fight his disease. ❞

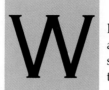hy do children like Danny develop different types of cancers than adults? Cancer in adults is often the result of dietary practices or habits such as smoking. Some adult-onset cancers, such as breast cancer, are the result of oncogenic responses to stimuli; that is, responses that stimulate cancerous changes in cells. Other cancers that occur in adults result from prolonged exposure to toxins such as coal dust and asbestos. In adults, prevention through general life-style changes is a major focus of interventions. However, in children, cancer is usually embryonic (occurring during development of the fetus) or oncogenic in origin. Thus, lifestyle changes have little effect on the incidence of childhood cancer.

Abnormal cellular growth can occur in any area of the body. Why are some growths called cancer and others not? Changes in cellular growth within the body are called **neoplasms** (new growth). A neoplasm is further classified as benign or malignant. **Benign** means that a growth does not endanger life or health. **Malignant** means that progressive growth of the tumor will, if not checked by treatment, result in spread to other parts of the body **(metastasis)**, ending in death. The common term for this type of cellular growth is cancer.

Anatomy and Physiology of Pediatric Differences

The major physiologic difference between adults and children that affects cellular growth involves the immune system and how well it functions in the defense of the body.

The immune system defends the body against foreign organisms and substances through two responses: nonspecific and specific. In a nonspecific response the components of the immune system attack a variety of targets. Nonspecific components include phagocytic (cell-destroying) cells such as mononuclear leukocytes, polymorphonuclear (PMN) leukocytes, natural killer (NK) cells, and complements (noncellular proteins) that work together to destroy invading cells and substances. During the first month of a child's life the nonspecific response is immature, so phagocytic cells have little ability to move toward cancer cells and fulfill their function. The nonspecific response is also impaired in stressed and small-for-gestational-age (SGA) infants. In a specific response, T lymphocytes and immunoglobulin (Ig) attack only one type of invader. The specific response capability also is immature in infants. B cell production of various proteins called immunoglobins (M, G, and A) is below adult levels, so that the infant is vulnerable to bacterial and viral infections. (For a discussion of immune function, see Chapter 9.)

■ GROWTH AND DEVELOPMENT CONSIDERATIONS

Adult levels of immunoglobulin M (IgM) are reached in a child at about 1 year of age; IgG adult levels are reached between 5 and 7 years of age; and IgA, between 10 and 14 years.[1]

Childhood Cancer

The care of children who have cancer is a challenging specialty in pediatric nursing. For several years the child undergoes aggressive treatments that may be life threatening and cause temporary illness. Although much of the child's treatment is provided on an outpatient basis, the periods of hospitalization are times of intense physical vulnerability for the child and intense emotional vulnerability for both the child and the family. To monitor the child closely, nurses need a sound knowledge of physiologic responses and medical interventions. Effective communication skills are necessary to support the child and family and promote realistic hope.

Incidence

Each year in the United States, cancer is diagnosed in approximately 6000 to 7000 children.[2] In children under 15 years of age, cancer is the leading cause

TABLE 16-1 Five-Year Relative Survival Rates for Childhood Cancers*

	Year of Diagnosis	
	1970–1973	1981–1987
All sites	45	66.8
Brain and central nervous system	45	57.7
Neuroblastoma	40	55.0
Wilms tumor	70	83.7
Bone	30	55.6
Acute lymphocytic leukemia	34	72.9
Hodgkin disease	90	86.8
Non-Hodgkin lymphoma	26	68.2

Data from National Cancer Institute, (1991). *Cancer statistics review 1973–1988*. NIH Pub. No. 91-2789.
*Numbers shown are percentages.

of disease-related death. In 1988, 1638 U.S. children died of cancer. Cancer was the third leading cause of death among black children 1 to 14 years of age in 1988.[3] National Cancer Institute data show that the incidence of childhood cancer increased 4.1% between 1973 and 1988. However, during the same period the mortality (death) rate from cancer decreased 38%. These data suggest that although cancer is diagnosed in more children each year, more children are also surviving cancer (Table 16–1).

Clinical Manifestations

Each type of childhood cancer signals its presence differently. Many presenting signs and symptoms of cancer are typical of common childhood illnesses.

■ **COMMON SIGNS OF CHILDHOOD CANCER**

Pain	Anemia
Cachexia	Infection

- *Pain* may be the result of a neoplasm either directly or indirectly affecting nerve receptors through obstruction, inflammation, tissue damage, stretching of visceral tissue, or invasion of susceptible tissue.
- *Cachexia is* a syndrome characterized by anorexia, weight loss, anemia, asthenia (weakness), and early satiety (feeling of being full).
- *Anemia* may be experienced during times of chronic bleeding or iron deficiency. In chronic illness the body uses iron poorly. Anemia is also present in cancers of the bone marrow when the number of red blood cells (RBCs) is reduced, in part because of the presence of large numbers of other bone marrow products.
- *Infection* is usually a result of an altered or immature immune system. In addition, infection occurs when bone marrow cancers inhibit maturation of normal immune system cells. Infection may also occur in children who are treated with corticosteroids. Because their immune response is altered, the normal signs of infection may not appear.

Etiology and Pathophysiology

Cellular growth changes in response to external and internal stimuli. Neoplasms are caused by one or a combination of three factors: (1) external stimuli that cause genetic mutations, (2) immune system abnormalities, and (3) chromosomal abnormalities.

External Stimuli. External stimuli may affect the child's general health and cause mutations in body cells. **Carcinogens** are chemicals or industrial processes that, when combined with genetic traits, result in cancer. Several carcinogens cause cancers that are diagnosed during childhood. Others cause cancers that begin in childhood but are not identified until adulthood. Some chemicals suspected of causing childhood cancer include diethylstilbestrol (maternal use of therapeutic estrogen hormones), anabolic androgenic steroids (cortisone), alkylating chemotherapy agents, immunosuppressants, and tobacco.[4]

Immune System Abnormalities. One critical function of a normal immune system is immune surveillance, in which phagocytic cells circulate throughout the body, detecting and destroying abnormal and cancerous cells. Children with congenital immune deficiencies, such as Wiskott-Aldrich syndrome, in which immune surveillance may fail,[5] are at high risk for cancer. A form of non-Hodgkin lymphoma develops in some children treated with immune system–suppressing drugs. This immunosuppression may be the result of virus-induced cellular changes.[5-7] Viruses stimulate certain genes **(protooncogenes)** in a way that helps them become **oncogenes** (cancer-producing genes). Protooncogenes have the latent ability to cause cancer by producing altered proteins that cause cells to proliferate.[8] In fact, viruses may be the second most important risk factor, after chemicals, for cancer development in humans.[9]

Chromosomal Abnormalities. Normal chromosomes undergo change as a part of the genetic process. Most of the changes are not harmful. However, some changes result in chromosomal abnormalities such as hyperploidy (more than the normal number of chromosomes), deletion, translocation, and breakage.

Some of these chromosomal abnormalities have been linked to an increased incidence of cancer. Children with Down syndrome have a 200 times higher incidence of leukemia than nonaffected children. Children who are missing a band of genetic material on their number 13 chromosome often have retinoblastoma. Similarly, Wilms tumor often develops in children missing part of the genetic material from their number 11 chromosome.[5,10]

Activation of Potentially Cancerous Cells. Many theories have been proposed to describe how potentially cancerous cells are activated to become cancerous. One theory suggests that cells must undergo two mutations to become malignant. The first mutation may be inherited, as in retinoblastoma. This mutation predisposes or readies the cell for the second mutation, which is triggered by a stimulus such as a virus or toxin. This second mutation causes the cell to multiply without control, or proliferate.[5,8] A second theory proposes that growth-promoting protooncogenes are counterbalanced by growth-constraining **tumor suppressor genes**.[11] As long as the balance is maintained, everything functions normally. If, however, mutation stimulates the activity of the protooncogene and the suppressor gene is lost or altered, malignant growth results. In this theory, many types of cells will not become malignant unless both types of change are present. Therefore the increased aggressiveness of cancer cells may reflect an accumulation of genetic changes that results in tumor growth.[9] Suppressor genes are not found in the chromosomes of children who have retinoblastoma, Wilms tumor, and neurofibromatosis.[11]

Regardless of the location of abnormal cellular growth, the pathophysiologic process is similar. The altered cell begins to multiply as directed by the altered genetic structure of its DNA and the absence or inactivation of tumor suppressor genes. Each new cell transmits the new or altered pattern to the next generation. As the abnormal cells replicate, the neoplastic mass grows. Normal cells usually die as the increased metabolic rate of the neoplastic cells depletes available nutrition. The altered DNA in the tumor cells may also cause the abnormal cells to invade adjoining tissue. Through continued

TABLE 16-2 Diagnostic Tests for Childhood Cancer

Test	Purpose	Normal Laboratory Values	Diagnostic Values
Bone marrow aspiration	Examines bone marrow	<5% blast cells (immature)	>25% blast cells in acute lymphoblastic leukemia, most with hypercellular marrow
Lumbar puncture	Examines cerebrospinal fluid	Cell count (mm^3) Polymorphonuclear leukocytes 0 Monocytes 0–5 RBCs 0–5	Presence of malignant cells indicates central nervous system involvement (unusual; occurs in < 5% of children)

Data from Gresik, M., Hawkins, E., and Finegold, M. (1991). Pathology. In Fernbach, D. & Vietti, T. (Eds.). *Clinical pediatric oncology* (4th ed.) (p. 69), St. Louis: Mosby–Year Book; Oski, F. (1990). *Pediatrics* (p.1569), Philadelphia: J.B. Lippincott; and Avery, M., and First, L. (1987). *Pediatric medicine* (pp. 549–593). Baltimore: Williams & Wilkins.
RBCs, red blood cells.

growth the mass expands until it enters and disrupts a major vessel or a vital organ, causing death.

Diagnostic Tests and Medical Management

The most common diagnostic tests performed on children with cancer are bone marrow aspiration, lumbar puncture (Table 16–2), peripheral blood studies, radiographic examination, magnetic resonance imaging (MRI), computed tomography (CT), ultrasound, and biopsy.

Cancer is treated with one or a combination of therapies: surgery, chemotherapy, radiation, immune therapy, and bone marrow transplantation. The choice of treatment is determined by the type of cancer, its location, and the degree of metastasis (spread to other sites in the body).

The goal of treatment may be curative, supportive, or palliative. Curative treatment rids the child's body of the cancer. Supportive treatment includes transfusions, pain management, antibiotics, and other interventions to help the body's defenses. Palliative treatment is designed to make the child as comfortable as possible.[12]

Surgery. Surgery is used to remove or debulk (reduce the size of) a solid tumor. An example of a cancer that is commonly treated with surgery is Wilms tumor. Surgery is also used to determine the stage and type of cancer.

Chemotherapy. **Chemotherapy** is the administration of specific drugs that kill both normal and cancerous cells (Fig. 16–1). The administration of various chemotherapeutic drugs (Table 16–3) is timed to achieve the greatest cellular destruction. The schedule is determined by the cell's cycle of replication. Several chemotherapeutic drugs are administered simultaneously to maximize their lethal impact on cells at all stages of activity. Whereas DNA in a normal cell can repair itself after chemotherapy, the DNA in a neoplastic cell cannot.

PROTOCOLS. Each type of cancer that is treated with chemotherapeutic drugs has a unique protocol. A protocol is a map or plan of action that directs treatment by identifying each drug, dose, and interval of administration. The protocol also specifies the action to take for side effects. It dictates the timing

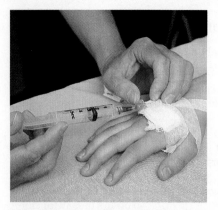

FIGURE 16-1 Chemotherapeutic drugs are given through intravenous infusion. Care should be taken to prevent leakage at the infusion site, since many drugs can cause blistering (extravasation).

TABLE 16-3 Chemotherapeutic Drugs and Their Actions

Class	Drugs	Mechanism of Action
Antimetabolites	Methotrexate, cytosine arabinoside (ARA-C) (CCS) hydroxyuria (CCS), 5-azacytidine (CCS) mercaptopurine (6-MP)	Interfere with function of nucleic acid, inhibiting synthesis of DNA or RNA
Alkylating agents	Nitrogen mustard (CCNS), cyclophosphamide (Cytoxan) (CCNS), chlorambucil (Leukeran) (CCNS), melphalan (PAM) (CCNS), busulfan (Myleran) (CCNS)	Prevent cancer cell division by cross-linkage of DNA strands, resulting in breakdown of chromosomal materials
Antibiotics	Daunorubican (CCS), doxorubicin (Adriamycin) (CCNS), actinomycin D, (CCNS), bleomycin (CCS)	Some interfere with synthesis of cellular proteins; others attack DNA by inhibiting synthesis or disrupting repair mechanisms
Mitotic inhibitors	Vincristine (CCS), vinblastine (CCS), etoposide (VP 16) CCNS)	Interfere with metabolic pathways of amino acids, affect cell energy production required for mitosis, and interfere with nucleic acid synthesis
Nitrosoureas	Lomustine (CCNS), carmustine(CCNS)	Highly lipid soluble and able to cross blood-brain barrier; inhibit several key enzymatic processes
Miscellaneous	L-Asparaginase	Enzyme that causes rapid depletion of exogenous asparagine needed by malignant cells
	Cisplatin	Produces intrastrand crosslinks in DNA

Data from Association of Pediatric Oncology Nurses,[13] McCance & Huether,[14] and Scherer.[15]
CCS, Cell cycle specific; CCNS, cell cycle nonspecific.

and type of laboratory tests and procedures. Some types of cancer, such as leukemia, have several protocols. The specific protocol that is chosen depends on the stage and cellular characteristics of the individual's cancer.

SIDE EFFECTS. The cells that normally divide rapidly are most sensitive to chemotherapeutic drugs. The mucosal tissue in the gastrointestinal tract (mouth, throat, intestines), the bone marrow, hair follicles, and reproductive tissue in pubescent children are examples of tissues containing such rapidly dividing cells.[16] This is why chemotherapy is often accompanied by hair loss, sores, diarrhea, and depletion of red and white blood cells and platelets.

The severity of chemotherapy-induced side effects depends on timing of the therapy. A point of maximum cellular damage is associated with each chemotherapy drug. There is also a point at which the body has not yet begun or is just starting to replace the damaged cells with healthy cells. When maximum cellular damage coincides with a low number of new healthy cells, side effects result.[16]

NURSING ASSESSMENT AND MANAGEMENT OF CHILDREN RECEIVING CHEMOTHERAPY. All children receiving chemotherapy are continually assessed for **extravasation** and inflammation of the bowel (neutropenic enterocolitis). Extravasation is damage caused by leakage of the drugs into the soft tissue surrounding the infusion site (peripheral intravenous infiltration). If

■ **SAFETY PRECAUTIONS**

The Occupational Safety and Health Administration (OSHA) mandates guidelines to protect health care providers from undue exposure to cytotoxic agents.

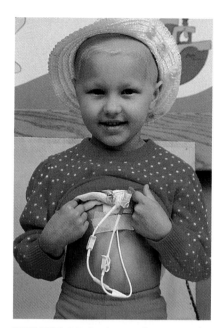

FIGURE 16-2 A vascular access device allows chemotherapeutic agents to be administered without the need for repeated "sticks" to the child.

the infiltrating substance is a vesicant (blistering agent) such as vinblastine or vincristine, the drug may cause cell lysis (dissolution), tissue sloughing, and a functional deficit at the infusion site. Placement of a central line or vascular access device (Fig. 16–2) is generally recommended to prevent this occurrence. Another advantage of these devices is that the child not only receives chemotherapy through this route, but also can have blood for laboratory evaluation drawn through the line. This reduces the number of times the child experiences arm or finger "sticks." These "sticks" are traumatic for the child and create an avenue for infection if the child is neutropenic.

Neutropenic enterocolitis is a complication of aggressive chemotherapy and resulting neutropenia. Chemotherapy damages the tissue of the bowel wall. The child's neutropenia then allows invasion of the bowel wall by bacteria. The result is an invasive infection leading to necrosis of several layers of the bowel wall. The terminal ileum and cecum are common sites for enterocolitis, but any part of the bowel may be involved.[17,18]

Management of common side effects of chemotherapy is summarized in Table 16–4. **Bone marrow suppression** occurs when reduced activity of the bone marrow stem cells results in reduced numbers of RBCs, white blood cells (WBCs), and platelets. The latest treatment for bone marrow suppression is the use of colony-stimulating factors (CSFs). CSFs are hormonelike glycoproteins that enhance growth of bone marrow (myelopoiesis), which increases production of WBCs and decreases the length and severity of **leukopenia** (reduced WBC production). Cloned CSFs are administered by subcutaneous injection. The most frequently reported side effect is bone pain. Temporary bruising and inflammation at the injection site have also been reported. Most patients, however, report no side effects.[24]

Radiation. **Radiation,** which involves the use of unstable isotopes that release varying levels of energy to destroy cells, has been used as a treatment method since the early 1900s. It is often used for local and regional control of cancer, as well as in combination with surgery and chemotherapy.

The area to be irradiated (treatment field) includes the tumor site and sometimes other involved areas, such as lymph glands. The total dose of radiation is divided (or fractionated) and given over several weeks. A common course of radiation treatment might be once daily 4 or 5 days per week for a period of 2 to 6 weeks.

Tumors that are highly sensitive to radiation include Hodgkin disease, Wilms tumor, retinoblastoma, and rhabdomyosarcoma. Tumors that have low sensitivity to radiation include osteosarcoma and soft tissue sarcomas. These low-sensitivity tumors require higher doses of radiation.

Radiation therapy presents several difficulties for children. The child must maintain a fixed and reproducible position during each therapy session. The session may take 10 to 20 minutes. Usually children over the age of 3 can learn to stay still during radiation treatments. It is helpful to have the child practice the required position before beginning radiation therapy.

Younger children, developmentally disabled children, and very anxious children may require sedation for radiation treatments. Drugs commonly administered for this purpose include chloral hydrate, fentanyl, and pentobarbital. The nurse should coordinate other tests needed by the child so that they are performed during the sedation period.[25]

Immune Therapy. **Immune therapy** is the use of biologic response modifiers, such as interleukin-2, lymphokine-activated killer cells, or radiolabeled monoclonal antibodies, to treat cancer. There are three major classes of biological response modifiers: (1) agents that restore, augment, or modulate the host's immunologic mechanisms, (2) agents that have direct antitumor activity, and (3) agents that have other biologic effects. The actions of many of

TABLE 16–4 Management of Common Side Effects of Chemotherapy

Side Effect	Medical Management	Nursing Interventions
Bone marrow suppression	Evidence of suppression usually appears 7–10 days after administration of chemotherapy; recovery is usually complete within 3–4 weeks Blood transfusions are administered when anemia is severe (Hgb <7 g/dL) Some institutions use a low-microbial diet to decrease the possibility that infectious organisms will colonize the intestine Septra is used for *Pneumocystis carinii* pneumonia prophylaxis; nystatin and oral vancomycin for antifungal and antibacterial prophylaxis; if a child does not become febrile, combination therapy using several intravenous antibiotics is initiated	Instruct the family and child about the importance of protecting the body from bruising during periods of mild to moderate thrombocytopenia (platelet count <500/mm^3) Careful handwashing is essential Encourage use of masks if family or staff have nasopharyngeal infections
Nausea and vomiting	Symptoms may occur immediately or 5–6 hours after administration of chemotherapy and may last 48 hours Antiemetics, such as ondansetron and compazine, are used to treat this side effect	Teach relaxation techniques, hypnosis, and systematic desensitization (a hypnotic process that progressively reduces reactions to objects that cause strong emotional or physical responses) to help to decrease the child's symptoms Encourage mild exercise and change of diet (eating only easily digestible foods) 12 hours before chemotherapy
Anorexia and weight loss	May occur at any time; hyperalimentation is necessary if dietary changes are unsuccessful in halting the child's weight loss	Pay careful attention to changes in taste that affect food preferences Referral to a dietician may be helpful to achieve successful modification of the child's diet
Mouth sores	The oral mucositis resulting from chemotherapy usually occurs within 3–4 days and is often a contributing factor in anorexia Antifungal agents, such as nystatin or clotrimazole, lessen the possibility of candidal infection	Promote good oral hygiene, use soft foam wand to clean teeth; commercial mouth washes are not recommended because they contain alcohol and increase drying of the oral cavity
Constipation	Stool softeners and laxatives are used to treat this side effect	Advise parents to increase fluids and fibrous foods in the child's diet
Pain	Acetaminophen, morphine, steroids, nonsteroidal antiinflammatory drugs, and antidepressants may be used to manage pain	Careful pain assessment is important; the location of the pain may provide a clue to its cause, for example, metastasis to the skull, infiltration of joints, or damage to soft tissue; pain associated with chemotherapy may also be related to oral mucositis, myalgia, or tumor embolization; painful polyneuropathy can follow treatment with vincristine or cisplatin Pharmacologic, nonhypnotic (deep breathing, self-control), and hypnotic methods of pain control may be used; the nonpharmacologic methods often prove helpful to children with pain from multiple etiologies

Data from Lilley,[16] Hogan, [19]Hutter, [20] Pervan, [21] Portenoy, [22] and Rostad.[23]

■ LEGAL AND ETHICAL CONSIDERATIONS

Consent is mandatory if a child is to be started on a medication that is considered a clinical trial drug.

these agents are not completely understood, and some agents have more than one effect. For example, interferon has both antiviral and antiproliferative effects on some malignant cells. Interferon and tumor necrosis factor are undergoing clinical trials to study their effectiveness and to develop protocols for their safe use against selected cancers. Because knowledge about these biologic response modifiers is limited, it is important that nurses record and report side effects that may occur when this therapy is administered according to a prescribed research protocol.

Allogenic Donor and recipient are of same species.
Autologous Donor and recipient are the same person.
Isogeneic or Syngeneic Donor and recipient are genetically the same.

■ LEGAL AND ETHICAL
CONSIDERATIONS

An objective child advocate whose role is to safeguard the rights and needs of a minor child involved in decisions about bone marrow harvests is frequently a part of the bone marrow transplant team.

■ NURSING ALERT

Watch for signs of septic shock: hyperthermia (or hypothermia), tachycardia, tachypnea, hypotension, mental changes (confusion, restlessness, irritability), peripheral cyanosis, and cold or clammy extremities.

Bone Marrow Transplantation. **Bone marrow transplantation** is used for treatment of leukemia, neuroblastoma, and some noncancerous conditions, such as aplastic anemia. The goal of therapy is to administer a lethal dose of therapy to kill the cancer, then resupply the body with bone marrow stem cells either from the child's own marrow previously removed and stored or from a compatible donor.

Bone marrow transplantation is the treatment of choice when a relapse occurs while the child is receiving another form of cancer therapy. First, a histocompatible donor must be located. The recipient then receives intensive chemotherapy, often followed by total body irradiation. This treatment kills all circulating blood cells and bone marrow contents. Following this treatment the recipient is transfused with the donor bone marrow. New blood cells usually form within 6 to 8 weeks.

Close monitoring and supportive treatment are needed until production of blood cells is adequate. Common complications immediately after transfusion include bacterial or fungal sepsis, interstitial pneumonia, massive vomiting, and diarrhea. Once the donor (allogenic or isogeneic) bone marrow is functioning, **graft-versus-host disease** (rejection) may occur. In graft-versus-host disease the new immune cells from the donor bone marrow identify the host cells as foreign and respond by defending the graft from the host cells and killing them. Symptoms of graft-versus-host disease include skin, liver, intestinal, and lymphoid reactions.

Oncologic Emergencies. Oncologic emergencies can be organized into three groups: metabolic, hematologic, and those involving space-occupying lesions.

METABOLIC EMERGENCIES. Metabolic emergencies result from the lysis (dissolving or decomposing) of tumor cells, a process called tumor lysis syndrome. This cell destruction releases high levels of uric acid, potassium, phosphates, and calcium into the blood and can lower serum sodium levels. These blood imbalances can be prevented or reduced by use of hydration, sodium bicarbonate, corticosteroids, allopurinol, and sodium polystyrene (Kayexalate).[12] In children, extensive cell destruction is most commonly seen in the treatment of leukemia and lymphoma.[26]

A second type of metabolic emergency is septic shock. During periods of immune suppression the child is vulnerable to overwhelming infection, resulting in circulatory failure, inadequate tissue perfusion, and hypotension. Septic shock can be fatal. Factors contributing to massive infection include inadequate neutrophil production, abnormal granulocytes (not able to be actively phagocytic), erosions through normal barriers such as blood vessels and mucous membranes, and altered bone marrow production caused by chemotherapy and some forms of radiation. The child's granulocyte counts should be monitored carefully because persistent and severe granulocytopenia (granulocyte count $<100/mm^3$) can be fatal.[27]

HEMATOLOGIC EMERGENCIES. Hematologic emergencies result from bone marrow suppression or neoplastic infiltration. Associated conditions include anemia, thrombocytopenia, disseminated intravascular coagulation (DIC), neutropenia, hyperleukocytosis (excessive numbers of WBCs), and acute graft-versus-host disease. These conditions, with the exception of graft-versus-host disease, are treated with transfusions.

Hemorrhage—either gastrointestinal or intracranial—is another potentially serious complication of cancer in children. Hemorrhage is usually caused by DIC and thrombocytopenia. A massive gastrointestinal hemorrhage may result in a loss of up to 15% of blood volume within minutes or hours. An intracranial hemorrhage is more likely to occur in a child with leukemia during diagnosis and relapse.

SPACE-OCCUPYING LESIONS. Extensive tumor growth may result in spinal cord compression, increased intracranial pressure, seizures, and superior vena cava syndrome (obstruction of the superior vena cava by tumor). These emergencies are often caused by neuroblastoma, medulloblastoma, astrocytoma, Hodgkin disease, or lymphoma. Treatment involves radiation therapy, chemotherapy, and corticosteroids.[12]

General Nursing Care of the Child with Cancer

Families of children with cancer require a complete understanding of their fears and needs. Communication skills are important, as is forthrightness about the child's condition, treatment, and prognosis. Families experience a devastating shock when cancer is diagnosed in their child. Many people still think that cancer is invariably fatal. It is important for the health care team to be composed of a variety of professionals to ensure direct intervention or referral of parents to community resources for the support they will need during the care of their child.

Effective communication is a major factor for families in which a child has cancer. Respect, honesty, and mutual caring are essential to effective communication. All family members should be encouraged to ask questions and express concerns. This can be done through standard communication techniques such as reflecting, restating, and observing nonverbal behaviors.

Initially most parents feel a need to protect the child from the emotional impact of the diagnosis. Open discussions between the health care team and the family will reduce the parents' fears about telling the child and siblings about the disease, its treatment, and the child's prognosis.

The family will be in a state of crisis following the diagnosis and will need crisis intervention techniques to support them. Although parents will not retain much information, large amounts of information must be given to them. Continual restatement and clarification of the information is a key responsibility of the health care team. Providing written and illustrated materials helps the parents to retain information and use it later. Some centers have devised simple handouts, containing definitions and basic information, that can be given to the family during the initial conference.

Most centers hold family conferences to encourage open communication between families and health care team members and within families. The parental role is reinforced by praise and acknowledgment of the parents' importance in the child's well-being. Many parents are concerned about what caused the cancer, and they may feel guilty in the mistaken belief that they contributed to its onset. Talking openly about this common feeling may aid parents to discuss their feelings.

Anticipatory guidance can assist the family in dealing with the challenges of hospital and home care. Role modeling can help with the problem of telling people outside the immediate family about the diagnosis.

The child also needs to learn about the disease. Age-appropriate drawings and stories assist children in learning not only about their disease but also how to cope with the disease. Focusing on activities the child can perform helps in building self-esteem and supports development.

A firm knowledge of development is essential to working with children who have cancer. Depending on the developmental stage, the child's fears may center on loss of parents (toddlers), abandonment and guilt (preschoolers), or loss of function and body image (school-age children and adolescents). Nurses can engage the child in play and distraction to support normal coping methods (see Chapter 4). Art and play therapy help the nurse to identify and resolve the child's fears (Fig. 16–3). A referral to a psychologist may be needed.

■ LEGAL AND ETHICAL CONSIDERATIONS

The nurse who cares for a child with cancer has an ethical responsibility to keep the child and family informed and to maintain privacy and confidentiality.

FIGURE 16-3 A child in a pediatric oncology clinic giving injections to a doll. This type of play therapy helps the child deal with fear and thus lower his or her stress level.

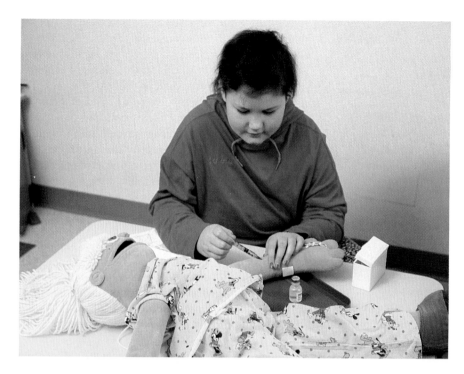

Education for both the family and the child should be continued throughout the treatment period. Praise and recognition of the family's and child's achievements in their daily life and in performing the treatment regimen are essential to supporting self-esteem and normal family development. Be alert to signs of closed family communication, including hesitancy to discuss issues with other family members, protective barriers to sharing of medical information, dishonesty about events or new information, or avoidance of other family members. Confrontation and role modeling are communication methods that may assist family members to increase communication. If these techniques are ineffective, referral to family therapy may be needed.

Nurses and other health care members must deal with their own feelings of sadness, grief, foreboding, and failure. Support from peers and support groups can help resolve these feelings. Opinions vary about how much these feelings should be shared between the nurse and the family. An overriding consideration is the family's well-being. Being open about feelings without adding to the burden the family already carries is a goal of open communication between the family and health care professionals.

The stressors in daily life are another area for communication. Problem solving, values clarification, and referral to social services are ways to help the family.

General guidelines on what to say and not to say to children are based on knowledge of normal developmental stages (see Chapter 2):

- *Infants* need nurturing and support.
- *Toddlers* need to express individuation and feel secure. Punishment and threats can be overwhelming when delivered by people the child perceives to have terrible powers, such as nurses with needles. A positive focus on getting better and use of distraction during stressful times are more effective.
- *Preschoolers* want to help and are open to learning ways to hold still or reduce pain. They can understand simple explanations about their bodies but are afraid of blood and "their insides." They may think that be-

ing "bad" caused them to get sick. They need reassurance that they did not cause the illness.

- *School-age children* seek knowledge and new skills. Drawings and discussions with peers are effective methods of expressing concerns and misconceptions. At this age children have unrealistic expectations of themselves and need objective evaluation from others to develop more appropriate goals and expectations.
- *Adolescents* are defining themselves as unique individuals. They are challenged by the natural changes in their bodies and distressed by the changes resulting from treatment. Insincere compliments and inappropriate joviality create communication barriers. Support of the grief process, along with continued empathy, respect, and genuineness, is an important approach for this age group.

Nursing Assessment

Physiologic Assessment. Physiologic assessment focuses on identifying signs and symptoms of cancer, and ongoing assessment of side effects of treatment (see earlier discussion). Specific assessment of children with different types of childhood cancer is presented later in the chapter.

Psychosocial Assessment. Assessment of body image, family stressors, knowledge, crises, coping mechanisms, family structure, support systems, and culture provides data that help determine the appropriate nursing interventions for the child with cancer and the family.

BODY IMAGE. Hair loss, surgical scars, and cushingoid changes are three common treatment-induced threats to body image.

Most children being treated for cancer experience hair loss (Fig. 16–4). Children who have cranial surgery lose hair as part of the surgical preparation. Chemotherapy frequently results in some degree of hair loss. The speed of hair loss is unique to the child and can be as rapid as overnight or slower, evidenced by hair left on the pillow and in the hairbrush.

A second challenge to the child's body image is surgery. The scars of cranial and neck surgery are obvious, as are amputation and limb salvaging.

FIGURE 16–4 One of the most common threats to a child's body image at any age is hair loss induced by chemotherapy.

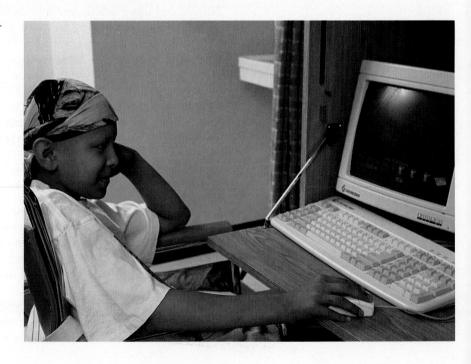

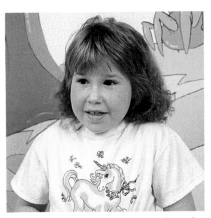

FIGURE 16–5 The child with cushingoid changes frequently has a rounded face and prominent cheeks.

Abdominal surgery for lymphoma is more easily concealed but is still a threat to the child's body image.

A third source of altered body image is the cushingoid features that result from use of corticosteroids. Cushingoid changes in the child with cancer are round and flushed face, prominent cheeks, double chin, and generalized obesity (Fig. 16–5). As the child's weight increases, stretch marks similar to those of pregnancy may occur. These stretch marks often remain after the corticosteroids are decreased.

The destruction of a previous self-image is necessary before the child can accept a new image. This process is based on the reactions of the child and others. Body image disturbances occur when a person cannot integrate new changes and continues to cling to old images despite their inconsistency with reality.[28] Common means for assessing body image are drawings, colored pictures cut out by the child to form a collage, and discussion and observation. Table 16–5 presents nursing interventions for the child with a body image disturbance.

FAMILY STRESSORS. One year after the diagnosis of childhood cancer, most families are coping well. The families who are not coping well have a high level of stress reflecting marital, family, or sibling problems or economic difficulties.[29] Concurrent stressors increase the family's difficulty in coping with childhood cancer. These stressors include illness or death of another family member, occupational changes, financial problems, relocation, and change in vacation plans. Therefore ongoing assessment includes exploration of additional stressors experienced by the family and encouragement to seek assistance for these problems.

KNOWLEDGE. People who are anxious tend to narrow their scope of attention and may read unintended messages into the behaviors of health care personnel. Anxiety also limits a person's ability to retain information.[30] For these reasons, be sure to repeat information and provide written materials to the family.

The child's knowledge of cancer and its treatment should be assessed throughout the treatment period. As the child matures cognitively, it is important to continue his or her education about the disease.

COPING MECHANISMS. There are two levels of coping. One level is the capacity to cope with opportunities, challenges, frustrations, and threats in the environment. The second level is the ability to maintain internal integration, that is, the capacity to manage one's reaction to the environment in a way that maintains the ability to function.[31] A person's perception of events is the basis for coping.

Destructive coping attempts to ward off anxiety without resolving the conflict. One method of coping is avoidance or evasion.[32] Avoidance-type coping is characterized by avoiding or denying the threatening aspects of an

---

TABLE 16-5 Nursing Interventions for the Child with a Body Image Disturbance

- Respect the child's need to avoid direct confrontation with the change.
- Be matter-of-fact when dealing with the affected area.
- Focus on the positive aspects of functioning that compensate for the loss.
- Use dolls and drawings to encourage expression of feelings about the altered part and to reinforce the positive aspects of the changes.
- Teach the child how to use camouflage or new equipment to compensate for any loss of function.
- Compliment the child on behaviors showing increased acceptance of change.
- Encourage general play to allow the child time to work through the changes.

upcoming event and being hesitant or unwilling to discuss thoughts about the event.[33]

Adolescents with cancer often delay, modify, or even stop their treatment because of its side effects.[34] Issues for teenagers include dealing with painful procedures and life-style changes, school reentry, changed appearance, loss of peer support, and attempts to balance independence and dependence. When these issues become overwhelming, teenagers may "break loose" to gain some emotional distance.[34]

The parents' adjustment to the child's chronic illness directly influences the child's adjustment. If the mother or primary caretaker is anxious and suspicious of the health care environment, the young child may reflect that anxiety through restlessness and irritability. How the parent performs the tasks associated with the chronic illness also directly influences the child's self-esteem.[35] Mothers who know what to expect experience less anxiety and expend less effort in coping with the stressful events during their child's hospitalization.[36]

FAMILY STRUCTURE. Some family structures are maladaptive. The stressors associated with cancer magnify a family's inability to cope adaptively. Thoroughly assess the coping strategies used by the family to meet the various challenges posed by the child's illness. This information helps to predict the success of various interventions, such as home care with intravenous medications, and to decide whether a referral for family therapy is appropriate.

SUPPORT SYSTEMS. To help the family during crises, assess family resources to identify support systems available to the family. Extended support systems include friends, jobs, insurance coverage, religious affiliations, cultural support systems, and the school system. Parents commonly lose contact with close friends following the diagnosis of cancer in a child. This is an additional stressor for the family.

Jobs are often a source of support because co-workers may have gone through the same experience. Jobs can also be a source of stress if employers are unsympathetic to the demands of the child's hospitalization and clinic or office visits.

Religious affiliations can be an important source of support. Transportation, food, money, and willing listeners are frequently found at church or synagogue. Spiritual beliefs can provide special solace. However, religious practices can also be a source of conflict with health care providers in decisions about treatment. For example, Jehovah's Witnesses do not allow the transfusion of blood products; this belief system may prohibit an anemic or neutropenic child from receiving much needed blood products during times of severe depletion. Parents should discuss these limitations with the oncology team.

The return to school may pose difficulties for the child with cancer. The school system may be reluctant to accept a medically vulnerable child into the classroom. Preparation of school officials, teachers, and classmates is often necessary for the child's successful reentry to school. Physicians and nurses from the cancer center can visit the classroom to discuss the cancer and its treatment before the child returns to school. Another approach is to show a videotape of the child while he or she is receiving treatment, as well as the child's hospital room and daily activities.[37] An interactive puppet show can be used to talk about the returning child's physical changes and ways to help him or her deal with hair loss and weight changes. Puppets encourage questions from the class. For high school students the use of slides, pamphlets, and discussion is effective.[38]

Children receiving cranial radiation will need continual scholastic evaluations. Memory deficits and selective attention deficits as well as decreased intelligence quotients may occur as long-term effects of treatment.[39] The academic environment will need to be modified to support the special needs of these children.

Developmental Assessment. Developmental assessment of children under 6 years of age should regularly be performed during treatment for cancer. Assessment of the child's physical and neurologic development helps in determining the progress made during treatment and provides a baseline for evaluating the long-term effects of treatment. Children under 6 years of age who have cancer should receive regular developmental assessment. Careful recording of height and weight is essential. Observations of gait and coordination are helpful and can be made during the physical examination, for example, by observing the child as he or she undresses and climbs onto the examining table.

Nursing Diagnosis

Children with cancer have common psychologic and physiologic problems, regardless of their specific type of cancer (Tables 16–6 and 16–7). They and their families are attempting to deal with a complex illness that will control their lives for several years. The impact of this experience extends into all areas of coping.

Nursing Management

The nursing care of children with cancer and their families includes immediate physiologic and psychologic support, along with anticipatory guidance

---

TABLE 16–6 Nursing Diagnoses for Common Psychologic Problems of the Child with Cancer

Anxiety related to actual or perceived loss of significant others, threat or change in health status, situational crises, unmet needs, threat of death, lack of knowledge, loss of control, disruptive family life

Body Image Disturbance related to effects of loss of body parts, effects of loss of body function

Ineffective Individual Coping related to effects of chronic or acute illness, loss of control over body part or function, lack of support system, low self-esteem, unrealistic perceptions, situational crises, knowledge deficit, sensory overload

Anticipatory Grieving related to actual or potential loss of significant other, health status

Altered Growth and Development related to environmental or stimulation deficiencies, prescribed dependence

Hopelessness related to grieving, depression, social isolation, prolonged activity restriction, role disruption

Knowledge Deficit (lack of exposure, information misinterpretation, denial)

Noncompliance related to denial, depression, knowledge deficit, lack of support system

Personal Identity Disturbance related to developmental crises, role changes

Powerlessness related to social isolation, lack of knowledge, health care environment

Altered Role Performance related to change in health status, developmental crises, role loss, loss of support group

Impaired Home Maintenance Management related to lack of knowledge, insufficient family organizing, inadequate support systems

Altered Health Maintenance related to knowledge deficit, dysfunctional grieving, ineffective coping, religious or cultural values, lack of support systems

Modified from Taptich.[40]

TABLE 16-7 Nursing Diagnoses for Common Physiologic Problems of the Child with Cancer

Activity Intolerance related to malnourishment, interrupted sleep, pain, fatigue, depression

Constipation related to pain or discomfort on defecation, effects of medication, immobility, effects of stress

Diarrhea related to effects of medications, radiation, surgical procedures, infectious process, nutritional disorders, stress, and anxiety

Altered Urinary Elimination related to stress, change in environment, effects of medications

Fluid Volume Excess related to compromised regulatory mechanisms, effects of medications, excessive fluid or sodium intake, low protein intake

Fluid Volume Deficit related to nausea and vomiting, dietary alterations

Ineffective Breathing Pattern related to decreased energy, fatigue, neuromuscular impairment, pain, anxiety

Impaired Tissue Integrity related to altered circulation, impaired mobility, nutritional deficit, fluid excess or deficit

Altered Oral Mucous Membrane related to effects of chemotherapy, radiation effects, inadequate oral hygiene, malnutrition, vomiting

Impaired Skin Integrity related to altered nutritional state, effects of medication, radiation, stress

Activity Imbalance related to malnourishment, interrupted sleep, pain, fatigue, lack of motivation

Fatigue related to decreased or increased metabolic energy production, overwhelming demands, altered body chemistry (chemotherapy)

Sleep Pattern Disturbance related to pain, diarrhea, nausea, stress, anxiety, unfamiliar environment

Diversional Activity Deficit related to effects of chronic illness, frequent lengthy treatments, isolation from peers

Impaired Swallowing related to mechanical obstruction (tumor), fatigue

Self-Care Deficit related to effects of loss of limb, fatigue, pain, presence of external devices, knowledge deficit, anxiety, dependence

Modified from Taptich.[40]

■ FAMILY TRANSITION MODEL[41]

Shattering of Reality Realization that the child's illness is malignant.

Limbo Waiting to see if the child will respond to the therapy and achieve a remission.

Reconstruction of Reality Seeking new strategies to deal with the changes in the family's life.

New Reality Using the new strategies to deal with demands of family life and a chronically ill child.

Readjusting Reality Therapy reaches a conclusion and the family readjusts to having a "cured" child.

---

about imminent and future medical interventions. Nursing care to support physiologic functioning centers on maintaining adequate nutrition and minimizing the side effects of treatment. Specific interventions for children with different types of childhood cancer are discussed later in the chapter.

Anticipatory guidance focuses on the purpose of medical or nursing interventions, what the child will experience, and what the child should do to help during the procedure or intervention. Information and direction for the parents on how they can assist their child during the event is also needed. All events regardless of their importance are communicated in advance to the parents and child to allow them to gather their coping resources and learn to deal with the event in a positive manner. Knowing what to do and being rewarded for doing as much to help as possible can support the child's self-esteem. Preparing the parents for their role during the event can further support their parental role and reduce their feelings of powerlessness.

Family Transition During the Child's Illness. To provide effective care, the nurse needs to understand the processes experienced by the family during the diagnosis and treatment of their child's cancer. Clarke-Steffan's family transition model[41] is helpful in understanding this process. This model also enables the nurse to provide appropriate education to the family during different stages of the transition process (Table 16–8).

As the course of treatment nears completion, the family often becomes anxious that the cancer will return after treatment is stopped. Once the treat-

TABLE 16–8 Parent and Family Teaching: Topics of Education for the Family of a Child with Cancer

Shattering of Reality Stage

- Discuss causes of childhood cancer as they differ from adult cancer.
- Describe general pathophysiology of child's cancer, if known.
- Describe purpose of tests.
- Discuss ways to help child cope during tests.

Limbo Stage

- Provide more specific information about tests, such as what is being tested and why.
- Provide information about treatment such as chemotherapy, for example, drug effects and immediate side effects.
- Discuss ways to help the child deal with immediate side effects.

Reconstruction of Reality Stage

- Inform the family of resources in the community and the hospital or agency for support.
- Repeat information about disease and treatment to clarify and fill in gaps in knowledge base.
- Problem-solve immediate anticipated problems.
- Problem-solve side effects, such as hair loss and appetite changes.

Reinduction Stage

- Review chemotherapy drugs and give information on any added drugs, effects, and side effects.

Maintenance Stage

- Review at-home regimen for medications.
- Problem-solve any potential family issues, such as safety.

---

ment ends, the family again experiences a period of transition, from having an ill child to having a "cured" child.

Impact of Relapse or Recurrence. Recurrence of the child's cancer during treatment is called a relapse. Relapse occurs because the remaining malignant cells have developed a high resistance to the chemotherapy already received. The nurse helps the family understand that this resistance cannot easily be overcome. Although different drugs may be used to regain remission, the resistant cells often break through, causing repeated relapses. When each treatment fails and relapse occurs, the child and family commonly respond with anger, guilt, fear, and resentment.[42] The family slowly begins to realize that the child may die. Each relapse reinforces the loss for the family until death finally occurs. Often the child's steadily deteriorating physical condition provides time for the family to let go of their protective denial slowly and to grieve with the child. Parents often benefit from referral to support groups such as the Candlelighter's Foundation (see Appendix F).

Both the child and the family feel anxiety throughout the course of treatment. Anxiety remains even after remission and cure are attained. This ever-present stress is increased whenever an unanticipated event occurs. One root of the anxiety is the parents' feelings of powerlessness to protect the child. The nurse can assist the parents with these feelings throughout treatment. Empowerment by including, informing, and supporting them can reduce the long-term effects of anxiety and powerlessness.

Impact of Being a Survivor. There are psychologic consequences even for the child who is a cancer survivor. Children cured of cancer report feeling different from other children their age. They feel that they missed part of their childhood because of the cancer treatment. Although the children describe the experience as difficult and painful, they also report that through it they gained a belief in themselves, an acceptance of death, and maturity.[43]

Goals of Nursing Care. For the nurse the broad goals of care change as the child progresses through the phases of treatment. During diagnosis the goal is to assist and support the parents through crises and to provide an initial level of education. As the family and child begin the reinduction and maintenance phases of chemotherapy, the nursing focus shifts to patient education and assisting the family with the demands on their time and energies. The final period before the end of therapy is a time of reorganization. The family no longer has the support of frequent contact with the hospital and familiar health care team members. They need reassurance and anticipatory problem solving during this period. If a relapse occurs, anticipatory grieving may begin. As death nears, hospice-type nursing care is provided.

Discharge Planning and Patient and Family Home Care Teaching. Preparation for home care of the child with cancer centers on creating a normal environment while supporting the body's response to the cancer and treatments. Education is the primary focus of discharge planning. Teach the parents about nutrition, signs of infection, protection from exposure to communicable diseases during times of neutropenia, administration of medications at home, and methods to handle pain and vomiting. Assist the parents and child to deal with any obstacles to normal development and functioning.

Home management of a vascular access device or central line, such as a Broviac (see Atlas of Pediatric Procedures), is an initial challenge for parents. An implanted port allows the child freedom to swim and engage in other activities. Before the child's discharge, parents will need information about cleaning the site and instilling heparin in the line or reservoir. Review instructions with parents and observe them perform the procedure before discharge.

It is important to stress the need for the child and family to have fun and be as normal as possible. Play distracts the child and is essential in reducing fears. The child, parents, and siblings often benefit from participation in cancer support groups. The family should be encouraged to take part in these groups and oncology camps. These activities create additional support systems, build the child's self-esteem, and enhance coping skills through role modeling.

Nursing care of the child with cancer at home and in the hospital is summarized in the accompanying care plans. These care plans are designed for the child who is past the cancer diagnosis phase and is receiving chemotherapy.

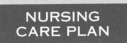

HOSPITAL CARE OF THE CHILD WITH CANCER

GOAL	INTERVENTION	RATIONALE	EXPECTED OUTCOME
1. Pain related to injuring agents			
Child will report lessened pain that is manageable.	Give analgesics. Teach relaxation, deep breathing, and distraction.	Adequate medications can reduce pain. Nonpharmacologic methods work with the medication to reduce pain.	Child experiences pain reduced to the level that allows child to interact appropriately and gain rest.
2. Sleep Pattern Disturbance related to physical discomfort, personal stress, family stress, environmental changes, or inactivity			
Child will sleep for hours appropriate to age. Child will report feeling rested.	Alter the environment to allow designated rest periods. Plan care to reduce frequency of interruptions during normal rest and sleep times.	A quiet environment encourages relaxation needed for resting. Reduced interruptions allow continuous sleep and rest.	Child rests and sleeps for age-appropriate amount of time per day.
3. Altered Nutrition: Less Than Body Requirements related to buccal cavity discomfort, altered taste sensation, anorexia, or emotional stress			
Child will maintain adequate nutritional intake.	Offer small feedings. Encourage home-type foods. Refer to dietician for special meals. Weigh daily.	Early satiety reduces food intake. Taste changes and mouth sores alter desire for food	Child maintains admission weight.
Child will experience reduced effects of chemotherapy (i.e., nausea and vomiting).	Teach child distraction and relaxation techniques. Give antiemetics according to orders.	Pharmacologic and nonpharmacologic methods are effective in helping to reduce nausea.	Child has minimal side effects of nausea and vomiting.
4. Constipation related to low-roughage diet, low fluid intake, decreased activity level, or absence of routine			
Child will reestablish normal bowel pattern.	Record all output by weight or size and description. Administer stool softeners. Obtain stool for guaiac assessment. Report changes in stool to physician.	Chemotherapy and tumor site may create constipation, diarrhea or blood in stool.	Child has normal bowel pattern.
5. Fluid Volume Excess related to excess fluid or sodium intake			
Child will be adequately hydrated.	Record all intake. Monitor intravenous rate and solution appropriate to chemotherapy. Test specific gravity of urine daily.	Cyclophosphamide necessitates high level of fluid intake to prevent bladder hemorrhage. Renal function may be affected by chemotherapy	Child demonstrates adequate hydration. Mucous membranes are hydrated. Specific gravity returns to normal after chemotherapy.

Continued.

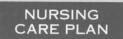
HOSPITAL CARE OF THE CHILD WITH CANCER— CONTINUED

GOAL	INTERVENTION	RATIONALE	EXPECTED OUTCOME
6. High Risk for Infection related to risk factors of inadequate primary defenses, inadequate secondary defenses, immunosuppression, insufficient knowledge, tissue destruction, invasive procedures, malnutrition, or pharmaceutical agents			
Child will remain free of infection.	Wash hands often.	Handwashing is effective in killing organisms.	Child remains infection free.
	Monitor temperature. Report elevation to physician.	Elevated temperature is a sign of infection.	
Child will return to normal, uninfected state.	Administer intravenous antibiotics as ordered. Monitor temperature. Use cooling mattress as ordered. Report elevations over 101° F to physician.	Multiple antibiotics are needed to deal with bacterial and fungal infections during neutropenia. Blood cultures may be taken to identify organism.	Child returns to normal, uninfected state.
7. Impaired Physical Mobility related to neuromuscular impairment (central nervous system tumor, increased intracranial pressure)			
Child will be managed with minimal complications.	Observe for changes in level of consciousness, seizure activity, and changes in gait.	Tumors and chemotherapy can can create changes in neurological status.	All changes in child's condition are reported promptly to the physician.
8. Ineffective Individual Coping related to changes in body integrity, altered affect (brain tumor), disruption of emotional bonds due to separation, or inadequate psychologic resources			
Child will demonstrate normal adaptive coping methods.	Encourage play, drawings and therapeutic play for expression of feelings. Provide structure for expression of angry feelings, such as hitting dolls and throwing sponge balls. Discuss how to behave during treatments.	Expression of feelings helps identify avoidance coping for further intervention. Play is normal way for child to express self and ideas. Misinterpretations can be corrected. Knowledge of appropriate and helpful behaviors supports self-esteem.	Child continues to use usual coping strategies expected for developmental stage.
9. Altered Health Maintenance related to new or complex treatment, misinterpretation of information, or lack of education			
Child will state understanding of treatments and procedures.	Use age-appropriate teaching methods. Content areas include child's cancer, medications (actions and side effects), how to deal with body changes, and how to deal with response of others to those changes. Correct misinterpretations. Anticipate upcoming events and teach child and family about them.	Education helps by increasing understanding, removing fantasy, and clarifying fears. Education promotes the use of new learning in all areas of life.	Child demonstrates an age-appropriate knowledge of the cancer, its treatments, and medications. Child has age-appropriate understanding of how to deal with changes in the body.

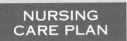

HOME CARE OF THE CHILD WITH CANCER

GOAL	INTERVENTION	RATIONALE	EXPECTED OUTCOME
1. High Risk for Infection related to immunosuppression, chemotherapy, presence of invasive lines			
Child will remain infection free.	Educate child and parents about meaning of blood counts.	Knowledgeable parents and child can protect themselves.	Child remains infection free.
	Encourage parents/family members to use masks when they are ill.	Masks help decrease airborne infection if used properly.	
	Encourage good handwashing at all times.	Handwashing is best prevention.	
	Inform teacher to tell parents if child is exposed to communicable illness at school.	Exposure can be reported to physician for possible use of acyclovir or admission for treatment.	All exposures are reported to physician immediately.
	Clean vascular access site and inject heparin per protocol. Observe for signs of infection. Report infection to physician.	Use of heparin maintains an open access route by preventing clotting.	
2. Altered Nutrition: Less Than Body Requirements related to hypermetabolic state, stomatitis			
Child will maintain adequate nutritional intake.	Encourage small and frequent meals. Encourage small bites of variety of foods.	Early satiety reduces intake. Taste changes and favorite foods may no longer be preferred.	Child maintains normal weight for height.
	Promote good oral hygiene and use of nonalcohol mouth washes.	Mouth sores interrupt eating. Alcohol stings open sores.	
3. Pain related to cancer, diagnostic tests, trauma			
Child will have reduced pain.	Teach methods of distraction, relaxation, hypnotic trance, nonpharmacologic measures.	Alteration of interpretation of pain signals allows rest.	Child's pain level is reduced to level that allows participation in activities of daily living and play.
4. Noncompliance related to increasing symptoms, side effects of therapy, complex therapy, knowledge deficit, concurrent stressors, poor self-esteem			
Child will comply with oral medication regimen.	Educate parents and child about the importance of taking medication as prescribed.	Understanding can assist parents and child in placing importance on medication intake.	Child takes all medications according to prescription.
	Set up calendar with dates, times, and medications clearly labeled.	Visual reminders can help them recall instructions.	
	Reward child for taking medications.	Reinforcing desired behaviors through rewards is effective with children.	

Continued.

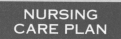
GOAL	INTERVENTION	RATIONALE	EXPECTED OUTCOME
5. Altered Growth and Development related to acute illness, prolonged pain, repeated illness, repeated hospitalizations, confinement for ongoing treatment, stress, inadequate parental support, loss of control over environment			
Child will demonstrate normal physical, emotional, and cognitive development	Encourage play appropriate to age.	Normal activities support self-esteem and self-knowledge.	Child continues to develop physically, emotionally, and cognitively at a normal pace.
	Encourage child to attend school.	School is the work of the child and promotes cognitive and social growth.	
	Encourage seeing peers when unable to attend school.	Peers' perceptions help child to have reality-based perceptions.	
	Work with teachers to support reentry to school. Use puppets, videotape, and discussion with classmates.	Classmates need to understand what has happened to their friend without asking the child directly.	
6. Fatigue related to fever, impaired oxygen transport (anemia), cancer, nutritional disorders, chemotherapy, stress, depression			
Child will maintain energy levels necessary for normal activities.	Problem-solve ways to save energy for play and school.	Child and parents are assisted to see school and play as important.	Child plans use of time effectively to maintain energy for school and play.
	Identify high-fatigue times associated with treatment.	They connect fatigue with treatment so that child will see it as a limited time.	Child conserves energy during times of increased fatigue.
	Plan with child for quiet activities during these times.	Child is empowered to select and plan own activities.	
7. Altered Family Processes related to illness of family member, time-consuming treatments, separation, conflict			
Child and family will demonstrate healthy adaptation.	Encourage open communication.	Open discussion allows problem solving and ego support.	Parents report better communication between themselves and the children.
	Suggest that all family members develop support networks.	Networks expand support systems.	Family members report an increase in friends with whom they can share feelings.
	Parents should be proactive with siblings about their feelings and needs.	Siblings feel valued and problems are confronted early.	
	Encourage attendance of all family members at oncology camps.	Oncology camps promote open discussion between peers for further support and fun.	Family report attending oncology camp and describe benefit of sharing with other families in same situation.

Brain Tumors

Central nervous system, or brain, tumors are the solid tumors most commonly occurring in children. Each year approximately 1100 children under the age of 15 years are diagnosed with tumors of the brain and central nervous system.[9] Brain tumors in children usually occur below the roof of the cerebellum and involve the cerebellum, midbrain, and brainstem (Fig. 16–6). In contrast, brain tumors in adults are usually located above the areas between the cerebrum and cerebellum.

The most common brain tumors in children are medulloblastoma, cerebral astrocytoma, and brainstem glioma. Less common tumors are cerebellar astrocytoma and ependymoma. These tumors usually involve the cerebellum, midbrain, and brainstem.

Clinical Manifestations and Pathophysiology

Medulloblastomas are brain tumors in the external layer of the cerebellum. They account for 25% of childhood brain tumors.[39] Common presenting symptoms are headache, vomiting, and ataxia.

Astrocytomas arise from glial cells and can be either above or below the area between the cerebrum and cerebellum. They comprise 47% of childhood brain tumors.[39] The symptoms include seizures, visual disturbances, or symptoms of increased intracranial pressure.

Brainstem gliomas are located in the pons and typically spread into the surrounding tissue.[9] They account for 10% of childhood brain tumors.[39] Chil-

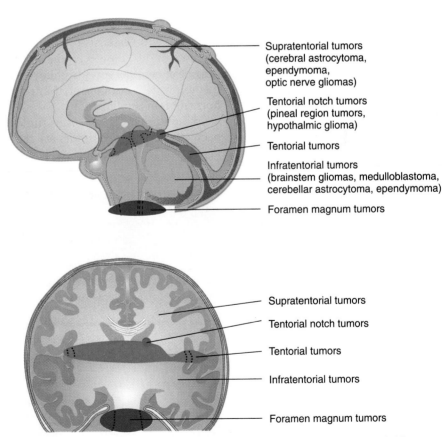

Supratentorial tumors
(cerebral astrocytoma,
ependymoma,
optic nerve gliomas)

Tentorial notch tumors
(pineal region tumors,
hypothalmic glioma)

Tentorial tumors

Infratentorial tumors
(brainstem gliomas, medulloblastoma,
cerebellar astrocytoma, ependymoma)

Foramen magnum tumors

Supratentorial tumors

Tentorial notch tumors

Tentorial tumors

Infratentorial tumors

Foramen magnum tumors

FIGURE 16–6 Sites of brain tumors in children. Approximately 1100 children under the age of 15 years annually are diagnosed as having tumors of the brain and central nervous system. The three most common brain tumors in children are medulloblastoma, cerebral astrocytoma, and brainstem glioma.

dren with brainstem gliomas have symptoms of cranial nerve and long tract (motor nerve) compression. Symptoms may include ataxia, unilateral (one-sided) paralysis of cranial nerves VI and VII, and vertical nystagmus.

Diagnostic Tests and Medical Management

Brain tumors are commonly diagnosed by means of computed tomography (CT) (Fig. 16–7A), magnetic resonance imaging (MRI) (Fig. 16–7B), myelography, and angiography. Neurophysiologic tests (electroencephalography and brainstem evoked potentials) are used to assess sensory pathway integrity and disease- or drug-related sensory dysfunction.[14] Other tests that may be performed are use of tumor markers and cerebrospinal fluid cytology.[39] Lumbar puncture is used to identify abnormal cells in the cerebrospinal fluid. Bone marrow aspiration identifies any extracranial primary neoplastic growth, since cancers in other sites can metastasize to the brain.[42]

Treatment depends on the type of brain tumor (Table 16–9). Surgery is a common treatment for brain tumors. Surgery may be performed to obtain a biopsy specimen, to debulk (reduce the tumor by partial removal) or excise the tumor, or to treat any hydrocephalus that may be present. The success of surgery is directly related to the use of state-of-the-art radiology equipment that allows the neurosurgeon to see computerized images of the brain while at the same time stimulating nerves to determine their functioning. These techniques provide rapid feedback to the neurosurgeon. Laser surgery, which has delicate precise control and accuracy, is used when tumors are close to sensitive neural or vascular structures.[39]

Use of radiation in combination with surgery and chemotherapy has improved the survival of children with medulloblastoma. Chemotherapy is improving the survival of children with astrocytoma and medulloblastoma. Children with extensive local tumor or metastatic disease benefit from chemotherapy.[39] However, the blood-brain barrier is a factor in the effectiveness of chemotherapy for children with brain tumors. For example, when methotrexate is administered intrathecally (in spinal canal), only 3% crosses normal brain capillaries.[44]

Immune therapy for brain tumors is being studied but to date has not been effective. Brain tumors are thought to produce substances that inhibit

FIGURE 16–7 Radiologic imaging of a child with a brain tumor.
Courtesy of Carlos Sivit, M.D., Children's National Medical Center, Washington, DC.

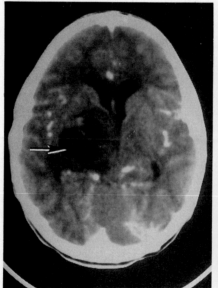
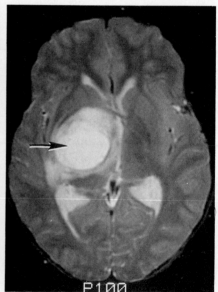

A, CT scan.   **B,** MRI.

TABLE 16-9 Comparison of Brain Tumors

Tumor	Site	Presenting Symptoms	Medical Management
Medullo-blastoma	External layer of cerebellum	Headache, vomiting ataxia	Surgery; chemotherapy with lomustine, vincristine, prednisone, cisplatin, radiation
Astrocytomas	Glial cells, supra-tentorial or infra-tentorial	Seizures, visual disturbances, increased intracranial pressure	Surgery; chemotherapy with vincristine, dactinomycin; radiation
Brainstem gliomas	Pons	Cranial nerve tract signs	Surgery

From Crist, W., & Kun, L. (1991). Common solid tumors of childhood. *The New England Journal of Medicine,* 324 (7), 461–471.

lymphocyte proliferation, which is normally enhanced by immune therapy. Autologous bone marrow transplant has not proved effective in recent studies of children with brain tumors but is still being investigated.[44]

Treatment of medulloblastoma centers on removal of the tumor followed by craniospinal irradiation. This treatment results in cure in approximately half the patients who receive it. High-risk patients also receive chemotherapy with lomustine, vincristine, and prednisone. Cisplatin-based therapy is improving cure rates.[9]

Long-term complications of treatment for children with brain tumors are significant. They include seizure activity, sensorimotor defects, hydrocephalus, and growth problems. Endocrine problems, such as growth hormone changes, hypothyroidism, and panhypopituitarism, may occur when the tumor is in the hypothalamic-pituitary area.[39] Treatment may also lead to a decrease in the intelligence quotient and frank mental retardation in some children. Memory deficits and selective attention deficits are the most common problems. Up to 68% of children less than 6 years old have intellectual deterioration.

Diabetes insipidus is a special consideration in children with midline brain tumors, such as those that compress the hypothalamus, pituitary stalk, or posterior pituitary gland. Manifestations of diabetes insipidus include voiding of large amounts of dilute urine with specific gravity less than 1.005.

Nursing Assessment and Management

The focus of physiologic assessment of the child with a brain tumor is determined by the clinical manifestations (Table 16–10). Presenting signs can be categorized as follows:

- Nonspecific signs related to increasing intracranial pressure
- Secondary signs related to displacement of intracranial structures
- Focal signs suggesting direct involvement of the brain and cranial nerves[42]

Thorough neurologic examination before surgery is essential to provide a record of baseline functioning. The neurologic examination also allows the evaluation of changing physiologic status before surgery. Measurement of head circumference and assessment of the anterior fontanel are necessary in children under the age of 18 months.[14]

TABLE 16–10 Physiologic Assessment of Brain Tumors

Clinical Manifestations	Assessment
Nonspecific signs: headache, morning vomiting, somnolence, irritability	Level of consciousness, pupil response pupil shape and size
Secondary signs: disturbances of cranial nerves; other signs depend on site of tumor	All cranial nerves
Focal signs: truncal ataxia (midline brain tumors), general nystagmus, head tilting	Motor ability, head positions when watching television or looking at people (double vision, sixth cranial nerve involvement)

TABLE 16–11 Parent and Family Teaching: The Child with a Brain Tumor

- Give general information about the purpose of radiation and chemotherapy. Most families will not retain details about these treatments because they are adjusting to the severity of their child's diagnosis.
- Give practical information about the location of the treatment center.
- Reassure parents that information is available from personnel at the treatment center.
- Focus on the benefits of the treatments. Avoid discussion of possible side effects at this time. (Because the postoperative healing process is not completed, it is too soon to know what effects the child may ultimately experience.)
- Teach parents to watch for an increase in voiding of dilute urine. This is a symptom of diabetes insipidus and should be reported immediately to the physician.
- Order equipment such as wheelchairs and bed rails before discharge so they are in the home when the child arrives. The American Cancer Society may be a source for loaner equipment (see Appendix F).

Psychosocial assessment should be ongoing (refer to the discussion earlier in the chapter).

For the nursing care of children immediately following surgery, refer to Chapter 4. In addition, close monitoring of neurologic status is needed postoperatively (refer to Chapter 14). Once the child is stable and ready for discharge, chemotherapy may begin.

Signs and symptoms of diabetes insipidus may also follow brain surgery. Nursing care includes hourly measurement of intake and output, measurement of serum sodium levels every 4 to 6 hours, accurate fluid replacement, and frequent assessment of neurologic status. An indwelling Foley catheter is useful for accurate measurement of urinary output.[45]

Topics for parent and family teaching and discharge planning are presented in Table 16–11.

Neuroblastoma

Neuroblastoma is the solid tumor most commonly occurring outside the cranium of children. It is responsible for 8% of childhood cancer and 15% of cancer deaths in children. The average age at onset is 20 months. The Childhood Cancer Study Group (CCSG) reports a lack of significant improvement in total survival for children older than 1 year with metastatic neuroblastoma.[46,47] Less than 20% of children with regional lymph node or distant metastasis survive for an extended period.[9]

Clinical Manifestations

Neuroblastoma is commonly a smooth, hard, nontender mass, most often in the flank area. The location of the mass determines the symptoms. Altered bowel and bladder function occur when the mass is retroperitoneal; characteristic signs are weight loss, irritability, fatigue, and fever. Dyspnea or infection may occur when the tumor is mediastinal. Neck and facial edema may result from vena cava syndrome if the tumor is mediastinal and large.

Etiology and Pathophysiology

Neuroblastoma originates in primitive neurocrest cells that form the adrenal medulla, paraganglia, and sympathetic nervous system of the cervical sympathetic chain and the thoracic chain. Of neuroblastomas, 40% develop in the adrenal medulla and 65% are retroperitoneal.[4] Other sites of origin include the pelvis, posterior mediastinum, and neck. Lymph node metastasis is common.[12]

Oncogenes are present in neuroblastoma cells in a DNA sequence known as n-*myc*. High levels of the n-*myc* oncogene are associated with rapid disease progression and a poorer prognosis.[46]

Diagnostic Tests and Medical Management

Diagnosis of neuroblastoma is based on radionuclide scanning with MIBG (^{131}I metaiodobenzylguanidine), detection of catecholamines in urine, and demonstration of neuroblastoma tissue in the primary site.

Vanillylmandelic acid (VMA) and homovanillic acid (HVA) levels are usually elevated in the urine. They are used initially to diagnose the disease and later to follow its progress. Areas of necrosis and calcification are readily identifiable with radiologic tests. These tests also help in the staging of the disease by identifying metastasis.

Routine blood cell counts may reveal anemia and thrombocytopenia (low platelet levels). There is no classic WBC response, although thrombocytopenia may occur in association with disseminated intravascular coagulation. **Leukocytosis** (elevated leukocyte count) and leukopenia have been observed with bone marrow involvement.

Bone marrow aspiration is performed to identify the presence of tumor cells. Neuroblastoma cells can form a classic rosette or cluster in the bone marrow aspirate.[46]

Neuroblastoma is classified by means of the Evans staging system (Table 16–12); the stage of the tumor determines the treatment protocol. Surgical excision, radiation, and chemotherapy are all used. The effectiveness of bone marrow transplantation is being studied. If the mass is localized, complete removal offers the best chance of survival. Neuroblastoma is radiosensitive and transiently chemosensitive. In children under 1 year of age, neuroblastoma often has a unique presentation and is much more responsive to treatment.[46]

Nursing Assessment and Management

The presenting site of the tumor, such as the face or abdomen, is assessed by observation and inspection. Palpation is contraindicated. Carefully document related functioning, such as bowel and bladder function. Specific assessments during treatment will depend on the treatment methods used (refer to the earlier discussions of chemotherapy and radiation treatment). Psychosocial assessment and emotional support should be ongoing.

The nursing management of the child with neuroblastoma encompasses

Radionuclide scan
24-Hour urine collection for catecholamine
Chest and abdominal radiographic studies
Computed tomography scan
Bone marrow aspiration

TABLE 16-12 Evans Staging System for Neuroblastoma

Stage	Description	Medical Management
I	Tumors confined to organ or structure of origin	Treated with surgery only
II	Tumors extending in continuity beyond other organs or structure of origin but not crossing the mid-line; regional lymph nodes on the homolateral side may be involved	Treated with surgery and chemo-therapy; may be treated with radiation
III	Tumors extending in continuity beyond the midline, with or with-out bilateral lymph node involve-ment, or bilateral extension of tumors arising in midline structures	Treated with surgery, postoperative radiation, and intensive chemotherapy
IV	Remote disease involving skeleton, organs, soft tissue, or distant lymph nodes	Treated with high-dose chemother-apy; autologous bone marrow transplantation is being studied
IV-S	Tumors that otherwise would be stage I or II but that are accom-panied by remote disease confined to one or more of the following sites: liver, skin, or bone marrow (without radiographic evidence of bone metastasis)	Same treatment as stage IV

Modified from Abelson[12] and Finkelstein.[46]

TABLE 16-13 Parent and Family Teaching: The Child with a Neuroblastoma

Chemotherapy Phase

- Frequently the child with neuroblastoma has a central line placed early in the chemotherapy phase. The central line greatly reduces the emotional trauma asso-ciated with chemotherapy and blood tests.
    Teach the child how to help the parents during cleaning of the central line.
    Teach the child how to protect the central line.
    Teach the parents how to clean and dress the site of the central line.
    Have the parents practice central line care with a model and then on the child before discharge to increase the parents' confidence.
    Give the parents written and illustrated information about care of a central line.
    Arrange for home care dressing supplies before discharge.
- Give the parents detailed chemotherapy information written at a tenth-grade com-prehension level.
- Refer the family to the American Cancer Society for coloring books for children receiving chemotherapy.
- Recommend the American Cancer Society as a resource for educational materials for the child.

Surgery Phase

- Teach the parent to observe for signs of infection at the wound site and to take child's temperature, if necessary.
- Advise parents to note bowel movements and report a lack of one for 3 days to the physician.
- Continue with progression to a regular diet.
- Encourage ambulation with active play.

Bone Marrow Transplantation

- Refer parents to the social worker at the transplant center.
- Encourage the family to talk with other families that have gone to the center for transplant procedures.
- Clarify inaccurate information the family may have based on the articles about bone marrow transplantations in the popular literature.

The nursing management of the child with neuroblastoma encompasses the three phases of medical treatment: chemotherapy, surgery, and bone marrow transplantation. Nursing care during the chemotherapy phase includes minimizing side effects, preventing infection, teaching parents about the medications their child is receiving, and monitoring physical and emotional growth and development of the young child. Specific postsurgical care depends on the size and site of the tumor. Normal postoperative care includes providing fluid support and respiratory care and preventing infection (see Chapter 4). Bone marrow transplantation care is usually performed at a special center. At such a center, specially trained nurses care for the children before the transplant and afterward until the graft begins to produce blood cells.

Topics for parent and family teaching and discharge planning are presented in Table 16–13. Many centers give notebooks with information on chemotherapy and other relevant treatment methods to families shortly after diagnosis. Information that is pertinent to the child is highlighted during the teaching sessions. Blank pages are included to encourage the parents to use the notebook for recording information, tests and results, and questions.

For children accepted for transplantation, the transplant centers give extensive information to the parents on arrival. Before going to the center for the transplantation, the family needs information about practical matters such as housing, transportation, and cost.

Wilms Tumor (Nephroblastoma)

Nephroblastoma, an intrarenal tumor that is commonly called Wilms tumor, is the second most common abdominal tumor of childhood. Each year the incidence is 7.6 cases per million children. Wilms tumor occurs most frequently between 2 and 5 years of age, but may also occur in adolescents and adults.[48]

Clinical Manifestations

Wilms tumor is usually an asymptomatic, firm, lobulated mass located to one side of the midline in the abdomen. Often a parent discovers the mass during the child's bath. Hypertension caused by increased renin activity related to renal damage is reported in 30% of cases. Bilateral Wilms tumors occur in 5% to 10% of cases.[9]

Etiology and Pathophysiology

Wilms tumor is associated with several congenital anomalies: aniridia (absence of the iris), hemihypertrophy (abnormal growth of one half of the body or a body structure), genitourinary anomalies, nevi, and hamartomas (benign, nodulelike growths). This connection suggests a genetic link. However, not all children with Wilms tumor have the same phenotype or have congenital anomalies.

Diagnostic Tests and Medical Management

The diagnosis of Wilms tumor is based on an intravenous pyelogram and is confirmed by surgical biopsy. Once the histopathologic features are known, CT scanning of the lungs, liver, spleen, and brain is performed to identify any metastasis. This information is used in staging the tumor (Table 16–14).

TABLE 16–14 National Wilms Tumor Study Staging System

Stage	Description
I	The tumor is limited to the kidney and completely excised. The surface of the renal capsule is intact. The tumor is not ruptured before or during removal. No residual tumor is apparent beyond the margins of excision.
II	The tumor extends beyond the kidney but is not completely excised. Regional extension of the tumor is present, i.e., penetration through the outer surface of the renal capsule into the perirenal soft tissues. Vessels outside the kidney substance are infiltrated or contain tumor thrombus. Biopsy may have been performed on the tumor, or local spillage of tumor confined to the flank has occurred. No residual tumor is apparent at or beyond the margin of excision.
III	Residual nonhematogenous tumor is confined to the abdomen. Any of the following may occur: Lymph nodes on biopsy are found to be involved in the hilus, the periaortic chains, or beyond. Diffuse peritoneal contamination by the tumor has occurred, such as by spillage of tumor beyond the flank before or during surgery, or by tumor growth that has penetrated through the peritoneal surface. Implants are found on peritoneal surfaces. The tumor extends beyond the surgical margins either microscopically or grossly. The tumor is not completely resectable because of local infiltration into vital structures.
IV	Hematogenous metastasis: deposits are present beyond stage II, e.g., lung, liver, bone and brain.
V	Bilateral renal involvement is present at diagnosis. An attempt should be made to stage each side according to the above criteria on the basis of extent of disease before biopsy.

From Abelson, H. (1990). Oncology. In Behrman, R., & Kliegman, T. (Eds.), *Nelson's essentials of pediatrics*, (p. 541). Philadelphia: W.B. Saunders Company.

▌WILMS TUMOR: CHEMOTHERAPEUTIC DRUGS

Vincristine
Dactinomycin
Doxorubicin

Treatment is multifaceted. Surgery, with a large transabdominal incision, is performed to examine the opposite kidney fully and to search for other sites of metastasis. Radiation may follow surgery. Children whose tumors are almost completely excised and who have a favorable prognosis do not require irradiation of the tumor bed.

Another approach, used in Europe and increasingly in the United States, is chemotherapy or radiation therapy, alone or in combination, before surgery to reduce tumor size and the risk of tumor spillage (release of tumor cells into the abdomen) during surgery. This approach is considered appropriate for large, nonremovable tumors thought to be Wilms tumor.[48] Children who have recurrent Wilms tumor are treated with chemotherapy using the drugs VP-16, cisplatin, and ifosfamide. An aggressive approach with chemotherapy, surgery, and radiation is used for recurrent Wilms tumor.[48]

Long-term complications of treatment include liver damage, portal hypertension, mild cirrhosis, and peliosis hepatica (mottling of the liver due to presence of blood in the tissues), which may occur in children treated for right-sided Wilms tumor. Radiation damage (such as thinning or weakening) to the skeleton, pelvis, and thorax has been reported. Kyphosis and scoliosis may occur from irradiation of vertebral bodies and the pelvis. Glomerular damage to the remaining kidney is also reported. Second malignancies in the original radiation field have occurred with orthovoltage radiation, but recent changes in radiation therapy have reduced this risk.[48]

Prognosis is determined by tumor stage and histologic findings. Children with classic histologic characteristics of nephroblastoma have an 88% survival rate, whereas those with anaplastic or sarcomatous variants have a 12% survival rate. In addition, children who are younger than 24 months at diagnosis and who have tumors that weigh less than 250 g have a more favorable prognosis.[12,48]

Nursing Management

Nursing management can be divided into two phases: the postrenal surgery phase and the chemotherapy phase. Drawings and special teaching dolls with removable kidneys can be used to teach young children about the surgery. Although chemotherapy may occur at two different times, before and after surgery, nursing management considerations remain the same.

Nursing care during the postrenal surgery phase focuses on pain management and close monitoring of fluid levels. The incision to remove a kidney is long, and the postoperative fluid shift may make the area uncomfortable for the child. Frequent repositioning of the child and use of noninvasive and pharmacologic pain interventions improve comfort. Gentle handling is important. Monitoring of fluids is necessary following surgery to prevent hypovolemia and assess the shift of fluids out of the third space and out of the body. Daily weight, intake and output (I&O), and urine specific gravity are assessed to monitor the function of the remaining kidney. Frequent blood pressure measurements are needed to watch for signs of shock and as another indication of the functioning of the remaining kidney.

During chemotherapy, close attention is given to side effects, potential for infection from the central line site, and continued functioning of the remaining kidney.

Bone Tumors

Osteosarcoma

Osteosarcoma is a rare, malignant bone tumor that occurs predominantly in adolescent boys. Its peak incidence is during the rapid growth years. The tumor is usually located at the epiphysis or metaphysis of the distal femur, proximal tibia, or proximal humerus.[9]

Clinical Manifestations

The common initial symptoms are pain and swelling.[14] Pulmonary metastasis is present in 10% to 20% of cases.

Etiology and Pathophysiology

Bone tissue produced by osteosarcoma never matures into compact bone. The exact cause of osteosarcoma is unknown, but a genetic link is suspected. Sixteen sets of siblings with the disease have been reported.[49] In addition, the incidence of osteosarcoma is 500 times greater for children with hereditary retinoblastoma.[12]

Diagnostic Tests and Medical Management

Diagnosis is made through radiographic tests (radiographic studies of the affected area, bone scan, CT scan of involved bone), blood test for serum alkaline phosphatase (level may be elevated), and tumor biopsy (to confirm the diagnosis). Arteriography may be performed if limb-sparing surgery is contemplated.

Treatment involves both surgery and chemotherapy. The surgery is either a limb-sparing procedure or limb amputation. In limb-sparing procedures the tumor is removed and an internal prosthesis is inserted. A limb-sparing procedure is possible if bone growth has taken place and a neurobundle (area where several nerves converge) is not involved in the tumor. If these two criteria are not met, limb amputation is necessary.[14,42] Aggressive chemotherapy following surgery has improved the survival rate.

Leukovorin (a water-soluble vitamin in the folate group) is used as an antidote to drugs that act as folic acid antagonists. It is given intravenously (a procedure termed leukovorin rescue) within 24 hours of administration of methotrexate or other strong folic acid inhibitors to avoid death of healthy cells from lack of folic acid.

A poor prognosis is indicated by age less than 10 years, male sex, tumor larger than 15 cm, osteoblastic cell type, involvement of the humerus, presence of symptoms for less than 2 months, and metastasis.[12]

Ewing Sarcoma

Ewing sarcoma is a malignant small cell tumor involving the diaphyseal portion of a long bone. The most common sites are the femur and pelvis, tibia, fibula, ribs, humerus, scapula, and clavicle, but any bone may be involved. Unlike osteosarcoma, Ewing sarcoma does not produce bone itself.

The symptoms are similar to those of osteosarcoma. They may include fever, high WBC count, and elevated erythrocyte sedimentation rate. Ewing sarcoma occurs in 2 children per million and is rare in black children.

A tumor biopsy is necessary for diagnosis. Diagnostic tests are the same as those for osteosarcoma.

Treatment for Ewing sarcoma is surgical removal of the entire bone or intensive high-dose irradiation of the entire bone, followed by chemotherapy. Aggressive treatment results in 80% to 90% likelihood of local control. Unfavorable features are soft tissue extension of the tumor, low lymphocyte count, and elevated serum lactate dehydrogenase level. Children have a better prognosis when the primary tumor is at a site other than the pelvis.[12,50]

Nursing Assessment and Management of Bone Tumors

Physiologic assessment of the child with a bone tumor includes assessment of the site before surgery and the wound following surgery. If a limb salvage procedure is performed, the child's extremity will be intact but it will not function as before because muscle insertion sites and mass have been removed with the tumor during surgery. Accurate charting of the condition of the surgery site and limb function is important.

Observe the wound postoperatively for infection and hemorrhage. Assess circulation above and below the operative site. If edema is found, elevate the limb.

If the limb has been amputated, assess the child for signs of disturbed body image[44]:

- Refusal to look at or touch the altered or missing body part
- Preoccupation with loss or change
- Feelings of shame or embarrassment, either verbalized or demonstrated
- Distorted perception of normal body (easily seen in the child's drawings of the body)
- Fears of rejection or unwanted attention from others
- Overexposure or hiding of the affected body part
- Actual or perceived change in the structure and function of the body or body parts[51]

TABLE 16–15 Parent and Family Teaching: The Child with a Bone Tumor

If the Child Underwent a Limb-Salvaging Procedure

- Educate the child and family about the safety hazards associated with the reduced functioning of the limb
- Demonstrate proper use of the adaptive devices such as splints to protect the limb from sores or restricted circulation.
- Reinforce the use of elevation with a pillow at night and as often as possible during the day.
- Contact the child's school to explain the need for elevation and the changes in functioning in that limb. Adaptive learning tools such as the computer are needed if the child's writing hand is impaired.

If the Child's Limb Is Amputated

- Educate the family about the care of the stump and the prosthesis.
- Teach how to wrap the stump, inspect for sores, and cleanse the prosthetic device.
- Provide written and illustrated instructions on care. Multiple temporary prostheses will be used until the stump is healed and in final form.
- Teach about chemotherapy and radiation as discussed earlier in the chapter.
- Remember that the child may experience multiple body image changes because of surgery, chemotherapy, and radiation. Referral to counseling may be beneficial before chemotherapy.

Psychosocial assessment of the child and family is discussed in the earlier section on General Nursing Care of the Child with Cancer.

Table 16–15 summarizes areas for parent and family teaching and discharge planning.

Leukemia

Leukemia is a condition characterized by a proliferation of abnormal white blood cells in the body. The three main forms are acute lymphocytic leukemia, acute nonlymphocytic leukemia, and acute myelogenous leukemia.

The most common form of leukemia is acute lymphocytic leukemia (ALL), which accounts for 68% of leukemias in children. The peak age at onset is between 2 and 5 years. Eighty-nine percent of children with ALL are Caucasian and 57% are male.

The second most common form of leukemia is acute nonlymphocytic leukemia (ANLL), which accounts for 15% to 20% of the leukemias diagnosed in children. Black and white children are affected equally, and there is no peak age at onset.

A third type of leukemia that occurs in children is acute myelogenous leukemia (AML), which accounts for 15% to 20% of pediatric leukemias. Danny, the boy described at the beginning of the chapter, has AML. AML is often considered a subset of ANLL.[12,52–55]

Clinical Manifestations

Children with ALL and ANLL usually have fever, pallor, overt signs of bleeding, lethargy, malaise, anorexia, and large joint or extremity pain. Petechiae, frank bleeding, and joint pain are cardinal signs of bone marrow failure. Enlargement of the liver and spleen (hepatosplenomegaly) and changes in the lymph nodes (lymphadenopathy) are common. If the leukemia has infiltrated the central nervous system (entered it by means of the circulatory or lymphoid system), the child will have such signs as headache, vomiting, papilledema, and sixth cranial nerve palsy (inability to move the eye laterally). These findings are caused by the leukemic cells massing and putting pressure on nerves. The testicle, spinal cord, and bone marrow are common sites for infiltration. The leukemic cells in the testicle become a mass that causes the testicle to enlarge, often painlessly.[12]

Etiology and Pathophysiology

The cause of leukemia is unknown. No specific etiologic agents have been found for ALL or ANLL of childhood. However, children with chromosomal defects such as Down syndrome have an increased incidence of ALL. Furthermore, ionizing radiation and chemical agents seem to have some role in the development of AML and ANLL.[52] Children with immune deficiency states, such as ataxia, telangiectasia, and Wiskott-Aldrich syndrome, also are at increased risk of ALL.

Leukemia occurs when the stem cells in the bone marrow produce immature WBCs that cannot function normally. They proliferate rapidly by cloning instead of normal mitosis, causing the bone marrow to fill with abnormal WBCs. These cells then spill out into the circulatory system where they steadily replace the normally functioning WBCs. As this occurs, the protective lymphocytic functions such as cellular and humeral immunity are reduced, leaving the body vulnerable to infections.

The malignant WBCs rapidly fill the bone marrow, replacing stem cells that produce erythrocytes (red blood cells) and other blood products such as platelets, thereby decreasing the amount of these products in circulation. The stem cells are replaced by leukemic clones, which eventually results in anemia. Patients with leukemia commonly experience abnormal bleeding because of the reduced amounts of platelets.

Diagnostic Tests and Medical Management

Diagnosis is based initially on blood counts and bone marrow aspiration. Blood counts reveal anemia, thrombocytopenia, and neutropenia. Bone marrow aspiration reveals immature and abnormal lymphoblasts and hypercellular marrow. Bone marrow aspiration is the differential test.

Treatment of ALL involves radiation and chemotherapy. Radiation is used for central nervous system prophylaxis and involvement and for testicular involvement. Chemotherapy is organized into three phases: (1) induction, (2) consolidation or reintensification, and (3) maintenance of remission.

Maximum cell death occurs during the induction phase. Cells that remain after that period are more resistant. After 3 to 4 weeks, when a remission has occurred, central nervous system prophylaxis begins. Drugs are used in combination with cranial irradiation. During the consolidation phase, chemotherapy with L-asparaginase and cyclophosphamide is administered. Treatment during the maintenance phase is aimed at destroying the remaining leukemic cells. Combinations of active drugs are used to prevent resistance. Occasionally other drugs are added to the regimen, such as vincristine, prednisone, cyclophosphamide, intravenous methotrexate, cytosine arabinoside, or anthracyclines.

The same general procedure is used for ANLL; however, it is less effective than for ALL.[12,52,53]

The prognosis for children with leukemia is much improved with current therapy. However, several risk factors affect the long-term outcome. The most favorable findings are[52]:

■ LEUKEMIA:
CHEMOTHERAPEUTIC DRUGS

Induction Phase
Prednisone
Vincristine
plus
L-Asparaginase, or cyclophosphamide, or doxorubicin

Central Nervous System Prophylaxis
Intrathecal methotrexate or cytosine arabinoside

Consolidation Phase
L-Asparaginase
Cyclophosphamide

Maintenance Phase
6-Mercaptopurine
Methotrexate

- Age at onset between 2 and 10 years
- Initial hemoglobin level less than 10 g/dL
- Low initial WBC count
- Lack of B or T cell antigens
- Absence of extramedullary (outside bone marrow or spinal cord) involvement
- Rapid response to chemotherapy

The most important factor is the initial leukocyte count. The higher the leukocyte count (over 50,000/mm^3), the worse the prognosis. For children in the low-risk group the probability of prolonged survival is as high as 90%. Infants under 12 months of age have a poor prognosis. Treatment is adjusted for each child, depending on that child's risk factor. More aggressive treatment is undertaken for those in the higher risk groups.[54]

Duration of treatment varies according to the risk factor. Typically, girls receive 2 years of treatment and boys 3 years. These periods have produced the best survival rates. Approximately 10% of children have a relapse within a year after completing treatment. After the second year, relapse occurs in about 1% of children; however, there have been recurrences as long as 9 years after treatment. It is unclear whether these late (and rare) events are true recurrences or a second malignancy.

Nursing Assessment and Management

Gentle physical assessment is mandatory. To avoid causing further bleeding, look carefully for new sites of bleeding. Once chemotherapy has begun, closely monitor renal functioning through specific gravity, intake and output (I&O), and daily weight measurement. Bone marrow suppression may necessitate protective isolation. Care of mouth sores and other side effects of chemotherapy is presented in the Nursing Care Plan for Hospital Care of the Child with Cancer, earlier in the chapter. Perform assessments every 8 hours or more often depending on the chemotherapy regimen. Many children are treated in an oncology clinic, staying in the hospital only on the day of IV drug administration, and receiving oral medications at home. Careful teaching is needed.

Special attention to renal function is needed when the child receives cyclophosphamide. Gross hematuria is a side effect of this drug. Hydration with intravenous fluids to attain specific gravity of less than 1.010 prevents or reduces the severity of hematuria. To achieve this specific gravity, the child receives intravenous fluids at 1½ times maintenance volume for at least 6 to 8 hours before and at least 1½ hours after administration of the drug. Careful monitoring of I&O is required to record the intravenous fluids and assess kidney functioning. Assess specific gravity every 8 hours, as well as before and during administration of the drug, and when the intravenous fluids are reduced to maintenance volume levels. Daily weight measurement documents the change resulting from adequate hydration for the chemotherapy.

Because leukemia can infiltrate the central nervous system, the system's functioning—including level of consciousness, irritability, vomiting, and lethargy—is assessed. However, these nonspecific signs can also be induced by the chemotherapeutic drugs and antiemetics.

The impact of a diagnosis of leukemia and the long-term nature of treatment can severely stress the coping abilities of both the child and the family. Ongoing psychosocial assessment and emotional support are essential (see the discussion earlier in the chapter). Referral to support groups and social services may be beneficial.

Hodgkin Disease

Hodgkin disease is a disorder of the lymphoid system. It usually arises in a single lymph node or an anatomic group of lymph nodes (Fig. 16–8). There are approximately 5.7 cases per million people, with the peak occurrence in adolescent boys. Hodgkin disease occurs most frequently between the ages of 15 and 30 years and after age 50. It rarely occurs before the age of 10 years.[12,42] The prognosis is good when the disease occurs in childhood.

Clinical Manifestations

The main symptom is nontender, firm lymphadenopathy, usually in the supraclavicular and cervical nodes but occasionally in a mediastinal area. Fever, night sweats, and weight loss occur in one third of the children and are associated with a more aggressive disease. Leukocyte count and erythrocyte sedimentation rate (ESR) may be elevated.

Etiology and Pathophysiology

Hodgkin disease occurs in clusters and is reported in families. This suggests that it is caused by an infectious agent.

Diagnostic Tests and Medical Management

Diagnosis is based on lymph node biopsy. Staging is done by using the Ann Arbor staging classification (Table 16–16). The basis for staging is data obtained from the history, physical examination, chest x-ray study (for metastasis), laboratory studies (complete blood count, erythrocyte sedimentation rate, serum copper level, liver function tests), CT scan of retroperitoneal nodes, radionuclide scans, and bone marrow biopsy.

■ CLINICAL TIP

An oral contrast medium is often given to children having CT scanning of the abdomen and pelvis. Mixing the contrast medium with fruit juice or punch makes it more palatable.

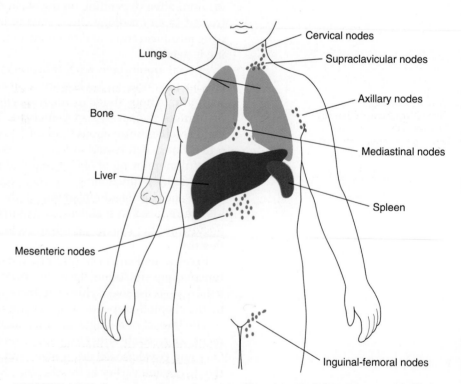

FIGURE 16–8 Lymph nodes and organs affected in Hodgkin disease in children.

TABLE 16-16 Ann Arbor Staging System for Hodgkin Disease

Stage	Description
I	Disease within a single lymph node region Disease within a single extralymphatic organ (I E)
II	Disease within two or more lymph node regions on same side of diaphragm Disease within extralymphatic organ, and of one or more lymph node regions on same side of diaphragm (II E)
III	Disease of lymph node regions on both sides of diaphragm Disease of lymph node regions on both sides of the diaphragm with involvement of extralymphatic organ (III 1) As in III, plus disease within spleen (III 2) As in III 2, plus disease within extralymphatic organ (III 3)
IV	Disseminated disease within one or more lymphatic organs with or without lymph node involvement

From Bonilla, J., & Healy, G. (1989). Management of malignant head and neck tumors in children. *Pediatric Clinics of North America, 36(6)*, 1443–1450.

■ HODGKIN DISEASE: CHEMOTHERAPEUTIC DRUGS

MOPP Drug Regimen
Mustargen (mechlorethamine)
Vinblastine
Procarbazine
Prednisone

ABVD Drug Regimen
Doxorubicin
Bleomycin
Vinblastine
Dacarbazine

■ COMPLICATIONS OF HODGKIN DISEASE THERAPY

Recurrent disease
Pneumococcal and *Haemophilus influenzae* sepsis
Growth retardation
Chronic immune deficiency
Amenorrhea
Development of secondary tumors
Thyroid, testicular, and ovarian dysfunction

Surgical staging, less commonly used, is performed during an exploratory laparotomy when multiple-node biopsy specimens are taken.[12,50] With surgical staging, however, as many as 25% of children with Ann Arbor stage I or II disease are reclassified upward to higher stages.[42]

Treatment is usually successful, with an 80% to 90% 5-year survival rate. To diminish side effects of radiation, radiation and chemotherapy are often used in combination, particularly in smaller children. Chemotherapy with two sets of four-drug combinations is often used to avoid emergence of resistant cells.

Three radiation fields are used in the treatment of children with Hodgkin disease: (1) a mantle including the neck, shoulders, and mediastinum; (2) a paraaortic field including the midline of the abdomen; and (3) an inverted Y involving the pelvic nodes.[12]

Non-Hodgkin Lymphoma

Non-Hodgkin lymphoma includes all lymphomas that are not classified as Hodgkin disease. These lymphomas are malignant tumors of lymphoreticular (internal framework of the lymph system) origin. The peak incidence for lymphomas is between the ages of 7 and 11 years, and they are three times more common in boys than in girls.

Children with non-Hodgkin lymphoma commonly have fever and weight loss. The lymph glands are usually enlarged or nodular, with the most frequent sites being the cervical, axillary, inguinal, and femoral nodes. However, the disease may be diffuse, without nodular glands. The anterior mediastinum is the primary site for T cell lymphomas. Tumors that occur in this area may compress the airway or superior vena cava.

Fifty percent of non-Hodgkin lymphomas are caused by T cell abnormalities. These abnormal T cells are diffuse, highly malignant, and very aggressive and do not mature. T cell lymphomas produced by these cells often occur in children with congenital or acquired immunodeficiency states, chronic immune stimulation, autoimmune disease, and Epstein-Barr virus–induced proliferation of the lymphoid tissue.

Diagnosis is by tissue biopsy. To date, no staging classification has been developed. Because systemic disease is present in 80% of children with non-Hodgkin lymphoma, the treatment is aggressive chemotherapy similar to

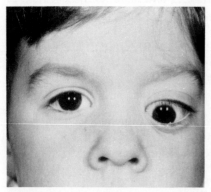

FIGURE 16-9 Rhabdomyosarcoma is characterized by ptosis and swelling.
From Vaughan, D., Asbury, T., & Riordan-Eva, P. (1992). *General ophthalmology* (13th ed.). Norwalk, CT: Appleton & Lange.

■ **RHABDOMYOSARCOMA: CHEMOTHERAPEUTIC DRUGS**

Vincristine
Dactinomycin
Doxorubicin
Cyclophosphamide

TABLE 16-17 Classification of Rhabdomyosarcoma

Group	Description
I	Localized, completely resected disease
II	Total gross resection with regional spread
III	Incomplete gross resection or biopsy
IV	Distant metastatic disease present

From Bonilla, J., & Healy, G. (1989). Management of malignant head and neck tumors in children. *Pediatric Clinics of North America, 36(6)*, 1443–1450.

that used for ALL. The induction phase of chemotherapy results in a 90% remission rate. Chemotherapy is administered to the central nervous system to prevent the spread of the disease. Treatment also includes localized radiation and surgery to remove the tumor mass. Between 50% and 75% of children with non-Hodgkin lymphoma have a good outcome. Children with local diseases have a more favorable prognosis.

Rhabdomyosarcoma

Rhabdomyosarcoma is a soft tissue cancer that is common in children. It occurs most often in the muscles around the eyes (extraorbital), in the neck, and less commonly in the abdomen and genitourinary tract. Among children under 15 years of age, rhabdomyosarcoma occurs four times more frequently in whites than in blacks.[56] Peak occurrence is between 2 and 4 years and again between 16 and 20 years.[57]

Tumors occurring close to the eye produce swelling, ptosis, visual disturbances, and eye movement abnormalities (Fig. 16–9). When the tumor occurs in the genitourinary tract, the result can be obstruction, hematuria, dysuria, vaginal discharge, and a protruding vaginal mass.[50] Rhabdomyosarcoma occurring in the abdomen may be asymptomatic. There is rapid metastasis to the lungs, bones, bone marrow, or distant lymph nodes.[42]

Diagnosis is based on CT, MRI, bone marrow aspiration, and biopsy. A useful biologic marker, Desmin, allows differentiation of rhabdomyosarcoma from other round cell tumors. Because 20% of children have metastatic disease at the time of diagnosis, chest and lung CT scans are necessary.

Treatment includes surgical removal of the tumor followed by wide-field radiation and chemotherapy. Prognosis depends on site, staging (Table 16–17), and histologic findings. Children with stage II or IV disease or abdominal tumors have a poor prognosis.

Retinoblastoma

Retinoblastoma is an intraocular malignancy of the retina. It may be bilateral (30%) or unilateral. In 10% to 15% of children the disease is inherited.[9,58–60]

The first sign of retinoblastoma is a white pupil, termed leukokoria or cat's-eye reflex (Fig. 16–10). Twenty percent of children with retinoblastoma have a fixed strabismus (a constant deviation of one eye from the other).

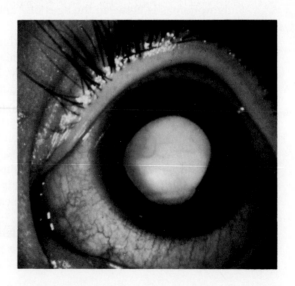

FIGURE 16-10 Retinoblastoma is characterized by leukokoria, a white reflection in the pupil.
From Hathaway, W.E., Hay, W.W. Jr., Groothuis, J.R., & Paisley, J.W. (1993). *Current pediatric diagnosis and treatment* (11th ed.). Norwalk, CT: Appleton & Lange.

Other signs include orbital cellulitis, glaucoma, and heterochromia (irises of different colors).[61]

Retinoblastoma is usually diagnosed when the child is between 1 and 2 years of age. The overall tumor-free survival rate is 90%, 5 to 10 years after diagnosis. Diagnostic tests include full ocular examination, computed tomography scan, bone marrow aspiration, and lumbar puncture.

Treatment for large tumors involves removal of the eye. Small tumors are treated with radiation (unilateral tumor) or a combination of radiation and chemotherapy (bilateral tumors). Recent studies advocate adding doxorubicin, cisplatin, and intrathecal methotrexate for local and metastatic disease.[50,62] Unfortunately, secondary sarcomas commonly develop, usually in the radiation treatment field.[9,42]

Nursing Assessment and Management of Soft Tissue Tumors

Physiologic assessment of the child with a soft tissue tumor, such as Hodgkin disease, non-Hodgkin lymphoma, rhabdomyosarcoma, and other lymphomas, focuses on the child's general condition. Accurate height and weight measurement is essential to provide a baseline against which to measure the growth process during treatment. Accurate height and weight are also necessary for calculation of chemotherapeutic drug dosages.

Observe the area of the tumor, such as the face, neck, and abdomen, and accurately describe any changes. Monitor respiratory status if the tumor is in the face or neck. Report any changes in respiratory pattern to the physician. Avoid palpation of any tumor site or enlarged area; metastasis can be influenced by injudicious palpation and manipulation of a tumor site. Notify the physician of a change in any lymph node or any other area of the body.

Gastrointestinal and genitourinary function can be altered by the presence of a tumor and by treatment such as chemotherapy and radiation. Accurate intake and output measurement is essential. Abdominal tumors may affect defecation, so notation of all bowel movements is important. Explain to the family and child why keeping accurate records is necessary.

Observe wounds closely for lack of healing as a result of chemotherapy or radiation. Examine mouth and extremities for wounds or ulcers. Nutritional changes caused by treatment will affect the body's ability to support healthy cells and heal wounds.

Assessment of the family's psychosocial status and coping mechanisms is an essential component of nursing care. Refer to the discussion under General Nursing Care of the Child with Cancer, earlier in the chapter.

Nursing management during chemotherapy and radiation is discussed in the earlier sections on these treatment measures and in the Nursing Care Plan for Hospital Care of the Child with Cancer, earlier in the chapter. Topics for parent and family teaching and discharge planning are similar to those previously presented (Table 16–18).

■ RETINOBLASTOMA: CHEMOTHERAPEUTIC DRUGS

Vincristine
Cyclophosphamide
Doxorubicin

■ CLINICAL TIP

To obtain an accurate weight measurement, use the same type of scale for all weights and have the child wear the same type of clothing (such as hospital gowns or lightweight nightwear, rather than street clothing). Chart whether the child had any intravenous lines or wound dressings in place when the weight was obtained. Weigh the child at the same time each day before a meal.

TABLE 16–18 Parent and Family Teaching: The Child with a Soft Tissue Tumor

- Teach the family about the chemotherapy drugs and their side effects.
- Special teaching on the care of venous access devices is done during the hospitalization for surgical placement.
- Provide written and illustrated information about the chemotherapy protocol(s).
- Radiation and surgery education are unique to the site of the tumor
- Assist the family to use nutrition resources such as dieticians to improve the child's nutritional status. This can be beneficial during periods of increased physical stress such as radiation and surgery.

REFERENCES

1 Bellanti, J., Boner, A., & Valletta, E. (1987). Immunology of the fetus and newborn. In Avery, G. (Ed.), *Neonatology: Pathophysiology and management of the newborn* (pp. 850–873). (3rd ed.). Philadelphia: J.B. Lippincott Company.

2 Boring, C., Squires, T., & Tong, T. (1992a). Cancer statistics. *CA—A Cancer Journal for Clinicians, 42*(1), 19–38.

3 Boring, C., Squires, T., & Heath, C. (1992b). Cancer statistics for African Americans. *CA—A Cancer Journal for Clinicians, 42*(1), 7–18.

4 Miller, R. (1989). Frequency and environmental epidemiology of childhood cancer. In Pizzo, P.A., & Poplack, D.G. (Eds.), *Principles and practice of pediatric oncology* (pp. 3–17). Philadelphia: J.B. Lippincott.

5 Sabio, H. (1985). Cancer in children. In Colon, A.R., & Ziai, T.M. (Eds.). *Pediatric pathophysiology* (pp. 449–460). Boston: Little, Brown & Co.

6 McGuire, P., & Moore, K. (1990). Recent advances in childhood cancer, advances in oncology nursing. *Nursing Clinics of North America, 25*(2), 447–460.

7 Waskerwitz, M., & Leonard, M. (1986). Early detection of malignancy: From birth to twenty years. *Oncology Nursing Forum, 13*(1), 50–57.

8 Crist, W., & Kun, L. (1991). Common solid tumors of childhood. *The New England Journal of Medicine, 324*(7), 461–471.

9 zur Hausen, H. (1991). Viruses in human cancers. *Science, 254*, 1167–1173.

10 Solomon, E., Borrow, J., & Goddard, A. (1991). Chromosome aberrations and cancer. *Science, 254*, 1153–1159.

11 Weinberg, R. (1991). Tumor suppressor genes, *Science, 254*, 1138–1146.

12 Abelson, H. (1990). Oncology. In Behrman, R.E., & Kliegman, R. (Eds.). *Nelson's essentials of pediatrics* (pp. 523–544). Philadelphia: W.B. Saunders.

13 Association of Pediatric Oncology Nurses. (1990). *Cancer chemotherapy* (p. 5). Richmond, VA: Author.

14 McCance, K., & Huether, S. (1990). *Pathophysiology: The biologic basis for disease in adults and children*. St. Louis: Mosby–Year Book.

15 Scherer, J. (1985). *Nurses' drug manual*. Philadelphia: J.B. Lippincott Company.

16 Lilley, L. (1990). Side effects associated with pediatric chemotherapy: Management and patient education issues. *Pediatric Nursing, 16*(3), 252–255.

17 Kinrade, L. (1988). Typhlitis: A complication of neutropenia. *Pediatric Nursing, 14*(4), 291–295.

18 Wade, D., Nava, H., & Douglass, H. (1992). Neutropenic enterocolitis. *Cancer, 69*(1), 17–22.

19 Hogan, C. (1990). Advances in the management of nausea and vomiting. Advances in Oncology Nursing. *Nursing Clinics of North America, 25*(2), 475–497.

20 Hutter, J. (1992). Principles of total care. In Fernbach, D., & Vietti, T. (Eds.), *Clinical pediatric oncology* (p. 245). (4th ed.). St. Louis: Mosby–Year Book.

21 Pervan, V. (1990). Practical aspects of dealing with cancer therapy–induced nausea and vomiting. *Seminars in Oncology Nursing, 6*(4) (Suppl. 1), 3–5.

22 Portenoy, R. (1992). Cancer pain: pathophysiology and syndromes. *Lancet, 339*, 1026–1036.

23 Rostad, M. (1991). Current strategies for managing myelosuppression in patients with cancer. *Oncology Nursing Forum, 18*(2) (Suppl.), 7–15.

24 Haeuber, D. (1991). Future strategies in the control of myelosuppression: The use of colony-stimulating factors. *Oncology Nursing Forum, 18*(Suppl. 2), 16–21.

25 Bucholtz, D. (1992). Issues concerning the sedation of children for radiation therapy. *Oncology Nursing Forum, 19*(4), 649–655.

26 Patterson, K., & Klopovich, P. (1987). Metabolic emergencies in pediatric oncology: The acute tumor lysis syndrome. *Journal of Pediatric Oncology Nursing, 4*(3&4), 19–24.

27 Mason, C. (1987). Septic shock. *Journal of Pediatric Oncology Nursing, 4*(3&4), 25–31.

28 Novotny, M. (1986). Body image changes in amputee children: How nursing theory can make a difference. *Journal of the Association of Pediatric Oncology Nurses, 3*(2), 8–12.

29 Moore, I., Kramer, R., & Perin, G. (1986). Care of the family with a child with cancer: Diagnosis and early stages of treatment. *Oncology Nursing Forum, 13*(5), 60–66.

30 Whitman, N., Graham, B., Gleit, C., & Boyd, M. (1992). *Teaching in nursing practice: A professional model*. Norwalk, CT: Appleton & Lange.

31 Murphy, L., & Moriarty, A. (1976). *Vulnerability, coping, and growth: From infancy to adolescence* (pp. 337–339). New Haven: Yale University Press.

32 Stuart, G., & Sundeen, S. (1991). *Principles and practice of psychiatric nursing* (4th ed.). (p. 78). St. Louis: Mosby–Year Book.

33 La Montagne, L. (1987). Adopting a process approach to assess children's coping. *Journal of Pediatric Nursing, 3*(3), 150–163.

34 Ellis, J. (1991). How adolescents cope with cancer and its treatment. *Maternal Child Nursing, 16*, 157–160.

35 Stullenbargar, B., Norris, J., Edgil, A., & Prosser, M.J. (1987). Family adaptation to cystic fibrosis. *Pediatric Nursing, 13*(1), 29–31.

36 Schepp, K. (1991). Factors influencing the coping effort of mothers of hospitalized children. *Nursing Research, 40*(1), 42–46.

37 Smith, S., & Cohen, D. (1992). Home movies as an intervention for school reentry. *Journal of Pediatric Oncology Nursing, 9*(2), 69.

38 Houlahan, K. (1991). School reentry program. *Journal of Pediatric Oncology Nursing, 8*(2), 70–71.

39 Finlay, J., Goins, S., Uteg, R., & Giese, W. (1987). Progress in the management of childhood brain tumors. *Hematology/Oncology Clinics of North America, 1*(4), 753–773.

40 Taptich, B., Iyer, P., & Bernocchi-Losey, D. (1989). *Nursing diagnosis and care planning*. Philadelphia: W.B. Saunders Company.

41 Clarke-Steffen, L. (1992). Waiting and not knowing: The diagnosis of cancer in a child. *Journal of Pediatric Oncology Nursing, 9*(2), 52–53.

42 Avery, M., & First, L. (1987). *Pediatric medicine* (pp. 549–593). Baltimore: Williams & Wilkins.

43 Moore, I., Glasser, M., & Ablin, A. (1987). The late psychosocial consequences of childhood cancer. *Journal of Pediatric Nursing, 3*(3), 150–158.

44 Baron, M. (1991). Advances in the care of children with brain tumors. *Journal of Neuroscience Nursing, 23*(1), 39–43.

45 Shiminski-Maher, T. (1991). Diabetes insipidus and syndrome of inappropriate secretion of antidiuretic hormone in children with midline suprasellar brain tumors. *Journal of Pediatric Oncology Nursing, 8*(3), 106–111.

46 Finkelstein, J. (1987). Neuroblastoma: The challenge and frustration. *Hematology/Oncology Clinics of North America, 1*(4), 675–689.

47 Kronreich, L., Horev, G., Kaplinsky, C., & Grunebaum, M. (1991). Neuroblastoma: Evaluation with contrast enhanced MR imaging. *Pediatric Radiology, 21*, 566–569.

48 Ganick, D. (1987). Wilm's tumor. *Hematology/Oncology Clinics of North America, 1*(4), 695–713.

49 Hansen, M. (1990). Molecular genetic considerations in osteosarcoma. *Clinical Orthopaedics and Related Research,* Sept. (270), 237–246.

50 Hockenberry, M., Coody, D., & Bennett, B. (1990). Childhood cancers: Incidence, etiology, diagnosis, and treatment. *Pediatric Nursing, 16*(3), 239–246.

51 Dickey, S. (1987). *A guide to the nursing of children* (p. 309). Baltimore: Williams & Wilkins.

52 Arena, F.P. (1991). Update on acute lymphocytic leukemia. *Hospital Medicine,* March, pp. 33–46.

53 Klopovich, P., & Cohen, D. (1984). An overview of pediatric oncology for the adult oncology nurse. *Oncology Nursing Forum, 11*(4), 56–63.

54 Steinherz, P. (1987). Acute lymphoblastic leukemia of childhood. *Hematology/Oncology Clinics of North America, 1*(4), 549–566.

55 Poplack, D. (1985). Acute lymphoblastic leukemia in childhood. *Pediatric Clinics of North America, 32*(3), 669–697.

56 Bonilla, J., & Healy, G. (1989). Management of malignant head and neck tumors in children. *Pediatric Clinics of North America, 36*(6), 1443–1450.

57 Prognostic factors in childhood rhabdomyosarcoma. (1989). *Lancet, 2*, 959–960.

58 Ville, R. (1989). Tumor suppressor genes: Loss of these genes may cause cancer. *British Medical Journal, 298*(6684), 1335–1336.

59 Benedict, W., Xu, H., Hu, S., & Takahashi, R. (1990). Role of the retinoblastoma gene in the initiation and progression of human cancer. *Journal of Clinical Investigation, 85*(4), 988–993.

60 Holladay, D., Holladay, A., Montebello, J., & Redmond, K. (1991). Clinical presentation, treatment, and outcome of trilateral retinoblastoma. *Cancer, 67*(3), 710–715.

61 Gallie, B., Dunn, J., Chan, H., Hamel, P., & Phillips, R. (1991). The genetics of retinoblastoma: Relevance to the patient. *Pediatric Clinics of North America, 38*(2), 299–315.

62 Zelter, M., Damel, A., Gonzales, G., & Schwartz, L. (1991). A prospective study on the treatment of retinoblastoma in 72 patients. *Cancer, 68*(8), 1685–1690.

SUGGESTED READINGS

Brophy, L., & Sharp, E. (1991). Physical symptoms of combination biotherapy: A quality-of-life issue. *Oncology Nursing Forum, 18*(1) (Suppl.), 25–30.

Dow, K.H., & Hilderley, L.J. (1992). *Nursing care in radiation oncology*. Philadelphia: W.B. Saunders.

Egan, A., Taggart, J., & Bender, C. (1992). Management of chemotherapy-related nausea and vomiting using a serotonin antagonist. *Oncology Nursing Forum, 19*(5), 791–795.

Foley, G.V., Fochtman, D., & Mooney, K.H. (Eds.). (1993). *Nursing care of the child with cancer* (2nd ed.). Association of Pediatric Oncology Nurses. Philadelphia: W.B. Saunders.

Gresik, M., Hawkins, E., & Finegold, M. (1991). Pathology. In D. Fernbach & T. Vietti (Eds.), *Clinical pediatric oncology* (4th ed.). St. Louis: Mosby–Year Book.

Mandall, L., & Wharam, M. (1991). Radiology. In D. Fernbach & T. Vietti (Eds.), *Clinical pediatric oncology* (4th ed.). St. Louis: Mosby–Year Book.

Rae, W., Worchel, F., Upchurch, J., Sanner, J., & Daniel, C. (1989). The psychosocial impact of play on hospitalized children. *Journal of Pediatric Psychology, 14*(4), 617–627.

Roth, M., & Foon, K. (1987). Biotherapy with interferon in hematologic malignancies. *Oncology Nursing Forum, 14*(6) (Suppl.), 16–22.

Sutters, K., & Miaskowski, C. (1992). The problem of pain in children with cancer: A research review. *Oncology Nursing Forum, 19*(3), 465–471.

Valente, S. (1991). Using hypnosis with children for pain management. *Oncology Nursing Forum, 18*(4), 699–704.

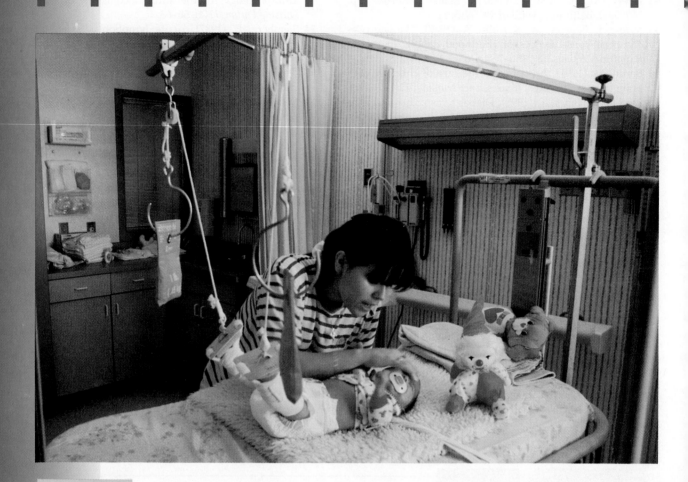

Carmen was born through breech delivery. When Carmen was 2 days of age, her physician noted that her left hip was easily dislocated; she had a dimple over her left hip and another at her knee, and her gluteal folds were more pronounced on the left side. Carmen was discharged with a Pavlik harness to keep her legs abducted as much as possible.

Carmen's parents, who are Hispanic, had many questions. A translator was used to perform teaching before discharge.

When Carmen returns for her 2-month examination, she is diagnosed as having developmental dysplasia of the left hip. She is admitted to the hospital and placed in bilateral Bryant traction to increase mobility and stretch her hip prior to a surgical reduction. The nurses reassure Carmen's parents that she is expected to have normal range of motion and activity as she grows older.

What are the risk factors for developmental dysplasia of the hip? What special needs do Carmen's parents have because of their inability to understand English? How can Carmen's parents and nurses meet her developmental needs during hospitalization?

ALTERATIONS IN MUSCULOSKELETAL FUNCTION

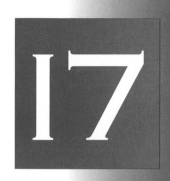

17

chondrolysis The breaking down and absorption of cartilage.

dislocation Displacement of a bone from its normal articulation with a joint.

dysplasia Abnormal development resulting in altered size, shape, and cell organization.

equinus A condition that limits dorsiflexion to less than normal; usually associated with clubfoot.

ossification Formation of bone from fibrous tissue or cartilage.

osteotomy Surgical cutting of bone.

subluxation Partial or complete dislocation of a joint.

valgus An abnormal position of a limb that involves bending away from the midline of the body.

varus An abnormal position of a limb that involves bending toward the midline of the body.

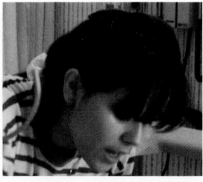

❝ When I first learned that Carmen has this condition, I wondered if she would be able to run and play like other children. It was sad to see my little baby in traction. But the doctor says that she really can have a normal childhood. ❞

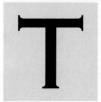

The musculoskeletal system helps the body to protect its vital organs, support weight, control motion, store minerals, and supply red blood cells. Bones provide a rigid framework for the body, muscles provide for active movement, and tendons and ligaments hold the bones and muscles together.

Musculoskeletal disorders may be congenital, such as clubfoot, or acquired, such as osteomyelitis, and may require short- or long-term management. Why do children develop certain musculoskeletal disorders? What impact do these disorders and their treatment have on a child's growth and development? How can nurses assist children and their families to cope with the mobility limitations imposed by the treatment of many of these disorders? This chapter will prepare you to answer these questions and will enable you to provide effective care for children who have musculoskeletal disorders.

Anatomy and Physiology of Pediatric Differences

Bones

Several differences exist between the bones of children and those of adults. Although primary centers of **ossification (bone formation)** are nearly complete at birth, a fibrous membrane still exists between the cranial bones (fontanels). The posterior fontanel closes between 2 and 3 months of age. The anterior fontanel does not close until approximately 18 months of age, allowing for growth of the brain and skull. In addition, the ends of the long bones (epiphyses) remain cartilaginous. Long bone growth continues until approximately age 20, when skeletal maturation is complete.

Secondary ossification occurs as the long bones grow. Cartilage cells at the epiphyses are replaced by osteoblasts (immature bone cells), resulting in deposition of calcium. Because growth takes place at these epiphyseal plates, injuries to this portion of a long bone are of particular concern in young children.

The long bones of children are porous and less dense than those of adults. For this reason, children's bones can bend, buckle, or break as a result of a simple fall.

In addition to the structural differences between the bones of children and adults, there are also functional differences in the skeletal system of children (see Fig. 3–1). Before birth, the thoracic and sacral regions of the spine are convex curves. As the infant learns to hold up its head, the cervical region becomes concave. When the child learns to stand, the lumbar region also becomes concave. Failure of the spine to assume these final curves results in abnormal curvature of the spine (kyphosis or lordosis).

Muscles, Tendons, and Ligaments

The muscular system, unlike the skeletal system, is almost completely formed at birth. As a child grows, muscles do not increase in number, but rather in length and circumference.[1] Until puberty, both tendons and ligaments are stronger than bone. When these structural differences are not recognized, a childhood fracture is sometimes mistaken for a sprain.

Disorders of the Feet and Legs

Metatarsus Adductus

Metatarsus adductus, the most common congenital foot deformity, is characterized by an inward turning of the forefoot at the tarsometatarsal joints (Fig.

FIGURE 17-1 Metatarsus adductus is characterized by convexity (curvature) of the lateral border of the foot, as shown by the red line.

From Staheli, L.T. (1992). *Fundamentals of pediatric orthopedics* (p. 5.7). New York: Raven Press.

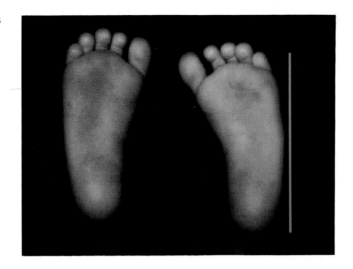

17–1). Often referred to as "intoeing," metatarsus adductus affects male and female infants equally and occurs in approximately 1 in 1000 births. This condition may be related to intrauterine positioning.[2,3]

Treatment depends on the degree of foot flexibility. If the foot can be readily maneuvered past the neutral position, simple exercises may correct the problem. Otherwise, serial casting is required. The feet are placed in a position as close to neutral as possible and are held secure with a cast. Casts are changed weekly until the desired correction is achieved.[4]

Nursing Management

Reassure parents that the child's condition can be corrected. If the child's deformity is mild, teach parents simple stretching exercises that can be performed at each diaper change. If casting is necessary, provide cast care as outlined in Table 17–1 and give parents instructions concerning cast care (Table 17–2).

Clubfoot

Clubfoot is a congenital abnormality in which the foot is twisted out of its normal position. It occurs in approximately 1 to 2 in 1000 births and affects boys nearly twice as often as girls.[3,4]

Clinical Manifestations

A true clubfoot (talipes equinovarus) involves three areas of deformity: the foot is directed downward (**equinus**) and inward (**varus**), with the forefoot adducted.[5] Most children have this combination of findings.

Clubfoot may be bilateral (Fig. 17–2) or unilateral. If the condition is unilateral, the left foot is usually affected. The foot is small with a shortened Achilles tendon. Muscles in the lower leg are atrophied, but leg lengths are generally normal.

Etiology and Pathophysiology

The exact cause of clubfoot is unknown; however, several possible etiologies have been proposed. Some authorities blame abnormal intrauterine positioning for causing the deformity. Other experts believe it has a genetic component. Drugs or irradiation during gestation may also play a role in causation.[4,6,7]

■ **CLINICAL TIP**

To perform stretching exercises for metatarsus adductus:
1. Hold the infant's foot securely in a natural position.
2. Move the forefoot away from the body with the other hand.
3. Hold the foot in this position for 5 seconds.
4. Repeat five times at every diaper change.

TABLE 17-1 Nursing Care of the Child in a Cast

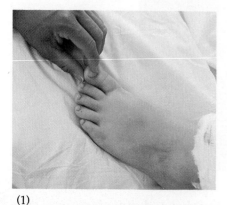
(1)

- A plaster cast takes anywhere from 24 to 48 hours to dry. When handling the cast, be gentle and use the palms of your hands as even fingertips can indent plaster and create pressure areas.
- After the cast is applied, elevate the extremity on a pillow above the level of the heart. Elevation helps to reduce swelling and increases venous return.
- If the cast is applied after surgery, there may be drainage or bleeding through the cast material. Circle the stain and note the date and time on the cast to provide a means of assessing the amount of fluid lost.
- Assess the distal pulses, and check the fingers and toes for color, warmth, capillary refill, and edema. Assess sensation as well as movement. Any deviation from normal may indicate nerve damage or decreased blood supply.
- During the first 24 hours, the casted extremity should be checked every ½ hour for 2 hours, then every 1 to 2 hours thereafter. The skin should be warm. It should blanch when slight pressure is applied and then return to its normal color within 3 seconds. (1) For the next 2 days, the casted extremity should be assessed at least every 4 hours.
- Check the edges of the cast for roughness or crumbling. If necessary, pull the inner stockinette over the edge and tape.
- The rough edges of the cast may also be alleviated by "petaling." This involves securing adhesive tape to the inside of the cast and pulling it over the edge, covering the jagged or broken pieces of plaster, and securing it to the outer surface of the cast. (2, 3, 4) Moleskin may be used on the cast as well.

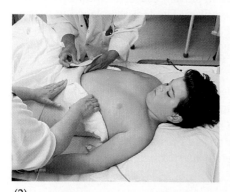
(2)

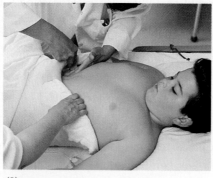
(3)

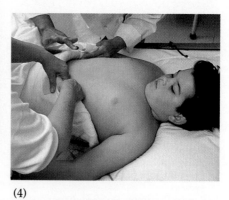
(4)

- Keep the cast as clean and dry as possible. Cover the cast with a plastic bag or plastic wrap when the child bathes or showers.
- The skin under the cast may itch; however, do not use powders or lotions near the edges or under the cast as they can cause skin irritation.
- Be sure that children do not put small objects between their casts and extremities, which can cause skin irritation as well as neurovascular compromise.

Nursing care of the child in a cast was provided by Marcia Wellington, RN, MS.

Diagnostic Tests and Medical Management

Diagnosis is made at birth on the basis of visual inspection. Radiographs are used to confirm the severity of the condition.

Early treatment is essential to achieve successful correction and reduce the chance of complications. Serial casting is the treatment of choice. Casting should begin as soon after birth as possible. Timing is critical because the short bones of the foot, which are primarily cartilaginous at birth, begin to ossify shortly thereafter.

The foot is manipulated to achieve maximum correction first of the varus deformity and then of the equinus deformity. A long leg cast is applied to hold the foot in the desired position. The cast is changed every 1 to 2 weeks.

TABLE 17-2 Discharge Teaching: Home Care Instructions for Casts

Care of Skin

- Check the skin around the cast edges for irritation, rubbing, or blistering. Skin should be clean and dry.
- You may cleanse the skin just under the cast edges and between the toes or fingers with a cotton-tipped applicator and rubbing alcohol. Avoid using lotions, oils, and powders near the cast as they may cause caking.
- Avoid poking sharp objects down inside casts as this may result in sores.

Care of Cast

- Keep the cast dry. Protect plaster with a cast shoe, thick sock, or sling.
- Allow a new, wet cast to air-dry for 24 hours.
- You may begin walking on leg casts only if your physician has given you permission to do so.

Things to Watch for

- Toes or fingers should be pink, not blue or white.
- Skin should be warm and the tips of toes or fingers should blanch when pinched.
- Raise the casted arm or leg above heart level to prevent or reduce any swelling.

Notify Your Health Care Provider if Any of the Following Occur

- Unusual odor beneath the cast; tingling, burning, or numbness in the casted arm or leg; drainage through the cast; swelling or inability to move fingers or toes; slippage of the cast; cast cracked, soft, or loose; sudden unexplained fever; unusual fussiness or irritability of an infant or child; fingers or toes that are blue or white; and pain that is not relieved by any comfort measures (i.e., repositioning or pain medication)

Adapted from Shriners Hospital for Crippled Children, Spokane, WA.

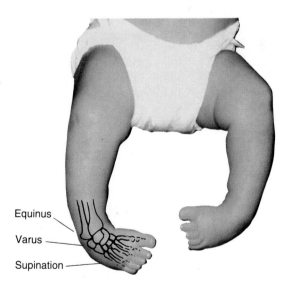

FIGURE 17-2 Bilateral clubfoot deformity. Parents who learn that their child has clubfoot will have many questions. Can the condition be treated? Will the child be completely normal after surgery? Will they need help caring for the infant? How much will it cost? Will any other children that they may have in the future possibly be affected with clubfoot?

Modified from Staheli, L.T. (1992). *Fundamentals of pediatric orthopedics* (p. 5.10). New York: Raven Press.

This regimen of manipulation and casting continues for approximately 12 weeks until maximum correction is achieved. If the deformity has been corrected, the child may begin wearing reverse or corrective shoes to maintain the correction. If the deformity has not been corrected, surgical intervention is required. Casting is maintained to hold position until the actual surgery date.

The age at which a child undergoes clubfoot surgery varies from surgeon to surgeon. However, most children have surgery between 4 and 12 months of age. The one-stage posteromedial release procedure,[8] which involves realignment of the bones of the foot and release of the constricting soft tissue, is most commonly performed. The foot is held in the proper position by a pin fixator. A cast is then applied with the knee flexed to prevent damage to the pin and discourage weight bearing. Casting continues for 6 to 12 weeks. The child may then need to wear a brace or corrective shoes, depending on the severity of the deformity and the surgeon's preference.

Nursing Assessment

Nursing assessment, which begins at birth and continues throughout the child's subsequent hospitalizations, includes genetic history, birth history, physical examination (position and appearance), motor development, and family coping mechanisms.

Nursing Diagnosis

Common nursing diagnoses for the child with a clubfoot deformity include the following:

- Impaired Physical Mobility related to cast wear
- High Risk for Impaired Skin Integrity related to cast wear
- Altered Parenting related to emotional reaction following birth of a child with a physical defect
- Knowledge Deficit (Parent) related to deformity, treatment, and home care

Nursing Management

Nursing management involves providing postsurgical care, providing cast and brace care, providing emotional support, and educating the family about home care.

Provide Postsurgical Care. Routine postoperative care after surgical correction includes neurovascular status checks every 2 hours for the first 24 hours and assessing for any swelling around the cast edges (see Table 17–1). Apply ice bags to the foot, and keep the ankle and foot elevated on a pillow for 24 hours. This promotes healing and helps with venous return. Check for drainage or bleeding. Administer pain medication routinely for 24 to 48 hours.

Provide Cast and Brace Care. Routine cast care is outlined in Table 17–1. After serial casting is complete, or following surgery, the child may progress to wearing a brace or special shoe for 6 to 12 months. Braces should fit snugly but should not interfere with neurovascular function. Before the child begins to wear a brace, check skin for any areas of redness or breakdown. Provide parents with guidelines for brace wear (Table 17–3). Emphasize that proper skin care is essential. If skin redness develops, arrange to have the brace modified.

TABLE 17–3 Guidelines for Brace Wear

- Braces should be as comfortable as possible and the child should have adequate mobility while wearing the brace.
- Begin wearing the brace for periods of 1 to 2 hours and then progress to 2 to 4 hours.
- Check skin at 1- to 2-hour intervals. If redness or breakdown is apparent, leave the brace off and allow the skin to clear.
- Always have the child wear a clean white sock, T-shirt, or other thin white liner beneath the brace. Be sure the liner is wrinkle-free under the brace. Avoid using powders or lotions that can cause skin to break down. Toughen any sensitive areas using alcohol wipes.
- Reapply the brace when the skin returns to its normal color.

Provide Emotional Support. Clubfoot is a condition that affects not only the child but also the family. The child's foot deformity is upsetting to parents, and they need emotional support to allay their fears. Helping parents understand the condition and its treatment is essential.

Encourage parents to hold and cuddle the child and to take an active role in the child's care to help promote bonding. Explain that, with treatment, the child will grow and develop normally.

Discharge Planning and Patient and Family Home Care Teaching. Give parents written instructions for cast care (see Table 17–2). In addition, assist them in the following ways:

- Demonstrate the use of a sponge bath to protect the cast.
- Discuss several options for clothing that accommodates a cast, for example, one-piece snap suits or sweatpants.
- Discuss potential safety hazards that may result from awkward positioning.
- Suggest that parents make an effort to place toys within the child's reach, since the movements of a child in a cast may be slowed.

■ SAFETY PRECAUTIONS

Advise parents that umbrella strollers may not be sturdy enough to support the infant's casted leg. Some infant swings do not provide a foot rest, and this can contribute to cast slippage or breakdown.

Genu Varum and Genu Valgum

Genu varum (bowlegs) is a deformity in which the knees are widely separated and the lower legs are turned inward **(varus)**. In genu valgum (knock-knees), the knees are close together and the ankles are directed outward **(valgus)**. Both conditions involve angular deformities of the tibiofemoral angle.

At certain stages of a child's development, the appearance of bowlegs or knock-knees is normal. However, the appearance of knock-knees beyond the age of 2 to 4 years necessitates further evaluation. Chapter 3 discusses the assessment of bowlegs and knock-knees in children.

Braces are often used to correct mild deformities that could worsen as the child grows. Braces for bowlegs are worn at night; those for knock-knees both day and night. Duration of brace wear is determined by the severity of the deformity, which is usually evaluated by radiographs. If the deformity continues to worsen, surgical intervention is necessary. An **osteotomy** (cutting of the bone) is performed and the tibiofemoral angle surgically corrected. The child is then placed in a cast for approximately 6 to 10 weeks, or until full healing has occurred.

Nursing Management

Reassure parents that both bowlegs and knock-knees are usually a normal part of a child's growth and development. Often these conditions resolve on their own and require no treatment other than continued observation.

Nursing care focuses on educating parents and child about the condition and its treatment. Provide the child and family with guidelines for brace wear, and teach them about brace maintenance (see Table 17–3).

Disorders of the Hip

Developmental Dysplasia of the Hip

Developmental dysplasia of the hip (DDH) refers to a variety of conditions in which the femoral head and the acetabulum are improperly aligned. These conditions include **dislocation** (displacement of the bone from its normal articulation with the joint), **subluxation** (partial dislocation), and acetabular **dysplasia** (abnormal development). In the past, DDH was referred to as congenital dislocated hip (CDH). The new name reflects the fact that many cases of dislocation, subluxation, and dysplasia occur well after the neonatal period and involve more than a simple dislocation.

DDH occurs in 1 to 2 in 1000 births, and affects girls six times as often as boys.[3,9] It is unilateral in three quarters of affected children, and the left hip is affected three times as often as the right.[3]

Clinical Manifestations

Common signs and symptoms include limited abduction of the affected hip, asymmetry of the gluteal and thigh fat folds, and telescoping or pistoning of the thigh (Fig. 17–3). Carmen, described at the beginning of this chapter, had signs of unilateral DDH. The older child walks with a significant limp, which results from telescoping of the femoral head into the pelvis. The longer the disorder goes untreated, the more pronounced the clinical manifestations become, and the worse the prognosis.

Etiology and Pathophysiology

Although the exact cause of DDH is unknown, genetic factors appear to play a role. DDH is 20 to 50 times more common in first-degree relatives of an in-

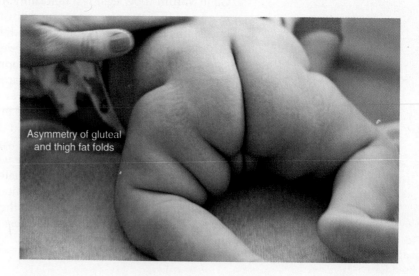

FIGURE 17–3 The asymmetry of the gluteal and thigh fat folds is easy to see in this child with developmental dysplasia of the hip.

Asymmetry of gluteal and thigh fat folds

PEDIATRIC NURSING

Infants positioned on cradle boards or traditionally swaddled, as in some Native American cultures, are 10 times more likely to have DDH than they would be otherwise. Where mothers carry their infants on their hips or their backs with the infant's legs abducted, as in some parts of Africa and Asia, the incidence of DDH is very low.[3,10]

fant with the condition than in the general population. If one child of a set of identical twins has DDH, the other twin is affected 30 to 40 percent of the time.

Prenatal conditions may affect the development of DDH. The left hip is involved more often than the right hip as a result of intrauterine positioning of the left side of the fetus against the mother's sacrum. Maternal estrogen may cause laxity of the hip joint and capsule, leading to joint instability. Cultural factors may also be associated with DDH.

Diagnostic Tests and Medical Management

Physical examination reveals Allis sign (one knee lower than the other when the knees are flexed), a positive Ortolani maneuver, and a positive Barlow test. Chapter 3 discusses the assessment of hip dislocations in newborns and infants. Radiographs should not be taken until approximately 6 weeks of age because the pelvis in a newborn infant is still primarily cartilaginous.

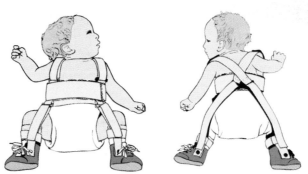

FIGURE 17-4 The most common treatment for DDH in a child under 3 months of age is a Pavlik harness.
From Staheli, L.T. (1992). *Fundamentals of pediatric orthopedics* (p. 7.10). New York: Raven Press.

Treatment plans vary according to the child's age. For infants younger than 3 months, the Pavlik harness is the most commonly used method for hip reduction (Fig. 17-4). For infants older than 3 months, skin traction is used. Correct positioning, which involves relocating the femoral head into the acetabulum while gently stretching the restrictive soft tissue, is essential. Surgery and the application of a spica cast may be necessary. In toddlers and children aged 3 to 6 years, surgery and casting are usually necessary and bracing may also be required (Fig. 17-5).

Early screening, detection, and treatment enable the majority of affected children to attain normal hip function.

Nursing Assessment

Assessment for DDH, which begins at delivery, continues through all well-child checkups and should include any specific family history or birth data that may indicate a high-risk infant. Instructions for performing the physical examination to assess the infant for DDH are given in Chapter 3.

Nursing Diagnosis

Several nursing diagnoses may apply to the child with DDH. They include:

- Impaired Physical Mobility related to treatment (Pavlik harness, traction, spica cast, brace)

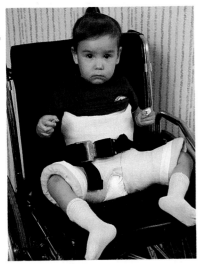

FIGURE 17-5 In children 3 to 6 years of age, a spica cast is most commonly used for DDH.

- High Risk for Impaired Skin Integrity related to treatment
- High Risk for Altered Urinary Elimination or Constipation related to immobility caused by treatment
- High Risk for Altered Nutrition related to immobility caused by treatment
- High Risk for Altered Growth and Development related to treatment
- Knowledge Deficit (Parent) related to disease process and treatment
- Knowledge Deficit (Parent) related to discharge planning and home care of child in brace or spica cast

Nursing Management

Nursing care varies according to the medical treatment and the child's age. Because treatment interferes with the child's normal development, the treatment plan should take into consideration the age and developmental stage of the child.

Ensure Proper Use of Pavlik Harness. Have parents demonstrate the proper application of the harness and care of the infant in the harness. The straps must be secure enough to provide hip flexion without being tight.

- Teach family members about daily care (bathing, dressing, and feeding) of the infant. Ideally, the harness is worn 23 hours per day and is removed only for skin checks and bathing. Hips and buttocks should be supported carefully when the infant is out of the harness. Demonstrate how to feed the infant in an upright position to maintain abduction and how to change a diaper without removing the harness.
- Instruct the parents to look for any reddened or irritated areas near the harness and to check toes frequently for proper circulation. Frequent repositioning reduces the risk for pressure sores or circulatory compromise.

Maintain Traction. Bryant skin traction is the most common form of traction used in the treatment of DDH. (Types of traction are discussed later in the chapter and presented in Table 17–11.) Check the traction apparatus frequently to ensure that proper alignment and healing occur.

Provide Cast Care. The principles of routine cast care presented in Table 17–1 apply to the care of spica casts. Special techniques should be used to help keep the cast clean and dry in children who are not toilet trained. Female and male urinals can be used for older children.

- Use a plastic lining to protect the cast edges and place a toilet paper "wick" on the perineum of girls to direct urine into the bedpan. For mobile children, use a small disposable diaper to cover the perineum, tucking edges beneath the cast. Be sure to change the diaper frequently.
- Help prevent skin irritation and breakdown. Use moleskin to provide protection from rough cast edges. Place tape around the perineal opening to prevent soiling.

Prevent Complications Resulting from Immobility. Immobilization from either traction or casting can cause alterations in physiologic functioning. Assess breathing patterns and lung sounds frequently for congestion or respiratory compromise. Perform skin and neurovascular assessments approximately every 2 hours. Use adequate padding and skin wrapping to avoid placing pressure on the popliteal space. Such pressure could lead to nerve palsy. For the child in a cast, change the child's position every 2 to 3 hours while awake to help avoid areas of pressure and promote increased circulation. The child can be placed either prone or supine on a spica board or positioned on the floor and supported with pillows.

Fluids and bulk or bran should be added to the child's diet, since a change in bowel or bladder status is commonly associated with immobility.

Permit limited mobility, if ordered by the physician, and release the child from traction for meals and daily care. The time out of traction should not exceed 1 hour per day. Encourage parents to hold and cuddle the child at this time to promote comfort and bonding.

Promote Normal Growth and Development. Engage the child in activities that stimulate the upper extremities and all five senses. Provide stimulating toys such as stacking blocks, brightly colored mobiles, Koosh balls, or musical toys. Position toys within the child's reach and interact with the child as much as possible. Use caution in selecting toys appropriate to the child's developmental stage. If the child is in a cast, be sure that the toys or their parts cannot be swallowed or stuck inside the cast.

Discharge Planning and Patient and Family Home Care Teaching. Parents need to be taught how to care for a child in a spica cast at home. The active participation of family members in the daily care of the child while hospitalized gradually increases their confidence in their ability to provide care once home. Home care needs should be identified and addressed well in advance of discharge. Before discharge, be sure the parents have:

- Information about general cast care (see Table 17–2), positioning, bathing, toileting, and age-appropriate diversional activities.
- Spica board materials and a bedpan available, if needed. Have parents demonstrate how to make a bed with a spica board and how to position the child in a spica cast on the board.
- Appropriate referrals for periodic assessment by a visiting nurse or home health nurse.
- Family resources to care for the child.

Before discharge, have parents demonstrate how to dress and feed a child in a spica cast. Ensure that safe travel arrangements have been made for the day of discharge. Encourage parents to let the child interact with other children at home. Children in casts should have plenty of opportunities for play and social activities.

Legg-Calvé-Perthes Disease

Legg-Calvé-Perthes disease is a self-limiting condition that involves avascular necrosis of the femoral head. The disease occurs in approximately 1 in 12,000 children and affects boys four time more often than girls. It usually occurs between the ages of 2 and 12 years.

Clinical Manifestations

Early symptoms of this disease include a mild pain in the hip or anterior thigh and a limp, which are aggravated by increased activity and relieved by rest. The child favors the affected hip and limits hip movement to avoid discomfort.

As the disease progresses, range of motion becomes limited and weakness and muscle wasting develop. The affected thigh is 2 to 3 cm smaller than the unaffected thigh. Over time, prolonged hip irritability may produce muscle spasms.

Etiology and Pathophysiology

The necrosis associated with Legg-Calvé-Perthes disease results from an interruption of blood supply to the femoral epiphysis. How and why this occurs is not completely understood, but several predisposing factors have been identified. The incidence of Legg-Calvé-Perthes disease is up to 20% higher in families with a history of the disease than in the general population, which suggests that genetic factors may play a role. In one quarter of the cases, onset of the disease is preceded by a mild traumatic injury. Trauma may cause a subchondral fracture, initiating the disease process.

Legg-Calvé-Perthes disease progresses through four distinct stages: synovitis, necrosis or collapse, fragmentation, and reconstitution. The disease generally lasts 1 to 2 years. The synovitis stage, which lasts approximately 1 to 3 weeks, is characterized by swelling of the synovial membrane, soft-tissue changes, and a painful limp. Decreased blood supply to the femoral head leads to necrosis. Once necrosis sets in, the bone weakens and dies, causing collapse. During the fragmentation stage, healing occurs as new bone forms and the necrotic bone is absorbed. Ossification occurs during the reconstruction phase, resulting in final healing.

Diagnostic Tests and Medical Management

Because the child's initial symptoms are so mild, parents often do not seek medical attention until symptoms have been present for several months. Diagnosis is made using standard anteroposterior and frog-leg radiographs. Radiographs taken early in the course of the disease may either be normal or show vague widening of the cartilage space.

Medical management and prognosis depend on the degree of femoral involvement. Early detection is important. The desired outcome is a pain-free hip that functions properly. To promote healing and prevent deformity, the femoral head must be contained within the hip socket until ossification is complete. Adequate containment will only be achieved if the hips remain in an abducted position. This is accomplished by using traction, Petrie casting, or surgical soft tissue releases such as adductor tenotomy, followed by bracing. Toronto (Fig. 17–6) and Scottish-Rite braces are most commonly used. Prognosis is good if the femoral head can be contained long enough for proper healing.

Nursing Assessment

Legg-Calvé-Perthes disease should be suspected in any child, especially a boy aged 2 to 12 years, who complains of hip discomfort accompanied by a limp. The school nurse may be the first person to observe the child with symptoms of Legg-Calvé-Perthes disease. The child may complain of pain and have to rest during physical education classes. Referral should be made to the health care provider immediately. Question the child who has an apparent limp about pain, and assess the child's range of motion.

Nursing Diagnosis

Nursing diagnoses, which center on altered activities and compliance, include the following:

- Impaired Physical Mobility related to brace or cast wear
- Knowledge Deficit related to complications of disease process if child is noncompliant
- High Risk for Noncompliance related to prolonged treatment period.

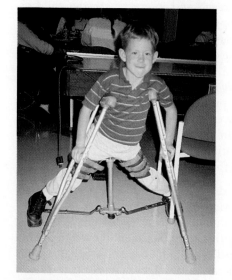

FIGURE 17–6 Although the Toronto brace may seem formidable for a child to wear, you can see by this photograph that, as usual, children adapt quite well to it.

Nursing Management

Helping the child and family comply with the prescribed treatment plan may
be challenging, since children with Legg-Calvé-Perthes disease are active,
may have little pain, and find immobilization difficult.

Promote Normal Growth and Development. Parents should be given suggestions to help redirect the child's energy within the limitations in mobility imposed by treatment. A return to school promotes a feeling of normalcy. Activities that involve peers also help the child achieve developmental
milestones.

Discharge Planning and Patient and Family Home Care Teaching. Both the child
and the family should be aware that treatment generally takes more than 2
years. Stress the importance of following the treatment plan to ensure adequate hip containment and proper healing. Changes in the treatment plan
should be kept to a minimum. Follow-up visits should be arranged at regular intervals.

Slipped Capital Femoral Epiphysis

Slipped capital femoral epiphysis (SCFE) occurs when the femoral head is
displaced from the femoral neck. This condition is commonly seen in adolescents between the ages of 10 and 17 years. Boys are affected two to three
times as often as girls.[3,10]

Clinical Manifestations

Symptoms include limp, pain, and loss of hip motion. The condition is categorized as acute, chronic, or acute-on-chronic, depending on the onset and
severity of symptoms.

    The child with an acute slip has sudden, severe pain and cannot bear
weight. An acute slip may be associated with traumatic injury.

    A chronic slip presents with persistent hip pain, which is generally aching
or mild and can be referred to the thigh, knee, or both. A limp and decreased
range of motion may also occur.

    When the child has had a chronic slip and then sustains a traumatic inci-
dent that causes further slippage of the femoral head, an acute-on-chronic
slip is said to occur. The child experiences sudden, severe pain.

Etiology and Pathophysiology

The cause of SCFE is unknown. Predisposing factors may include obesity, increased obliqueness of the growth plate angle, or decreased strength of the
growth plate. SCFE is also associated with rapid growth spurts resulting
from hormonal changes, which suggests the influence of endocrine alterations.

    The growth plate abnormalities occur prior to slippage. When acute
trauma or chronic weight-bearing stress is added, displacement inevitably
occurs. Slippage continues until the growth plate stabilizes, naturally or with
surgical treatment.

Diagnostic Tests and Medical Management

A precise history will usually reveal the extent of the slip. Radiographs are
used to confirm the diagnosis.

The goal of medical management is to stabilize the femoral head while keeping displacement to a minimum and retaining as much hip function as possible. Treatment may be either medical or surgical. Medical treatment includes non-weight-bearing regimens, bed rest, spica casts, and traction. Surgical stabilization of the femoral head may be necessary in severe cases.

Prognosis is related to the severity of the deformity and the occurrence of complications, such as avascular necrosis of the femoral head or **chondrolysis** (the breaking down and absorption of cartilage).[7,11]

Nursing Assessment

The child usually presents with hip pain and limited mobility. A thorough history is therefore needed to assess for injury or trauma as a cause. Assess the child's range of motion, pain, and limp, if apparent.

Nursing Diagnosis

Several nursing diagnoses may apply to the child with SCFE. They include the following:

- Impaired Physical Mobility related to non-weight-bearing treatment regimen
- Pain related to displacement of the femoral head or surgery
- High Risk for Body Image Disturbance related to treatment regimen or surgery
- High Risk for Altered Growth and Development related to mobility restrictions of treatment regimen
- High Risk for Altered Nutrition: More than Body Requirements related to immobility
- Knowledge Deficit (Child and Parent) related to disease process and treatment

Nursing Management

Nursing management involves caring for the child in traction or after surgery, maintaining mobility, providing adequate nutrition, educating the child and family about the disorder, and promoting compliance with the treatment plan.

Encourage Appropriate Nutritional Intake. A growing adolescent needs increased amounts of proteins, carbohydrates, and calcium to promote skeletal healing. Provide written instructions about nutritional requirements necessary to promote bone healing and maintain an ideal body weight. If a child is overweight, encourage weight loss, which decreases pressure on the femoral epiphysis and also leads to a more positive self-image.

Provide Emotional Support. The onset of SCFE is usually sudden, and the child and family who face surgery may be taken by surprise. Explain the treatment plan simply and thoroughly. Reassure the child that with proper compliance treatment should be successful.

Discharge Planning and Patient and Family Home Care Teaching. Follow-up visits are necessary until the child's epiphyseal plates close. It is not uncommon for SCFE to occur in the opposite hip. Make sure the child and family are aware of symptoms such as decreased range of motion or pain that could indicate onset of the disorder in the opposite hip. Tell parents to contact their health care provider immediately if these symptoms occur.

Disorders of the Spine

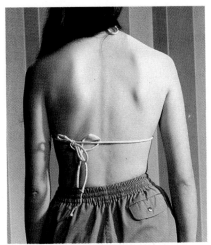

FIGURE 17–7 A child may have varying degrees of scoliosis. For mild forms, treatment will focus on strengthening and stretching. Moderate forms will require bracing. Severe forms may necessitate surgery and fusion. Clothes that fit at an angle, such as this teenage girl's shorts, and anatomic asymmetry of the back provide clues for early detection.

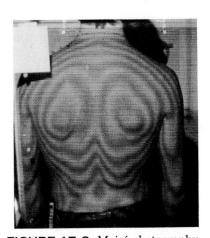

FIGURE 17–8 Moiré photography is sometimes used to document the degree of spinal asymmetry.

From Staheli, L.T. (1992). *Fundamentals of pediatric orthopedics* (p. 8.12). New York: Raven Press.

Scoliosis

Scoliosis is a lateral S- or C-shaped curvature of the spine that is often associated with a rotational deformity of the spine and ribs. It may be structural or functional in origin. Up to 10% of school-age children exhibit some degree of spinal curvature, and 2% to 3% have curvatures of more than 10 degrees. Curvatures of 15 degrees or more are considered significant. Scoliosis occurs most often in girls, especially during the growth spurt between the ages of 10 and 13 years.[3]

Clinical Manifestations

The classic signs of scoliosis include truncal asymmetry, uneven shoulders and hips, a one-sided rib hump, and a prominent scapula. The child does not complain of pain or discomfort. The child with structural scoliosis has a fixed or rigid spinal curvature with no visible correction during bending. In contrast, the child with functional scoliosis has a flexible spine, and the deformity is not apparent when the child bends toward the convex side (outside of the curve).

Etiology and Pathophysiology

The cause of scoliosis is complex. Structural scoliosis may be congenital, idiopathic, or acquired (associated with neuromuscular disorders such as muscular dystrophy or myelodysplasia, or secondary to spinal cord injuries). Functional scoliosis is usually a result of poor posture.

In idiopathic structural scoliosis (the most common type), the spine for unknown reasons begins to curve laterally, with vertebral rotation. As the curve progresses, structural changes occur. The ribs on the concave side (inside of the curve) are forced closer together, while the ribs on the convex side separate widely, causing narrowing of the thoracic cage and formation of the rib hump. The lateral curvature affects the vertebral structure. Disk spaces are narrowed on the concave side and spread wider on the convex side, resulting in an asymmetric vertebral canal (Fig. 17–7).

Diagnostic Tests and Medical Management

Generally, observation and radiographic examination are used to diagnose scoliosis. Additional diagnostic studies include magnetic resonance imaging, computed tomography, and bone scanning, which are used occasionally to assess the degree of curvature. Moiré photography using a special screen and a point light source documents spinal asymmetry (Fig. 17–8).

The goal of medical management is to limit or stop curve progression. Early detection is essential to successful treatment. Adequate treatment and follow-up maximize the child's chances for proper spinal alignment. The treatment regimen chosen depends on the degree and progression of the curvature and the reaction of the child and family to medical management.

Treatment of children with mild scoliosis (curvatures of 10 to 20 degrees) consists of exercises to improve posture and muscle tone and to maintain, or possibly increase, flexibility of the spine. Emphasis is placed on bending strength toward the outside of the curve while stretching the inside of the curve. These exercises are not a cure, however, and the child should be seen by a physician at 3-month intervals, with radiographic evaluation every 6 months.

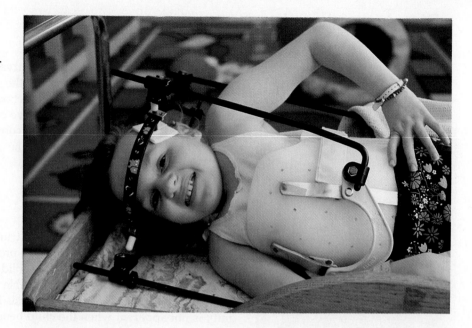

Medical management of moderate scoliosis (curvatures of 20 to 40 degrees) includes bracing with either a Boston, Milwaukee, or halo brace (Fig. 17–9). The goal of brace wear is to maintain the existing spinal curvature with no increase. Brace wear begins immediately on diagnosis. To achieve maximum effectiveness, the brace should be worn 23 hours per day. Brace treatment is lengthy and requires a high degree of compliance, which is often difficult for adolescents, for whom body image or sports involvement is often important.

Electrical stimulation is occasionally used as an alternative treatment. Electric current stimulates the back muscles to help correct the spinal curvature. This treatment, which is performed at night, eliminates the need for bracing.

Children with severe scoliosis (curvatures of 40 degrees or more) require surgery, which involves spinal fusion. The majority of spinal fusions are performed using instrumentation. The Harrington rod, Luque wire, or Coutrel-Dubosset (CD) instrumentation may be used. The Harrington rod has the fewest complications but is less stable than the Luque wire or CD instrumentation, requiring prolonged immobilization in a cast or halo brace.

Nursing Assessment

School nurses may screen children for scoliosis, generally beginning in the fifth grade. Children should be examined every 6 to 9 months thereafter. If scoliosis is detected, the child's brothers and sisters should be examined and observed closely. Chapter 3 discusses screening children for scoliosis.

Once scoliosis has been identified, the nurse's focus becomes education and follow-up. Any child with scoliosis should have a neurologic examination, since spinal structure and neurologic function are integrally linked.

Nursing Diagnosis

The following nursing diagnoses may apply to the child with scoliosis who is not undergoing surgery:

- High Risk for Noncompliance with exercise program related to knowledge deficit and lack of motivation

- Activity Intolerance related to brace wear
- Impaired Physical Mobility related to brace wear
- High Risk for Impaired Skin Integrity related to brace wear, or electrodes from electrical stimulation therapy
- High Risk for Knowledge Deficit (Child and Parent) related to disease process

Common nursing diagnoses for the child who is having surgery can be found in the accompanying Nursing Care Plan.

Nursing Management

An important aspect of nursing care is patient education. Patient compliance is critical to the success of treatment. Children and their families need to understand the condition and the stages of treatment. Children or adolescents facing surgery require education, reassurance, and support. The accompanying Nursing Care Plan summarizes nursing care for the child undergoing surgery for scoliosis.

Promote Compliance with the Treatment Plan. Provide instructions about exercises that will help to decrease the severity of the spinal curvature. Demonstrate the exercises, and explain their purpose (i.e., to strengthen back muscles).

Help the child adjust to wearing a brace. Adolescents, in particular, may be reluctant to wear an external device such as a brace. To promote a sense of control, allow the adolescent to chose when to exercise and when to be out of the brace, within the treatment guidelines. Provide reassurance and encouragement and promote interaction with peers. Suggesting that the adolescent work with a peer support person who is being treated for scoliosis or has had the condition in the past may be beneficial.

Discharge Planning and Patient and Family Home Care Teaching. Home care needs should be identified and addressed well in advance of discharge. The child will need to learn to adapt to a new set of body mechanics. Show the child how to do simple tasks *without bending or twisting the torso*. Have the child demonstrate the ability to perform daily activities before discharge from the hospital.

Activities allowed for the child who has had spinal surgery are limited (Table 17–4). Restrictions usually remain in place for 6 to 8 months, depend-

---

TABLE 17–4 Discharge Teaching: Postoperative Activities After Spinal Surgery

Recommended

Lying
Sitting
Standing
Walking (including normal stair climbing)
Swimming, gentle (not with a cast); diving is *not* permitted

Not Recommended

Bending or twisting at the waist
Lifting more than 10 pounds
Household chores such as vacuuming, unloading groceries, mowing the lawn, taking out garbage
Sports such as bicycle riding, horseback riding, skiing, roller blading, skating
Physical education classes

---

ing on the type of surgery and the surgeon. Emphasize the importance of compliance to both the child and the family. Give written discharge instructions to the child and family. The child and parent often agree to follow the physician's instructions by signing a written contract.

Follow-up visits are important. The child should be seen 4 to 6 weeks after discharge, then every 3 to 4 months for 1 year, and every 1 to 2 years thereafter.

Several organizations provide information and assistance to families of children with scoliosis (see Appendix F). The National Scoliosis Foundation is concerned with early detection and prevention of spinal curvature; the Scoliosis Association is a self-help group. The Scoliosis Research Society, a group of physicians and scientists, has published an informative book, *Scoliosis: A Handbook for Patients*.

Kyphosis and Lordosis

Kyphosis (hunchback) and lordosis (swayback) are two other types of spinal curvature that may occur in children (Table 17–5). Like scoliosis, these curvatures may be structural or functional in origin. Functional curvatures are usually a result of poor posture. Structural curvatures may be congenital or acquired. Medical management depends on the cause and degree of the curvature, and the age of the child at onset.

■ **GROWTH AND DEVELOPMENT CONSIDERATIONS**

Postural lordosis is a characteristic finding in toddlers but should disappear by the school-age years.

TABLE 17–5 Kyphosis and Lordosis: Clinical Manifestations and Treatment

Condition	Diagnostic Tests and Medical Management	Nursing Management
Kyphosis		
Excessive posterior curvature of the spine *Clinical manifestations:* Visible hunchback or rounded shoulders; shortness of breath or fatigue; abdominal creases and tight hamstrings in severe cases	*Diagnostic tests:* Spinal curvature is assessed by having the child bend 90 degrees at waist and looking at the scapular area from side. Diagnosis is confirmed by radiograph. *Medical management:* Bracing is the treatment of choice.	*Nursing management:* Provide support. Encourage diligent brace wear. Help child to deal with the psychological stress of altered body image.
Lordosis		
Inward curvature of the spine with an angle of more than 60 degrees. Most common in prepubescent girls and American blacks. *Clinical manifestations:* Presence of swayback; prominent buttocks; hip flexion contractures; tight hamstrings	*Diagnostic tests:* Spinal curvature is assessed by looking at the standing child from the side. Lumbar lordosis is confirmed by visualizing the spine on standing, lateral radiograph. *Medical management:* Treatment focuses on exercises and postural awareness. Bracing and surgery are rarely prescribed.	*Nursing management:* Provide support. Reassure child and family that condition is often outgrown as child matures. Encourage physical conditioning exercises and follow-up examinations on a yearly basis.

THE CHILD UNDERGOING SURGERY FOR SCOLIOSIS

GOAL	INTERVENTION	RATIONALE	EXPECTED OUTCOME
1. Knowledge Deficit (Child and Parents) related to disease process and surgical procedure			
The child and parents will verbalize understanding of the disease, its treatment, and the surgical procedure.	Teach the child and family about the course of the disease, its signs and symptoms, and its treatment. Provide appropriate handouts. Encourage the child and parents to ask questions.	Understanding and involvement increase motivation and compliance while reducing fear.	The child and family accurately verbalize knowledge about the disease and its treatment. The child and family ask appropriate questions about postoperative care.
	Begin preoperative teaching at the time of admission. Orient the child to hospital and postoperative procedures. Before surgery, have the child demonstrate logrolling, range of motion exercises in extremities, and use of an incentive spirometer. Discuss pain management.	Preoperative teaching and familiarity with hospital procedures reduces the stress related to surgery and reduces postoperative complications.	
2. Ineffective Breathing Pattern related to administration of analgesics and operative procedure			
The child will show no signs of respiratory compromise.	Monitor respiratory status, especially after the administration of analgesics.	Evaluation of the child's respiratory condition anticipates and avoids complications. Analgesics such as morphine may increase or potentiate respiratory compromise.	The child has no respiratory complications.
	Administer oxygen if ordered.	Oxygen increases peripheral oxygen saturation to 95% to 100%.	
	Have the child use an incentive spirometer.	Spirometry increases lung expansion and aeration of alveoli.	
	Monitor intake and output.	Good hydration promotes loose secretions and helps prevent infection.	
	Elevate the head of the bed.	Repositioning reduces breathing difficulties.	
3. High Risk for Injury related to neurovascular deficit secondary to instrumentation			
The child's neurovascular system will remain intact as evidenced by circulation, sensation, and motor checks. The child will feel no numbness or tingling.	Monitor the child's color, circulation, capillary refill, warmth, sensation, and motion in all extremities. Perform neurovascular checks every 2 hours for first 24 hours and then every 4 hours for next 48 hours. Record presence of pedal and distal tibial pulses every hour for 48 hours.	When the spinal column is manipulated during surgery, altered neurovascular status, thrombus formation, and paralysis are possible complications. Postoperative risks include loss of bowel or bladder control, weakness or paralysis, and impaired vision or sensation.	The child evidences only temporary alteration (pale skin, faint pulse, and edema occur but then resolve within the initial postoperative phase). The child returns to the preoperative baseline state by discharge.

Continued.

GOAL	INTERVENTION	RATIONALE	EXPECTED OUTCOME
3. High Risk for Injury related to neurovascular deficit secondary to instrumentation—Continued			
	Have the child wear antiembolism stockings until ambulatory. The stockings may be removed for 1 hour per shift.	Antiembolism stockings prevent blood clots and promote venous return. Thrombus formation is a postoperative risk.	
	Check for any pain, swelling, or a positive Homan sign in the legs. Record any evidence of edema	Swelling may indicate a tight dressing and tissue damage. Positive Homan sign and. pain may indicate thrombus formation.	
	Monitor input and output.	Abnormalities may indicate a fluid shift problem.	
	Encourage and assist the child with range of motion exercises, both passive and active.	Activity promotes mobility and reduces risk of thrombus formation.	
4. Pain related to spinal fusion with instrumentation			
The child will verbalize an adequate level of comfort or show absence of pain behavior within 1 hour of a specific nursing intervention.	Assess the level of pain and initiate pain management strategies as soon as possible. Use patient-controlled analgesia if ordered.	Adequate pain management allows for faster healing and a more cooperative patient. Patient-controlled analgesia may be effective.	The child experiences pain relief early in the postoperative period.
	Administer pain medication around-the-clock to help ensure pain relief, especially during the first 48 hours.	Medicating around-the-clock helps to maintain this level of comfort.	
	Use nonpharmacologic pain management techniques, such as imagery, relaxation, touch, music, application of heat and cold, and reduced environmental stimulation to supplement medications (see Chapter 5).	Alternative treatments also interrupt the pain stimulus and provide relief. Nonpharmacologic methods can be an effective adjunct to pain management.	
	Document pain assessment, interventions, and the child's reactions.	Proper documentation guides the nurse to select the most effective means of pain control.	
	Reassure the child that some pain is expected and not all pain will "disappear" with medications or other interventions.	Realistic expectations decrease anxiety and give the child a sense of control.	

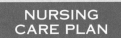
GOAL	INTERVENTION	RATIONALE	EXPECTED OUTCOME
5. Impaired Physical Mobility related to surgical procedure, pain management, or muscle spasms			
The child will maintain proper body alignment and progress with activity as ordered by the physician. If no anteroposterior shell bracing is required, the child will have active mobility by the third to fifth postoperative day.	Reposition the child every 2 hours using the log-roll technique. Support the back, feet, and knees with pillows.	Proper positioning prevents twisting or turning of the spine.	The child is as mobile as appropriate to condition within 3 to 5 days after surgery.
	Have the child do passive and active range of motion exercises every 2 hours for 48 hours and then every 4 hours while awake. Have the child dangle the legs at the bedside by the second to fourth postoperative day. Begin ambulation by the third to fifth postoperative day. Note any complaints of dizziness, pallor, etc. Proceed slowly.	Exercises help maintain strength, circulation, and muscle tone. If the spine is stable and the physician has ordered no external support, the child may progress to full ambulation as tolerated. If the spine is not stable, great care must be taken until external supportive devices are used.	
6. High Risk for Body Image Disturbance related to brace or cast wear or surgery			
The child will verbalize feelings about body image and self-esteem in relation to the disease and its treatment. The child will be informed about available support services and use them as needed.	Encourage independence in daily activities within allowable limits. Use positive reinforcements. Encourage the child to participate in community activities, if possible. Involve the child in scoliosis support groups.	Involvement in activities demonstrates that a "normal" life is realistic.	The child has a positive self-image and is involved in community activities or support groups.
	Provide contact with a peer resource person who has undergone treatment for scoliosis.	Peers are an effective means of support.	
7. High Risk for Knowledge Deficit (Child and Parent) related to discharge planning and home care			
The child and family will verbalize reduced anxiety about home care. The child will demonstrate knowledge of self-care and permitted activities.	Teach cast or brace care as appropriate (see Tables 17–2 and 17–3). Provide oral and written instructions and a list of activity limitations (see Table 17–4). Have the child and family demonstrate adequate knowledge.	Providing education decreases anxiety and increases compliance with treatment plan. Demonstration reinforces the learning process.	The child and family demonstrate home care and implementation of discharge teaching.
	Arrange for follow-up appointments as ordered by the physician. Encourage the child and family to notify the nurse or physician with any questions or concerns.	Follow-up visits help the nurse and physician evaluate the effectiveness of the treatment plan and patient compliance.	

Disorders of the Bones and Joints

Osteomyelitis

Osteomyelitis is an infection of the bone, most often one of the long bones of the lower extremity. It may be acute or chronic and may spread into surrounding tissues. Although osteomyelitis may occur at any age, it is most common in children between the ages of 1 and 12 years. Boys are affected four times as often as girls, primarily because they have a greater incidence of trauma.[3]

Clinical Manifestations

Symptoms include pain and tenderness with swelling, redness, decreased mobility of the infected joint, and fever. Onset of acute osteomyelitis is generally rapid, and symptoms should not be ignored.

Etiology and Pathophysiology

Osteomyelitis is caused by a microorganism, which is usually bacterial but can be viral or fungal. *Staphylococcus aureus* is the most common causative pathogen, followed by *Escherichia coli, Pseudomonas, Klebsiella,* and *Salmonella.*

The infecting organism is spread by the bloodstream or via penetrating injury to the bone, where it becomes established, usually in the bone cortex or marrow cavity. Inflammation and abscess formation may be followed by interruption of the blood supply to the underlying bone and, ultimately, by necrosis if the infection is left untreated.

Diagnostic Tests and Medical Management

Laboratory evaluation shows leukocytosis and an elevated erythrocyte sedimentation rate (ESR). The degree of ESR elevation is directly related to the severity of the infection.

Medical management begins with antibiotic therapy even before culture results are available. A broad-spectrum antibiotic is administered. If there is no clinical response within 48 hours, an abscess or lesion is likely and surgical drainage is required.[2]

Prompt diagnosis and treatment usually result in complete resolution of the infection. Prognosis is related to the initiation of therapy—the earlier treatment begins, the better the outcome.

Nursing Assessment

A thorough history, including information about the onset of symptoms and a history of recent infections or puncture wounds, is essential. Assess the affected area for signs of swelling and tenderness.

Nursing Diagnosis

Several nursing diagnoses may apply to the child with osteomyelitis. They include:

- Pain related to disease process or surgical drainage of abscess
- Impaired Physical Mobility related to disease process, destruction of bone, or joint tenderness
- High Risk for Infection related to presence of infecting organism
- High Risk for Altered Nutrition related to disease process

■ GROWTH AND DEVELOPMENT CONSIDERATIONS

Osteomyelitis in a newborn is of great concern, since before 18 months of age the blood vessels still cross the growth plates. This creates a higher risk of epiphyseal involvement with resultant limb length discrepancy.

- High Risk for Noncompliance related to long course of antibiotic therapy
- Knowledge Deficit (Child and Parent) related to disease process

Nursing Management

Nursing management focuses on administering antibiotics, maintaining traction, protecting from further infection, and encouraging a well-balanced diet. Universal precautions should be used.

Administer Medications. Antibiotics are administered as prescribed, usually for 7 to 10 days. Children who require surgical drainage and those with chronic osteomyelitis will require IV antibiotic therapy followed by an extended course of oral antibiotics. In the early stages of the infection, analgesics are prescribed to relieve the associated pain and joint tenderness.

Maintain Traction. Rest with traction is often utilized for immobilization. The affected extremity should be moved cautiously, to avoid any further insult to the joint.

Protect from Further Infection. Strict aseptic technique and universal precautions should be used during all dressing changes. Children and family members should avoid direct contact with any dressings or drainage. Teach good hygiene practices, including handwashing, in order to maintain infection control.

Encourage a Well-Balanced Diet. Educate both the child and the parents about healthy dietary choices that promote the healing process. Providing a high-protein diet and extra vitamin C will contribute to this process. Encourage increased fluid intake to provide adequate hydration and circulation.

Discharge Planning and Patient and Family Home Care Teaching. Emphasize the importance of completing the full course of antibiotic therapy, especially for children who have undergone surgical drainage of an abscess or lesion. Failure to follow the prescribed antibiotic therapy may result in chronic infection.

Skeletal Tuberculosis and Septic Arthritis

Skeletal tuberculosis and septic arthritis are two other infections that, although infrequent, may affect children and adolescents. Table 17–6 summarizes clinical manifestations, diagnostic tests, and medical and nursing management for these infections.

Osteogenesis Imperfecta

Osteogenesis imperfecta, also known as brittle bone disease, is a connective tissue disorder that primarily affects the bones. Children with this condition have fragile bones that are more likely to fracture. Osteogenesis imperfecta occurs in 1 in 20,000 live births and affects boys and girls equally.

Clinical manifestations include multiple and frequent fractures; blue sclerae; thin, soft skin; increased joint flexibility; enlargement of the anterior fontanel; weak muscles; soft, pliable, brittle bones; and short stature.

The underlying disorder is a biochemical defect in the production of collagen. The disease is genetically transmitted with an autosomal dominant inheritance pattern. The disease is classified into four types. In children with

TABLE 17–6 Skeletal Tuberculosis and Septic Arthritis: Clinical Manifestations and Management

Condition	Diagnostic Tests and Medical Management	Nursing Management
Skeletal Tuberculosis		
Rare microbacterial infection that can be very destructive. The spine is the most frequent site of infection. May be associated with other diseases (e.g., Pott disease) *Clinical manifestations:* Pain, limp, severe muscle spasms, muscle atrophy, "doughy" swelling of joints, decreased joint motion, changes in reflexes, low-grade fever	*Diagnostic tests:* Diagnostic studies include tuberculosis skin test, complete blood count, synovial fluid analysis, and radiographs of affected limb or joint. *Medical management:* Antibiotic therapy (using combination of drugs) for 6 to 9 months is the treatment of choice. Disease may become resistant to these drugs, and additional therapy may be necessary.	*Nursing management:* Educate the child and family about the disorder and stress the importance of complying with long-term antibiotic therapy.
Septic Arthritis		
Joint infection most often caused by *Haemophilus influenzae, Staphylococcus,* and *Escherichia coli.* The most common site of infection is the knee, followed by the hip, ankle, and elbow. *Clinical manifestations:* Pain and local inflammation, joint tenderness, loss of spontaneous movement	*Diagnostic tests:* Diagnosis is made based on joint aspiration findings. Radiographic changes may not be evident until later in the disease process. *Medical management:* Prompt treatment is essential. Treatment involves joint aspiration, open drainage, and irrigation, followed by antibiotic therapy. If the full course of antibiotic treatment is not completed, the child risks recurrent infection and further degeneration of the infected joint.	*Nursing management:* Educate the child and family about the disorder and emphasize the importance of proper antibiotic therapy. Practice careful management of the painful joint.

type I disease, fractures tend to occur once ambulation begins but show a marked decrease during puberty. Children with type II disease are stillborn or die within the first year. Type III is the classic form of the disease. Children with type III disease have severe osteoporosis and progressive deformities of the long bones. They are often wheelchair bound by adulthood but have a normal life span. Fractures occur later in life in children with type IV disease.

Diagnosis of osteogenesis imperfecta is often made only with delay in walking or on the basis of a fracture. Radiographic evaluation may detect old as well as new fractures. This may lead to an erroneous diagnosis of battered child syndrome.

Osteogenesis imperfecta has no cure. Medical management consists primarily of fracture care. The goal is to maximize the child's independence and mobility while minimizing the risk of fractures. Treatment includes physical therapy; casting, bracing, or splinting; and surgical stabilization.

Nursing Management

Nursing care is primarily supportive and focuses on educating the parents and child about the disease and its treatment.

To prevent fractures, children must be handled gently. The trunk and extremities should be supported whenever the child is moved. Such tasks as bathing and diapering may cause fractures and should be performed carefully.

Emphasize the importance of maintaining normal patterns of growth and development. Toddlers should be helped to explore and interact safely with their environment. Socialization is essential during the school-age and adolescent years. Encourage exercise, such as swimming, to improve muscle tone and prevent obesity. Independent functioning is promoted by the use of adaptive equipment and motorized wheelchairs.

The Osteogenesis Imperfecta Foundation provides information about the disease and can put families in touch with others who have the disease (see Appendix F). Parents should receive genetic counseling.

Muscular Dystrophies

The muscular dystrophies are a group of inherited diseases characterized by muscle fiber degeneration and muscle wasting. These disorders can begin early or late in life, and onset can be at birth or gradual.

Many kinds of muscular dystrophies affect children and adults (Table 17–7 and Fig. 17–10). The most common form of childhood muscular dystrophy is Duchenne muscular dystrophy (pseudohypertrophic). Pseudohypertrophy refers to enlargement of the muscles as a result of their infiltration with fatty tissue.

Diagnosis and classification are most often based on clinical signs and the pattern of muscle involvement. Children with muscular dystrophy have generalized muscle weakness. They compensate for weak lower extremities by using the upper extremity muscles to raise themselves to a standing position (Gower maneuver) (Fig. 17–11). Biochemical examinations such as serum enzyme assay, muscle biopsy, and electromyography confirm the diagnosis.

There is no effective treatment for childhood muscular dystrophy. Progressive weakness and muscle deformity result in chronic disability. The goal of medical management is to provide support and prevent complications such as infection or spinal deformities. The team approach to managing the child with muscular dystrophy ensures a comprehensive management plan. Team members should include physicians (pediatrician, orthopedic surgeon, neurologist), nurses, physical and occupational therapists, a nutritionist, and a social worker.

Nursing Management

Nursing care focuses on promoting independence and mobility and providing psychosocial support that helps the child and family deal with this progressive, incapacitating disease.

Encourage the child to be as independent as possible for as long as possible. Concentrate on what the child can accomplish and do not ask the child to complete tasks that may prove frustrating. Reading books to the child, lis-

The section on muscular dystrophies was provided by Marcia Wellington, RN, MS.

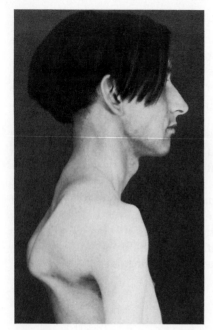

FIGURE 17-10 Scapulohumeral muscular dystrophy is characterized by atrophy of the upper limb muscles and winged scapulae.

From Walton, J. (1981). *Disorders of voluntary muscle* (4th ed.) (p. 449). Essex, England: Longman Group UK Ltd.

TABLE 17-7 Muscular Dystrophies of Childhood

Type of Dystrophy	Clinical Manifestations	Treatment and Prognosis
Duchenne Muscular Dystrophy		
X-linked recessive disorder; however, 30% to 50% of affected children have no family history Onset: within the first 5 years of life	Delayed walking; frequent falls; easily tired when walking, running, or climbing stairs; hypertrophied calves; waddling gait; lordosis; Gower maneuver; mental retardation frequently seen	Supportive care; physical therapy and braces to help maintain mobility and prevent contractures Most children are wheelchair bound by age 10 to 12 years; death usually occurs during adolescence
Becker Muscular Dystrophy		
X-linked recessive disorder Onset: usually after 5 years	Symptoms are similar to those of Duchenne muscular dystrophy, but delayed; child is mobile until late teens; normal intelligence	Supportive care; same as for Duchenne muscular dystrophy Slow progression (same as for Duchenne muscular dystrophy); death usually occurs in adulthood
Fascioscapulohumeral (Landouzy-Dejerine) Muscular Dystrophy		
Autosomal dominant disorder Onset: late childhood and adolescence (as early as 5 years; as late as 50 years; usually between 20 and 30 years)	Face, shoulder girdle, lower limbs affected; unable to raise arms over head; lordosis; cannot close eyes, whistle, smile, or drink from a straw because of inability to move face; characteristic appearance includes facial weakness, winging of the scapula, thin arms, well-developed forearms	Physical therapy Slow progression except infantile form (rapidly progressive severe myopathy); confined to wheelchair as older adult, but usually attains normal life span
Limb-girdle Muscular Dystrophy		
Autosomal recessive disorder Onset: late childhood to adulthood	Weakness of muscles in shoulder and pelvic girdle; waddling gait; lordosis; difficulty climbing stairs	Physical therapy; weight control Mildly progressive; spreads from lower to upper extremities; death usually occurs in middle to late adulthood
Congenital Muscular Dystropies		
Autosomal recessive disorder Onset: present at birth	Muscle weakness present at birth; motor development delay; contractures and joint deformities; hypotonia	Correction of skeletal deformity (orthosis or surgery) Usually nonprogressive; life expectancy is variable

Provided by Marcia Wellington, RN, MS.

tening to tapes, and watching television offer the child stimulation during hospitalization. Exercise as tolerated contributes to muscle strength. Physical therapy helps the child ambulate and prevents joint contractures. It is important to provide good back support and posture by keeping the child's body in alignment when confined to a wheelchair.

Parents may exhibit feelings of guilt and hopelessness. Encourage parents to express their feelings. Genetic counseling is recommended for the entire

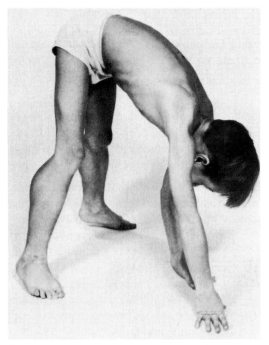

A

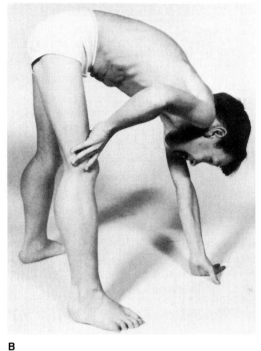

B

FIGURE 17-11 Since the leg muscles of children with muscular dystrophy are weak, these children must perform the Gower maneuver to raise themselves to a standing position. **A,** The child first maneuvers to a position supported by arms and legs. **B,** The child next pushes off the floor and rests one hand on the knee. **C,** The child pushes himself upright.

Courtesy of the Division of Pediatric Neurology, University of Minnesota Medical School. From Swaiman, K.F., & Wright, F.S. (1982). *Practice of pediatric neurology* (2nd ed.). St. Louis: Mosby–Year Book.

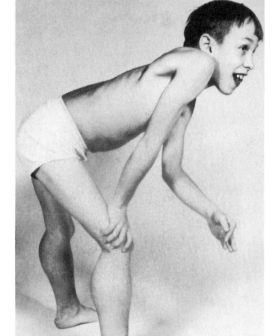

C

family. Siblings may feel neglected because their brother or sister is receiving so much attention. Encourage the parents to involve siblings in the child's care to reassure them of their importance.

Refer family members to resource and support groups such as the Muscular Dystrophy Association (see Appendix F).

Injuries to the Musculoskeletal System

Musculoskeletal injuries are classified according to the mechanism, the location, and the force of the injury. Strains, sprains, dislocations, and fractures are the most common musculoskeletal injuries in children. Distinguishing among these injuries is often difficult. Table 17–8 summarizes management of strains, sprains, and dislocations. A detailed discussion of fractures follows.

Fractures

A fracture is a break in a bone that occurs when more stress is placed on the bone than the bone can withstand. Fractures, which may occur at any age, occur frequently in children because their bones are less dense than those of adults.[7,11] Table 17–9 outlines several types of fractures.

Clinical Manifestations

Signs and symptoms of fractures vary depending on the location, type, and nature of the causative injury. Fractures are generally characterized by pain, abnormal positioning, edema, immobility or decreased range of motion, ecchymosis, guarding, and crepitus. Childhood fractures most often involve the clavicle, tibia, ulna, and femur. Epiphyseal (growth plate) injuries are

---

TABLE 17–8 **Strains, Sprains, and Dislocations**

Strain

- Stretching or tearing of either a muscle or a tendon, usually from overuse (example: back strain resulting from improper or overly heavy lifting).
- Clinical manifestations vary according to the type and severity of the strain. Pain can be acute or chronic.
- Management involves rest and support of the injured part until the muscle or tendon heals and normal activity can occur.

Sprain

- Stretching or tearing of a ligament, usually caused by falls, sports injuries, or motor vehicle crashes.
- Clinical manifestations include edema, joint immobility, and pain.
- Management (generally continued for 24 to 36 hours) includes
  Rest
  Ice
  Compression, and
  Elevation

Dislocation

- Complete displacement of an articular joint surface, usually associated with falls, sports injuries, or motor vehicle crashes. Although almost any joint may be dislocated, most dislocations occur in the shoulder, knee, and hip.
- Clinical manifestations include pain and tenderness, swelling and obvious deformity, and instability of the joint.
- Management varies according to the site and severity of the injury, and consists of:
  Shoulder: Open or closed reduction followed by sling.
  Knee: Closed reduction with gentle traction, then immobilization with a splint.
  Hip (posterior): Immediate closed reduction or possibly open reduction, traction, or hip spica cast.
  Hip (anterior): Immediate closed reduction, extension traction, and hip spica cast.

TABLE 17-9 Classification and Types of Fractures

Classification	Type

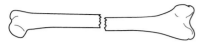

Classification

Complete (transverse) fracture

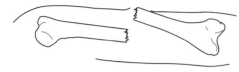

Break across entire section of bone, resulting in two or more fragments

Open fracture

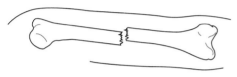

Broken bone protrudes through skin, leaving path to fracture site; high risk of infection exists

Closed fracture

Broken bone does not protrude through skin

Type

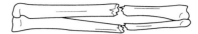

Spiral fracture

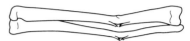

Associated with twisting force; fracture coils around bone

Greenstick fracture

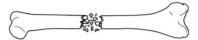

Caused by compression force; often seen in young children

Comminuted fracture

Associated with high impact forces; bone breaks into three or more segments

Additional types of fractures include: *incomplete*, in which the break occurs in only one side of the cortex; *transverse*, in which the bone breaks at a right angle to the bone shaft; *oblique*, in which the fracture slants across the long axis of the bone; *compression*, in which two bones are jammed together (usually occurs in spinal area); and *compacted*, in which one bone fragment is wedged into another.

■ **NURSING ALERT**

Fractures involving the epiphyseal plate disrupt the growth process in children who are still growing. If not treated properly, such injuries often cause limb length discrepancies, joint incongruities, or angular deformities.

also common in children. These injuries are described using the Salter-Harris classification system (Fig. 17–12).

Etiology and Pathophysiology

Fractures in children may result from direct trauma to a bone (falls, sports injuries, abuse, motor vehicle crashes) or bone diseases (osteogenesis imperfecta) that result in weakening of the bone.

Diagnostic Tests and Medical Management

Radiographs are useful for determining the exact location and type of the fracture. Medical management consists of two basic steps: (1) reduction to realign displaced or fragmented bones, and (2) immobilization so that healing can take place.

A closed reduction aligns the bone by manual manipulation or traction. An open reduction requires surgical alignment of the bone, often using pins,

FIGURE 17-12 The Salter-Harris classification system is based on the angle of the fracture in relation to the epiphysis.

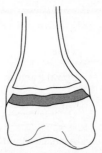

Type I
Common
Growth plate undisturbed
Growth disturbances rare

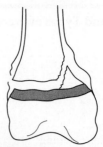

Type II
Most common
Growth disturbances rare

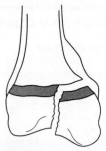

Type III
Less common
Serious threat to growth
and joint

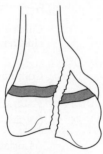

Type IV
Serious threat to growth

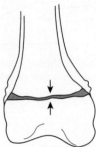

Type V
Rare
Crush injury causes cell death in growth plate,
resulting in arrested growth and limited
bone length
If growth plate is partially destroyed, angular
deformities may result

plates, wires, or screws. Casting is the most common external method of immobilization. Other external methods include traction and splinting.

Healing of fractures is influenced by factors including age, size of the involved bone, and fracture site. Fractures heal in less time in children than in adults. Immobilization is essential for the bone healing process to take place. If a fracture is properly reduced, complications should be minimal (Table 17–10).

Nursing Assessment

When dealing with an injured child, be alert to the signs and symptoms of fractures before moving the child. Try to identify the cause of the injury by asking the child, parents, or other family members what happened. When a child is admitted to the hospital, nursing assessment includes the extent of the injury, the degree of pain, and the child's vital signs (respiratory status, pulse, blood pressure).

Nursing Diagnosis

Several nursing diagnoses may apply to the child with a fracture. They include:

- Pain related to fracture, trauma, or muscle spasm
- High Risk for Impaired Skin Integrity related to trauma, traction, cast, or splint
- High Risk for Infection related to open fracture or trauma

TABLE 17-10 Complications of Fracture Reduction

Complication	Medical Management

Infection
  Acute (may occur with open
    fractures)
  Chronic (osteomyelitis)
	Debridement, drainage, culture, and treatment
	  with antibiotics

Neurovascular injury resulting from physical nerve damage	Nerve repair
Vascular injury	Vascular repair, amputation, tendon lengthen- ing

Malunion (undesired healed align-
  ment of bone) or delayed union
	Corrective osteotomy; prolonged immobiliza-
	  tion

Nonunion	Surgical intervention; internal fixation
Leg length discrepancy	Shoe lift

- Impaired Physical Mobility related to cast, splint, or traction
- Knowledge Deficit with increased anxiety related to unknown course of treatment

Nursing Management

Nursing care focuses on care of the child before and after fracture reduction, encouraging mobility as ordered, maintaining skin integrity, preventing infection, and teaching parents and child care of the fracture. When caring for a child who has undergone fracture reduction, it is important to be aware of the signs of complications. Notify the physician immediately if these signs occur.

Maintain Proper Alignment. Immobilization is used to maintain proper alignment of fractures. Casts and traction are methods used for immobilizing an injured child. Cast care guidelines are included in Table 17–1.

Different types of traction are used, depending on the location and type of fracture (Table 17–11). Nursing care for the child in traction is described in Table 17–12.

Monitor Neurovascular Status. Monitor the child's sensation to touch, strength of the pulse in the extremity distal to the injury, and capillary refill time.

Promote Mobility. The amount of mobility the child is allowed is ordered by the physician and restrictions depend on the extent and site of the fracture. Fractures of the hip or pelvis may involve body casts, and providing wheeled carts makes mobility possible. Children with leg fractures can move around with crutches, walkers, or wheelchairs.

Discharge Planning and Patient and Family Home Care Teaching. Most fractures can be easily managed at home. Activities are generally limited for approximately 8 weeks. Teach parents and child cast care and activity restrictions (see Table 17–2). Help parents to identify any modifications that may be needed at home and school. The child who has to manage steps at home or school may need special training with crutches or a temporary ramp. Refer parents to home health nurses or home teaching services if indicated.

■ **NURSING ALERT**

Compartment syndrome may occur with a crush injury or when a fracture is reduced. Swelling associated with inflammation reduces blood flow to the affected area, and casting causes further constriction of blood flow. Deep pain unrelieved by analgesia is the diagnostic sign. Notify the physician immediately to remove any constricting dressings or casts to prevent progressive neurologic damage.

TABLE 17-11 Types of Traction

Type

Skin Traction

Pull is applied to the skin surface, which puts traction directly on the bones and muscles. Traction is usually attached to the skin with adhesive materials or straps.

Dunlop Traction
(can be either skeletal or skin)

Used for fracture of the humerus. The arm, which is flexed, is suspended horizontally with straps placed on both the upper and lower portions for pull from both sides.

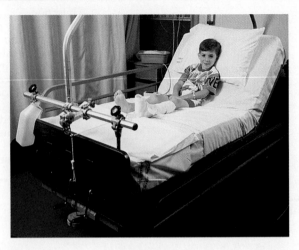

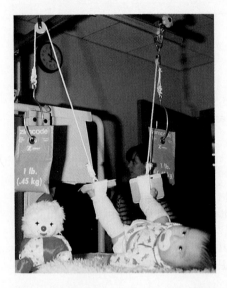

Bryant Traction

Used specifically for the child under 2 years of age and weighing less than 12 to 14 kg, who has developmental dysplasia of the hip or a fractured femur. This bilateral traction is applied to the child's legs and kept in place by wrapping the legs from foot to thigh with elastic bandage. The hips are flexed at a 90-degree angle, with knees extended. This position is maintained by attaching the traction appliance to weights and pulleys, which are suspended above the crib. The buttocks do not rest on the mattress, but are slightly elevated off the bed.

Buck Traction

Used for knee immobilization; to correct contractures or deformities; or for short-term immobilization. It keeps the leg in an extended position, without hip flexion.

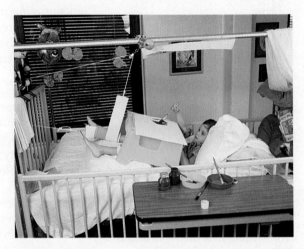

Russell Traction

Used for fractures of the femur and lower leg. Traction is placed on the lower leg while the knee is suspended in a padded sling. The hips and knees, which are slightly flexed, are immobilized.

Information on types of traction was provided by Marcia Wellington, RN, MS.

TABLE 17-11 Types of Traction—Continued

Type

Skeletal Traction

Pull is directly applied to the bone by pins, wires, tongs, or other apparatus that have been surgically placed through the distal end of the bone.

Crutchfield Tongs

Used for cervical spine injuries to reduce fractures and dislocations. Tongs are placed in the skull with burr holes. Weights are attached to the apparatus with a rope and pulley system to the hyperextended head.

Halo Traction

Used to immobilize the head and neck after cervical injury or dislocation. Also used for positioning and immobilization after cervical injury.

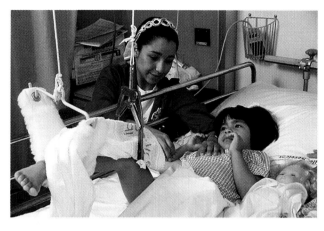

90-90 Traction

Used for fractures of the femur or tibia. A skeletal pin or wire is surgically placed through the distal part of the femur, while the lower part of the extremity is in a boot cast. Traction ropes and pulleys are applied at the pin site and on the boot cast to maintain the flexion of both the hip and knee at 90 degrees.

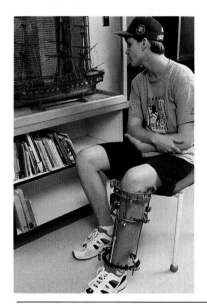

External Fixators

These devices can be used in the treatment of simple fractures, both open and closed; complex fractures with extensive soft tissue involvement; correction of bony or soft tissue deformities; pseudoarthroses; and limb length discrepancy. They are attached to the extremity by percutaneous transfixing of pins or wires to the bone.

TABLE 17-12 Nursing Care of the Child in Traction

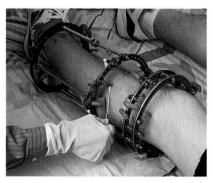

Providing pin care

1. Assess the child in traction by first checking the equipment. Make sure that the equipment is in the proper position. Observe both the body appliance and the attached weights and pulleys. Make certain that the child's body is in proper alignment.
2. Assess the skin under the straps and pin insertion sites for any signs of erythema, edema, or skin breakdown.
3. Assess the extremity by checking neurovascular status frequently (check warmth, color, distal pulses, capillary refill time, movement, sensation).
4. Provide pin care when ordered. Clean the area surrounding the pin with cotton-tipped applicators saturated with normal saline or half-strength hydrogen peroxide. Clean the area again with sterile water or more saline. Apply an antibacterial ointment, if ordered, using another cotton-tipped applicator.
5. Traction equipment should be removed every 4 hours, and the child should be given skin care if orders permit.
6. Place a sheepskin pad under the child's extremity if orders permit.

Amputations

Amputation—the complete absence of a body extremity—can be either congenital or acquired. Approximately two thirds of amputations in children are congenital and one third are acquired. Congenital amputations can be caused by constrictive amniotic bands, drugs, or irradiation. Acquired amputations are generally associated with trauma or a result of a disease or disorder.

The child with an absent limb should be fitted with a prosthesis as soon as feasible. This fosters a positive body image, independence, and self-confidence, and also ensures that motor skills develop as normally as possible. The prosthetic device should be reevaluated as the child progresses physically and developmentally.

Frequent stump reconstructions are often necessary in children with traumatic amputations because as children grow, so do their bones, and the skin tends to adhere to the bone. Bone may need to be cut and soft tissue added to keep the stump rounded. Joint fusions or stump lengthenings may also be needed to allow for effective use of the prosthesis.

Nursing Management

Nursing care focuses on providing emotional support regarding altered body image, maintaining skin integrity, and encouraging maximal independent functioning.

Provide Emotional Support. Recovering from the loss of a limb is one of the most difficult challenges facing a child. Emphasize what the child can do rather than what he or she cannot do. Good listening skills are important.

Maintain Skin Integrity. The child usually begins wearing the prosthetic device for 1- to 2-hour intervals. Check the skin for any redness or breakdown. If redness or breakdown develops, leave the prosthesis off and allow the skin to clear before reapplying. Have the prosthesis adjusted if necessary, and increase wearing time as tolerated by the child.

Maximize Independent Functioning. Children with amputated limbs quickly learn how to accommodate to the prosthetic device. Make use of physical therapy programs that are specifically designed to help the child perform activities of daily living.

Discharge Planning and Patient and Family Home Care Teaching. Answer any questions concerning the prosthesis, activity restrictions, and general prognosis. Instruct parents about care of the prosthetic device and skin checks. Encourage parents to allow the child to participate in peer activities that are physically and emotionally challenging. Sporting activities that enable the child to participate using modified equipment are a good way to build self-confidence and motivation. Several ski resorts offer programs that teach children with physical disabilities how to ski. Assess the need for counseling and offer referrals as appropriate.

REFERENCES

1 Hole, J.W. (1993). *Human anatomy and physiology.* (6th ed.). Dubuque, IA: Brown.
2 Avery, M.E., & First, L.R. (1991). *Pediatric medicine.* Baltimore: Williams & Wilkins.
3 Salmond, S.W., Mooney, N.E., & Verdisco, L.A. (1991). *Core curriculum for orthopaedic nursing* (2nd ed.). Pitman, NJ: Anthony J. Jannetti.
4 Tachdijan, M. (1985). *The child's foot.* Philadelphia: Saunders.
5 Kyzer, S.P. (1992). Congenital idiopathic clubfoot. *Orthopaedic Nursing, 10*(4), 11–18.
6 Behrman, R.E., & Vaughn, V.C. (1987). *Nelson textbook of pediatrics* (13th ed.). Philadelphia: Saunders.
7 Staheli, L.T. (1992). *Fundamentals of pediatric orthopedics.* New York: Raven Press.
8 Turco, V. (1971). Surgical correction of the resistant club foot. *The Journal of Bone and Joint Surgery, 53-A,* 477–497.
9 Shoppee, K. (1992). Developmental dysplasia of the hip. *Orthopaedic Nursing, 11*(5), 30–36.
10 Morrisy, R.T., & Selman, S. (1991). Slipped capital femoral epiphysis. *Orthopaedic Nursing, 10*(1), 11–20.
11 Wenger, D.R., & Rang, M. (1992). *The art and practice of children's orthopaedics.* New York: Raven Press.

SUGGESTED READINGS

Bender, L.H. (1991). Osteogenesis imperfecta. *Orthopaedic Nursing, 10*(4), 23–32.
Drummond, D.S. (1991). A perspective on recent trends for scoliosis correction. *Clinical Orthopaedics and Related Research,* (March) 90–101.
Fox, M.J. (1989). *Standards of care: Osteogenesis imperfecta.* Twin Cities Unit, Shriners Hospital for Crippled Children.
Fox, M.J. (1989). *Standards of care: Osteomyelitis.* Twin Cities Unit, Shriners Hospital for Crippled Children.
Gershwin, M.E., & Robbins, D.L. (1983). *Musculoskeletal diseases of children* (2nd ed.). New York: Grune & Stratton.
Maroteaux, P. (1989). *Bone diseases of children.* Philadelphia: Lippincott.

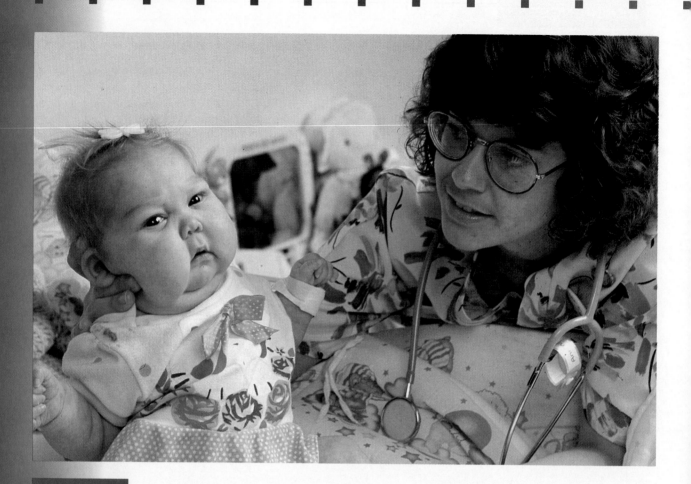

A lexis, 6 months old, was born with a major congenital anomaly of the kidney. She seemed healthy at birth, but during the first few weeks of life she was constantly irritable, ate poorly, and spit up after feeding. At Alexis's 2-week examination, the pediatrician found that she had gained little weight since birth. She continued to show poor weight gain at her 1-month follow-up visit.

Subsequent laboratory evaluation revealed altered serum electrolyte levels, lowered pH, and increased blood urea nitrogen (BUN) level. A 24-hour urine collection showed an increased creatinine level and proteinuria. An abdominal ultrasound was ordered, which revealed congenital absence of one kidney and a second kidney remnant. Alexis was diagnosed with end-stage renal disease (ESRD), the most advanced form of chronic renal failure, resulting from congenital kidney atresia.

Beginning at 1 month of age, Alexis began undergoing hemodialysis at a tertiary care referral center. Because she continued to be a poor feeder, naso-gastric feedings were given at night to supplement her oral intake during the day. Alexis's growth has been poor. Because of the adverse effects of ESRD on growth and development, renal transplantation is planned as soon as a donor kidney becomes available.

ALTERATIONS IN GENITOURINARY FUNCTION

TERMINOLOGY

azotemia   Accumulation of nitrogenous wastes in the blood.

dialysate   The solution used in dialysis.

hydronephrosis   Collection of urine in renal pelvis as a result of obstructed outflow.

oliguria   Diminished urine output (less than 0.5 to 1 mL/kg/hr).

stent   A device used to maintain patency of the urethral canal after surgery.

uremia   Toxicity resulting from the buildup of urea and nitrogenous waste in the blood.

vesicoureteral reflux   The backflow of urine from the bladder into the ureters during voiding.

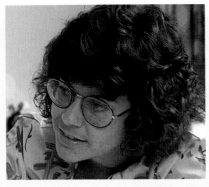

❝ As we wait for a kidney donor, Alexis's condition needs to be monitored closely. Two major goals are to prevent infection and to make sure that Alexis's nutritional needs are being met fully. ❞

What are the consequences of urinary and renal disorders such as chronic renal failure in children? What specific and nonspecific signs alert parents and health care professionals to suspect these disorders? End-stage renal disease is uncommon in infancy, and laboratory and diagnostic evaluation was required to confirm the diagnosis in Alexis's case. With congenital kidney atresia, dialysis is the only treatment option until renal transplantation can be performed.

Many infections, structural disorders, and disease processes alter genitourinary function. Because the kidneys and other urinary system organs perform several essential body functions, including removal of waste products and maintenance of fluid and electrolyte balance, disorders that affect these organs pose a significant threat to the health of children.

Although the reproductive system is functionally immature until puberty, disorders involving these organs may also have a significant impact on the health of children. Structural defects, if uncorrected, and sexually transmitted diseases can have both psychologic and physiologic implications.

■ Anatomy and Physiology of Pediatric Differences

The genitourinary system is made up of the urinary and reproductive organs. The urinary system—kidneys, ureters, bladder, and urethra (Fig. 18–1)—functions to excrete wastes and maintain fluid and electrolyte balance. The reproductive system consists of internal and external organs that at maturity function to promote the conception and healthy development of a fetus.

■ GROWTH AND DEVELOPMENT CONSIDERATIONS

Urinary output per kilogram of body weight decreases as the child ages because the kidney becomes more efficient at concentrating urine. Expected output:

Infants:	2 mL/kg/hr
Children:	0.5–1 mL/kg/hr
Adolescents:	40–80 mL/hr

■ CLINICAL TIP

A child's bladder capacity (in ounces) can be estimated by adding 2 to the child's age. For example, normal bladder capacity of a 4-year-old is 6 ounces.

Urinary System

The kidneys grow gradually during childhood, reaching full size by age 10. Most renal growth occurs during the first 5 years of life. This increase in size is due primarily to enlargement of the nephrons. The efficiency of the kidney also increases with age. Because the kidney is less able to concentrate urine in infancy, urine output per kilogram of body weight is higher at that time than in later childhood or adolescence.

Bladder capacity increases with age from 20 to 50 mL at birth to 700 mL in adulthood. Stimulation of "stretch receptors" within the bladder wall initiates urination. Simultaneous contraction of the bladder and relaxation of the internal and external sphincters result in emptying of the bladder. Children less than 2 years of age cannot maintain bladder control because of insufficient nerve development.

The shortness of the urethra in children results in a greater incidence of urinary tract infection because bacteria ascend the urethra more readily than in adults.

Reproductive System

The reproductive system in children is functionally immature until puberty. Throughout childhood the genitalia (with the exception of the clitoris in girls) enlarge gradually. Anatomic and functional development accelerates with the hormonal changes of puberty (see Figs. 3–37 and 3–38). In girls the mons pubis becomes more prominent and hair begins to grow. The vagina lengthens, and the epithelial layers thicken. The uterus and ovaries enlarge,

The editors wish to thank Lynda Frassetto, M.D., for her valuable contributions to this chapter.

FIGURE 18-1 The kidneys are located between the twelfth thoracic (T-12)and third lumbar (L-3) vertebrae.

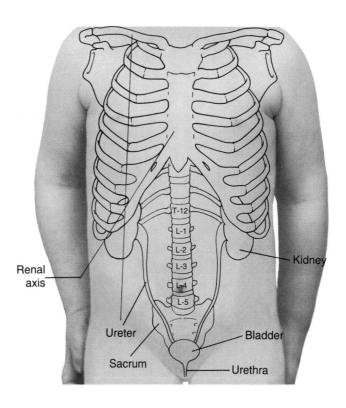

and the musculature and vascularization of the uterus also increase. In boys downy hair begins to appear at the base of the penis and the scrotum becomes increasingly pendulous. The penis increases in length and width.

Structural Defects

Bladder Exstrophy

Bladder exstrophy is a rare defect in which the posterior bladder wall extrudes through the lower abdominal wall (Fig. 18–2). Failure of the abdominal wall to close during fetal development results in eversion and protuberance of the bladder wall and a wide separation of the symphysis pubis.[1] The defect occurs in approximately 1 in every 30,000 live births and is more common in boys than girls.[2] The bladder mucosa appears as a mass of bright red tissue, and urine continually leaks from an open urethra. Females have a bifid clitoris. Males have a short, stubby penis, and the glans is flattened with dorsal chordee and a ventral prepuce. Epispadias and bilateral inguinal hernias are also common.

Because the penis is usually paired and very small, the possibility of changing the boy's gender to female is often discussed with the parents.[2]

Treatment is surgical reconstruction, which is performed in several stages. The initial stage (bladder closure) is usually completed within 48 hours after birth but may be deferred up to 6 months after birth. Epispadias repair is usually begun when the infant is 9 months of age. Reconstruction of the bladder neck is performed when the child is 2 to 3 years of age. The goals of surgical reconstruction are (1) bladder and abdominal wall closure; (2) urinary continence, with preservation of renal function; and (3) creation of functional and normal-appearing genitalia. Some children require permanent urinary diversion because urinary continence is not always achieved.

Because the bladder epithelium is abnormal, it is prone to neoplasms. Yearly cystoscopy after the age of 20 years is recommended to evaluate for possible malignancies.[3]

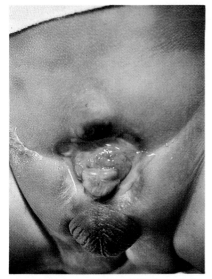

FIGURE 18-2 This child has bladder extrophy, noted by extrusion of the posterior bladder wall through the lower abdominal wall.

Nursing Management

Preoperative nursing care centers on preventing infection and trauma to the exposed bladder. The bladder mucosa is covered in plastic wrap to prevent trauma, and the surrounding area is cleaned daily and protected from leaking urine with a skin sealant.

Postoperatively the wound and pelvis are immobilized to facilitate healing. External immobilization is achieved by use of modified Bryant traction (see Chapter 17). Nursing care includes maintaining proper alignment, monitoring peripheral circulation, and providing meticulous skin care. Abduction of the infant's legs should be avoided.

Renal function is monitored by assessment of the adequacy of urine output and blood and urine chemistries. Observe for any indications of obstruction in the drainage tubes such as increased intensity of bladder spasms, decreased urine output, or urine or blood draining from the urethral meatus.

Parents require emotional support to help them cope with the disfiguring nature of the infant's defect and the uncertainty of complete repair. To promote parent-infant bonding, encourage parents to participate in all aspects of the infant's care, including bathing, feeding, and wound care. Discharge teaching should include instructions about dressing changes and diapering and the need for immediate reporting of any signs of infection or change in renal function. Emphasize the need for routine follow-up visits after surgery to assess urinary function and to ensure that the next stages of surgery are performed at the appropriate time and age in the child's development.

Hypospadias and Epispadias

Hypospadias and epispadias are congenital anomalies involving the location of the urethral meatus in males (Fig. 18–3). Both defects result from failure of the urethral folds to fuse completely over the urethral groove.

In hypospadias, which occurs in 8 of 1000 live male births, the urethral meatus can be located anywhere along the course of the anterior urethra on the ventral surface of the penile shaft, from the perineum to the tip of the glans. The defect may range from mild (with the meatus slightly off center

FIGURE 18–3 **A,** In hypospadias the urethral canal is open on the under surface of the penis. **B,** In epispadias the canal is open on the upper surface.

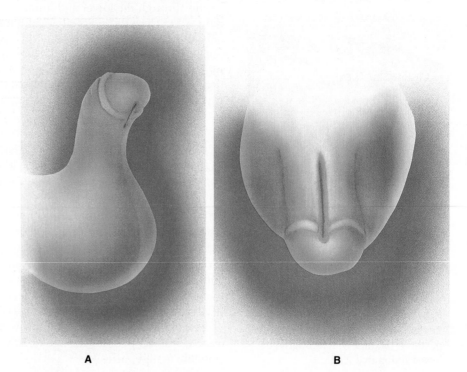

A

B

TABLE 18–1 Parent Teaching: Hypospadias and Epispadias Repair

- Use the double-diapering technique to protect the stent (the small tube that drains the urine).
- Restrict the child from activities (e.g., playing on riding toys) that put pressure on the surgical site.
- Encourage the child to drink fluids to ensure adequate hydration. Provide fluids in a pleasant environment, for example, by giving a tea party or using a special cup. Offer fruit juice, fruit-flavored ice pops, fruit-flavored juices, flavored ice cubes, and gelatin.
- Be sure to give the complete course of prescribed antibiotics to avoid infection.
- Watch for signs of infection: fever, swelling, redness, pain, strong-smelling urine, or change in flow of the urinary stream.

from the tip of the penis) to severe (with the meatus on the scrotum). Hypospadias often occurs in conjunction with congenital chordee, a fibrous line of tissue that results in ventral curvature of the penile shaft.

In epispadias the meatal opening is located on the dorsal surface of the penile shaft. Epispadias often occurs in conjunction with exstrophy of the bladder.

Diagnosis is made at birth. The infant should not be circumcised because the dorsal foreskin tissue will be used for surgical repair. The defects are corrected surgically, usually during the first year of life, to minimize psychologic effects when the child is older. Surgery may be performed in a single operation or as a multistage procedure. The goals of surgical repair are (1) restoration of normal urination (enabling the child to void in a standing position); (2) release of chordee; (3) assurance of a sexually adequate penis; and (4) placement of the urethral meatus at the end of the glans penis.

Analgesics and muscle relaxants may be prescribed to relieve any postoperative pain.

Nursing Management

Addressing parents' concerns is a key part of nursing care. Preoperative teaching can relieve some of the anxiety about the future appearance and functioning of the penis.

Postoperative care focuses on protecting the surgical site from injury. The infant or child returns from surgery with the penis wrapped in a pressure dressing and a urethral **stent** (device used to maintain patency of urethral canal) in place to keep the new urethral canal open. Use of arm and leg restraints prevents inadvertent removal of the stent. A bed cradle may be used to keep bed linens from touching the operative site.

Encourage fluid intake to maintain adequate urinary output and patency of stents. Accurate documentation of intake and output is essential. Observe for signs of decreasing urinary output or pain, which may be an indication of kinks in the system or partial obstruction by sediment and must be corrected. Administer prescribed pain medications, and notify the physician.

Discharge teaching should include instructions for parents about care of the reconstructed area, fluid intake, medication administration, and signs and symptoms of infection (Table 18–1). Caution parents to avoid holding the infant or child straddled on the hip.

Cryptorchidism

Cryptorchidism (undescended testes) occurs when one or both testes fail to descend through the inguinal canal into the scrotum. Normally the testes de-

■ CLINICAL TIP

After surgery for hypospadias or epispadias repair, it is important to protect the surgical site from injury. A double diaper can be created by cutting a hole in one diaper to fit over the pressure dressing. This inner diaper is secured by using a second (outer) diaper, applied in the usual way.

scend during the seventh to ninth month of gestation. Cryptorchidism may be the result of a hormonal deficiency, an intrinsic abnormality of a testis, or a structural problem such as a narrow inguinal canal, short spermatic cord, or adhesions. The disorder occurs in 3% to 4% of term male infants and in approximately 30% of premature infants.[1] Because proper function of the testes depends on a temperature cooler than 98.6° F (37° C), failure to descend by early childhood can result in serious complications.

Cryptorchidism is usually detected during the newborn examination when palpation of the scrotum fails to reveal one or both testes (see Fig. 3–39). It is not unusual for boys with cryptorchidism to have an inguinal hernia as well. In 75% of cases the testes descend spontaneously by 9 to 12 months of age. If descent does not occur within the first year, human chorionic gonadotropin may be prescribed to induce testicular descent. An orchiopexy is performed, preferably by 3 years of age, if hormone therapy is ineffective. In this procedure the testis is positioned in the scrotal sac by use of a traction device such as a button on the scrotal surface or an elastic band attached to the thigh. Surgery must be performed early in life, since the warm temperature in the abdomen will lead to sterility in the male if the testis is allowed to remain in the abdomen. If the testis has atrophied, it may be surgically removed to decrease the risk of later malignancies and a prosthesis may be placed in the scrotum.[4]

Nursing Management

Preoperative nursing care includes preparing the parents and child for the procedure and addressing parents' concerns about the postsurgical outcome. Orchiopexy is often performed as an outpatient procedure. If the child is hospitalized, postoperative nursing care focuses on maintaining comfort and preventing infection. Encourage bed rest, and monitor voiding. Apply ice to the surgical area, and administer prescribed analgesics to relieve pain. A bed cradle can be used to keep bed linens off the surgical site.

Discharge instructions should include demonstration of proper wound cleansing and dressing changes. Teach parents to identify signs of infection such as redness, warmth, swelling, and discharge. The child's activity should be restricted for 3 to 7 days following surgery to promote healing and prevent injury.

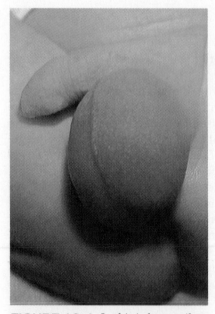

FIGURE 18–4 In this infant, unilateral hydrocele was noted at birth. Transillumination was done to confirm the diagnosis.

From Zitelli, B.J., & Davis, H.W. (Eds.) (1987). *Atlas of pediatric physical diagnosis* (p. 2.10). New York: Mosby–Year Book Europe Ltd.

Hydrocele

A hydrocele (Fig. 18–4) is a fluid-filled mass that occurs when the processus vaginalis fails to close at birth, allowing peritoneal fluid to enter the scrotum. It is often associated with an inguinal hernia.

Diagnosis is made by physical examination. On palpation of the scrotum, a round, smooth, nontender mass is noted.

Most hydroceles close by the time an infant is 1 year of age and the fluid reabsorbs. If surgical repair is needed, it is usually performed on an outpatient basis, lessening the stress for both the child and the family. The prognosis is generally excellent.

If a hydrocele is large, bowel may slip into the inguinal canal, forming an inguinal hernia. Prompt surgical repair is necessary to avoid incarceration, which is a medical emergency.

Nursing care for hydrocele and inguinal hernia include explaining the disorder and its treatment and providing preoperative and postoperative teaching and care. Inform parents that the scrotum may be edematous and may appear bruised after surgery. Care of the incision involves application of a protective sealant; no dressing is applied.

Obstructive Uropathy

Obstructive uropathy refers to structural or functional abnormalities of the urinary system that interfere with urine flow. Obstruction results in urinary stasis, which promotes the growth of bacteria. The pressure caused by urine backup compromises circulation within the kidney and can result in areas of ischemia and atrophy within the renal parenchyma.

Obstruction may be congenital or acquired, unilateral or bilateral, complete or partial. It may occur at any point in the upper or lower urinary tract. Boys are affected more often than girls. Clinical manifestations vary, depending on the cause and location of the obstruction. Characteristic findings include difficulty urinating, abdominal pain, bacteriuria, failure to thrive, poor urinary outflow (dribble or drip versus stream), and hematuria.

Obstructive uropathy may be caused by a wide variety of lesions and congenital defects, including ureteropelvic junction obstruction, posterior urethral valves (PUVs), **hydronephrosis** (accumulation of urine in renal pelvis as a result of obstructed outflow), myelomeningocele, neoplasms, and prune-belly syndrome. The ureteropelvic junction is the most common site of obstruction of the upper urinary tract in infants and children. PUVs (abnormal folds of mucosa at the male urethral opening) are the most common cause of anatomic bladder outlet obstruction. PUVs occur in approximately 1 in 5000 to 8000 live male births. In this defect the valves themselves obstruct the urethral conduit, interfering with voiding. Infants with PUVs have vomiting, diarrhea, sepsis, flank or abdominal pain, and failure to thrive.

Early diagnosis and surgical correction of or urinary diversion around the obstruction are necessary to prevent kidney damage and deterioration of renal function. Diagnostic evaluation may include ultrasound, radionuclide scan, voiding cystourethrogram, and measurement of serum creatinine. The goals of surgical correction or diversion are to lower the pressure within the collecting system, which prevents parenchymal damage, and to prevent stasis, which decreases the risk of infection. Surgical correction may necessitate pyeloplasty (removal of an obstructed segment of the ureter and reimplantation into the renal pelvis) or valve repair or reconstruction, depending on the cause of the obstruction. Urinary incontinence resulting from sphincter weakness is a common problem after surgery.

PRUNE-BELLY SYNDROME

Prune-belly syndrome, also known as Eagle-Barrett syndrome, is a congenital defect characterized by failure of the abdominal musculature to develop. The skin covering the abdominal wall is thin and resembles a wrinkled prune. Other characteristics include urinary tract anomalies, enlarged bladder, and bilateral cryptorchidism. Prune-belly syndrome occurs predominantly in males, with an incidence of 1 in 35,000 to 1 in 50,000 births.

Nursing Management

Preoperative nursing care focuses on preparing the parents and child for the procedure and addressing parents' concerns about the postsurgical outcome. Provide parents with an opportunity to discuss concerns about the effect of the disorder on the child's long-term renal functioning.

Postoperative care involves monitoring vital signs and intake and output and observing for signs of urine retention, such as decreased output and bladder distention. Many children are discharged with stents or catheters. Teach parents how to change dressings, care for catheters, and recognize signs of possible obstruction or infection. Parents should encourage the child to participate in age-appropriate activities. However, contact sports should be avoided because of their potential to injure the bladder.

Urinary Tract Infection

A urinary tract infection (UTI) is an infection of bacterial, viral, or fungal origin that occurs in the urinary tract. A lower UTI involves the urethra or bladder; an upper UTI involves the ureters, renal pelvis, and renal parenchyma. UTIs can be acute or chronic (recurrent or persistent).

■ **NURSING ALERT**

Rule out a urinary tract infection in any child under 2 years of age with a fever of unknown origin.

■ **NURSING ALERT**

The American Academy of Pediatrics currently recommends that a radiologic evaluation be performed on all children who have had one documented urinary tract infection.

UTIs are the second most common infections in children. What accounts for the high incidence of these infections? Among newborns most infections occur in boys.[1] These infections are usually associated with structural defects that predispose the infant to infection (e.g., obstructive uropathy). Among older infants and children the incidence of UTIs is higher in girls. This is attributed to the shorter female urethra (2 cm in young girls) and its proximity to the anus and vagina, which increases the risk of contamination by fecal bacteria. The incidence of UTI is also increased in teenage girls who are sexually active.[5]

Clinical Manifestations

Symptoms depend not only on the location of the infection, but also on the age of the child (Table 18–2). Symptoms in the newborn period tend to be nonspecific. Not until the toddler years are the more "classic" symptoms of lower urinary tract infection—urinary frequency, dysuria, urgency, and enuresis—observed. Upper urinary tract infections are characterized by fever, abdominal pain, and flank pain.

Etiology and Pathophysiology

Most UTIs are caused by *Escherichia coli*, a common gram-negative enteric bacterium. Other causative organisms include *Staphylococcus, Klebsiella, Proteus,* and *Pseudomonas. Proteus* and *Pseudomonas* are more likely to be associated with nosocomial infections.[1]

Urinary stasis enhances the risk of UTI. Stasis may be caused by abnormal anatomic structures or abnormal function. Another cause of UTI is **vesicoureteral reflux,** the backflow of urine from the bladder into the ureters during voiding. This creates a reservoir for bacterial growth. Vesicoureteral reflux can be the result of abnormal insertion of the ureters into the bladder, or it may be transient. Transient vesicoureteral reflux occurs during and immediately after an acute UTI as a result of mucosal edema of the bladder and impaired peristaltic action of the ureters.

Infrequent voiding, which is common in school-age girls, also increases the risk of UTI. Children normally void four to six times a day. Some children, however, develop the habit of urinating only once or twice a day, which results in incomplete emptying of the bladder and urinary stasis.

Diagnostic Tests and Medical Management

A urine culture is examined to confirm the presence of bacteria. Radiologic studies reveal structural abnormalities in approximately 1% to 2% of girls and 10% of boys with UTIs.[6] The intravenous pyelogram (IVP) and voiding cystourethrogram (VCUG) are the most commonly administered tests. An IVP involves the intravenous injection of radiographic contrast media to visualize the kidneys, renal pelvis, ureters, and bladder. The VCUG is used to assess the structure and function of the bladder and to visualize vesicoureteral reflux.

Antibiotic therapy is initiated as soon as urine samples have been collected. Sulfisoxazole or ampicillin is commonly prescribed for uncomplicated infection. For children with recurrent infections, intermittent or long-term, low-dose antibiotic prophylaxis may be used. Follow-up cultures should be obtained 48 hours after drug therapy has started, then 1 to 3 weeks after antibiotics are discontinued, and every 1 to 3 months thereafter until the child has been free of infection for 1 year.[7] Subsequent infections may be asymptomatic.

Children with uncomplicated UTIs usually have a complete recovery. With recurrent UTIs the prognosis depends on the underlying cause. If a structural defect is identified, surgical correction may be necessary to prevent recurrent infections that could lead to renal damage.

Nursing Assessment

Physiologic Assessment. A history of urinary symptoms is obtained, and the abdomen is palpated for masses, tenderness, and distention. Observe the urinary stream if possible and perform a urinalysis, including specific gravity. Proper collection of the urine specimen is essential. A clean-catch urine specimen may be obtained if the child is able to cooperate. (See the Atlas of Pediatric Procedures.) If not, a catheterized sample is obtained. An early morning urine specimen is preferred because the urine is more concentrated.

Psychosocial Assessment. Sexually active adolescents may deny having symptoms because they fear disclosure of their sexual activity to their parents. Careful questioning may be necessary to elicit these concerns. The nurse must be open and approachable and allow the patient and family the opportunity to address their concerns.

Nursing Diagnosis

Common nursing diagnoses for the child with a UTI include:

- Altered Urinary Elimination related to dysuria and recurrent infections
- Pain related to infection
- High Risk for Ineffective Management of Therapeutic Regimen related to lack of knowledge of preventive measures (adequate fluid intake, proper hygiene, signs and symptoms of recurrence)
- High Risk for Fluid Volume Deficit related to fever and inadequate intake
- Knowledge Deficit (Parent) related to lack of information about diagnostic procedures and management

Nursing Management

Children with UTIs are usually cared for at home unless the infection has been caused by another condition that necessitates hospitalization. Nursing care for the hospitalized child centers on administering prescribed medications, encouraging fluid intake (offer frequent small quantities of liquids, flavored ices, and juices) and frequent voiding, and teaching parents and older children how to minimize the risk of future infection (see Table 18–3).

TABLE 18–3 Discharge Teaching: Preventive Strategies for Urinary Tract Infections

- Teach proper perineal hygiene. Girls should always wipe the perineum from front to back after voiding.
- Encourage the child to drink plenty of fluids and avoid long periods of "holding urine."
- Caution against tight underwear; children should wear cotton rather than nylon underwear.
- Discourage bubble baths, which can irritate the urethra.
- Instruct sexually active adolescent girls to void after sexual intercourse to prevent urinary stasis and flush out bacteria introduced during intercourse.

Administer antibiotics and antipyretics as prescribed to maintain therapeutic drug levels and reduce fever. Encourage fluid intake to dilute the urine and flush the bladder.

Frequent voiding minimizes urinary stasis. Postvoid catheterization may be needed to determine the amount of residual urine left after urinating. Palpate or percuss the bladder after voiding to evaluate bladder emptying.

Because bladder training is such an important milestone for young children, any disorder that affects voiding may have developmental implications. A toddler who has been potty trained may regress following a UTI and require diapers temporarily. Reassure parents that this is normal and that they should offer the toddler support rather than disapproval. A preschooler may perceive the infection as punishment of an imagined wrong such as masturbation. Provide support and reassurance that the child is not being punished for any actions.

Discharge Planning and Patient and Family Home Care Teaching. Discharge teaching focuses on instructing parents, older children, and adolescents in preventive strategies (Table 18–3). The most common cause of recurrent infection is noncompliance with the medication regimen. Emphasize to parents and adolescents that antibiotics must be taken for the full course.[9] Teach parents to recognize the signs and symptoms of recurrent infection (see Table 18–2).

■ Enuresis

Enuresis refers to involuntary micturition by a child who has reached an age at which bladder control is expected. This is usually considered to be between 4 and 5 years of age. Three types of enuresis are distinguished: primary, intermittent, and secondary (Table 18–4). Nocturnal enuresis (nighttime bedwetting) occurs two to three times more often in boys, whereas diurnal enuresis (daytime bedwetting) is more common in girls.

Enuresis may result from neurologic or congenital structural disorders, illness, or stress. Nocturnal enuresis occurs with high frequency in children whose parents or siblings have a history of bedwetting.[10] In most children with primary enuresis the bladder has a smaller functional capacity and neuromuscular maturation of the inhibitory fibers is delayed. Minor abnormalities of the bladder neck and urethra are also associated with enuresis. Some children sleep more deeply than others and may fail to respond to bladder signals.

Enuresis is the initial symptom in 15% of children with UTIs.[11] Diabetes mellitus or renal insufficiency should be ruled out in children with both enuresis and polyuria or oliguria. Prolonged hospitalization, family stressors, and preoccupation with school concerns also have been associated with enuresis.

Laboratory evaluation includes urinalysis and urine culture. A multitreatment approach is usually most effective. Fluid restriction, bladder training, and enuresis alarms are common approaches (Table 18–5). Approximately one third of children with nocturnal enuresis are treated with medications, primarily oxybutynin (Ditropan), an anticholinergic. Imipramine (Tofranil), an antidepressant, is often used but requires close monitoring because of its effects on myocardial function.

TABLE 18-4 Types of Enuresis

Primary enuresis: Child has never had a dry night; attributed to maturational delay and small functional bladder.

Intermittent enuresis: Child has occasional nights or periods of dryness.

Secondary enuresis: Bedwetting that occurs in a child who has been reliably dry for 1 year; associated with infections, pinworm infestations, stress, and sleep disorders.

Nursing Management

Enuresis is managed as an outpatient problem. A thorough history can help identify potential causes of bedwetting (Table 18–6). Asking about the child's

TABLE 18-5 Treatment Approaches for Enuresis

Approach	Description
Fluid restriction	Fluid intake is limited in the evening and before the child goes to bed.
Bladder stretching exercises	Child drinks a large amount and then holds urine as long as he or she can. Exercises should continue for at least 6 months.
Bladder training	Parents are instructed to take the child to the toilet and ensure voiding every half hour on day 1; this interval is increased by a half hour each day until an interval of 3 to 4 hours is achieved. The child should be taken to the toilet before bed, and then again before the parents go to bed.
Enuresis alarms	Two types of alarms are available: (1) a urine-sensitive pad that is inserted between bottom sheet and mattress, and (2) a detector strip that is attached to the child's pants. The alarm sounds a buzzer that alerts the child when wetting occurs.
Reward system	Set realistic goals for the child and reinforce dry days or nights with stars and stickers on a chart.

TABLE 18-6 Questions to Ask When Taking an Enuresis History

Family History
- Is there a family history of bedwetting?
- What happens when the child wets? How is the child treated? (Who gets up and changes sheets?)

Toilet Training
- Did the child have a difficult time with toilet training?
- What method of toilet training was used?

Stressors
- How is the child doing in school?
- Are any stressors present in the child's life?

Risk Factors
Diabetes
- Does the child void often or have urgency?
- Is the child frequently thirsty?
- How long is the child's longest dry period, and when does it occur?

Urinary Tract Infection
- Does the child experience burning on urination?
- Has the child had a urinary tract infection before?

Other
- Does the child have a history of constipation?
- Does the child have encopresis?

■ CLINICAL TIP

Enuretic children often have a history of constipation. Rectal pressure on the posterior bladder wall stimulates the bladder to empty.

elimination patterns and developmental milestones and the parents' methods of toilet training can provide essential information (see Table 2–18).

Teach the child and parents about the causes and treatment of enuresis, and address feelings of guilt or blame. Assess parents' knowledge of developmental milestones in bladder training, and provide necessary information

TABLE 18-7 Milestones in the Development of Bladder Control

Age	Developmental Milestone
1 ½ years	Child passes urine at regular intervals.
2 years	Child announces when he or she is voiding.
2 ½ years	Child makes known need to void; can hold urine.
3 years	Child goes to the bathroom by himself or herself; holds urge if preoccupied with play.
2 ½ to 3 ½ years	Child achieves nighttime control.
4 years	Child shows great interest in going to bathrooms when away from home (shopping centers, movies).
5 years	Child voids approximately 7 times a day; prefers privacy; is able to initiate emptying of bladder at any degree of fullness.

(Table 18–7). Psychosocial support is an essential part of care. Provide emotional support to the parents and child, and encourage the child's participation in the treatment plan. Refer the child for counseling or therapy if appropriate.

Renal Disorders

Nephrotic Syndrome

Nephrotic syndrome refers not to a specific disease, but rather to a clinical state characterized by edema, massive proteinuria, hypoalbuminemia, hyperlipidemia, and altered immunity (Table 18–8). Nephrotic syndrome is classified as congenital, primary, or secondary. Congenital nephrotic syndrome, an autosomal recessive disorder, is extremely rare. Primary nephrotic syndrome results from a disease, such as glomerulonephritis, that affects only the kidney. Secondary nephrotic syndrome results from a disease, such as diabetes, with multisystem effects.

Approximately 80% of children with nephrotic syndrome have a type of primary disease called minimal change nephrotic syndrome (MCNS). MCNS

TABLE 18-8 Summary of Common Renal Disorders

	Minimal Change Nephrotic Syndrome	Acute Renal Failure	Chronic Renal Failure	Hemolytic-Uremic Syndrome	Acute Poststreptococcal Glomerulonephritis
Severity and prognosis	Generally good prognosis	Variable	Serious	Serious; variable recovery	Generally good prognosis
Age	2 to 7 years Males > females	Variable	Congenital	6 months to 3 years	6 to 7 years Male/female ratio 2:1
Onset	Over weeks	Days to weeks	Months to years	Days to weeks	Days to weeks
Clinical manifestations	Edema, abdominal pain, nausea and vomiting, fatigue, respiratory distress	Nausea and vomiting, lethargy, edema	No symptoms until disease far advanced, then uremic syndrome	Pallid coloring, easy bruising, petechiae, decreased urine output	Tea-colored urine, periorbital edema, anorexia, lethargy
Etiology	Unknown	Multifactorial	Multifactorial	Drugs, viral or bacterial origin, immunologic reactions	Immunologic reaction to group A beta-hemolytic streptococci

usually occurs in children between the ages of 2 and 7 years and is approximately twice as common in boys as in girls.[12] MCNS derives its name from the fact that the glomeruli appear normal or show only minimal changes on light microscopic evaluation. Because MCNS is the most common form of nephrotic syndrome, it is the focus of the following discussion.

Clinical Manifestations

In most children, edema develops gradually over several weeks. Children may have a history of periorbital edema on waking that resolves during the day and nonspecific malaise.[7] Medical treatment often is not sought until generalized edema develops on the child's extremities, abdomen, or genitals (Fig. 18–5).

Massive edema resulting in a dramatic weight gain and abdominal pain, with or without vomiting, may occur, depending on the amount of albumin lost and the amount of sodium ingested. Edema of the interstitial mucosa may cause diarrhea or anorexia. Children with marked edema appear pale and fatigued, and respiratory distress may occur in severe cases.

Etiology and Pathophysiology

What accounts for the dramatic symptoms of altered renal functioning in children with nephrotic syndrome? Why do proteinuria, hypoalbuminemia, hyperlipidemia, and altered immunity develop in these children?

The cause of MCNS is unknown, and its pathophysiology is not completely understood. Normally only a minute amount of protein is present in the urine. In MCNS, however, increased permeability of the glomerular membrane permits large, negatively charged molecules such as albumin to pass through the membrane and be excreted in the urine. Proteinuria results in decreased oncotic pressure and the development of edema, since fluid remains in the interstitial spaces instead of being pulled back into the vascular compartment. These changes cause hypoalbuminemia.

Because the kidney reabsorbs salt and water, edema develops. Immunoglobulins are lost, resulting in altered immunity. The liver, stimulated by hypoalbuminemia or decreased osmotic pressure, responds by increasing synthesis of lipoprotein (cholesterol), resulting in hyperlipidemia.

Diagnostic Tests and Medical Management

Diagnosis is based on the history, physical examination, presence of characteristic symptoms, and laboratory findings. Serum albumin and other blood studies may be ordered. In children, edema begins to develop when the serum albumin concentration falls below 27 g/L.[12] Urinalysis reveals massive proteinuria (50 mg/kg/day), the primary indicator of nephrotic syndrome. Microscopic hematuria may also be present.

Medical management focuses on decreasing proteinuria, relieving edema, managing associated symptoms, and preventing infection. Corticosteroids (such as prednisone), the drugs of choice, are prescribed to decrease proteinuria. In most children, urine protein levels fall to trace or negative values within 10 to 15 days of the start of corticosteroid therapy. Children who respond successfully to therapy continue to take corticosteroids daily until protein has been absent from the urine for 3 days. The drug dosage is then gradually decreased and discontinued over a 4-week period.[12]

Approximately 80% of children experience complete remission with corticosteroid therapy. Repeat therapy is administered to children who have a re-

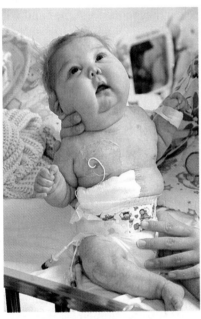

FIGURE 18–5 This infant has generalized edema, a characteristic finding in nephrotic syndrome.

lapse after drug therapy is discontinued. Alkylating agents such as chlorambucil and cyclophosphamide have been effective in children with frequently recurring nephrotic syndrome, but they have serious side effects, including carcinogenesis. If steroid therapy is ineffective, a renal biopsy is performed to identify other causes for the child's symptoms.

To reduce massive edema, intravenous administration of albumin or oral diuretics may be ordered. Since diuretics can precipitate hypovolemia, hyponatremia, and hypokalemia, electrolyte levels should be carefully monitored. Broad-spectrum antibiotics are prescribed to treat any infections.

A diet that is normal for the child's age is recommended. No attempt should be made either to restrict or to increase protein intake. A "no added salt" diet is recommended.

Nursing Assessment

Physiologic Assessment. Careful assessment of the child's hydration status and edema is essential. Monitor intake and output and vital signs and record accurately. Perform a careful respiratory assessment to check for pleural effusion (see Chapter 10). Test urine for proteinuria and specific gravity at least once each shift.

Psychosocial Assessment. Children and parents are often fearful or anxious on admission. Because edema often develops gradually, parents may feel guilty if they did not seek medical attention immediately. School-age children with generalized edema are often concerned about their appearance. Careful questioning may be necessary to elicit these concerns. The child who is hospitalized for a recurrence of nephrotic syndrome may be frustrated or depressed. Assess individual and family coping mechanisms, support systems, and level of stress.

Nursing Diagnosis

Common nursing diagnoses for the child with MCNS include:

- High Risk for Infection related to increased susceptibility and lowered resistance secondary to corticosteroid therapy
- High Risk for Impaired Skin Integrity related to edema, lowered resistance to infection and injury, immobility, and malnutrition
- Fluid Volume Excess related to sodium and water retention
- Altered Nutrition: Less Than Body Requirements related to anorexia and protein loss in urine
- Fatigue related to fluid and electrolyte imbalance, albumin loss, and altered nutrition
- High Risk for Altered Family Processes related to child's hospitalization
- Knowledge Deficit (Parent) related to treatment regimen

Nursing Management

Nursing care is mainly supportive and focuses on administering medications, preventing infection, preventing skin breakdown, meeting nutritional and fluid needs, promoting rest, and providing emotional support to the parents and child.

Administer Medications. It is important to give prescribed medications at the scheduled times. Watch for side effects of corticosteroids such as moon face, increased appetite, increased hair growth, abdominal distention, and mood swings. If the child is receiving albumin intravenously, monitor closely for hypertension or signs of volume overload caused by fluid shifts.

Prevent Infection. Children with MCNS are at risk for infection because of the loss of immunoglobulins in the urine and other alterations of the immune system associated with renal failure. Careful handwashing is important. Strict aseptic technique during invasive procedures should be used. Monitor vital signs carefully to detect early signs of infection that may be masked by corticosteroid therapy. Caution parents and children to avoid exposure to individuals with respiratory infections and communicable diseases.

Prevent Skin Breakdown. Meticulous skin care is essential to prevent skin breakdown and potential infection. Perform repeated skin assessments, turn the child frequently, and use therapeutic mattresses (e.g., egg crate, airflow) to help prevent skin breakdown. Keep the skin clean and dry.

Meet Nutrition and Fluid Needs. Keep the child's food preferences in mind when planning menus. Encourage the child to eat by presenting attractive meals with small portions. Mealtimes should center on pleasurable socialization. Encourage the child to eat meals with other children on the unit.

Carefully monitor intake and output. Weigh the child daily using the same scale, and measure abdominal girth to monitor changes in edema and ascites (see Fig. 7–12). Vital signs should be monitored every 4 hours to watch for signs of respiratory distress, hypertension, or circulatory overload.

Promote Rest. Provide opportunities for quiet play as tolerated, such as drawing, playing board games, listening to tapes, and watching videos. Adjust the child's daily schedule to allow rest periods after activities. Signs of fatigue may include irritability, mood swings, or withdrawal. Inform parents and child about the importance of rest. Limiting visitors during the acute phase of the illness may be necessary. Telephone contacts may be encouraged as an alternative to visitors. To provide a sense of control, encourage the child to set his or her own limits on activity.

Provide Emotional Support. Parents and children often need support to cope with the development of this potentially chronic disease. Provide parents with thorough explanations about the child's disease and treatment regimen. Parental anxiety in combination with the prolonged hospitalization may interfere with the child's independence. Assist parents to promote the child's independence by allowing the child to fill in the menu or complete the daily activity schedule. This gives the child some sense of control.

Children with MCNS may have a distorted body image because of sudden weight gain and edema. Behavioral manifestations may include refusal to look in the mirror, refusal to participate in care, and decreased interest in appearance. Encourage children to express their feelings. Help them maintain a normal appearance by promoting normal grooming routines. Encourage children to wear their own pajamas rather than hospital gowns. Scarves or hats may be used to lessen the child's edematous appearance.

Discharge Planning and Patient and Family Home Care Teaching. Home care needs should be identified and addressed well in advance of discharge. Provide parents and school-age children with explanations of the disease process, prognosis, and treatment plan. Ensure that parents know how to administer medications and can identify potential side effects. Instruct the par-

■ **NURSING ALERT**

Traditionally, a high-protein, low-salt diet was recommended for children with MCNS. Current data, however, suggest that the high-protein diet increases urinary protein loss and may accelerate the development of renal failure.[8]

ents about the need to monitor urine daily for protein, and have them keep a diary to record results.

Tutoring may be required for a short period after discharge. However, parents should be encouraged to allow the child to return to normal activities once the acute episode has resolved. Emphasize the importance of avoiding contact with individuals who have infectious diseases because of the child's reduced immunity. Reinforce to parents that as long as the child is on corticosteroid therapy or shows signs of MCNS, the "no added salt" diet should be followed.

Parents, school-age children, and adolescents need to be able to recognize the signs of relapse. Be sure that parents know when to contact a health care professional about worsening symptoms (fever, chest pain, dyspnea, respiratory distress).

Renal Failure

Renal failure occurs when the kidney is unable to excrete wastes and concentrate urine. There are two types of renal failure: acute and chronic. Acute renal failure occurs suddenly (over days or weeks), whereas in chronic renal failure, kidney function diminishes gradually over months or years.

Both types of renal failure are characterized by **azotemia** (accumulation of nitrogenous wastes in the blood) and sometimes **oliguria** (urine output less than 0.5 to 1 mL/kg/hr). The degree of renal impairment is estimated by the degree of azotemia and the increase in serum creatinine level. **Uremia** occurs when there is an excess of urea and other nitrogenous waste products in the blood.

Acute Renal Failure

Acute renal failure (ARF), which occurs when kidney function abruptly diminishes, is characterized by a sharp rise in the blood urea nitrogen (BUN) level. It occurs most frequently in neonates who are critically ill with asphyxia, shock, and sepsis. It can also be a postoperative complication of cardiac surgery or may result from drug toxicity.[2, 7]

Clinical Manifestations

Characteristically, a healthy child suddenly becomes ill with nonspecific symptoms, including nausea, vomiting, lethargy, edema, and hypertension (see Table 18–8). These symptoms are a result of electrolyte imbalances (Table 18–9), uremia, and fluid overload. The child appears pale and lethargic.

Hyperkalemia is the most life-threatening electrolyte disorder associated with ARF. An increase in serum potassium adversely affects the electrical conductivity within the heart. Hyponatremia affects central nervous system function, resulting in symptoms that range from fatigue to seizures. Edema occurs as a result of sodium and water retention. (Refer to Chapter 7 for a discussion of these fluid and electrolyte alterations.) Children with ARF are also more susceptible to infection because of depressed immune functioning.

Etiology and Pathophysiology

ARF may be caused by prerenal, postrenal, or intrinsic factors.

Prerenal ARF is a result of decreased perfusion to an otherwise normal kidney. Hemorrhage, dehydration, sepsis, or hypoxia may precipitate prerenal ARF. This is the most common type of ARF in infants and young children.

Intrinsic ARF results from primary damage to the parenchymal cells of the kidneys. Damage can be caused by infection, diseases such as hemolytic-uremic syndrome or acute glomerulonephritis, cortical necrosis, nephrotoxic

The following factors increase the risk of acute renal failure:

Newborn
Critically ill neonate
Dehydration
Hemolytic-uremic syndrome

Toddler
Accidental poisoning (e.g., acetaminophen, mushrooms)

School-Age Child and Adolescent
Trauma

TABLE 18-9 Clinical Manifestations of Electrolyte Imbalances in Acute Renal Failure

Hyperkalemia

Results from inability to adequately excrete potassium derived from diet and catabolized cells. In metabolic acidosis there is also movement of potassium from intracellular fluid to extracellular fluid.
- Peaked T waves, widening of QRS on ECG
- Dysrhythmias: ventricular dysrhythmias, heart block, ventricular fibrillation
- Diarrhea
- Muscle weakness

Hyponatremia

In acute oliguric phase, hyponatremia is related to the accumulation of fluid in excess of solute.
- Change in level of consciousness
- Muscle cramps
- Anorexia
- Abnormal reflexes, depressed deep tendon reflexes
- Cheyne-Stokes respirations
- Seizures

Hypocalcemia

Even when hypocalcemia is severe, the following common clinical manifestations may not be seen because of hyperkalemia and metabolic acidosis:
- Muscle tingling
- Change in muscle tone
- Seizures
- Muscle cramps and twitching
- Positive Chvostek sign (contraction of facial muscles after tapping facial nerve just anterior to parotid gland)

There is also phosphate retention (hyperphosphatemia) that depresses serum calcium concentration. Calcium is deposited in injured cells.

Data from Chan, J.C.M., Alon, U., & Oken, D.E. (1992). Acute renal failure. In Edelman, C.M., Jr. (ed.). *Pediatric kidney disease*, (2nd ed.) (pp. 1923–1940). Boston: Little, Brown.

■ NEPHROTOXIC DRUGS

Antimicrobials: aminoglycosides, cephalosporins, tetracycline, sulfonamides
Radiographic contrast media with iodine
Heavy metals: lead, barium, iron
Nonsteroidal antiinflammatory drugs: indomethacin, aspirin

drugs, or accidental ingestion of drugs or poisons. The structure most susceptible to damage is the kidney tubule. Injury to the tubule resulting in acute tubular necrosis is the most frequent cause of intrinsic renal failure in children.

Postrenal ARF, which is caused by obstruction of the urinary flow from the kidneys, is uncommon in children.

Reversible ARF commonly progresses through three phases: oliguric, diuretic, and recovery. The oliguric phase is characterized by a decrease in urinary output and lasts approximately 10 days. The oliguria is a sign of the degree of renal damage. BUN and creatinine levels are elevated. The diuretic phase is characterized by a sudden increase in urinary output because of the inability of the kidney tubules to conserve water. The excessive losses of sodium and potassium result in electrolyte imbalance. The recovery phase is signaled by a decrease in serum creatinine followed by a decrease in BUN as the kidney tubule function begins to return to normal. Signs and symptoms of diminished renal function resolve quickly, although polyuria may persist for days or weeks.[7] Children who recover from ARF may have residual kidney damage and compromised renal function.

Diagnostic Tests and Medical Management

Diagnosis of renal failure is based primarily on urinalysis and blood chemistry results, including BUN, serum creatinine, sodium, potassium, and calcium levels (Table 18–10).

TABLE 18-10 Diagnostic Tests for Renal Failure

Test	Normal Values	Findings in ARF
Urinalysis		
pH	4.5-8.0	Lowered
Osmolarity	50-1400	>500 prerenal
		<350 intrinsic
Specific gravity	1.001-1.030	High: prerenal ARF
		Low: intrinsic ARF
		Normal: postrenal ARF
Protein	Negative	Positive
Blood Chemistry		
Potassium	3.5-4.5 mEq/L	Elevated
Sodium	135-145 mEq/L	Normal or low
Calcium	8-10.5 mg/dL	Low
Phosphate	2.5-4.5 mg/dL	High
Blood urea nitrogen	5-20 mg/dL	Increases by 20-25 mg/dL
Creatinine	0.7-1.5 mg/dL	Progressive increase
pH	7.35-7.45	Low acidic

ARF, Acute renal failure.

TABLE 18-11 Medications Used to Treat Complications of Acute Renal Failure

Complication	Medication	Action or Indication	Nursing Implications
Hyperkalemia (>5 mEq/L)	Kayexalate	Exchanges sodium for potassium	May require up to 4 hours to take effect
	Calcium gluconate 10%	Counteracts potassium-induced increased myocardial irritability	Monitor for electrocardiographic (ECG) changes. Intravenous (IV) infiltration may result in tissue necrosis.
	Sodium bicarbonate	Helps correct acidosis by exchanging hydrogen for potassium	*Do not mix with calcium.* Complications include fluid overload, hypertension, and tetany.
Hypocalcemia (<7 mg/dL)	Calcium gluconate 10%	Used in presence of tetany; provides ionized calcium to restore nervous tissue function	Administer slowly to prevent bradycardia. Monitor for ECG changes.
Hypertension (blood pressure >95% for age)	Sodium nitroprusside, nitroglycerin	Relaxes smooth muscle in peripheral arterioles	Administer by continuous IV infusion; fall in blood pressure is seen within 10-20 minutes.

Treatment depends on the underlying cause of the renal failure. The goal of treatment is to minimize or prevent permanent renal damage by restoring and maintaining fluid and electrolyte balance and managing complications (Table 18–11). Initial emergency treatment of children with fluid depletion focuses on fluid replacement at 20 mL/kg of saline or lactated Ringer solu-

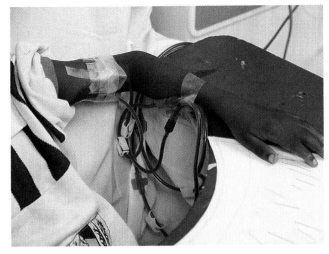
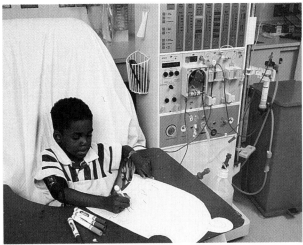

A

B

FIGURE 18–6 Child undergoing dialysis. **A,** A surgically implanted vascular graft is being used here. One needle is placed in the arterialized end of the graft (red tubing), and one needle is placed in the venous end (blue tubing) for blood return. **B,** The child is able to draw or perform other quiet activities during dialysis treatment. Note that the child's blood pressure is monitored carefully throughout the treatment.

■ CLINICAL TIP

Carefully monitor fluid balance in the child undergoing hemodialysis. Check vital signs and blood pressure every half hour. Monitor oral intake and urinary output on the dialysis equipment every half hour. Weigh the child before and after the dialysis to determine any fluid imbalances that must be adjusted in the next hemodialysis session.

tion given rapidly or over 5 to 10 minutes to ensure renal perfusion. Albumin may also be administered when blood loss is the cause of circulatory depletion. If oliguria persists after restoration of adequate fluid volume, intrinsic renal damage is suspected. Children with fluid overload, like those with pulmonary edema, need diuretic therapy or dialysis.

Fluid requirements are calculated to maintain zero water balance. Intake should equal output. Antibiotics are prescribed for infection. Nephrotoxic antibiotics such as aminoglycosides are avoided.

Some children with ARF require dialysis to correct electrolyte imbalances and cleanse the blood of waste products (Fig. 18–6). A calcium ion exchange resin may be administered to decrease the potassium level. However, hemodialysis is the treatment of choice for renal failure that results from dehydration and drug toxicity. Because of advances in techniques for peritoneal dialysis, this method is now being used to treat some children with ARF.

In hemodialysis a cannula is inserted into a large vein (e.g., the femoral or jugular vein) or through an arteriovenous shunt or fistula. Blood circulates out of the body through an artificial semipermeable membrane and into a dialyzer where waste products are filtered out. A **dialysate** (dialysis solution) is pumped in the direction opposite blood flow. Differences in osmolarity and concentration between the child's blood and the dialysate alter the intravascular electrolyte concentration and reduce the intravascular volume.

Hemodialysis is more efficient than peritoneal dialysis but requires close monitoring for symptoms related to rapid changes in fluid and electrolyte balance (nausea and vomiting, dizziness, muscle cramps). It is usually performed three times a week, with each treatment lasting approximately 3 to 4 hours.

In peritoneal dialysis a catheter is inserted into the peritoneal cavity. Buretrols or graduated cylinders are used to monitor the volume of fluid exchanged. Because peritoneal dialysis removes fluid at a slower rate then hemodialysis, complications resulting from rapid fluid and electrolyte shifts are less likely. However, other potential complications include peritonitis, pain, leakage of fluid, and respiratory symptoms (Table 18–12). Peritoneal dialysis can be performed manually or mechanically (using automated peritoneal dialysis cyclers).

Prognosis depends on the cause of ARF. When renal failure results from drug toxicity or dehydration, the prognosis is generally good. However, ARF that results from diseases such as hemolytic-uremic syndrome or acute glomerulonephritis may be associated with residual kidney damage.

TABLE 18-12 Complications of Peritoneal Dialysis

Complication	Cause
Peritonitis	
Cloudy dialysate, abdominal pain, tenderness, leukocytosis, fever (neonatal hypothermia), constipation	*Staphylococcus aureus, Staphylococcus epidermidis,* fungal infections, gram-negative rods (risk is proportional to duration of dialysis and inversely proportional to age)
Pain	
During inflow	Too rapid a rate of infusion, too large a volume of dialysate, encasement of catheter in a false passage, extremes in temperature of dialysate
During outflow at end of emptying	Omentum entering catheter at end of outflow
Leakage	
Fluid around catheter, edema of penis or scrotum secondary to leakage into abdominal subcutaneous tissue	Overfilling of abdomen, catheter that has migrated from peritoneal cavity
Respiratory symptoms	
Shortness of breath, decreased breath sounds in lower lobes, inadequate chest expansion	Abdominal fullness that compromises diaphragm movement, hole in diaphragm allowing dialysate into chest cavity

Nursing Assessment

A complete history and physical examination are necessary to identify progression of symptoms and possible causes for renal failure.

PHYSIOLOGIC ASSESSMENT. Assessment of vital signs, level of consciousness, and other neurologic indicators helps to identify clinical signs of electrolyte imbalance (see Table 18–9). Measurement of the child's weight on admission provides a baseline for evaluating changes in fluid status. Monitor urine culture results and blood studies. Inspect urine for color (Fig. 18–7).

FIGURE 18-7 A color wheel, such as the one shown here, can be used as a guide in standardizing descriptions of urine color. Normal urine is pale yellow. Changes in urine color can indicate the following alterations: *yellow*—concentrated urine; *amber*—bile in urine; *orange*—alkaline or concentrated urine; *red orange*—acid pH, medications; *red*—blood, menses; *pink*—dilute blood; *burgundy*—laxatives; *tea*—melanin, hematuria; *dark gray*—medications, dyes; *blue*—dyes, medications.

Copyright © 1993 Connie Cooper, R.N., M.S.N.

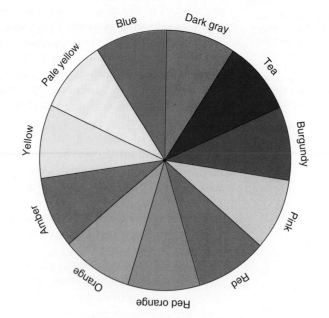

Cloudy urine may indicate infection; tea-colored urine suggests hematuria. Assess urine specific gravity and intake and output.

PSYCHOSOCIAL ASSESSMENT. The unexpected and acute nature of the child's hospitalization creates anxiety for both parents and child. Assess for feelings of anger, guilt, or fear associated with the hospitalization. Such feelings are likely if ARF developed as a result of dehydration, a preventable injury, or poisoning. Assess coping mechanisms, family support systems, and level of stress.

Nursing Diagnosis

Nursing diagnoses depend on the cause of renal failure and accompanying complications. Several nursing diagnoses may apply to the child with ARF, including:

- Altered Renal Tissue Perfusion related to hypovolemia, sepsis, or drug toxicity
- Fluid Volume Excess related to sodium and water retention
- Altered Nutrition: Less Than Body Requirements related to anorexia, nausea, and vomiting
- High Risk for Infection related to invasive procedures and diminished immune functioning
- Anxiety (Child and Parent) related to sudden hospitalization and uncertain prognosis
- Noncompliance related to lack of knowledge of treatment plan

Nursing Management

Nursing care focuses on preventing complications, maintaining fluid balance, administering medications, meeting nutritional needs, preventing infection, and providing emotional support to the child and parents.

PREVENT COMPLICATIONS. Complications of impaired renal function include hypertension, anemia, osteodystrophy (defective formation of bone), and uremic syndrome (discussed later in the section on chronic renal failure). Complications are best prevented by ensuring compliance with the treatment plan. Careful monitoring of vital signs, intake and output, serum electrolytes, and level of consciousness can alert the nurse to changes that indicate potential complications.

MAINTAIN FLUID BALANCE. Estimate the child's fluid status by monitoring weight (on the same scale), intake and output, and blood pressure two or three times a day. Also monitor serum chemistry values, especially for sodium. The aim of fluid balance is to achieve a stable serum sodium concentration and a decrease in body weight by 0.5% to 1% a day.

ANURIC OR OLIGURIC PHASE. Fluid intake, including parenteral nutrition, is limited to replacement of insensible water loss from the lungs, skin, and gastrointestinal tract (about one-third the daily maintenance requirements in afebrile children). If the child is febrile, increase fluid administration by 12% for each centigrade degree of temperature elevation.

DIURETIC PHASE. Fluid replacement should precisely match urine excreted if the child was not previously overloaded. As renal function returns to normal, replacement fluids are gradually decreased.[13]

ADMINISTER MEDICATIONS. Because the kidney's ability to excrete drugs is impaired in ARF, dosages of all medications should be adjusted. The actual dosage of the drug can be reduced or the time interval between doses can be increased. Check drug levels to monitor for drug toxicity. Be aware of signs of drug toxicity for each medication the child is receiving.

MEET NUTRITION NEEDS. Children are at risk of malnutrition because of a high metabolic rate. Parenteral alimentation or enteral feeding may be used

■ CLINICAL TIP

If serum sodium concentration rises and weight falls, insufficient fluids are being administered. If the serum sodium level falls and the weight increases, excessive fluids are being administered.

initially to minimize protein catabolism. The diet is tailored to the individual child's need for calories, carbohydrates, fats, and amino acids or protein hydrolysates. Depending on the degree of renal failure, sodium, potassium, and phosphorus may be restricted. Oral feeding is initiated as soon as the child can tolerate it.

PREVENT INFECTION. The child with ARF is extremely susceptible to nosocomial infections as a result of altered nutritional status, compromised immunity, and numerous invasive procedures. Thorough handwashing is imperative to decrease the risk of infection. Sterile technique should be used for all invasive procedures and when caring for lines. Drainage from catheter sites should be cultured to check for the presence of infectious organisms. Assess vital signs and lung sounds frequently.

PROVIDE EMOTIONAL SUPPORT. The sudden onset of ARF presents parents with an unexpected threat to their child's life. Both the child and the parents experience anxiety because of the unexpected hospitalization and the uncertainty of the prognosis. Parents often feel guilty, regardless of the cause of renal failure. This guilt is intensified when renal failure is a result of dehydration or poisoning. Encourage parents to verbalize their fears and assist them in working through feelings of guilt. Explain procedures and treatment measures to decrease anxiety. Encouraging parents and older siblings to participate in the child's care can increase their sense of control.

DISCHARGE PLANNING AND PATIENT AND FAMILY HOME CARE TEACHING. Home care needs should be identified and addressed well in advance of discharge. Encourage parental involvement early in the child's hospitalization. Be sure that parents understand the importance of administering medications correctly. Instruct family members in the proper technique for measuring blood pressure so they can monitor the child's hypertension, if ordered. Have them provide a return demonstration.

Diet counseling is a key component of discharge planning and is usually performed by a renal dietitian. Depending on the degree of renal failure, the child's diet may include restrictions on protein, water, sodium, potassium, and phosphorus. The parents should be given written guidelines listing appropriate food choices to assist in menu planning. Ethnic and cultural preferences should be considered in listing menu options.

Referral to support groups can be helpful for both parents and children. The National Kidney Foundation is a source of numerous publications (see Appendix F).

Chronic Renal Failure

Chronic renal failure (CRF) is a progressive, irreversible reduction in kidney function. CRF is rare in children, occurring in 3.5 to 6 per million.[3]

Clinical Manifestations

Children with CRF frequently have mild symptoms initially. More severe symptoms do not appear until the child is in advanced renal failure (see Table 18–8). In the early stages the child may appear pale and complain of headache, nausea, and fatigue. As the disease progresses, the child experiences a loss of appetite and complications of renal impairment, including growth retardation, dental and skeletal deformities (renal osteodystrophy, rickets), and delayed sexual maturation.

Growth retardation is caused by hyperparathyroidism; disturbances in metabolism of calcium, phosphorus, and vitamin D; and decreased caloric intake. Osteodystrophy results in bone demineralization, increasing the child's risk for spontaneous fractures.

■ CULTURAL CONSIDERATIONS

Special effort is often needed to reduce the sodium in the diet of an Asian child. Sauces and seasonings for foods (soy sauce, mustards, monosodium glutamate, and garlic salt) are sodium rich even though the foods seasoned (rice, vegetables, shrimp, and chicken) are low in sodium. The child may ingest up to 18 g of sodium a day with these added sauces and seasonings when 4 g a day is the goal. Individualized counseling and motivation are needed to encourage families to reduce the child's sodium intake. Encourage the family to use spices low in sodium when preparing rice, vegetables, and meats.

In end-stage renal disease (ESRD), the most advanced form of CRF, all body systems are adversely affected by renal failure. Uremic syndrome occurs when various clinical and biochemical disturbances appear as a result of the progressive renal deterioration that has taken place with CRF.

Etiology and Pathophysiology

In children, CRF usually results from developmental abnormalities of the kidney or urinary tract. Alexis, described at the beginning of the chapter, had ESRD resulting from bilateral kidney atresia. It may also be caused by hemolytic-uremic syndrome, glomerulonephritis, or other renal diseases.[7]

The gradual, progressive loss of functioning nephrons ultimately results in ESRD. ESRD is characterized by minimal renal function (less than 5% of normal), uremic syndrome, anemia, and abnormal blood values. In ESRD the kidneys can no longer maintain homeostasis and the child requires dialysis.

The kidneys function to excrete excess acid in the body and to regulate the body's fluid and electrolyte balance. Renal failure upsets this fluid and electrolyte balance. As renal failure progresses, metabolic acidosis occurs because the kidneys cannot excrete the acids that build up in the body. Retention of excessive sodium and water is a common cause of the elevated blood pressure associated with CRF. Calcium and phosphorus retention leads to uremic bone disease. Since the kidneys are the site of production of erythropoietin (the growth factor responsible for the production and maturation of red cells), lack of erythropoietin and progressive renal disease are the underlying causes of the anemia of CRF.

Diagnostic Tests and Medical Management

Laboratory evaluation, including serum electrolyte, phosphate, BUN, and creatinine levels and pH, is used to confirm the diagnosis of CRF. A urine sample is collected for culture, and a 24-hour urine sample is obtained to quantify creatinine and protein excretion.

The goals of treatment are to slow the progression of renal disease and to prevent complications. Treatment includes a combination of dietary management, drug therapy, and, in ESRD, dialysis.

Dietary management focuses on maximizing caloric intake for growth while limiting demands on the kidneys and minimizing fluid and electrolyte disturbances. Some children require tube feedings to achieve optimal protein intake. Sodium bicarbonate (Bicitra) is used for treatment of metabolic acidosis. Restricting sodium to as little as 2 g/day may be necessary if the child is hypertensive or edematous. If the child has hyponatremia, a sodium supplement of up to 10 mEq/kg is given three or four times a day. As renal failure progresses, potassium and phosphate restrictions become necessary.

Diuretics are given to reduce the edema associated with renal failure. Antihypertensives are prescribed to reduce blood pressure and prevent the progression of renal disease. As in ARF, medication dosages are adjusted because of the reduced glomerular filtration rate. Supplementation of vitamins (pyridoxine and folic acid) is usually necessary to offset deficiencies. Ergocalciferol and calcitriol (vitamin D) are given to increase calcium absorption. Ascorbic acid is administered to enhance iron absorption. Erythropoietin is given to stimulate increased production of red blood cells in children undergoing dialysis.

Children who progress to ESRD require dialysis treatments, which may be performed either in an outpatient dialysis center or in the home. (Refer to the earlier discussion of medical management of ARF.)

In continuous ambulatory peritoneal dialysis (CAPD) the dialysate is infused into the peritoneal cavity and left in place for 4 to 6 hours. An attached bag is folded under the child's clothes, permitting normal activity. After the allotted time the dialysate is drained by hanging the bag lower than the pelvis. This process is repeated four to six times a day.

Two other types of dialysis are continuous cycling peritoneal dialysis (CCPD), which is given 24 hours a day, and intermittent peritoneal dialysis (IPD), in which the dialysis exchange is done at night by an automatic cycling dialysis machine.

Renal transplantation provides the only alternative to long-term dialysis for children with ESRD. Because of the adverse effects on growth and development resulting from delaying transplantation, children are given some priority over adults awaiting transplantation. After transplantation the child must take immunosuppressive medications such as prednisone, azathioprine, and cyclosporine to suppress rejection. This therapy places the child at risk for infection.

CRF is irreversible. However, the course of the disease is variable. Some children progress quickly to renal failure, necessitating dialysis. Other children are managed with a combination of medication and diet therapy for some time before significant renal impairment occurs. Frequent modifications in the treatment plan are often necessary to address the child's changing status.

Nursing Assessment

PHYSIOLOGIC ASSESSMENT. The initial and ongoing assessment of the child focuses on identifying complications of renal failure. Observe for signs of edema, osteodystrophy, and anemia. Assessment of vital signs helps to identify electrolyte alterations (see Table 18–9).

PSYCHOSOCIAL ASSESSMENT. As renal disease progresses, the number of stressors on the child and family increases. Denial and disbelief are commonly the first reactions. A thorough family assessment can help to identify particular needs of the child and family (Table 18–13).

TABLE 18–13 Family Assessment: The Child with Chronic Renal Failure

- What coping strategies have worked before in stressful situations for the child? For the family? Can those strategies be used or modified to deal with the current situation?
- Who offers support within the family? In the community? In the health care system?
- Who cares for the child? (Identify people and specific responsibilities.)
- Who coordinates follow-up health care?
- If renal transplantation is an option, who are potential donors? Are they willing donors? Have they been tested for compatibility? What impact will this donation have on the donor? What is the donor's goal for the recipient?

DEVELOPMENTAL ASSESSMENT. Compare the child's height and weight to age norms to identify growth retardation. Assess the adolescent for signs of delayed sexual maturation and, in girls, amenorrhea. School-age children and adolescents are often embarrassed about being perceived as different from peers. Ask the child how he or she feels about the need to follow a special diet, take medications, and undergo dialysis treatments.

■ RENAL TRANSPLANTATION

An alternative to lifelong dialysis for children with chronic renal failure is renal transplantation. The donor kidney can be obtained from a living related donor or from a cadaver donor. Cadaver kidneys are matched with recipients through a computerized list of potential recipients.

Nursing Diagnosis

Nursing diagnoses for the child with CRF are similar to those previously listed for ARF. Additional diagnoses include:

- Altered Growth and Development related to decreased caloric intake and metabolic disturbances
- Self-Esteem Disturbance related to impaired growth and perception of being "different"
- Activity Intolerance related to headaches and fatigue
- Altered Family Processes related to life-threatening illness of child
- Ineffective Management of Therapeutic Regimen related to lack of knowledge of home dialysis plan

Nursing Management

Children with CRF are usually hospitalized for initial diagnostic evaluation, to monitor problems that develop in the treatment plan, or to treat infection or another concurrent problem. Nursing care for the hospitalized child with CRF focuses on monitoring for side effects of medications, preventing infection, meeting nutritional needs, and providing emotional support and anticipatory teaching.

MONITOR FOR SIDE EFFECTS OF MEDICATIONS. Watch for signs of electrolyte imbalance such as weakness, muscle cramps, dizziness, headache, and nausea and vomiting in children who are taking diuretics. Supervise the child's activities closely to prevent falls resulting from dizziness, especially at the beginning of diuretic therapy. If antihypertensive medications such as hydralazine are being administered, monitor the child's weight to detect excessive gain resulting from water and sodium retention.

PREVENT INFECTION. The child with CRF is extremely susceptible to infections. Be alert for signs of infection, such as elevated temperature; cloudy, strong-smelling urine; dysuria; changes in respiratory pattern; or productive cough. Emphasize to the child and family the importance of good hand-washing practices.

MEET NUTRITION NEEDS. Maintaining adequate nutritional intake in a child with CRF is challenging. A renal dietitian usually assists the child to make food selections, taking into account the child's likes and dislikes and cultural background. Provide small, frequent feedings and present meals attractively to encourage the child to eat.

PROVIDE EMOTIONAL SUPPORT. Development of progressive CRF requires a total life-style change for the child and family. The parents and child need opportunities to express and work through their feelings related to the disease, prognosis, and treatment restrictions. Children can be assisted to express their feelings through drawings or therapeutic play.

The need for ongoing dialysis treatments and the wait for a suitable donor kidney are stressful for both parents and child. Identification of effective coping methods and family support systems is needed. The National Kidney Foundation and local support groups for kidney disease can provide the family with information or additional support (see Appendix F).

PROVIDE ANTICIPATORY TEACHING. Supply the parents with information about the disease process, dialysis treatments, issues related to renal transplantation, and possible behavioral responses to dietary restrictions and limitations imposed by the treatment plan. School-age children may not understand the consequences of noncompliance with dietary restrictions and may perceive these restrictions as punishment. Adolescents often resent the dietary restrictions and ongoing dialysis treatments, which pose a threat to their independence and evolving sense of self. Noncooperation, depression,

■ CLINICAL TIP

Dilute liquid doses of iron supplement in juice or water, and have the child drink through a straw to prevent staining of teeth.

and hostility are common responses. Encouraging older children and adolescents to be responsible for self-care may help them cope with the disease.

DISCHARGE PLANNING AND PATIENT AND FAMILY HOME CARE TEACHING. Home care needs should be identified and addressed well in advance of discharge. Parents need to understand the necessity of long-term treatments and follow-up care. Help the family develop a schedule for medication administration that fits with their routine. Stress the importance of consistency in administration times. Teach parents how to recognize side effects and complications.

Appropriate referrals should be made to the local visiting nurse association and to home care nursing agencies. Home care nurses will help the parents care for the child on dialysis as well as provide necessary support and reassurance. Parents of children receiving dialysis at home should be taught how to perform the treatment and how to identify complications (see Table 18–12). Strict aseptic technique is necessary to prevent infection at the catheter site.

Review any dietary restrictions with parents. Provide sample menus for meal planning to help parents incorporate dietary changes into daily meals.

To minimize the psychologic consequences of coping with a chronic disease, encourage parents to promote the child's participation in age-appropriate activities. Attendance at school and contacts with peers promote normal growth and development.

Hemolytic-Uremic Syndrome

Hemolytic-uremic syndrome (HUS) is a relatively rare, acute renal disease that occurs primarily before 3 years of age (see Table 18–8). The syndrome is characterized by a classic triad of signs: (1) hemolytic anemia, (2) thrombocytopenia, and (3) ARF.

HUS usually follows an episode of mild gastroenteritis, upper respiratory infection, or urinary tract infection. The acute stage occurs when the child suddenly appears pale and develops petechiae, bruising, or bloody stools (Table 18–14). Urine output is decreased. Signs of central nervous system involvement include irritability, lethargy, gait changes, and convulsions. Edema and ascites resulting from renal failure may also be apparent.

The etiology of HUS is multifaceted. Suggested causes include bacterial and viral agents, genetic factors, and immunologic responses. Damage to the lining of the glomerular arterioles results in swelling of the endothelial cells. In response, clotting mechanisms deposit fibrin in the renal arterioles and capillaries. This partial occlusion damages the red blood cells, resulting in hemolysis and subsequent anemia. Platelet agglutination occurs in areas of vascular endothelial damage, causing thrombocytopenia. ARF develops as a consequence of blood clotting in the arterioles as well as the toxic effect of hemoglobin on renal tubular cells leading to acute tubular necrosis.

A peripheral blood smear with fragments of red blood cells, fibrin split products, and a decreased platelet count ($<140,000/mm^3$) confirms the diagnosis. Treatment focuses on the complications of ARF and includes fluid restrictions, antihypertensive medications, and a high-calorie, high-carbohydrate diet that is low in protein, sodium, potassium, and phosphorus. (Refer to the earlier discussion of ARF.) Dialysis may be necessary, depending on the degree of renal failure. Transfusions of fresh packed red blood cells may be ordered to prevent anemia and hyperkalemia. Transfusions should be administered carefully to prevent hypertension caused by hypervolemia. Plasmapheresis is sometimes helpful, but the reason for its success is unknown. In this technique, blood is withdrawn, its cellular components are reconstituted in an isotonic solution, and the solution is then reinfused.

TABLE 18–14 Clinical Manifestations of Hemolytic-Uremic Syndrome

Prodromal Stage (1–7 days)

Upper respiratory illness
Abdominal pain with nausea, vomiting, and bloody diarrhea
Pallor
Fever
Irritability
Lymphadenopathy
Skin rash
Edema

Acute Stage

Severe gastroenteritis with bloody diarrhea
Hemolytic anemia
Hypertension
Purpura
Neurologic involvement (irritability, seizures, stupor, coma, lethargy)
Oliguria or anuria
Edema and ascites

LABORATORY FINDINGS IN HEMOLYTIC-UREMIC SYNDROME

Red blood cells: fragmented on smear (schistocytes)
Hemoglobin: 2 to 10 g/dL (levels depend on the degree of hemolytic anemia)
Elevated white blood cell count
Platelet count: $<140,000/mm^3$
Elevated serum creatinine level
Elevated blood urea nitrogen concentration

Data from Feeg, V., & Harbin, R.E. (1991). *Pediatric core curriculum and resource manual.* Pitman, NJ: Anthony J. Jannetti.

Nursing Management

Nursing care is the same as that for the child with ARF, described earlier. Careful monitoring of fluid balance is essential. The child must be observed carefully for signs of progressive renal impairment. Discharge planning focuses on teaching parents about medications and dietary and fluid restrictions. Follow-up visits are necessary to evaluate the effectiveness of the treatment plan.

Acute Poststreptococcal Glomerulonephritis

Glomerulonephritis is an inflammation of the glomeruli of the kidneys. In children it is most often a response to a group A beta-hemolytic streptococcal infection. The incidence of acute poststreptococcal glomerulonephritis (APSGN) is highest in children who are 6 to 7 years of age, and it is twice as common in boys as in girls (see Table 18–8). Early antibiotic therapy for streptococcal infection does not seem to prevent the development of APSGN.

Clinical Manifestations

Onset is usually abrupt. Hematuria and mild periorbital edema are usually the first clinical signs.[1] Hypertension is the next sign to appear. As the disease progresses, the child becomes lethargic and feverish and may complain of abdominal pain, headache, and costovertebral tenderness (related to stretching of the renal capsule from edema). Gross hematuria, resulting in tea-colored urine, is a classic symptom. Other symptoms include oliguria, hypertension, anorexia, and generalized edema.

Etiology and Pathophysiology

The child with APSGN usually becomes ill after a group A beta-hemolytic streptococcal infection of the upper respiratory tract or the skin. Often the child becomes ill with strep throat, recovers, and then develops symptoms of APSGN after an interval of 1 to 2 weeks.

Glomerular damage occurs as a result of an immune complex reaction. Antibody-antigen complexes become lodged in the glomeruli, leading to inflammation and obstruction. Damage to the glomerular membrane allows red blood cells and red cell casts to be excreted. Sodium and water are retained, expanding the intravascular and interstitial compartments. This process results in the characteristic finding of edema.

Diagnostic Tests and Medical Management

■ **URINALYSIS RESULTS IN APSGN**

Decreased pH
Hematuria
Proteinuria: trace to 2+
Discoloration (reddish brown to rusty color secondary to red blood cell and hemoglobin content)
Leukocyturia
Urine specific gravity greater than 1.020

Blood tests reveal elevated BUN and creatinine concentrations only when there is an 80% decrease in the glomerular filtration rate, which is relatively uncommon. The erythrocyte sedimentation rate is increased in the acute phase, and serum lipid levels are increased in about 40% of cases. An elevated antistreptolysin O (ASO) titer reflects the presence of antibodies from a recent respiratory infection, but the ASO level associated with a recent skin infection is low. The anti-DNAse titer is helpful for detecting antibodies associated with recent skin infections. Anemia is common in the acute phase and is generally caused by dilution of the serum by the extracellular fluid. The hemoglobin level and hematocrit value may decrease during the late phase as a result of hematuria. The white blood cell count may be normal or slightly elevated.

Treatment focuses on relief of symptoms and supportive therapy. Bed rest is a key component of the treatment plan during the acute phase. Hypertension is managed with a combination of an antihypertensive medication (such as hydralazine [Apresoline]) and a diuretic (such as furosemide [Lasix]). Mild to moderate hypertension should be treated with fluid and salt restriction. Corticosteroids are prescribed to decrease the inflammatory response. Penicillin is given to ensure eradication of streptococcal infection.

Fluid requirements are determined by careful monitoring of urinary output, weight, blood pressure, and serum electrolytes. Initially only insensible losses are replaced until the status of renal function is known. The degree of dietary restriction is determined by the severity of edema. Sodium and potassium intake is restricted. With severe azotemia, protein intake may have to be limited.

The prognosis for the majority of children with APSGN is good. Most children recover completely within a few weeks. Recurrences are rare.

Nursing Assessment

Assess edema, which may be periorbital and dependent and shifts as the child's position is changed. Assess for circulatory congestion (crackles, dyspnea, and cough). Monitor blood pressure, which can rise as high as 200/120 mm Hg. The initial elevation is highest; then it decreases for a few days and is increased again for 1 to 2 weeks. When hypertension is present, assess for signs of central nervous system problems (headache, blurred vision, vomiting, decreased level of consciousness, confusion, and convulsions).

Nursing Diagnosis

The accompanying Nursing Care Plan lists several nursing diagnoses that may apply to the child with APSGN.

Nursing Management

As with other renal disorders, care of the child with APSGN requires careful monitoring of vital signs and fluid-electrolyte balance to evaluate renal functioning and identify complications. Bed rest is required during the acute phase. Immediate emergency care is needed for severe hypertension with cerebral dysfunction; diazoxide or hydralazine is administered intravenously. Nursing care focuses on monitoring fluid status, preventing infection, preventing skin breakdown, meeting nutritional needs, and providing emotional support to the child and family. The Nursing Care Plan summarizes nursing care of the child with APSGN.

Monitor Fluid Status. Monitor vital signs, fluid and electrolyte status, and intake and output. Hypovolemia can occur as a result of fluid shifting from vascular to interstitial spaces despite the outward clinical signs of excess fluid retention. Monitor the degree of ascites by measuring abdominal girth. Document urine specific gravity.

Prevent Infection. Impaired renal function and corticosteroid therapy place the child at risk for infection. Monitor for signs of infection, including fever, increased malaise and an elevated white blood cell count. Instruct the family in good handwashing technique. Limit visitors, and screen for upper respiratory infections.

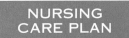

THE CHILD WITH ACUTE POSTSTREPTOCOCCAL GLOMERULONEPHRITIS

GOAL	INTERVENTION	RATIONALE	EXPECTED OUTCOME
1. High Risk for Fluid Volume Excess related to decreased glomerular filtration			
Child will regain normal fluid balance.	Assess for edema (periorbital or dependent areas).	Sodium and water retention leads to edema.	Child maintains normal urine output of 0.5 to 1 mL/kg/hr.
	Calculate fluid intake and plan amounts to offer throughout the day.	An intake/output ratio of 1:1 reflects normal hydration and kidney function.	Child receives appropriate fluid each day.
	Document intake and output.	Prevents excessive fluid intake.	
	Perform daily weight measurement on the same scale at the same time of day.	Weight gain is an early sign of fluid retention. Weight loss indicates improvement in condition.	
	Administer prescribed medications (diuretics and antihypertensives).	Diuretics cause excretion of excess fluid by preventing reabsorption of water and sodium. Antihypertensives increase excretion of water and sodium and cause vasodilation.	
2. High Risk for Infection related to renal impairment and corticosteroid therapy			
Child will be infection free.	Assess temperature every 4 hours. Observe for signs of infection.	Child is at risk for secondary infection.	Child's temperature remains within normal limits and child is free of secondary infection.
	Obtain throat and other cultures as ordered.	Culture can identify causative microorganism in secondary infection or presence of residual streptococcal infection.	
3. High Risk for Impaired Skin Integrity related to tissue edema			
Child will be free of skin breakdown.	Assess skin for breakdown secondary to edema and bed rest.	Ensures early identification and implementation of preventive measures.	Child has unimpaired skin integrity.
	Encourage position changes every 1 to 2 hours. Provide skin care. Use a therapeutic mattress.	Prolonged pressure leads to skin breakdown.	
4. Altered Nutrition: Less Than Body Requirements related to anorexia			
Child will maintain adequate caloric intake.	Maintain meal schedule similar to that at home. Serve food in age-appropriate servings. Assess for food likes and dislikes. Provide favorite foods, as possible.	Normal routine and preferred food choices help to encourage the child to eat.	Child maintains weight and tolerates daily intake that meets nutritional requirements.

Continued.

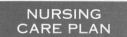

THE CHILD WITH ACUTE POSTSTREPTOCOCCAL GLOMERULONEPHRITIS—CONTINUED

GOAL	INTERVENTION	RATIONALE	EXPECTED OUTCOME
5. Activity Intolerance related to fluid and electrolyte imbalance, infectious process, and altered nutrition			
Child will progress in activity tolerance without excess fatigue as the disease process improves.	Maintain bed rest during acute stage. Encourage gradual activity increase as the condition improves. Provide for quiet play according to the developmental stage of the child (e.g., coloring books, music, videotapes, television).	Rest decreases the production of waste materials, which place increased stress on the kidneys. Quiet activities minimize energy expenditures and stress on the kidneys.	Child avoids fatigue and exhibits the ability to tolerate activity for longer periods.
6. Knowledge Deficit (Parent) related to child's medication schedule and treatment regimen after discharge			
Parents will state knowledge of child's treatment regimen after discharge.	Assess parents' understanding of need for compliance with medication schedule. Describe best schedule for giving medications to match child's and family's routines. Inform parents about potential side effects of prescribed medications and signs and symptoms of complications. If antibiotics are prescribed, instruct parents to administer complete course.	Diuretics and antihypertensives are central to treatment plan. Improves compliance. Allows early intervention to prevent side effects. Offers best chance to cure infection.	Parents administer medications as prescribed.

Prevent Skin Breakdown. Dependent areas or areas prone to pressure are vulnerable to skin breakdown. Turn the child frequently. Pad bony prominences or susceptible areas with sheepskin, or protect skin with a transparent dressing. Make sure the child's bed is free of crumbs or sharp toys. Keep sheets tight and free of wrinkles.

Meet Nutritional Needs. A team approach (including the nurse, renal dietitian, parents, and child) is often needed to meet the child's nutritional needs. In most cases a "no added salt" diet is implemented. Anorexia presents the greatest challenge to meeting daily nutritional requirements during the acute phase of the disease. Encouraging parents to bring the child's favorite foods from home, serving foods in age-appropriate quantities, and allowing the child to eat with other children or with family members may increase the child's appetite.

Provide Emotional Support. Guilt is a common reaction of parents of a child with APSGN. Parents may blame themselves for not responding more quickly to the child's initial symptoms or may believe they could have prevented the development of glomerular damage. Discuss the etiology of the disease and the child's treatment, and correct any misconceptions. Emphasize that APSGN develops in only a few children with streptococcal infection.

Discharge Planning and Patient and Family Home Care Teaching. Discharge planning focuses on teaching parents about the medication regimen, potential side effects of medications, dietary restrictions, and signs and symptoms of complications. Teach parents how to take the child's blood pressure and how to test urine for albumin, if ordered. Have them demonstrate these procedures. Emphasize that it is important to avoid exposing the child to individuals with upper respiratory tract infections. Recommend family screening for streptococcal infection. After discharge, parents should allow the child to return to his or her normal routine and activities, with periods allowed for rest.

Sexually Transmitted Diseases

Over the past 10 years, sexually transmitted diseases (STDs) have become a major national public health concern. There are presently more than 20 organisms of bacterial and viral origin, including human immunodeficiency virus (HIV), that are identified as causative agents of STDs.[14] (Refer to Chapter 9 for a discussion of acquired immunodeficiency syndrome [HIV infection].)

It is the combined responsibility of the federal, state, and local health departments to control and prevent STDs. On a national level the Centers for Disease Control and Prevention (CDC) and the National Institutes of Health (NIH) coordinate control plans, provide surveillance, and fund basic science and clinical research.

State and local health departments are responsible for controlling the spread of STDs through health promotion programs, staff training, reporting systems, diagnosis, treatment, patient counseling, and the notification of sex partners.[15]

Children and adolescents can become infected with sexually transmitted organisms through sexual experimentation, sexual play, molestation, and sexual abuse. Adolescents are considered an at-risk population because of their inexperience and lack of knowledge about STDs. They may disregard the importance of using barriers, may have multiple sexual partners, and often do not seek medical treatment until symptoms are well advanced.

Approximately 50% of adolescents who are 16 years of age have had sexual intercourse. This number increases to 70% by 19 years of age. More than half of the STDs reported occur in adolescents and young adults under the age of 25 years.[2] The most frequently diagnosed STDs are chlamydia, gonorrhea, herpes simplex (type 2), and syphilis (Table 18–15). Adolescents represent 1% of the population infected with HIV.

Complications of STDs include pelvic inflammatory disease, infertility, high risk for ectopic pregnancy, and genital cancer. HIV infection is invariably fatal.

The nurse usually encounters the child, adolescent, and family in the emergency department, outpatient clinic, or nursing unit. Since adolescents are often afraid of the consequences of reporting symptoms, it is important

Instruct parents to delay immunizations until the child's corticosteroid treatment has been discontinued for 3 months and no proteinuria is present. Because corticosteroids suppress immune function, the immunization may not be effective.

■ NURSING ALERT

When a child less than 10 years of age is found to have gonorrhea, consider the possibility of sexual abuse. Any time anorectal symptoms are found, suspect molestation.

■ LEGAL CONSIDERATIONS

When a child is found to have an STD, the law requires that a report be made to social services and the local health department and that an investigation take place.

TABLE 18–15 Sexually Transmitted Diseases

Disease	Clinical Manifestations	Medical and Nursing Management
Chlamydia Causative organism: *Chlamydia trachomatis* Incubation period: 5 to 10 days Reportable: In most states	*C. trachomatis* is most frequent cause of nongono-coccal urethritis. Common symptoms include: Adolescent females: yellow-green mucopurulent endocervical discharge, cervicitis, salpingitis, pelvic inflammatory disease (PID). Adolescent males: urethritis, yellow-white discharge, dysuria, proctitis, epididymitis.	Recommended drug therapy includes doxycycline, tetracycline, erythromycin, or sulfisoxazole for 7 days. Sexual partners should be treated if adolescent has had sexual contact within 30 days of onset of symptoms. Encourage use of condoms.
Genital herpes Causative organism: Herpes simplex virus (HSV-2) Incubation period: 2 to 12 days Reportable: No	Presentation can be variable and ranges from no symptoms to systemic involvement. A single lesion or a small cluster of papules appears anywhere on the genitalia, buttocks, or thighs. Papules develop into vesicles and pustules, and eventually ulcers. Ulcers can appear between vaginal folds, in posterior cervix, on glans penis or shaft of penis, in rectum, or in anus. Intense itching is followed by pain when ulcers break. Ulcers heal within 12 days. Lymph nodes closest to lesions are frequently enlarged.	Recommended drug therapy is acyclovir given for 7 to 10 days. Occasionally acyclovir is applied directly to lesions. Discourage oral sex if ulcers are present in mouth, on lips, in vagina, or on penis. Discourage anal sex when lesions are active. Encourage use of condoms.
Gonorrhea Causative organism: *Neisseria gonorrhoeae* Incubation period: 2 to 7 days Reportable: Mandatory	Symptoms and severity vary from mild to severe and are different for males and females. In females, areas that can be infected include urethra, cervix, fallopian tubes, and Bartholin and Skene glands. In males, areas include urethra, prostate, seminal vesicles, epididymis, and Littre and Cowper glands. Classic sign is discharge from vagina or urethra; however, infections involving conjunctivae, pharynx, and anus are also seen. Prepubescent girls: thick green or creamy vaginal discharge, vulvovaginitis. Adolescent girls: purulent vaginal discharge, cervicitis, PID. Fallopian tube involvement can lead to sterility. Prepubescent and adolescent boys: yellow puslike urethral discharge, erythematous meatus, frequency, dysuria.	Recommended drug therapy includes ceftriaxone or spectinomycin IM given once and followed by 7-day course of doxycycline. For *N. gonorrhoeae* that is non-penicillin resistant, amoxicillin and probenecid are given followed by doxycycline. Sexual partners should be treated. Follow-up cultures should be done 4 to 7 days after treatment. Encourage use of condoms.
Syphilis Causative organism: *Treponema pallidum* Incubation period: 3 weeks Reportable: Mandatory	Appearance of classic signs and symptoms of syphilis depends on stage of disease. *Primary stage* manifests as single lesion that appears at invasion site approximately 2 weeks to 3 months after infection. Lesion appears as ulcer that has indurated border and smooth base (chancre). It is painless and can appear on labia, within vagina, on glans penis, in anus, or on lips or tongue. Lymphadenopathy is usually present. Lesion spontaneously heals within 5 weeks. *Second stage* appears up to 10 weeks after initial infection. Child develops fever, sore throat, lymphadenopathy, malaise, and diffuse rash.[2] Lesions of rash can be macular, papular, papulosquamous, or bullous. Flat mucous patches called condylomata appear on genitals.[16,17] *Latent stage* follows beginning of second stage by about 6 weeks. Latent phase can last for several years or be lifelong.[18]	Recommended drug therapy includes single IM injection of benzathine penicillin G. For children allergic to penicillin, erythromycin is given by mouth for 15 days. Saline compresses and a topical antibiotic are often used to treat lesions on skin.[17] Treat all sexual contacts. Encourage use of condoms.

TABLE 18-16 Patient Education: Preventing STDs

- Limit the number of sexual contacts.
- Always use condoms for vaginal and anal intercourse.
- Refrain from oral sex if partner has active sores in mouth, vagina, or anus or on penis.
- Reduce high-risk sexual behaviors.

for the nurse to develop good assessment skills, particularly when asking questions about sexual activity, partners, and the possibility of abuse.

Nursing care focuses on identifying the cause and the organism, providing appropriate treatment, preventing transmission and complications, and educating the child, adolescent, and family (Table 18–16). When counseling the adolescent, the nurse should reinforce the importance of treating all sexual partners involved and modifying high-risk sexual behaviors. Be supportive and understanding—never judgmental.

REFERENCES

1 Behrman, R.E. (Ed.). (1992). *Nelson's textbook of pediatrics* (14th ed.). Philadelphia: W.B. Saunders.

2 Rudolph, A.M., Hoffman, J.I.E., & Rudolph, C.D. (1991). *Rudolph's pediatrics* (19th ed.). Norwalk, CT: Appleton & Lange.

3 Feeg, V., & Harbin, R.E. (1991). *Pediatric core curriculum and resource manual*. Pitman, NJ: Anthony J. Jannetti.

4 Tanagho, E.A., & McAninch, J.W. (1992). *Smith's general urology* (13th ed.). Norwalk, CT: Appleton & Lange.

5 Weir, M.R., & Lampe, R.M.F. (1984). Urinary tract infections in children. *American Family Physician, 29,* 149.

6 Edelmann, C.M. (1988). Urinary tract infection and vesicoureteral reflux. *Pediatric Annals, 17,* 9.

7 Hathaway, W.E., Hay, W.W., Jr., Groothuis, J.R., & Paisley, J.W. (1993). *Current pediatric diagnosis and treatment* (11th ed.). Norwalk, CT: Appleton & Lange.

8 Sobata, A.E. (1984). Inhibition of bacterial adherence by cranberry juice, potential use for the treatment of urinary tract infections. *Journal of Urology, 131,* 1013.

9 Edelmann, C.M., Jr. (1992). *Pediatric kidney disease* (2nd ed). Boston: Little, Brown.

10 Castiglia, P.T. (1987). Nocturnal enuresis. *Journal of Pediatric Health Care, 1,* 280.

11 Standfeld, J.M. (1973). Enuresis and urinary tract infection. *Clinics in Developmental Medicine, 49,* 102.

12 Kelsch, R.C., & Sedman, A.B. (1993). Nephrotic syndrome. *Pediatrics in Review, 14,* 33.

13 Long, S., Gaudio, K.M., & Siegel, N.J. (1992). Nondialytic treatment of acute renal failure. In Edelmann, C.M., Jr. (Ed.). *Pediatric kidney disease* (2nd ed.) (pp. 801–814). Boston: Little, Brown.

14 Last, J.M., & Wallace, R.B. (1992). *Public health and preventive medicine* (13th ed.). Norwalk, CT: Appleton & Lange.

15 Centers for Disease Control and Prevention, Division of Sexually Transmitted Diseases. *Annual report,* 1989 (1990). Atlanta: Author.

16 Bondi, E.E., Jesothy, B.V., & Lazarus, C.S. (1991). *Dermatology: Diagnosis and therapy.* Norwalk, CT: Appleton & Lange.

17 Habif, T.P. (1990). *Clinical dermatology: A color guide to diagnosis and therapy* (2nd ed). St. Louis: Mosby–Year Book.

18 Grimes, D. (1991). *Infectious diseases.* St. Louis: Mosby–Year Book.

SUGGESTED READINGS

Bernhardt, J. (1986). Percutaneous nephrostomy tubes in the neonate with obstructive uropathy. *Neonatal Network, 4,* 51–53.

Coleman, E.A. (1986). When the kidneys fail. *RN, 49,* 28–38.

Denson, C.E., & Terry, W.J. (1988). Hypospadias repair. *AORN Journal, 47,* 906–923.

Frauman, A.C., & Gilman, C.M. (1990). Care of the family of the child with end stage renal disease. *ANNA Journal, 17,* 383–386.

Horton, H.M., Crutchfield, P., & Garrison C. (1990). Hypospadias: When baby boys need surgery. *RN, 53,* 48–51.

Radebough, L.C. (1986). Nursing care of the infant with bladder exstrophy. *AUAA Journal, 2,* 14–15.

Strupp, T.W. (1988). Post shock resuscitation of the trauma victim: Preventing and managing acute renal failure. *Critical Care Nurse Quarterly, 11,* 1–9.

Thomas, C.K. (1982). Childhood urinary tract infection. *Pediatric Nursing, 8,* 114–119.

Wilson, D., & Killion, D. (1989). Urinary tract infections in the pediatric patient. *Nurse Practitioner, 14,* 38–42.

Wiseman, K.C. (1991). Nephrotic syndrome: Pathophysiology and treatment. *ANNA Journal, 188,* 469–476.

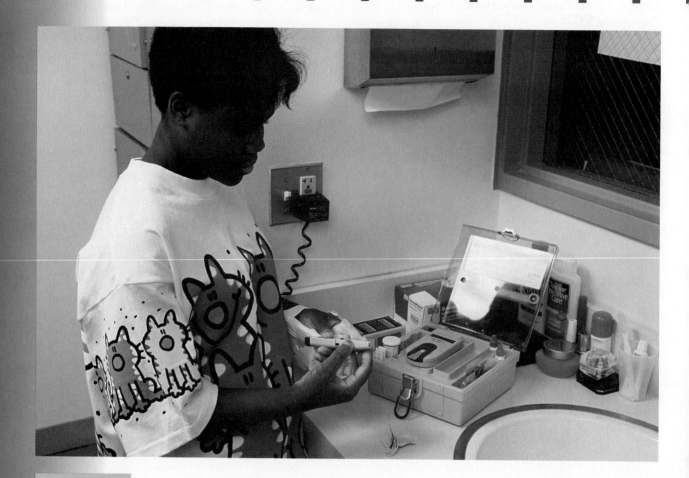

D anielle, 12 years old, has been vomiting sporadically for approximately 12 hours and is severely dehydrated and disoriented when she is brought to the emergency department. Her parents state that Danielle has complained of being constantly thirsty and hungry for the past week. Despite this she has lost 10 pounds. She had a viral illness about 1 month ago but has been well since. Her mother says that Danielle has seemed lethargic for about 3 days.

Danielle's pulse is rapid, and her respirations are shallow and labored. Routine laboratory evaluation reveals abnormal values for potassium and sodium and a glucose level of 762 mg/dL. Her urine contains large amounts of ketones and glucose. An intravenous infusion of one-quarter normal saline and an insulin drip are started to begin rehydration and to lower her blood glucose level.

Danielle has diabetic ketoacidosis, a complication of insulin-dependent diabetes mellitus. What causes diabetes? What treatment will Danielle require? What are the long-term implications of her diagnosis? During Danielle's hospitalization the nurses answer these questions and address other concerns raised by Danielle and her parents. They teach Danielle how to test her blood glucose level and administer insulin, and they reassure her that she can live a normal life despite her disease.

ALTERATIONS IN ENDOCRINE FUNCTION

TERMINOLOGY

glycosuria Abnormal amount of glucose in the urine.

goiter Enlargement of the thyroid gland.

hormone A chemical substance that is produced by a gland or organ and carried in the bloodstream to another part of the body where it has a regulatory effect on particular cells.

karyotype A microscopic display of the 46 chromosomes in the human body lined up from the largest to the smallest. The human female is 46,XX and the human male is 46,XY.

polydipsia Excessive thirst.

polyphagia Excessive or voracious eating.

polyuria Passage of a large volume of urine in a given period.

pseudohermaphroditism Ambiguous development of the external genitalia.

puberty Period of life when the ability to reproduce sexually begins; characterized by maturation of the genital organs, development of the secondary sex characteristics, and (in females) the onset of menstruation.

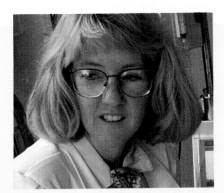

❝ It will be important for Danielle to take responsibility for performing diabetes self-care activities, such as testing blood glucose and administering insulin, to minimize episodes of hyperglycemia and hypoglycemia. **❞**

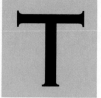

The endocrine system controls the cellular activity that regulates growth and body metabolism through the release of hormones. **Hormones** are chemical messengers secreted by various glands that exert controlling effects on the cells of the body. The general functions of the endocrine system include the following:

- Differentiation of the reproductive and central nervous systems in the fetus
- Stimulation of growth and development throughout childhood and adolescence
- Coordination of the male and female reproductive systems, enabling sexual reproduction
- Maintenance of an optimal level of hormones for body functioning

Endocrine disturbances result in alterations in metabolism, growth and development, and behavior that may have significant implications for children.

Inborn errors of metabolism—inherited biochemical abnormalities of the urea cycle and amino acid and organic acid metabolism—often have a significant impact on the endocrine system's ability to support growth and development. Some chromosomal abnormalities also result in disturbances in growth and sexual development. For these reasons inborn errors of metabolism and chromosome disorders are included in this chapter.

Most endocrine malfunctions are present at birth. They are often observed at birth or during the routine newborn assessment or detected by health care providers within the first year of life. If not diagnosed and treated early, these conditions can result in delays in growth and development, mental retardation, and, occasionally, death. However, treatment, which usually consists of supplementation of missing hormones, adjustment of hormone levels, or dietary measures, allows most children to live a normal life.

Most children with endocrine and metabolic disorders are treated on an outpatient basis. Children may be admitted to the hospital in cases of acute metabolic disturbance that occur before diagnosis or when treatment is inadequate. Children may also be admitted to the hospital for other acute problems even though their endocrine disorder is well controlled.

Anatomy and Physiology of Pediatric Differences

The endocrine glands include the hypothalamus, pituitary gland, thyroid gland, parathyroid glands, adrenal glands, ovaries, testes, and islets of Langerhans in the pancreas (Fig. 19–1). These glands secrete hormones into the bloodstream that are carried to target organs or tissues, enabling them to function properly (Table 19–1).

Endocrine glands usually regulate secretion of hormones by negative feedback to maintain an optimal internal environment. Negative feedback occurs when a gland receives a message that an adequate amount of hormone has been received by the target cells. The gland responds by inhibiting further secretion. Secretion is not resumed until the gland receives another message indicating that levels of the hormone are low.

The endocrine system is responsible for sexual differentiation during fetal development (Fig. 19–2) and for stimulating sequential growth and development during childhood and adolescence. This includes stimulating development of the reproductive system in both sexes.

Puberty (sexual maturation, lasting 2 to 3 years) occurs when the gonads secrete increased amounts of the sex hormones estrogen and testosterone. At the average age of 10 years in girls and 11 years in boys, the hypothalamus

FIGURE 19–1 Major organs and glands of the endocrine system.
Reproduced with permission from *Medical terminology: A programmed text*, 6th ed., by Genevieve Love Smith, Phyllis E. Davis, & Jean Tannis Dennerll. Albany, NY: Delmar Publishers, Inc., copyright 1991.

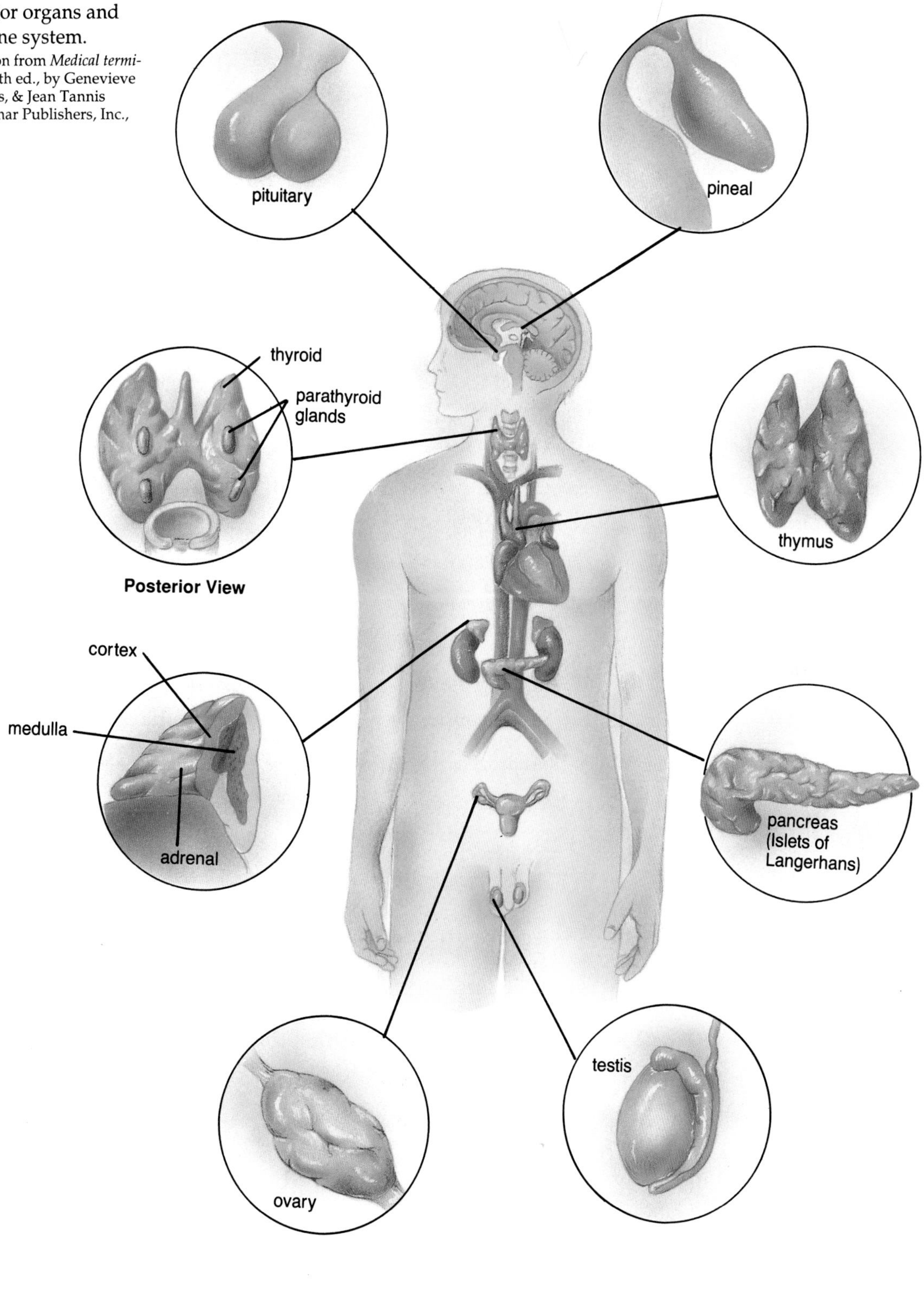

pituitary

pineal

thyroid

parathyroid glands

Posterior View

thymus

cortex

medulla

adrenal

pancreas (Islets of Langerhans)

ovary

testis

produces increased amounts of gonadotropin-releasing hormone. This hormone stimulates the anterior pituitary gland to increase the production of luteinizing hormone (LH) and follicle-stimulating hormone (FSH). These hormones in turn stimulate the gonads to secrete more sex hormones (Fig. 19–3), resulting in the development of primary and secondary sex characteristics.

TABLE 19-1 Endocrine Glands and Their Functions

Gland/Hormone	Function
Pituitary	
Growth hormone	Stimulates growth of all body tissues
Thyroid-stimulating hormone (TSH)	Stimulates thyroid hormone secretion
Adrenocorticotropic hormone (ACTH)	Stimulates secretion of glucocorticoids and androgens
Follicle-stimulating hormone (FSH)	Stimulates secretion of estrogen
Luteinizing hormone (LH)	Stimulates secretion of androgens in males and progesterone in females
Prolactin	Stimulates secretion of milk during lactation
Melanocyte-stimulating hormone (MSH)	Stimulates skin pigmentation
Antidiuretic hormone (ADH)	Stimulates permeability of renal tubules
Oxytocin	Stimulates uterine contractions and let-down reflex
Thyroid	
Thyroxine (T_4) and triiodothyronine (T_3)	Stimulates cellular growth rate
Thyrocalcitonin	Stimulates bone ossification and development
Parathyroid	
Parathyroid hormone	Stimulates reabsorption of calcium and excretion of phosphorus
Adrenal	
Aldosterone	Stimulates reabsorption of sodium and excretion of potassium
Androgens	Stimulates bone development and secondary sexual characteristics
Cortisol	Stimulates antiinflammatory reactions, among many other functions
Epinephrine	Activates sympathetic nervous system; stimulates increase in blood pressure and blood glucose levels
Pancreas (Islets of Langerhans)	
Insulin	Stimulates cellular glucose utilization
Glucagon	Stimulates hyperglycemia
Somatostatin	Stimulates inhibition of insulin and glucagon secretion; inhibits growth hormone; inhibits gastric acid secretion
Ovaries	
Estrogen	Stimulates development of breasts and ova
Progesterone	Stimulates breast glandular development; acts to maintain pregnancy
Testes	
Testosterone	Stimulates production of sperm, development of secondary sexual characteristics, and closure of epiphysis

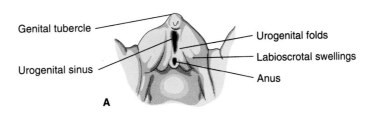

Undifferentiated

Genital tubercle

Urogenital folds

Labioscrotal swellings

Urogenital sinus

Anus

A

7 weeks

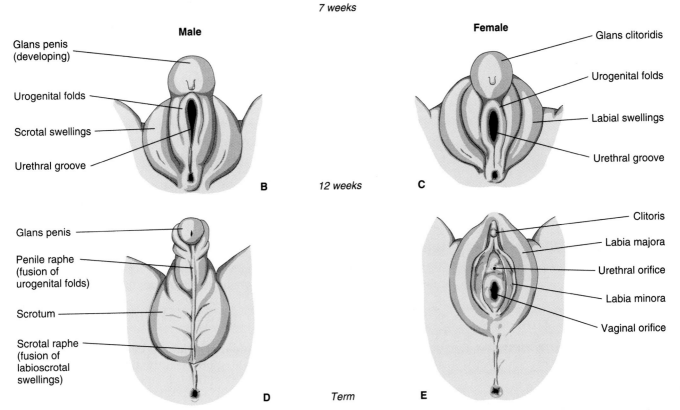

Male

Glans penis (developing)

Urogenital folds

Scrotal swellings

Urethral groove

B

12 weeks

Female

Glans clitoridis

Urogenital folds

Labial swellings

Urethral groove

C

Glans penis

Penile raphe (fusion of urogenital folds)

Scrotum

Scrotal raphe (fusion of labioscrotal swellings)

D

Term

Clitoris

Labia majora

Urethral orifice

Labia minora

Vaginal orifice

E

FIGURE 19–2 Sexual differentiation. **A,** At 7 weeks' gestation, male and female genitalia are identical (undifferentiated). **B** and **C,** By 12 weeks' gestation, noticeable differentiation begins to occur. **D** and **E,** Differentiation continues until birth but is almost complete at term stage.

FIGURE 19–3 Feedback mechanism in hormonal stimulation of the gonads during puberty.

Feedback mechanism

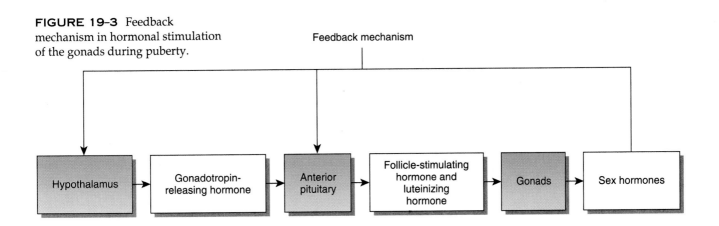

Hypopituitarism (Growth Hormone Deficiency)

Hypopituitarism is a disorder caused by decreased activity of the pituitary gland. Because most children with this disorder secrete inadequate amounts of growth hormone, the term "hypopituitarism" is often used interchangeably with "growth hormone deficiency." An estimated 1 in 4000 school-age children has growth hormone deficiency.[1]

Children with hypopituitarism are of normal weight and length when born. By the age of 1 year, however, they are below the third percentile on the growth chart. They characteristically grow at a rate of less than 5 cm per year. Other characteristic findings in infants include hypoglycemic seizures, neonatal jaundice, micropenis, and undescended testicles.[1] Children with hypopituitarism tend to be overweight and to have youthful facial features, delayed dentition, "ripply" abdominal fat, delayed skeletal maturation, delayed sexual maturation, and hypoglycemia.[1,2]

The release of growth hormone from the anterior pituitary gland is controlled by the hypothalamus, which secretes releasing and inhibitory factors. Growth hormone stimulates the growth of all body tissues. It also stimulates the synthesis of proteins in the liver, among them the somatomedins or insulin-like growth factors (IGFs), which promote glucose utilization by the cells and cell proliferation.

Infection, infarction of the pituitary gland (related to sickle cell disease), central nervous system disease, and tumors of the pituitary gland or hypothalamus (primarily craniopharyngiomas and gliomas) may cause hypopituitarism or growth hormone deficiency by interfering with the production or release of growth hormone. In approximately 80% of affected children, however, the cause is unknown. In these cases it is suspected that the pituitary gland or hypothalamus became damaged or malformed during fetal development or at birth.[1]

Any child whose height is 3 standard deviations below the mean height for age or whose measurement is falling off the normal growth chart should be evaluated for short stature. A child whose screening tests reveal low levels of IGF-1 requires further evaluation by a pediatric endocrinologist. A careful history, physical examination, and radiologic studies are necessary to rule out familial short stature, constitutional growth delay, skeletal dysplasias, or psychosocial dwarfism. Provocative growth hormone testing, in which various medications (arginine, clonidine, glucagon, insulin, L-dopa) are administered to stimulate release of growth hormone, is the definitive diagnostic test in most children.

Treatment depends on the cause of the deficiency. In most cases treatment consists of replacement of the missing growth hormone and outpatient follow-up to monitor the child's growth. The development of a synthetic form of growth hormone has greatly increased the supply of this medication. Most children receive subcutaneous injections three times a week. Replacement therapy is continued until the child achieves an acceptable height or fails to respond to treatment. Early diagnosis and treatment are important to ensure attainment of maximum adult height potential.

Nursing Management

Nursing care consists of monitoring growth, teaching the child and family about the disorder and its treatment, and providing emotional support. The child's height and weight are carefully measured (see Atlas of Pediatric Procedures) and plotted on a growth chart (see Appendix A).

■ PSYCHOSOCIAL DWARFISM

Psychosocial dwarfism is a syndrome of emotional deprivation that causes suppression of production of pituitary hormones. Treatment involves removal of the child from the stressful environment and normal dietary intake. Pituitary secretion is usually restored, and dramatic catch-up growth in height is observed.

■ ETHICAL CONSIDERATIONS

The increased availability of synthetic growth hormone has led to questions about the use of this medication for children who are below average for height but not growth hormone deficient. The medication is expensive (up to $20,000 per year), and its long-term effects are still being investigated.

■ CULTURAL CONSIDERATIONS

In the United States, tall stature is associated with positive attributes, including success, wealth, and power. This has resulted in societal discrimination against many short children and adults. Be alert to hidden value judgments and assumptions regarding height.[3]

Teach the parents and child about the growth hormone replacement therapy and provide the parents with educational resources (Table 19–2). Since replacement therapy is expensive and usually is not covered by insurance, parents may need help with finances. National organizations such as the Human Growth Foundation and the Short Stature Foundation (see Appendix F) are sources of additional information.

Children with growth hormone deficiency may have academic problems resulting from learning disabilities and below-average intelligence.[3] Before the child enters school, a comprehensive evaluation should be performed to identify potential problems.

People often treat short children on the basis of their size rather than their age, and such children experience social prejudice related to height.[3] Teasing is a common problem. The teenage years may be particularly stressful because of the preoccupation with body image characteristic of adolescence.

Encourage parents and teachers to treat the child in an age-appropriate manner. The child should dress in clothing that reflects chronologic age. Emphasize the child's strengths, support independence, and encourage participation in age-appropriate activities to aid in the development of a positive self-image. Suggest that the child take part in sports in which ability does not depend on size (e.g., swimming, wrestling, martial arts). Identifying positive role models, short individuals who are successful in accomplishing their goals, is another approach that promotes a positive image.[3] Refer the child for counseling if appropriate.

Hyperpituitarism

Hyperpituitarism, a disorder in which excessive secretion of growth hormone increases the growth rate, is rare in children.

Oversecretion of growth hormone is usually caused by a pituitary adenoma. Another possible cause is a tumor of the hypothalamus. Affected children can grow to 7 or 8 feet in height when oversecretion occurs before closure of the epiphyseal plates.

Because tall stature is valued in our society, assessment of children (particularly boys) with accelerated growth is often delayed.[4] Any child whose predicted height exceeds that consistent with parental height should be evaluated for possible growth problems and underlying pathologic conditions.

A complete history is obtained, and physical examination and laboratory testing are performed. Increased levels of IGF-1 establish the diagnosis of hyperpituitarism. A bone scan is usually obtained to determine whether the epiphyseal plates have begun to fuse. Radiologic studies are used to detect a tumor. Thorough evaluation is required to differentiate hyperpituitarism from familial tall stature.

Treatment depends on the cause of the excessive growth and may involve surgical removal of a tumor, radiation therapy, or oral administration of bromocriptine, which suppresses secretion of growth hormone.

Nursing Management

Tall stature, like short stature, can be stressful for children. Tall children are often treated as if they are older than their chronologic age. Tall adolescents may have problems with self-image, and girls in particular may worry about their appearance.

Nursing care focuses on teaching the parents and child about the disorder and its treatment, providing emotional support, and, if surgery is required, providing preoperative and postoperative teaching and care (see Chapter 4).

Diabetes Insipidus

Diabetes insipidus, a rare disorder of the posterior pituitary gland, is characterized by a deficiency of antidiuretic hormone (ADH), or vasopressin. ADH facilitates concentration of the urine by stimulating reabsorption of water from the distal tubule of the kidney. When ADH is inadequate, the tubules do not resorb, leading to polyuria. Two forms of diabetes insipidus occur in children: true (or central) ADH deficiency and nephrogenic diabetes insipidus, in which the kidneys are unable to respond to the ADH that is present.

Polyuria (large volume of urine) and **polydipsia** (excessive thirst) are the cardinal signs of diabetes insipidus. The child is thirsty even at night and becomes irritable when fluid is withheld. Nocturia and enuresis may occur in the previously toilet-trained child. Constipation, fever, and dehydration also may occur because body fluid is depleted or thirst is not satisfied. Although the onset of symptoms is usually sudden, diagnosis is often delayed. Children who are able to quench their thirst may not complain to parents about symptoms.

True ADH deficiency in children is usually familial or idiopathic. Secondary causes include tumors of the hypothalamus, infiltrative diseases such as histiocytosis or leukemia, and in occasional cases inflammatory conditions such as encephalitis or meningitis, neurosurgical trauma, and autoimmune disorders.[5] Nephrogenic diabetes insipidus may be familial, with either an X-linked or an autosomal recessive form, or it may result from drug toxicity or recurrent infection.

Dehydration usually precipitates diagnosis. Serum sodium concentration and osmolality increase rapidly to pathologic levels. Often an unconscious child is admitted to the emergency department with dehydration accompanied by hypernatremia.

Serum electrolytes and both serum and urine osmolalities are tested. Diagnosis is confirmed by a water deprivation test, which is usually conducted in the hospital or in a carefully controlled outpatient setting. Parents should be advised that the child will be frustrated and irritable from thirst. No one should drink in front of the child during the testing period. Fluids are restricted until the child has lost 3% to 5% of body weight. During this time, urine output and specific gravity are measured. The child's output will exceed intake and urine will not be excessively concentrated; more concentrated urine is normally seen with fluid restriction.

Treatment of true ADH deficiency consists of the intranasal or intramuscular administration of desmopressin, or DDAVP (1-deamino-8-D-arginine vasopressin), a synthetic analogue of vasopressin. DDAVP reduces urinary output, enabling the child to live a more normal life with a decrease in thirst, urinary output, and nocturia. DDAVP is not effective in controlling nephrogenic diabetes insipidus. Children with nephrogenic diabetes insipidus are treated with diuretics and a salt- and protein-restricted diet. The child's sodium and potassium levels must be carefully monitored to prevent hypernatremia and hypokalemia (see Chapter 7).

Nursing Management

Nursing care centers on administering medications and teaching parents how to manage the condition and recognize signs of altered fluid status. Parent education is of primary importance. Infants usually need fluid intake even during the night. Many infants have coexisting brain damage and decreased thirst and require nasogastric or gastrostomy feeding to maintain adequate hydration.

Teach parents to recognize signs of inadequate fluid intake (see Chapter 7) and to adjust the child's fluid intake to prevent dehydration. When an acute illness occurs, the child's physician should be notified immediately because the increase in metabolic activity will necessitate administration of additional fluid to prevent dehydration.

Parents may need assistance to manage the child's care. Arrangements for a visiting nurse, a home health nurse, or respite care may be needed.

Precocious Puberty

Puberty normally occurs between 8 and 13 years of age in girls and between 9½ and 14 years of age in boys. Precocious puberty is defined as breast development with growth of pubic hair before age 8 in girls or testicular growth greater than 3 cm in diameter with development of pubic hair before age 9 in boys.[6] Precocious puberty is nine times more common in girls than in boys.[2] Early puberty is inherited in 5% to 10% of boys.[7]

Early secretion of the normal hormones responsible for pubertal changes usually is not associated with abnormalities. However, a benign hypothalamic tumor may be present. Other causes include cerebral trauma, central nervous system disorder, infection, chronic adrenal insufficiency, and severe hypothyroidism.[4] Children with precocious puberty have premature skeletal maturation and may appear unusually tall for their age. Their growth ceases prematurely, however, as the hormones stimulate closure of the epiphyseal plates, resulting in short stature.[2]

Because the cause of the condition usually cannot be treated, management focuses on altering hormonal balance. A synthetic form of luteinizing hormone–releasing factor (Leuprolide) is used to slow or arrest the progression of puberty. The medication is administered either monthly by intramuscular injection or daily by subcutaneous injection. Treatment is continued until the child reaches a more appropriate age for puberty. Hormone levels are monitored to ensure maintenance of prepubertal levels, which results in regression or cessation of accelerated physical development.

Nursing Management

Nursing care centers on teaching the child and parents about the condition and its treatment and providing emotional support. The child should be informed in age-appropriate terms that physiologic changes are normal but occurring at an earlier than usual age. The child should be dressed in a manner appropriate to his or her chronologic age, even though the child may look older.

Children with precocious puberty become self-conscious as body changes occur. Provide privacy during examinations. Encourage the child to express his or her feelings about the changes. The child may need to practice role playing as a coping mechanism to manage teasing by other children.

Boys may become more aggressive and develop a sex drive as a result of hormonal changes. Parents should be advised that they may need to discuss issues of sexuality with the child. Refer the child for counseling if appropriate.

Disorders of Altered Thyroid Function

Hypothyroidism

Hypothyroidism is a disorder in which levels of active thyroid hormones are decreased. It may be congenital or acquired. Congenital hypothyroidism occurs in approximately 1 in 4000 live births and is twice as common in girls as in boys.[5] It is less prevalent in black infants but more frequent in Hispanic infants (1 in 2000 births). It also occurs more commonly in children with Down syndrome. Acquired hypothyroidism occurs after the child is 2 years old and is more common in girls than in boys.

Clinical Manifestations

Infants with congenital hypothyroidism have few clinical signs of the disorder in the first weeks of life. The characteristic cretinoid features (thickened protuberant tongue, thick lips, dull appearance) appear during the first few months of life in untreated infants. These signs are rarely seen today because routine screening within a few days of birth identifies most infants with the disorder, enabling early treatment. Other signs of congenital hypothyroidism include prolonged neonatal jaundice, hypotonia, bradycardia, cool extremities, mottling, umbilical hernia, a posterior fontanel larger than 1 cm in diameter, difficulty feeding, and a hoarse cry.

Children with acquired hypothyroidism have many of the same signs as adults: decreased appetite, dry skin, coarse hair or hair loss, depressed deep tendon reflexes, bradycardia, constipation, and an enlarged thyroid gland or a goiter. Manifestations unique to children include growth retardation, delayed bone age, muscle hypertrophy with muscle weakness, and either delayed or precocious puberty.[5]

Etiology and Pathophysiology

Congenital hypothyroidism is usually caused by a spontaneous gene mutation, an autosomal recessive genetic transmission of an enzyme deficiency, failure of the central nervous system–thyroid feedback mechanism to develop, or iodine deficiency. Acquired hypothyroidism can result from autoimmune thyroiditis, late-onset thyroid dysfunction, isolated thyroid-stimulating hormone (TSH) deficiency, an inborn error of thyroid hormone synthesis, or exposure to drugs or substances such as lithium that interfere with thyroid hormone synthesis.

The thyroid hormones are important for growth and development and for the metabolism of nutrients and energy. When the thyroid hormones are not available for stimulation of other hormones or specific target cells, growth is delayed and mental retardation develops.

Diagnostic Tests and Medical Management

Congenital hypothyroidism is usually detected during newborn screening of thyroxine (T_4) and TSH levels. If the T_4 level is below normal and the TSH level is increased, the synthetic thyroid hormone levothyroxine (Synthroid) is prescribed. The dose is increased gradually as the child grows to ensure a euthyroid (normal thyroid) state. Treatment is monitored by a pediatric endocrinologist. Periodic evaluation of T_4 serum level and bone age and careful monitoring of growth parameters are necessary to assess for signs of excess or inadequate thyroid hormone.

To ensure an adequate growth rate and prevent mental retardation, the hormone must be taken throughout life. Children with congenital hypothyroidism that is diagnosed before 3 months of age have the best prognosis for optimal mental development. Children with acquired hypothyroidism usually have normal growth following a period of catch-up growth.

Nursing Assessment

Routine neonatal screening may be performed before discharge from the hospital to evaluate levels of circulating thyroid hormones. However, many newborns are currently discharged before 24 hours of life. Nurses frequently make home visits a few days later to assess the health of the mother and infant. Neonatal screening may be performed at that visit (Table 19–3). Alternatively, T_4 and TSH screenings may be performed in a health care facility soon after birth.

Accurate measurement and recording of height and weight are performed at each follow-up visit. The child is assessed for signs of inadequate thyroid hormone to monitor compliance with medication or need for additional dosage with growth.

Nursing Diagnosis

Common nursing diagnoses for the child with hypothyroidism include the following:

- Altered Nutrition: Less Than Body Requirements related to poor appetite or inability to utilize nutrients fully
- Hypothermia related to lowered metabolic rate
- Constipation related to decreased bowel motility
- Fatigue related to an imbalance in energy production
- High Risk for Altered Health Maintenance related to parental knowledge deficit of treatment regimen

Nursing Management

Nursing care focuses on teaching the parents and child about the disorder and its treatment and monitoring the child's growth rate. When the cause is

---

TABLE 19-3 Blood Collection Tips for Neonatal Screening

To reduce errors in collection of blood for neonatal screening:
1. Collect blood before 72 hours of age. If blood is collected before 24 hours of age, repeat screening before 14 days of age.
2. Perform a heel stick and collect one large drop on the infant's heel.
3. Fill the entire circle on a clean filter paper. Apply blood to only one side of the filter paper.
4. Allow the paper to air dry at room temperature in a horizontal position.
5. Make sure all patient information is provided on the screening form to ensure that the infant can be found if the result is abnormal.
6. Mail the specimen to the laboratory within 24 hours of collection.

genetic, a referral for genetic counseling should be made. Explain how to administer thyroid hormone (e.g., tablets can be crushed and mixed in a small amount of formula or applesauce). Advise parents that the child may experience temporary sleep disturbances or behavioral changes in response to therapy. Teach the parents how to assess for increased pulse, which can indicate the presence of excess thyroid hormone, and to report problems such as fatigue, which may indicate improper drug dose.

Caution parents to dress the child appropriately for the season to prevent hypothermia. Modify the child's diet by increasing the amount of fruits and bulk if constipation is a problem.

Reassure the family that the child will develop normally with hormone replacement therapy. Reinforce the importance of follow-up visits to assess growth rate and response to therapy and to regulate drug dosages as the child grows. Parents should be informed that therapy will be lifelong and is needed to promote the child's mental development.

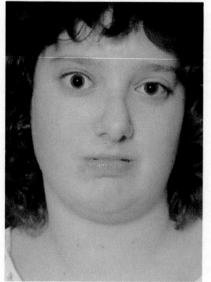

FIGURE 19–4 Exophthalmos and an enlarged thyroid in an adolescent with Graves disease.

From Zitelli, B.J., & Davis, H.W. (Eds.) (1987). *Atlas of pediatric physical diagnosis* (p. 9.6). New York: Mosby–Year Book Europe Ltd.

Hyperthyroidism

Hyperthyroidism occurs when thyroid hormone levels are increased (thyrotoxicosis). It is most common in adolescent girls and is almost always due to Graves disease.

Clinical Manifestations

Characteristic findings include **goiter** (an enlarged, nontender thyroid gland), prominent or bulging eyes (exophthalmos) (Fig. 19–4), tachycardia, nervousness, irritability, increased appetite, weight loss, emotional lability, heat intolerance, and muscle weakness. The thyroid gland may be slightly enlarged or grow to three to four times its normal size, feel warm, soft, and fleshy, and have an auditory bruit on auscultation. Onset is subtle, and the condition often goes unrecognized for 1 to 2 years.

Children with Graves disease usually manifest behavioral problems and declining performance in school. They become easily frustrated in the classroom and overheated and fatigued during physical education class. It is difficult for them to relax or sleep. These symptoms usually prompt parents to seek medical treatment for them.

Etiology and Pathophysiology

Graves disease is an autoimmune disorder in which the body produces antibodies that attack the cells of the thyroid gland. It has a high familial incidence. Immunoglobulins produced by the B lymphocytes stimulate oversecretion of thyroid hormones, resulting in the clinical symptoms. Signs and symptoms such as tachycardia, tremor, excessive perspiration, irritability, and emotional lability are caused by hyperactivity of the sympathetic nervous system.

Other, more unusual forms of hyperthyroidism result from thyroiditis and thyroid hormone–producing tumors, including thyroid adenomas and carcinomas, and pituitary adenomas.

Diagnostic Tests and Medical Management

Diagnostic studies include laboratory evaluation of serum T_3 (triiodothyronine), T_4, and TSH levels and a thyroid scan. Blood studies are also performed to detect autoantibodies specific for the various thyroid disorders.

The goal of medical management is to inhibit excessive secretion of thy-

Propylthiouracil therapy can cause temporary side effects, including mild itching and lymphadenopathy. If fever or sore throat develops, the child should be evaluated by a health care professional to rule out leukopenia.

roid hormones. Treatment may include antithyroid drug therapy, surgery, or radiation therapy. Drug therapy is most often used as the initial treatment modality. Propylthiouracil (PTU) and methimazole (Tapazole) are given to inhibit thyroid hormone secretion. Treatment continues for 18 months to 2 years or until the disease runs its course. Symptoms usually improve within weeks of starting treatment. If drug therapy is ineffective, thyroidectomy or radiation therapy using radioactive iodide (^{131}I) may be used. Removal or destruction of the thyroid gland results in permanent hypothyroidism, necessitating hormone replacement therapy.

Nursing Assessment

Assess the child's vital signs, since blood pressure and pulse may be elevated. Keep a record of food intake. Accurate measurement and recording of height and weight are important to establish baselines and identify patterns of growth. Observe the child's behavior, activity, and level of fatigue.

Nursing Diagnosis

Common nursing diagnoses for the child with hyperthyroidism include the following:
- Ineffective Thermoregulation (Elevated) related to excessive activity of the sympathetic nervous system
- Altered Nutrition: Less Than Body Requirements related to increased metabolic rate
- Body Image Disturbance related to presence of prominent eyes, excessive perspiration, and tremors
- Fatigue related to imbalance in energy production, muscle weakness, and sleep disturbance
- Self-Concept Disturbance related to declining school performance and behavior problems

Nursing Management

Nursing care focuses on teaching the child and parents about the disorder and its treatment, promoting rest, providing emotional support, and, if the child requires surgery, providing preoperative and postoperative teaching and care. Promote increased caloric intake by providing five or six moderate meals per day. Encourage the child and family to express their feelings and concerns about the disorder. Pointing out even slight improvements in the child's condition increases compliance with therapy. Children with hyperthyroidism are easily fatigued. Rest periods should be scheduled at school and home and physical activities kept to a minimum until symptoms resolve. Encourage parents to provide a cool environment, and allow the child to wear fewer clothes until symptoms subside.

Children who have partial or total removal of the thyroid gland receive antithyroid drugs, such as iodide, for approximately 2 weeks before surgery. Teach the child and parents about drug therapy and instruct parents to watch for side effects of antithyroid drugs, including fever, urticaria, and lymphadenopathy. Provide preoperative teaching (see Chapter 4). Young children, in particular, may be fearful about having their throat "cut." Postoperatively, observe for signs of severe thyrotoxicosis (thyroid "storm") and hypercalcemia, which can be life threatening. Treatment includes administration of antithyroid drugs and propranolol. Monitor the child's surgical site. Assess the child for bleeding, hoarseness, and difficulty breathing, which may be signs of inflammation.

■ NURSING ALERT

Thyroid storm may occur when thyroid hormone is suddenly released into the bloodstream during surgery. The child experiences fever, diaphoresis, and tachycardia, progressing to shock and, if untreated, death.

Disorders of Altered Parathyroid Function

Hyperparathyroidism

Hyperparathyroidism is a rare disorder in children. It is characterized by overproduction of parathyroid hormone. Hyperparathyroidism is most often a primary condition caused by adenoma or hyperplasia of the parathyroid gland. Familial hyperparathyroidism, which occurs infrequently, may be transmitted by autosomal dominant inheritance.[5] Hyperparathyroidism may also occur secondary to chronic renal disease and rickets.

Parathyroid hormone acts on the kidney, bone, and intestine to increase calcium reabsorption. Thus excessive levels of parathyroid hormone result in signs of hypercalcemia. Clinical manifestations include generalized weakness and hypotonicity of muscles, behavioral changes, nausea, vomiting, constipation, abdominal pain, and weight loss. Bone pain and bone changes also may occur. Polydipsia and polyuria may be renal responses to hypercalcemia. (Refer to Chapter 7 for additional discussion of hypercalcemia.)

Diagnosis is based on the clinical findings, laboratory evaluation, which reveals elevated serum calcium levels and decreased phosphorus levels, and radiographic studies, which show destructive changes in bones and may reveal a parathyroid tumor. Renal function studies also may be performed. Surgery to remove a majority of the parathyroid gland is the treatment of choice for primary hyperparathyroidism. Secondary hyperparathyroidism is managed by treating the underlying disease, usually with a low-phosphorus diet and medications (calcium, vitamin D, and aluminum hydroxide [binds with dietary phosphorus and is excreted in feces; decreases amount of phosphorus in urine]).

FOODS THAT CONTAIN HIGH LEVELS OF PHOSPHORUS

Meat
Fish
Poultry
Milk
Soft drinks

SAFETY PRECAUTIONS

Surgical removal of the parathyroid glands can result in hypocalcemia. Observe for signs of anxiety, neuromuscular excitability, and tetany. Be sure that calcium gluconate is available for emergency use.

Nursing Management

Nursing care focuses on teaching the parents and child about the disorder, promoting compliance with the diet and medication regimen, and providing emotional support for the child and family. The parents may be referred for genetic counseling and family studies. For children undergoing surgery, provide preoperative and postoperative teaching and care (see Chapter 4). Frequent blood calcium measurements are essential postoperatively.

Disorders of Altered Adrenal Function

Cushing Syndrome

Cushing syndrome, also called adrenocortical hyperfunction, is characterized by a group of symptoms resulting from excess levels of glucocorticoids (especially cortisol) in the bloodstream. It is uncommon in children and occurs more often in girls than boys.[2] During infancy and childhood, most cases are due to malignant adrenal tumor. After 8 years of age more than half of the cases are due to secretion of adrenocorticotropic hormone (ACTH) by a pituitary adenoma.[9]

The initial sign in most children is generalized obesity. The affected child has the characteristic "cushingoid" appearance, which includes a moon face (chubby cheeks and a double chin) and fat pads over the shoulders and back (buffalo hump). Other signs and symptoms include hypertension, weight gain with distribution primarily on the trunk, striae on the abdomen, buttocks, and thighs, muscle weakness and wasting, bruising, osteoporosis, growth failure with delayed bone age, and delayed puberty.

CLINICAL TIP

Cushingoid features may also be noted in children being treated with high doses of corticosteroids for other diseases. Corticosteroids suppress adrenal function when given long term. These children do not have Cushing syndrome.

Causes of Cushing syndrome include tumors of the pituitary gland that result in an overproduction of ACTH (which stimulates cortisol secretion), tumors of the adrenal glands, and hyperplasia of one or both adrenal glands.

Increased secretion of cortisol alters metabolism, resulting in catabolism of protein, leading to capillary weakness and poor wound healing; decreased absorption of calcium from the intestines, leading to demineralization of the bone and osteoporosis; an increased appetite, leading to the accumulation of fat; and salt-retaining activity of cortisol, leading to an increase in blood volume and hypertension.

Diagnosis is based on characteristic physical findings and laboratory values, including reduced serum levels of potassium and phosphorus; elevated serum calcium concentration; increased urinary levels of free cortisol, 17-hydroxycorticosteroid (17-OHC), and 6β-hydroxycortisol; and loss of diurnal rhythm in serum cortisol (usually elevated at night).

The adrenal suppression test is used for initial screening of children with suspected adrenocortical hyperfunction. When adrenal cortisol output is not suppressed overnight after a dose of dexamethasone, further diagnostic testing is necessary to determine the cause of hypercortisolism. Computed tomography (CT) and magnetic resonance imaging (MRI) are used to detect tumors in the adrenal and pituitary glands.

Surgical removal is the current treatment of choice for adrenal tumors or pituitary adenomas. Cortisol replacement is required when both adrenal glands are removed. The prognosis for children with malignant adrenal tumors is poor.

Nursing Management

The nurse usually encounters a child with Cushing syndrome when the child is hospitalized for diagnostic evaluation or surgery. Nursing assessment includes monitoring the child's vital signs and fluid and nutritional status. Assess muscle strength and endurance during hospital play activities.

Teach the child and family about the disorder and its treatment, and, for children undergoing surgery, provide preoperative and postoperative teaching and care. Answer any questions the child and family have and explain all laboratory and diagnostic tests. Explain to parents that the child's cushingoid appearance is reversible with treatment. Provide nutritional guidance to the child and parents or referral to a nutritionist to promote maintenance of an appropriate weight.

Preoperative and postoperative teaching and care are similar to those for the child undergoing surgery (see Chapter 4). Refer to Chapter 16 for general nursing care of the child with cancer.

For children who require cortisol replacement therapy, administering the drug early in the morning or every other day causes fewer symptoms than daily administration and mimics the normal diurnal pattern of cortisol secretion. Cortisol replacement in the postoperative period must be explained carefully to parents. Hydrocortisone (Cortef, Solu-Cortef, cortisone acetate) comes in liquid, tablet, or injectable form. Teach parents how and when to administer the injectable hydrocortisone. The oral preparations of cortisone have a bitter taste and can cause gastric irritation. Giving the dose at mealtimes and using antacids help reduce these side effects.

Teach parents to be alert to the signs of acute adrenal insufficiency during the withdrawal of corticosteroid therapy. They must inform all health care providers of the child's condition and medication.

Congenital Adrenal Hyperplasia

Congenital adrenal hyperplasia, sometimes called adrenogenital syndrome, adrenocortical hyperplasia, or congenital adrenogenital hyperplasia, is an autosomal recessive disorder that causes a deficiency of various enzymes necessary for the synthesis of cortisol. It occurs in 1 in 12,000 live births.[8]

■ **NURSING ALERT**

Signs of acute adrenal insufficiency may include increased irritability, headache, confusion, restlessness, nausea and vomiting, diarrhea, abdominal pain, dehydration, fever, loss of appetite, and lethargy. If untreated, the child will go into shock.

More than 80% of children with congenital adrenal hyperplasia have partial or complete 21-hydroxylase enzyme deficiency. Another 10% have 11-hydroxylase deficiency. The remainder have deficiencies in five other enzymes. In its most severe form the disorder can be life threatening.

Clinical Manifestations

Congenital adrenal hyperplasia is the most common cause of **pseudohermaphroditism** (ambiguous genitalia) in newborn girls. The female infant is born with an enlarged clitoris and labial fusions (Fig. 19–5). The male may be born with an enlarged penis and hyperpigmented scrotum. Partial enzyme deficiency produces less obvious symptoms. Precocious puberty and tall stature for age may be noted later. Recurrent vomiting, dehydration, metabolic acidosis, hypotension, and hypoglycemia are characteristic signs of the salt-wasting form of the disorder. Hypertension with hypokalemic alkalosis is alternately found in children with 11-hydroxylase deficiency.

Etiology and Pathophysiology

In all forms, increased secretion of ACTH occurs in response to diminished cortisol levels. In cases of 21-hydroxylase enzyme deficiency, there is usually deficient aldosterone synthesis leading to excess renal excretion of salt (salt wasting).

During fetal development the lack of cortisol results in excessive secretion of ACTH, which causes continued androgen secretion by the adrenal glands. Female virilization of the external genitalia causes sexual ambiguity at birth. In boys the external genitalia may appear normal to the examiner. If untreated, the overproduction of androgens results in accelerated height, early closure of the epiphyseal plates, and premature sexual development.

Diagnostic Tests and Medical Management

Diagnosis in infants and children is usually confirmed by laboratory evaluation of serum 17-hydroxyprogesterone (17-OHP) level. Routine newborn

FIGURE 19–5 Newborn girl with ambiguous genitalia.
Courtesy of Patrick C. Walsh, M.D.

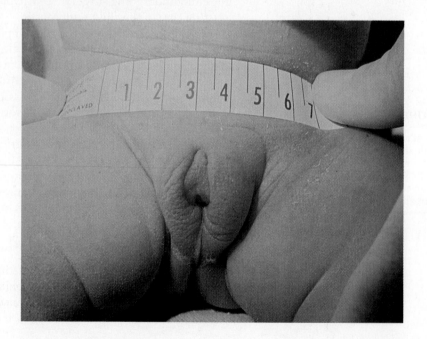

screening for congenital adrenal hyperplasia is performed in six states.[8] In instances of ambiguous genitalia a **karyotype** (chromosome study) is obtained to determine the sex of the infant. Ultrasonography may be used to visualize pelvic structures. In the salt-wasting form of the disorder the child may have hyponatremia, hyperkalemia, a high urine sodium level, and low serum and urinary aldosterone levels.

The goal of treatment is to suppress adrenal secretion of androgens by replacing deficient hormones. This is accomplished by oral administration of glucocorticoids (hydrocortisone). The glucocorticoid replacement results in reduced ACTH release and overstimulation of the adrenal cortex. Excessive adrenal androgen production is suppressed. Growth parameters and sexual development are closely monitored to watch for return to a more normal rate. If the infant has the salt-wasting form of the disorder, salt is added to the infant's formula and a mineralocorticoid (Florinef) is given to replace the missing hormone. Hormone dosage must be increased during acute illnesses and for surgery.

Reconstructive surgery of the enlarged clitoris is often performed on girls during the first year of life.[2] Vaginal reconstruction is performed in a later procedure.

Nursing Assessment

Assess the infant and child for signs of dehydration, electrolyte imbalance, and shock in the salt-wasting form of the disease. Monitor vital signs and assess peripheral perfusion (capillary refill, distal pulses, color and temperature of the extremities) frequently to detect early changes in condition.

Assess the parents for their emotional response to a child with ambiguous genitalia. Explore their values and beliefs regarding gender roles and sexuality while awaiting results of the karyotype.

Nursing Diagnosis

Common nursing diagnoses for the child with congenital adrenal hyperplasia include:
- High Risk for Altered Parenting related to child with congenital defect
- High Risk for Caregiver Role Strain related to care of a child with a chronic, potentially life-threatening condition
- High Risk for Fluid Volume Deficit related to excess excretion of salt by the kidneys
- Altered Growth and Development related to premature development of secondary sex characteristics and accelerated growth

Nursing Management

Nursing care of the newborn with congenital adrenal hyperplasia focuses on teaching parents about the disorder and its treatment, giving emotional support, and providing preoperative and postoperative teaching for parents of infants undergoing reconstructive surgery.

It is often difficult for parents to accept that their infant, whose genitalia look male, is really female. With medication and surgery the genitalia assume a female appearance and all organs necessary for future childbearing are usually functional. Nurses can assist parents in educating the child's siblings, grandparents, other family members, and babysitters about the condition. In the newborn nursery the infant should be referred to as "your beautiful infant," not "your son" or "your daughter," until gender identity is confirmed.

Explain the medication regimen and teach parents how to administer intramuscular injections of hydrocortisone. Make sure the parents have an emergency kit of injectable hydrocortisone at home to be used when the child is vomiting or has diarrhea. Teach parents about the special problems that develop in the salt-wasting forms of the disease during acute illness. The child may become dehydrated quickly and need intravenous fluid replacement in addition to higher doses of hydrocortisone.

Inform parents that genetic counseling should be provided for the child during adolescence. Parents considering a future pregnancy should also be informed that prenatal testing may detect congenital adrenal hyperplasia in the fetus. Refer the family for counseling if indicated.

Addison Disease

Addison disease, also known as chronic adrenocortical insufficiency, is a rare disorder in childhood characterized by a deficiency of glucocorticoids (cortisone) and mineralocorticoids (aldosterone). It may be acquired after trauma or fungal infections that cause destruction of the adrenal glands or as the result of an autoimmune process. Adrenal failure has also been found in acquired immunodeficiency syndrome (AIDS).

Adrenal insufficiency usually develops slowly as the adrenal glands deteriorate. The early signs may not be noticed but include weakness with fatigue; anorexia and salt craving; weight loss; hyperpigmentation at pressure points, lip borders and buccal mucosa, nipples, body creases, and scarred areas of the body; abdominal pain; vomiting; and diarrhea. Symptomatic hypoglycemia may also be present. If the child experiences a stressful period, acute adrenal insufficiency may occur. Signs of an adrenal crisis include weakness, fever, abdominal pain, hypotension, dehydration, and shock.

Serum cortisol and urinary 17-hydroxycorticoid levels are measured in the early morning. Low levels are associated with adrenal insufficiency. The ACTH stimulation test is used to detect adrenal gland reserve. Electrolyte values generally reveal low serum sodium, elevated serum potassium, and low fasting blood glucose levels. CT may be used to visualize the adrenal glands.

Treatment involves replacement of the deficient hormones. Oral hydrocortisone is given in the lowest therapeutic dose to control symptoms and promote normal growth. Additional hydrocortisone is required during acute illness and stress. Fludrocortisone acetate (Florinef) is administered to replace the missing mineralocorticoid in children with aldosterone deficiency.

Nursing Management

Nursing management focuses on patient teaching, supporting the child and family, and caring for the child during acute episodes. See the earlier discussion of congenital adrenal hyperplasia for further detail.

Pheochromocytoma

Pheochromocytoma is a tumor that usually originates in the chromaffin cells of the adrenal medulla. In most cases these tumors are benign and curable. They occur in a familial pattern (autosomal dominant trait) with a 3:2 male to female ratio.[1] Most tumors are diagnosed in children between the ages of 6 and 14 years.

Clinical manifestations include labile hypertension with a systolic reading that may reach 250 mm Hg, tachycardia, profuse sweating with cool extremities, headache, nausea and vomiting, weight loss, visual disturbances, polydipsia, and polyuria. Because release of catecholamines (norepinephrine and epinephrine) from the tumor is not continuous, these symptoms occur intermittently.

Diagnosis is based on 24-hour urine studies to detect the presence of catecholamines and CT, MRI, and ultrasound studies to localize the tumor. The treatment of choice is surgical removal of the tumor; however, the procedure is dangerous and may result in sudden death.[2] Alpha-adrenergic blocking agents to control hypertension are given for 2 weeks prior to surgery. Postoperatively, a 24-hour urine collection is measured for catecholamines to determine if all of the tumor sites were removed. With successful removal of all of the tumor sites, the prognosis is generally good. Follow-up is important to assess for recurrence.

Nursing Management

Nursing care is mainly supportive. Provide preoperative and postoperative teaching and care (see Chapter 4). Preoperatively, monitor vital signs and observe for signs of complications associated with hypertension (encephalopathy, seizures). Administer antihypertensives and watch for any signs of hyperglycemia (see Table 19–4). Postoperatively, monitor blood pressure and observe for signs of shock.

Disorders of Altered Pancreatic Function

Diabetes Mellitus

Diabetes mellitus, the most common endocrine disease in children, is a disorder of glucose metabolism. There are two main types of diabetes.

The majority of children with diabetes have insulin-dependent diabetes mellitus (IDDM), or type I. Formerly this condition was known as juvenile diabetes. In the United States about 1 to 2 children per 1000 have IDDM. There are 12 to 16 new cases per 100,000 children per year.[5] The peak ages of occurrence are between 5 and 7 years and at puberty.

Non-insulin-dependent diabetes mellitus (NIDDM), or type II, is usually contracted as an adult and is associated with being overweight. NIDDM that occurs in adolescents is referred to as maturity-onset diabetes of youth (MODY). Diet, exercise, and oral hypoglycemic drugs are used to treat non-insulin-dependent diabetes.[2]

TABLE 19–4 Comparison of the Signs and Symptoms of Hyperglycemia and Hypoglycemia

Hyperglycemia	Hypoglycemia
Gradual onset	Rapid onset
Lethargic, slowed responses, confusion	Irritable, nervous, difficulty concentrating or speaking
Deep, rapid breathing	Shallow breathing
Weak pulse	Tachycardia
Flushed skin	Pallor, sweating
Dry mucous membranes, thirst, dehydration	Moist mucous membranes, hunger
Weakness	Tremors, shaky feeling
Abdominal pain, nausea, vomiting	Headache, dizziness
Fruity or acetone breath	Normal breath odor

Because the majority of children with diabetes have IDDM, the remainder of the discussion focuses on this form of the disease.

Clinical Manifestations

The classic signs of IDDM are polyuria, polydipsia, and **polyphagia** (excessive appetite) with significant weight loss. Unexplained lethargy and occasional enuresis may also occur in a previously toilet-trained child. Adolescent girls may have vaginitis caused by *Candida,* which thrives in the hyperglycemic tissues. Symptoms develop gradually and insidiously but have usually been present less than a month.

In severe cases diabetic ketoacidosis (DKA), a type of metabolic acidosis, may develop. Characteristic signs of DKA include dehydration, tachycardia, Kussmaul respirations, acetone breath, depressed level of consciousness, and hypotension. Children complain of abdominal or chest pain, begin to vomit, have labored breathing, and can slowly slip into a semiconscious state. Hyperglycemia, **glycosuria** (abnormal amount of glucose in the urine), and ketonuria are also present. Several of these symptoms were experienced by Danielle in the vignette at the beginning of this chapter.

Etiology and Pathophysiology

It is thought that IDDM is caused by a genetic component, environmental influences, and an autoimmune response. IDDM has strong familial tendencies but does not show any specific pattern of inheritance. The child inherits a susceptibility to the disease rather than the disease itself.

Environmental factors such as viruses or chemicals in the diet are believed to play an important role in damaging the beta cells in the islets of Langerhans. These are the cells responsible for insulin production. The incidence of onset of IDDM is increased during winter when viral diseases are more prevalent. Often the child has a history of a viral infection 1 to 2 months before the onset of symptoms.

The presence of circulating antibodies in pancreatic islet cells indicates that the body is having an immunologic response to an inflammatory process. As the beta cells are destroyed, the level of circulating antibodies falls.

Insulin helps transport glucose into the cells so that this carbohydrate can be used as an energy source. It also prevents the outflow of glucose from the liver to the general circulation. In IDDM over 90% of the beta cells in the islets of Langerhans are destroyed. The remaining beta cells are unable to produce sufficient insulin to maintain a normal blood glucose level, defined as 80 to 120 mg/dL. Lack of insulin results in a rise in blood glucose level and a decrease in the glucose level inside the cells. When the renal threshold for glucose (160 mg/dL) is exceeded, glycosuria occurs. Up to 1000 calories per day can be lost in the urine.

When glucose is unavailable to the cells for metabolism, an alternate source of energy is provided by free fatty acids. They are metabolized at an increased rate by the liver, producing acetyl coenzyme A (CoA). The by-products of acetyl CoA metabolism (ketone bodies) accumulate in the body, resulting in a state of metabolic acidosis, or ketoacidosis. (Refer to Chapter 8 for discussion of metabolic acidosis.)

Diagnostic Tests and Medical Management

Diagnosis is based on the presence of classic symptoms. A 2-hour postprandial blood glucose level above 200 mg/dL is indicative of IDDM. A glucose tolerance test is not required when these findings are present. A careful his-

GENETIC CONSIDERATIONS

Specific genetic markers associated with an increased risk for IDDM are located in the major histocompatibility complex (MHC) II on chromosome 6. Susceptibility to the development of IDDM may be increased when a child inherits markers from both parents.

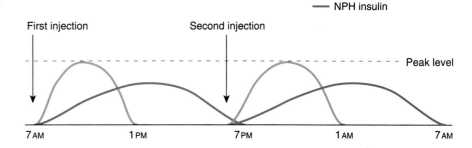

tory is necessary to rule out the presence of stress-related illness, corticosteroid usage, fracture, acute infection, cystic fibrosis, pancreatitis, or liver disease. DKA is present when the following findings are present: blood glucose level greater than 300 mg/dL, ketones in the serum, acidosis (pH less than or equal to 7.30 and bicarbonate less than 15 mEq/L), glycosuria, and ketonuria.

Therapy for IDDM combines insulin, dietary management, an exercise regimen, and physiologic support. Initial insulin therapy is designed to lower blood glucose levels to normal and to treat the DKA, which is a sign of inadequate glucose utilization. Long-term insulin therapy is calculated to maintain a blood glucose level as close to the normal range as possible and to minimize episodes of hyperglycemia and hypoglycemia (see Table 19–4). Insulin therapy must be balanced by the child's dietary intake and exercise level. Stress, infection, and illness increase insulin needs.

The most common insulin regimen consists of daily administration of a combination of a short-acting (regular) insulin and an intermediate-acting insulin (NPH or Lente) or long-acting insulin (Ultralente) before breakfast and before the evening meal (Fig. 19–6 and Table 19–5). However, other routines are preferred by some physicians. Insulin is usually provided in prepackaged doses of 100 units/mL. Diluted insulin prepared by a pharmacist may be used for infants and toddlers who require a small insulin dosage.[1]

Daily blood glucose levels are tested and recorded before meals and at bedtime. Laboratory evaluation of glycosylated hemoglobin (HbA$_{1C}$) levels should be performed every 2 to 3 months.[1] This provides an objective measurement of glycemic control because it represents the amount of glucose irreversibly attached to the hemoglobin molecule over an extended period (the life span of the red blood cell, approximately 120 days).

Physical activity is associated with increased insulin sensitivity. Regular exercise and fitness improve metabolic control with a lower insulin dose.

■ RESEARCH DEVELOPMENTS

The insulin pump is an alternative to subcutaneous insulin injections. The pump is about the size of a calculator and can provide insulin at a slow steady rate or in a bolus dose. It delivers insulin through a plastic syringe or reservoir attached to a catheter and needle inserted in the subcutaneous tissue, usually in the abdomen.[10]

TABLE 19-5 Insulin Action (Subcutaneous Route) in Hours

Type	Onset	Peak	Duration
Short Acting			
Regular	½–1	2–4	6–8
Intermediate Acting			
NPH	1–2	6–12	18–26
Lente	1–2	6–12	24–26
Long Acting			
Ultralente	4–6	14–24	28–36

Blood lipid levels are also positively affected. However, the child must have an adequate caloric intake to prevent hypoglycemia.

Long-term complications of IDDM (retinopathy, heart disease, renal failure, and peripheral vascular disease) result from vascular changes. Despite careful management, approximately 30% to 40% of diabetic children develop renal failure and loss of vision in adulthood.[2] Careful management is important, however, to delay or lessen the side effects of the disease.

Nursing Assessment

Physiologic Assessment. Children are generally admitted to the hospital at the time of diagnosis and with acute episodes of DKA. Assess the child's physiologic status, focusing on vital signs and level of consciousness. Assess hydration by checking mucous membranes, skin turgor, and urine output. Blood initially is collected hourly to monitor blood gases, glucose, and electrolytes. Once the child is stable, assess dietary and caloric intake and the ability of the child or family to manage care.

For follow-up visits, ask the child or parents about signs indicating problems of diabetic control (Table 19–6). Record growth parameters and vital signs in the child's chart. Review typical dietary intake and exercise regimens.

Psychosocial Assessment. Parents may feel guilty at the time of diagnosis if they waited to seek care until the child began to experience symptoms of DKA. Assess coping mechanisms, ability to manage the disease, and educational needs of both the child and parents. Adolescents should be assessed for their potential to comply with insulin therapy, blood glucose testing, diet, and exercise regimen. Adolescents perceive IDDM as a disability and often deny having the disease so they can be like their peers when eating and exercising.

Developmental Assessment. Assess the child's developmental level, particularly fine motor skills and cognitive level. The child will need to learn how to obtain and read a blood glucose sample and how to draw up and administer insulin. Children are usually able to perform some of these tasks with supervision by 6 to 8 years of age. Self-management is the eventual goal, and the child's responsibilities are gradually increased.

Talk with the adolescent to evaluate motivation to manage diet and insulin therapy. Although the adolescent is cognitively able to manage self-care, the desire to be like peers often interferes with compliance.

TABLE 19–6 Questions to Ask to Identify Problems in Diabetic Control

- Is the child hungry at meals? Between meals?
- How much fluid is the child drinking?
- Has the child been going to the bathroom frequently or had episodes of bedwetting?
- Does the child have dry skin?
- Are there sores on the feet? Do scratches or scrapes take a long time to heal?
- Has the child had any skin infections?
- Does the child have changes in mood (depression, unexplained sadness, irritability) or energy level from day to day or throughout the day?

Nursing Diagnosis

Several diagnoses that may apply to the child newly diagnosed with IDDM are provided in the accompanying Nursing Care Plan. Additional diagnoses that may be appropriate include the following:

- High Risk for Fluid Volume Deficit related to glycosuria
- Ineffective Breathing Pattern related to effort to compensate for metabolic acidosis
- Powerlessness related to presence of a chronic illness requiring a tight dietary, exercise, and medication regimen
- Noncompliance related to denial of chronic condition

Nursing Management

Nursing care focuses on teaching the child and parents about the disease and its management, managing dietary intake, providing emotional support, promoting self-care, and providing anticipatory guidance. Refer to the accompanying Nursing Care Plan, which summarizes nursing care for the child with newly diagnosed IDDM.

Provide Education. The nurse is an important member of the management team (physician, nurse, nutritionist, and social worker) and is usually responsible for educating the child and family. Teaching often is performed in the home setting, since children may be only briefly hospitalized following diagnosis.

The timing and amount of information provided are especially important in the first days following diagnosis. Both the child and parents are often in a state of shock and disbelief; information presented during this period may need to be repeated. This time should be used to assess learning needs, as described in the Nursing Care Plan, and answer the family's questions. Initial teaching focuses on the skills necessary for home management (insulin administration, blood glucose testing, urine testing, record keeping, and the recognition and treatment of both hypoglycemia and hyperglycemia).

Explain the goals of insulin therapy. Teach the child and parents how to administer insulin and test blood glucose (Fig. 19–7). Rotating the injection

FIGURE 19–7 This mother is being taught how to test her child's blood glucose level.

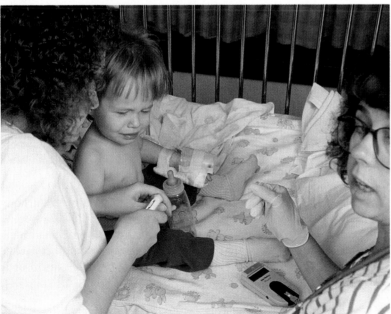
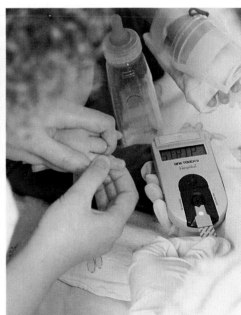

FIGURE 19–8 Insulin injection sites.

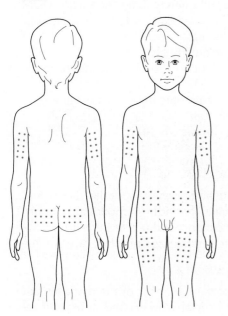

sites is important to decrease the chances of lipodystrophy (development of fibrotic tissue that interferes with absorption of insulin) (Fig. 19–8). An understanding of the different types of insulin and their actions is essential. Once the child and parents demonstrate understanding of this information, guidelines for managing episodes of hyperglycemia during acute illness using a sliding scale are taught. A sliding scale indicates specific insulin dosages appropriate for a particular blood glucose level.

Caution parents to check the blood glucose level of a toddler who is extremely sleepy or irritable, since these can be signs of either hypoglycemia or hyperglycemia.

Manage Dietary Intake. The preferred diet for children with IDDM is a low-fat, low-sodium diet that avoids concentrated sugars. The child should have adequate calories to reach or maintain a desirable body weight. Usually at the time of diagnosis the child needs to regain lost weight, so extra calories may be recommended.

Dietary intake should include three meals per day, eaten at consistent intervals, plus a midafternoon carbohydrate snack and a bedtime snack high in protein. The American Diabetes Association's exchange lists facilitate dietary management by suggesting portions and types of foods and noting allowed substitutions.

Provide Emotional Support. The diagnosis of IDDM often comes as a shock to the family. If there is a familial history, parents may be feeling guilty about having caused the disease. Parents may need counseling to allay guilt feelings.

The diagnosis of a chronic disease that requires daily management can be difficult to accept. Give parents information about diabetes education programs, put them in touch with parents of other diabetic children, and help them to learn the role they can play in managing the disease.

Support for the child depends on age and developmental stage. Encourage the child to express feelings about the disease and its management. The adolescent may benefit from contact with other adolescents who have IDDM. Summer camps and other programs for diabetic children are often helpful in providing support.

Promote Self-Care. Assist children to assume responsibility for self-care. The child's developmental stage and cognitive level influence his or her readiness to take on responsibility for self-care.[11]

The preschool child's need for autonomy and control can be met by allowing the child to choose snacks or to pick which finger to stick for glucose testing and by helping parents to gather necessary supplies. Preschool children do not understand explanations about food intake and restrictions.[11]

School-age children can learn to test blood glucose, administer insulin, and keep records. They should be taught how to select foods appropriate for dietary management and how to plan an exercise program. School-age children need to be able to recognize the signs of hypoglycemia and hyperglycemia, and they should carry a rapidly absorbed sugar product for treatment.

Adolescents should take on total responsibility for self-care. Although adolescents understand explanations about potential complications of diabetes, they are present oriented and may rebel against the daily regimentation of insulin injections and dietary management. Successful self-care depends in part on the adolescent's adjustment to the chronic nature of the disease and feelings of being different from peers.

Provide Anticipatory Guidance. Children with IDDM often learn manipulating behaviors, using their disease to obtain something they want. Advise parents to be alert to signs of manipulation, such as helpless, demanding, or whining behaviors, and any evidence of poor coping. Referral for counseling may be appropriate for some families.

Discharge Planning and Patient and Family Home Care Teaching. Home care needs should be identified and addressed before discharge. This is often difficult because of the short hospitalization of children with newly diagnosed diabetes. Home health or visiting nurses should be notified to visit the family within 24 hours of discharge. The goal of the teaching plan is to enable the child and family to assume the necessary responsibility for home care and to reduce the number of episodes of DKA.

Make every effort to incorporate the diabetic regimen (insulin administration, diet, blood glucose monitoring, and exercise) into the family's present life-style. The fewer the changes the family has to make, the greater the chance of compliance. For the child admitted for treatment of DKA, evaluate the child's and family's ability to perform diabetic care. Assist them to make modifications necessary to meet care recommendations.

The child with IDDM may have circulatory and neurologic changes that make skin breakdown a greater risk than normal. If signs of infection occur, the parents should seek medical care.

Emphasize the importance of good foot care, for example, wearing clean white cotton socks; changing socks and shoes when they are damp; washing, drying, and powdering feet; and keeping toenails short.

Provide written materials and refer parents to books and other materials for teaching the child about the disease (see Table 19–7). The American Diabetes Association is a good source of information (see Appendix F).

Tell the parents that the child should wear some type of medical alert identification. Notify the school nurse of the child's disease, and educate the child's teacher about signs of hypoglycemia or hyperglycemia and its emergency management.

Hypoglycemia

Hypoglycemia can develop within minutes in children with diabetes mellitus. Symptoms outlined in Table 19–4 may occur when there is a sudden drop in blood glucose levels. Common causes include an error in insulin dosage, inadequate calories because of missed meals, or exercise without a corresponding increase in caloric intake.

Hypoglycemia can be diagnosed on the basis of the sudden onset of signs and symptoms. A blood glucose reading should be taken to confirm the diagnosis, since signs of hyperglycemia and hypoglycemia may be difficult to distinguish. Give glucose immediately in the form of a carbohydrate-containing snack or drink, cake frosting, or glucose paste. In the hospital setting, administer an intravenous infusion of dextrose to prevent progression of symptoms. If the child becomes unconscious, cake frosting or glucose paste can be squeezed onto the gums.

Nursing Management

Teach parents and children to recognize the signs of hypoglycemia and take appropriate action. Reinforce the importance of dietary intake, insulin, and exercise and the need to balance all three every day.

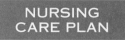

THE CHILD WITH NEWLY DIAGNOSED DIABETES MELLITUS

GOAL	INTERVENTION	RATIONALE	EXPECTED OUTCOME
1. Knowledge Deficit (Child and Parents) related to diabetic management in the newly diagnosed child			
Child and parents will state diabetic home management regimen.	Assess child's developmental level and select an educational approach and self-care activities to match.	Learning goals for the child must match knowledge and skill expectations appropriate for developmental stage.	Child and parents will demonstrate proper technique for blood glucose monitoring, urine testing for ketones, insulin administration, and record keeping.
	Teach blood glucose monitoring, insulin administration, urine testing for ketones, and record keeping.	These diabetic management skills are needed for initial home management.	
	Use demonstration/return demonstration until family and child are comfortable with procedures.	Evaluation permits positive reinforcement and guidance for modification of techniques.	
2. High Risk for Injury related to periods of hypoglycemia and diabetic ketoacidosis			
Child will experience few episodes of hypoglycemia and no episodes of diabetic ketoacidosis during hospitalization.	Assess child at least every 2 hours for signs of hypoglycemia (see Table 19–4). If hypoglycemia exists, check blood glucose to verify and administer source of quick sugar (sugar cube, hard candy).	Hypoglycemia commonly occurs during hospitalization because of change in diet, lack of food intake, or illness.	Child and staff will manage episodes of hypoglycemia without a crisis developing.
	When the child is NPO for a special procedure, withhold morning insulin and verify with physician when food, fluids, and insulin are to be given or if an intravenous infusion with dextrose is to be given.	Giving insulin in absence of food can lead to hypoglycemia. Intravenous dextrose and insulin can be used when the child must be NPO.	
	Have glucose paste or 50% dextrose solution readily available.	Dextrose is used for emergency IV treatment of severe hypoglycemia. Glucose paste is used for oral treatment.	
	If signs of hyperglycemia are present, check blood glucose to verify and administer insulin as ordered. Be prepared with intravenous equipment.	If the child's condition is severe, insulin, fluid, and electrolyte therapy may be required.	
	Check blood glucose three to four times daily, before each insulin dose.	Allows for consistent measurement and establishment of patterns.	
	Administer insulin doses on time and not more than 30 minutes before meals.	Prevents hyperglycemia and hypoglycemia.	
	Have insulin doses checked by a second nurse.	Doses are frequently small, and the possibility of error is great.	
Child and parents will recognize signs and symptoms of poor glucose control.	Teach signs and symptoms of hypoglycemic and hyperglycemic reactions.	Recognition of and treatment of poor glucose control will prevent progression of symptoms.	Child and family describe symptoms of hypoglycemia and hyperglycemia.

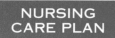
THE CHILD WITH NEWLY DIAGNOSED DIABETES MELLITUS—CONTINUED

GOAL	INTERVENTION	RATIONALE	EXPECTED OUTCOME
Child and parents will demonstrate emergency management of hypoglycemia.	Identify sources of glucose to give in case of hypoglycemic reaction. Tell child and parent to carry candy with them at all times.	Access to sources of glucose and its rapid administration are important for emergency care.	Child and family identify several glucose sources for emergencies. Child and family will have candy or another source of glucose with them at each visit.
	Teach child and family to test blood glucose and urine for ketones with acute symptoms and notify the physician.	Appropriate doses of insulin may be prescribed to prevent progression of hyperglycemia to ketoacidosis.	Child's hyperglycemic episodes do not progress to ketoacidosis.

3. High Risk for Altered Nutrition: Less Than Body Requirements related to glycosuria

Child will eat a well-balanced diet and maintain normal height and weight proportions.	Encourage and serve meals and snacks at the same time each day. Assess height and weight regularly and plot on growth chart.	Keeps blood glucose levels stable, which reduces sequelae of disease. Method of evaluating growth accurately.	Child demonstrates normal growth without fluctuations in height, weight, and blood glucose level.
Child and parents will state understanding of dietary management of diabetes mellitus.	Make an appointment with a nutritionist who can assess child's favorite foods and promote their utilization in the child's diet. Reinforce dietary information taught. Provide sample menus and food exchanges.	The nutritionist can develop dietary recommendations that fit the specific needs of the child and include favorite foods, thereby increasing compliance with the diet. Assists family in diet planning.	The child and family describe nutritional needs of the child and dietary management to meet those needs.
	Make sure the child and family understand the importance of regularly spaced meals and snacks every day. Encourage them to keep a food diary.	Nutritional intake should be balanced with insulin administration and exercise to prevent hypoglycemia.	Diet records indicate meals eaten at consistent times each day with appropriate distribution of carbohydrates, protein, and fats.

4. High Risk for Impaired Skin Integrity related to poor healing of injuries

Child will maintain intact skin.	Assess skin thoroughly each shift, especially extremities, mouth, and pressure areas.	Diabetic patients may have decreased circulation and sensation, which can lead to skin breakdown.	Child's skin is free of any lesions.
	Report and record any changes.	Allows for close observation of changes.	
	Keep lesions clean, keep them covered if draining, and check every 2 hours.	Prevents infection or worsening of lesion.	
	Take temperature at least every 4 hours.	Temperature elevation can indicate infection.	
	Administer antibiotics if prescribed.	Diabetic patients may heal slowly because of circulatory changes and thus are more prone to infection. Antibiotics may be needed for treatment.	

Continued.

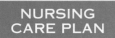

THE CHILD WITH NEWLY DIAGNOSED DIABETES MELLITUS—CONTINUED

GOAL	INTERVENTION	RATIONALE	EXPECTED OUTCOME
5. Altered Family Processes related to management of a chronic disease			
Child and family will manage medications, dietary modifications, and exercise regimen.	Assess family's life-style. Attempt to fit the child's care needs to the family's schedule. Discuss the family's routines for special occasions and vacations. Identify ways to modify the child's management for these occasions.	Fitting the care to the family's life-style promotes compliance with regimen. It is important for the child to participate in special events with family and peers as a normal child to promote psychologic development.	Child and family make minimal changes in usual life-style while managing diabetes.
6. Body Image Disturbance related to perceived loss of health			
Child will demonstrate enhanced coping skills.	Ask how the child has solved problems in the past. Review possible problems the child may encounter. Together evaluate the effectiveness of solutions. Suggest other solutions to consider.	Children's success in mastering maturational conflicts and daily psychosocial problems will influence their pattern of coping.	Child demonstrates enhanced coping skills and expresses positive attitude toward self. Child displays warmth and affection toward family.
Child will develop positive self-esteem.	Encourage the child to express feelings about disease to those he or she trusts.	Expressing feelings decreases anxiety.	
	Encourage child to continue previous social activities and hobbies. Praise all endeavors.	Increased social interaction, especially in group sessions, improves self-esteem.	
	Reassure child that friends cannot see overt evidence of disease.	Self-esteem is closely linked to body image, especially during adolescence.	
7. Altered Role Performance (Child) related to need to begin self-management of chronic disorder			
Child will develop independent ability to manage diabetes care.	Allow child to perform as many self-care procedures as possible at each developmental stage.	Normal growth and development are ensured if the child is encouraged to participate in care from the beginning.	Child is able to perform as many diabetic care techniques as possible for age.
	Encourage the child to make decisions regarding care. Review decisions and discuss possible alternative solutions. Role play possible scenarios. Provide 24-hour access to physician or diabetes nurse educator. Encourage the child to seek help early.	Feelings of trust are developed when children sense that their decisions are respected or at least considered by others.	

TABLE 19–7 Teaching Tools for Children with Diabetes Mellitus

Understanding Insulin Dependent Diabetes, by Peter Chase, M.D.; Pink Panther; for parents and adolescents

Kids, Food and Diabetes, by Gloria Loring; Chicago: Contemporary Books, 1986; for parents

The Truth About Stacy, one of The Babysitters Club books; excellent resource for girls age 9–12 years

Grilled Cheese at Four O'Clock in the Morning, an American Diabetes Association publication (see Appendix F); excellent for boys age 10–14 years

Several pamphlets and dolls are available that illustrate anatomy and physiology, provide step-by-step instructions on injecting insulin, and allow the child to practice injections.

Disorders of Altered Gonadal Function

Gynecomastia

Gynecomastia is the presence of unilateral or bilateral enlarged breast tissue in males. It is a common finding during adolescence and is sometimes confused with subcutaneous fat pads in obese boys. The condition usually disappears in 1 to 2 years.

Nursing care focuses on reassuring the boy and his parents that gynecomastia is a transient condition. Because of the concerns about body image that are common during adolescence, embarrassment is a frequent problem. Alerting the teen's teachers may be necessary if teasing becomes a problem.

Amenorrhea

Amenorrhea, or lack of menstruation, may be primary or secondary. Primary amenorrhea is defined as the failure to have menstrual periods by the age of 16 to 18 years.[14] Primary amenorrhea is differentiated from delayed menarche, which is associated with well-developed secondary sexual characteristics and a strong family history of late menarche.[15] Secondary amenorrhea is the cessation of menstrual periods after menstruation has begun; it is characterized by absence of spontaneous bleeding for at least 120 days. Pregnancy is the most common cause of secondary amenorrhea in adolescents.

Primary amenorrhea is most often caused by structural defects of the reproductive system, chromosomal abnormalities (such as Turner syndrome), or hypothalamic, pituitary, or ovarian failure. In approximately 30% of adolescents no underlying pathologic condition is found.[14]

A thorough history, physical examination, and laboratory evaluation are required to determine the cause. The history focuses on asking questions about recent excessive weight loss or gain; excessive physical activity or sports training; chronic illness; use of illegal drugs, birth control pills, or phenothiazines; and emotional problems, all of which may result in absence or cessation of menses.

The physical examination focuses on evaluating the adolescent's stage of sexual development (see Chapter 3). A bone scan is performed to determine bone age, and hormone levels are evaluated (estrogen, LH, FSH, and prolactin).

Treatment of amenorrhea depends on the specific cause. The most common approach is to give birth control pills containing both estrogen and progesterone. Athletic teenagers are encouraged to eat a well-balanced, high-calorie diet. Nursing management centers on patient education and emotional support. The goal is to maintain normal growth and development.

Dysmenorrhea

Dysmenorrhea (menstrual pain or cramping) is the most common complaint of adolescent girls.[2] It is usually caused by increased secretion of prostaglandins. Dysmenorrhea usually occurs following the beginning of ovulation and ends on the second day of the menstrual cycle. The pain can be mild or severe. Other symptoms may include nausea, vomiting, diarrhea, and urinary frequency.

Nonprescription analgesics, relaxation techniques, and application of a heating pad may relieve mild discomfort. Nursing care centers on providing patient education and emotional support.

Disorders Related to Sex Chromosome Abnormalities

Turner Syndrome

Turner syndrome is a genetic condition that occurs in girls who have a missing or abnormal X chromosome. It occurs in approximately 1 in 2000 to 1 in 5000 live female births.[5] The cause of the chromosomal error is unknown.

Characteristic clinical findings include significant short stature; undeveloped ovaries; short, webbed neck with a low posterior hairline; cubitus valgus (increased angle at the elbow); broad chest with widely spaced nipples; lymphedema; hyperconvex fingernails; dark, pigmented nevi; amenorrhea; and infertility (Fig. 19–9). Few girls have all of these features.

Several conditions that may be associated with Turner syndrome are listed in Table 19–8. Kidney abnormalities are present in 25% to 30% of girls.

Growth usually proceeds at a normal rate for the first 2 to 3 years of life and then slows. Breast tissue, which begins to bud at about 10 to 12 years, fails to develop fully. Only in rare instances will a girl with Turner syndrome menstruate spontaneously or be able to conceive. Final height is approximately 4 feet 8 inches.

The presence of characteristic physical findings may alert health care providers to suspect Turner syndrome. Some infants, however, have few of

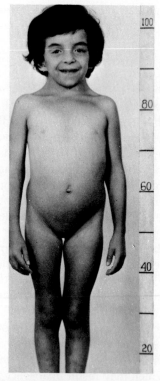

FIGURE 19-9 What characteristic physical manifestations of Turner syndrome can you identify in this 8-year-old girl?

From Grumbach, M.M., & Barr, M.L. (1958). *Recent Progress in Hormone Research, 14,* 255.

TABLE 19-8 Conditions Associated with Turner Syndrome

Congenital heart disease (most commonly atrial septal defect or pulmonic stenosis)
Structural abnormalities of the kidney (horseshoe shape, unusual position)
Hypothyroidism or thyroiditis
Diabetes mellitus
Chronic or recurrent otitis media
Ptosis (drooping eyelids), myopia, or amblyopia (lazy eye)
Malformation of intestinal blood vessels
Inflammatory bowel disease (Crohn disease, ulcerative colitis)

Modified from Rieser, P.A., & Underwood, L.E. (1989). *Turner syndrome: A guide for families.* Copyright © 1989 the Turner's Syndrome Society, Wayzata, MN; supported by an educational grant from Genentech, Inc.; and prepared by Mason Medical Communications, Inc.

these characteristics. In some instances diagnosis is made only when short stature and delayed puberty become apparent in the teenage years. The condition is diagnosed definitively by a karyotype, which reveals the classic 45,XO chromosome pattern or 46,XX pattern with one misshapen X chromosome.

Treatment involves carefully monitoring the child's growth. A growth chart made especially for girls with Turner syndrome is available. Low-dose estrogen therapy is usually begun between 13 and 15 years of age, with dosage increases for the next 2 to 3 years. This treatment produces pubertal changes such as breast development and pubic hair. Progesterone is added to the estrogen therapy to initiate menstrual periods.

Some controversy exists over when to begin estrogen treatment because estrogen replacement advances bone maturation. Health care providers in collaboration with the family must determine which is more important, attaining maximum stature or initiating normal pubertal changes (breast tissue, menstruation, and pubic hair).

Nursing Management

The lack of growth and sexual development associated with Turner syndrome presents problems not only for physical growth but also for psychosocial development. Children's self-image, self-consciousness, and self-esteem are affected by their perception of their bodies and how they differ from peers.

In the United States, cultural values place importance on attaining normal to tall stature. Short children tend to be treated according to their size rather than their age. Emphasis is also placed on sexual maturity. Television, advertisements, and movies encourage adolescents to dress and behave in a sexually mature manner. Girls with Turner syndrome are often self-conscious and easily embarrassed and suffer from low self-esteem. They also have a higher incidence of learning problems because of visual-spatial deficits that affect performance on mathematical and manual dexterity tasks.[3]

The nurse can be instrumental in helping the child adapt to the condition and gain self-esteem. Be an active listener and reinforce abilities and skills that the girl exhibits. Encourage parents to provide support. The Turner Syndrome Society (see Appendix F) can provide additional information about the disorder for parents and adolescents.

Klinefelter Syndrome

Klinefelter syndrome is a genetic condition that occurs in boys who have an extra X chromosome (usually 47,XXY). It occurs in approximately 1 in 1000 male births[1] and is the single most common cause of hypogonadism (decreased secretory activity of the gonad) and infertility in males.

Most infants appear normal at birth. The condition is usually diagnosed during the school-age years when the boy's behavior becomes a problem in the classroom. Boys with Klinefelter syndrome may have emotional problems because of delayed language development and auditory processing problems that are frustrating to the child. Intelligence quotient (IQ) scores are often 10 to 15 points below those of unaffected siblings, and IQs below 80 are not uncommon. Boys with Klinefelter syndrome are tall and thin, with overly long arms and legs. The onset of puberty is often delayed with decreased growth of testes. Development of the penis and pubic hair may be normal. Gynecomastia is a characteristic finding.

Diagnosis is confirmed by chromosomal analysis revealing one or more extra X chromosomes. The goal of treatment is to stimulate masculinization and the development of secondary sex characteristics when adolescence is delayed. Testosterone replacement is begun when the boy is 11 or 12 years of age. Depo-Testosterone is given by intramuscular injection every 3 to 4 weeks to maintain serum testosterone levels within the normal range. The dose is increased gradually until an adult dose is reached between 15 and 17 years of age.

Nursing Management

Nursing care consists of educating the parents and child about the syndrome, evaluating the child's and family's coping mechanisms, assisting with school problems, and capitalizing on the child's strengths. Encourage parents to channel their son's energy into areas that will provide opportunities for success and productive experiences. Emphasize the importance of rewarding the boy's successes in school, sports, or hobbies. Make genetic counseling available to adolescents because sexual functioning and fertility may be impaired.

Inborn Errors of Metabolism

Inborn errors of metabolism are inherited biochemical abnormalities of the urea cycle, amino acid, and organic acid metabolism. Individually they are rare disorders; however, as a group they are a significant health problem in infancy.

Clinical manifestations usually occur within days or weeks of birth. Signs and symptoms may include lethargy and poor feeding, persistent vomiting, abnormal muscle tone and seizures, apnea and tachycardia, and an unusual urine or body odor (musty, sweet odor of maple syrup or burnt sugar, or cheesy or sweaty feet).

The biochemical defect usually causes an abnormal chemical by-product to accumulate in the blood, urine, or tissues or results in a decreased amount of normal enzymes. Most disorders are associated with a protein intolerance, with symptoms developing shortly after formula or breast milk feedings are begun.

In many states neonatal screening is used to detect several of these conditions before symptoms develop. However, most inborn errors of metabolism are not detected until signs and symptoms are present. Initial laboratory tests include measurement of serum glucose, electrolytes, blood gases, and serum ammonia. Results of these tests make it possible to classify the disorder by the presence of hypoglycemia, metabolic acidosis, hyperammonemia, or liver dysfunction. Further diagnostic laboratory tests are then performed.

Treatment, when available, focuses on replacing or reducing the amount of the substance causing the biochemical abnormality.

Two of the more common inborn errors of metabolism, phenylketonuria and galactosemia, are presented here. Congenital hypothyroidism and congenital adrenal hyperplasia, also considered inborn errors of metabolism, were previously discussed in this chapter.

■ CULTURAL CONSIDERATIONS

Phenylketonuria is rare in African, Jewish, and Japanese populations. It is more commonly found in isolated communities with numerous intermarriages between families over several generations.

Phenylketonuria

Phenylketonuria (PKU) is an inherited disorder of amino acid metabolism that affects the body's utilization of protein. Children with PKU have a deficiency of the liver enzyme phenylalanine hydroxylase, which breaks down the essential amino acid phenylalanine into tyrosine. As a result, phenylalanine accumulates in the blood, causing a musty body odor, musty urine odor, irritability, vomiting, hyperactivity, seizures, and an eczema-like rash. Persistence of elevated phenylalanine for 2 to 3 years results in a seizure disorder and mental retardation. PKU is inherited as an autosomal recessive disorder. The incidence is 1 in 14,000 children.[16]

Screening for PKU is required by state law in all 50 states. For best results the newborn should have begun formula or breast milk feeding before specimen collection. Newborns who are screened within 24 hours of birth should have the screening test repeated. If the test shows elevated levels of plasma phenylalanine, a repeat test is performed. If the second test is positive, the family is referred to a treatment center and treatment is begun on an outpatient basis.

PKU is treated using special formulas and a diet low in phenylalanine to keep plasma phenylalanine levels between 2 and 8 mg/dL. The diet must also meet the child's needs for optimal growth. High-protein foods (meats and dairy products) and aspartame are avoided because they contain large amounts of phenylalanine. The low-phenylalanine diet should be maintained until late school age or adolescence. Affected adolescent girls and women who become pregnant should resume the low-phenylalanine diet before they conceive to prevent congenital defects (low birth weight, mental retardation, microcephaly) in the fetus.

Nursing Management

Nursing care is mainly supportive and focuses on teaching parents about the disorder and its management. Serum levels of phenylalanine should be measured periodically. When the child begins to eat solid foods, parents need to watch the amount of phenylalanine consumed by the child daily and should not allow it to exceed the amount prescribed by the physician.

The low-phenylalanine diet is a rigid, strict diet that excludes many foods. Parents and children need a great deal of support to promote compliance. Like children with diabetes mellitus, children with PKU may rebel against the dietary limitations in an effort to be like their peers. For this reason the low-phenylalanine diet may be discontinued during the late school-age years or adolescence. If the child has problems concentrating or sitting still, resumption of the low-phenylalanine diet may be recommended.

Parents of an affected child who are considering a future pregnancy and adolescents with the disorder should be referred for genetic counseling.

Galactosemia

Galactosemia is a disorder of carbohydrate metabolism that results from a deficiency of the liver enzyme galactose-1-phosphate uridyltransferase. This is one of three enzymes needed to convert galactose to glucose. Galactosemia has an autosomal recessive inheritance pattern and occurs in 1 in 60,000 to 80,000 live births.[17] If left untreated, galactosemia results in feeding problems, vomiting, weight loss, jaundice, enlarged liver, mental retardation, sepsis, lethargy, and coma leading to death.

Routine newborn screening for galactosemia is performed in 37 states.[8] Infants in other states are identified once they become symptomatic. Infants with galactosemia are placed on a lactose-free formula (usually a soy formula), which remains the child's milk substitute for life. A galactose-free diet (no milk or cheese products) is prescribed when the infant is ready for solids. In spite of compliance with the diet, complications (learning disabilities, speech defects, ovarian failure, and neurologic syndromes) develop in many children.

Nursing management focuses on educating the parents and child about the disorder and required diet, assessing coping abilities, and providing emotional support. Refer the family to a nutritionist for diet counseling. Advise parents that several galactose-free cheeses are sold commercially. Because the disorder is inherited, the family should be referred for genetic counseling.

REFERENCES

1 Rudolph, A.M., Hoffman, J.I.E, & Rudolph, C.D. (Eds.). (1991). *Rudolph's pediatrics* (19th ed.). Norwalk, CT: Appleton & Lange.

2 Hathaway, W.E., Hay, W.W. Jr., Groothuis, J.R., & Paisley, J.W. (Eds.). (1993). *Current pediatric diagnosis & treatment* (11th ed.). Norwalk, CT: Appleton & Lange.

3 Rieser, P.A. (1992). Educational, psychologic, and social aspects of short stature. *Journal of Pediatric Health Care, 6*(5), 325–332.

4 Connaughty, M.S. (1992). Accelerated growth in children. *Journal of Pediatric Health Care, 6*(5), 316–324.

5 Kaplan, S.L. (1990). *Clinical pediatric endocrinology*. Philadelphia: W.B. Saunders.

6 Wheeler, M.D., & Styne, D.M. (1990). Diagnosis and management of precocious puberty. *Pediatric Clinics of North America, 37*, 1255–1271.

7 Office of Research Reporting, National Institute of Child Health and Development (1989). *Facts about precocious puberty*. Washington, DC: National Institutes of Health.

8 Buist, N.R.M., & Tuerck, J.M. (1992). The practitioner's role in newborn screening. *Pediatric Clinics of North America, 39*(2), 199–211.

9 Lifshitz, F. (1990). *Pediatric endocrinology: A clinical guide* (2nd ed.). New York: Marcel Dekker.

10 Clark, L.M., & Plotnick, L.P. (1990). Insulin pumps in children with diabetes. *Journal of Pediatric Health Care, 4*(1), 3–10.

11 Giordano, B.P., Petrila, A., Banion, C.R., & Neuenkirchen, G. (1992). The challenge of transferring responsibility for diabetes management from parent to child. *Journal of Pediatric Health Care, 6*(5), 235–239.

12 American Diabetes Association Task Force on Nutrition (1987). Nutritional recommendations and principles for individuals with diabetes mellitus: 1986. *Diabetes Care, 10*, 126–132.

13 Drash, A.L., & Becker, D.J. (1993). Nutritional considerations in the therapy of the child with diabetes mellitus. In Suskind, R.M., & Lewinter-Suskind, L. (Eds.), *Textbook of pediatric nutrition* (2nd ed.). New York: Raven Press.

14 Murata, J. (1989). Primary amenorrhea. *Pediatric Nursing, 15*(2), 125–129.

15 Tuttle, J.I. (1991). Menstrual disorders during adolescence. *Journal of Pediatric Health Care, 5*(4), 197–203.

16 Bradburn, J.M., & Shapira, E. (1993). Nutritional treatment of children with inborn errors of metabolism. In Suskind, R.M., & Lewinter-Suskind, L. (Eds.), *Textbook of pediatric nutrition* (2nd ed.). New York: Raven Press.

17 Strobel, S.E., & Keller, C.S. (1993). Metabolic screening in the NICU population: A proposal for change. *Pediatric Nursing, 19*(2), 113–117.

SUGGESTED READINGS

Amer, K., August, G.P., & Robnett, M.A. (1991). *The nursing perspective: Monitoring and evaluation of growth*. Califon, NJ: Gardiner-Caldwell Syner Med.

Anderson, R., Nowacek, G., & Richards, F. (1988). Influencing the personal meaning of diabetes: Research and practice. *The Diabetes Educator, 14*(4), 297–302.

Austin, J. (1990). Assessment of coping mechanisms used by parents and children with chronic illness. *American Journal of Maternal-Child Nursing, 15*(2), 98–102.

Balik, B., Haig, B., & Moynihan, P. (1986). Diabetes and the school-aged child. *American Journal of Maternal-Child Nursing, 11*, 324–330.

Brandt, P.A., & Magyary, D.L. (1993). The impact of a diabetes education program on children and mothers. *Journal of Pediatric Nursing, 8*(1), 31–40.

Daniels, D. (1988). A guide to pediatric diabetes for the home health nurse. *Home Healthcare Nurse, 6*(5), 22–26.

Davidson, A. (1992). Management and counseling of children with inherited metabolic disorders. *Journal of Pediatric Health Care, 6*(3), 146–152.

Edwards, D. (1987). Initial psychosocial impact of insulin-dependent diabetes mellitus in the pediatric client and family. *Issues in Comprehensive Pediatric Nursing, 10*, 199–207.

Gray, D.P. (1990). Mechanisms of hormone regulation. In McCance, K.L., & Huether, S.E. (Eds.), *Pathophysiology: A biologic basis for disease in adults and children* (pp. 564–593). St. Louis: Mosby–Year Book.

Henry, J., & Giordano, B. (1992). Assessment of growth in infants and children: Normal and abnormal patterns. *Journal of Pediatric Health Care, 5*(2), 289–334.

Kushion, W., Salisbury, P., Seitz, K., & Wilson, B. (1991). Issues in the care of infants and toddlers with insulin-dependent diabetes mellitus. *The Diabetes Educator, 17*(2), 107–110.

Lipman, T., Difazio, D., Meers, R., & Thompson, R. (1989). A developmental approach to diabetes in children: School age–adolescence. *American Journal of Maternal-Child Nursing, 14*, 330–332.

Robnett, M.A., et al. (1992). *Pediatric endocrinology nursing resource manual.* Los Angeles: Pediatric Endocrinology Nursing Society.

Rosenfeld, R.G. (1989). *Turner syndrome: A guide for physicians.* Wayzata, MN: The Turner's Syndrome Society.

Saudek, C.D. (1992). Use of implanted insulin pumps to treat IDDM. *Journal of Pediatric Endocrinology, 5*(4), 217–227.

Yoos, L. (1987). Chronic childhood illness: Developmental issues. *Pediatric Nursing, 13*(1), 25–28.

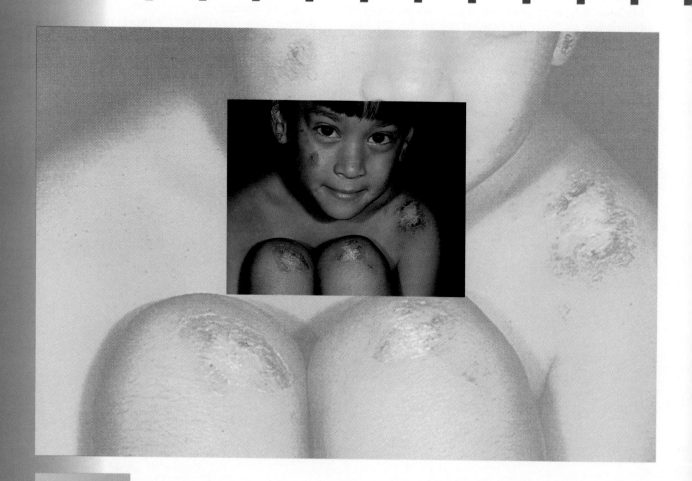

A woman brings her 6-year-old daughter Luisa to your clinic. She says that 2 weeks ago "sores" started developing on Luisa's fingers and have since spread to her face, shoulder, and knees. They started out as flat, red patches and have become crusted-over scabs. Luisa complains of itching. Her mother has noted no fever or flulike symptoms. Luisa, her mother, and her three siblings live in a two-room apartment and share bathroom facilities with three other families.

What common skin disorders should you consider as you begin your assessment of Luisa? Many skin disorders are characterized by lesions or itching; however, the appearance of these "sores" and the history suggest that Luisa has impetigo, an infectious disorder that is easily transmitted among children who live in crowded conditions.

What treatment will be necessary? Based on the family's socioeconomic situation, what will be your focus in providing education for Luisa's mother? This chapter will prepare you to answer these and other questions about pediatric skin disorders, enabling you to provide effective care to Luisa and other children.

Photograph of child with impetigo (above) from Habif, T.P. (1990). *Clinical dermatology: A color guide to diagnosis and therapy* (2nd ed.) (p. 159). St. Louis: Mosby–Year Book.

ALTERATIONS IN SKIN INTEGRITY

20

TERMINOLOGY

atopy A hereditary allergic tendency.

debridement Removal of dead tissue to speed the healing process.

dermatophytoses Fungal infections that affect primarily the skin but may affect the hair and nails.

eschar Slough or layer of dead skin or tissue.

escharotomy Incision into constricting dead tissue of a burn injury to restore peripheral circulation.

lichenification Thickening of the skin.

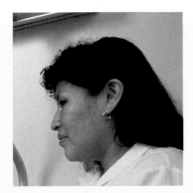

❝ I had never seen sores like Luisa's before. They appeared so suddenly and seemed to get worse each day. The nurses told me that Luisa's sores are caused by an infection that children can easily give to one another. ❞

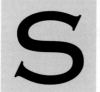kin disorders are seen frequently by nurses who work in outpatient clinics, emergency departments, and pediatric units of hospitals. Many of these disorders are not unique to children, but children are at greater risk for some skin conditions for reasons that are discussed in this chapter.

The skin is the largest organ in the body. It performs several essential functions, among them perception, protection, temperature regulation, vitamin D synthesis, and excretion. The skin enables us to perceive pain, heat, and cold and protects underlying tissues from invasion by microorganisms and from trauma.

Temperature regulation of the body is achieved by dilation or constriction of blood vessels and sweat glands that act under the control of the central nervous system. The skin also supplements the body's intake of vitamin D by synthesizing this vitamin from ultraviolet light. Excretion is performed by the sweat glands, which secrete a solution of water, electrolytes, and urea, thus helping to rid the body of toxins.

Anatomy and Physiology of Pediatric Differences

The skin is made up of three distinct layers: the epidermis, the dermis, and the subcutaneous fatty layer that separates the skin from the underlying tissue (Fig. 20–1). Within the dermis are nerves, muscles, connective tissue, hair follicles, sebaceous and sweat glands, lymph channels, and blood vessels.

At birth the skin is thin with little underlying subcutaneous fat. Because of this the infant loses heat more rapidly, has greater difficulty regulating body

FIGURE 20–1 Layers of the skin with accessory structures.

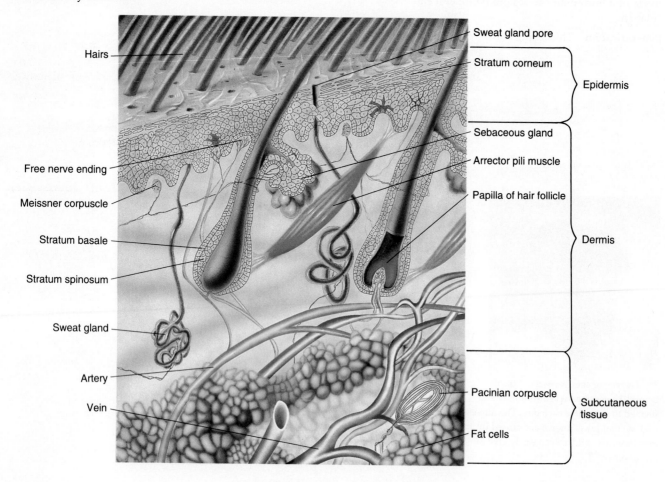

temperature, and becomes easily chilled. The thinner skin also leads to increased absorption of harmful chemical substances. The newborn's skin contains more water than an adult's and has loosely attached cells. As the infant grows, the skin toughens and becomes less hydrated, making it less susceptible to bacteria.

The accessory structures of the skin (hair, sebaceous glands, eccrine glands, and apocrine glands) are present at birth. Like other body structures, however, they are still immature.

At birth the infant may have soft, downy hair, called lanugo, on the shoulders and back. Lanugo is usually shed by 2 to 3 weeks of age. The amount of hair on the head varies. Scalp hair usually is shed within a few months and replaced, sometimes with hair of a different color.

Sebaceous glands function at birth, although somewhat immaturely. They vary in size and appear all over the body except on the hands and soles of the feet. Sebum, a lipid substance produced and secreted into the hair follicle or directly onto the skin, provides lubrication to the skin and hair.

Eccrine glands, located in the dermis, open onto the skin surface. They secrete an odorless, watery fluid, primarily in response to emotional stress. They also respond to changes in body temperature. As body temperature increases, the glands increase production of sweat. The result is decreased heat as the sweat evaporates. Because the eccrine sweat glands usually are not fully functional until middle childhood, infants and young children are unable to regulate temperature as effectively as older children and adults.

Apocrine glands, located mainly in the axillary and genital areas, do not function until puberty. Decomposition of the fluid secreted by these glands leads to body odor. Their biologic function, however, is unknown.

Skin Lesions

Skin lesions vary in size, shape, color, and contents. The two major types of skin lesions are primary lesions and secondary lesions. Primary lesions arise from previously healthy skin and include macules, patches, papules, nod-

TABLE 20–1 **Common Secondary Skin Lesions and Associated Conditions**

Lesion Name	Description	Example
Crust	Dried residue of serum, pus, or blood	Impetigo
Scale	Thin flake of exfoliated epidermis	Dandruff, psoriasis
Lichenification	Thickening of skin with increased visibility of normal skin furrows	Eczema (atopic dermatitis)
Scar	Replacement of destroyed tissue with fibrous tissue	Healed surgical incision
Keloid	Hypertrophied scar	Healed skin area following traumatic injury
Excoriation	Abrasion or scratch mark	Scratched insect bite
Fissure	Linear crack in skin	Tinea pedis (athlete's foot)
Erosion	Loss of superficial epidermis; moist but does not bleed	Ruptured chicken pox vesicle
Ulcer	Deeper loss of skin surface; bleeding or scarring may ensue	Chancre

ules, tumors, vesicles, pustules, bullae, and wheals (see Table 3-7). Secondary lesions result from changes in primary lesions. They include crusts, scales, **lichenification** (thickening of the skin), scars, keloids, excoriation, fissures, erosion, and ulcers (Table 20–1). It is important for the nurse to be able to identify and describe the primary and secondary skin lesions and understand their underlying cause and treatment.

Wound Healing

Wound healing is a process that occurs in three overlapping phases: inflammation, proliferation, and maturation (Table 20–2).

Inflammation, the initial response at the injury site, lasts approximately 3 to 5 days. This phase prepares the injury site for the repair process. Vasodilation, which occurs shortly after injury, allows leukocytes to travel to the injury site, where they ingest bacteria and debris. Fibroblasts deposit fibrin throughout the site, assisting in clot formation.

Proliferation, the second phase, may last from 5 days to 4 weeks, depending on the extent of the injury. During this phase, fibroblasts secrete collagen into the meshwork of fibrin, creating highly vascular granulation tissue. A fine layer of epithelial cells forms over the site.

Maturation, the third phase, involves continued collagen production. Contraction of the healing area leads to closure of the wound. Scarring can then occur. Maturation can take months to years, depending on the extent of the injury.

Dermatitis

Many skin disorders occur in early childhood. Most are easily treated and do not have long-term consequences. Dermatitis is a condition in which changes occur in the skin in response to external stimuli. The four most common types of dermatitis that occur in infants, children, and adolescents are contact dermatitis, diaper dermatitis, seborrheic dermatitis, and eczema. It is important for the nurse to understand that these skin disorders bring with them emotional problems for the family and child. Be sympathetic and remember that the family and child can see the skin condition and need to be reassured that the child is not infectious.

TABLE 20–2 Phases of Wound Healing

Inflammation (3 to 5 Days)
Clotting
Phagocytosis
Epithelialization

Proliferation (5 Days to 4 Weeks)
Epithelialization
Fibroblast migration and capillary budding
Collagen synthesis
Granulation

Maturation (Months to Years)
Remodeling
Contraction

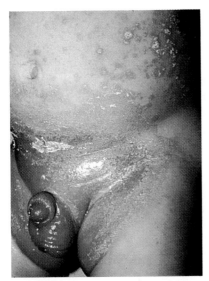

FIGURE 20–2 Diaper dermatitis. Courtesy of the Centers for Disease Control, Atlanta, GA.

■ NURSING ALERT

Avoid using such products as baby wipes on an infant with diaper dermatitis. The alcohol content in the wipes may exacerbate the condition.

Contact Dermatitis

Contact dermatitis is an inflammation of the skin that occurs in response to an allergen or irritant. Common allergens include poison ivy, poison oak, rubber, shoe leather, and nickel. Common irritants include soaps, detergents, bleaches, lotions, urine, and stool. Reactions to latex, which can be found in many types of hospital equipment (gloves, intravenous equipment, airway equipment, plastic syringes, adhesive tape) also have been reported.[1]

Symptoms of allergic contact dermatitis can develop up to 18 hours after contact, peak between 48 and 72 hours, and can last up to 3 weeks. In contrast, irritant contact dermatitis usually develops within a few hours of contact, peaks within 24 hours, and quickly resolves.

Diaper Dermatitis

Diaper dermatitis, the most common irritant contact dermatitis, occurs in approximately one third of young children, usually in a mild form.[3] It is most common in infants from 4 to 12 months of age.

The rash is characterized by erythema, edema, vesicles, papules, and scaling that appear in areas in direct contact with the diaper, usually the perineum, genitals, buttocks and skin folds (Fig. 20–2). In severe cases, the infant develops a rash that is fiery red, raised, and confluent. Pustules with tenderness can also be present.

Urine, stool, baby wipes, and detergents can irritate the perianal area. The warm, moist environment of the wet or soiled diaper is conducive to bacterial and fungal growth and is a mechanical irritant to the infant's delicate skin. *Candida albicans* is frequently the underlying cause of severe diaper rash. Diaper candidiasis often occurs simultaneously with oral candidiasis (see later discussion).

Treatment for mild diaper dermatitis involves application of 1% hydrocortisone cream with each diaper change for 5 to 7 days and good basic hygiene. Diaper candidiasis is treated with alternating applications of 1% hydrocortisone cream and antifungal creams (nystatin) applied to the affected areas at diaper change. Fluorinated topical corticosteroids should not be used.

Nursing Management

Severe diaper dermatitis can be a major source of stress for parents who must deal with a child in constant discomfort. The goal of treatment is to identify and remove the cause of the irritation. It is important to instruct parents to change the diaper as soon as the infant is wet. Most disposable diapers contain fibers to increase their absorbency. However, this should not be an excuse for waiting until the diaper is saturated to change it. Tell parents to avoid using plastic pants. A & D ointment, zinc oxide, Desitin, and Balmex can be used to protect the skin from the acidity of urine and stool.

Advise parents to wash the perianal area with warm water and a mild soap (such as Dove or Tone) with every diaper change. Exposing the diaper area to air helps with healing. Allowing the child to go without a diaper, while lying on an absorbable pad or cloth, is also beneficial.

Seborrheic Dermatitis

Seborrheic dermatitis is a recurrent inflammatory skin condition of unknown etiology. It is found over the areas of the body where sebaceous glands are most plentiful: scalp (cradle cap), forehead, and postauricular and periorbital areas. It may also occur on the skin of the eyelids, inguinal area,

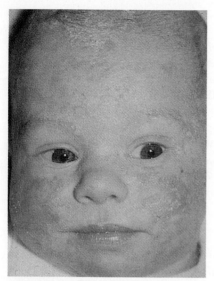

FIGURE 20–3 Seborrheic dermatitis.

or nasolabial folds. The condition is frequently seen in infants and adolescents.

Common symptoms are pruritus and scaling of the scalp (or "dandruff"). Dry or greasy, yellow scales or crusts may be present, typically on the scalp and face, behind the ears, and on the upper chest (Fig. 20–3).

Treatment for seborrheic dermatitis consists of daily shampooing with a mild baby shampoo, followed by removal of the crusts from the scalp. The shampoo is left on the scalp for a few minutes to soften crusts. The hair is then rinsed thoroughly, and a fine-toothed comb is used to remove loosened crusts from the hair. Treatments are continued for several days after the lesions disappear. Shampoos such as Head and Shoulders or Selsun Blue are used for adolescents. Topical steriods are used to treat seborrhea that is not on the scalp.

Nursing Management

Seborrheic dermatitis can usually be prevented with proper scalp hygiene. Teach new parents that the infant's hair should be washed daily. Reassure parents that gentle cleansing will not harm the infant's "soft spot." Follow-up is seldom necessary, since the condition resolves with treatment.

Drug Reactions

Adverse reactions to over-the-counter or prescription medications are not uncommon. Children with drug allergies usually have reactions after ingestion (aspirin, antibiotics, sedatives), injection (penicillin), or direct skin contact. Drug sensitivities may result from variations in an individual's ability to tolerate a particular drug or concentration of a drug or from allergic responses.

Sensitivity reactions to a drug not previously administered may take up to 7 days to develop. If the child has been sensitized to a drug, the reaction is almost immediate. The most common reactions in children are the development of erythematous macules and papules or urticaria, which may be pruritic. The nurse should be alert to the possibility of an anaphylactic reaction, which is a medical emergency.

The treatment of choice for most drug sensitivity reactions is discontinuation of the causative drug. Supportive measures should be taken to decrease the intensity of the reaction. An antihistamine may be used to block the release of histamine, which causes the rash. Topical steroids, cool compresses, and baths may also be prescribed.

Nursing Management

Nurses can play an important role by teaching parents to be alert to the signs of drug sensitivity reactions. Obtain a careful history of the child's past reactions to medications before starting new therapies. If a reaction occurs, discontinue the medication until the physician is notified. Prominently mark the child's records so that all allergies are easily identified.

Eczema (Atopic Dermatitis)

Eczema, also called atopic dermatitis, is a chronic, superficial inflammatory skin disorder characterized by intense pruritus. The condition affects infants, children, and adolescents. It is a common skin condition, although the exact incidence is difficult to estimate because most mild cases go untreated.

Clinical Manifestations

Acute eczema is characterized by pruritus and erythematous patches with vesicles, exudate, and crusts. Symptoms of chronic eczema are pruritus, dryness, scaling, and lichenification (Fig. 20–4). Inflammation usually occurs on the face, upper arms, back, upper thighs, and back of the hands and feet.

Eczema occurs in three forms: infantile (ages 2 months to 2 years), childhood (ages 2 years to puberty), and adolescent (Table 20–3). In infantile eczema, lesions are exudative and crusted. Vesicles and erythema are common. Itching frequently interrupts the child's sleep patterns. In childhood eczema, lesions are drier, scaly, pruritic, well circumscribed, and rarely exudative. Lesions in adolescent eczema are similar to those in the childhood form; however, larger plaques and lichenification may also be present.

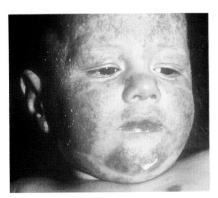

FIGURE 20–4 Chronic eczema.

Etiology and Pathophysiology

The etiology of eczema is unknown, but the disorder tends to occur in children with hereditary allergic tendencies **(atopy).** If one parent has allergies (e.g., hay fever, asthma, or contact dermatitis), the child has a 60% greater chance of having allergies. This increases to 80% if both parents have allergies. A family history of asthma or hay fever frequently predisposes a child to eczema. Eczema may be intensified by dry skin, irritating clothing, abrasive detergents, perspiration, emotional stress, cosmetics and perfumed lotions and soaps.

Diagnostic Tests and Medical Management

Eczema is distinguished from other forms of dermatitis by its history and clinical manifestations. Eczema is more likely to have a generalized distribution with no known exposure to an allergen.

TABLE 20-3 Types of Eczema

Type	Clinical Manifestations	Outcome
Infantile (2 months to 2 years)	Exudative, crusty, papulovesicular, and erythematous lesions on cheeks, scalp, forehead, arms, and legs; intensely pruritic	50% of cases resolve by age of 2 to 3 years
Childhood (2 years to puberty)	Erythematous, dry, scaly, well-circumscribed, papular, more thickened and lichenified pruritic lesions on wrist, hands, neck and antecubital and popliteal fossae	75% of cases have no recurrence after adolescence
Adolescent (puberty on)	Much the same as childhood eczema; large plaques thickened and lichenified on face, neck, back, hands, feet, and upper arms	May recur often

Goals of treatment are to hydrate and lubricate the skin, reduce pruritus, and minimize inflammatory changes. The cardinal principle of topical therapy for oozing or weeping is "wet on wet." If lesions are weeping, wet compresses (cotton cloths) soaked in aluminum acetate solution sometimes are used. Lubrication is achieved by applying lotion after bathing to trap moisture and prevent drying of skin. Noninflamed areas are treated with emollients such as Eucerin.

Topical corticosteroids are used to reduce inflammation. Ointments are preferred over creams because of their occlusive effect, which ensures a stronger barrier and absorption into the skin. Hydrocortisone 1% or triamcinolone 0.1% is usually the drug of choice. Corticosteroids are used one to three times daily for 4 to 5 days. Systemic antibiotics are given only if the child has a superimposed infection.

Antipruritic agents such as hydroxyzine (Vistaril and Atarax) can be given to relieve itching. Methods to reduce pruritus include environmental controls, such as humidification in the winter and air conditioning in the summer. Use of a humidifier counteracts dryness of the surrounding air, minimizing loss of skin moisture. Air conditioning limits unnecessary sweating that can exacerbate inflamed areas.

Nursing Assessment

A thorough history, including family history of allergy, any environmental or dietary factors, and past exacerbations, is necessary. Note distribution and type of lesions.

Nursing Diagnosis

Common nursing diagnoses for the child with eczema include:

- Impaired Skin Integrity related to open vesicles and open lesions as a result of scratching
- High Risk for Infection related to breaks in skin barrier
- Body Image Disturbance related to presence of noticeable skin lesions
- Self-Esteem Disturbance related to peer reaction to visible skin disorder

Nursing Management

Nursing management focuses on education and emotional support. Although no "cure" has been found for eczema, the condition can be controlled. Advise parents that the lesions are not contagious and will not result in scarring.

Instruct parents or adolescents to avoid using harsh or perfumed soaps. Aveeno or oatmeal baths to control itching and "weeping" or use of a mild soap (Dove or Tone) is recommended. Wool clothing should be avoided because it can increase skin irritation and pruritus. Encourage the wearing of cotton clothing. Hot water can exacerbate the condition and increase itching. Colloidal baths with Aveeno can help reduce itching. Recommend tepid baths and air drying afterward.

Teach parents and adolescents appropriate application of topical ointments or creams. Instruct parents to place clean cotton gloves or socks over the infant or young child's hands and to keep the child's fingernails cut short to decrease scratching and reduce the chance of secondary infection.

Eczema produces visible changes that can affect a child's self-confidence and self-esteem. Children need to be educated about the disorder and its treatment. Emphasize the importance of following the treatment plan to promote healing of existing lesions and to reduce the risk of secondary infections.

Infectious Disorders

Impetigo

Impetigo is a highly contagious, superficial infection caused by streptococci, staphylococci, or both. The most common sites are the face, around the mouth, the hands, the neck, and the extremities.

Clinical manifestations include pruritus, burning, and secondary lymph node involvement. The lesion begins as a macule that changes rapidly to form a small, thin-walled vesicle with an erythematous halo. The initially serous vesicular fluid becomes cloudy, and the vesicle ruptures, leaving a honey-colored crust covering an ulcerated base (Fig. 20–5). When the infection is caused by staphylococci, the initial macule may form small, thin-walled pustules or the larger bullae of bullous impetigo.

Infection occurs more commonly in children who are in close physical contact with one another. This was illustrated in the case of Luisa, described at the beginning of the chapter. Children frequently pass the infection to one another in pre-school or day care settings.

Local treatment involves removal of the crusts and application of a topical antibiotic. Crusts are soaked in warm water and gently scrubbed with an antiseptic soap (pHisoHex). A topical bactericidal ointment (such as neosporin, bacitracin, or mupirocin) is applied for 5 to 7 days. Children with multiple lesions may require systemic antibiotics.

Nursing Management

Advise parents that oral or topical medication must be continued for 7 to 10 days. Caution parents that an infected child should not share towels or toiletries with others and that all linens and clothing used by the child should

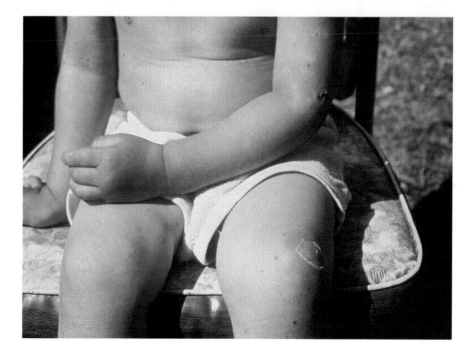

FIGURE 20–5 Characteristic lesions of impetigo.
Courtesy of the Centers for Disease Control, Atlanta, GA.

be washed separately in hot water. Fingernails should be kept short and clean to prevent the spread of infection from scratching.

Pediculosis Capitis (Lice)

Pediculosis capitis is an infestation of the hair and scalp with lice. Head lice live and reproduce only on humans and are transmitted by direct contact such as sharing of brushes, hats, towels, and bedding. The female louse lays her eggs (nits) on the hair shaft, close to the scalp (see Fig. 3-8). The incubation period is 8 to 10 days.

Clinical manifestations include intense pruritus and complaints of "dandruff" that sticks to the hair (actually the nits) and "bugs" in the hair. Secondary effects of scratching include inflammation, pustules, and bacterial infection. Nits are found most commonly behind the ears and at the back of the head. Occipital nodes are frequently palpable.

Infestation occurs among children of all socioeconomic levels. The presence of lice may be noted by parents or teachers, or by health care providers during routine examination of the child (see Chapter 3). Outbreaks occur periodically among preschool and school-age children, particularly those in day care and elementary school.

Treatment involves use of a pediculicide shampoo, such as lindane (Kwell [contraindicated for children less than 2 years of age]), or an ovicidal rinse, such as permethrin (Nix). Lindane shampoo is applied to the hair and scalp and is worked into a lather with a small amount of water. The lather is rubbed into the scalp for 4 to 5 minutes, then rinsed out thoroughly. The hair is towel dried, and the nits are removed with a fine-toothed comb. Vinegar compresses applied to the hair for 15 minutes will help remove the nit shells. The treatment is repeated in 7 days.

Permethrin is used for children under 2 years of age or pregnant adolescents. The preparation is applied, left in place for 10 minutes, and then rinsed. The hair is then towel dried. This treatment is effective in 99% of cases.[4]

Nursing Management

Infestation with lice can be upsetting for both the child and family. Emphasize to the family that anyone can get lice. Thorough interventions and education are essential for effective treatment.

Although lice can survive for only about 48 hours away from a human host, nits that are shed are capable of hatching 8 to 10 days later. For this reason, bedding and clothing used by the child should be changed daily, laundered in hot water with detergent and dried in a hot dryer for 20 minutes. Nonessential bedding and clothing can be stored in a tightly sealed bag for 10 days to 2 weeks and then washed. Hairbrushes and combs should be discarded or soaked in boiling water for 10 to 15 minutes or washed with pediculicide shampoo. Furniture should be vacuumed and treated with a hot iron when possible. Use of an insecticide is usually not recommended in households containing young children. All contacts of the child should be examined for infestation and should be treated as necessary.

Scabies

Scabies is a highly contagious infestation caused by the mite *Sarcoptes scabiei*. Symptoms include a rash, severe pruritus that worsens at night, and restlessness. Lesions are usually located in the webs of the fingers, in the intergluteal folds, around the axillae, or on the palms, wrists, head, neck, legs,

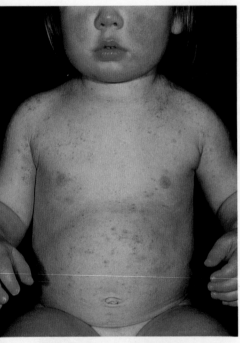

FIGURE 20–6 Diffuse scabies in an infant. The lesions are most numerous around the axillae, chest, and abdomen.

From Habif, T.P. (1990). *Clinical dermatology: A color guide to diagnosis and therapy* (2nd ed.) (p. 298). St. Louis: Mosby–Year Book.

buttocks, chest, abdomen, and waist (Fig. 20–6). In infants the palms, soles, and head and neck can be affected. Lesions appear as linear, threadlike, grayish burrows 1 to 10 cm in length, which may end in a pinpoint vesicle.

Children of all ages and both sexes can be affected. The female mite burrows into the outer layer of the epidermis (stratum corneum) to lay her eggs. The larvae hatch in approximately 2 to 4 days and proceed toward the surface of the skin. The cycle is repeated 14 to 17 days later. The intense pruritus is caused by sensitization to the ova and mite feces, which occurs approximately 1 month after infestation. Because the mite usually takes at least 45 minutes to burrow into the skin, transient contact is unlikely to cause infestation.

Diagnosis is confirmed by examination of scrapings from a burrow under the microscope, which reveals eggs or nits. Treatment involves application of a scabicide, such as lindane lotion (Kwell, Scabene), over the entire body from the neck down.

Application of lotion is preceded by a warm soap and water bath. Skin must be cool and dry before the lotion is applied. The lotion is left in place for 4 to 6 hours. Usually only one application is necessary; however, 2- or 3-day treatment cycles are sometimes recommended. All members of the household should be treated at the same time.

It is recommended that Eurax lotion be used for children under 2 years of age. The child is thoroughly bathed with soap and water using a rough washcloth. The cream is then applied to the entire body and to face and scalp lesions if present. Reapplication is needed 24 hours later. The child is bathed 48 hours after the last application to remove any residual medication. An oral antihistamine (Benadryl, Atarax) may be prescribed to help relieve itching.

Nursing Management

Advise parents that all clothing, bedding, and pillowcases used by the child should be changed daily, washed with boiling water, and ironed before reuse. Parents and siblings should avoid touching the affected child until after treatment is completed. If contact is made, hands should be washed well.

Scabies, like pediculosis, can be embarrassing or upsetting for the child. Educate children, as well as parents, about the condition, its spread, and treatment measures to prevent recurrence.

Fungal Infections

Oral Candidiasis (Thrush)

Oral candidiasis (moniliasis or thrush) is a fungal infection that occurs as an acute condition in newborns (usually acquired during birth from the vaginal canal of an infected mother) and a chronic condition in young children (often when a child is receiving antibiotics and the normal flora is disturbed, allowing growth of the fungus).

Thrush is characterized by white patches that look like coagulated milk on the oral mucosa (Fig. 20–7). The infant may refuse to nurse or feed because of discomfort and pain.

Treatment involves oral nystatin suspension, which is given after feedings. Older children are instructed to swish the solution around in the mouth before swallowing it. For infants, parents should use a swab to apply the suspension to the buccal mucosa and tongue surfaces, allowing the infant to swallow the remaining suspension.

If infection is severe, occurs in the esophagus, or invades other body systems, oral fluconazole or intravenous amphotericin B may be prescribed.

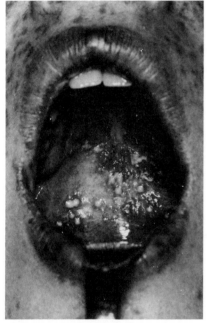

FIGURE 20–7 Thrush, an acute pseudomembranous form of oral candidiasis, is a common fungal infection in infants and young children.
From Orkin, M., Maibach, H.I., & Dahl, M.V. (1991). *Dermatology* (p. 575). Norwalk, CT: Appleton & Lange.

■ CLINICAL TIP

The white patches of candidiasis are easily differentiated from coagulated milk. Milk residue can be removed from the oral mucosa with gentle swabbing. With candidiasis, however, attempts at gentle removal are unsuccessful. (Avoid scraping the patches, since this will result in bleeding.)

Dermatophytoses (Ringworm)

Dermatophytoses are fungal infections that affect the skin, hair, or nails. Children of all ages may be affected. Dermatophytoses may be spread from person to person or from animal to person. The most common infections are tinea capitis, tinea corporis, tinea cruris, and tinea pedis. Table 20–4 compares and contrasts these infections.

Diagnosis is confirmed through microscopic examination of the scrapings using a potassium hydroxide (KOH) wet mount to reveal hyphae (threadlike fungal bodies). A Wood's lamp is also useful in identifying some forms of tinea that fluoresce under ultraviolet light. Treatment involves application of an antifungal lotion, cream, or shampoo (see Table 20–4).

Nursing Management. Advise parents that lotion and cream should be applied to the entire lesion, as well as to approximately 1 cm surrounding the lesion. Teach parents and older children or teenagers that fungi are found in soil and animals and are transmitted through direct contact. Household pets should be examined for signs of infection.

Since person-to-person transmission is common, personal contact with hair and the sharing of hair care products should be avoided. For children with tinea cruris, encourage the use of loose-fitting undergarments to promote dryness. With tinea pedis, feet should be kept clean and dry and nails clipped short. Discourage the wearing of occlusive footwear or nylon socks, which trap moisture.

TABLE 20–4 Types of Tinea Infection

Site	Clinical Manifestations	Incidence	Treatment
Tinea capitis (scalp)	Hair loss (one or several patches); broken hairs; thickened, white scales; fine scaling	Usually postpubertal adolescents	Griseofulvin cream and 2.5% selenium sulfide shampoo; apply daily; extended treatment may be necessary (2–3 months)
Tinea corporis (trunk)	One or several circular erythematous patches; may be scaly or erythematous throughout	Children or adolescents	Topical cream (clotrimazole) twice a day until clear (usually 2–4 weeks)
Tinea cruris ("jock itch") (inner thighs, inguinal creases)	Scaly, erythematous eruption; possibly elevated lesions; possible papules or vesicles	Rare before adolescence	Same as for tinea corporis
Tinea pedis ("athlete's foot") (feet and toes)	Vesicles or erosions on instep or between toes (fissures, red scaly)	Usually postpubertal adolescents	Same as for tinea corporis and cruris

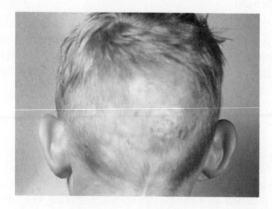

Tinea capitis

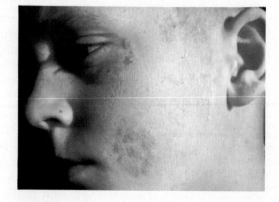

Tinea corporis

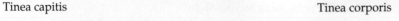

Photographs of *tinea capitis* and *tinea corporis* courtesy of the Centers for Disease Control and Prevention, Atlanta, GA.

Parents of children with tinea capitis should be told that hair regrowth is slow and may take 3 to 6 months. In some cases hair loss is permanent, which can be particularly stressful for older children or adolescents. Provide emotional support.

Cellulitis

Cellulitis is an acute inflammation of the skin and subcutaneous fat characterized by red or lilac, tender, edematous skin that may have an ill-defined, nonelevated border.[5] The condition usually occurs on the face and extremities as a result of trauma or compromise of the skin barrier.

Clinical Manifestations

Children with cellulitis appear ill and are commonly febrile. Classic signs and symptoms include erythema, edema of the face or infected limb, warmth, and tenderness around the infected site (Fig. 20–8). Other symptoms include chills, malaise, and enlargement and tenderness of regional lymph nodes.

Etiology and Pathophysiology

Children with cellulitis often have a history of trauma, impetigo, folliculitis, or recent otitis media.[6] Common causative organisms are *Staphylococcus aureus* and *Streptococcus pyrogenes*. Onset is usually rapid.

Diagnostic Tests and Medical Management

Blood studies may show an increase in white blood cells. Cultures are taken by needle aspiration, if possible, to identify the causative organisms. If the face is involved, antibiotic therapy is used to avoid serious complications. (Periorbital cellulitis is discussed in Chapter 11.)

FIGURE 20–8 Characteristic appearance of cellulitis.
From Ben-Amitai, D., & Sahkenazi, S. (1993). Common bacterial skin infections in children. *Pediatric Annals, 22*(4), 226. Photograph courtesy of Dr. Aryeh Metzker.

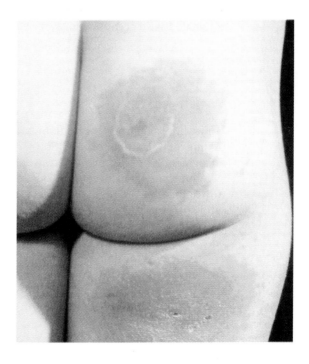

Children with cellulitis on the trunk, limbs, or perianal area may be treated on an outpatient basis with oral antibiotics. Recovery begins within 48 hours, but therapy should continue for at least 10 days.

Children with severe cases or a large affected surface area are hospitalized to prevent sepsis. Systemic antibiotics are administered. Untreated cellulitis or cellulitis that does not respond to treatment can lead to osteomyelitis or arthritis.

Nursing Assessment

Assessment centers on recognition of infection, documentation of location and related symptoms, and monitoring of vital signs.

Nursing Diagnosis

Common nursing diagnoses for the child with cellulitis include:

- Impaired Skin Integrity related to the inflammatory process and presence of infection
- Pain related to swelling and inflammation of the skin
- Knowledge Deficit (Parent or Child) related to care of the infected area

Nursing Management

Because of the risk of sepsis, cellulitis should be managed carefully. Supportive care includes warm compresses to the affected area four times daily, elevation of the affected limb, and bed rest. Outpatient follow-up is crucial.

Advise parents about possible complications, such as abcess formation. Instruct parents of children who are treated as outpatients to contact their health care provider if the child has any of the following signs: (1) spread of the infected area in the 24- to 48-hour period after the start of treatment, (2) temperature over 101° F, or (3) increased lethargy. Reinforce to parents the importance of compliance with the treatment regimen and the seriousness associated with complications.

▣ Folliculitis

Folliculitis is a superficial inflammation of the pilosebaceous follicle caused by infection, trauma, or irritation. The condition is common in children and teenagers because of increased sweat production.

Symptoms include tenderness, localized swelling, and the formation of tiny dome-shaped, yellowish pustules and red papules at follicular openings with surrounding erythema. Lesions are usually seen in clusters on the face, scalp, and extremities. The causative organism is usually *Staphylococcus aureus*.

Treatment of inflamed follicles consists of washing the affected area with soap and water, followed by application of hot compresses for 20 minutes, four times a day. Complications are rare. If lesions do not resolve within a week, the child may need antibiotics and, if the infection is deep, incision and drainage.

Nursing Management

Nursing management focuses on educating the parents and child about prevention. Advise children to shower daily and shortly after exercise, to cleanse with an antibacterial soap, and to wear loose cotton clothing.

Acne

Acne, a disorder of the pilosebaceous unit (hair follicle and sebaceous gland), is the most common skin disorder in the pediatric population. The prevalence in adolescents aged 15 to 17 years is estimated to approach 85%. Acne may also occur in neonates in response to maternal androgen hormones. This form of acne usually develops between 2 and 4 weeks of age and resolves by 4 to 6 months of age.

Clinical Manifestations

There are three main types of acne: comedomal (characterized by open and closed comedones), papulopustular (characterized by papules and pustules) (Fig. 20–9), and cystic (characterized by nodules and cysts). Lesions occur most often on the face, upper chest, shoulders, and back. In adolescents the major complaint is an increase in the number of closed (blackhead) or open (whitehead) comedones, pimples, and red papules that are tender to touch. Cystic acne may result in permanent scarring and disfiguration.

Etiology and Pathophysiology

Obstruction of the sebaceous follicle opening, usually by keratin and sebum, produces the comedones that are seen most commonly in acne. Papules, pustules, and cysts result from rupture of the follicle walls. Although familial trends are recognized, hard data to define the pattern of inheritance are not conclusive.

Diagnostic Tests and Medical Management

Treatment depends on the type of lesion. Most adolescent acne is treated with topical and oral medications, alone or in combination. Table 20–5 out-

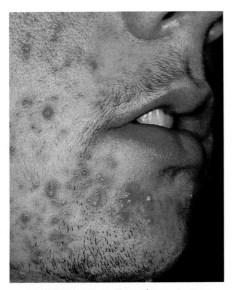

FIGURE 20-9 Pustular acne can have a significant effect on an adolescent's self-esteem.

From Habif, T.P. (1990). *Clinical dermatology: A color guide to diagnosis and therapy* (2nd ed.) (p. 113). St. Louis: Mosby–Year Book.

TABLE 20-5 Treatment Protocols for Acne

Appearance	Treatment
Comedomal acne (comedones only)	Retinoic acid 0.025% cream and 10% benzoyl peroxide daily
Papulopustular acne	
Red papules, few pustules	Retinoic acid in morning and 10% benzoyl peroxide in evening
Red papules, many pustules	Follow above regimen with addition of oral antibiotics (tetracycline or erythromycin, 500 mg twice a day)
Cystic acne (red papules, many pustules, cysts, and nodules)	Retinoic acid and benzoyl peroxide twice a day, with oral antibiotics (tetracycline or erythromycin, 1–1.5 g daily)

From Weston, W.E. (1985). *Practical pediatric dermatology* (2nd ed.). (p.32). Boston: Little, Brown.

THE ADOLESCENT WITH ACNE

GOAL	INTERVENTION	RATIONALE	EXPECTED OUTCOME
1. Impaired Skin Integrity related to destruction of skin layers, multiple pustules, papules, and secretions			
Adolescent will verbalize proper hygiene, nutrition, and treatment of acne.*	Teach good skin care: • Wash skin with mild soap and water. • Do not use astringents. • Avoid vigorous scrubbing. • Praise good habits.	Good hygiene and appropriate skin care reduce surface oils that build up on the skin, exacerbating acne lesions.	Adolescent exhibits habits of good hygiene.
	Advise adolescent to wash hair with antiseborrheic shampoo, avoid oil-based cosmetics or lotions.	Treats seborrhea, which frequently accompanies acne. Oil-based preparations can obstruct sebaceous glands, exacerbating acne.	
	Encourage a balanced diet, exercise, and adequate rest. Encourage adolescent to keep a diary of health and diet habits.	Adequate nutrients and exercise promote healthy skin.	Adolescent keeps diary for one week to support healthy habits.
2. Knowledge Deficit related to treatment of acne			
Adolescent will verbalize understanding of treatment regimen.	Educate adolescent about medications (action, side effects, dosage, method of application) and duration of treatment.	Proper application of medication enhances healing of lesions.	Adolescent states understanding of treatment regimen, resulting in a noticeable reduction in lesions.
3. Body Image Disturbance related to visible facial lesions as evidenced by decreased interest in self and self-degrading comments			
Adolescent will demonstrate increased self-confidence and self-esteem.	Establish a rapport with adolescent.	A trusting relationship promotes verbalization of concerns and fears.	Adolescent freely discusses concerns and fears.
	Provide education about the disease process and therapy modalities.	Providing information better enables adolescent to take control of the disease process.	Adolescent demonstrates active involvement in own care.
	Encourage adolescent to be responsible for treatment and follow-up, and give positive reinforcement when compliance is noted.	Responsibility reinforces sense of self-esteem.	
	Encourage adolescent to become involved with school activities and peers.	Involvement in activities helps to enhance self-esteem and allows adolescent to explore new experiences and friendships.	Adolescent shows increased confidence, as demonstrated by involvement in extracurricular activities.

*The care described for goal 1 also applies to goal 2.

lines specific treatment protocols for comedomal, papulopustular, and cystic acne. The goal of treatment is to prevent infection and scarring and minimize psychologic distress.

Nursing Assessment

Physical assessment should include documentation regarding distribution, type, and severity of acne lesions. The child and parents should be assessed for their knowledge about the cause and treatment of acne.

Nursing Diagnosis

Common nursing diagnoses are presented in the Nursing Care Plan for the Adolescent with Acne.

Nursing Management

Nursing care for the adolescent with acne is summarized in the accompanying Nursing Care Plan. Nursing management focuses on educating the child and parents about acne and its treatment. Advise adolescents not to touch the affected areas, avoid picking at lesions, avoid using any cosmetics or cleansing products that have a greasy base, shampoo hair regularly (to treat seborrhea that can accompany acne), expect flare-ups despite treatment, and eat a well-balanced diet.

Emphasize that treatment is often long term. Significant improvement may not be seen until at least 4 weeks after the start of treatment.

Correct misconceptions about dietary causes. (For example, there is no evidence that chocolate causes acne.) Teach parents and children that increased sweating, as well as heat and humidity, may exacerbate acne. Emotional stress may increase adrenal androgen production, resulting in increased sebum production and acne flare-ups.

Caution patients who are taking vitamin A preparations (Retin-A) that these medications can make their skin sensitive to sunlight, resulting in sunburns with even minimal exposure. Teach correct procedures for taking other prescribed drugs, such as tetracycline, and discuss possible side effects.

Psychologic support is an important aspect of care. Because adolescents are preoccupied with peer relationships and body image, they find acne embarrassing. Encourage expression of feelings and refer for counseling, if necessary.

Injuries to the Skin

Burns*

Burns are the second leading cause of injury deaths (after motor vehicle crashes) in children between 1 and 14 years of age.[7] Boys between the ages of 1 and 4 years are twice as likely as girls to be burned. However, the national average age of pediatric burn patients is 32 months. Each year in the United States alone there are over 2 million injuries and thousands of deaths related to burns.

There are four main types of burns: thermal, chemical, electrical, and radioactive. Thermal burns, the most common burns in children, may occur through exposure to flames or hot liquids (such as coffee or grease). Chemical burns occur when children touch or ingest caustic agents. Electrical burns occur from exposure to direct or alternating current in electrical wires, appli-

---

*Material for the discussion of burns was provided by Amy Burke, R.N., B.S.N., Children's National Medical Center, Washington, DC.

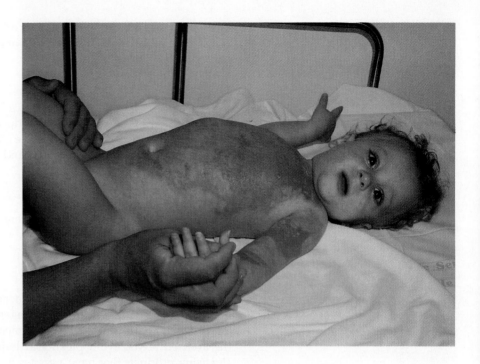

FIGURE 20–10 Thermal (scald) burns are the most common burn injury in infancy.

ances, or high-voltage wires. Radiation burns result from exposure to radioactive substances or the sun.

Etiology

Children at different developmental stages are at risk for different types of burns:

- Infants are most often injured by thermal burns (scalding liquids, house fires) (Fig. 20–10). They are also at risk for sunburn.
- Toddlers are at risk for thermal burns (pulling hot liquids or grease onto themselves), electrical burns (biting electrical cords) (Fig. 20–11), and chemical burns (ingesting cleaning agents and other substances) associated with exploring the environment.
- Preschool-age children are most often injured by scalding or contact with hot appliances (curling irons, ovens).
- School-age children are at risk for thermal burns (playing with matches), electrical burns (climbing high-voltage towers, climbing trees, and contact with electrical wires), and chemical burns (combustion experiments) associated with their curiosity and interest in experimentation.
- Adolescents also experience thermal, chemical, and electrical burns.

Medical Management

Assessment of Burn Severity. Burn severity is determined by the depth of burn injury, percentage of body surface area (BSA) affected, and involvement of specific body parts. Burn depth may be defined as first degree, second degree (superficial and deep), or third degree (Table 20–6). Because the skin is thin in young children, second- and third-degree burns are more common. Burn depth can also be defined as partial thickness or full thickness. Partial-thickness burns, in which the injured tissue can regenerate and heal,

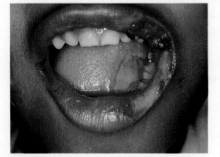

FIGURE 20–11 Electrical burn caused by biting an electrical cord.
Courtesy Dr. Lezley McIlveen, Department of Dentistry, Children's National Medical Center, Washington, D.C.

TABLE 20–6 Classification of Burns

First degree (superficial)	Second degree (partial thickness)	Third degree (full thickness)
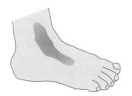	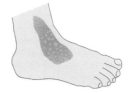	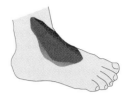
Skin red, dry	Blisters; skin moist, pink or red	Charring: skin black, brown, red
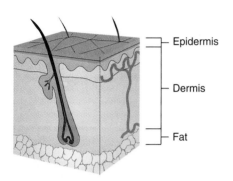	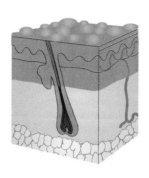	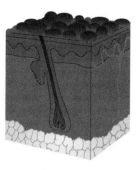
Damages only outer layer of skin; burn is painful and red; heals in a few days (example: sunburn)	Involves epidermis and upper layers of dermis; painful (partial thickness) and sensitive to cold air; results in blisters that blanch with pressure; heals in 10–14 days	Involves all of epidermis and dermis; may also involve underlying tissue; skin brown, black, or deep cherry red; usually no pain because nerve endings have been destroyed; injured area may appear sunken; requires skin grafting

encompass first- and second-degree burns. Full-thickness burns, in which the injured tissue cannot regenerate, are also known as third-degree burns.

A Lund and Browder chart with BSA distributions for various body parts at different ages is used to calculate the area affected by the burn injury (Fig. 20–12). Once the affected BSA is calculated, the burn can be classified as minor (less than 5% of BSA), moderate (10% to 15% of BSA), or major (greater than 15% of BSA). Children with moderate and major burns require hospitalization.

The involvement of specific body parts or specific burn distributions increases the burn severity, regardless of BSA affected. Burns to the face, hands, feet, or perineal area are treated as major because of the potential for functional impairment. Circumferential burns (injury completely surrounding the thorax or an extremity), anterior chest burns, and smoke inhalation are also classified as major burns.

Initial Treatment. The first step is to stop the burning process by removing any jewelry and all clothing. Emergency treatment of major burns is based on the ABCs of basic life support (*a*irway patency, *b*reathing, and *c*irculation). Assessment and treatment are necessary to ensure airway patency, es-

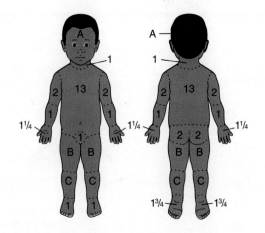

Relative Percentages of Areas Affected by Growth

Area	Age in Years					
	0	1	5	10	15	Adult
A = ½ of head	9½	8½	6½	5½	4½	3½
B = ½ of one thigh	2¾	3¼	4	4½	4½	4¾
C = ½ of one lower leg	2½	2½	2¾	3	3¼	3½

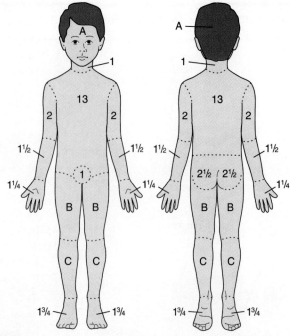

FIGURE 20–12 Lund and Browder chart for determining percentage of body surface area in pediatric burn injuries.

Adapted from Artz, C.P., & Moncrief, J.A. (1969). *The treatment of burns* (2nd ed.). Philadelphia: W.B. Saunders.

pecially when signs of smoke inhalation or burns to the face and neck are present. The child is assessed for other potential injuries when the mechanism of injury also includes a fall or explosion. Identify signs of respiratory distress and any potential bleeding source.

A weak, thready pulse, tachycardia, and pallor are important signs of early shock that may provide clues of an internal injury. Fluid replacement is necessary to prevent hypovolemic shock in cases of major burn injury. Fluid shifts from the vasculature to the interstitial spaces (third spacing) occur soon after the burn. Vascular integrity is usually restored after the first 24 hours.

Fluid replacement for the first 24 hours after the injury is based on a fluid volume formula calculated from the child's body weight, affected BSA, and normal maintenance needs. Several formulas exist for this calculation. Lactated Ringer's solution is the preferred fluid. Half of the total volume calculated for the 24-hour period is infused over the first 8 hours, and the remainder is distributed evenly over the next 16 hours. Resuscitation efforts are also focused on maintaining the child's temperature because heat is lost rapidly through burned skin.

Treatment of Minor Burns. For minor burns, exposure to cool, running water is the best treatment. This stops the burning process and helps to alleviate pain. Ice is contraindicated. All jewelry and clothing are removed, and the burn area is placed under running water. A topical antibiotic (Neosporin) may then be applied, if desired. If acid is the burning agent, neutralization in the emergency department is often required. Any open blisters are debrided, and a thin layer of silver sulfadiazine is applied over the burn. The burn is then covered with one or two layers of gauze. Burn dressings should be changed twice daily. This involves cleaning the burn and reapplying antibiotic cream.

Instruct parents that the child will need to increase fluid intake to compensate for loss of fluid through damaged skin. A high-calorie, high-protein

PEDIATRIC NURSING

diet is necessary to meet the increased nutritional requirements of healing. Acetaminophen (Tylenol) with codeine is often given, especially before dressing changes. Infection is a common complication. The child should be seen within 48 hours of treatment to monitor progress. Reinforce to parents the importance of follow-up appointments.

Treatment of Major Burns. Children with major burns are monitored closely for hyperthermia and usually require more aggressive wound management. Intravenous narcotics are often necessary to alleviate pain from treatment. Intake and output must be monitored closely. Intravenous fluids are administered to replace fluid lost through the skin. A Foley catheter may be inserted to enable close monitoring of urine output.

Hyperthermia is a normal, expected outcome of any significant thermal injury. Infection of the burned area is a frequent complication. Frequent checks of vital signs are necessary. Treatment may include analgesics, ice packs, cooling blankets, or cool hydrotherapy sessions. Enteral feedings are initiated within 24 hours of the burn injury to support the child's increased nutritional requirements.

Special consideration is needed when burns involve certain areas of the body:

- Dependent edema is common with burn injuries. Elevation of the burned extremity helps to minimize edema. Check pulse every hour in the burned extremity (distal to the circumferential or nearly circumferential burn). Any decrease, change, or absence of pulse requires immediate notification of the physician, since an **escharotomy** (incision into the constricting tissue) may be necessary to restore peripheral circulation.
- Facial burns usually cause significant edema. Care must be taken to ensure airway patency. For burns to the eye, an ophthalmologist should be consulted to assess damage. If damage has occurred, the affected eye should be covered with a dressing saturated with sterile saline solution. If the lips are burned, an infant may be unable to suck.
- Burns of the hands require careful management to maintain function. Special splinting and physical therapy are usually necessary.
- Perineal burns are at higher risk for infection because of frequent contamination with urine and stool. Perineal burns are treated with bacitracin on the urethral meatus and silvadene on the rest of the burn. The area is then wrapped with a burn pack and secured with a diaper. Frequent dressing changes are required. A Foley catheter is usually inserted but is removed once hydration status is stable to minimize the risk of urinary tract infection.

Treatment of Burn Wounds. Wound management is the most important aspect of caring for the burned child. Burn wound care has three main goals: (1) to speed wound debridement, (2) to protect granulation tissue and new grafts, and (3) to conserve body heat and fluids. Several treatment regimens are used to achieve these goals.

The entire body is bathed to initiate debridement. Hair should be shaved or cut away from burned areas because it can harbor bacteria. Intact blisters provide a natural, pain-free, sterile dressing. If blisters break open, the tissue should be carefully cut away. After initial cleansing, antibacterial agents, such as silvadene, are applied to prevent bacterial infection and dressings are added to cover the burned area (Table 20–7).

Dressing changes are performed at least twice daily. These changes are often very painful. When an old dressing is removed, a layer of **eschar** (the

TABLE 20-7 **Burn Wound Care**

Preparation

1. Check the physician's orders. Since burn care is often a painful procedure, check for pain medication orders and administer medication at least ½ hour before starting burn care.
2. Wash your hands. Gather supplies, including gloves (clean and sterile), a basin, sterile normal saline solution, a large supply of 4 × 4 gauze pads, forceps, scissors, a sterile tongue blade, the prescribed topical medication, tape, and an absorbent pad.
3. You may need an assistant to hold the child and the burned extremity during care.

Procedure

1. Place the absorbent pad under the area to be cleaned. Put on clean gloves. Soak the wound for about 10 minutes in normal saline solution, or apply wet dressing to the area. This will soften the wound. Remove the gloves.
2. After approximately 10 minutes, put on sterile gloves and wash the burn with the gauze pads using a *firm*, circular motion, moving from the inside to the outer edges. As you do this, be sure to remove any medication or crusting. Bleeding may occur, but this is a sign of healing, healthy tissue. Rinse with more normal saline solution. Pat dry with sterile gauze.
3. Remove (per physician's orders) any loose or dead skin around the edges of the burn by gently lifting it with the forceps and snipping it. This is not painful to the child. You may rinse and dry again.
4. Place a thin layer of prescribed medication (about ⅛ inch thick) on the burn with gauze or a tongue blade. Cover with a dry, sterile dressing.

Burn wound care written by Marcia Wellington, R.N., M.S.

tough leathery scab that forms over severely burned areas) is also removed, resulting in **debridement** (removal of necrotic tissue from a burned area). Children should be given analgesics before debridement procedures.

Hydrotherapy (whirlpool) baths are given before debridement to loosen eschar. Hydrotherapy is performed twice daily to increase vasodilation and circulation and to speed healing (Fig. 20–13). As a rule, tap water is used for debridement. Gentle washing is necessary to protect new epithelial cells. Granulation tissue forms as a result of daily debridement.

Skin grafting is necessary with any deep second- or third-degree burns that (1) have an impenetrable leathery layer of eschar that is preventing

FIGURE 20-13 A whirlpool bath is being used to increase this child's circulation and speed the healing of his burns.

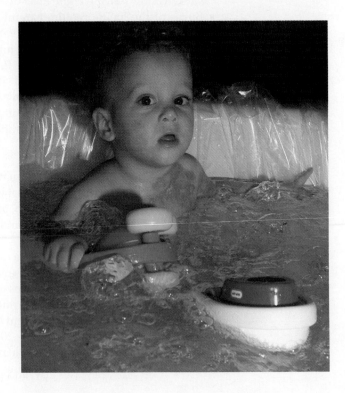

PEDIATRIC NURSING

spontaneous regeneration of skin or (2) are so deep that not enough skin structures are left to permit spontaneous growth. The graft is placed only after the area is excised to reveal healthy bleeding tissue. Wet-to-dry dressings may be used for a few days preoperatively to prepare an area for the graft. However, these dressings are very painful, and the child will need analgesics and emotional support.

Four types of grafts are available: autografts, allografts, xenografts, and synthetic grafts. In an autograft, healthy skin is taken from a nonburned area of the child's body and placed on the burned area. This type of graft is permanent. The donor site (where the autograft was harvested) is a new wound, causing pain and requiring close monitoring for signs and symptoms of infection.

Temporary grafts include allografts (use of skin of the same species, for example, cadaver), xenografts (use of skin from another species, such as pig skin), and synthetic grafts (artificial skin substitutes). Temporary grafts are used to promote epithelial stimulation in partial-thickness burns and to cover healing granulation tissue. They usually slough off in 4 to 5 weeks as a result of tissue rejection. These grafts provide the functions of the skin that were lost in the burn (temperature regulation, pain control, fluid loss, infection barrier). Often they are used as a test to determine whether an autograft is likely to succeed in a burned area. The potential risk of HIV infection associated with homografts needs to be considered.

Nursing Assessment

Obtain information about the type of burn (thermal, electrical, chemical), as well as a complete history. Thorough documentation is essential to rule out child abuse. Be alert to signs of abuse (glove and stocking burns, contact burns from cigarettes or irons, zebra burn lines on the legs). If a burn injury was preventable, parents may be emotionally stressed by feelings of guilt. Caution is needed to avoid sounding accusatory when questioning parents about the injury.

Physical assessment should be thorough, including frequent monitoring of vital signs and daily weight measurement. A head-to-toe assessment is performed at the beginning of every shift followed by system-specific assessments, depending on clinical findings and changes in the child's status.

Nursing Diagnosis

Common nursing diagnoses for the child with a burn are included in the accompanying Nursing Care Plan. Additional nursing diagnoses for the child with a major burn include:

- Impaired Physical Mobility related to limb immobilization, contractures, and pain
- Body Image Disturbance related to possible disfigurement
- Altered Nutrition: Less Than Body Requirements related to hypermetabolic state
- Anxiety related to crisis, memory of trauma experience, and threat of death or disfigurement

Nursing Management

Nursing care focuses on performing burn care, preventing complications, and providing emotional support. Care of the burned child involves various treatments designed to promote healing and prevent complications. These include dressing changes, hydrotherapy, antibiotic therapy, analgesic support, physical therapy, play therapy, and possibly skin grafting.

The accompanying Nursing Care Plan summarizes nursing care of the child with a major burn. Severe morbidity is likely with major burns. Severe scarring may occur regardless of autografting. Contractures and loss of function are also possible. If fluid replacement is inadequate, irreversible renal damage or cardiac damage may ensue, necessitating close follow-up unrelated to the actual burn injury. Children with major burns require comprehensive follow-up, sometimes involving repeated hospitalizations for surgery to release burn contractures, perform new grafting, or provide scar revision.

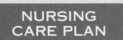

THE CHILD WITH A BURN INJURY

GOAL	INTERVENTION	RATIONALE	EXPECTED OUTCOME
1. Pain related to destruction of tissues and edema			
Child will verbalize adequate relief from pain and will be able to perform activities of daily living (ADLs).	Assess level of pain frequently using pain scales (see Chapter 5).	Pain scale provides objective measurement. Pain is always present, but changes in location may indicate complications.	Child verbalizes adequate relief from pain and is able to perform ADLs.
	Cover burns as much as possible.	Temperature changes or movement of air causes pain.	
	Change child's position frequently. Perform range of motion exercises.	Reduces joint stiffness and prevents contractures.	
	Elevate burned extremities.	Helps reduce swelling and pain.	
	Encourage verbalization about pain.	Provides an outlet for emotions and helps child cope.	
	Provide diversional activities.	Helps to lessen focus on pain.	
	Promote uninterrupted sleep with use of medications.	Sleep deprivation can increase pain perception.	
	Use analgesics before all dressing changes and burn care.	Helps to prevent pain and decreases anxiety for subsequent dressing changes.	
2. High Risk for Infection related to destruction of skin barrier, traumatized tissue, multiple indwelling catheters			
Child will be free of infection during healing process.	Take vital signs frequently.	Increased temperature is an early sign of infection	Child is free of secondary infection.
	Use protective isolation (gown, gloves, mask) when wounds are exposed for any major burn. Change dressings daily using sterile technique. Limit visitors (no one with an upper respiratory infection or other contagious disease).	Reduces risk of contamination.	
	Shave or clip hair around burns.	Hair harbors bacteria.	
	Debride necrotic tissue.	Promotes formation of granulation tissue, which aids healing.	
	Apply topical antibacterial agents.	Helps to reduce the number of bacteria present on the burn.	

GOAL	INTERVENTION	RATIONALE	EXPECTED OUTCOME
3. High Risk for Fluid Volume Excess or Deficit related to loss of fluid through wounds, hemorrhagic losses			
Child will maintain normal vital signs and urine output.	Monitor vital signs, central venous pressure, capillary refill time, pulses.	Child is at risk initially for going into shock and requires fluid resuscitation (see Chapter 7).	Child maintains normal vital signs and urine output.
	Monitor intake and output carefully.	Child has potential for fluid overload during hydration and edema in the tissues at the burn site.	
	Administer intravenous and oral fluids as ordered.	Careful calculation of fluid needs and ensuring proper intake helps to keep child properly hydrated.	
	Estimate insensible fluid losses.	Losses are increased during the first 72 hours after burn injury; may need replacement. Plasma is lost through burn site because of capillary damage.	
	Weigh child daily.	Significant weight loss or gain can help determine amount of fluid needed. Weight gain is normal during the first 72 hours.	
	Insert Foley catheter.	Helps maintain accurate intake and output measurements.	
	Monitor for hyponatremia and hyperkalemia (see Chapter 7).	Sodium is lost with burn fluid and potassium is lost from damaged cells, causing electrolyte imbalances.	
4. Altered Peripheral Tissue Perfusion related to edema of burned extremities			
Child will have reduced edema in burned extremities.	Elevate extremities. Perform hourly distal pulse checks. Notify physician of decreased or absent pulses.	Elevation helps to reduce dependent edema. Dependent edema can constrict peripheral circulation.	Child has reduced edema.
5. High Risk for Ineffective Breathing Pattern related to hypervolemia, smoke inhalation, airway edema			
Child will maintain or demonstrate improvement in breathing pattern.	Closely monitor quality of respirations, breath sounds mucus secretions, pulse oximetry.	Excess fluid replacement can cause pulmonary edema.	Child has regular and unlabored breathing pattern.
	Provide thorough pulmonary care.	Carbon monoxide and cyanide produced when plastics and fabrics burn can damage lung tissue. Pulmonary care assists in removal of resultant secretions to prevent infection.	
	Elevate head of bed. Keep intubation tray at bedside.	Dyspnea, nasal flaring, air hunger (respiratory distress) may develop.	
	Administer corticosteroids, as prescribed.	Reduces airway edema.	

Continued.

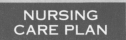

GOAL	INTERVENTION	RATIONALE	EXPECTED OUTCOME
6. Impaired Physical Mobility related to burns involving joints			
Child will maintain maximum range of motion.	Arrange physical and occupational therapy twice daily for stretching and range of motion exercises. Splint as ordered. Encourage independent ADLs.	Good positioning, range of motion exercises, and alignment prevent contractures	Child maintains maximum range of motion without contractures.
7. Altered Nutrition: Less Than Body Requirements related to hypermetabolic burn wound state			
Child will maintain weight and demonstrate adequate serum albumin and hydration.	Provide opportunity to choose meals. Offer a variety of foods. Provide snacks. Encourage child to have meals with other children.	Encourages intake. General malaise and anorexia lead to poor healing.	Child maintains weight, adequate hydration, normal serum albumin.
	Substitute milk and juices for water.	Provides additional calories.	
	Provide multivitamin supplement.	Vitamin C aids zinc absorption; zinc aids in healing.	
	Provide nasogastric feedings as ordered.	A child with a burn greater than 10% of BSA cannot usually meet nutrition requirements without assistance.	
	Weigh child daily.	Provides objective evaluation.	
8. Anxiety (Child) related to hospitalization and painful interventions			
Child will verbalize reduced anxiety.	Provide continuity of care providers.	Helps to build a trusting relationship.	Child states reduced anxiety.
	Encourage parents to stay with child; calls from home; pictures from classmates.	Familiar surroundings, people, and items encourage relaxation.	
	Group tasks and activities.	Reduces overstimulation and encourages rest.	
9. Anxiety (Parent) related to child's hospitalization and fear			
Parents will verbalize decreased anxiety.	Provide educational materials about healing, grafting expectations, and so on.	Knowledge reduces anxiety.	Parents state decreased anxiety.
	Be flexible when teaching parents wound care.	Adults learn in many different ways.	
	Provide referral to social services or parent support group.	Allows for venting of fears and guilt feelings, and provides exchange of ideas on dealing with hospitalization and long-term care.	

Prevent Complications. Severe complications of burns include infections, pneumonia, and renal failure, as well as possible irreversible loss of function of the burned area. The goal of the health care team is to prevent complications. Parents need to be involved in their child's care and to learn how to change dressings, assess for infection and dehydration (see Chapter 7), and perform range of motion exercises to aid in the child's recovery.

Provide support and encouragement to parents when they are learning how to care for the burned child. Many parents find it difficult to do "hurtful" things to their child. Outline specific guidelines so that parents and health care team members will have the same focus. Parents should first observe care being performed and then provide two repeat demonstrations.

Play therapy is encouraged for children, even if they can only observe initially. Play therapy serves several purposes for the child with a major burn:

- It provides an outlet for frustration, independence, and creativity.
- It promotes activities that challenge range of motion.
- It normalizes the child's daily routine.
- It encourages the child, who sees the progress that other children make day by day.

Provide Emotional Support. Burned children have received a profound insult to their body and their self-image. Fear and anxiety related to disfigurement and scarring are common responses, especially among adolescents. Increased stress occurs as a result of the shock and pain of the injury, as well as the unfamiliar surroundings and presence of health care providers.

An attitude of genuine interest and concern on the part of the nurse is essential. The child should be oriented to his or her surroundings frequently and given ample preparation for procedures, when possible. Continuity of care providers is important in developing a trusting relationship with the child. Encourage the child to voice concerns, and show understanding and support.

Families are at risk for emotional stress. They should be forewarned about the expected edema and resulting gross changes on the child's body. Parents often feel guilty and responsible for the child's injury. It is important to help parents focus on recovery rather than past actions. Fear usually results from lack of knowledge about the severity of the burn and the child's status, especially in the early stages of burn care and admission to the hospital ICU. Include the family in the child's care whenever possible. The family needs to be given information and frequent updates. This promotes the development of trust between the family and the health care team.

Autografting procedures enable the child to recover from major burns, but the operation leaves visible scarring. Psychologic support is therefore essential to the child's recovery. Social workers, chaplains, art therapists, child life specialists, and play therapists are all trained to help a child and family deal with the stressors of recovery. Appropriate referrals should be made to ensure that the child and family receive necessary services.

Discharge Planning and Patient and Family Home Care Teaching. Home care needs should be identified and addressed well in advance of discharge. Thorough assessment is necessary to identify the family's needs related to the child's discharge home or to a rehabilitation facility.

Discharge planning may include instructing parents in nutrition and diet needs, safety in the home, burn wound care, and range of motion exercises to prevent contractures.

Long-term care commonly involves the wearing of an elasticized (Jobst) garment and scar management. The Jobst garment may present a threat to the child's body image, but it is an important means of decreasing scarring. Scar management may be handled through drug injections or surgery (i.e., revision, grafting, or Z-plasty).

Continued physical therapy and occupational therapy are often needed to increase strength and dexterity in performing activities of daily living (ADLs) and to prevent contractures. Emphasis is placed on returning to normal ADLs as soon as possible. This includes return to the school as soon as health permits. Some children have home tutors for a while to decrease their risk of exposure to infection.

School reentry is often a traumatic experience, especially for older children and adolescents, because of fear of rejection, decreased self-esteem, and impaired body image. The child's primary nurse, social worker, and child life specialist may visit the school of a child with a burn injury—bringing photographs of the child, pressure garments, or other items—to desensitize the class and allow them to explore their emotions relating to the child's burn injury.

Several communities offer support groups for families and children with burn injuries. Referral to these groups may be beneficial.

Sunburn

Sunburn is a burn injury to the outer layer of skin caused by ultraviolet rays. It occurs more often in fair-skinned children, who have less melanin (skin pigment) to protect their skin against these harmful rays.

Erythema and skin tenderness usually develop between 30 minutes and 4 hours after exposure to the sun. Prolonged exposure can result in edema, vesiculation, bullae, or ulceration. Secondary complaints include insomnia (because of skin tenderness), fatigue, headaches, and chilling (because of rapid heat loss).

Treatment is generally supportive. Pain can be relieved by cool compresses followed by the application of a topical corticosteroid to relieve discomfort. Children with severe sunburn may require antiinflammatory drugs, such as ibuprofen.

Nursing Management

Educate parents and children about ways to prevent sunburn (Table 20–8). Advise that repeated sunburns may lead to permanent skin damage and skin cancer. Recommend to parents that children use sunscreens, wear protective clothing, and limit the amount of time they spend in the sun.

Hypothermia

Hypothermia is a condition in which the body temperature falls below 95° F (35° C). This occurs when the heat produced by the body is less than the heat lost. Hypothermia is a life-threatening emergency.

TABLE 20-8 Parent Teaching: Preventing Sunburn

- Keep children out of direct sunlight as much as possible.
- When outdoors, minimize exposed areas by wearing hats and long-sleeved clothing and pants: wear T-shirts while swimming.
- Be aware that water, concrete, and sand reflect sunlight and increase exposure up to 90%.
- Avoid scheduling outdoor activities during the hours of maximum exposure (10 AM to 2 PM).
- Use sunscreen (preferably 15 SPF [sun protection factor]). Apply liberally to all exposed areas. Reapply every 2 hours as needed.
- Use a waterproof sunscreen when swimming; this provides protection in water for approximately 60 to 80 minutes. Then reapply.
- Remember that a child can be burned even on a cloudy day.
- If the child is taking any medications, check with your health care practitioner before exposure (some medications cause hypersensitivity to sunlight).

Hypothermia is associated with near-drowning episodes because body heat is lost quickly in water, as compared with air. Children are at greater risk for hypothermia because of their thinner skin, limited subcutaneous fat, and high surface area to body mass ratio. As the body temperature falls, the body tries to conserve the core temperature at the expense of the extremities. Shivering occurs to try to rewarm the blood before it returns to the core of the body.

Symptoms of hypothermia include depressed respirations, slow pulse, low blood pressure, pale or cyanotic color, shivering, dilated pupils, and confusion. Profound hypothermia (body temperature below 84° F [28° C]) may result in absence of respirations and pulse and loss of consciousness.

Treatment focuses on resuscitation, if necessary, and gradual rewarming of the body. The child who has been immersed in cold water for a long time (up to 30 to 45 minutes) should receive CPR until the body temperature returns to normal because the diving reflex may preserve vital organs. Body temperature is assessed with a rectal thermometer. For mild hypothermia (temperature above 95° F [35° C]), external heat lamps, immersion in warm water, and an electric blanket may be all that are necessary. More aggressive techniques are required for profound hypothermia. These may include use of humidified, warm oxygen; warmed intravenous fluids; hemodialysis; or application of warmth to core circulation areas (axilla, groin, and posterior neck).

If a child becomes hypothermic during an outing such as a camping trip, a warm person should get into a sleeping bag (or under the blankets) next to the child. This action will warm the child and prevent further heat loss.

Nursing Management

Monitor vital signs and urine output during rewarming. Prevention is geared toward educating parents to layer clothes in cold climates, recognize signs of hypothermia, decrease time of exposure to cold, and be aware of actions to take for mild hypothermia.

Frostbite

Frostbite is an extreme form of hypothermia that results from overexposure to extremely low temperatures. Areas of the body at high risk for frostbite include the hands, feet, cheeks, nose, and ears. Skin cells have a high concentration of water; thus exposure to cold can result in cellular damage or rupture as water within the cells freezes.

Clinical manifestations depend on the severity of the cellular damage. The skin at first appears pale and is numb. Rapid rewarming causes a flush. The extent of injury usually is not apparent initially.

If frostbite is suspected, loosen all constricting clothing and remove any wet clothes. Obtain health care as soon as possible. Rewarming is done slowly to decrease the chance of cellular damage. Immerse the affected part for 10 to 15 minutes in water warmed to between 100° and 105° F (37.8° and 40.5° C). Analgesics may be given to manage pain. Elevate the affected part, if possible, to improve venous return. Encourage the child to drink warm fluids. This will help to warm the child slowly. Because the frostbitten area is numb, extreme caution is needed to protect it from any trauma.

The child may complain of tingling, burning, or prickling in the affected area during rewarming. These are signs that sensation is returning.

Amputation is sometimes necessary when tissues are permanently damaged.

Nursing Management

As with hypothermia, the goal of management is prevention. Teach parents to layer children's clothing for warmth and to pack extra blankets and clothing if cold temperatures are expected during outdoor activities. Wet clothing should be changed quickly. Early care is instrumental in minimizing permanent injury. Severe frostbite will require hospitalization, with fluid management, dressing changes, antibiotic therapy, and careful attention to diet.

Bites

Animal Bites

■ LEGAL CONSIDERATIONS

If a child sustains an animal bite, a complete and accurate history is essential. Include:
- Circumstances surrounding the attack
- Present location of the animal
- Attempts to assess the animal's health
- Extent of the injury

■ RABIES PROPHYLAXIS

Rabies immune globulin (RIG) or antirabies serum (ARS) should be given to all children bitten by wild animals in which rabies cannot be excluded, as well as to children bitten by domestic animals (cats and dogs) suspected or proved to be rabid.

Each year 1 million people are bitten by animals and require medical attention.[6] Children are at higher risk for animal bites, and boys seem to be bitten more frequently than girls.

Assessment includes noting location and number of bites, any breaks in the skin, redness or swelling at entry sites, redness extending out from site (possible cellulitis), and any drainage related to the bite. Check for any nerve, muscle, tendon, or vascular damage. Findings should be carefully documented. Head and neck bites require x-ray examination to rule out associated injury, such as trauma to airway or breathing structures or a depressed skull fracture.

Initial treatment involves irrigating the wound with large quantities of sterile saline solution and then debriding any necrotic tissue. A clean pressure dressing is applied, and the affected part is elevated to reduce bleeding. Severe bites sometimes require surgical closure or reconstruction. Puncture wounds should not be sutured.

Dog bites tend to be crushing, rather than clean, sharp lacerations. The major complication of dog bites is infection. Early treatment of the wound can greatly decrease this sequela. Cat bites are also dangerous because they tend to be puncture wounds. Check the child's immunization record to determine whether a tetanus booster is necessary. (Refer to the immunization schedule in the Atlas of Infectious and Communicable Diseases.) Instruct parents how to care for the wound. Dog bites should be reported to the police, and the dog should be observed for 10 days for signs of rabies.

Human Bites

Human bites are more common than most people realize. They usually occur in toddlers and other young children. Because the mouth harbors many bacteria, infection is fairly common. Antibiotics may be prescribed to prevent systemic complications. Initial treatment includes irrigating with sterile saline and debridement. Instruct parents how to care for the wound. Follow-up is important to watch for infection.

Nursing Management

Educate parents about ways to prevent animal and human bites and the importance of teaching children appropriate behavior around other children and animals (Table 20–9).

Children who receive traumatic animal bites often experience significant psychologic trauma. They may develop a fear of strange animals and a decreased capacity to enjoy the presence of household pets. Counseling and follow-up may be necessary to evaluate such concerns.

TABLE 20-9 Parent Teaching: Preventing Animal Bites

- Teach children the following rules:
  Avoid all unfamiliar animals.
  Avoid contact with all wild animals.
  Do not touch an animal when it is eating or sleeping.
  Never overexcite an animal, even in play.
  Never tease an animal.
  Never put your face close to an animal.
- If an animal is sick or acting strangely, notify the health department.
- Never leave a child alone with an animal.
- Do not buy a pet unless you are confident of your child's ability to respect it.

Insect Bites and Stings

Insect bites and stings occur frequently in children and usually are not a cause for concern. Exceptions include bites or stings by insects that carry parasites or communicable diseases (ticks, mosquitos), those of venomous insects (spiders), and those that produce an allergic reaction. (For a discussion of Lyme disease and Rocky Mountain spotted fever, see the Atlas of Infectious and Communicable Diseases.)

Reactions to insect bites can be localized or systemic. Local reactions include discrete, red papules and edema at the bite site, as well as itching and pain. Local inflammation results from injected foreign protein or chemicals. Most bites produce minimal discomfort. Systemic reactions can include wheezing, urticaria, laryngeal edema, and shock.

Treatment is usually supportive and focuses on relieving itching and reducing inflammation. Pruritus is treated with cold compresses or ice applied to the site and an antihistamine. In children who are sensitized to insect bites, pruritic wheals and bullae tend to develop with repeat exposure. In rare cases exposure can lead to an anaphylactic reaction. If large wheals, swelling of extremities, or respiratory difficulty occurs, emergency medical treatment is needed.

Black widow spider bites are characterized by a stinging sensation at the time of the bite followed by swelling, redness, and pain at the site. Red fang marks can be seen. Systemic symptoms can occur 15 minutes to 2 hours after the bite and include dizziness, severe abdominal pain (abdominal muscle rigidity) and weakness. Muscle cramps begin near the bite and can involve all skeletal muscles. If large doses of venom are absorbed, the bite may lead to paralysis and death. A neurotoxin produced by the spider is responsible for the symptoms. The black widow spider can be recognized by the red and orange hourglass-shaped markings on its underside. It usually bites in self-defense and avoids light areas. Treatment involves cleansing the wound and immediately applying ice packs. Sedatives, antivenom, analgesics, or muscle relaxants may be prescribed. Hydrocortisone may decrease the inflammatory response. Symptoms can progress for 24 hours and gradually decrease over 2 to 3 days.

The brown recluse spider bite is characterized by a sharp pain resembling a sting. Most bites are mild and cause only minimal edema and mild erythema. Severe bites can become necrotic within 4 hours. The child experiences mild to severe pain and tenderness. Within 3 to 4 days a purple, star-shaped area forms at the site. This is followed by necrotic ulceration in 7 to 14 days. Severe progressive reactions may include associated fever, restlessness, malaise, joint pain, and nausea and vomiting. The wound usually heals with scar formation. The brown recluse spider is recognized by the fiddle-shaped marking on its head. It is usually unaggressive and bites only when

■ **CLINICAL TIP**

A dash of meat tenderizer (papain powder) and a drop of water massaged into the skin for 5 minutes quickly relieves the pain of most insect bites and stings. Ice is also effective.

provoked. Treatment involves antibiotics, analgesics, application of cool compresses to the site, and corticosteroids for inflammation. In some cases a skin graft is needed.

Nursing Management

The goal of nursing care is prevention. Children should be taught to avoid spiders and other biting or stinging insects. Many commercial repellents (OFF, Cutter's, Deep Woods OFF) are available. Most products contain DEET (diethyltoluamide) and are effective against many insects including mosquitos, fleas, ticks, and chiggers. DEET does not repel stinging insects. Warn parents against using heavily perfumed shampoos, powders, or lotions, or dressing children in bright clothing when outdoors, since these may attract insects. Household pets may be a source of fleas or ticks. Encourage frequent inspection of pets and preventive treatments against fleas and ticks before pets are allowed prolonged contact with children.

Contusions

Contusions are soft tissue injuries that result from a variety of causes. Often it is difficult to assess whether an injury has caused underlying tissue damage. An injury does not have to break the skin to result in internal damage. X-ray examination may be necessary to rule out broken bones or further tissue damage. Signs and symptoms that indicate a need for treatment include swelling that does not subside within 72 hours, intense pain, inability to move the injured part, and infection.

Ice should be applied as soon as possible after injury. This can reduce inflammation and swelling in the area.

Foreign Bodies

Many skin injuries result in penetration of foreign particles. Common substances include gravel from abrasions, bee stingers, and splinters. Treatment of superficial foreign bodies involves irrigating the wound to try to forcibly dislodge the debris. A deeply embedded foreign body is best removed under medical supervision to avoid permanent injury or scarring.

REFERENCES

1 Fritsch, D.F., & Fredrick Pilat, D. (1993). Exposing latex allergies. *Nursing '93, 23*(8), 46–48.
2 Vermont Department of Health, Agency of Human Services (1993). Update: Latex in the home and community. *Vermont EMS Today,* December, 8.
3 Farrington, E. (1992). Diaper dermatitis. *Pediatric Nursing, 18*(1), 81–82.
4 Boynton, R.W., Dunn, E.S., & Stephens, G.R. (1988). *Manual of ambulatory pediatrics.* Chicago: Scott, Foresman, & Co.
5 Ben-Amitai, D., & Ashkenazi, S. (1993). Common bacterial skin infections in childhood. *Pediatric Annals, 22*(4), 226–227.
6 Hoekelman, R.A., Blatman, S., Friedman, S.B., Nelson, N.M., & Seidel, H.M. (1987). *Primary pediatric care.* St. Louis: Mosby–Year Book.
7 Weston, W.E., & Lane, A.T. (1991). *Color textbook of pediatric dermatology.* St. Louis: Mosby–Year Book.
8 Rustad, O.J. (1992). Outdoors and active: Relieving summer's siege on skin. *Physician and Sportsmedicine, 20*(5), 162–168, 171–176, 178.

Arendt, D.L., & Arendt, D.B. (1992). Rescue operations for snakebites. *American Journal of Nursing, 92*(7), 26–32.

Beschorner, J., Gray, W., Luu, L., Marriott, M., & Colwell, J. (1991). Managing skin breakdown complicated by candida infection [letter]. *Oncology Nursing Forum, 18*(1), 135.

Callaham, M.L. (1988). When an animal bites. *Emergency Medicine, 20*(11), 118–122, 124–126, 131.

Children's National Medical Center, Burn Unit Staff. (1990). *Burn wound care.* Washington, DC: Children's National Medical Center.

Committee on Infectious Diseases (1991). *Report of the Committee on Infectious Diseases.* Elk Grove Village, IL: American Academy of Pediatrics.

Cuzzell, J.Z. (1990). Derm detective clues: Itching and burning in skin folds. *American Journal of Nursing, 90*(1), 23–24.

DeWitt, S. (1990). Nursing assessment of the skin and dermatologic lesions. *Nursing Clinics of North America, 25*(1), 234–245.

Frey, C. (1992). Frostbitten feet: Steps to treatment and prevention. *Physician and Sportsmedicine, 20*(1), 67–72, 76.

Kieltyka, E.G. (1992). Pediatric management problems . . . chronic vaginal and oropharyngeal candidiasis. *Pediatric Nursing, 18*(4), 376–377.

Kizer, K.W. (1991). Treating insect stings, *Physician and Sportsmedicine, 19*(8), 33–34, 36.

Kohn, S.R. (1988). Acute skin problems of summer. *Emergency Medicine, 20*(13), 132–134, 137–138, 140.

Koo, J.Y.M., & Smith L.L. (1991). Psychologic aspects of acne. *Pediatric Dermatology, 8*(3), 185–188.

Lamb, C. (1987). Fungal infections from head to toe. *Patient Care, 21*(11), 62–66, 72, 74.

LaVoy, K. (1985). Emergency!: Dealing with hypothermia and frostbite. *RN, 48*(1), 53–56.

Rasmussen, J.E. (1989). Advances in nondietary management of children with atopic dermatitis. *Pediatric Dermatology, 6*(3), 210–215.

Ritchie, S.R. (1992). Primary bacterial skin infections. *Dermatology Nursing, 4*(4), 261–268.

Surkitt-Parr, D. (1989). The removal of foreign bodies. *Nursing, 3*(35), 11–13.

Thompson, J. (1990). Eczema, *Community Outlook*, August, 16–18.

Wilson, P.A. & Dallas, M.J. (1990). Diaper performance: Maintenance of healthy skin. *Pedicatric Dermatology, 7*(3), 179–184.

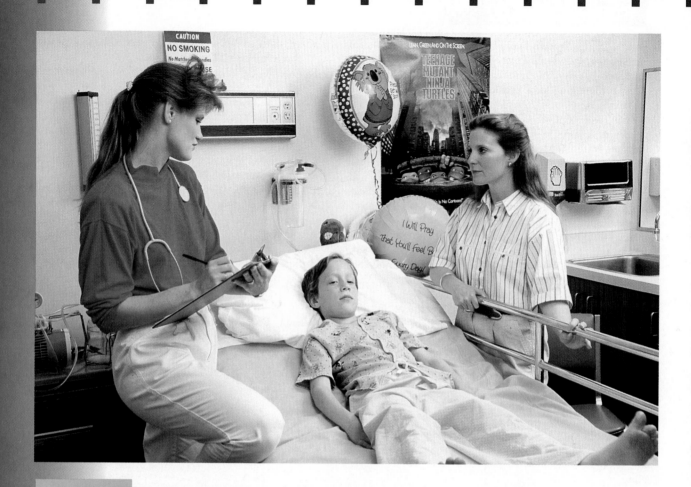

R obby, 8 years old, has been hospitalized for an insulin reaction. At age 6 he was brought to the child evaluation center because of his inability to sit in his seat at school, follow directions, or complete tasks at the same level as other pupils. Attention deficit hyperactivity disorder (ADHD) was diagnosed, and twice-daily administration of methylphenidate (Ritalin), a central nervous system stimulant, was prescribed. Since that time Robby has been repeatedly suspended for fighting in school. Academically he is performing on a first-grade level.

Compounding Robby's difficulties is his insulin-dependent diabetes mellitus (IDDM), which was diagnosed when he was 3 years of age. He requires two insulin injections a day and is expected to test his blood glucose three times a day. He is supposed to follow a constant carbohydrate diet with no added sugar. Because Robby's family has lived in a state of chaos for many years, he has not had appropriate parental supervision.

Robby has been hospitalized twice before for problems related to poor control of his diabetes. During his current admission, he is observed to be anxious. He is constantly fidgeting and makes only fleeting eye contact with the nurse.

ALTERATIONS IN PSYCHOSOCIAL FUNCTION

21

TERMINOLOGY

affect Outward manifestation of feeling or emotion; the tone of a person's reaction or response to people or events.

behavior modification A technique used to reinforce desirable behaviors, helping the child to replace maladaptive behaviors with more appropriate ones.

cognitive therapy A therapeutic approach that attempts to help the person recognize automatic thought patterns that lead to unpleasant feelings.

play therapy Therapeutic intervention often used with preschool and school-aged children. The child reveals conflicts, wishes, and fears on an unconscious level while playing with dolls, toys, clay, and other objects.

stereotypy Repetitive, obsessive, machine-like movements, commonly seen in autistic or schizophrenic children.

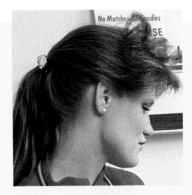

❝ I feel overwhelmed by the problems faced by Robby and his family. It's no wonder this child has such poor control of his diabetes. I'll need to work with several different health care professionals to help Robby and his family.❞

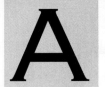s the nurse evaluating Robby, how would you begin to develop a nursing diagnosis and a plan of care? Clinical situations are often complex with many factors that must be considered, as illustrated by the preceding situation. The purpose of this chapter is to give you the knowledge and tools that can help you provide appropriate care for children like Robby with alterations in psychosocial functioning. Because much of this care will be provided by psychiatric–mental health specialists, the nurse's role often centers on identification, teaching, and referral.

Psychotherapeutic Management of Children and Adolescents

The primary treatment goal in management of children and adolescents with psychosocial disorders is to assist the child and family to achieve and maintain an optimal level of functioning through interventions designed to reduce the impact of stressors. Therapeutic interventions and communications are based on the principle that one must look at the feelings behind the behaviors. Parents and others close to the child often fall into the habit of reacting to the child's behaviors rather than trying to find out what feelings may be precipitating the undesirable actions.

Treatment Modes

Three basic treatment modes are used: individual, family, and group therapy.[1] The choice of treatment mode must take into account the child's age and developmental stage. Various strategies may be used within these modes, as discussed below. Most therapists incorporate several strategies simultaneously. Different strategies are more or less effective and appropriate for children and adolescents in various stages of development. Thorough knowledge and understanding of developmental needs, expectations, and abilities are therefore essential.

Individual Therapy

Individual therapy involves only the child and the therapist. Treatment of specific emotional problems or disorders may involve various techniques such as play therapy, psychodrama, art therapy, and **cognitive therapy** (a technique used to help a person recognize automatic negative thinking). Individual therapy may be short term (four to six sessions) or long term (lasting for several years).

Family Therapy

Family therapy involves the exploration of a particular emotional problem and its manifestations among the family members. Family therapy is based on the idea that the emotional symptoms or problems of an individual are an expression of emotional symptoms or problems in the family. The focus is on the relationships among the family members, not the psychologic conflict of each individual member.

Group Therapy

Group therapy involves an ongoing or limited number of sessions in which several patients participate. The emphasis is on the interpersonal styles of re-

The editors wish to acknowledge the contribution of Jo Trilling, RN, MS, Intercollegiate Center for Nursing Education, Spokane, WA, in supplying information for this chapter.

lating to one another in the group. Group therapy is particularly effective with adolescents because of the importance of the peer group at this age. An advantage of group therapy is that stimuli and feedback come from multiple sources (the group members) instead of just one person (the therapist).

Therapeutic Strategies
Play Therapy

Play is often called the language or work of the child. From a developmental perspective, children progressively learn to express feelings and needs through action, fantasy, and finally language. The special quality of play buffers children against the pressures and demands of daily life. Play facilitates mastery of developmental stages by strengthening physical and neurologic processes. Play also assists in cognitive learning, setting the stage for problem solving and creativity.

Play therapy is a technique that reveals problems on a fantasy level through the use of toys, dolls, clay, art, and other creative objects. It is often used with preschool and school-age children who are experiencing anxiety, stress, and other specific nonpsychotic mental disorders. Play therapy encourages the child to act out feelings, such as anger, hostility, sadness, and fear. It also provides the opportunity for the therapist to help the child understand, on a conscious and unconscious level, his or her own responses and behavior in a safe, supportive environment.

Art Therapy

Children who may be apprehensive about playing can sometimes be encouraged to participate in art therapy, using brief drawing exercises. This technique is appropriate for children of all ages, including adolescents. The drawings can help the therapist gain information about the child, the family, and the interactions between the child and family. However, children's drawings should never be used solely to form a definitive diagnosis.

When used in conjunction with a thorough history and appropriate psychologic testing information, art therapy can guide the child's treatment. These drawing exercises provide an opportunity to help in the healing process. The therapist can assist the child to release feelings of anger, pain, or fear onto paper where they can be examined objectively. Figures 21–1 to 21–4 present several examples of this technique.

Behavior Therapy

Behavior modification is a therapeutic technique that uses stimulus and response conditioning to alter inappropriate behaviors. It is used to reinforce desirable behaviors, helping the child to replace maladaptive behaviors with more appropriate ones. It is based on the assumption that any learned behavior can be unlearned. Thus, if parents, nurses, teachers, and other adults consistently reinforce desirable behaviors, the child will eventually alter or discontinue undesirable behaviors. Behavior modification may include (1) removing the child from the home to a more structured environment, such as a hospital, for a brief time and (2) teaching the parents, teachers, and other appropriate adults to be agents of behavioral change.[1] This may require several ongoing sessions with the adults involved, using role play and other techniques. Consistency is the most important principle in successful use of behavior modification.

PLAY THERAPY

Play therapy, a technique used with children who have psychosocial disorders, is different from *therapeutic play,* which may be used with many hospitalized children (see Chapter 4). Although some techniques overlap, only a specialist is qualified to provide play therapy.

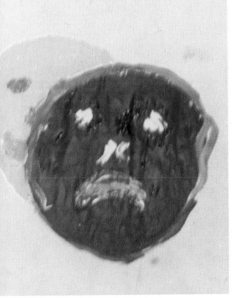

FIGURE 21–1 "Me." Drawn by a 14-year-old girl with major depression, anxiety, and school phobia who had experienced multiple losses over several years. Her mother had severe chronic lung problems and diabetes, and the girl had stopped attending school for fear that something would happen to her mother. This drawing represents the girl's obvious feelings of sadness and depression but also indicates a glimmer of hope (represented by yellow mask coming from behind dark mask of depression).

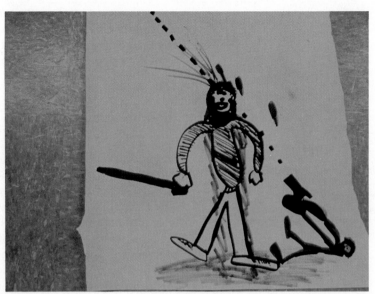

FIGURE 21–2 "Self-Portrait." Drawn by a 15-year-old boy who was admitted through the emergency department after a failed suicide attempt by hanging. He had a psychiatric diagnosis of depression and polysubstance abuse (including inhalants and alcohol) and insisted that he was a member of a satanic cult in his hometown. Most of his drawings depicted a preoccupation with violence and suicide. The boy said that he always felt a "darkness" like a shadow that followed him around and wanted him dead. His family history was significant for depression and suicide on both his mother's and his father's side. His father also had a lengthy history of polysubstance abuse and alcoholism. The boy was discharged to a long-term residential treatment facility for adolescents.

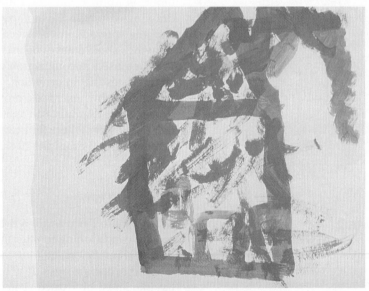

FIGURE 21–3 "An Activity." Drawn by a 8-year-old boy who was initially admitted to the medical-surgical floor of a pediatric hospital for dehydration resulting from vomiting and diarrhea. Psychiatric evaluation was ordered for extreme anxiety. These drawings, completed during the initial interview, led to further investigation, which revealed that the child had started a house fire in which his grandmother (his primary caretaker at the time) was killed. The family's home and all their belongings were lost. No one had known that the child had set the fire. Further sessions indicated that he had been setting neighborhood garage fires frequently and watching them burn from a distance.

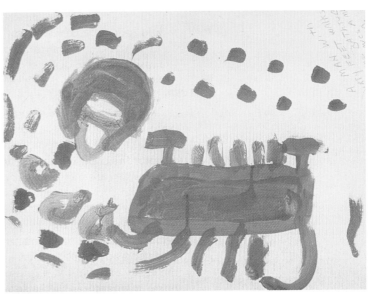

FIGURE 21–4 "A Family Activity." By the same boy who drew Fig. 21–3. This drawing depicts a recurring incident of physical and emotional abuse by his mother's live-in boyfriend. It shows the family bathtub with feces and blood smeared on the floors and walls. The boy reported that when either he or his 3-year-old brother had a toileting accident, the boyfriend would make them go into the bathroom and stand in the bathtub while he smeared the feces on the walls. He would then hit the children and make them clean up the mess. The boy had been removed from the mother's custody previously for neglect. He was transferred from the medical-surgical area to the inpatient children's psychiatric unit, where he received a diagnosis of depression, overanxious disorder, and child abuse (physical and emotional). Charges were filed against the mother's boyfriend, and custody of both children was temporarily revoked.

Visualization and Guided Imagery

The techniques of visualization and guided imagery begin with specific directions for progressive relaxation according to the child's ability. This form of therapy uses the child's own imagination and positive thinking to reduce stress and anxiety, decrease the experience of pain or discomfort, and promote healing. The techniques are especially useful in the management of anxiety disorders and chronic pain. It is not easy for every child to use his or her imagination in this way, so the technique may not work or be appropriate for everyone.

Hypnosis

Hypnosis involves varying degrees of suggestibility and deep relaxation effects. This technique is useful for children and adolescents because they can usually be hypnotized more easily than adults. Hypnosis is especially helpful in treating physical symptoms with a psychologic component, anxiety, and phobias and in managing severe physical symptoms or discomfort (pain or nausea) associated with a physiologic disorder or its treatment (e.g., cancer or juvenile rheumatoid arthritis).

Nurse's Role

Although many psychosocial disorders are managed effectively with medication on an outpatient basis, some necessitate admission to an inpatient psychiatric setting. The nurse also may encounter the child with a psychosocial disorder during hospitalization for a concurrent physiologic problem. If a child is hospitalized for a concurrent problem, the nurse needs to assess the child's current level of functioning in relation to the psychosocial disorder. In the case of Robby, described in the opening vignette, the nurse would assess his current attention deficit behaviors by observing Robby during admission and the entire hospital stay.

Nursing assessment also focuses on identifying medications being taken, common abnormal behaviors (what triggers them, what reduces them), and routines to maintain appropriate behaviors. The nurse then considers how to support the child within the hospital environment.

Nursing care includes carrying out the prescribed treatment plan and administering psychotropic medications. The child's medication regimen should be evaluated for administration schedule, dosage, side effects, and effectiveness. Inform the therapist of the child's hospitalization if the child has been hospitalized for a concurrent condition, and consult with the therapist regarding appropriate approaches for the child. Provide supportive care for the child and family. Continuation of family involvement is critical. The nurse frequently is the liaison between the family and the therapist in making follow-up arrangements.

Autism

Autism is a complex childhood disorder that involves abnormal emotional, social, and linguistic development. The essential features of autism typically become apparent by the time a child is 3 years of age. For every 10,000 births, 4 to 5 children are found to have autism. The disorder occurs four times more often in boys than in girls.[2]

Clinical Manifestations

Autistic children may manifest disturbances in rate or sequence of development. Characteristically the child engages in repetitive behaviors, including head banging, twirling in circles, biting himself or herself, and flapping the hands or arms. Frequently the child's behavior is self-stimulating or self-destructive. Responses to sensory stimuli are frequently abnormal and include extreme aversion to touch, loud noises, and bright lights.

Difficulties or delays in speech, language, and cognitive abilities are common and may correspond to intellectual deficits. Abnormal communication patterns include both verbal and nonverbal communication. Autistic children may eventually learn to talk, in some cases well, but their speech is likely to show certain abnormalities: use of "you" in place of "I"; echolalia (a compulsive parroting of what is heard); repeating questions rather than answering them; and fascination with rhythmic, repetitive songs and verses.

Autistic children often find it difficult or impossible to relate to people, events, and objects.[3] Emotional lability is common. The child may cry at one moment and giggle or laugh at the next.

Etiology and Pathophysiology

The cause of autism is unknown. Brain dysfunction is probably a predisposing factor.[4] Genetic transmission and biochemical imbalances may also be involved. Autistic children are usually cognitively impaired and demonstrate a wide range of intellectual ability and functioning. Sixty percent of autistic children have an intelligence quotient (IQ) below 50; 20% have an IQ between 50 and 70; and only 20% have scores greater than 70.[5]

Medical Management

Diagnosis is based on the presence of specific DSM-III-R criteria, as outlined in Table 21–1.

Treatment focuses on behavior modification to reward appropriate behaviors, foster positive or adaptive coping skills, and model appropriate behaviors. The goals of treatment are to reduce rigidity or **stereotypy** (repetitive, obsessive, machine-like movements) and decrease maladaptive behaviors. Often the child must be physically restrained from aggressive or self-destructive behaviors for his or her safety.

The overall prognosis for autistic children to become functioning members of society is guarded. The extent to which adequate adjustment is achieved varies greatly. Successful adjustment is more likely for children with higher IQs, adequate speech, and access to specialized programs.

Nursing Assessment

The nurse may encounter the autistic child when parents seek care for a suspected hearing impairment or developmental delay. Parents may report abnormal interaction such as lack of eye contact, disinterest in cuddling, minimal facial responsiveness, and failure to talk. Initial assessment focuses on language development, response to others, and hearing acuity (see Chapters 3 and 11).

When a child with a diagnosis of autism is hospitalized for a concurrent problem, the nurse obtains a history from the parents regarding the child's routines, rituals, and likes and dislikes, as well as ways to promote interaction and cooperation. Ask about the child's behaviors as well as observing them on admission. Obtain a history of acute and chronic illnesses and injuries.

Autistic children may carry a special toy or object that they play with during times of stress. Ask parents about these objects and their use.

Nursing Diagnosis

Nursing diagnoses must be tailored to fit the individual needs of the child. Examples of nursing diagnoses for autistic children include the following:

- Impaired Verbal Communication related to poor language skills
- Impaired Social Interaction related to slow developmental maturation
- Impaired Adjustment related to disruption of daily routine
- Altered Thought Processes related to abnormal response to environmental cues
- Sleep Pattern Disturbance related to hyperactivity and hypermobility
- High Risk for Injury related to cognitive impairment
- High Risk for Caregiver Role Strain related to child's delayed development, need for constant care, and inability to relate to caregivers
- Ineffective Family Coping: Compromised or Disabling related to child who does not become integrated into family

Nursing Management

Nursing care focuses on decreasing environmental stimuli, providing supportive care, maintaining a safe environment, giving the parents anticipatory guidance, and providing emotional support.

Decrease Environmental Stimuli. Autistic children interpret and respond to the environment differently from other individuals. Sounds that are not distressing to the average person may be interpreted by autistic children as

TABLE 21-1 DSM-III-R Diagnostic Criteria for Autistic Disorder

At least eight of the following sixteen items are present, these to include at least two items from A, one from B, and one from C.

Note: Consider a criterion to be met *only* if the behavior is abnormal for the person's developmental level.

A. Qualitative impairment in reciprocal social interaction as manifested by the following: (The examples within parentheses are arranged so that those first mentioned are more likely to apply to younger or more handicapped—and, in the later ones, to older or less handicapped—persons with this disorder.)

1. Marked lack of awareness of the existence or feelings of others (e.g., treats a person as if he or she were a piece of furniture; does not notice another person's distress; apparently has no concept of the need of others for privacy)
2. No or abnormal seeking of comfort at times of distress (e.g., does not come for comfort even when ill, hurt, or tired; seeks comfort in a stereotyped way, e.g., says "cheese, cheese, cheese" whenever hurt)
3. No or impaired imitation (e.g., does not wave bye-bye; does not copy mother's domestic activities; mechanical imitation of others' actions out of context)
4. No or abnormal social play (e.g., does not actively participate in simple games; prefers solitary play activities; involves other children in play only as "mechanical aids")
5. Gross impairment in ability to make peer friendships (e.g., no interest in making peer friendships; despite interest in making friends, demonstrates lack of understanding of conventions of social interaction, for example, reads phone book to uninterested peer)

B. Qualitative impairment in verbal and nonverbal communication, and in imaginative activity, as manifested by the following: (The numbered items are arranged so that those first listed are more likely to apply to younger or more handicapped—and, in the later ones, to older or less handicapped—persons with this disorder.)

1. No mode of communication, such as communicative babbling, facial expression, gesture, mime, or spoken language
2. Markedly abnormal nonverbal communication, as in the use of eye-to-eye gaze, facial expression, body posture, or gestures to initiate or modulate social interaction (e.g., does not anticipate being held, stiffens when held, does not look at the person or smile when making a social approach, does not greet parents or visitors, has a fixed stare in social situations)
3. Absence of imagination activity, such as playacting of adult roles, fantasy characters, or animals; lack of interest in stories about imaginary events
4. Marked abnormalities in the production of speech, including volume, pitch, stress, rate, rhythm, and intonation (e.g., monotonous tone, question-like melody, or high pitch)
5. Marked abnormalities in the form or content of speech, including stereotyped and repetitive use of speech (e.g., immediate echolalia or mechanical repetition of television commercial); use of "you" when "I" is meant (e.g., using "You want cookie" to mean "I want cookie"); idiosyncratic use of words or phrases (e.g., "Go on green riding" to mean "I want to go on the swing"); or frequent irrelevant remarks (e.g., starts talking about train schedules during a conversation about sports)
6. Marked impairment in the ability to initiate or sustain a conversation with others, despite adequate speech (e.g., indulging in lengthy monologues on one subject regardless of interjections from others)

C. Markedly restricted repertoire of activities and interests, as manifested by the following:

1. Stereotyped body movements, e.g., hand-flicking or -twisting, spinning, head-banging, complex whole-body movements
2. Persistent preoccupation with parts of objects (e.g., sniffing or smelling objects, repetitive feeling of texture of materials, spinning wheels of toy cars) or attachment to unusual objects (e.g., insists on carrying around a piece of string)
3. Marked distress over changes in trivial aspects of environment, e.g., when a vase is moved from usual position
4. Unreasonable insistence on following routines in precise detail, e.g., insisting that exactly the same route always be followed when shopping
5. Markedly restricted range of interests and a preoccupation with one narrow interest, e.g., interested only in lining up objects, in amassing facts about meteorology, or in pretending to be a fantasy character

D. Onset during infancy or childhood.

Specify if childhood onset (after 36 months of age)

From American Psychiatric Association (1987). *Diagnostic and statistical manual of mental disorders* (3rd ed., rev.). Washington, DC: Author.

louder, more frightening, and overwhelming. The child needs orientation to his or her hospital room and may adjust best to a room with only one other child. Encourage parents to bring the child's favorite objects from home, and try to keep these objects in the same places because the child does not cope well with changes in the environment.

Provide Supportive Care. Developing a trusting relationship with the autistic child is often difficult. Adjust communication techniques and teaching to the child's developmental level. Ask parents about the child's usual home routines, and maintain these routines as much as possible. Because self-care abilities are often limited, the child may need assistance to meet basic needs. When possible, schedule daily care and routine procedures at consistent times to maintain predictability. Encourage parents to remain with the child and to participate in daily care planning. Identify rituals for naptime and bedtime, and maintain them to promote rest and sleep.

■ SAFETY PRECAUTIONS

If the autistic child or adolescent is particularly aggressive or self-abusive, bike helmets and mitts can be the least restrictive method used for the safety of the autistic child, other patients, and staff. This may enable the child to participate in activities and engage in the social environment (to the degree capable) with specially trained professionals.

Maintain a Safe Environment. Monitor autistic children at all times, including bathtime and bedtime. Close supervision is needed to ensure that the child does not obtain any harmful objects or engage in dangerous behaviors.

Provide Anticipatory Guidance. Approximately half of the children with autism require lifelong supervision and support. This is especially true if autism is accompanied by mental retardation. Some children may grow up to lead independent lives, although they will be socially inept and their social and interpersonal relationships will be limited. Encourage parents to promote the child's development through behavior modification and specialized educational programs. The overall goal is to provide the child with the guidance, education, and support necessary for optimal functioning.

Provide Emotional Support. Families of autistic children need a great deal of support to cope with the challenges of home care. The parent or primary caretaker often has difficulty obtaining respite care. Family support programs are available in some states to provide assistance to parents.

Local support groups for parents of autistic children are available in most areas. Parents can also be referred to the Autism Society of America (see Appendix F) for information.

Attention Deficit Hyperactivity Disorder

Attention deficit hyperactivity disorder (ADHD) is characterized by a triad of developmentally inappropriate behaviors: inattention, impulsiveness, and hyperactivity. The disorder affects approximately 9% to 10% of boys and 3% of girls.[2]

Clinical Manifestations

Children with ADHD have problems related to decreased attention span, impulsiveness, or increased motor activity. Symptoms may be mild, moderate, or severe. ADHD often coexists with various developmental learning disabilities. The child has difficulty completing tasks, fidgets constantly, is frequently loud, and interrupts others. Because of these behaviors the child often has difficulty developing and maintaining social relationships and may be shunned or teased by other children. This only increases the anxiety of the already compromised child, whose behavior is set on a downward-spiraling course.

Typically girls with ADHD show less aggression and impulsiveness than boys, but far more anxiety, mood swings, social withdrawal, rejection, and cognitive and language problems. Girls tend to be older at the time of diagnosis.

Etiology and Pathophysiology

The results of research have dramatically changed the thinking about ADHD in the last 40 years. Although a variety of physical and neurologic disorders can result in ADHD, children with identifiable causes represent a small proportion of this population. Probably there are many types of attention deficit, resulting from several different brain mechanisms.[2]

The most common causative neurologic disorders are seizures and cerebral palsy. These are diagnosed in 5% of children with ADHD.[2] ADHD occurs more frequently in some families than in the general population and is especially prevalent in males. There is no evidence, however, of a single gene defect or a specific mechanism of genetic transmission.

Medical Management

Children are usually brought for evaluation when behaviors escalate to the point of interfering with the daily functioning of teachers or parents. This was the case with Robby, described in the opening vignette. When children have learning disabilities or anxiety disorders, the problem is commonly misdiagnosed as ADHD without further evaluation of the child's symptoms. Therefore obtaining an accurate diagnosis by a pediatric mental health specialist is important.

Specific diagnostic criteria (Table 21–2) vary among children. Treatment depends on the severity of the disorder and may include environmental changes, behavior modification, and/or pharmacotherapy.

Children with milder cases of ADHD often benefit from environmental changes. Decreasing stimulation, for example, by turning off television, keeping the environment quiet, and maintaining an orderly and clutter-free desk or study area without distraction, may help the child to stay on task. Another relatively simple change is appropriate classroom placement, preferably in a small class with a teacher who can provide close supervision and a structured daily routine.

Children with moderate to severe ADHD are treated with pharmacotherapy. Methylphenidate (Ritalin) is most often prescribed. It acts mainly on the central nervous system to inhibit impulsiveness and hyperactivity while generally improving attention.[6] Usually a favorable response (a decrease in impulsive behaviors and an increase in the ability to sit still and attend to an activity for at least 15 minutes) is seen in the first 10 days of treatment and frequently within the first few doses.[2]

Approximately 20% of children do not respond to stimulants such as methylphenidate. Other medications that have been shown effective include antidepressants such as desipramine (Norpramin) and bupropion (Wellbutrin); carbamazepine (Tegretol), an anticonvulsant; magnesium pemoline (Cylert), a dopamine agonist; and lithium, an antimanic drug that is used occasionally in children with a coexisting conduct disorder.[7]

ADHD is primarily a disorder of childhood. During adolescence, attention span lengthens and impulse control generally improves.

■ NURSING ALERT

Children receiving magnesium pemoline (Cylert) should continue to receive the drug during hospitalization. If the medication is stopped during hospitalization, the child may have behavioral problems for weeks after discharge.

TABLE 21-2 DSM-III-R Diagnostic Criteria for Attention Deficit Hyperactivity Disorder

Note: Consider a criterion met *only* if the behavior is considerably more frequent than that of most people of the same mental age.

A. A disturbance of at least six months during which at least eight of the following are present:
1. Often fidgets with hands or feet or squirms in seat (in adolescents, may be limited to subjective feelings of restlessness)
2. Has difficulty remaining seated when required to do so
3. Is easily distracted by extraneous stimuli
4. Has difficulty awaiting turn in games or group situations
5. Often blurts out answers to questions before they have been completed
6. Has difficulty following through on instructions from others (not due to oppositional behavior or failure of comprehension), e.g., fails to finish chores
7. Has difficulty sustaining attention in tasks or play activities
8. Often shifts from one uncompleted activity to another
9. Has difficulty playing quietly
10. Often talks excessively
11. Often interrupts or intrudes on others, e.g., butts into other children's games
12. Often does not seem to listen to what is being said to him or her
13. Often loses things necessary for tasks or activities at school or at home (e.g., toys, pencils, books, assignments)
14. Often engages in physically dangerous activities without considering possible consequences (not for the purpose of thrill seeking), e.g., runs into street without looking

Note: The above items are listed in descending order of discriminating power based on data from a national field trial of the DSM-III-R criteria for disruptive behavior disorders.

B. Onset before the age of seven.
C. Does not meet the criteria for a pervasive developmental disorder.

Criteria for severity of ADHD:

Mild: Few, if any, symptoms in excess of those required to make the diagnosis **and** only minimal or no impairment in school and social functioning.

Moderate: Symptoms or functional impairment intermediate between "mild" and "severe."

Severe: Many symptoms in excess of those required to make the diagnosis **and** significant and pervasive impairment in functioning at home/school and with peers.

From American Psychiatric Association (1987). *Diagnostic and statistical manual of mental disorders* (3rd ed., rev.). Washington, DC: Author.

Nursing Assessment

The nurse may encounter the child with ADHD in the hospital when parents bring the child for treatment of an injury (e.g., fracture) or other problem. Explore the parent's report of the child's attention span in detail. Usually within 15 minutes in an unstructured setting or waiting area, the child with ADHD becomes restless and searches for distraction.[8] Gather information about the child's activity level and impulsiveness. Be alert for information that reveals a serious problem, such as hurting animals or other children. Obtain information about distractibility, attention deficit in activities of daily living, characteristic ways of reacting, and the extent of impulsiveness when the child is receiving medication.

Nursing Diagnosis

Examples of nursing diagnoses for children with ADHD include the following:
- Impaired Verbal Communication related to inattention

- Impaired Social Interaction related to chronic episodes of impulsive behavior
- Chronic Low Self-Esteem related to lack of positive feedback and lack of success in social interactions
- Anxiety related to mood swings and concern about ability to behave in a socially appropriate manner
- High Risk for Injury related to high level of impulsiveness, excitability, and low impulse control
- High Risk for Caregiver Role Strain related to unpredictable nature of child's moods and difficulty in managing high-energy child

Nursing Management

Nursing care for the hospitalized child with ADHD focuses on administering medications, providing emotional support to the child and family, and promoting self-esteem.

Administer Medications. Methylphenidate and other medications increase the child's attention span and decrease distractibility. Be alert for the common side effects of these medications, including anorexia, insomnia, and tachycardia. Administering medication early in the day helps to alleviate insomnia. Anorexia can be managed by giving medication at mealtimes. Careful monitoring of weight, height, and blood pressure is necessary.

Provide Emotional Support. Children with ADHD offer a special challenge to parents, teachers, and health care providers. Parents must cope simultaneously with managing the difficult needs and demands of a hard-to-handle child, obtaining appropriate evaluation and treatment, and understanding and accepting the diagnosis, even when the child exhibits different behaviors with different people.[9] Family support is essential. Educate both the parents and the child about the importance of appropriate expectations and consequences of behaviors.

Promote Self-Esteem. Help the child to understand the disorder at an appropriate developmental level, and facilitate a trusting relationship with health care providers. Assist the child with social skills through the use of role-play, playing in small groups, and modeling. Promote the child's self-esteem by pointing out the positive aspects of behavior and treating instances of negative behavior as learning opportunities. Help the child to develop ego strengths (the consciousness to be able to screen outside stimuli and control internal demands), which will result in better impulse control and thus increase self-esteem over time.

Discharge Planning and Parent and Family Home Care Teaching. Discharge planning focuses on educating the child, parents, and other family members about the disorder and its management. Be sure that parents understand how to administer prescribed medications and how to manage common side effects.

Emphasize the importance of a stable environment, at home as well as at school. At home the child may have difficulty staying on task. Parents need to consider age and developmental appropriateness of tasks, give clear and simple instructions, and provide frequent reminders to ensure completion.

Behavior modification programs may help to reduce specific impulsive behaviors. An example is setting up a reward program for the child who has completed a homework assignment. The rewards may be daily as well as weekly or monthly, depending on the child's age. (For example, one completed homework assignment is rewarded with 30 minutes of basketball or a bike ride; assignments completed for a week are rewarded with participation in an activity of the child's choice on the weekend.)

If punishment is necessary, parents need to be certain they correct the behavior while supporting the child as a person. Punishment should follow the offense quickly because the child quickly forgets what he or she did.

The nurse can serve as a liaison to teachers and school personnel. Special classrooms or periods of instruction free from the distractions of the entire class may enable the child to improve school performance. Parents may have difficulty understanding the need for these approaches because the child often tests with above-average intelligence. Reinforce the importance of providing a structured environment free from unnecessary external stimuli.

Mental Retardation

Mental retardation is defined as significantly subaverage intelligence (IQ below 70 on the Wechsler Intelligence Scale for Children–Revised [WISC–R] or below 69 on the Stanford-Binet test) that occurs in association with developmental delays. Retardation may be mild (IQ of 50 to 69), moderate (IQ of 30 to 49), or profound (IQ <30).[10] Moderate to profound retardation accounts for approximately 15% of all cases of mental retardation[11] and is more common in boys than in girls.

Children who are mentally retarded manifest delays in all areas of development: motor, language, and adaptive behavior. Sensory impairment, speech problems, motor and orthopedic disabilities, and seizure disorders are commonly associated with mental retardation.

Mental retardation may result from genetic, familial, and fetal and birth-related factors and from acquired conditions. Genetic factors include inborn errors of metabolism or chromosomal abnormalities such as congenital hypothyroidism and Down syndrome. Examples of fetal and birth-related factors are fetal alcohol syndrome, maternal infections, intrauterine growth retardation, asphyxia, prematurity, hyperbilirubinemia, and intraventricular hemorrhage. Familial factors include low family intelligence or environmental deprivation. Acquired conditions are exemplified by meningitis, lead poisoning, and traumatic brain injury.

■ NURSING ALERT

Prematurity places the child at risk of displaying below-normal cognitive development. The premature infant needs frequent, thorough neurologic and developmental examinations, particularly in the first year of life.

Approximately 10% of affected children (usually those who are moderately to profoundly retarded) are identified during infancy or the toddler period because of significant developmental delays. The remainder are identified after they have entered school. Most mentally retarded children have a history of normal development in the first 2 years with a subsequent decline in developmental competency. Careful individualized testing is required to distinguish mentally retarded children from those who are autistic or have only a sensory impairment.

A goal of medical management is early recognition of the child with potential for mental retardation, such as during hospitalization for prematurity or meningitis or during screening for metabolic disorders. Children diagnosed with mental retardation should be enrolled in education and habilitation programs to maximize their functioning. Simultaneous treatment of associated physical, emotional, and behavioral problems must be done. Depending on the severity of the child's condition, special education programs and physical and occupational therapy programs may be necessary. Children who are profoundly retarded usually require continuous care.

Nursing Management

Nurses may be involved in identifying mentally retarded children through developmental screening during early childhood (see Chapter 3). Nursing care focuses on determining the impact of the child's condition on the family, educating parents about the child's condition, and providing supportive care and appropriate referrals.

Talk with the parents honestly and show empathy. Parents may be in an acute or chronic stage of grief (over the loss of a perfect child), depending on how long they have known about the child's diagnosis. The family faces a series of challenges, such as accepting the child's lack of educational success and the continual comparisons between the accomplishments of other children with their retarded child.

Teach parents about the child's educational potential and any physical disabilities. Provide guidance about the care needed to promote the child's optimal development and appropriate social behavior. Effective methods to teach self-care activities (e.g., toileting, dressing, feeding, and hygiene) are provided when the child is developmentally ready.

Health professionals in early intervention programs, such as Zero to Three, can provide direct services and educate families about the child's care. Appropriate school experiences, beginning with preschool, promote optimal development and socialization. As the child reaches adolescence, education should be directed toward a vocation, issues of sexuality, and the goal of independent living. Parents can be referred to agencies such as the Association for Retarded Citizens of the United States for additional information (see Appendix F).

Additional nursing measures are needed to provide appropriate care to a mentally retarded child during hospitalization. Talk with the parents to identify the child's abilities and special needs and to determine how the family manages the child's care at home. Perform a functional assessment of the child that includes toileting, dressing, and feeding skills. Support efforts to maintain these skills. Assess language, sensory, and psychomotor functioning. Determine whether the child has any self-stimulating or self-injurious behaviors that need to be monitored.

Involve the parents in the child's care as much as they desire. Interact with the child at his or her cognitive level, especially when preparing the child for procedures (see Chapter 4). Promote socialization by encouraging interaction between the child and his or her peers in the playroom. Use appropriate language and communication techniques.

Use the opportunity during hospitalization to assess whether there are gaps in the child's treatment. Encourage parents to take over the role of coordinating comprehensive care for the child, and provide information and resources to enable them to learn needed skills (see Chapter 4).

■ Eating Disorders

Three major eating disorders affect children, particularly adolescents: anorexia nervosa, bulimia nervosa, and compulsive overeating (obesity). The psychologic and physiologic alterations associated with these disorders create increasing difficulty in family and social relationships for the child or adolescent. The results are depression, isolation and withdrawal, and other self-destructive behaviors.

Eating symbolizes many things. On a basic level, eating represents parental nurturing. The act of being fed or cared for by a parent is the model for all future intimate relationships. For some individuals, however, eating creates anxiety related to a negative association with unpleasant or unsatisfactory parent-child interactions.[12]

Control is an issue central to the development of many eating disorders. Adolescent resentment of authority plays a role in the commonly observed manipulative behaviors of patients with eating disorders. Often the family history indicates overprotectiveness and overcontrol. The family is unwilling to allow the adolescent to operate as independently as possible. This serves only to reinforce the adolescent's patterns of self-doubt and inability to accept responsibility for his or her behaviors.

A multidisciplinary team, including the pediatrician, pediatric mental health specialist (psychiatrist, child psychologist, clinical nurse specialist, or social worker), family therapist, and nutritionist, assesses the child's physical, developmental, mental health, familial, and nutritional status. Because nutritional deficiencies often accompany eating disorders, physical assessment focuses on identifying possible associated problems (e.g., anemia). The overall strengths and weaknesses of the child and family must be evaluated to identify the various factors contributing to the child's inadequate or excessive caloric intake and caloric expenditure. Treatment is then designed to address these factors.

Anorexia Nervosa

Anorexia nervosa is a potentially life-threatening eating disorder that occurs almost exclusively in young women and affects an estimated 5% to 18% of young women in the United States.[13] The typical patient is white and from a middle- to upper middle-class family. Age at onset varies, and incidence peaks at 13 to 14 years and 17 to 18 years.[14]

Clinical Manifestations

Anorectic adolescents are characterized by extreme weight loss accompanied by a preoccupation with weight and food, excessive compulsive exercising, peculiar patterns of eating and handling food, and distorted body image. They may prepare elaborate meals for others but eat only low-calorie foods.[15] Characteristically the fear of becoming fat does not decrease with continued weight loss. Accompanying signs and symptoms of depression, crying spells, feelings of isolation and loneliness, and suicidal thoughts and feelings are common.

Physical findings include cold intolerance, dizziness, constipation, abdominal discomfort, bloating, cessation of menses, and malnutrition (Fig. 21–5). Lanugo (fine, downy body hair) may be present. Fluid and electrolyte imbalances, especially potassium imbalances, are common. The child or adolescent is usually energetic despite significant weight loss. Extreme weight loss often leads to cardiac dysrhythmias (bradycardia).

Etiology and Pathophysiology

It is thought that many individuals with anorexia nervosa, as well as those with other eating disorders, have basic problems with body image. Cultural overemphasis on thinness may contribute to the overconcern with dieting and fear of becoming fat experienced by many adolescents.

Genetics may also play a role in the incidence of eating disorders, as evidenced by their increased incidence in relatives of anorectic and bulimic individuals.[2] Chemical changes have been found in the brain and blood of anorectic patients. However, it is not clear whether these changes are a cause or an effect of the disorder.[16]

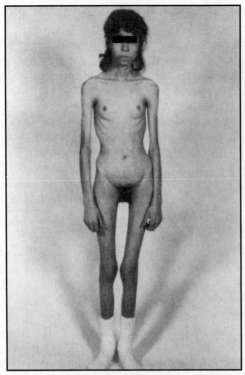 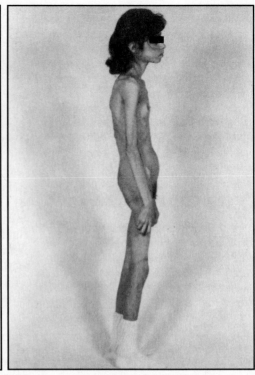

FIGURE 21-5 Characteristic physical appearance of an adolescent girl with anorexia nervosa.

From Rawlings, R.P., Williams, S.R., & Beck, C.K. (1992). *Mental-health psychiatric nursing* (3rd ed.). St. Louis: Mosby–Year Book.

Often a significant life stress, loss, or change precedes the onset of anorexia. Some research suggests that anorexia nervosa may be a form of a serious depressive disorder.[16]

Many authorities view anorexia as a family problem. Intrafamilial conflicts and dysfunctional family patterns may occur when parents are over-controlling and perfectionistic. The adolescent's eating behaviors may be an attempt to exercise independence and resolve internal psychologic conflicts.

The adolescent may engage in lengthy and vigorous exercise (up to 4 hours daily) to prevent weight gain. Laxatives or diuretics may be used to induce weight loss. As the disorder progresses, the adolescent perceives the ever-thinner body as becoming more beautiful. The body responds to the abnormal eating behaviors as if starvation were occurring. Leukopenia, electrolyte imbalance, and hypoglycemia develop as a result of protein-calorie malnutrition.[15] Once the body mass decreases to a critical level, menstruation ceases.

Medical Management

Diagnosis is based on a comprehensive history, physical examination revealing characteristic clinical manifestations, and the DSM-III-R criteria included in Table 21-3.

The goal of treatment is to address the physiologic problems associated with malnutrition, as well as the behavioral and cognitive components of the disorder. A firm focus is placed on reaching a targeted weight with a gradual weight gain of 0.1 to 0.2 kg/day. Enteral feedings or total parenteral nutrition (TPN) may be necessary to replace lost fluid, protein, and nutrients. However, the adolescent often perceives these feedings as a punitive measure.

TABLE 21-3 DSM-III-R Diagnostic Criteria for Anorexia Nervosa

A. Refusal to maintain body weight over a minimal normal weight for age and height, e.g., weight loss leading to maintenance of body weight 15% below that expected; or failure to make expected weight gain during period of growth, leading to body weight 15% below that expected.
B. Intense fear of gaining weight or becoming fat, even though underweight.
C. Disturbance in the way in which one's body weight, size, or shape is experienced, e.g., the person claims to "feel fat" even when emaciated, believes that one area of the body is "too fat" even when obviously underweight.
D. In females, absence of at least three consecutive menstrual cycles when otherwise expected to occur (primary or secondary amenorrhea). (A woman is considered to have amenorrhea if her periods occur only following hormone, e.g., estrogen, administration.)

From American Psychiatric Association (1987). *Diagnostic and statistical manual of mental disorders* (3rd ed., rev.). Washington, DC: Author.

Individual treatment and family therapy are used to address dysfunctional family patterns and assist the family to accept and deal with the adolescent as an independent and less than perfect individual. Family involvement is crucial to effect a lasting change in the adolescent.

Long-term outpatient treatment, in either an individual or a group setting, is frequently necessary. Counseling may be continued for 2 to 3 years to ensure that weight gain and self-image are maintained. Antidepressant drugs such as imipramine (Tofranil) or desipramine (Norpramin) may be prescribed for coexisting conditions such as depression, anxiety, or obsessive-compulsive disorders.

Indications for hospitalization include loss of 25% to 30% of body weight, fluid and electrolyte imbalances or dysrhythmias, or the need to provide a more intense period of therapy if outpatient treatment fails to produce improvement.[2] Behavior modification techniques are used extensively in combination with counseling and other methods in care of the hospitalized anorectic adolescent.

Nursing Assessment

Obtain a thorough individual and family history. Ask about usual eating patterns, daily caloric intake, exercise patterns, and menstrual history. Is there a family history of eating disorders? Assess for signs of malnutrition. Obtain height and weight measurements, and compare with norms for the general population.

Nursing Diagnosis

Common nursing diagnoses for the adolescent with anorexia nervosa include the following:

- Altered Nutrition: Less Than Body Requirements related to distorted beliefs about food requirements, inadequate food intake, or refusal to eat
- High Risk for Fluid Volume Deficit related to inadequate fluid intake or overuse of laxatives and diuretics
- High Risk for Altered Body Temperature related to excessive weight loss and absence of subcutaneous fat
- Constipation related to inadequate food intake and overuse of laxatives
- Body Image Disturbance related to distorted perception of body size and shape

- Self-Esteem Disturbance related to dysfunctional family dynamics
- Ineffective Family Coping: Compromised or Disabling related to parental tendency to be overcontrolling and perfectionistic

Nursing Management

Nursing care centers on meeting nutritional and fluid needs, preventing complications, administering medications, and providing referral to appropriate resources. Specific treatment measures vary depending on physical complications, length and degree of illness, emotional symptoms accompanying the disorder, and family dynamics. Resistance to treatment is common, and nurses who care for anorectic adolescents must deal with their own feelings of frustration and anger.

Meet Nutritional and Fluid Needs. Monitor nutritional and fluid intake, encourage consumption of food, and observe eating behaviors at mealtime. Elimination patterns may be altered as a result of increased intake during hospitalization. Monitor for possible problems, including abdominal distention, constipation, or diarrhea. Daily monitoring of serum electrolytes is necessary.

If TPN is administered, watch for complications such as circulatory overload, hyperglycemia, or hypoglycemia. Use strict aseptic technique when changing tubing or dressings.

Administer Medications. Monitor vital signs if the adolescent is receiving antidepressants. Watch for signs of hypertension and tachycardia. Administering medications after meals helps to prevent gastric irritation.

Provide Referral to Appropriate Resources. Refer parents and other family members to the American Anorexia and Bulimia Association, National Anorectic Aid Society, and National Association of Anorexia Nervosa & Associated Disorders for further information about the disorder and a list of support groups in their area (see Appendix F).

Bulimia Nervosa

Bulimia nervosa is an eating disorder characterized by binge eating (a compulsion to consume large quantities of food in a short period of time). Usually the episodes of bingeing are followed by various methods of weight control (purging), such as self-induced vomiting, large doses of laxatives or diuretics, or a combination of methods. Like anorexia, bulimia affects mainly adolescents and young women who are white and in the higher socioeconomic classes. The disorder usually begins in middle to late adolescence, frequently emerging in the first year of college.

Clinical Manifestations

Bulimic adolescents, like anorectic ones, are preoccupied with body shape, size, and weight. They may appear overweight or thin and usually report a wide range of average body weight over the years. Physical findings depend on the degree of purging, starvation, dehydration, and electrolyte disturbance. Erosion of tooth enamel, increased dental caries, and gum recession, which result from vomiting of gastric acids, are common findings. Abdominal distention is often seen. Esophageal tears and esophagitis may also occur.

Etiology and Pathophysiology

Causes of bulimia nervosa are similar to those of anorexia nervosa: sensitivity to social pressure for thinness, body image difficulties, and long-standing dysfunctional family patterns. Many bulimic individuals experience depression. It is not clear whether the depression is a cause or a result of the bulimic individual's inability to control the bingeing and purging cycles. A bulimic adolescent often binges after any stressful event.[16]

Bingeing usually occurs in secret for several hours until the individual is stopped by abdominal discomfort, by another person, or by vomiting. At first the episodes of binge eating are pleasurable. Immediately following the binge episode, however, feelings of guilt, shame, anger, depression, and fear of loss of control and weight gain arise. As these feelings intensify, the bulimic adolescent becomes increasingly anxious. This usually initiates the purge behaviors.

Purging eliminates the discomfort from bloating and also prevents weight gain. This relieves the feelings of depression and guilt, but only temporarily. Adolescents with bulimia commonly practice the binge-purge cycle many times a day, losing their ability to respond to normal cues of hunger and satiety.[2]

Medical Management

A comprehensive history is necessary because most bulimic adolescents appear normal in weight or only slightly underweight. Laboratory evaluation may identify signs of altered electrolyte and hematologic status. The diagnosis is confirmed by the presence of specific DSM-III-R criteria (Table 21–4).

Treatment includes management of physiologic problems, behavior modification, and psychotherapy. Behavior modification focuses on modifying the dysfunctional eating patterns and restoring a normal pattern. Until the episodes of bingeing and purging are under control, feelings of discouragement and hopelessness prevail. Thus the focus early in treatment is on initiating an immediate behavioral change. Specific treatment measures may include the following:

- Educating the adolescent about good nutrition (including food choice and caloric content)
- Encouraging the adolescent to keep a log or food journal and assisting the adolescent to make connections between emotional states and stress and the impulse to binge or purge
- Setting up a daily dietary routine of three meals and three snacks a day (using the same foods for each meal and snack every day to change mis-

---

TABLE 21-4 DSM-III-R Diagnostic Criteria for Bulimia Nervosa

A. Recurrent episodes of binge eating (rapid consumption of a large amount of food in a discrete period of time).
B. A feeling of lack of control over eating behavior during the eating binges.
C. The person regularly engages in either self-induced vomiting, use of laxatives or diuretics, strict dieting or fasting, or vigorous exercise in order to prevent weight gain.
D. A minimum average of two binge eating episodes a week for at least three months.
E. Persistent overconcern with body shape and weight.

From American Psychiatric Association (1987). *Diagnostic and statistical manual of mental disorders* (3rd ed., rev.). Washington, DC: Author.

conceptions about the weight-gaining potential of certain foods and to decrease anxiety about what food must be eaten at the next meal).

Once these initial measures have been taken, the underlying psychosocial issues are explored.[13] The goals of therapy are to provide the bulimic adolescent with adaptive coping skills and to improve self-esteem.

Most bulimic adolescents do not require hospitalization. Serious abnormalities in fluid and electrolyte levels caused by uncontrollable cycles of bingeing and vomiting, accompanied by depression or suicidal activity, are indications of the need for hospitalization. The prognosis is good with long-term therapy.

Nursing Assessment

Obtain a thorough individual and family history, including daily dietary intake and exercise patterns. Inquire about problems such as abdominal pain or distention, which may indicate an abnormal eating or elimination pattern. Assess the oral mucosa for signs of damage to tooth enamel caused by purging.

Nursing Diagnosis

Common nursing diagnoses for the adolescent with bulimia nervosa include the following:

- Altered Nutrition: Less Than or More Than Body Requirements related to binge-purge behaviors, vomiting, or laxative use
- High Risk for Fluid Volume Deficit related to excess vomiting or laxative use
- Altered Oral Mucous Membrane related to damaging effects of vomited gastric acids
- Knowledge Deficit (Child) related to health risks of excessive use of laxatives and diuretics
- Anxiety related to weight gain and loss of control over eating behavior
- Self-Esteem Disturbance related to dysfunctional family dynamics
- Ineffective Individual Coping related to life stressors

Nursing Management

Nursing care includes monitoring nutritional intake and elimination patterns, preventing complications, and providing appropriate referrals.

During hospitalization a food diary is kept by the patient. Be alert to the adolescent who hides, gives away, or discards food from the tray or who exits to use the bathroom after meals. Withdrawal from laxatives and diuretics is managed with careful observation for alterations in fluid and electrolyte status. Cardiac monitoring may be necessary if potassium levels are seriously altered. Esophageal tearing or esophagitis is managed with symptomatic treatment.

Bulimic adolescents and their families can be referred to various organizations for assistance and information about the disorder (see Appendix F).

Compulsive Overeating and Obesity

Obesity is usually defined as an excessive accumulation of body fat. Whether obesity should be classified as an eating disorder is a matter of considerable discussion and disagreement, since many obese individuals appear to be well adjusted. However, a number of these persons have low self-esteem,

■ CLINICAL TIP

Monitor bulimic adolescents for at least a half hour after each meal to ensure that they do not attempt purging behaviors. These patients should not be allowed to go into their rooms alone. One technique is to contract with the adolescent to sit at the nurse's station during this period.

poor body image, difficulty in relationships, and recurring bouts of anxiety and depression.

Abnormal eating patterns may begin in childhood or adolescence. Obese children and adolescents may use compulsive overeating to make up for a lack of parental love and nurturance or in an attempt to relieve stress.[12]

Treatment usually combines behavioral modification with dietary modifications and an exercise program. Family involvement in the treatment plan is essential.

Nursing Management

Obesity alone rarely necessitates hospitalization. Most often the nurse encounters the obese child when he or she is hospitalized for an orthopedic problem or recurrent abdominal pain. Nursing care focuses on meeting the child's nutritional needs, managing related problems, and promoting self-esteem. Nurses can use mealtimes to educate the child and family about nutritionally sound food choices. Referral to a nutritionist is usually appropriate. Caloric count and portion control need to be emphasized.

The child and family can be referred to local organizations that are devoted to education and support.

Substance Abuse

Substance abuse occurs in children and adolescents of all socioeconomic levels and is a growing health problem. It is important to keep in mind that the use of any drug can pose a serious psychologic and physical risk to children and adolescents.

Although a decline in the daily use of marijuana by adolescents has been reported, abuse of other substances, particularly alcohol, cocaine, crack, and heroin, remains high.[17] Synthetic drugs such as phencyclidine (PCP) (commonly referred to as "designer" drugs) mimic other narcotics, stimulants, and hallucinogens and are also dangerous.

Over-the-counter medications are legal substances that are frequently abused. Easily obtainable at grocery stores and drugstores, these drugs include antihistamines, atropine, bromides, caffeine, ephedrine, pseudoephedrine, phenylpropanolamine, and amphetamine-like substitutes.[18] Volatile inhalants, such as glues, are dangerous substances of abuse, and their use appears to be rising among school-age children and adolescents. Anabolic steroids are relatively new drugs of abuse.

Clinical Manifestations

Substance abuse in children and adolescents is commonly overlooked and underdiagnosed by health care providers. This is due in part to the wide range of clinical presentations, which vary according to type of drug abused, amount, frequency, time of last use, and severity of drug dependence (Table 21–5).

Common physical manifestations include alterations in vital signs, weight loss, chronic fatigue, chronic cough, respiratory congestion, red eyes, and general apathy and malaise. The mental status examination may reveal alterations in level of consciousness, impaired attention and concentration, impaired thought processes, delusions, and hallucinations. Low self-esteem, feelings of guilt or worthlessness, and suicidal or homicidal thoughts are also common.

TABLE 21-5 Commonly Abused Drugs and Their Effects

Drug	Potential for Dependence	Effects of Intoxication
Depressants		
Alcohol, barbiturates (amobarbital, pentobarbital, secobarbital)	*Physical and psychologic:* High; varies somewhat among drugs	*Physical:* Decreased muscle tone and coordination, tremors *Psychologic:* Impaired speech, memory, and judgment; confusion; decreased attention span; emotional lability
Stimulants		
Amphetamines (e.g., Benzedrine), caffeine, cocaine	*Physical:* Low to moderate *Psychologic:* High; withdrawal from amphetamines and cocaine can lead to severe depression	*Physical:* Dilated pupils, increased pulse and blood pressure, flushing, nausea, loss of appetite, tremors *Psychologic:* Euphoria; increased alertness, agitation, or irritability; hallucinations; insomnia
Opiates		
Codeine, heroin, meperidine (Demerol), methadone, morphine, opium, oxycodone (Percodan)	*Physical and psychologic:* High; varies somewhat among drugs; withdrawal effects are uncomfortable but rarely life threatening	*Physical:* Analgesia, depressed respirations and muscle tone (may lead to coma or death), nausea, constricted pupils *Psychologic:* Changes in mood (usually euphoria), drowsiness, impaired attention or memory, sense of tranquility
Hallucinogens		
Lysergic acid diethylamide (LSD), mescaline, phencyclidine (PCP)	*Physical:* None *Psychologic:* Unknown	*Physical:* Lack of coordination, dilated pupils, hypertension, elevated temperature; severe PCP intoxication can result in seizures, respiratory depression, coma, and death *Psychologic:* Visual illusions and hallucinations, altered perceptions of time and space, emotional lability, psychosis
Volatile Inhalants		
Glues, typing correction fluid, acrylic paints, spot removers, lighter fluid, gasoline, butane	*Physical and psychologic:* Varies with drug used	*Physical:* Impaired coordination, liver damage (in some cases) *Psychologic:* Impaired judgment, delirium
Marijuana	*Physical:* Low *Psychologic:* Usually low; occasionally moderate to high	*Physical:* Tachycardia, reddened conjunctiva, dry mouth, increased appetite *Psychologic:* Initial anxiety followed by euphoria; giddiness; impaired attention, judgment, and memory

Based on information in Finke, L. (1992). Nursing interventions with children and adolescents experiencing substance abuse. In West, P., & Sieloff Evans, C.L., (Eds.), *Psychiatric and mental health with children and adolescents* (pp. 244–246). Gaithersburg, MD: Aspen Publications, Exhibit 17–1; and Lahmeyer, H.W., Channon, R.A., & Francis Schlemmer, R., Jr. (1993). Psychoactive substance abuse. In Flaherty, J.A., Davis, J.M., & Janicak, P.G. (Eds.), *Psychiatry: Diagnosis & therapy* (2nd ed.) (pp. 268–283). Norwalk, CT: Appleton & Lange.

Poor school performance and changes in mood, sleep habits, appetite, dress, and social relationships are nonspecific characteristics of the substance-abusing child.

Etiology and Pathophysiology

In most cases substance abuse represents a maladaptive coping response to the stressors of childhood and adolescence. A child may begin using drugs or alcohol to deal with stress because family members or peers do so. Children in families with a history of substance abuse are at higher risk of abusing drugs and alcohol. Other risk factors include rebelliousness, aggressiveness, low self-esteem, dysfunctional parental relationships, lack of adequate

Initial experimentation with alcohol or drugs may be unpleasant. With continued use, however, the adolescent learns to "achieve the high," an illusion of power and well-being.[17] The adolescent wants the high more frequently and actively seeks alcohol or drugs. Tolerance to the substance occurs with continued use, and ever-increasing amounts are required to achieve a pleasurable high. Physical and psychologic dependence ensues as the body's tissues require the substance to function properly.[16] Withdrawal symptoms occur when the child or adolescent is deprived of the substance.

Medical Management

Multiple psychiatric diagnostic criteria exist for each drug class. Children and adolescents who have other psychosocial disorders commonly use or abuse drugs or alcohol. Treatment should therefore focus not only on the substance use or abuse, but also on the issues underlying the problem. Intervention includes the family as well as the substance-abusing child or adolescent.

The primary goal of treatment is to teach and support the child and other family members to develop and sustain positive coping patterns. Most treatment programs offer inpatient and outpatient services, as well as after-care programs. These programs usually consist of peer support focusing on the development of a life-style free of drugs or alcohol, healthy family relationships, and positive coping skills. Family involvement is strongly encouraged. Hospitalization is required if the physical dependence is significant and withdrawal places the child at risk for complications such as seizures, depression, or suicidal behavior.

Nursing Assessment

Nurses may encounter the substance-abusing child or adolescent in the emergency room or outpatient clinic or during hospitalization for an injury or other acute problem. Nursing assessment includes taking a thorough history from the parents and child, observing the child's behavior, and performing a physical examination. The history should include the age at which drug use began, pattern of use, length of time the drug has been used, amount of drug used, and psychologic state while on drugs.

Physiologic Assessment. Look for physical signs and symptoms of substance abuse, including bloodshot eyes, dilated pupils, slurred speech, and weight loss. The adolescent may appear sleepy or restless or may show signs of clumsiness.

Psychologic Assessment. Changes in social habits may indicate substance abuse. Parents may report a drop in the school-age child's or adolescent's grades or decreased interest in school activities. New friends are not introduced to parents, and the adolescent has less contact with parents, teachers, and other adults who were previously important.

Nursing Diagnosis

Common nursing diagnoses for children and adolescents who abuse drugs or alcohol include the following:

- Impaired Social Interaction related to substance abuse behaviors and effects of drugs

- Self-Esteem Disturbance related to dysfunctional family and social relationships
- High Risk for Injury related to altered perceptions and sensorium
- High Risk for Violence: Self-Directed or Directed at Others related to physiologic dependence on drugs or alcohol and lack of concern about behaviors or actions necessary to obtain the next dose

Nursing Management

Care of children and adolescents who abuse drugs and alcohol is challenging and often frustrating. Long-term mental health counseling may be necessary to resolve underlying issues and foster life-style and behavioral changes.

Prevention is the most desirable intervention. The nurse can play a major role in teaching children and their families about substance abuse. Education should begin in primary school. Nurses also can play a major role in community education. Various prevention programs have been developed by federal and private organizations.

Referral to support organizations may be beneficial for the child, parents, and other family members (see Appendix F). Self-help groups, which are available in most communities, include Alcoholics Anonymous, Narcotics Anonymous, Al-Anon, Nar-Anon, and Ala-Teen.

Depression and Anxiety

Both depression and anxiety can be seen as symptoms or disease states. *Symptoms* include both subjective feelings and physiologic manifestations of distress. A *disease state* is diagnosed when a pattern of symptoms exists as a result of an identified cause.[19]

Depression

Only in recent years has depression in children been recognized as a clinical condition. Many children referred to child guidance centers and mental health professionals because of behavioral difficulties or poor achievement actually suffer from depression. The incidence of major depression is estimated to be about 2% in prepubertal children and about 5% in adolescents. Before puberty, depression is more common in boys than girls. Depressive symptoms and disorders increase with age, as does the female/male ratio.[14]

Clinical Manifestations

Characteristic findings of major depression in children and adolescents include declining school performance; withdrawal from social activities; sleep disturbance (either too much or too little); appetite disturbance (too much or too little); multiple somatic complaints, especially headaches and stomachaches; and various conduct and behavioral problems.

Etiology and Pathophysiology

Many theories have been proposed to explain the cause of depression in children and adolescents. Depression may be biologic in origin or a result of learned helplessness, cognitive distortion, social skills deficit, or family dysfunction.[14] Childhood depression sometimes occurs secondary to parental depression because the parental depression deprives the child of effective parenting. Abuse and neglect predispose children to depression, especially very young children.

Medical Management

Treatment may include psychotherapy in combination with psychotropic medication. Often a combination of individual, family, and group therapy provides the greatest benefits for young children and adolescents. Involving parents and other family members in the treatment plan is essential. Group therapy is an effective treatment measure for adolescents because of the importance of peer group relationships during the teenage years. Cognitive therapy may be used with adolescents, and play therapy with younger children (see discussion earlier in this chapter).

Antidepressant medications, most commonly imipramine (Tofranil), desipramine (Norpramin), and amitriptyline (Elavil), may be prescribed.

Nursing Assessment

A thorough history and physical examination, including observation of behavior, are obtained at the time of admission. Assess the child for common risk factors for depression and anxiety (Table 21–6).

Nursing Diagnosis

Common nursing diagnoses for the child or adolescent hospitalized with depression are included in the accompanying Nursing Care Plan. Other diagnoses that might be appropriate include the following:

- Altered Health Maintenance related to inability to perform or lack of interest in activities of daily living (ADLs)
- Altered Nutrition: More Than Body Requirements related to coping mechanism of compulsive eating
- Powerlessness related to overwhelming sense of doom or inability to cope
- Self-Esteem Disturbance related to dysfunctional family dynamics

Nursing Management

Nursing care of the child hospitalized for depression includes administering medications and providing supportive care. Monitor vital signs of children receiving antidepressant medications. Watch for common side effects, including hypertension and tachycardia. Refer to the Nursing Care Plan for specific nursing interventions for the child or adolescent hospitalized with depression.

Discharge Planning and Patient and Family Home Care Teaching. Teaching parents to recognize signs and symptoms of anxiety and depression is essential. Assisting parents to recognize normal behaviors in children provides es-

---

TABLE 21–6 Risk Factors for Depression and Anxiety in Children and Adolescents

Parental neglect, abuse, or loss
Stressful social relationships
Academic pressures and underachievement
Dysfunctional family relationships
Family history of depression, suicide, substance abuse, alcoholism, or other psychopathology
Chronic illness and frequent hospitalization

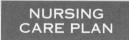

THE CHILD OR ADOLESCENT HOSPITALIZED WITH DEPRESSION

GOAL	INTERVENTION	RATIONALE	EXPECTED OUTCOME
1. Hopelessness related to fear and anxiety			
Child or adolescent will discuss feelings of hopelessness.	Encourage open expression of feelings. Explore hopeless, sad, or lonely feelings. Point out the connection between feelings and behavior. Assess child or adolescent to identify the precipitating event when feelings of sadness arise.	Expressing feelings may help to relieve sadness, loneliness, despair, and hopelessness. An accepting and nonjudgmental attitude must be maintained regarding any feelings expressed by child.	By discharge, child or adolescent expresses an interest in the future.
	Encourage child or adolescent to take part in self-care and unit activities. Use routines to establish feelings of control.	An active role in self-care and treatment helps child or adolescent to feel more in control.	
	Medicate as ordered and document results.	Antidepressants modify mood to a more hopeful outlook.	
2. Ineffective Individual Coping related to dysfunctional family system			
Child or adolescent will use effective coping skills.	Teach positive, effective coping strategies such as guided imagery and relaxation. Assist child or adolescent in focusing on strengths rather than weaknesses.	Therapeutic techniques can help child or adolescent to replace negative thoughts and images with more positive and effective beliefs and images.	Child or adolescent verbalizes and demonstrates ability to cope appropriately for his or her age.
	Assist child or adolescent to identify friends, family members, and others who are positive and supportive.	Helps the child or adolescent to become aware that people can be caring and supportive (thus validating self-esteem).	

sential knowledge and perspective. Parents should also be taught dosages and side effects of any prescribed medications.

Suicide

Suicide is the third leading cause of death between 15 and 19 years of age. Over the past 30 years, teenage suicide has increased by more than 250%.[20] Suicide rates among children under age 12 have doubled.

Boys die as a result of suicide four times more often than girls. This statistic is reversed for suicide attempts, perhaps because boys use lethal methods such as guns, hanging, and jumping more often than girls, who use drug overdose and wrist cutting.

It is not unusual for health care professionals and parents to label suicide attempts by children and adolescents "accidents." Adults may have difficulty believing that young children, in particular, would have any reason to want to end their lives. Because of this, many children who are brought to the emergency room with indications of a suicide attempt are classified as unin-

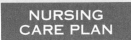

THE CHILD OR ADOLESCENT HOSPITALIZED WITH DEPRESSION—CONTINUED

GOAL	INTERVENTION	RATIONALE	EXPECTED OUTCOME
3. Impaired Social Interaction related to low self-esteem and negative body image			
Child or adolescent will participate in and initiate activities and conversation.	Assist child or adolescent to identify topics and activities of interest.	The more child or adolescent focuses on areas of interest, the less he or she will focus on internal anxiety and depression.	By discharge, child or adolescent initiates conversation and activities with staff and peers.
	Encourage interaction with peers and staff.	Each positive interaction reinforces feelings of success. Each success reinforces the desire for future social interaction.	
	Facilitate visits from family and friends.	Reinforces positive and rewarding relationships.	
	Provide guidance to family regarding interaction that promotes self-esteem.	Family often has existing negative interaction style.	
4. Altered Nutrition: Less Than Body Requirements related to loss of appetite secondary to depression			
Child or adolescent will consume adequate daily intake to maintain optimal nutritional status.	Offer nutritious finger foods, sandwiches, and high-calorie liquid supplements frequently throughout the day.	Convenient easy-to-eat foods encourage child or adolescent to eat and maintain nutritional status.	Child or adolescent consumes adequate daily intake to maintain optimal nutritional status by discharge.
	Offer easy-to-carry drinks that are high in vitamins, minerals, and calories.	Convenient method for meeting hydration and electrolyte needs.	

TABLE 21-7 Risk Factors for Suicide in Children and Adolescents

School problems
Pregnancy
Drug use or abuse
Problems with a romantic relationship
Feelings of anxiety
History of chronic family problems
Chronic illness
Physical, emotional, or sexual abuse
History of suicide in a family member
History of depression
Chronic low self-esteem

tentional injury victims and released without arrangements for appropriate follow-up care.

Many risk factors for suicide exist in children and adolescents (Table 21–7). The most common precursor to adolescent suicide is depression. Common signs or symptoms of an underlying depression that could lead to suicide include boredom, restlessness, problems with concentration, irritability, lethargy, intentional misbehavior, preoccupation with one's own body or health, and excessive dependence on or isolation from others (especially adults or caregivers).

The child or adolescent found to be at high risk for suicide is generally admitted to a psychiatric unit for care. Treatment may include individual, group, or family therapy. Negotiating a "no suicide" contract is one method that may be used with a suicidal youth. In the contract the child agrees that he or she will not attempt suicide during a specified time period.

Many more threats, gestures, and attempts are made than actual suicides are carried out. Although many adolescents make suicidal gestures out of anger or in an attempt to manipulate others, these gestures must be recognized as involving an element of desperation. If indeed the threats are manipulative or an expression of anger, the idea of hospitalization is usually enough to stop the adolescent from using them as a habitual method. On the other hand, if a threat is assumed to be manipulative and is not taken seriously, the adolescent is challenged to prove that he or she is not bluffing.

Nursing Management

Nursing care centers on taking appropriate precautions to ensure the child's safety. Both the child and the hospital environment are monitored for any object that could be used for self-harm. All potentially harmful objects, such as shoestrings, belts, pantyhose, and hair ribbons, are removed. All personal care items (including toothbrush and shampoo) are kept locked at the nursing station and monitored constantly when used by the child.

Children or adolescents who are considered at high risk for suicidal behaviors are attended by a nursing staff member at all times, including while using the bathroom and sleeping. It may be necessary for the child to dress in a plain hospital gown, be kept in a visually monitored seclusion room, or (if seriously impaired and self-abusive) be medicated or physically restrained for a period of time. Restraints are used only when ordered by the physician and interdisciplinary team caring for the child.

Hospitalization continues as long as the child's behavior is self-destructive. Children are referred for intensive individual and family therapy. Encourage parents to keep follow-up clinic appointments, to watch for self-destructive behaviors, and to administer any prescribed medications according to the treatment schedule.

Separation Anxiety and School Phobia

Anxiety is a subjective feeling that affects every person at some time. It can be defined as a feeling of apprehension or dread, usually accompanied by central nervous system signs, including restlessness, trembling, perspiration, and rapid pulse.[21]

Separation anxiety disorder is characterized by an extreme state of uneasiness when in unfamiliar surroundings and often by refusal to visit friends' homes or attend school. This disorder occurs in approximately 3% of children and in twice as many girls as boys.[2]

Children with separation anxiety disorder tend to be perfectionistic, overly compliant, and eager to please. They appear to cling to the parent or caretaker. They may use physical complaints such as headaches, abdominal pain, nausea, and vomiting in an attempt to avoid being away from the parent. Depression frequently accompanies separation anxiety disorder. The resulting avoidant behaviors often interfere with personal growth and development, academic achievement, and social functioning.

School phobia (also called school avoidance or school refusal) is a persistent, irrational, or excessive fear of attending school. The child may fear being harmed or losing control. School phobia is common in children between 5 and 12 years of age but can occur in children up to age 16.[22] The child's avoidance of school is often a manifestation of his or her fear of leaving the parent or primary caretaker (usually the mother). Children commonly report that teachers and peers "pick on them." Somatic complaints are similar to those seen in children who have separation anxiety disorder. Characteristically symptoms are present only on school days and not on weekends or holidays.

Treatment of children with separation anxiety disorder or school phobia must include the family as well as the child. Establish firm limits defining the behavioral expectations and consequences for the child. Antidepressant medications (such as imipramine [Tofranil]) or antianxiety medications (such as lorazepam [Ativan] or clonazepam [Klonopin]) are often helpful in decreasing the child's overwhelming sense of anxiety.

Prompt intervention is needed in cases of school absenteeism. The longer the child is out of school, the greater the likelihood that a chronic, treatment-resistant condition will result. Referral for psychiatric evaluation is indicated if symptoms persist.

Nursing Management

Nursing care centers on educating parents about the disorder and management techniques. Children with separation anxiety disorder benefit from a predictable routine and environment during hospitalization. Advise children in advance of any specific testing or procedures to be performed. Explaining the procedure fully also helps to minimize anxiety.

Recurrent Abdominal Pain

■ **CLINICAL TIP**

Children commonly hold their feelings in their "tummies." When interviewing children to find out how they are feeling inside, you only need to ask, "What's your tummy feel like today? Right now? Yesterday when that happened?"

Recurrent abdominal pain is a frequent problem among young children and adolescents. It is the most commonly reported symptom of children who have been sexually abused or traumatized in some way (Fig. 21–6) and is often a complaint of anxious or depressed children and adolescents. The abdominal distress may be due in part to the anxiety response. Parents and health care professionals should not dismiss the child's pain just because the cause is unknown or unidentified.

Commonly children and adolescents are admitted to the hospital and un-

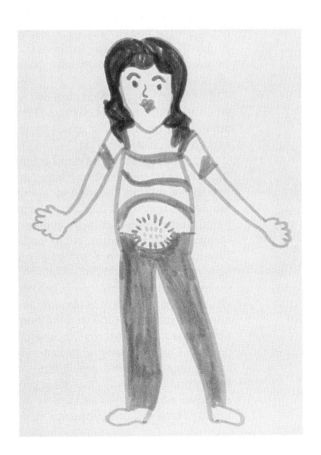

FIGURE 21–6 "Self-Portrait." Drawn by a 12-year-old girl during her third hospitalization in 4 months for recurrent abdominal pain. Upper and lower gastrointestinal series and other invasive procedures were conducted but produced negative findings. As a last resort, before discharge a psychiatric consultation was ordered. This drawing was the first in a series of pictures. After several sessions the girl disclosed that she had been sexually abused by her stepfather for several years.

dergo an array of painful and expensive procedures in an attempt to find the cause of the pain. An underlying psychosocial problem may be identified only after the test results come back negative and the child continues to complain of pain. At other times symptoms subside and the child is released from the hospital with instructions to take antacid medication, follow a restrictive diet, and return to the physician's office or clinic for follow-up. In these instances hospitalization may provide the respite needed to reduce or eliminate symptoms of abdominal discomfort and pain for a brief period. However, once the child returns to the source of the anxiety, the pain resurfaces, much to the dismay of parents and physician. Thus the cycle of searching for the cause begins again.

Nursing Management

Nursing care includes supporting the child during assessment and diagnostic testing. Children with continuing or recurrent abdominal pain should be referred to a mental health professional while in the hospital.

Encopresis

Encopresis is an abnormal elimination pattern characterized by the recurrent soiling or passage of stool at inappropriate times by a child who should have achieved bowel continence. It occurs in approximately 1% to 5% of school-age children and is three times as common in boys as in girls. Children with primary encopresis have never achieved bowel control. Children with secondary encopresis have been continent of stool for several months.

Encopresis is usually associated with voluntary or involuntary retention of stool in the lower bowel and rectum, leading to constipation or diarrhea. Soiling may occur during the day or night and usually takes place when the child is under stress. The child may be ridiculed by peers because of his or her offensive body odor. This rejection leads to withdrawal and behavioral problems, often resulting in altered school performance and attendance. Parents commonly seek health care, believing that the child has diarrhea or constipation.

The underlying constipation that leads to encopresis may be caused by the stress of environmental changes (birth of a sibling, moving to a new house, attending a new school), issues of control related to bowel training, or a genetic predisposition.

A thorough history, physical examination, and diagnostic studies (including barium enema, lead screening, and thyroid function tests) are necessary to rule out organic causes and anatomic abnormalities. A mental status examination may be indicated. Information about the child's toilet-training habits and parents' attitudes concerning those habits is obtained. A dietary history, including eating habits and types of foods eaten, is often helpful. Physical examination commonly reveals a nontender mass in the lower quadrant of the abdomen.[23]

Treatment may include behavior modification techniques, dietary changes, use of lubricants to clear the bowel of impacted stool and encourage normal defecation, and psychotherapy. Behavior modification programs that reward and reinforce appropriate toileting habits are moderately successful. Dietary changes include incorporating high-fiber foods such as fruits, vegetables, and cereals into the diet. Limiting intake of refined and highly processed foods and dairy products also may be helpful. Psychotherapy involving the child and family may be indicated in instances of dysfunctional parent-child relationships.

Nursing Management

Nursing care centers on educating the child and parents about the disorder and its treatment and providing emotional support. Explain the treatment plan, including dietary changes and use of laxatives or stool softeners. Reassure the child that he or she has a healthy body and, with treatment, will achieve normal functioning.[15] Prevention is the goal. Nurses are in a position to offer anticipatory guidance about bowel training to parents with young children (see Chapter 2). Encourage realistic expectations and developmentally appropriate toileting practices.

Childhood Schizophrenia

Schizophrenia is a psychotic disorder that is seen more commonly in boys than girls.[2] Although it is relatively rare in young children and adolescents, it can occur in children as young as 5 years of age. The prevalence of schizophrenia increases after puberty and reaches adult levels by late adolescence (approximately 1% of the population).

Clinical manifestations depend on the individual's coping abilities and defense mechanisms. Characteristic behaviors include social withdrawal, impaired social relationships, flat **affect** (outward appearance of feeling or emotion), regression, loose associations (thought characterized by speech in which ideas shift from one subject to another that is unrelated), delusions, and hallucinations.

The cause of childhood schizophrenia is unknown, but genetic predisposition may play a role in its occurrence. The disorder most often becomes manifest between 15 and 20 years of age. Onset may be sudden or insidious. Most often the child demonstrates restlessness, poor appetite, and social withdrawal over several weeks to months. Some children, however, become psychotic without any warning over a few days.

During adolescence, acute schizophrenia is likely to begin while the teenager is making plans to leave home and family in order to attend college, marry, or work in another area.[16] Onset of symptoms may be triggered by an important loss (death of a significant other, parent, child, or friend).

Treatment of childhood schizophrenia is multifaceted, including individual psychotherapy, family therapy, and various psychotropic medications (antipsychotics such as haloperidol [Haldol], antianxiety agents such as lorazepam [Ativan], and antidepressants such as imipramine). Drugs are only moderately effective at controlling hallucinations and delusions, and responses vary considerably among individuals. Side effects will determine what drugs are used and for how long. Antipsychotic medication often must be continued for several months or years after recovery from an acute schizophrenic episode.

Most episodes of acute schizophrenia require several weeks to months of inpatient hospitalization on a psychiatric unit. Treatment may include an intensive school-based program in a structured, supervised setting with specially trained professionals. The goal of treatment initially is to reduce or control psychotic episodes and provide a safe, structured environment for the child or adolescent, enabling the child to live each day at an optimal level of functioning.

Most children require long-term treatment, including intermittent periods of hospitalization. Children or adolescents whose symptoms are difficult to control and who present a safety risk to themselves or others may require long-term residential treatment.

Nursing Management

The nurse usually encounters the child or adolescent with schizophrenia during hospitalization for an acute episode or for treatment of another problem. Nursing care centers on providing education and supportive care to the child and parents.

Educating the child and parents about the risk of recurrence and methods to alleviate side effects of prescribed medications may increase compliance with the treatment plan. Because many schizophrenic children return home after hospitalization for an acute episode, family education and involvement in the treatment plan are essential. The nurse may also need to communicate with school personnel in order to ensure understanding of the child's condition.

Conversion Reaction

Conversion reaction is a disorder in which a disturbance or loss of sensory, motor, or other physical functions suggests neurologic or other somatic disease. The disturbance or loss cannot be explained by any known pathophysiologic mechanism. Instead, psychologic factors are involved.

Clinical manifestations include altered sensations, such as blindness or deafness; paralysis or ataxia, including inability to stand or walk and loss of ability to speak (aphonia); involuntary movements, such as pseudoepileptic convulsions; and constant complaints of pain with no physical basis (psychogenic pain). The onset of conversion symptoms is usually dramatic and sudden. Symptoms often appear to be neurologic, but on careful examination obvious discrepancies are found. Often the child or family members appear indifferent or unconcerned over what health care providers consider an overwhelming physical disability.

Children suspected of having a conversion reaction require a complete physical and neurologic evaluation to rule out any possible physiologic basis for the symptoms. Individual and family therapy is usually necessary to identify the source of the psychologic conflict, pain, or need resulting in the conversion symptoms.

Child Abuse

Awareness of the problem of child abuse is increasing. More cases are being reported; however, these are probably only a small percentage of the total. Approximately 4% of children between the ages of 3 and 17 years—about 2 million children—are physically abused each year.[24]

Physical abuse is only one part of a larger problem. The definition of child abuse has expanded over the past 10 years to include physical neglect, emotional abuse and neglect, verbal abuse, and sexual abuse, as well as physical abuse. Many children who are sexually abused are under the age of 5 years, some as young as 3 months of age. The average age for sexual molestation is 4 years.[25]

An abused child is one whose parent or another person legally responsible for his or her care:

- Inflicts or allows another to inflict physical or emotional pain or injury, or
- Creates or allows another to create a significant risk of serious physical or emotional pain or injury, or
- Commits or allows another to commit an act of sexual abuse, as defined by law, against the child

Abuse generally involves an act of commission, that is, actively doing something to a child physically, emotionally, or sexually, such as hitting, belittling, or molesting. Neglect more often involves an act of omission, such as not providing adequate nutrition, emotional contact, or necessary physical care. Because the evidence is often not visible, emotional abuse and neglect are more difficult to identify and prove than physical abuse or neglect. Risk factors for abuse and neglect are listed in Table 21–8.

Types of Abuse

Physical Abuse. Physical abuse is the deliberate maltreatment of another individual that inflicts pain or injury and may result in permanent or temporary disfigurement or even death. Common methods of physical abuse in children are listed in Table 21–9.

Physical Neglect. Physical neglect is the deliberate withholding of or failure to provide the necessary and available resources to the child. Behaviors constituting physical neglect include failure to provide for the following basic needs: adequate nutrition and hydration, hygiene (e.g., clean diapers and

---

TABLE 21-8 Risk Factors for Child Abuse and Neglect

Factors Increasing Risk for Physical Abuse

Low socioeconomic status
Prematurity
Unrelated male primary caretaker
Parents who were abused as children
Age less than 3 years
Handicap or condition that requires a great deal of care (e.g., mental retardation, attention deficit hyperactivity disorder)
Parental substance abuse or social isolation

Factors Increasing Risk for Sexual Abuse

Absence of natural father or having a stepfather
Being female
Mother's employment outside the home
Poor relationship with parent
Parental relationship characterized by conflict
Parental substance abuse or social isolation

Compiled from Rudolph, A.M., Hoffman, J.I.E., & Rudolph, C.D. (Eds.) (1991). *Rudolph's pediatrics* (19th ed.) (pp. 839–840). Norwalk, CT: Appleton & Lange.

TABLE 21-9 Methods of Physical Abuse in Children

Hitting, slapping, kicking, or punching
Whipping with belts, shoes, or electrical cords
Inflicting burns with a lit cigarette or lighter
Immersing child or body part in scalding water (commonly legs, perineal area, hands, or feet)
Shaking the child violently ("shaken child" syndrome)
Tying the child to a fence, bed, tree, or other object
Throwing the child against a wall, down stairs, or against a window
Choking or gagging the child
Fracturing the legs, arms, ribs, or skull
Deliberately administering excessive doses of prescribed or nonprescribed drugs
Deliberately withholding prescribed medication

---

clothes, bathing and toileting facilities), shelter (e.g., warmth in winter), and appropriate health care (e.g., immunizations, dental care, medications, eyeglasses).

Emotional Abuse. Emotional abuse usually involves shaming, ridiculing, embarrassing, or insulting the child. It can also include the destruction of a child's personal property, such as tearing up the child's favorite family photographs or letters or harming, killing, or giving away the child's pet. These actions are frequently used as a means of frightening or controlling the child.

Verbal abuse is a common method of emotional abuse. Words can be a violent and volatile weapon against a child, eroding the child's fragile sense of self and destroying self-esteem. Common examples of verbal abuse include yelling obscenities at the child, calling the child names, threatening to "put the child away" or to give away or kill the child's pet, telling the child "I wish you were never born" or "You're worthless," and using words to humiliate, shame, or degrade the child.

Emotional Neglect. Emotional neglect is characterized by the caretaker's emotional unavailability to the child. The usual style of interaction is cold and lacking in sensitive personal attention. The child suffers from a lack of nurturance and failure of the parent or caretaker to meet basic dependency needs.

■ COMMON FORMS OF SEXUAL ABUSE

- Oral-genital contact
- Fondling and caressing the genitals
- Anal intercourse
- Sexual intercourse
- Rape
- Sodomy
- Prostitution

Sexual Abuse. Child sexual abuse is the exploitation of a child for the sexual gratification of an adult. Between 100,000 and 500,000 children in the United States are sexually abused each year.[25] Approximately 75% to 80% of child sexual abusers are immediate family members, other relatives, friends, or neighbors. Male perpetrators make up 92% to 98% of all abusers.[25] Abusers often threaten to harm or kill the child or another family member if the child discloses the abuse.

Clinical Manifestations

Manifestations of physical abuse include but are not limited to:
- Multiple bruises in various stages of healing
- Scald burns with clear lines of demarcation and in a glove or stocking distribution
- Rope, belt, or cord marks, usually seen on the mouth, buttocks, back, legs, and arms
- Burn scars in various stages of healing
- Multiple fractures in various stages of healing
- Shortness of breath and distress upon being moved, indicating chest contusions and possible rib fractures
- Sedation from overmedication
- Exacerbation of chronic illness (such as diabetes or asthma) because of withholding of medication

Behaviors inconsistent with developmental stage may also be apparent. For example, the toddler or preschool child may be indiscriminantly friendly with unfamiliar adults, including health care providers, rather than demonstrating shyness or anxiety.

Manifestations of physical neglect include undernourishment (evidenced by constantly feeling hungry, hoarding or stealing food, and being underweight), unclean clothes and body, poor dental health (extensive cavities or generally poor condition of teeth), and inappropriate clothing for the season.

Manifestations of emotional abuse, verbal abuse, and emotional neglect include fear, poor physical growth, and failure to meet appropriate develop-

TABLE 21-10 Physical and Behavioral Manifestations of Sexual Abuse in Children and Adolescents

Vaginal discharge
Bloodstained underpants or diaper
Genital redness, pain, itching, or bruising
Difficulty walking or sitting
Urinary tract infection
Sexually transmitted disease
Somatic complaints, such as headaches and stomachaches
Sleeping problems, such a nightmares or night terrors
Bedwetting
Unwillingness to go to babysitter, family member, neighbor, or other person
Fear of strangers
New or excessive sexual curiosity or play
Constant masturbation
Curling into fetal position
Excessively seductive behavior
Phobias about particular places, people, or things
Abrupt changes in school performance and attendance
Changes in eating habits
Abrupt changes in behavior (especially withdrawal)
Child or adolescent acts like a wife or mother

---

mental milestones. The child may have difficulty relating to adults, impaired communication skills, and developmental delays.

Children who have been sexually abused may exhibit a variety of physical and behavioral signs and symptoms (Table 21–10). However, sexual abuse does not always result in apparent injury. Among the many long-term consequences of child sexual abuse are ongoing feelings of shame, guilt, anger, and hostility; decreased self-esteem, which leads to increased self-destructive behavior and risk of suicide; recurrence of victimization experiences; substance abuse; and eating disorders. Factors associated with greater psychologic harm to the child include (1) a long period of abuse, (2) use of violent force or threat of violence, (3) abuse involving penetration (intercourse or oral-genital sex), and (4) abuse involving family members, especially the father or stepfather (Fig. 21–7).

FIGURE 21-7 These drawings illustrate, from the child's point of view, what it is like to live in an abusive home environment. The artist is a woman who was sexually abused by her father and suffered physical and emotional abuse by both parents as a child.

From Harris, P. (1993). *A child's story: Recovering through creativity* (pp. 10 & 15). St. Louis: CRACOM Corp.

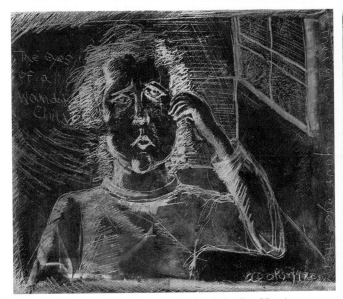

"The Eyes of a Wounded Child" by Pat Harris
Oil pastel and paintstick on paper (24" × 20"), 1989

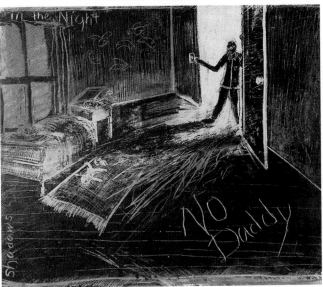

"No Daddy" by Pat Harris
Oil pastel and paintstick on paper (24" × 20"), 1989

Etiology and Pathophysiology

Regardless of the type of abuse, the most common abuser is the child's parent or guardian or the boyfriend of the child's mother. Risk factors associated with abusive behavior in adults include the following:

- *Psychopathology*, such as drug addiction or alcoholism, low self-esteem, poor impulse control, and other personality disorders
- *Poor parenting experiences*, such as abuse in the abuser's own childhood, rejection by the abuser's own parent(s), lack of knowledge of alternative methods of discipline, strong belief in or family tradition of harsh discipline, and lack of parental affection
- *Marital stressors and problems with partners*, such as hostile-dependent, abusive, or nonsupportive relationships, and one-sided decision making
- *Environmental stressors*, such as legal, financial, medical, or housing problems
- *Social isolation*, such as few friends and limited use of sitters, family, or other resources
- *Inappropriate expectations* for the developmental level of the child

Medical Management

Diagnosis of abuse is made on the basis of a careful history and thorough physical examination. X-ray studies may be ordered to identify signs of recurrent abuse (e.g., healed fractures). Some children are admitted directly to the hospital with the diagnosis of suspected abuse or neglect. Less obvious as a victim of abuse is the child admitted with a skull fracture who "fell off a chair."

Neglect, which is more difficult to define and identify, frequently requires hospitalization with a comprehensive medical, social, and psychiatric evaluation. Five basic categories must be considered when attempting to diagnose neglect: (1) medical care neglect (lack of necessary medical care), (2) gross safety neglect (lack of appropriate supervision), (3) physical neglect (lack of food and shelter), (4) emotional neglect, and (5) educational neglect.

All 50 states have extensive and complex statutes regarding reporting of child abuse and neglect. A specialist must be consulted, especially if the child's testimony will be used in court.

Children do not routinely make false allegations of abuse. If indeed there is reason to believe the allegations are false, a child and adolescent therapist (psychiatrist, psychologist, psychiatric clinical nurse specialist, or social worker) with special expertise should be consulted to determine the truth. Keep in mind that children who withdraw their accusations have often been threatened or coerced into doing so.

Because children who have been physically, emotionally, or sexually abused are at risk for major depression, they require skilled care by mental health professionals who are specially trained in this area. Initially the treatment goals include prevention of self-destructive or other dangerous acts. Children must be encouraged to express their fears and feelings in a safe and supportive environment. Equally important is the child's need to build coping skills and self-esteem. The child must be reassured and convinced that he or she is in no way responsible or to blame for what happened.

Individual treatment with art therapy is used initially because it is the least threatening method in the early stages of treatment, it can easily be tailored to meet the child's individual needs, and it prepares the child for other forms of treatment such as family and group therapy. Family or group therapy may be of benefit in exploring the child's concerns and feelings. Anger is

■ CULTURAL CONSIDERATIONS

Traditional treatment practices are sometimes mistaken for signs of physical abuse. The Chinese practice of cupping, which involves heating a bamboo cup and placing it on the skin, is a traditional treatment for headaches or abdominal pain. The Vietnamese practice of *caogio* (rubbing out the wind), in which a coin or the fingers are forcefully rubbed on the chest, back, or neck, is used to treat minor ailments.

■ LEGAL CONSIDERATIONS

Every state has a child abuse law specifying the particular behaviors that define every type of abuse. Any professional who works with children and reasonably suspects that a child has been abused is required to report his or her suspicions to the local agency for child protective services. Reports made in good faith are not liable to countersuits. However, professionals who suspect abuse and do not report it may be held responsible by the courts.

common, especially in children who were abused by a trusted adult such as the father or stepfather.

Nursing Assessment

Nursing assessment in instances of suspected child abuse or neglect requires a comprehensive history and physical examination, with documentation of findings. Consultation with social service agencies in the community is important if the family is receiving services.

Obtaining the history can be stressful for both the nurse and the parent. Use of therapeutic communication techniques and a quiet, unhurried environment are helpful. Maintaining a nonjudgmental attitude at all times is essential. Obtaining information about abusive and neglectful behaviors requires the nurse to establish a trusting relationship with parents who are often afraid to trust any professional.

The health history sequence should include (1) parental concerns, (2) general family history, and (3) specific child history. This sequence begins with nonthreatening topics and allows the nurse to demonstrate concern before asking about abuse-related concerns. Obtain details about how injuries occurred. The parents' and child's own words should be documented verbatim using quotation marks. Compare reports obtained from each family member for lack of consistency and details that change over time.

It is desirable to interview the parent and child separately as well as together. Parent-child interaction during an intensive history-taking session provides an opportunity to observe the child's behavior and the parent's method of handling and responding to the child.

Data gathered during history-taking are particularly important in light of physical findings. Are there discrepancies between the history and physical assessment data? Do the parents give a history of an uncontrollable, inattentive toddler when the nurse observes a child who is attentive throughout a 15-minute examination? Assess the child's general appearance, including dress and behavior during the assessment. How do the child's affect, behavior, and development compare with those of other children the same age?

Documentation of findings is important in all situations but is essential in cases of suspected child abuse and neglect. Physical findings should be recorded as observed. Figure diagrams should be used to document skin injuries. Photographs are taken to document the location, nature, and extent of injuries.[26]

Nursing Diagnosis

Common nursing diagnoses for the physically abused or neglected child include the following:

- Pain related to inflicted injuries
- Impaired Skin Integrity related to inflicted injuries
- Altered Growth and Development related to lack of supportive parenting and environment
- Altered Nutrition: Less Than Body Requirements related to inadequate caloric intake
- Altered Health Maintenance related to lack of parental provision of child's essential needs
- Fear related to actual physical harm or repeated risk of injury
- High Risk for Injury related to physical abuse
- High Risk for Violence (Parent) related to inability to manage anger

Additional diagnoses that may apply to the emotionally abused or neglected child include the following:

- Defensive Coping related to belittling or verbal threats by parents
- Chronic Low Self-Esteem related to lack of appropriate emotional support from parents
- Disabling Family Coping related to dysfunctional family dynamics and pattern of physical abuse

Diagnoses that may apply to the sexually abused child include the following:

- Anxiety related to potential separation from parent
- Rape-Trauma Syndrome related to sexual exploitation of child
- Altered Role Performance related to expectation of meeting adults' sexual gratification needs
- Personal Identity Disturbance related to disturbance of usual child activities and decreased self-esteem

Nursing Management

Nursing care focuses on helping to remove the child from an abusive environment, preventing further injury, providing supportive care, and reinforcing the importance of follow-up care and counseling.

Prevent Further Injury. Work with social services and community agencies to assess the child's home environment, individuals living in the home, and the actions surrounding the abuse. Assist in removing the child from the home to temporary custody of the court or foster care of another relative, if indicated. Counsel family members about abuse and refer for appropriate therapy.

Provide Supportive Care. Protect and treat the child's injuries (e.g., fractures, burns). Include parents in the child's treatment plan, and keep them informed about the child's progress. Even if suspected of inflicting injuries to the child, the parent is still the child's primary caretaker. Talk with the parent as you would with any parent. Be supportive of any guilt expressed. Encourage the parent to assist with the child's care. Observe parent-child interactions and document supportive behaviors and the child's response to the parent versus other care providers.

Interacting nonjudgmentally with a parent suspected of abusing his or her child can be difficult. Talk with a colleague about any anger you feel toward the parents or about the child's injuries or specific actions surrounding the abuse. Use team meetings to develop strategies that enable you to work with the parents and child.

Discharge Planning and Patient and Family Home Care Teaching. If there is any question about the child returning to a potentially dangerous situation, support the child's removal from the situation. After discharge the child may receive supervised care in the home by court order. Day care, home nursing, and social worker visits may be arranged. Parents should be referred to parent effectiveness classes, family therapy, and support groups as necessary.

Munchausen Syndrome by Proxy

Munchausen syndrome by proxy is a potentially deadly form of child abuse that involves the fabrication of signs and symptoms of a health condition in a child.[27] Usually it is the mother who creates these fictitious signs in her child (the proxy). The victim is usually under 6 years of age. Frequently the child's symptoms of illness are used to gain entry into the medical system in order to meet the abuser's own needs.

The issues of abuse are multidimensional. The child is a victim of the feigned illness, repeated hospitalizations, and invasive procedures. Equally disruptive is the deprivation of the child's daily routine caused by the periodic medical crises.

Munchausen syndrome by proxy should be suspected when unexplained, recurrent, or extremely rare conditions occur; illness is unresponsive to treatment; and the history and clinical findings are inconsistent. The most commonly reported signs and symptoms are central nervous system dysfunction, apnea, diarrhea, vomiting, fever, seizures, signs of bleeding (in urine or stool), and rashes. The symptoms always occur in the presence of the same caretaker and disappear when the child is separated from that caretaker.

The child often appears uncooperative, extremely anxious, fearful, and negative. The caretaker, who in contrast appears very cooperative, competent, and loving, often expresses a desire for the child to recover. The caretaker may even suggest diagnostic procedures to try to determine "what's wrong." Characteristically the caretaker thrives in the health care environment.[27]

The cause of Munchausen syndrome by proxy is often complex and rooted in the caretaker's own abusive or neglectful childhood. The disorder occurs in all socioeconomic classes. Often the perpetrator has some type of health care background, such as nursing or another allied health profession.[28]

A suspicion of Munchausen syndrome by proxy requires a coordinated evaluation by an interdisciplinary team. Members of the team must organize and communicate a strategic plan regarding collection of evidence, confrontation of the abuser, and management of the hospitalized child. The child's safety is the ultimate concern.[29] The case must also be reported to the appropriate child protective services.

Nursing Management

Special care should be taken to maintain a trusting relationship with the caretaker so that he or she does not become suspicious and leave the hospital. Often the best person on the team to function in the role of "trusted other" is a member of the psychiatric consultation team.

Careful documentation of parent-child interactions, presence or absence of symptoms, and other pertinent observations is essential. The child must be closely monitored. When enough evidence is collected to prove Munchausen syndrome by proxy, the caretaker is confronted.

Failure to Thrive

■ CULTURAL CONSIDERATIONS

Each child should maintain a height and weight growth curve similar to the population standard. Asian-American children may normally be below the fifth percentile on standard growth charts and not have FTT. Suspect FTT when the infant or child falls 1 standard deviation below *his or her own* curve as established by several prior measurements.

Failure to thrive (FTT) describes a syndrome in which an infant or child experiences a failure in physical growth along with signs of malnutrition. This disorder accounts for 1% to 5% of pediatric hospitalizations.[2] The growth of children with FTT consistently falls below the third percentile for age or decreases rapidly from a higher percentile. The child commonly has delays in reaching developmental milestones.

The symptoms may be caused by organic or nonorganic factors or by a combination of both. Nonorganic FTT is most common. Organic causes include congenital acquired immunodeficiency syndrome (AIDS), inborn errors of metabolism (see Chapter 19), neurologic disease, and various congenital or structural problems. The most common cause of organic FTT in infants with no structural abnormality is gastroesophageal reflux (see Chapter 15).

Nonorganic FTT includes the pathologic refusal of food, sleep and feeding disorders, and social and emotional factors that interfere with adequate nutrition. Nonorganic FTT may reflect intrauterine growth retardation or a lack of adequate maternal care and warmth.[30] Infants and children whose parents or caretakers suffer from depression, substance abuse, mental retardation, or psychosis are therefore at risk. The parents are frequently uneducated, poor, and socially and emotionally isolated.

A thorough history and physical examination are needed to rule out any chronic physical illness. The infant or child may be hospitalized so that health care providers can establish a routine for feeding and sleeping. The goals of treatment are to provide adequate caloric and nutritional intake, promote normal growth and development, and assist parents in developing nurturing feeding routines and responding to the infant's cues of physical and psychologic hunger.

Nursing Management

Nursing care centers on observing parent-child interactions during feeding times and providing necessary teaching to enable parents to respond appropriately to their child's needs. Often nurses feed the child to determine if he or she is eating, how much food is eaten, and the amount of time it takes to eat. Parents need to be taught how to feed the infant and provide other basic infant care in a warm, loving, attentive environment.

REFERENCES

1 Herrick, C.A., Goodykoontz, L., & Herrick, R.H. (1992). Selection of treatment modalities. In West, P., & Sieloff Evans, C.L. (Eds.). *Psychiatric and mental health with children and adolescents* (pp. 98–115). Gaithersburg, MD: Aspen Publications.

2 Dulcan, M., & Popper, C. (Eds.) (1991). *Child and adolescent psychiatry* (pp. 16–41, 45–91). Washington, DC: American Psychiatric Press.

3 Stanley, S. (1992). Nursing interventions in children and adolescents experiencing communication disabilities. In West, P., & Sieloff Evans, C.L. (Eds.). *Psychiatric and mental health with children and adolescents* (pp. 199–211). Gaithersburg, MD: Aspen Publications.

4 Taylor, C.M. (1990). Populations at risk: Children and adolescents. In Taylor, C.M. (Ed.). *Essentials of psychiatric nursing* (13th ed.) (pp. 369–393). St. Louis: Mosby–Year Book.

5 Kozloff, M.A. (1973). *Reaching the autistic child: A parent training program.* Champaign, IL: Research Press.

6 Rapport, M.D., Stoner, G., & Dupaul, G.J. (1985). Methylphenidate in hyperactive children: Differential effects of doses on academic learning and social behavior. *Journal of Abnormal Psychology, 13,* 227–244.

7 Greenhill, L.L. (1991). Attention-deficit hyperactivity disorder. In Weiner, J.M. (Ed.). *Textbook of child and adolescent psychiatry* (pp. 261–275). Washington, DC: American Psychiatric Press.

8 Clunn, P. (1991). *Child psychiatric nursing.* St. Louis: Mosby–Year Book.

9 Yearwood, E. (1992). Nursing interventions with children experiencing attention and motor difficulties. In West, P., & Sieloff Evans, C.L. (Eds.). *Psychiatric and mental health with children and adolescents* (pp. 169–181). Gaithersburg, MD: Aspen Publications.

10 Hathaway, W.E., Hay, W.W., Jr., Groothuis, J.R., and Paisley, J.W. (1993). *Currrent pediatric diagnosis and treatment* (11th ed.). Norwalk, CT: Appleton & Lange.

11 American Psychiatric Association (1987). *Diagnostic and statistical manual of mental disorders* (3rd ed., rev.). Washington, DC: Author.

12 Chitty, K. (1992). Eating disorders. In Wilson, H.S., & Kneisl, C.C. (Eds.). *Psychiatric nursing* (pp. 468–483). Redwood City, CA: Addison-Wesley.

13 Deering, C.G. (1992). Nursing interventions with children and adolescents experiencing eating difficulties. In West, P., & Sieloff Evans, C.L. (Eds.). *Psychiatric and mental health with children and adolescents* (pp. 343–358). Gaithersburg, MD: Aspen Publications.

14 Kashani, J.H., & Eppright, T.D. (1991). Mood disorders in adolescents. In Weiner, J.M. (Ed.). *Textbook of child and adolescent psychiatry* (pp. 248–260). Washington, DC: American Psychiatric Press.

15 Rudolph, A.M., Hoffman, J.I.E., & Rudolph, C.D. (Eds.). (1991). *Rudolph's pediatrics* (19th ed.). Norwalk, CT: Appleton & Lange.

16 Greenberg, H.R. (1989). *Emotional illness in your family: Helping your relative, helping yourself.* New York: Macmillan.

17 Finke, L. (1992). Nursing interventions with children and

adolescents experiencing substance abuse. In West, P., & Sieloff Evans, C.L. (Eds.). *Psychiatric and mental health with children and adolescents* (pp. 242–254). Gaithersburg, MD: Aspen Publications.

18 Pentel, P. (1984). Toxicity of over-the-counter stimulants. *Journal of the American Medical Association, 252,* 1898–1903.

19 Brantly, D.K., & Takacs, D.J. (1991). Anxiety and depression in preschool and school-aged children. In Clunn, P. (Ed.). *Child psychiatric nursing* (pp. 351–364). St. Louis: Mosby–Year Book.

20 Valente, S. (1992). Nursing interventions with children and adolescents experiencing self-destructive tendencies. In West, P., & Sieloff Evans, C.L. (Eds.), *Psychiatric and mental health with children and adolescents* (pp. 315–327). Gaithersburg, MD: Aspen Publications.

21 Flaherty, J.A., Davis, J.M., & Janicak, P.G. (Eds.) (1993). *Psychiatry: Diagnosis and therapy* (2nd ed.). Norwalk, CT: Appleton & Lange.

22 Rapoport, J. (1989). The biology of obsessions and compulsions. *Scientific American,* March, 83–89.

23 West, P., & Sieloff Evans, C.L. (Eds.). (1992). *Psychiatric and mental health nursing with children and adolescents.* Gaithersburg, MD: Aspen Publications.

24 U.S. Bureau of the Census (1992). *Statistical abstract of the United States: 1992* (112th ed.). Washington, DC: Author.

25 Fontaine, K. (1992). Rape and intrafamily abuse and violence. In Wilson, H.S., & Kneisl, C.R. (Eds.). *Psychiatric nursing* (pp. 508–544). Redwood City, CA: Addison-Wesley.

26 Campbell, J., & Humphreys, J. (1993). *Nursing care of survivors of family violence.* St. Louis: Mosby–Year Book.

27 Crouse, K. (1992). Munchausen syndrome by proxy: Recognizing the victim. *Pediatric Nursing, 18*(3), 249–252.

28 Rosenberg, D. (1987). Web of deceit: A literature review of Munchausen syndrome by proxy. *Child Abuse and Neglect, 11,* 547–563.

29 Sheridan, M. (1989). Munchausen syndrome by proxy. *Health and Social Work, 14*(1), 53–58.

30 Chatoor, I. (1991). Eating and nutritional disorders of infancy and early childhood. In Weiner, J.M. (Ed.). *Textbook of child and adolescent psychiatry* (pp. 351–361). Washington, DC: American Psychiatric Press.

SUGGESTED READINGS

Bailey, G. (1991). Substance use and abuse. In Weiner, J.M. (Ed.). *Textbook of child and adolescent psychiatry* (pp. 351–361). Washington, DC: American Psychiatric Press.

Bluestein, J., & Collins, M.A. (1989). *Parents in a pressure cooker: A guide to responsible and loving parent/child relationships.* Rosemont, NJ: Modern Learning Press.

Castiglia, P. (1993). School phobia-school avoidance. *Journal of Pediatric Health Care, 7*(5), 229–232.

Clark, L. (1989). *The time-out solution: A parent's guide for handling everyday behavior problems.* Chicago: Contemporary Books.

Dreikurs, R., & Cassel, P. (1990). *Discipline without tears: A reassuring and practical guide to teaching your child positive behavior.* New York: Dutton.

Eminson, D.M., & Postlethwaite, R.J. (1992). Factitious illness: Recognition and management. *Archives of Disease in Childhood, 67,* 1510–1516.

Fiesta, J. (1992). Protecting children: A public duty to report. *Nursing Management, 23*(7), 14–15.

Glenn, H.S., & Nelson, J. (1989). *Raising self-reliant children in a self-indulgent world: Seven building blocks for developing capable young people.* Rocklin, CA: Prima Publishing.

Greenspan, S., & Greenspan, N.T. (1989). *The essential partnership: How parents and children can meet the emotional challenges of infancy and childhood.* New York: Penguin Books.

Humphreys, J., & Campbell, J.C. (1989). Abusive behavior in families. In Gillis, C.L., et al., (Eds.). *Toward a science of family nursing* (pp. 394–417). Redwood City, CA: Addison-Wesley.

Olshaker, B. (1989). *What shall we tell the kids? What kids want to hear from their parents.* New York: Lynx Communications.

Straus, M.A., Gelles, R.J., & Steinmetz, S.K. (1980). *Behind closed doors: Violence in the American family.* New York: Anchor Books/Doubleday Publishing.

Weinhaus, E., & Friedman, K. (1988). *Stop struggling with your teen: A complete, easy-to-use guide for parents of preteens and teens.* New York: Penguin Books.

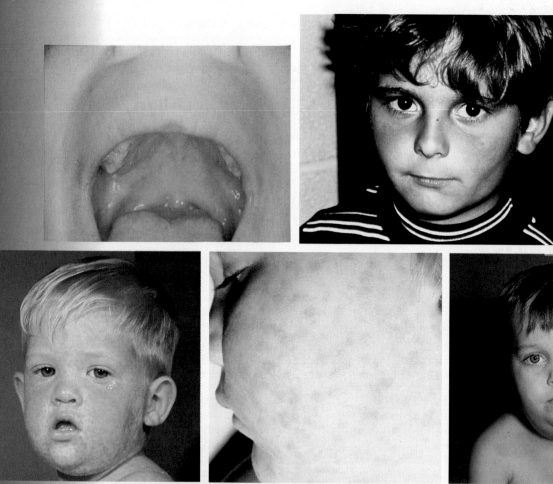

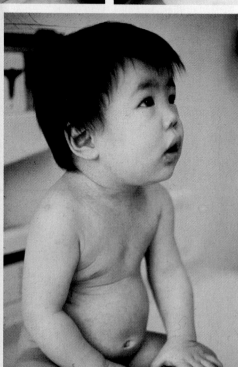

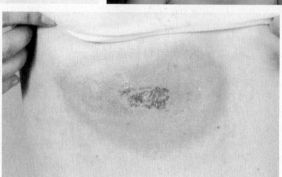

Bottom right: Photograph by L. Zemel, courtesy of Pfizer Central Research, Groton, CT. All other photographs courtesy of Centers for Disease Control and Prevention, Atlanta, GA.

ATLAS OF INFECTIOUS AND COMMUNICABLE DISEASES

TERMINOLOGY

acellular vaccine Uses proteins from the microorganism to stimulate the process of active immunity.

active immunization Stimulation of antibody production without causing clinical disease.

communicable disease Illness that is directly or indirectly transmitted from one person to another.

killed virus vaccine Contains the microorganism that has been killed but is still capable of inducing the human body to produce antibodies to the disease.

direct transmission Passage of infectious disease by physical contact between source of pathogen and new host.

indirect transmission Passage of infectious disease involving survival of pathogens outside humans before invasion of new host.

infectious disease Illness, caused by a microorganism, that is commonly communicated from one host (human or otherwise) to another.

live virus vaccine Contains the microorganism in live but attenuated, or weakened, form.

nosocomial infection Infection acquired in the hospital, not present at the time of admission.

passive immunization Immunity produced through introduction of specific antibodies to the disease, which are usually obtained from the blood serum of immune persons and animals. *Does not confer lasting immunity.*

toxoid Toxin that has been treated (by heat or chemical) to weaken its toxic effects but retain its antigenicity.

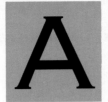

An **infectious disease** is an illness caused by microorganisms that are commonly communicated from one host (human or otherwise) to another. A **communicable disease** is an illness that is directly or indirectly transmitted from one person to another. Communicable diseases are a major cause of the morbidity and mortality of infants and children in the United States.[1]

For a communicable disease to occur, the following need to be present (Fig. D–1):

- An infectious agent, or pathogen
- An effective means of transmission
- A susceptible host

An effective chain of transmission for infection requires a suitable habitat, or reservoir, for the pathogen. A reservoir may be living or nonliving. Transmission may be direct or indirect. **Direct transmission** involves physical contact between the source of the infection and the new host. **Indirect transmission** occurs when pathogens survive outside humans before causing infection and disease.

A susceptible host is also necessary for the occurrence of infectious disease. Young children whose immune systems are not fully developed, and who have not yet developed antibodies to many agents, cannot defend against disease as well as older children. Other characteristics, such as immunodeficiency and poor health, may increase a child's risk of contracting an infectious disease.

Control of communicable diseases is usually directed at interrupting the chain of transmission or eliminating one or more of the habitats or reservoirs (e.g., spraying insecticide to kill mosquitoes that carry malaria). Isolating an infected individual interferes with disease transmission, and killing the pathogen eliminates the causal agent. Public health authorities monitor pat-

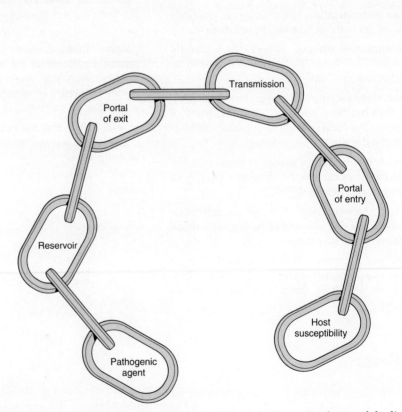

FIGURE D–1 The chain of infection. To achieve infection control, one of the links in the chain needs to be broken.

terns of disease occurrence, and health care workers are required to report cases of many infectious diseases to state health officials.

As a result of major public health programs and scientific advances such as safer drinking water, better sanitation, improved standards of living, immunization, and advanced medical treatment, communicable diseases have decreased in occurrence but remain a significant source of morbidity and mortality in infants and children, especially in developing countries.

Special Vulnerability of Children

The capability and function of the immune system, especially of infants, is poorly understood. Infants are particularly vulnerable to infectious diseases because their immune responses are immature, passively acquired maternal antibodies are decreasing, and disease protection through immunization is as yet incomplete. As children grow, they develop immunity through immunization or exposure to the natural disease. As children mature and become more active, they interact more frequently in play groups and day care settings, which increases their exposure to infectious agents. Transmission is facilitated by the close environment and the difficulty in monitoring the hygiene habits of young children (e.g., covering the mouth when coughing, thorough washing after toileting) without very close supervision. The fecal-oral and respiratory routes are the most common sources of transmission in children (Fig. D–2). As healthy children are exposed to more infections, they develop antibodies naturally. Thus subsequent infections with the same type of organism may be less severe or avoided.

FIGURE D–2 Infectious diseases are easily transmitted in settings such as day care centers where children handle common objects.

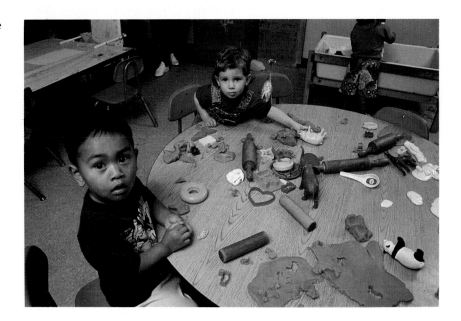

Fever

Fever in a child is often a sign of infectious disease. Why does fever develop in response to certain illnesses and infections? What methods can be used to manage fever in children? Table D–1 provides guidelines for evaluating fever in children.

Many Latino and Asian cultures subscribe to the hot and cold theory of disease causation. Fever, a hot condition, is treated by giving the patient cold substances (foods or medicines). "Hot" and "cold" do not refer to temperature but to categories. Cold foods include vegetables, fruits, and fish. Cold medicines include orange flower water, linden, and sage.

TABLE D-1 Parent Teaching: Guidelines for Evaluating Fever in Children

Call your health care provider immediately if:

- The child is under 2 months old or has a fever over 104.2° F (40.1° C).
- The child is crying inconsolably or whimpering.
- The child cries when moved or otherwise touched by the parent or other family members.
- The child is difficult to awaken.
- The child's neck is stiff.
- There are any purple spots present on the skin.
- Breathing is difficult and no better after the nose is cleared.
- The child is drooling saliva and is unable to swallow anything.
- The child has a convulsion.
- The child acts or looks very sick.

Call your health care provider within 24 hours if:

- The child is 2 to 4 months old (unless fever occurs within 48 hours of a DTP shot and the infant has no other serious symptoms).
- The fever is between 101° F and 104.2° F (39° C and 40.1° C) (especially if the child is under 2 years old).
- The child complains of burning or pain with urination.
- The fever has been present more than 24 hours without an obvious cause or location of infection.

Modified from Hathaway, W.E., Hay, W.W., Jr., Groothuis, J.R., & Paisley, J.W. (1993). *Current pediatric diagnosis and treatment* (11th ed.). Norwalk, CT: Appleton & Lange.

Physiologic Response

The hypothalamus is the control center for the regulation of body temperature and is frequently compared to a thermostat because of its regulatory function. When the blood circulates through the hypothalamus, the hypothalamus regulates body temperature by directing body systems to conserve heat or dissipate heat, depending on the blood temperature.

If body temperature is lower than normal, vasoconstriction occurs to conserve heat. The adrenal glands produce epinephrine and norepinephrine, which cause an increase in metabolism, more vasoconstriction, and more heat production. Shivering or chills may occur, which in turn may increase heat production.

One degree of temperature elevation causes an increase in respiratory rate by four breaths per minute and increases oxygen need by 7%.

When excess heat is produced, the body responds with an increase in temperature. With the increase in temperature, vasodilation occurs. In response, the child may become lethargic and irritable. The skin flushes and becomes warm to the touch. The heart rate and respiratory rate increase. As the temperature decreases, the child may start to perspire, the heart rate and respiratory rate return to normal, and the child becomes more active.

Elevated temperature can be a helpful mechanism. It helps to eradicate organisms that thrive at lower body temperatures and mobilizes the immune response. Fever is not inherently harmful until it reaches 41° C (105.9° F). If not managed, it can result in febrile seizures, which usually have no long-term sequelae. Parents often fear fevers and need information and reassurance. Nursing care for treatment of fever includes administering antipyretics, removing unnecessary clothing, encouraging increased fluid intake, and giving tepid baths or sponging.

▨ Immunization

The development and widespread availability of immunizations has been one of the great breakthroughs of modern medicine. Immunization intro-

TYPES OF VACCINES

killed virus vaccine Contains a microorganism that has been killed but is still capable of inducing the human body to produce antibodies. EXAMPLE: inactivated poliovirus vaccine.

live virus vaccine Contains a microorganism in live but attenuated, or weakened, form. EXAMPLE: live poliovirus vaccine

toxoid A toxin that has been treated (by heat or chemical) to weaken its toxic effects but retain its antigenicity. EXAMPLE: tetanus toxoid.

LEGAL CONSIDERATIONS

Federal legislation requires consent to be obtained before administration of vaccines. In most institutions it is the nurse's responsibility to inform parents, supply literature, and obtain the parents' written consent before the vaccine is administered.

The nurse is required to record the (1) lot number of the immunization given, (2) site of administration, (3) route of administration, and (4) name and address of the person who administers the vaccine. In addition, the nurse is obligated to report any severe immunization reactions to the state health department.

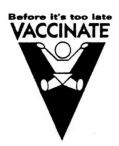

Courtesy of the National Immunization Campaign.

duces an antigen (foreign substance that triggers an immune response) into the body, allowing immunity against disease to develop naturally. In **active immunization** an antigen is given in the form of a vaccine. However, a child may need antibodies faster than the body can develop them. **Passive immunization** with antibodies (proteins capable of reacting specifically to an antigen) produced in another host, not in the child, is given to high-risk children after a single exposure to prevent the disease from occurring or to reduce its severity. For example, if a child who has never had a tetanus immunization steps on a rusty nail, the child needs immediate protection (passive immunity) from tetanus. Antibodies from the tetanus immune globulin injection combat the tetanus toxin produced by the bacterial spores introduced by the nail. The process of antibody development (active immunity) is then initiated with administration of tetanus toxoid.

Since vaccines were first developed in the late 1800s, many diseases have decreased dramatically in incidence. The introduction of vaccines against childhood diseases such as measles (rubeola), mumps, rubella, polio, diphtheria, and *Haemophilus influenzae* type b has greatly improved the quality of life for children and adults.

Improvements in vaccine technology continue to increase the safety and efficacy of immunization against an increasing number of diseases. Immunizations should be given to all children on specific schedules. There are now major national, state, and private initiatives to immunize all children on schedule. Nurses should be strong advocates for immunization. Being well informed about immunizations, their potential side effects, and recommended schedules assists immunization efforts.

Vaccines should be administered at specific ages. Timing is determined by the age at which transplacental immunity (passive immunity) transferred from mother to infant decreases or disappears and the infant or child develops the ability to make antibodies in response to the vaccine. The recommended schedule for immunization has changed to reflect new vaccines and knowledge about the length of time immunity lasts. Vaccines and vaccine theory are still considered as recent developments, and refinements continue to occur. Two reliable sources for current immunization recommendations for both children and adults are the Centers for Disease Control and Prevention (CDC) and the American Academy of Pediatrics (AAP). The AAP recommendations are given in Table D–2.

Supplemental immunizations for influenza, meningococcal, and pneumococcal infections are recommended for certain children (Table D–3). Figure D–3 shows a sample vaccine administration record.

Recent outbreaks of measles and the increased incidence of congenital rubella syndrome in infants born in the United States have resulted from a decline in immunization compliance. The effectiveness of vaccines depends on the immunization of all susceptible individuals. Currently, efforts to initiate, complete, and monitor immunizations in children are increasing. Influences on lower immunization rates of children include economic factors, poor access to sources of health care, inadequate education regarding the importance of immunization, religious prohibitions, and belief that any drug intake is wrong or not healthful.

Worldwide immunization efforts are focused on increasing the vaccine supply and distribution and decreasing the cost.[2] In many developing countries, communicable diseases, even those that can be prevented by immunization, cause significant morbidity and mortality because of unavailability of vaccine and inadequate medical facilities, staff, and medication.

The nurse should have up-to-date information about common pediatric immunizations (Table D–4).

The pertussis vaccine is given in combination with the diphtheria and tetanus toxoids (DTP). Pertussis immunization has been associated with neurologic events. Questions about pertussis and other vaccines led to the passage of the National Childhood Vaccine Injury Act of 1986, which provides compensation if a link between immunization and serious effect is determined. Recently a new acellular, highly refined pertussis vaccine has become available. It is recommended for the fourth and fifth doses and has less potential for causing serious side effects.

■ NURSING ALERT

The CDC recently revised its recommendation for the third polio dose to be given at 6 months. Recommendations are updated periodically, and practitioners should contact their state department of health to check for changes in this information.

TABLE D-2 Recommended Schedule of Vaccinations for All Children

2 Mo	4 Mo	6 Mo	12 Mo	15 Mo	4–6 Yr	11–12 Yr	14–16 Yr
DTP	DTP	DTP		DTP* or DTaP	DTP or DTaP		Td†
Polio	Polio			Polio*	Polio		
				MMR‡		MMR§	
Hib ‖ or Hib	Hib Hib	Hib	Hib	Hib			

Birth	1–2 Mo	4 Mo	6–18 Mo
HB	HB¶ HB¶	HB¶	HB¶ HB¶

Modified from American Academy of Pediatrics. (1991). *Report of the Committee on Infectious Diseases* (pp. 313–315). Elk Road Village, IL: Author. Used with permission of the American Academy of Pediatrics.
DTP, Diphtheria, tetanus, and pertussis vaccine; *DTaP,* diphtheria, tetanus, and **acellular** pertussis **vaccine;** *Td,* diphtheria-tetanus adult; *Polio,* live oral polio vaccine (OPV) drops or killed (inactivated) polio vaccine (IPV) shots; *MMR,* measles, mumps, and rubella vaccine; *Hib, Haemophilus influenzae* b conjugate vaccine; *HB,* hepatitis B vaccine.
*Many experts recommend these vaccines at 18 months.
†Repeat every 10 years.
‡In some areas this dose of MMR vaccine may be given at 12 months.
§Unless second dose previously given.
‖ Hib vaccine is given in either a four-dose schedule or a three-dose schedule, depending on the type of vaccine used.
¶Hepatitis B vaccine can be given simultaneously with DTP, polio, MMR, and *Haemophilus influenzae* b conjugate vaccine at the same visit.

TABLE D-3 Supplemental Immunizations

Vaccine	Recommendation
Influenza	For children with chronic pulmonary disease, cardiac disease, sickle cell disease or other hemoglobinopathies, diabetes, metabolic disease, HIV infection or those undergoing immunosuppressive therapy or chronic aspirin therapy. Administered annually in autumn.
Meningococcal	For children older than 2 years with asplenia. Vaccine duration is 3 years or longer.
Pneumococcal	For children older than 2 years with sickle cell disease, asplenia, nephrotic syndrome, renal failure, HIV infection or CSF leaks or those undergoing immunosuppressive therapy. Vaccine is administered one time, not to be repeated.

■ CLINICAL TIP

Read the package inserts of vaccines to determine proper storage conditions. Some vaccines are frozen, and others are refrigerated. When reconstituting vaccines, it is important to use the solution provided or follow the manufacturer's directions. Write the date and time on the bottle if it is a multidose vial. Many reconstituted vaccines do not have a long shelf life.

Proper storage and delivery are necessary to ensure that vaccines are effective. An improperly stored vaccine or poorly administered vaccine may make it ineffective and prevent the child from developing immunity.

Certain reactions following immunization are reportable by law to the U.S. Department of Health and Human Services (Table D–5).

Many parents have fears about immunization based on stories they have heard about reactions and experiences that others have had. It is important for the nurse to understand parents' concerns and to be able to explain the risks and benefits of each immunization. Today's vaccines are safer and are often produced synthetically by means of recombinant DNA technology or genetic engineering. Parents have the right to refuse immunizations for their child on the basis of religious beliefs. However, they must sign a waiver not-

Vaccine Administration Record

Patient Name _____

Birthdate _____

Record # _____

<table>
<tr><td colspan="3">Clinic Name/Address</td></tr>
<tr><td></td><td></td><td></td></tr>
</table>

"I have been provided a copy, and have read or have had explained to me, information about the diseases and the vaccines listed below. I have had a chance to ask questions that were answered to my satisfaction. I believe I understand the benefits and risks of the vaccines cited, and ask that the vaccine(s) listed below be given to me or to the person named above (for whom I am authorized to make this request)."

Vaccine	Date Given m/d/y	Age	*Site	Vaccine Manufacturer	Vaccine Lot Number	**Handout Publ. Date	***Initials	Signature of Parent or Guardian
DTP 1								
DTP 2								
DTP 3								
DTP/DTaP4								
DTP/DTaP5								
DT								
DTP/Hib1								
DTP/Hib2								
DTP/Hib3								
DTP/Hib 4								
Td								
OPV/IPV 1								
OPV/IPV 2								
OPV/IPV 3								
OPV/IPV 4								
MMR 1								
MMR 2								
Hib 1								
Hib 2								
Hib 3								
Hib 4								
Hep B 1								
Hep B 2								
Hep B 3								

*** Initials	Signature of Vaccine Administrator
_____	_____
_____	_____
_____	_____

(Use reverse side if more signatures are needed)

*Site Given Legend

RA = Right Arm
LA = Left Arm
RT = Right Thigh
LT = Left Thigh
O = Oral

** If required by state law

American Academy of Pediatrics

Copyright©1992
Rev 7/93

HE0116

FIGURE D–3 Sample vaccine administration record.

Courtesy of American Academy of Pediatrics. Copyright © 1992 American Academy of Pediatrics.

TABLE D-4 Common Pediatric Immunizations

Immunization Type	Side Effects	Contraindications	Nursing Considerations
Diphtheria and Pertussis Vaccines and Tetanus Toxoid (DTP)			
Route: Intramuscular *Dosage:* 0.5 mL *Age(s) Given:* 2, 4, 6, 15 to 18 months; 4 to 6 years (five doses) *Storage:* Store in body of refrigerator at 2 to 8° C (35 to 46° F).	*Common:* Redness, pain, nodule at injection site; temperature up to 101° F; drowsiness; fussiness; anorexia *Serious:* Anaphylaxis; shock or collapse; residual seizure disorder; fever above 102° F	Occurrence of a serious side effect after previous administration of DTP Administration to be delayed for 1 month after immunosuppressive therapy and until febrile illnesses have resolved Administration of immune serum globulin within last 90 days	Prior to immunization, ask about previous reactions to immunization. Ask for history of seizures or neurologic diseases. Shake vaccine before drawing. Solution will be cloudy. If pertussis only is withheld, give DT (for use in children under 7 years) and Td (for use in adults and children over 7 years of age). Acellular pertussis preparation is recommended for fourth and fifth doses.
Trivalent Oral Polio Vaccine (TOPV)			
Route: Oral *Dosage:* 0.5 mL, or drops, or entire contents of single-dose dispenser *Age(s) Given:* 2, 4, 15 to 18 months; 4 to 6 years (four doses) *Storage:* Keep frozen at −10° C (14° F). Refreeze thawed container if temperature did not exceed 8° C (46° F) during thaw period. Vial can go through maximum of 10 thaw/freeze cycles. Alternatively, thawed vial can be stored in refrigerator from 2 to 8° C (35 to 46° F) for maximum of 30 days.	*Common:* None *Serious:* Paralytic polio disease in child or caregiver	Immunosuppression or lack of acquired immunity of infant or caregiver If family member is immunosuppressed, infant can be immunized with injectable inactivated polio vaccine rather than TOPV.	Prior to immunization, ask if child or family members are immunosuppressed or have been immunized. Live virus vaccine must be handled carefully. Wipe spill from surface. Instruct parents that caregivers must wash hands carefully after diaper changes for first month to avoid transmission of live virus from infant's stool to nonimmunized caregiver.
Measles, Mumps, Rubella Vaccines (MMR)			
Route: Subcutaneous *Dosage:* 0.5 mL *Age(s) Given:* 12 to 15 months; 11 to 12 years (two doses) *Storage:* Store in body of refrigerator at 2 to 8° C (35 to 46° F). When reconstituted, keep refrigerated and away from light; discard if unused within 8 hours.	*Common:* Elevated temperature; redness or pain at injection site; noncontagious rash; joint pain *Serious:* Anaphylaxis; encephalopathy; residual seizure disorder	Allergy to neomycin, eggs Immunosuppression Administration of immune serum globulin in past 90 days Pregnancy	Prior to immunization, ask if child has allergy to eggs or neomycin. Immunosuppression Instruct adolescents of childbearing age to avoid pregnancy for 3 months after immunization.

Data from Bindler, R., & Howry, L. (1991). *Pediatric drugs and nursing implications.* Norwalk, CT: Appleton & Lange.

TABLE D-4 Common Pediatric Immunizations—Continued

Immunization Type	Side Effects	Contraindications	Nursing Considerations
Hepatitis B Vaccine (HB)			
Route: Intramuscular *Dosage:* Engerix B: 0.5 mL Recombivax: 0.25 mL (If mother is HBsAg+, give infant 0.5 mL) *Age(s) Given:* 2 weeks; 1 month after first dose; 6 months after first dose (three doses total) *or* 1 to 2, 4, and 6 to 18 months (three doses total). *Storage:* Store in body of refrigerator at 2 to 8° C (35 to 46° F).	*Common:* Pain or redness at injection site; headache; photophobia; altered liver enzymes *Serious:* Anaphylaxis	Prior anaphylaxis, liver abnormalities	Prior to immunization, check on status of mother's hepatitis B test and presence of other liver disease. *Note:* If mother is HBsAg+, vaccine must be given to infant within 12 hours of birth. Shake vaccine before withdrawing. Solution will appear cloudy.
Haemophilus Influenza Type B (Hib)			
Route: Intramuscular *Dosage:* 0.5 mL *Age(s) Given:* 2, 4, 6, 12 to 15 months (four doses for HbOC* and PRP-T*) *or* 2, 4, 12 to 15 months (three doses for PRP-OMP*) *Storage:* Store in body of refrigerator at 2 to 8° C (35 to 46° F).	*Common:* Pain, redness, or swelling at site *Serious:* Anaphylaxis (extremely rare)	Prior anaphylactic reaction to this vaccine	Prior to immunizations, ask if child is immunosuppressed. Since schedules for products of different companies vary, it is important to read package insert carefully. A new preparation, Tetramune, has become available recently. It combines DTP and Hib.

*Trade name.

TABLE D–5 Reportable Events Following Immunization*

Vaccine/Toxoid	Event	Interval from Vaccination
DTP, polio, DTP/poliovirus combined	A. Anaphylaxis or anaphylactic shock	24 hours
	B. Encephalopathy (or encephalitis)†	7 days
	C. Shock-collapse or hypotonic-hypo-responsive collapse†	7 days
	D. Residual seizure disorder†	See note†
	E. Any acute complication or sequela (including death) of above events	No limit
	F. (See package insert)‡	(See package insert)
Measles, mumps, and rubella; DTaP, Td, tetanus toxoid	A. Anaphylaxis or anaphylactic shock	24 hours
	B. Encephalopathy (or encephalitis)†	15 days for measles, mumps, and rubella vaccines; 7 days for DTaP, Td, and tetanus toxoids
	C. Residual seizure disorder†	See note†
	D. Any acute complication or sequela (including death) of above events	No limit
	E. (See package insert)‡	(See package insert)
Oral poliovirus vaccine	A. Paralytic poliomyelitis	
	In a nonimmunodeficient recipient	30 days
	In an immunodeficient recipient	6 months
	In a vaccine-associated community case	No limit
	B. Any acute complication or sequela (including death) of above events	No limit
	C. (See package insert)‡	(See package insert)
Inactivated poliovirus vaccine	A. Anaphylaxis or anaphylactic shock	24 hours
	B. Any acute complication or sequela (including death) of above event	No limit
	C. (See package insert)‡	(See package insert)

From Centers for Disease Control and Prevention (1990). Vaccine Adverse Event Reporting System—United States: Requirements. *MMWR, 39*:730–732.
*Events listed are required by law to be reported to the U.S. Department of Health and Human Services; however, the Vaccine Adverse Event Reporting System (VAERS) will accept *all* reports of suspected adverse events after the administration of any vaccine. Call 1-800-822-7967.
DTP, diphtheria, tetanus, and pertussis vaccine; *DTaP*, diphtheria, tetanus, and acellular pertussis vaccine; *Td*, diphtheria-tetanus adult.
†Aids to interpretation:
■ Shock-collapse or hypotonic-hyporesponsive collapse may be evidenced by signs or symptoms such as decrease in or loss of muscle tone, paralysis (partial or complete), hemiplegia, hemiparesis, loss of color or change of color to pale white or blue, unresponsiveness to environmental stimuli, depression of or loss of consciousness, prolonged sleeping with difficulty arousing, or cardiovascular or respiratory arrest.
■ Residual seizure disorder may be considered to have occurred if no other seizure or convulsion unaccompanied by fever or accompanied by a fever of <102° F occurred before the first seizure or convulsion after the administration of the vaccine involved, *and*, if in the case of measles-, mumps-, or rubella-containing vaccines, the first seizure or convulsion occurred within 15 days after vaccination *or* in the case of any other vaccine, the first seizure or convulsion occurred within 3 days after vaccination, *and*, if two or more seizures or convulsions unaccompanied by fever or accompanied by a fever of <102° F occurred within 1 year after vaccination.
■ The terms "seizure" and "convulsion" include grand mal, petit mal, absence, myoclonic, tonic-clonic, and focal motor seizures and signs.
■ Encephalopathy means any substantial acquired abnormality of, injury to, or impairment of brain function. Among the frequent manifestations of encephalopathy are focal and diffuse neurologic signs, increased intracranial pressure, or changes lasting ≥ 6 hours in level of consciousness, with or without convulsions. The neurologic signs and symptoms of encephalopathy may be temporary with complete recovery, or they may result in various degrees of permanent impairment. Signs and symptoms such as high-pitched and unusual screaming, persistent unconsolable crying, and bulging fontanel are compatible with an encephalopathy, but in and of themselves are not conclusive evidence of encephalopathy. Encephalopathy usually can be documented by slow wave activity on an electroencephalogram.
‡Refer to the *contraindication* section of the manufacturer's package insert for each vaccine.

ing their decision. If there is an outbreak of a disease, the nonimmunized child must be kept out of school. Local, city, or state courts decide how to settle any conflicts.

The nurse needs to give written materials about immunization to the parents. When teaching parents about immunizations, the nurse must explain the risks and benefits of immunization, risks of disease, and common side effects and treatments. The nurse should record the child's history carefully, specifying any previous reactions to immunizations, allergies, and immune diseases.

Antibiotics

Before the introduction of antibiotics, children were often unable to fight infection and died as the result of overwhelming sepsis. Antibiotics have been responsible for decreases in morbidity and mortality from infections among children. However, strains of bacteria and viruses that are resistant to antibiotics have developed. Children with chronic illnesses such as cystic fibrosis, sickle cell disease, and acquired immunodeficiency syndrome (AIDS) are particularly susceptible to infections by drug-resistant pathogens.

Infection Control

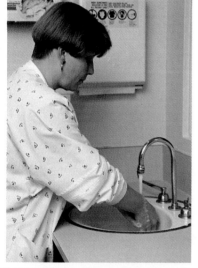

FIGURE D–4 Thorough handwashing by the nurse is an important measure for infection control.

Children are often admitted to the hospital for treatment of severe infections. Each year, countless numbers of **nosocomial** (hospital-acquired) **infections** occur.

The fecal-oral and respiratory routes are the most common sources of preventable infections in children. The most important link in infection control is good handwashing by health care professionals. Handwashing should be done before providing care to another child and after all diaper changes (Fig. D–4).

Isolation

Consult the infection control manual in your hospital when caring for a child in isolation, and bring any questions and concerns to your hospital's infection control nurse. (See the Atlas of Pediatric Procedures for more detailed information.)

Universal Precautions

Universal precautions are essential to decrease the transmission of diseases by blood and body fluids. Refer to the Atlas of Pediatric Procedures for more detailed information.

Nursing Management

Nursing care of children with infectious diseases focuses on preventing spread of infection, treating infection, administering antibiotics, and educating parents. Antibiotics should be given on schedule. Blood tests are used to monitor antibiotic levels and to ensure appropriate results from the antibiotic.

Involve the parents by allowing them to assist with their child's care. Correct any misconceptions they may have about the occurrence or cause of the infectious disease in their child. The parents may feel that they have exposed their child to certain germs or bacteria.

Infectious and Communicable Diseases in Children

The epidemiology, clinical manifestations, treatment, prevention, and nursing care of selected infectious and communicable diseases of childhood are described in Table D–6.

TABLE D–6 Selected Infectious and Communicable Diseases in Children

Disease	Clinical Manifestations

CHICKENPOX (VARICELLA)*

Causal agent: Varicella-zoster, a member of the herpesvirus group.
Epidemiology: Peak occurrence is in the late fall, winter, and spring. Maternal antibodies disappear 2 to 3 months after birth.
Transmission: Direct contact or airborne spread of secretions.
Incubation period: 14 to 21 days.
Period of communicability: As long as 5 days before the onset of the rash to a maximum of 6 days after the appearance of the first group of vesicles. This period may be prolonged after passive immunization or in immunodeficient children.

The onset of symptoms is acute. Mild fever, malaise, and irritability occur. The rash begins as a macule on an erythematous base and progresses to a papule and then to a clear, fluid-filled vesicle. Lesions are often described as a "teardrop on a rose petal." Lesions of all stages may be present at any one time. Crusts may remain for 1 to 3 weeks.
Complications: Complications are rare but can include infected lesions, encephalitis, varicella pneumonia, thrombocytopenia, arthritis, meningitis, and Reye syndrome. This disease may cause very significant illness or death to immunocompromised children.

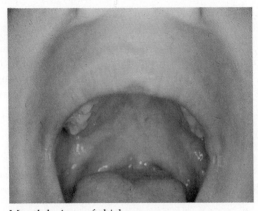

Mouth lesions of chickenpox.
Courtesy of Centers for Disease Control and Prevention, Atlanta, GA.

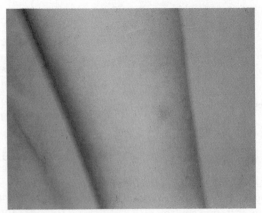

Skin lesions of chickenpox.
Courtesy of Centers for Disease Control and Prevention, Atlanta, GA.

COXSACKIEVIRUS

Causal agent: Coxsackieviruses cause a wide group of acute diseases that range from minor and self-limiting to potentially fatal.
Epidemiology: Occurs worldwide, most commonly in the summer and early fall. Sporadic outbreaks are seen, especially among children in out-of-home settings. Illnesses include the common cold; pharyngitis; pneumonia; hand, foot, and mouth disease; and herpangina. Immunity probably occurs after clinical or subclinical infection, but the duration of the immunity is unknown.
Transmission: Fecal-oral route and possibly respiratory route.
Incubation period: 3 to 6 days.
Period of communicability: During the acute illness and for several weeks after symptoms appear, as the virus is shed in the stool.

Each of the coxsackieviruses is responsible for a different set of manifestations. Herpangina is an acute, self-limiting viral disease characterized by the sudden onset of fever, sore throat, and small, discrete, grayish papulovesicular pharyngeal lesions that gradually increase in size. In hand, foot, and mouth disease the lesions are more diffuse and may occur on the buccal surfaces of the cheeks, gums, and sides of the tongue. Papulovesicular lesions occur on the hands and feet and last for 7 to 10 days. Children may be irritable and have fever, anorexia, dysphagia, and a sore throat.

NOTE: An asterisk (*) after the disease name indicates that a vaccine or antitoxin is available for use in high-risk or as-needed situations. A dagger (†) indicates that the disease currently has a safe and effective vaccine.

Treatment

There is no cure for chickenpox. Medical management is supportive.

Prognosis: Most children recover fully. Giving the antiviral agent acyclovir to healthy children results in less severe illness. However, the cost of acyclovir has made this treatment controversial.[3] Children who are immunocompromised must be treated aggressively.

Prevention: Isolation of children during the contagious stage is the only control method available. A varicella vaccine has been approved and may be available soon.[4]

■ NURSING ALERT

Chickenpox can be fatal in immunocompromised children. For example, children who are undergoing chemotherapy, steroid treatment, or transplant therapy should be carefully monitored after exposure to the disease. Varicella-zoster immune globulin is usually administered as soon as possible after exposure. A chickenpox vaccine is available for prophylactic use in immunocompromised children.

There is no specific treatment.

Prognosis: Recovery is generally good with supportive care.

Prevention: Avoid contact with infected persons early in the disease.

Nursing Management

Maintain strict isolation of hospitalized children while they are contagious (usually a period before the lesions appear until all lesions are dry). Hospitalization is generally reserved for children with complications or other illnesses. Varicella history, especially recent exposure in susceptible children, should be obtained for all children entering the hospital. Children who have been exposed to varicella and require admission should be placed in isolation as a means of protecting immunocompromised patients. Nurses caring for the child should have a varicella titre done to be certain of their immune status if they have not had a documented case of chickenpox.

Most children are treated at home. While contagious, they should be isolated from all susceptible individuals, especially medically fragile or immunocompromised children or women early in pregnancy. The school or child care facility should be notified of the child's illness.

Give nonaspirin antipyretics to control fever.

Give oral antihistamines for relief of discomfort from itching. Oatmeal and Aveeno baths are soothing. Caladryl lotion applied in moderation to lesions may also provide relief.

Observe the child closely for drowsiness and dehydration.

Keep the child's fingernails short and clean. Young children may need to wear soft cotton mittens to prevent infection when itching cannot be controlled. Observe the skin closely for evidence of secondary infection.

Change bed linens frequently. Linen should be washed in mild soap and rinsed well.

Watch for symptoms of complications. Disorientation and restlessness may indicate viral encephalitis.

Reassure the child that the lesions are temporary and will go away. Children, especially of school age, may fear disfigurement.

Isolate the child while contagious.

Use enteric precautions if the child is hospitalized.

Apply topical lotions and give systemic medications as ordered to lessen the pain and relieve any irritation.

Offer cool drinks and soft, nonacidic foods. Swallowing may be painful.

Observe for dehydration.

Provide reassurance and support to parents.

Continued.

Disease	Clinical Manifestations

DIPHTHERIA†

Causal agent: *Corynebacterium diphtheriae,* a bacterium.

Epidemiology: Occurs mostly during colder months in temperate zones in unimmunized children under 15 years of age and among adults with lapsing immunity.[5] In tropical areas, cases of cutaneous and wound diphtheria occur sporadically. Maternal immunity lasts as long as 6 months after birth.

Transmission: By contact with an infectious patient or carrier or, less commonly, indirectly by contact with contaminated articles. Unpasteurized milk has also served as a vehicle.

Incubation period: 2 to 5 days, sometimes longer.

Period of communicability: Varies but is usually 2 to 4 weeks.

Symptoms can be mild or severe. Low-grade fever, anorexia, malaise, rhinorrhea, cough, and pharyngitis may be present. In more severe cases the membranes of the tonsils, pharynx, and larynx are affected. The characteristic membranous lesion is a thick, bluish white to grayish black patch that covers the tonsils. It can spread to cover the soft and hard palates and the posterior portion of the pharynx. Attempts to remove the membrane result in bleeding.

Complications: Myocarditis and neuritis have been recorded.

ERYTHEMA INFECTIOSUM (FIFTH DISEASE)

Causal agent: Human parvovirus B19.

Epidemiology: Occurs worldwide, most often in winter and spring. The disease also occurs in epidemics, with peak activity every 6 years. The incidence is highest in children between the ages of 5 and 14 years.

Transmission: Respiratory secretions and blood.

Incubation period: Usually 7 days (range: 7 to 18 days).

Period of communicability: Unknown; believed to be highest before the onset of the disease.

The first sign of illness is the red rash, which appears in three stages. It begins on the cheeks as an erythematous, maculopapular rash that coalesces, giving the "slapped face" appearance. The rash is accompanied by circumoral pallor. In 2 to 4 days the second stage develops. A lacelike, symmetric, erythematous, maculopapular rash appears on the trunk and limbs and spreads from proximal to distal surfaces of the body. During the third stage, which lasts 1 to 3 weeks, the rash fades but can reappear if the skin is irritated or exposed to cold or heat. The rash may be mildly pruritic.

Complications: Children with diseases such as hemolytic anemia may have hematologic complications.

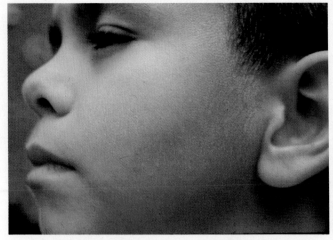 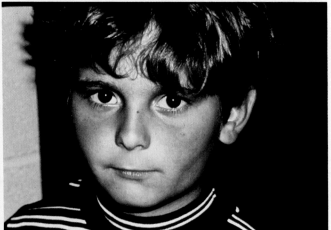

Characteristic facial rash of erythema infectiosum (Fifth disease).
Courtesy of Centers for Disease Control and Prevention, Atlanta, GA.

Administration of antitoxin and antibiotics within 3 days of the onset of symptoms. When diphtheria is strongly suspected, antibiotic therapy (penicillin or erythromycin) should be initiated without waiting for laboratory results.

Prognosis: With treatment, prognosis is good. If untreated, diphtheria can cause death from airway obstruction.

Prevention: Diphtheria is a vaccine-preventable disease. The immunization series is initiated at 2 months of age and is usually given in combination with tetanus and pertussis. Diphtheria-tetanus (Td) is administered to children over the age of 7.

Maintain strict isolation.

Monitor closely for signs of increasing respiratory distress.

Have emergency airway equipment readily available.

Administer antibiotics. Give no medications containing caffeine or other stimulants.

Use oral suction gently as necessary.

Allow children to use mouthwash if desired. Gargling is not permitted because it can irritate the back of the throat.

Encourage liquids as tolerated. Intravenous fluids may be necessary.

Provide emotional support to the family.

There is no specific treatment, and recovery is spontaneous.

Children are rarely hospitalized unless they have preexisting diseases.

Antipyretics (acetaminophen) may be given to control fever.

Use soothing oatmeal-based commercial bath products (Aveeno) if the rash is pruritic. Antipruritics may also help to relieve itching.

Encourage rest and offer frequent fluids.

Keep children out of direct sunlight if possible. Provide protective, light, loose clothing if exposure to sunlight cannot be avoided.

Provide quiet diversionary activity.

Explain to parents the three stages of rash development.

Continued.

TABLE D-6 Selected Infectious and Communicable Diseases in Children—Continued

Disease	Clinical Manifestations

HAEMOPHILUS INFLUENZAE TYPE B (H-INFLUENZAE TYPE B; H-FLU TYPE B)†

Causal agent: Coccobacilli *H. influenzae* bacteria, which has several serotypes and can be encapsulated or nonencapsulated.

Epidemiology: Occurs most often in the spring and summer. Most commonly affected are infants and young children who are black, Native American, Eskimo, or members of group settings such as day care centers. Low-birth-weight children and children with chronic illnesses also have increased susceptibility. The epidemiology is currently being altered with the introduction of the Hib vaccine.

Transmission: Direct person-to-person contact or droplet inhalation. The organism is frequently asymptomatically colonized in the respiratory tract.

Incubation period: Unknown.

Period of communicability: 3 days from onset of symptoms.

H. influenzae type B can cause several severe illnesses, including meningitis, epiglottitis, pneumonia, septic arthritis, and cellulitis. It is also a cause of sepsis in infants. Other illnesses include sinusitis, otitis media, bronchitis, and pericarditis. Each disease has very specific clinical manifestations.

Complications: Illness caused by *H. influenzae* type B responds to antibiotic therapy. Left untreated, severe sequelae and death, especially in young infants, can occur.

HEPATITIS B†

Causal agent: Hepatitis B virus (HBV), a member of the family Hepadnaviridae.

Epidemiology: Occurs worldwide. In the United States, hepatitis B is seen in greater frequency among certain high-risk groups and among immigrants from areas of high incidence. High-risk groups include intravenous drug users; homosexual men; women with multiple sexual partners; medical and dental personnel; household contacts of HBV carriers; patients who are receiving hemodialysis or have received multiple blood transfusions, especially before blood product screening began; inmates in correctional facilities; and children in long-term care facilities.[6]

Transmission: Primarily by body fluids, particularly blood, semen, saliva, and vaginal secretions. Exposure to blood or blood products and use of unsterilized needles. Sexual transmission is one of the most common methods of transmission.[7] Perinatal transmission is a significant source of infection in the newborn.

Incubation period: 45 to 160 days (average: 60 to 90 days).

Period of communicability: During incubation period and throughout clinical course of disease.

Onset is insidious, with malaise and weakness. Muscle aches, anorexia, nausea, vomiting, and vague abdominal discomfort may occur.

Complications: Because diagnosis can be made only by serologic testing, hepatitis B may go undiagnosed and lead to chronic active hepatitis, which can severely affect the liver and eventually cause liver failure.

■ **CLINICAL TIP**

Hepatitis B can be transferred from mother to infant, and infection in the newborn often results in a chronic carrier state. An infant born to an infected mother should be immunized within 12 hours of birth with both hepatitis B immune globulin and hepatitis B vaccine.

Treatment consists of antibiotic therapy.

Prognosis: With rapid diagnosis and treatment, the outlook for recovery is good but highly dependent on the disease the organism has caused. When treatment has been delayed, the prognosis for full recovery becomes much more guarded.

Prevention: Immunization is now available for *H. influenzae* type B as part of the recommended childhood immunization series beginning at 2 months of age. Although the vaccine has been available for only a few years, there have already been dramatic declines in illness caused by this organism.

The child is put in respiratory isolation until 24 hours after the initiation of antibiotics.

Antibiotic therapy is administered intravenously for severe infections. Infections such as otitis media can be managed at home with oral antibiotics.

Children under the age of 4 years who have not been immunized are at increased risk for developing disease from *H. influenzae*. Specific prophylactic measures for susceptible children may be ordered by the physician.

Administer antipyretics to help the child feel more comfortable.

Closely monitor IV sites for patency and infiltration.

Perform nursing care measures specific to the illness.

There is no cure for hepatitis B. Treatment is supportive.

Prognosis: Children may become lifelong carriers even if they have shown no signs of the illness.

Prevention: Hepatitis B is a vaccine-preventable disease. The hepatitis B vaccine is now recommended for all children. All health care workers should be immunized. Blood supplies in the United States are now screened for HBV.

Children with acute hepatitis B are usually not hospitalized.

If the child is hospitalized, maintain strict isolation.

Use universal precautions when obtaining specimens and performing care.

Encourage the child to rest.

Observe sclera for change from white to yellow.

Observe closely for prolonged or unusual bleeding. Watch for bruising.

Provide high-calorie liquids and encourage small, frequent feedings.

Provide diversionary activity.

Educate parents about transmission.

(Refer to Chapter 15 for further discussion of acute hepatitis.)

Continued.

Disease	Clinical Manifestations

LYME DISEASE

Causal agent: *Borrelia burgdorferi,* a spirochete, which is transmitted by ixodid ticks.

Epidemiology: Distribution in the United States correlates highly with the distribution of the various tick carriers (vectors). Animals such as dogs and cats can also have the disease. Lyme disease occurs year round, with the highest risk of infection in summer. Infection does not induce immunity.

Transmission: Tick bite. The tick transmits the infected spirochete when it draws blood. The tick must feed for 36 hours to transmit the disease.

Incubation period: 3 to 32 days after an infected tick bite.

The most typical early symptom is a slowly expanding red rash, called erythema migrans, at the site of the bite. The rash starts as a flat or raised red area and may progress to partial clearing, develop blisters or scabs in the center, or have a bluish discoloration. Early symptoms include malaise, fatigue, headache, stiff neck, mild fever, and muscle and joint aches. The most common late symptom of untreated disease is pain and swelling of the joints, most commonly the knee (Lyme arthritis). Neurologic and cardiac abnormalities may occur in 3 to 4 weeks. These may become chronic.

Complications: Left untreated, Lyme disease can cause significant neurologic deficits, including arm and leg weakness, numbness, tingling, arthritis, and sometimes depression.

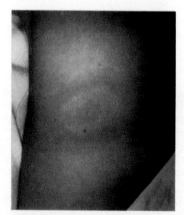 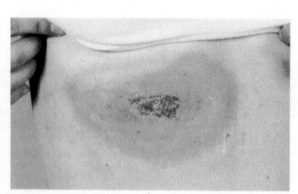

The appearance of the erythema migrans rash may vary in early Lyme disease.
From Pfizer Central Research. (1989). *Lyme disease.* Groton, CT: Author.

MONONUCLEOSIS

Causal agent: Epstein-Barr virus (EBV), a member of the herpesvirus group.

Epidemiology: Occurs worldwide. In developing countries the disease occurs in young children and may be asymptomatic or mild. In developed countries the disease is more common in older children and adolescents.

Transmission: Direct contact with infected oropharyngeal secretions (saliva, kissing). EBV can also be transmitted by blood transfusion.

Incubation period: 30 to 50 days.

Period of communicability: Virus is shed for up to 18 months after the clinical course of the disease.

In very young children mononucleosis may be asymptomatic. In older children the disease is characterized by malaise, fatigue, and fever, followed by lymphadenopathy and sore throat. Splenomegaly may occur. Pain from swelling of the tonsils and lymph nodes may be significant.

Complications: Rare side effects include central nervous system symptoms such as encephalitis, aseptic meningitis, Guillain-Barré syndrome, splenic rupture, and hematologic complications. In immunodeficient children, fatal infections or lymphomas can occur.

Treatment

Antibiotics are the treatment of choice. Penicillin or erythromycin is most often used in children 8 years of age or younger. Doxycycline or tetracycline is given to children over the age of 8 years. Intravenous antibiotics are often required in the later stages of the disease.

Prognosis: Lyme disease does not cause acute, life-threatening illness, but it may result in significant morbidity, especially when chronic.

Prevention: Avoid areas that are heavily tick infested, and wear protective clothing. Check for ticks (especially hidden in hair) after every outing. Remove ticks as soon as possible. If symptoms develop, seek medical attention promptly for a child who has been bitten.

Nursing Management

Children with early disease are usually treated at home. Children with progressive symptoms may be hospitalized.

Administer antibiotics. Nonaspirin analgesics and antipyretics may provide relief of mild fevers, headaches, and muscle and joint aches.

Allow children to rest. Children with Lyme disease may tire easily. Vigorous activities may be difficult.

Educate parents and children about the disease.

Provide emotional support.

▮ TICK REMOVAL

To remove a tick, first smother it with petroleum jelly or a few drops of rubbing alcohol to make it withdraw, then, using tweezers, gently pull the tick away from the skin.

There is no specific treatment. Corticosteroids may be used to control tonsillar swelling and pain.[8]

Give antipyretics and analgesics for fever and sore throat.

Offer soft foods and encourage fluids.

Maintain bed rest.

Give adolescents a sense of responsibility by involving them in decisions about care whenever possible. Be sure to include parents and adolescent in discussions.

Adolescents may be worried about keeping up with schoolwork if they are absent from school for a prolonged period. Help to arrange hospital or home teaching.

Continued.

Disease	Clinical Manifestations

MUMPS (PAROTITIS)†

Causal agent: Myxovirus group.

Epidemiology: Occurs worldwide in unvaccinated children, most often in winter and spring. Infection and vaccination induce lifelong immunity. Maternal immunity begins to disappear in infants at the age of 12 to 15 months. Vaccine failure and lack of immunization have been implicated in cases occurring in vaccinated populations.[9]

Transmission: Saliva droplets and direct contact.

Incubation period: 2 to 3 weeks.

Period of communicability: 7 days before parotid swelling until 2 to 3 days after swelling subsides.

Malaise; low-grade fever; and earache, especially with chewing; followed by bilateral or unilateral parotid gland swelling. Swelling peaks around the third day. Meningeal signs (stiff neck, headache, photophobia) occur in about 15% of patients.

Complications: Orchitis (most often unilateral) may occur in postpubertal males; sterility is relatively rare.[10] Oophoritis, pancreatitis, aseptic meningoencephalitis, and unilateral permanent deafness are sometimes seen.

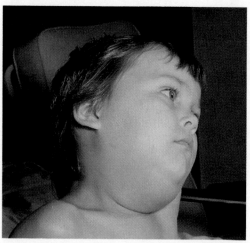 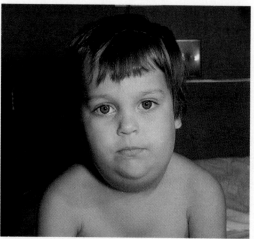

This child has mumps with diffuse lymphedema of the neck. **A,** Side view. **B,** Front view.
Courtesy of Centers for Disease Control and Prevention, Atlanta, GA.

PERTUSSIS (WHOOPING COUGH)†

Causal agent: *Bordetella pertussis.*

Epidemiology: Occurs worldwide. Predominantly a childhood disease, pertussis also occurs in health care workers or adults who may have weakened or incomplete immunity. Adults may become only mildly ill but can spread the disease to unimmunized children.

Transmission: Respiratory droplets and direct contact with discharge from the respiratory membranes.

Incubation period: 7 to 21 days (commonly 7 to 10 days).

Period of communicability: Begins approximately 1 week after exposure. Pertussis is communicable for 5 to 7 days after the initiation of antibiotic therapy. The disease is most contagious before the paroxysmal cough stage.

The onset is insidious. The disease begins with a runny nose, followed by an irregular, nonproductive cough. The cough becomes more severe at night and changes into spasms of paroxysmal coughing followed by inspiration, stridor, or "whooping." (Young infants do not manifest the "whooping.") May be accompanied by flushing, cyanosis, and vomiting. Coughing may last 1 to 4 weeks or more.

Complications: Pneumonia, atelectasis, otitis media, and seizures.

Treatment	Nursing Management

There is no specific treatment. Therapy is supportive.

Prognosis: Mumps is usually self-limiting.

Prevention: Mumps is a vaccine-preventable disease. The vaccine is usually administered in combination with the measles and rubella vaccines (MMR) at 15 months of age and again at either 4 to 6 years or before grade 6.

Children are generally uncomfortable but are rarely very ill. They seldom require hospitalization.

Maintain strict respiratory isolation of hospitalized children while contagious. If children are treated at home, attendance at day care or school exposure to immunocompromised individuals or participation in activities where susceptible persons might be present should not be allowed.

Give nonaspirin analgesics and antipyretics to control fever and pain. Give steroids if ordered.

Encourage fluid intake. Swallowing and chewing may be painful. Offer soft and blended foods. Acidic foods and beverages should be avoided.

Talking may be painful. Provide a bell or other attention-getting device.

Apply warm or cool compresses, whichever is preferred, to the parotid area.

Be alert for signs of complications. Headache, stiff neck, vomiting, or photophobia may indicate meningeal irritation.

Provide scrotal supports if testicular swelling occurs.

Reassure children who may be upset about the facial swelling that it will go away.

Encourage diversional activities.

Treatment consists of antibiotics, corticosteroids, if ordered, and supportive care.

Prognosis: The disease is most severe in infants under 1 year of age, and most deaths occur in this age group.

Prevention: Pertussis is a vaccine-preventable disease. Active immunization should be given in early infancy. Health care professionals who are in close contact with infected children before diagnosis may need antibiotics to prevent transmission.

Maintain strict respiratory isolation until 5 to 7 days after the initiation of antibiotics. Most hospitalized cases occur in children under the age of 5 years.

Closely monitor respiration and oxygen saturation. The smaller the child, the greater the risk for respiratory distress and apnea. Remain with the child during coughing spells, when apneic episodes are most likely. Have emergency equipment readily available.

Provide humidification. Gentle suctioning may be necessary.

Give antipyretics as needed for fever.

Encourage frequent rest periods.

Allow the child to eat desired foods.

Encourage the child to take fluids.

Provide emotional support to parents.

Continued.

TABLE D–6 Selected Infectious and Communicable Diseases in Children—Continued

Disease	Clinical Manifestations

POLIOMYELITIS†

Causal agent: There are three serotypes of poliovirus.

Epidemiology: Occurs worldwide. Polio primarily affects children, although some of the cases involve transmission to immunocompromised or non–polio-protected adults caring for infants who have received the live polio virus vaccine. The disease can be mild or severe. Because of the widespread availability of polio vaccine, the disease is no longer a public health concern in the United States and other industrialized countries. The vaccine induces lifelong immunity.

Transmission: Primarily by the fecal-oral route.

Incubation period: Usually 7 to 24 days (range: 3 to 36 days).

Period of communicability: Unknown. Infectious for up to several weeks before symptoms develop. The virus is shed in pharyngeal secretions for a few days and in the stool for several weeks.

Affects the central nervous system. Less severe infections may be limited to fever and stiffness in the neck or back, headache, vomiting, and sore throat. Paralysis results from damage to neurons.

Complications: Motor paralysis.

RABIES (HYDROPHOBIA)*

Causal agent: Rhabdoviridae, two types (urban, in dogs; wild, in wildlife).

Epidemiology: Occurs worldwide. Urban rabies is generally controlled by vaccination of domestic animals susceptible to the infection, especially dogs and cats. Rural rabies can occur in many wild animals, particularly bats, foxes, skunks, and raccoons.

Transmission: Infected saliva from bite of rabid animal. Virus enters the wound and travels along the nerves from point of entry to the central nervous system.

Incubation period: Highly variable (average 6 weeks). This period depends on the amount of virus in the saliva, how close to the brain or major nerves the bite occurred, and how deeply the saliva penetrated the skin.

Children may be free of symptoms during the long incubation period. Initial acute symptoms include headache, fever, loss of appetite, and malaise. Painful contractures in the muscles used in swallowing lead to hydrophobia, a reflex contraction at the sight of liquid. Neurologic symptoms such as hallucinations, disorientation, periods of excitability (mania) and quiet, and seizures later occur. Usually results in death.

■ CLINICAL TIP

Any animal suspected of having rabies should be quarantined, if possible.[11] Rabies is diagnosed on the basis of history and clinical symptoms. The importance of history cannot be underestimated. Diagnosis is usually confirmed by fluorescent antibody staining of the dead animal's brain tissue.

Treatment

There is no specific treatment. No chemotherapeutic agents that directly kill the polio virus are available.

Prognosis: Respiratory complication is life-threatening and involves 5% to 10% of all cases. Respiratory paralysis may lead to death.

Prevention: Poliomyelitis is a vaccine-preventable disease. Children should be immunized with the live oral poliovirus vaccine (OPV) or, if contraindicated, with the inactivated poliovirus vaccine (IPV). OPV is excreted in the stool for about 1 month after administration. Young children should be kept away from immunocompromised, elderly, or unimmunized persons for 7 to 10 days after receiving OPV.

Nursing Management

Maintain strict isolation in hospital.

Observe closely for respiratory paralysis. Have emergency equipment at bedside.

Administer sedatives as ordered to allow for rest.

Encourage fluids.

Position the child to promote body alignment.

Perform range of motion exercises to prevent contractures.

Provide emotional support.

Animal bites should be washed thoroughly with soap and water and irrigated well. Suturing should be avoided if possible. Rabies immune globulin (RIG) or antirabies serum (ARS) should be given to all persons bitten by animals that may be rabid.[8] The vaccine is of no value once rabies symptoms are present.

Prognosis: Without prompt treatment, rabies is fatal.

Prevention: Immunization with RIG or ARS should begin as soon as possible after exposure. Expert advice on the administration of these vaccines can be supplied by state and local health officials. Prevention also includes immunizing all domestic animals against rabies and avoiding contact with wild animals.

Administer RIG and ARS as ordered.

Maintain isolation.

Institute universal precautions. The virus is transmitted primarily in the saliva and cerebrospinal fluid.

Make the child as comfortable as possible.

Keep liquids out of sight of the hydrophobic child.

Use caution in the late stages of the disease when children are usually combative. Various medications, paralyzing agents, and sedatives may be used to provide relief. Coma and death occur after an exhaustive period of excitement and agitation that may last for days.

Provide emotional support to the family.

Continued.

Disease	Clinical Manifestations

ROCKY MOUNTAIN SPOTTED FEVER (TICKBORNE TYPHUS FEVER, SÃO PAULO TYPHUS)

Causal agent: *Rickettsia rickettsii,* a bacterium that is transmitted by infected ticks.

Epidemiology: Rocky Mountain spotted fever (RMSF) occurs in most of the United States, southwestern Canada, and Mexico. In the United States most cases have been reported from the south Atlantic and south central states. Generally occurs between April and September. Most infections occur in children who are less than 15 years of age. Infection induces immunity.

Transmission: Transmitted by bites of ticks, principally dog ticks. There is no evidence of person-to-person transmission.

Incubation period: 3 to 14 days (most commonly 7 days) after bite of an infected tick.

RMSF is a multisystem disease that can be mild, moderate, or severe. Onset may be gradual or rapid. Children may be very ill. Sudden onset is characterized by a moderate to high fever that ordinarily lasts for 2 to 3 weeks, significant malaise, deep muscle pain, severe headache, chills, and conjunctival injection. The characteristic rash, which usually appears between the third and fifth days, starts on the extremities, including the palms and soles, and moves to the trunk. Initially the rash is maculopapular and blanches with pressure. It later becomes petechial and more defined; it is rarely pruritic.

In severe cases bleeding from disseminated intravascular coagulation (DIC) can be significant. Gastrointestinal symptoms often occur early in the disease.

Complications: Pulmonary complications, especially pneumonitis, are common and can become life threatening. Central nervous system involvement can cause significant encephalitis and overall severe neurologic dysfunction. Cardiac and renal complications can also occur, leading to shock in severe cases.

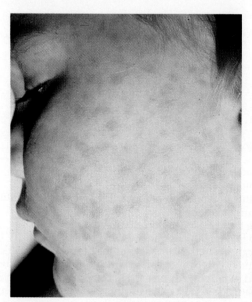

Facial rash of Rocky Mountain spotted fever.

Courtesy of Centers for Disease Control and Prevention, Atlanta, GA.

ROSEOLA (EXANTHEM SUBITUM)

Causal agent: Herpesvirus type 6.

Epidemiology: Occurs worldwide, primarily in children 6 to 24 months of age.

Transmission: Unknown.

Incubation period: Appears to be 5 to 15 days.

Period of communicability: Unknown.

Sudden, high fever for 3 to 5 days, followed by characteristic erythematous, maculopapular rash, which starts on the trunk and spreads to the face, neck, and extremities. The rash can last for 1 to 2 days.

Complications: Children may have febrile seizures.

Treatment	Nursing Management

Treatment consists of antibiotics, such as chloramphenicol, tetracycline, and rifampin.

Prognosis: Without early recognition and treatment, morbidity is significant and mortality ranges from 5% to 7%.[12] If the rash occurs late or not at all, the disease is likely to be more severe.

Prevention: Avoid areas that are heavily tick infested, and wear protective clothing. Check for ticks and if found remove promptly. Seek medical attention promptly for a child who has been bitten and becomes symptomatic.

Children may require prolonged hospitalization, including monitoring in the intensive care unit.

Have hemodynamic monitoring equipment and emergency supplies readily available.

Administer antibiotics as ordered.

Observe for any abnormal bleeding.

Make the child as comfortable as possible. If the child is unconscious, support the extremities and keep the eyes closed and lubricated.

Provide quiet diversional activities.

Provide emotional support, and keep parents informed about their child's condition.

Roseola is self-limiting, and there is no treatment other than supportive care.

Prognosis: Roseola is benign in most cases.

Children are rarely hospitalized.

Give nonaspirin antipyretics to control fever.

Observe closely for any seizure activity, especially during the acute febrile periods.

Encourage fluids.

Reassure parents that the rash will disappear in a few days.

Continued.

Disease	Clinical Manifestations

RUBELLA (GERMAN MEASLES)†

Causal agent: Rubella virus, a member of the family Togaviridae.

Epidemiology: Occurs worldwide and is most prevalent in the winter and spring. Children are susceptible after loss of transplacentally acquired maternal antibodies about 6 to 9 months after birth. Natural infection or vaccination induces lifelong immunity. Congenital rubella syndrome, which has been increasing in frequency, is most likely the result of lack of immunization rather than vaccine failure.[13]

Transmission: Droplet spread, direct contact with infected persons, or contact with freshly soiled articles.

Incubation period: 14 to 21 days (most commonly 16 to 18 days).

Period of communicability: From about 7 days before until about 4 days after the onset of the rash. Infants with congenital rubella may shed the virus for months after birth and should not be exposed to or cared for by persons who are not immune to the disease.

Rubella is generally a mild disease with a characteristic pink, nonconfluent, maculopapular rash. The rash appears on the face and progresses to the neck, trunk, and legs. Symptoms include low-grade fever, headache, malaise, coryza, sore throat, and anorexia. Generalized lymphadenopathy involving the postauricular, suboccipital, and posterior cervical areas is common.

■ NURSING ALERT

Congenital rubella syndrome occurs in at least 25% of infants born to women who acquired rubella during the first trimester of pregnancy. Infants can be born with cardiac defects, ophthalmologic disturbances (blindness, cataracts), mental and physical retardation, deafness, and neurologic complications.

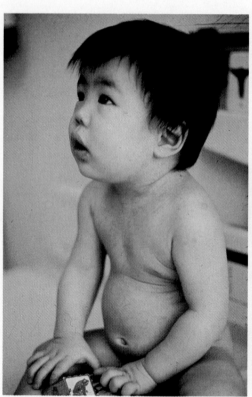
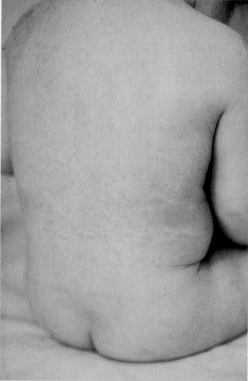

A   B

Eleven-month-old child with rubella. **A,** Front view. Nondescript macular rash. **B,** Posterior view. Discrete maculopapular erythematous rash.
Courtesy of Centers for Disease Control and Prevention, Atlanta, GA.

Treatment

Treatment is supportive. Rubella is generally self-limiting in children.

Prognosis: Disease is usually mild and benign. Major risk is for the fetus if the mother is infected. Abortion, stillbirth, or death under 6 months are common (10% die after birth). Many other anomalies may be present, such as cardiac, ear, and eye deficits.

Prevention: Rubella is a vaccine-preventable disease. It is important that females of childbearing age be immunized because of the severe complications rubella poses to the fetus during the first trimester. All health care workers should have documented immunity.[14,15]

Nursing Management

Children are usually treated at home and rarely require hospitalization. They should not attend school or day care while contagious, and they should be isolated from pregnant women. School and child care facilities should be notified of the child's illness.

Maintain respiratory and enteric isolation of contagious children.

Give nonaspirin analgesics and antipyretics for any pain and fever.

Allow children to choose what they would like to eat and drink. Encourage fluids.

Provide quiet activities.

Continued.

Disease	Clinical Manifestations

RUBEOLA (MEASLES)†

Causal agent: Measles virus, a member of the paramyxovirus group.

Epidemiology: Occurrence peaks in the late winter and early spring. In developed countries measles occurs mostly in outbreaks among adolescents, which are largely the result of lack of immunization or possibly declining immunity. Maternal immunity is active in the infant until the age of approximately 12 to 15 months. Vaccination induces life-long immunity. In developing countries measles remains largely an endemic problem and is a significant cause of infant and childhood morbidity and mortality.

Transmission: Airborne; respiratory droplets and contact with infected persons.

Incubation period: Approximately 8 to 12 days.

Period of communicability: Begins during the prodromal phase and ends about 2 to 4 days after the rash appears.

Children are quite ill in the prodromal phase, with symptoms including high fever, conjunctivitis, coryza, and cough. Small, irregular, bluish white spots on a red background, called Koplik spots, appear on the buccal mucosa about 2 days before and after the onset of the rash. The characteristic red, blotchy, maculopapular rash usually appears approximately 14 days after infection and 2 to 4 days after onset of prodromal phase. The rash begins on the face and spreads to the trunk and extremities. Symptoms gradually subside in 4 to 7 days. Other symptoms include anorexia, malaise, fatigue, and generalized lymphadenopathy.

Complications: Diarrhea, otitis media, bronchopneumonia, bronchiolitis, laryngotracheitis, and encephalitis. Complications and sequelae occur most often in children who are malnourished, medically fragile, and immunosuppressed. The younger the child, the greater the risk for complications.

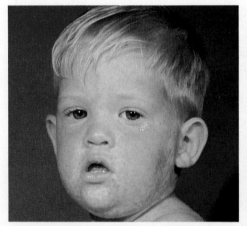
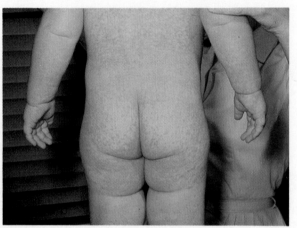

A

B

Rubeola (measles), third day of rash. **A,** Facial rash. **B,** Posterior view.
Courtesy of Centers for Disease Control and Prevention, Atlanta, GA.

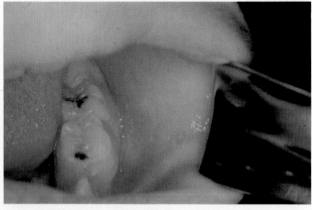

Koplik spots on oral mucosa, fifth day of rash.
Courtesy of Centers for Disease Control and Prevention, Atlanta, GA.

Treatment

There is no cure for measles. Treatment is supportive.

Prognosis: Recovery is generally good with supportive care.

Prevention: Measles is a vaccine-preventable disease. The measles vaccine is available alone (M), in combination with the rubella vaccine (MR), or in combination with the rubella and mumps vaccines (MMR). Immune globulin, administered up to 6 days after exposure, may be helpful in preventing the disease in susceptible persons (immunocompromised children, infants less than 1 year of age, pregnant women).

All health care workers should have documented immunity.[14,15]

Nursing Management

If the child is hospitalized, maintain strict respiratory isolation during the contagious period.

Use a cool-mist vaporizer to help clear respiratory passages.

Suction nose and oral cavity very gently as necessary.

Give antipyretics for fever and antipruritics for itching.

Assess lungs carefully, especially in young children, in whom pneumonias are a common complication. Antitussives may be ordered to control coughing.

If the child has conjunctivitis, remove crusting around eyes with tepid water.

Keep lights dim, and cover windows if necessary.

Elevate the head of the bed. Keep the room cool with good air circulation. Provide light, nonirritating blankets.

Keep skin clean and dry. No soaps should be used.

Offer cool liquids frequently in small amounts. Blended, pureed, and mashed foods are most easily tolerated.

Maintain bed rest. Visitors should be immune to measles.

Provide diversions such as music, stories, and favorite toys.

Continued.

Disease	Clinical Manifestations

SCARLET FEVER

Causal agent: Group A beta-hemolytic streptococci.

Epidemiology: The incidence of scarlet fever has decreased in recent years, and the disease is now less severe. It occurs primarily in children between the ages of 2 and 8 years.[8]

Transmission: Airborne respiratory droplets.

Incubation period: Usually 2 to 4 days (range: 1 to 7 days).

Period of communicability: Not communicable.

Onset is abrupt, with a sore throat, malaise, high fever, chills, and anorexia. The characteristic erythematous rash appears on the neck 12 to 48 hours after onset of symptoms and spreads to the trunk and extremities. It is more intense in skin folds. In 3 to 4 days the rash begins to fade and the tips of the toes and fingers begin to peel. A beefy red pharynx with exudate (strep throat), tender cervical nodes, and a strawberry tongue are also characteristic of scarlet fever.

Complications: If scarlet fever is untreated, acute rheumatic fever and glomerulonephritis can occur.

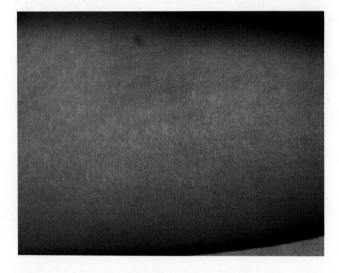

Skin rash of scarlet fever.
Courtesy of Centers for Disease Control and Prevention, Atlanta, GA.

TETANUS

Causal agent: *Clostridium tetani* or tetanus bacillus.

Epidemiology: The bacillus is common and exists as a spore in soil, dust, and animal excretions.

Transmission: The organism is transmitted to humans through wounds in the skin from contact with contaminated soil or implements. Newborns can acquire tetanus via the umbilical cord if they are born in an unclean area or if a contaminated implement is used to cut the cord.

Incubation period: 3 days to 3 weeks (average 8 days).

Period of communicability: Not communicable to other individuals except through skin wounds.

Stiffness of the neck and jaw, facial spasm; eventual rigidity of abdomen and trunk; difficulty breathing.

Complications: Laryngospasm, death.

Treatment	Nursing Management

Prompt antibiotic treatment is effective. Penicillin is the drug of choice. Erythromycin is used if the child is allergic to penicillin.

Prognosis: Recovery is usually good with antibiotic therapy.

Prevention: None.

Children are usually not hospitalized.

If the child is hospitalized:

Monitor vital signs, especially temperature.

Encourage fluids.

Provide cool, clear liquids. Swallowing may be difficult. Avoid acidic beverages.

Administer antibiotics as ordered.

Give antipyretics to control fever.

Make sure the child has a bell or attention-getting device to signal for assistance. Loud talking may be difficult.

Explain to parents the importance of the child's taking antibiotics for the full number of days prescribed.

Tetanus immune globulin is given. Intensive care is provided with cardiorespiratory monitoring, IV penicillin G, and supportive care.

Prognosis: 30% mortality; much higher in newborns.

Prevention: Tetanus immunizations are routinely given. They must be updated every 10 years, or, if a potentially contaminated wound occurs, in 5 years.

Prevent disease by checking immunization records and administering immunizations as necessary.

Give immune globulin and penicillin for treatment.

Monitor the child's condition.

Offer skin and respiratory care.

Provide feedings via total parenteral nutrition or feeding tube.

Prepare family for possible poor prognosis.

Continued.

Disease	Clinical Manifestations

TUBERCULOSIS

See Chapter 10.

TYPHOID FEVER†

Causal agent: *Salmonella typhi,* a Gram-negative bacterium.

Epidemiology: Occurs worldwide but is very rare in developed countries. Between 1% and 4% of patients who recover from typhoid fever become carriers. In underdeveloped countries the disease is a significant source of morbidity and mortality, especially in school-age children. Clinical illness confers immunity.

Transmission: Fecal-oral route; ingestion of food and water contaminated with human waste. Transmission to the neonate from either the mother or medical personnel can occur at delivery.

Incubation period: 1 to 3 weeks.

Period of communicability: Variable. Typhoid fever is communicable as long as bacteria are excreted, usually from the first week until disease recovery.

Initial symptoms are malaise, fever, anorexia, and abdominal pain. Constipation occurs more frequently than diarrhea. Older children may complain of muscle aches and headaches. Generalized lymphadenopathy, spleen and liver enlargement, bradycardia, conjunctival irritation, and abdominal distention and tenderness may occur. During the second week of the disease, discrete, rose-colored spots (caused by bacterial emboli in the skin capillaries) may appear on the trunk.

Complications: Intestinal perforation and hemorrhage, cholecystitis, and hepatitis are the most common severe complications.

REFERENCES

1 Hinman, A.R. (1988). Control of communicable diseases. In: Wallace, H.M., Ryan, G., & Oglesby, A.C. (Eds.), *Maternal and child health practices* (3rd ed.). Oakland, CA: Third Party Publishing.

2 Torrigiani, G. (1993). Communicable diseases: A major burden of morbidity and mortality. *Vaccine, 11*(5), 570–572.

3 Asano, Y., et al. (1993). Postexposure prophylaxis of varicella in family contact by oral acyclovir. *Pediatrics, 92*(2), 219–222.

4 Gershon, A.A. (1993). What's new in chickenpox (varicella-zoster) infection. *Western Journal of Medicine, 158*(2), 180.

5 Karzon, T.D., & Edwards, K.M. (1988). Diphtheria outbreaks in immunized populations. *New England Journal of Medicine, 318,* 41–43.

6 Alter, M.J., Hadler, S.C., & Margolis, H.S. (1990). The changing epidemiology of hepatitis B in the United States: Need for alternative vaccination strategies. *Journal of the American Medical Association, 263,* 1218–1222.

7 Alter, M.J., & Margolis, H.S. (1990). The emergence of hepatitis B as a sexually transmitted disease. *Medical Clinics of North America, 74*(6), 1529–1541.

8 Last, J.M., & Wallace, R.B. (Eds.). (1992). *Maxcy-Rosenau-Last public health and preventive medicine* (13th ed.). Norwalk, CT: Appleton & Lange.

9 Hersh, B.S., et al. (1991). Mumps outbreak in a highly vaccinated population. *Journal of Pediatrics, 119*(2), 187–193.

10 Shulman, A., et al. (1992). Mumps orchitis among soldiers: Frequency, effect on sperm quality, and sperm antibodies. *Fertility and Sterility, 57*(6), 1344–1346.

11 Centers for Disease Control and Prevention. (1992). Human rabies, California, 1992. *Morbidity and Mortality Weekly Reports, 41*(26), 461–463.

12 Hathaway, W.E., Hay, W.W., Groothuis, J.R., & Paisley, J.W. (Eds.). (1993). *Current pediatric diagnosis and treatment* (11th ed.). Norwalk, CT: Appleton & Lange.

13 Centers for Disease Control and Prevention. (1991). Increase in rubella and congenital rubella syndrome, United States, 1988–1990. *Morbidity and Mortality Weekly Reports, 40,* 93–95.

14 Atkinson, W.L., Markowitz, L.E., Adams, N.C., & Seastrom, G.R. (1991). Transmission of measles in medical settings, United States, 1985–1989. *American Journal of Medicine, 91*(suppl 3B), 320S–324S.

15 Farizo, K.M., Stehr-Green, P.A., Simpson, D.M., & Markowitz, L.E. (1991). Pediatric emergency room visits: A risk factor for acquiring measles. *Pediatrics, 87,* 74–79.

Antimicrobial drugs of choice are chloramphenicol, trimetho-prim/sulfamethoxazole, cephalosporins, and ampicillin.

Prognosis: With treatment the prognosis is good.

Prevention: Vaccines against typhoid fever are available. Immunization is advised for travelers to areas where typhoid incidence is high.

Maintain strict enteric precautions. Wash hands after contact with excreta from the child. Proper disposal of gloves and gowns is necessary. Separate toilet facilities are necessary.

Monitor vital signs, and examine chest and abdomen frequently. Observe for respiratory problems and intestinal perforation.

Monitor intake and output. Encourage fluids. Administer intravenous fluids as necessary.

Administer antibiotics.

Maintain bed rest. Keep room quiet.

Provide diversionary activities such as board games and videos when the child is feeling better.

Instruct visitors not to use the child's toilet facility.

Provide emotional support to the parents and family.

The school or child care facility should be notified of the child's illness.

SUGGESTED READINGS

Adcoch, L.M. (1992). A new look at measles. *Infectious Disease Clinics of North America, 6*(1), 133–147.

American Academy of Pediatrics (1991). *Report of the Committee on Infectious Diseases* (22nd ed.). Elk Grove Village, IL: Author.

Benenson, A.S. (Ed.). (1990). *Control of communicable diseases in man* (15th ed.). Washington, DC: American Public Health Association.

Feigen, R.D., & Cherry, J.D. (1992). *Textbook of pediatric infectious diseases* (3rd ed.), vols. 1 & 2. Philadelphia: W.B. Saunders.

Gildea, J.H. (1992). When fever becomes an enemy. *Pediatric Nursing, 18*(2), 165–167.

Grimes, D. (1991). *Infectious diseases.* St. Louis: Mosby–Year Book.

Groleau, G. (1992). Rabies. *Emergency Medicine Clinics of North America, 10*(2), 361–368.

Kamper, C. Treatment of Rocky Mountain spotted fever. (1992). *Journal of Pediatric Health Care, 5,* 216–222.

Massachusetts Medical Society. *Morbidity and Mortality Weekly Report* [general source]. Waltham, MA: Author.

Strebel, P.M., et al. (1992). Epidemiology of poliomyelitis in the United States one decade after the last reported case of indigenous wild virus–associated disease. *Clinical Infectious Diseases, 14,* 568–579.

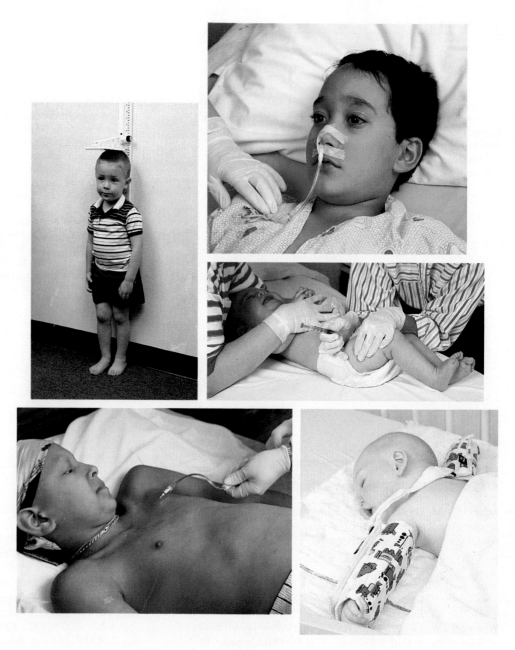

C hildren undergo a number of procedures during diagnostic evaluation and hospitalization. These procedures, although similar to procedures performed on adult patients, may differ in several ways. Nurses must therefore be knowledgeable about variations in preparation, equipment, positioning, and specific steps when performing procedures on children.

Preparation for procedures must take into account a child's developmental stage and cognitive ability (see the discussion in Chapter 4). General guidelines for preparing the child are outlined in the accompanying box. Follow these guidelines before beginning any procedure. After the procedure, provide emotional support and comfort the child.

ATLAS OF PEDIATRIC PROCEDURES

GENERAL GUIDELINES

- Explain the procedure to the child and family.
- Ask if they have any questions about the procedure (refer to Table 4–8).
- If the parent agrees to hold the child, demonstrate exactly what you want done. Make sure that the parent feels comfortable about assisting with the procedure.
- Be familiar with the equipment.
- If the parent will not be present, reassure the child that the parent will return after the procedure has been completed.

Each procedure included here is concisely presented to emphasize essential information. Many procedures begin with brief lists of equipment and preparatory actions. These lists are not meant to be all-inclusive. Rather, they are intended to highlight equipment and information that is most important when performing the procedure on a child.

The procedures themselves are presented in a condensed format unlike the comprehensive approach used to teach basic skills. It is understood that students have already learned the basic steps involved in performing these procedures on an adult patient. *The intent of this presentation is, therefore, to highlight essential steps and pediatric variations with which the nurse should be familiar.* Students should consult their hospital or institution procedure manual or a pediatric procedure manual for more specific information.

Several steps should be taken when performing any procedure. These steps are listed in the accompanying box. Clean (nonsterile) gloves should be worn during any procedure that may involve contact with blood or body fluids. A glove symbol is

Clean   Sterile   One clean, one sterile

used to denote procedures that require the use of clean or sterile gloves.

The procedures that follow are grouped into several categories for ease of reference:

- Informed consent
- Positioning and restraint
- Transport
- Protective precautions
- Physical assessment
- Specimen collection
- Administration of medication
- Intravenous access
- Cardiorespiratory care
- Nutrition
- Elimination
- Irrigation

Many commonly performed procedures have not been included because they do not differ significantly when performed on an adult or pediatric patient.

PROCEDURAL STEPS

1. Identify yourself to the child and parents.
2. Check the physician's orders.
3. Identify the child.
4. Give instructions and explanation to the child and parent.
5. Wash your hands.
6. Gather the necessary equipment.
7. Put on gloves.*
8. Begin the procedure.
9. Document findings.

*Gloves should be worn when it is likely that contact with mucous membranes, nonintact skin, or moist body substances will occur. Gloves should be changed between different patient contacts.

Informed consent involves obtaining written permission from the parent (or legal guardian) or the patient to perform specific procedures. Both legally and ethically necessary, informed consent requires that the parent/legal guardian or patient clearly understand the procedure or treatment to be performed and any risk factors involved as well as alternate methods available to achieve the same end. Without this permission for medical management, the physician and/or nurse could be found guilty of assault and battery.

General Guidelines

Certain guidelines have been established to ensure informed consent:

1. Information must be presented to the individual responsible for making the decision to allow him or her to weigh the benefits of the proposed treatment or procedure against the potential for complications. This information should be presented in simple, easy-to-understand terms. All questions and concerns should be answered honestly. If appropriate, an interpreter should be used to ensure clear communication.
2. The person making the decision must be over the age of majority (i.e., the age at which full civil rights are accorded) and must be competent (i.e., he or she must be able to make a decision based on the information received). The person needs to understand the proposed medical management and any risks.
3. The decision reached must be voluntary. The person making the decision must not be coerced, forced, or placed under duress while considering the options.

Although general written consent for care is obtained within the hospital setting during the admission process, specific consent must be obtained for procedures or treatments that include:

- Major surgery
- Minor surgery such as a cutdown, incision and drainage, closed reduction of a fracture, or fracture pinning
- Invasive diagnostic tests such as lumbar puncture, bone marrow aspiration, biopsy, cardiac catheterization, or endoscopy
- Treatments that may involve high risk, such as radiation therapy, chemotherapy, or dialysis
- Any procedure or treatment that falls under the auspices of research
- Photographing patients, even when done for educational purposes

Pediatric Considerations

Informed consent for the child involves the following additional considerations that must be addressed:

When the child is a minor (under the age of 18 years), his or her parent or legal guardian must give consent for all procedures or treatments.

If the parent is unavailable, the person in charge of the child (e.g., relative, baby-sitter, teacher, or camp counselor) may give consent for emergency treatment if the person has signed written permission from the parent to authorize care in his or her absence.

If the parent can be contacted by telephone, verbal consent can be obtained with two witnesses listening simultaneously. The consent should be recorded for later signature.

If the child is an emancipated minor (under the age of 18 years), that is, if his or her parents cannot meet their responsibilities or if the teenager is married, is in the military, is living apart from his or her parents and is financially independent, or is a parent himself or herself, the child may give informed consent as a mature minor.

POSITIONING AND RESTRAINT

When a child must be held in position for a procedure, it is important to try to use an assistant rather than a mechanical restraint for this purpose. The parent can both comfort and restrain the child. With the parent nearby, the child will be far less anxious and will not feel that he or she is being punished. If the parent does not feel comfortable about holding the child, another person should do so. If this is not possible, a papoose or mummy restraint can be used.

Human Restraint

For Intravenous Access/Injection

Procedure

- Place the child in a supine position on a bed or stretcher.
- Have the parent, a nurse, or an assistant lean over the child to restrain the child's body and extend the extremity to be used for access or injection.

For Lumbar Puncture

Procedure

- Place the child on side with knees pulled to abdomen and neck flexed to chin.
- The *infant* can be held in this position easily by holding the neck and thighs in your hands (Fig. P–1).

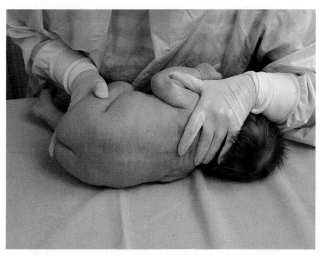

FIGURE P–1

- The *older child* can be quite strong, and someone with enough strength will be needed to hold him or her in this position. Lean over the child with your entire body, using your forearms against the thighs and around the shoulders and head.

■ NURSING ALERT

Lumbar puncture requires that the child be held still. It is advisable to have an experienced staff member hold the child in position for the procedure.

Mechanical Restraint

Use of a Papoose

The papoose consists of a board and cloth wrappings with Velcro fasteners (Fig. P–2). Two sizes are available—one for infants and toddlers and one for larger children.

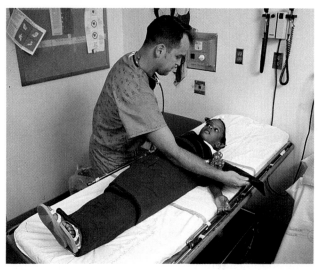

FIGURE P–2

Preparation

Explain to the child and parents why the restraint is being used. Compare the feeling of the papoose to a hug.

Procedure

- Place a towel or sheet over the board.
- Have the child lie supine on the board, with the head at the top.
- Place the fabric wrappings around the child, and secure the Velcro fasteners.

Some papooses come with openings for arms. If the child is positioned for a venipuncture, the arm can fit through the opening in the vest and then the remaining fabric pieces can be secured.

Use of a Mummy Restraint

Preparation

- Use a blanket or sheet large enough to hold the child in place. Put the blanket (or sheet) on the bed or examination table.
- Explain to the child and parents why the restraint is being used.

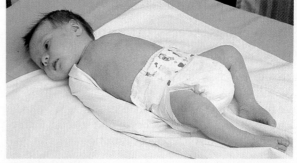
FIGURE P–3A

Procedure

Infant

- Fold down one corner until it reaches the middle of the blanket.
- Place the infant in a diagonal position with his or her neck on the folded edge.
- Bring one side of the blanket over the infant's arm. Tuck that edge under the other arm and around the back (Fig. P–3A).
- Bring the other side of the blanket around the body and tuck underneath the body (Fig. P–3B).
- Bring the bottom corner of the blanket up and over the abdomen (Fig. P–3C).

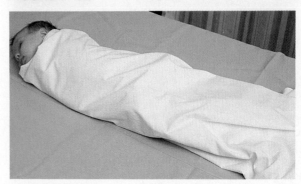
FIGURE P–3B

Toddler and Older Child

- Place the child on the blanket, positioning so that there is sufficient material to wrap the knees and lower legs. If necessary, fold down the top edges of the blanket to the shoulders.
- Bring one side of the blanket over the arm, body, and legs, and tuck it under the other arm and around the back and legs.
- Bring the other side of the blanket up and around the body, and tuck underneath the back and legs.

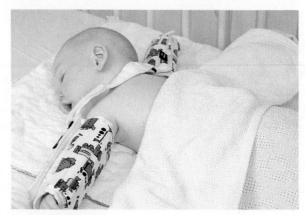
FIGURE P–3C

Use of Elbow Restraints

Elbow restraints (Fig. P–4) are used to prevent the infant or child from reaching his or her face or head. Although the ready-made type is available commercially, an elbow restraint can be devised easily from a piece of muslin that has vertical pockets sewn into it.

- Wrap the muslin around the arm from axilla to wrist.
- Place tongue depressors in the vertical pockets of the muslin wrap so that the arm cannot be bent.
- Secure the restraint with pins or tape.
- Remove the restraints at least every 2 hours to assess skin and circulation.

FIGURE P–4

Safety is the most important aspect of transporting infants and children. In determining the best method of transporting a child, the developmental stage must be taken into consideration.

Transport of the Infant

The infant who is lying down, either on the side or supine, can be placed in a bassinet or crib for transport. If the bassinet has a bottom shelf, it can be used for carrying the IV pump or monitor. A wagon may also be used, and the IV pole can be pushed along with it (Fig. P–5). The infant is kept covered with a blanket to avoid hypothermia resulting from a cool environment.

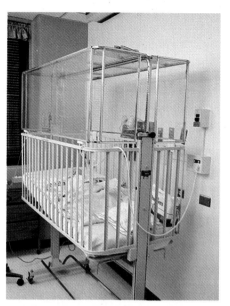

FIGURE P–6

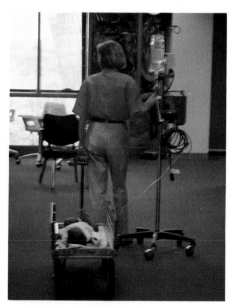

FIGURE P–5

Transport of the Disabled or Immobile Child

For the older child who is unable to walk because of a disability or whose mobility must be restricted, a specially designed wagon (Fig. P–7) can be used for transport.

Transport of the Toddler

The toddler should be transported in a high-top crib (also used for infants, as shown in Fig. P–6), with the siderails up and the protective top in place. The child may be sitting or lying down. Stretchers should not be used because the mobile toddler may roll or fall off.

A stroller or wheelchair may also be used, if available. Be sure to secure the child in the stroller with the seat safety strap. If a wheelchair is used, have the parent (if available) sit in the wheelchair and hold the toddler securely on his or her lap.

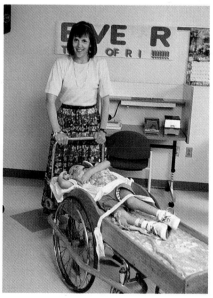

FIGURE P–7

Isolation

Isolation techniques are used to protect others from the bacteria or viruses shed by the child with an infection (Fig. P–8). Conversely, reverse, or protective, isolation protects the immunosuppressed child from the bacteria and normal body flora shed by staff members, family members, and visitors.

Check the infection control policy manual for the protective precautions necessary for different diseases or conditions. Explain the techniques to the child and parents. Be sure the family understands the technique since they, too, will need to don and remove protective garb. Advise them of strict orders for handwashing and monitor when they enter and leave the child's room.

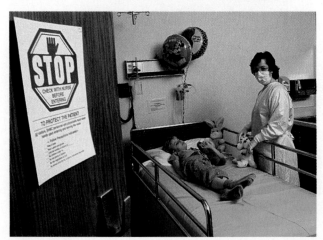

FIGURE P–8

Body Substance Isolation

Body substance isolation (BSI) has two goals: (1) to decrease nosocomial transmission of infectious agents to patients, and (2) to reduce exposure of health care workers to viral and bacterial pathogens. This technique requires that all personnel put on clean gloves immediately before contact with mucous membranes or nonintact skin of *all* patients. In addition, health care workers should wear protective aprons or other barriers as needed to keep their skin and clothing clean.

Whenever possible, health care workers should receive immunizations against influenza or hepatitis. If immunization is not possible, masks should be worn to protect staff against airborne pathogens.

Special care should be used in handling trash and linen (double-bagging is required). Sharps need special

attention. Do not recap needles. Place in a puncture-proof receptacle for disposal.

BSI guidelines are recommended for *all* patients, not only those diagnosed as infectious.

Universal Precautions

Universal precautions require health care workers to protect themselves from diseases transmitted by blood and body fluid by using protective barriers such as gowns, gloves, masks, and goggles (Fig. P–9).

Soiled linen and trash that needs to be double-bagged is labeled for laundering or disposal, as appropriate. Sharps are to be disposed of in a puncture-proof container; recapping of needles is to be avoided.

Equipment and Methods

Isolation Equipment

Isolation equipment consists of protective barriers (masks, gloves, gowns, protective eyewear) that should be kept on a cart just outside the child's room for easy access.

Masks

Masks are used for protection from pathogens that are shed through respiratory droplets.

Gloves

Gloves are used to protect the skin from contact with pathogens. They protect the nurse and the child from cross contamination. Gloves should be worn when it is likely that contact with mucous membranes, nonintact skin, or moist body substances will occur. They should be changed between different patient contacts.

Gowns

Gowns are used for protection against contact with pathogens. They should be worn when it is likely that body substances will come in contact with your clothing. Gowns should be changed between different patient contacts.

Protective Eyewear

Goggles or face shields should be worn if there is a risk of blood or body fluid being splattered. They should be

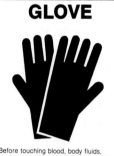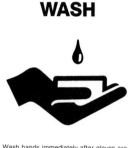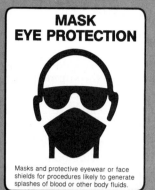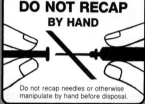

FIGURE P–9
Courtesy of BREVIS Corporation.

worn (1) when there is a chance that your eye, nose, or mouth may be splashed with body substances or (2) when you are working in close proximity to any open skin lesions.

Isolation Methods

The type of isolation required determines what kind of protective measures are necessary:

Isolation Type	Equipment
Strict	Mask, gown, gloves
Respiratory	Mask; gown and gloves may be worn
Contact	Gown and gloves; mask with shield is worn for close contact with child
Drainage/ secretions	Gloves if touching infectious material; gown and gloves if soiling is likely
Blood/body fluids	Gloves if touching infectious material; gown and gloves if soiling is likely; mask and goggles may be worn
Enteric	Gloves if touching infectious materials; gown and gloves if soiling is likely
Tuberculosis	Mask if coughing; gown and gloves if soiling is likely

Reverse (Protective) Isolation

Reverse isolation is used to protect the immunosuppressed child from environmental bacteria that might be harmful.

Good handwashing techniques are critical when caring for an immunosuppressed child. In addition, a clean or sterile gown, gloves, and mask must be donned by anyone, either staff or visitor, entering the child's room and must be removed when leaving.

Removal of Objects from Child's Room

Objects should be completely covered before they are removed from the child's room. All items should be double-bagged and marked "contaminated."

Equipment Taken into Child's Room

Any equipment taken into the child's room should be disposable or able to be sterilized or cleaned with bacterostatic cleaner. Disposable equipment should be discarded appropriately according to hospital policy. Equipment to be sterilized or cleaned should be double-bagged before removal.

Growth Measurements*

Length

Until a child is 2 years of age, length is measured with the child in the supine position (Fig. P–10). Because of the normally flexed posture of the infant, the body must be extended to obtain an accurate measurement. Hold the infant's head in the midline and gently push down on the knees until the legs are straight.

If a measuring board is used, place the infant's head against the top of the board and position the heels of the feet on the footboard. If such a device is not available, place the infant on a paper sheet. Make one mark at the vertex of the head and another at the heel. Then measure the distance between the two marks.

Record length in centimeters or inches.

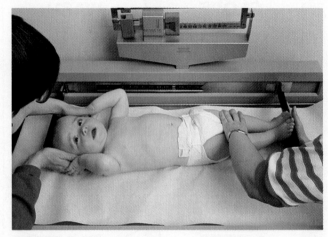

FIGURE P-10

Height

After the age of 2 to 3 years, height is measured with the child standing upright against a wall (Fig. P–11). The child's shoes are removed, and he or she is asked to stand straight with head erect and in the midline position. Shoulders, buttocks, and heels should touch the wall. Place a flat surface such as a ruler on top of the child's head. Make a mark where the ruler's edge hits the wall. Measure the distance from the mark to the floor. In the older child, height is measured using a platform scale with an attached stature-measuring device.

Record height in centimeters or inches.

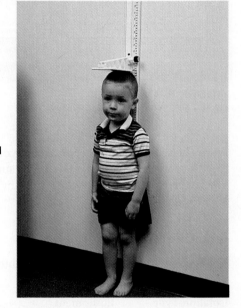

FIGURE P-11

Weight

Infants are weighed on a platform scale (Fig. P–12), either in a supine or sitting position, depending on their age. Check the balance of the scale before placing the infant on it, and put a paper cover on the scale. Care should be taken to ensure the infant's safety. Infants should be nude when they are weighed. Remember to change the paper covering after weighing.

The older child's weight can be measured on a standing scale. Toddlers should be weighed in their underclothes. Older children can remain in their street clothes with sweaters and shoes removed. Keep the room warm for comfort and provide privacy of the older child and adolescent.

Record weight in kilograms or pounds.

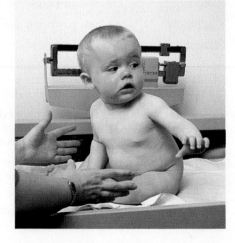

FIGURE P-12

For a complete discussion of pediatric physical assessment, see Chapter 3.

*For physical growth charts for boys and girls, see Appendix A.

Head Circumference

Head circumference is usually measured at regular intervals until the child's first or second birthday. Measure the head at its greatest circumference, just above the brow, just above the pinna of the ears, and around the occipital prominence (Fig. P–13). Use a paper tape measure, and record the circumference in inches or centimeters.

Chest Circumference

Chest circumference is often measured until 1 year of age. Measure the chest with a tape measure placed just under the axilla, over the nipple line (Fig. P–14).

Record circumference in centimeters or inches.

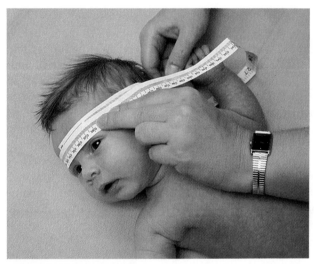

FIGURE P-13

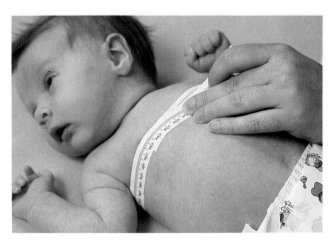

FIGURE P-14

▇ Vital Signs*

Heart Rate

The apical heart rate is preferred in children. To count the rate, place the stethoscope on the anterior chest at the fifth intercostal space in a midclavicular position. Each "lub-dub" sound is one beat. Count the beats for 1 full minute.

While auscultating the heart rate, note whether the rhythm is regular or irregular. Also record whether the pulse is normal, bounding, or thready. Compare the distal and proximal pulses for strength.

Pulse rates may be checked at sites other than the apex, for example, the carotid, brachial, radial, femoral, and dorsal pedis sites.

The range of normal heart rates based on age is as follows:

Age	Range (beats/min)
Newborn	100–170
6 mo–1 yr	90–130
3 yr	80–120
5 yr	70–110
10–14 yr	60–100

Respiratory Rate

The procedure for measuring a child's respiratory rate is essentially the same as for an adult. However, keep in mind these points:

- Since a child's respirations are diaphragmatic, observe abdominal movement to count respirations.
- Abdominal movement in a child will be irregular.

Count breaths for 1 full minute.

The range of normal respiratory rates based on age is as follows:

Age	Range (breaths/min)
Newborn	30–80
6 mo	24–36
1 yr	20–40
3 yr	20–30
6 yr	16–22
10 yr	16–20
17 yr	12–20

*Assessment of vital signs is also discussed in Chapter 3.

Blood Pressure

Blood pressure measurement for the child is basically the same as for an adult. Whether manual or electronic equipment is being used, the size of the blood pressure cuff is determined by the size of the child's arm or leg. Generally, the bladder of the cuff is two thirds of the width of the extremity used (Fig. P–15). If the bladder is too small, the pressure will be falsely high; if it is too large, the pressure will be falsely low.

If electronic equipment is being used, place the cuff around the desired extremity and activate the equipment according to the manufacturer's recommendations.

If a manual cuff is being used, wrap the cuff around the desired extremity. Close the air escape valve. Palpate for the pulse, and place the stethoscope over the pulse area. Pump the cuff with the bulb until the mercury rises and no beat is auscultated; continue pumping until the mercury rises another 20 to 30 mm. Slowly release the air through the valve at 2 to 3 mm/sec while watching the falling column of mercury. Note the number at which the first return of a pulse is heard; this is the systolic pressure. Continue releasing the air to determine the diastolic pressure: if the child is less than 12 years, a muffled sound will be heard; if the child is older than 12 years, all sound will disappear. Note that number. Blood pressure is read as systolic over diastolic pressure (Table P–1).

If the pulse cannot be auscultated, blood pressure can still be measured by touch. Wrap the cuff around the desired extremity, close the air valve, and palpate for the pulse. Keeping your fingers on the pulse, pump the cuff with the bulb until the pulse is no longer felt. Slowly open the air valve, watching the column of mercury, and note the number at which the pulse is again palpated. This is the palpated systolic blood pressure read as the number over "P."

Systolic pressure can also be measured by using Doppler ultrasonography (Fig. P–16). With this technique, the frequency of ultrasonic waves is reflected by movement of the surface of the blood vessels, which differs slightly from that of other structures in the same area. Pressure is recorded as the number over "D."

TABLE P–1 Median Systolic and Diastolic Blood Pressure Values for Children of Different Ages*

Age	Systolic (mm Hg)	Diastolic (mm Hg)
Newborn	73	55
1 mo	86	52
6 mo	90	53
1 yr	90	56
3 yr	92	55
6 yr	96	57
9 yr	100	61
12 yr	107	64
15 yr	114	65
18 yr	121	70

Adapted from the Normal Blood Pressure Readings for Boys from the Second Task Force on Blood Pressure Control in Children, National Heart, Lung, and Blood Institute (1987), Bethesda, MD. Normal blood pressure readings for girls are very similar to those for boys at all age groups.
*Readings show 50th percentile.

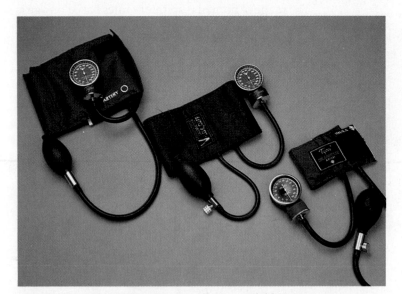

FIGURE P–15 Blood pressure cuffs are available in various types and sizes for pediatric patients.

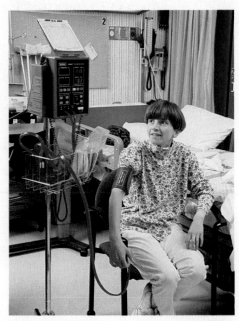

FIGURE P–16

Body Temperature

Body temperature can be measured in two scales: Fahrenheit or centigrade.

If an electronic thermometer is being used, follow the manufacturer's guidelines. There is no documented "universal" agreement on the length of time that a mercury thermometer should be kept in place. Follow the guidelines of your hospital or institution.

The four routes for measuring body temperature are tympanic, oral, rectal, and axillary.

Tympanic Route

The tympanic route (Fig. P–17) is advised for patients over 3 months of age.

Make sure the thermometer tip is aimed toward the tympanic membrane to ensure accuracy. Always use a clean probe tip for each child.

If you are using the child's right ear, hold the thermometer in your right hand. For the child's left ear, hold the thermometer in your left hand.

Procedure

CHILD YOUNGER THAN 1 YEAR
- Place the infant in a supine position on a flat surface.
- Stabilize the infant's head.
- Turn the infant's head 90 degrees for easy access.
- Pull the pinna of the ear straight back.
- Approach the ear from behind to direct the tip anteriorly.
- Place the probe in the ear as far as possible to seal the canal.
- Turn on the scanner.
- Leave the probe in the ear according to the manufacturer's recommendations.

- Remove the probe.
- Record the temperature.

CHILD OLDER THAN 1 YEAR
- Have the parent hold the child on his or her lap, keeping the child's head against his or her chest for support. The child's arms and legs may need to be held.
- Pull the pinna up and back.
- Place the probe and continue as described in the preceding section.
- Record the temperature.

Oral Route

The oral route may be used for the child over 3 years of age. (An electronic nonbreakable probe is preferred.)

Procedure

- Place the appropriate probe (with protective sheath) or the thermometer under the tongue and have the child close his or her mouth.
- If electronic equipment is being used, it will tone or beep when finished.
- If you are using a glass thermometer, keep it in place for approximately 5 minutes; then read the temperature based on the column of mercury.
- Record the temperature.

Rectal Route

The rectal route should be used only when no other route is possible. It is not recommended because of the potential for rectal perforation. The rectal temperature is one degree higher than the oral temperature.

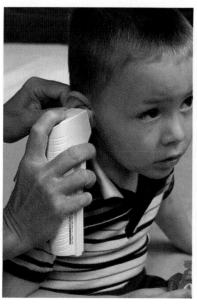

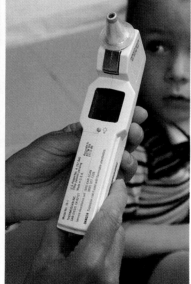

A

B

FIGURE P-17 A, Position for inserting thermometer when tympanic route is used. **B,** Digital readout of temperature appears within 1 minute.

Procedure

- Place the infant or child prone on a bed or the parent's lap; turn the older child on the side.
- Cover the tip of the probe (with protective sheath) or the thermometer with a water-soluble lubricant.
- For the infant, place the tip ¼ to ½ inch into the rectum.
- For the child, place the tip 1 inch into the rectum.
- Hold the thermometer in place for 3 to 5 minutes.
- Record the temperature.

Axillary Route

The axillary route (Fig. P–18) is often used for children who are seizure-prone, unconscious, or immunosuppressed, or who have a structural abnormality that precludes an alternate route. The axillary temperature is one degree lower than the oral temperature.

Procedure

- The probe (with sheath) or the thermometer (rectal or oral) is held in place in the axilla, with the child's arm pressed close to his or her side.
- If you are using an electronic probe, wait for the tone before removing it to read the temperature. If you are using a glass thermometer, keep it in place for a minimum of 5 minutes before reading it.
- Record the temperature.

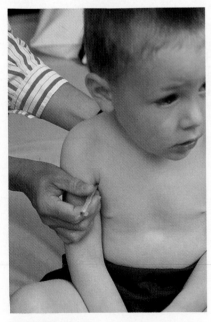

FIGURE P-18

■ Oxygen Saturation: Pulse Oximetry

Pulse oximetry is a simple noninvasive means of measuring the oxygen saturation of the blood (SaO_2).

Preparation

Emphasize that pulse oximetry is a pain-free procedure.

Procedure

- Assess the child's condition before attaching the sensor. Check respiratory status, including heart rate, respiratory rate, skin color, and respiratory effort.
- The sensor may be placed on the fingertip over the nail (Fig. P–19), on the toe over the nail, or on the ear lobe (if the child is cold or has poor perfusion).
- Probes come in two sizes: infant and pediatric. Size is determined by the size of the child and/or the placement site.
- Turn on the oximeter. Set parameters for alarms according to physician's orders. Attach the sensor to the machine. Watch for readout of pulse rate and oxygen saturation.
- You may leave the oximeter on for continuous readouts.
- If frequent, but not continuous, monitoring is indicated, leave the sensor on the child but disconnect it from the machine.
- If the sensor is removed, place it on the plastic backing for further use.
- Always remove the sensor from the extremity at least every 2 hours to check skin condition.

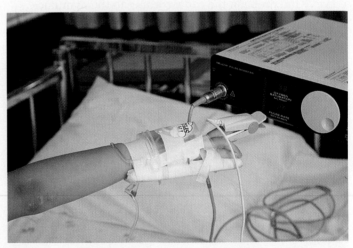

FIGURE P-19 Pulse oximetry.

Cardiorespiratory Monitoring Equipment

The standard cardiorespiratory monitor measures heart rate and respiratory rate. The high and low limits are set according to the age of the child. Usually a 15- to 20-second period of apnea will set off the alarm.

An apnea monitor (Fig. P–20) is used to monitor for abnormal or irregular breathing.

Procedure

- Place leads on the infant's or child's chest: one on the right side, one on the left, and one (ground) on the lateral side of the abdomen (Fig. P–21).
- If the monitor sounds, check the child immediately. Assess breathing and heart rate.
- If the child is not in distress, silence the alarm, check the connections and leads, and reset the alarm.

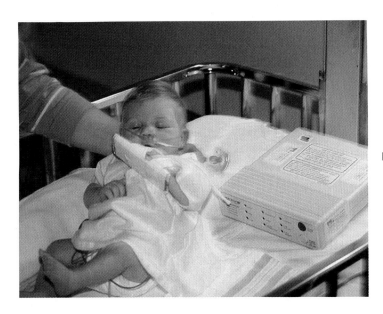

FIGURE P–20 Apnea monitor.

FIGURE P–21 Placement of leads in cardiorespiratory monitoring.

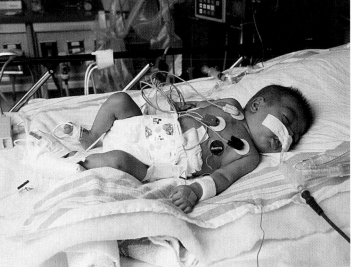

Visual Acuity

If the child stands 20 feet from the visual acuity chart and can correctly read the line designated "20 feet," vision is described as "20/20." However, if the child can read only the line designated "40 feet" from a 20-foot distance, vision is described as "20/40."

Snellen E Chart

For toddlers and children who have not yet mastered the alphabet, the Snellen E chart (Fig. P–22A) or picture chart may be used. In the E chart the capital letter E is shown in different directions. The child is asked to point in the direction of the "legs" of the E. Another option is to give the child a paper with an E on it and have the child turn it in the direction the E is pointing on the chart.

Picture Chart

The picture chart (Fig. P–22B) shows commonly identified silhouettes (e.g., house, apple, umbrella) lined up. The child is asked to identify the picture.

Snellen Letter Chart

The Snellen letter (alphabet) chart (Fig. P–22C) is the most commonly used assessment tool for visual acuity. It consists of lines of letters in decreasing size.

Procedure

- With the toddler, make a game of identifying the direction of the E or the picture.
- Assess each eye separately and then both together.
- While one eye is being tested, use the child's hand, a patch, or a piece of cardboard to cover the other eye. Tell the child to keep the covered eye open during the testing.
- Observe for squinting, moving the head forward (to be closer to the chart), excessive blinking, or tearing during the examination.

Normal visual acuity based on age is as follows:

Age (years)	Normal Visual Acuity
3	20/50
4	20/40
5	20/30
6	20/20

- Record the last line the child read correctly, either 3 of 4 or 4 of 6 letters or symbols.

Referrals

When the child's vision is not found to be within the normal limits for his or her age, make the appropriate referral to the child's private pediatrician, ophthalmologist, or optometrist.

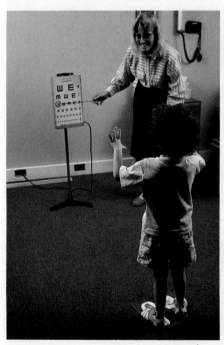
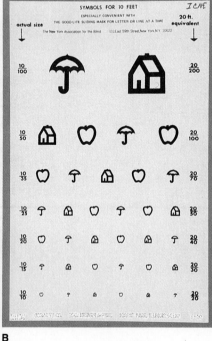
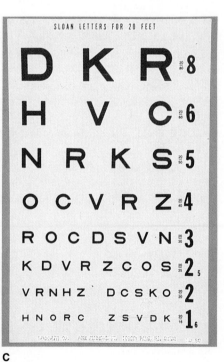

A B C

FIGURE P–22 Visual acuity charts. A, Snellen E chart. B, Picture chart. C, Snellen letter chart.
Courtesy of the National Society to Prevent Blindness, Schaumburg, IL.

Fluid and Electrolyte Balance: Intake and Output

Intake and output (I and O) is a measurement of fluid and electrolyte balance in the body.

Input is a measurement of what is delivered to the child through parenteral or oral routes. It is recorded in cubic centimeters (cc) or milliliters (mL). Output is a measurement of what is expelled, drained, secreted, or suctioned from the body. Output sources include urine, stool, vomitus, sweat, drainage from wounds, and nasogastric suction. Output can be measured easily in a graduated cylinder and is recorded in cubic centimeters (cc) or milliliters (mL).

Accurate measurement of I and O needs to be documented if the child is receiving IV fluids, has had major surgery, suffers from renal disease or kidney damage, is oliguric, is in congestive heart failure, has diabetes mellitus, is dehydrated, is hypovolemic, has suffered severe thermal burns, is taking medications such as diuretics or corticosteroids, or has a head injury, meningitis, or signs of increased intracranial pressure.

Infant

For the infant, there are two methods of measuring urine or stool output:

1. Diapers can be weighed dry and then again after the infant has voided/stooled. For each 1-gram increase in weight of the diaper, 30 mL of liquid has been excreted by the infant. Disadvantages to this system include the inability to differentiate between urine and stool weights since the two substances may mix in the diaper, and the evaporation of urine that takes place after 30 minutes. Counting diapers is also used since the amount of micturation is fairly standard during infancy and early toddlerhood.

2. A urine bag (see discussion of specimen collection that follows) may be used to obtain a more accurate measurement. Be aware of any leakage.

Toddler and Older Child

For the toddler and older child, urine and stool output can be measured in a bedpan.

SPECIMEN COLLECTION

In the collection of any type of specimen, it is the nurse's responsibility to be sure that the specimen is labeled correctly and sent to the laboratory.

Blood Samples

There are two methods of obtaining blood samples in children: venipuncture and capillary puncture. For both methods the following preparation is necessary:

- Prepare the child and parents emotionally for the procedure.
- Have another nurse, an assistant, or the parent ready to restrain the child.

Refer to Table 4–9 for communication strategies for a toddler undergoing venipuncture.

Venipuncture

Venipuncture, or the puncturing of a vein, is used to obtain a sample for complete blood count, blood culture, sedimentation rate, blood type and crossmatch, blood clotting times, drug screen, ammonia level, or fibrinogen level.

Selected Equipment

20- to 27-gauge needle with attached syringe (slightly larger than volume of blood needed)
Large-bore (19-gauge) needle
Appropriate blood collection tubes

Preparation

Choose the appropriate site. The veins of the antecubital fossa or forearm are usually the best choice because of their accessibility. However, the dorsum of the hand or foot also may be used.

Procedure

- Place a tourniquet proximal to the desired vein to distend it. If necessary, hold the extremity below heart level, gently rub or tap the vein, or apply a warm compress to promote dilation of the vein.
- Locate the vein by inspection (wiping with alcohol will make the vein shine) or palpation.
- Once the vein has been located, clean the skin with alcohol or povidone-iodine, using an outward circular motion. Let dry.
- With your nondominant hand, hold the skin taut, gently pulling with your thumb just under the site of the puncture.
- Puncture the skin with the needle, beveled up at a 15-degree angle and directed toward the vein. When blood appears in the tube, gently pull back on the syringe.
- Release the tourniquet after all the blood has been collected. Remove the needle at the same angle used for entry and apply pressure to the site with gauze (alcohol will sting).
- Have the assistant or parent maintain pressure for a few minutes until the bleeding has stopped, at which point an adhesive bandage can be placed. Meanwhile, remove the butterfly needle from the syringe.
- Attach the large-bore (19-gauge) needle, and expel blood into the appropriate collection tubes as soon as possible.

Capillary Puncture

Capillary puncture may be used to obtain a sample for complete blood count, reticulocyte count, platelet count, or blood chemistries such as electrolyte, glucose, or drug levels.

Selected Equipment

Lancet
Appropriate micro-size blood collection tubes

Preparation

Choose the appropriate site. Puncture sites include the plantar surface of the heel (Fig. P–23) (for newborns and children under the age of 1 year), the great toe (for children over 1 year), and the palmar surface of the tip of the third or fourth finger.

Procedure

Finger Stick. Hold the child's hand with your nondominant hand (or have an assistant hold it), keeping the finger to be used extended and pointed down.

- Make sure the tourniquet is tight enough to restrict venous (but not arterial) blood flow.
- Keep the level of the needle up. Do not draw back too hard on the syringe since the vein will collapse.
- If blood fails to enter the tubing, the needle may not be placed correctly in the vein. Advance the needle slightly.
- If a flash was seen but blood no longer appears, the butterfly needle may be located incorrectly in the vein. Gently draw back on the needle.

Heel Stick. Hold the child's foot in your nondominant hand, supporting the dorsum of the foot with your thumb and the ankle with your other fingers.

Toe Stick. Grasp the child's foot across the dorsum with your nondominant hand, supporting the toe with your thumb on the plantar surface.

- Clean the site.
- Using your dominant hand, pierce the skin with the lancet.
- Wipe the first drop of blood away with the gauze.
- Using a milking motion, gently squeeze the site and direct the blood into the appropriate tube.
- When collection is complete, have an assistant hold the gauze on the site until the bleeding has stopped. Apply an adhesive bandage.

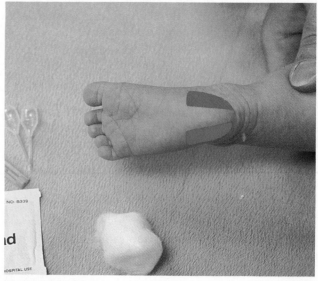

FIGURE P–23

PEDIATRIC NURSING

Urine Samples

A urine sample is obtained to assess for infection and to determine levels of blood, protein, glucose, acetone, bilirubin, drugs, hormones, metals, and electrolytes. Urine can also be evaluated for concentration/specific gravity, pH, and crystals or other substances.

Clean-Catch Collection

A collection bag is used to obtain a urine sample from an infant. After being given clear instructions, older children are usually capable of collecting their own urine. Younger children will need assistance from the nurse or their parents.

Infant

The urine bag is designed to collect urine from the infant or child who is not yet toilet trained. The bags come in two sizes: newborn and pediatric.

Procedure

TO PLACE THE BAG CORRECTLY
- Remove the diaper and clean the skin around the meatus (as described below).
- Attach the bag with the adhesive tabs (Fig. P–24): for girls, around the labia; for boys, around the scrotum.
- Make sure the seal is tight to prevent leakage.
- Check the bag frequently for urine.

TO REMOVE THE BAG CONTAINING URINE
- Gently pull bag away from the skin and pour urine into a sterile container.
- Cap the container tightly.

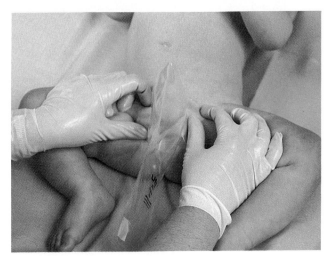

FIGURE P-24

Older Child

Procedure

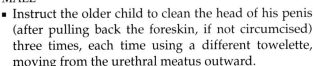

MALE
- Instruct the older child to clean the head of his penis (after pulling back the foreskin, if not circumcised) three times, each time using a different towelette, moving from the urethral meatus outward.
- Have the child urinate a small amount into the toilet, stop the flow, then urinate into the sterile container.
- Cap the container tightly.

FEMALE
- Instruct the child to sit back on the toilet as far as possible with her legs apart. Have her spread her labia with her fingers and wipe each side with a separate towelette using a front-to-back stroke. Tell the child to use a third wipe to clean the meatus, repeating the front-to-back motion.
- Have the child urinate a small amount into the toilet, stop the flow, then urinate into the sterile container.
- Cap the container tightly.

Stool Culture

Stool cultures are used to detect the presence of bacteria in the intestinal tract. A sample for culture can be obtained from stool collected in a cup, from a diaper, or from a swab that has been gently inserted into the child's rectum.

Selected Equipment

Two culturette swabs

Procedure

- Open one culturette swab, holding it in your dominant hand while keeping the cover in your nondominant hand.
- Dip the swab into the stool. Replace the cover. Squeeze the bottom of the closed culturette to release the culture medium.
- Repeat with the second culturette.

Wound Culture

A culturette swab is used to obtain samples for microscopic examination from a wound or body site such as throat, ears, nose, eyes, rectum, or vagina.

Selected Equipment

One culturette swab

Procedure

- Open the culturette, holding it in your dominant hand while keeping the cover in your nondominant hand.
- Gently swab the infected area.
- Cover the swab and release the culture medium.

Throat Culture

A culturette swab is used to obtain a sample from the throat for examination.

Selected Equipment

Two culturette swabs

Procedure

- Using the technique described in the preceding section, open the culturette. Gently swab the back of the throat along each tonsillar area with a separate culturette.
- Cover the swabs and release the culture medium.

Respiratory Secretions

Secretions are obtained to detect bacteria that cause respiratory infections. Different techniques are used for infants and older children. The infant will need suctioning. The older child can cooperate and cough into the provided container.

Infant

Selected Equipment

Sterile suction catheter
Sterile normal saline
Lukin's trap

Procedure

- According to the manufacturer's guidelines, attach the Lukin's trap to low wall suction (60 mm Hg).
- Suction the child's nose (see section on suctioning), using a small amount of sterile normal saline to clear the tubing.
- Close the trap.

Child

Selected Equipment

Sterile specimen container

Procedure

- Encourage the child to take several deep breaths, then cough up sputum into the cup (Fig. P–25).
- Close the cup.

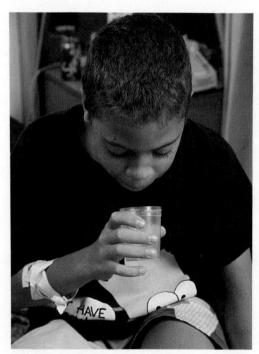

FIGURE P–25

PEDIATRIC NURSING

Administering medications to children presents a number of challenges: deciding which drugs to use, determining dosages, choosing methods and sites, and taking into account implications based on the child's development.

Although the drug and the dosage are determined by the physician, it is imperative that the nurse observe the "Five Rights" of medication administration (see box) before any medication is given.

When a medication is given, record the name of the drug, the route, the date and time, and, if appropriate, the site.

Explain all procedures or treatments to the child and parents, based on the child's developmental stage and the level of understanding of both parties. Answer all questions before giving the medication.

Oral Medication

Preparation

Measure the medication accurately to ensure that the dose is correct. If the medication is liquid (especially if less than 5 mL), it should be measured in a syringe or calibrated small medicine cup or dropper (Fig. P–26).

If a tablet or pill needs to be crushed, place it between two paper medicine cups and crush it with a pestle. Once the tablet or pill has been pulverized, mix the powdered medication with a small amount of flavored substance such as juice, applesauce, or syrup.

"FIVE RIGHTS" OF MEDICATION ADMINISTRATION

1. Right medication
   - Compare the name of the drug on the medication sheet with the name of the drug on the label of the drug container three times.
   - Know the action of the drug.
   - Identify the potential side effects of the drug.
   - Use the pharmacy, hospital, or other drug formulary as a reference for medications with which you are unfamiliar.
2. Right patient
   - Verify the name on the medication sheet against the name on the child's identification band.
3. Right time
4. Right route of administration
5. Right dose
   - Calculate the ordered dose based on the child's weight in kilograms.
   - If in doubt about what constitutes an appropriate dose, compare to the pharmacy, hospital, or other drug formulary guidelines for recommended dose.
   - Question order if dose is outside of recommended amounts.

Procedure

Infant

- A syringe or dropper provides the best control.
- Place small amounts of liquid along the side of the infant's mouth. To prevent aspiration or spitting out, wait for the infant to swallow before giving more.
- Alternative method: Have the infant suck the liquid through a nipple.

Toddler or Young Child

- Place the child firmly on your lap or the parent's lap in a sitting or modified supine position (Fig. P–27).
- Administer the medication slowly with a syringe or small medicine cup.

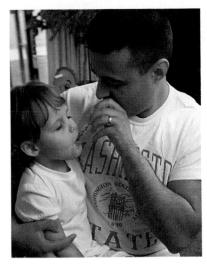

FIGURE P–27

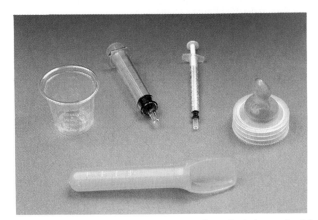

FIGURE P–26 Oral medications can be administered with various types of equipment, depending on the child's age.

▪ Intramuscular Injection

Selected Equipment

Syringe filled with medication

Preparation

Select the syringe size according to the volume and dose of medication to be delivered. The needle must be long enough to penetrate the subcutaneous tissue and enter the muscle. Needles with a length of 0.5 to 1 inch (25 to 21 gauge) are recommended for infants and children.

The site of injection (Fig. P–28) depends on the age of the child, the amount of muscle mass, and the density and volume of medication to be administered. Small infants may not tolerate volumes greater than 0.5 mL in a single site, whereas older infants or small children may

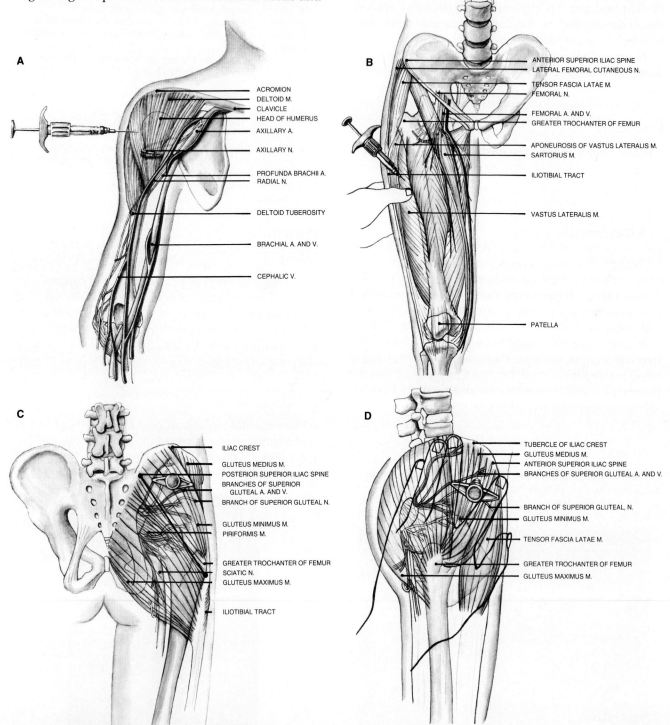

FIGURE P–28 Intramuscular injection sites. **A,** Deltoid. **B,** Vastus lateralis. **C,** Dorsogluteal. **D,** Ventrogluteal.
From Bindler, R., & Howry, L. (1991) (pp. 38–41). *Pediatric drugs and nursing implications*. Norwalk, CT:Appleton & Lange.

be able to tolerate 1 mL per site. As the child grows, greater volumes can be administered. Remember: The larger the volume of medication, the larger the muscle to be used. If possible, avoid areas that involve major blood vessels or nerves.

The preferred site for the infant is the vastus lateralis muscle (Fig. P–29), which lies along the lateral aspect of the thigh. After the child has been walking for 1 year, the dorsogluteal site can be used. However, since these muscles are poorly developed, they are not the ideal choice for a child less than 5 years old.

For the older child and adolescent, the sites are the same as for the adult: the vastus lateralis, deltoid, and ventrogluteal muscles.

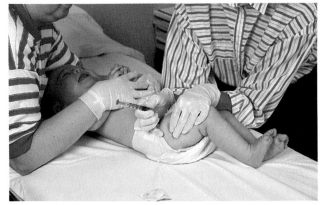

FIGURE P–29

Procedure

- Have another nurse, an assistant, or the parent restrain the child during the injection (Fig. P–30).
- Locate the site. Clean with alcohol or povidone-iodine using an outward circular motion.
- Grasp the muscle between your thumb and fingers for stabilization.
- Remove the cap from the syringe. Insert the needle quickly at a 90-degree angle. Pull back the plunger.
- If no blood is aspirated, inject the medication, withdraw the needle, massage the area with a gauze pad (alcohol will sting), and return the child to a position of comfort.
- Do not recap the needle. Discard in a puncture-resistant container according to universal precaution recommendations.

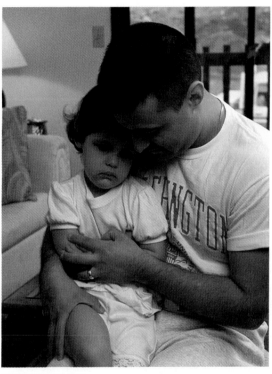

FIGURE P–30

▋ **SAMPLE DOCUMENTATION**

September 6, 1993, 1400 hours: 250 mg (1 mL) Ceftriaxone injected into the right deltoid. No redness, swelling noted. September 6, 1993, 1420 hours: No reaction to medication noted at this time. Patient discharged to home with instructions to return immediately if he has difficulty breathing or the area becomes red or swollen.

▋ Subcutaneous Injection

Selected Equipment

Syringe filled with medication

Preparation

Select the syringe size based on the volume or dose of medication to be delivered.

The needle must be just long enough to penetrate the subcutaneous tissue, which lies below the skin and fat surface and above the muscle. Needles with a length of $\frac{3}{8}$ to $\frac{5}{8}$ inch (26 to 25 gauge) are recommended for infants and children.

The site of injection depends on the age of the child. Usually the dorsum of the upper arm or the anterior thigh is used for newborns, infants, and toddlers.

Procedure

- Have another nurse, an assistant, or the parent restrain the child while the injection is being given.
- Locate the site. Clean with alcohol or povidone-iodine using an outward circular motion.
- Pinch the skin between your thumb and index finger.
- Remove the cap from the syringe. Insert the needle quickly at about a 45-degree angle. Release the skin and pull back the plunger.
- If no blood is aspirated, inject the medication, withdraw the needle at the angle at which it was inserted, massage the area with a gauze pad (alcohol will sting), and return the child to a position of comfort.
- Do not recap the needle. Discard it in a puncture-resistant container according to universal precaution recommendations.

Intravenous Medication

Preparation

Assess the IV for patency.

Remember that the effect of most IV medications is almost immediate. If you are administering narcotics or benzodiazepines, have antagonists and ventilation equipment at the bedside.

Many drugs have specific dilution recommendations. Some medications are compatible with only specific fluids such as normal saline. Other medications must be given very slowly. Still other drugs can be administered quickly. Know your institution's or pharmacy's standards for IV push (less than 10 minutes) versus intermittent medication administration. Recognize that many medications are incompatible with one another and therefore the IV line will need to be flushed between administrations.

Special Considerations

It is recommended that IV medications for infants and children be put in a Soluset or Metriset with the diluent and placed on an electronic pump for accurate administration. Set the pump for the volume to be infused and the rate of infusion. Flush the line after the infusion to ensure that all medication has been administered, since some medication will remain in the distal tubing.

Some medications can be given as a bolus, by injecting the drug directly into a port of the IV tubing. Check with your pharmacy, the manufacturer's insert, or a resource book for recommendations about which port to use, distal or proximal to the child, and the rate of infusion.

Optic Medication

Selected Equipment

Medication

Procedure

- Have another nurse, an assistant, or the parent restrain the child in a supine position with the child's head extended.
- Use your nondominant hand to pull the child's lower lid down while your other hand rests on the child's head (Fig. P–31).
- Instill the drops or ointment into the conjunctival sac that has formed.
- Alternative method: Pull the lower lid out far enough to form a reservoir in which the medication can be instilled.
- After the medication has been instilled, close the child's eyelids to prevent leakage.
- Have the child lie quietly for a minimum of 30 seconds.
- Dry the inner canthus of the eye.
- Keep the child's head in the midline position to prevent medication contamination of the other eye.

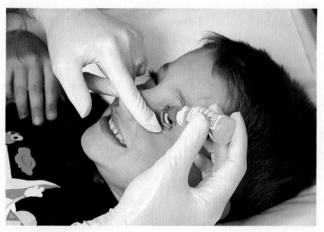

FIGURE P–31

Otic Medication

Selected Equipment

Medication
Cotton ball

Procedure

- Have another nurse, an assistant, or the parent restrain the child in a supine position with the head turned as appropriate for administration (Fig. P–32).

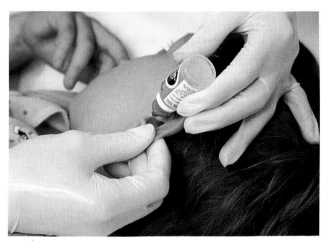

FIGURE P–32

Aerosol Therapy

Aerosol therapy is used when medication needs to be deposited directly into the airway. Bronchodilators, steroids, and antibiotics can be administered to children in aerosol form.

Selected Equipment

Assembled kit with mask
Mouthpiece or blow-by tubing (depending on child's age)

Preparation

The dose of the medication is based on the child's weight. The medication is placed in the cup of the aerosol kit; 2 to 3 mL of normal saline can be added as a diluent if ordered.

Perform a baseline assessment, including heart and respiratory rates, breath sounds, and respiratory effort.

Procedure

- Place the mask on the child.
- Give the parent the tubing for blow-by, or have the child put the mouthpiece in his or her mouth (P–33).
- Attach the oxygen tubing to the oxygen flowmeter at 6–7 L/min.
- Have the child take deep breaths during the treatment.
- The aerosol administration should last about 10 minutes. Reassess the child's condition after the therapy.
- Document medication, dose, and child's response to therapy.

- *For the child less than 3 years of age:* Gently pull the pinna straight back and downward to straighten the ear canal.
- *For the older child:* Pull the pinna back and upward.
- When the pinna is in the proper position, instill the drops into the ear.
- Keep the child in the same position for a few minutes. Gently rub the area just anterior to the ear to facilitate drainage of the medication into the ear canal. If desired, a cotton ball may be loosely placed in the ear to promote retention of the medication.

Nasal Medication

Selected Equipment

Medication

Procedure

- Place the child in a supine position with the head hyperextended over the parent's lap or over the edge of the examination table or bed.
- Instill the drops into the nostrils.
- Keep the child in the same position for at least 5 minutes to allow the medication to contact the nasal mucosa.

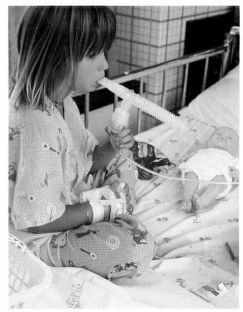

FIGURE P–33

■ Per Rectum

Rectal administration is sometimes used when the oral route is contraindicated. Although absorption is less reliable than with oral preparations, many medications, such as acetaminophen, aspirin, antiemetics, analgesics, and sedatives, come in suppository form.

Selected Equipment

Water-soluble lubricant
Suppository

Preparation

If the suppository is to be halved, cut it lengthwise.

Procedure

- Have another nurse, an assistant, or the parent hold the child in a side-lying or (if small enough) a prone position on the parent's lap.
- Slightly lubricate the tapered tip of the suppository. Using either the index or little finger (depending on the child's age), gently insert the suppository into the child's rectum, just beyond the sphincter.
- Hold the buttocks together for 5 to 10 minutes, until the urge to expel the medication has passed.

■ Calculation of Medication Doses

It is the nurse's responsibility to calculate the dosage of the medication to determine if the dosage is within the normal range for the child's height and weight.

Dosages can be calculated using the child's weight (written as mg/kg) or total body surface area. This is determined by plotting the child's height and weight on a nomogram (see Appendix E). Draw a line connecting the two columns and note the results at the point where the drawn lines cross the center column. The dosage is ordered as mg/m^2.

Example 1

The physician orders **morphine (10 mg/mL)** for a 3-year-old child who weighs 15 kg. The recommended dose for children is 0.1 **mg/kg**. What dose is appropriate for the child's weight? How much volume should be drawn?

ANSWER

Recommended dose × Weight = Dose for patient
0.1 mg/kg × 15 kg = 1.5 mg

$$\frac{\text{Dose desired}}{\text{Dose on hand}} \times \text{Quantity in mL} = \text{Volume to be administered}$$

$$\frac{1.5 \text{ mg}}{10 \text{ mg}} \times 1 \text{ mL} = 0.15 \text{ mL to be administered}$$

Example 2

The physician orders phenobarbital (65 mg/mL) for a 5-year-old child who weighs 20 kg. The recommended loading dose for the child is 10 to 20 mg/kg. The physician orders 250 mg to be infused over 30 minutes. Is this dose appropriate for the child's weight? How much volume should be drawn? How do you set the infusion pump?

ANSWER

Recommended dose × Weight = Desired dose
10 mg/kg × 20 kg = 200 mg
20 mg/kg × 20 kg = 400 mg

Dose of 250 mg is within recommended range.

$$\frac{\text{Dose desired}}{\text{Dose on hand}} \times \text{Quantity in mL} = \text{Volume to be administered}$$

$$\frac{250 \text{ mg}}{65 \text{ mg}} \times 1 \text{ mL} = 3.85 \text{ mL}$$

Pump set up

The nurse determines the volume for the setup is 50 mL.

$$\frac{50 \text{ mL}}{30 \text{ min}} \times \frac{60 \text{ min}}{1 \text{ hr}} = \frac{\text{mL}}{\text{hr}} = 100 \text{ mL/hr}$$

Rate = 100 mL/hr

Peripheral Vascular Access

Veins of the extremities are used for venous access of both infants and children, whereas those of the scalp may be used in infants.

Over-the-needle catheters (19 to 27 gauge) are preferred for infants and children. The size of the catheter is determined by the size of the child and size of the vein. For example, a 24-gauge catheter is used for a newborn; a 20- to 22-gauge catheter is used for an older infant, toddler, or school-aged child. A butterfly needle (23 gauge) may be used in certain situations, such as when accessing a scalp vein in an infant or during an emergency for peripheral access in a toddler. Use of a butterfly needle should be considered a temporary measure, with continued effort made to achieve more stable and secure venous access.

Choice of Site

Scalp

Scalp veins are used when other access cannot be obtained (Fig. P–34). Protect the site by covering it with a plastic medication cup secured with tape.

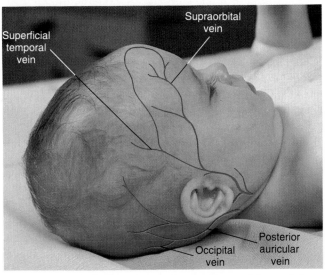

FIGURE P–34 Scalp veins are frequently used for peripheral vascular access in infants.

Extremities

Veins of the antecubital fossa or forearm are usually the best sites for venous access because they are highly visible; however, the dorsum of the hand and foot also may be used.

Special Considerations

- Avoid using the foot veins as a site in children who are walking.
- Avoid using the child's dominant hand or the hand used by an infant for finger sucking or blanket holding.
- If two sites are needed, do not use both antecubital veins because the child will be rendered helpless.
- Use padded armboards as splints to decrease mobility of the extremity.
- Use gauze under tape or tape over tape to decrease skin contact with adhesive tape.

Selected Equipment

Different sized armboards
IV catheter (depends on size of vein)
T connector that has been flushed and attached to normal saline–filled syringe

Preparation

- Place and maintain the child in a supine position with the help of an assistant. Have the person assisting you lean over the child to control the child's body and extend the extremity to be used. An alternative to human restraint is to use a papoose board (see procedures for IV placement and use of a papoose).
- If a scalp vein is to be used, place a rubber band around the infant's head to serve as a tourniquet to distend the veins. If the extremities are to be used, place the tourniquet proximal to the desired vein to distend it. If necessary, hold the extremity below heart level, gently rub or tap the vein, or apply a warm compress to promote dilation of the vein.
- Locate the vein by inspection (wiping with alcohol will make the vein shine) or palpation.
- If you are using an extremity, apply an armboard or footboard. Relocate the vein.

- *If using the antecubital fossa:* Slightly hyperextend the child's elbow and pronate arm. Secure arm to armboard by applying tape above the elbow and at the wrist.
- *If using the dorsum of the hand:* Place the child's hand on the armboard, palmar side down, with the fingers wrapped around the distal edge (Fig. P–35). Apply tape over the fingers, then around the thumb separately. Next apply tape at the wrist. A gauze roll may be placed under the wrist to increase flexion.
- *If using the foot:* Apply the footboard to the child's foot, which is dorsiflexed. Apply tape across the toes, instep, and ankle. Use gauze as needed under the lateral malleolus.

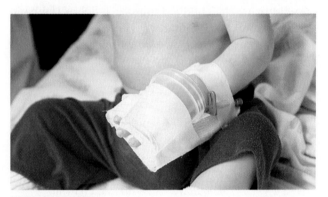

FIGURE P–35

Procedure

- Clean the skin with alcohol or povidone-iodine using an outward circular motion. Let each area dry before continuing. Hold the skin taut, gently pulling with your thumb just distal to the site of the puncture.
- Puncture the skin with the catheter, with the bevel side up, positioned at a 15-degree angle and aimed at the vein in the direction of the blood flow. When blood appears, gently slide the catheter into the vein. Remove the stylette. Release the tourniquet.
- Attach the normal saline–filled T connector and attempt to flush the catheter. If it flushes easily, tape the catheter in place, using a V pattern around the catheter itself. Further secure the catheter with gauze and tape (taking care not to cover the area proximal to the site completely) or a transparent dressing (to allow observation for signs of infiltration or phlebitis). Write the date, time, catheter size, and your initials on a piece of tape and place on the dressing.

At this point the T connector can be hooked up to a heparin lock or used immediately for fluid or medication infusion.

Heparin Lock

Attachment of Heparin Lock Cap

Selected Equipment

To connect the heparin lock (catheter) cap (male adapter) to a T connector after starting an IV infusion, add the following equipment to the IV start list in the previous procedure:

Syringe filled with 1 mL of prepackaged heparin flush solution
Luer-lok catheter cap

Procedure

- Tape the IV line securely in place (Fig. P–36*A*).
- With the normal saline–filled syringe, flush the IV line through the T connector to ensure its patency and placement. Remove syringe.

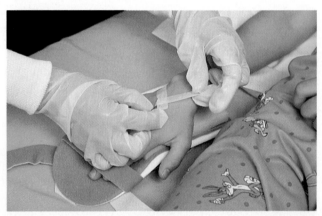

A

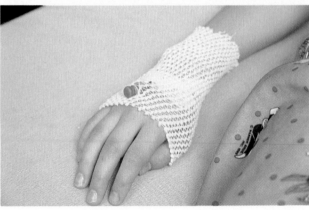

B

FIGURE P–36 A, Taping IV line for placement of heparin lock. **B,** Heparin lock in place.

- Attach the syringe containing the heparin flush solution; slowly infuse the solution through the IV tubing. Remove syringe.
- Place a primed catheter cap on the T connector. Secure with tape (Fig. P–36B).

Infusion of Medication: Heparin Lock in Place

Selected Equipment

19- to 27-gauge needle
Two syringes filled with normal saline
Syringe with 1 mL of heparin flush solution

Procedure

- Clean the catheter cap with either alcohol or povidone-iodine.
- Check the patency of the IV by flushing it with normal saline.
- Insert the needle (attached to the distal end of the IV tubing) through the cap after cleaning its surface.
- Secure the needle in place with tape.
- Begin the infusion of medication according to the physician's orders.
- After completion of the infusion, discard needle into a puncture-proof container according to universal precaution recommendations. Cover the IV tubing with a clean needle if it is to be used again.
- Clean the catheter cap with alcohol.
- Flush first with normal saline and then with heparin flush solution (as in preceding procedure).

IV Push Bolus of Medication: Heparin Lock in Place

Selected Equipment

Two 2 mL syringes filled with normal saline covered with 19- to 27-gauge needles
Syringe filled with 1 mL of heparin flush solution covered with 19-gauge needle
Medication in syringe covered with 19- to 27-gauge needle

Procedure

- Clean the catheter cap with alcohol or povidone-iodine.
- Pierce the catheter cap with a normal saline–filled syringe.
- Flush the line with 2 mL of normal saline to check patency.
- Remove syringe and needle.
- Insert the medication syringe through the catheter cap and give the medication according to physician's orders. Check a resource book or call your hospital

pharmacy to determine rate of administration. When medication is finished, remove the syringe.
- Flush the line with the second normal saline–filled syringe, followed by the heparin flush solution.
- Discard the needles and syringe in a puncture-proof container according to universal precaution recommendations.

Intravenous Infusion

Fluid Administration

The amount of fluid to be administered to a child is based on the child's weight and pathophysiologic state. It is recommended that fluids be given to the infant or child via an infusion pump (Fig. P–37), since this device allows more accurate setting of flow rates than gravity does. Maintenance fluid requirements are based on the child's weight as follows:

Weight (kg)	Fluid requirements
0–10	100 mL/kg/24 hr
10–20	1000 mL + 50 mL/kg/24 hr for each kg between 11 and 20
20–70	1500 mL + 20 mL/kg/24 hr for each kg between 21 and 70
Over 70	2500 mL/24 hr (adult requirement)

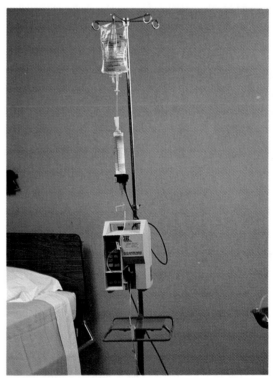

FIGURE P–37 IV setup with infusion pump.

Pumps

An infusion pump can be used to control the administration of small volumes of fluid, blood, medication, and total parenteral nutrition. A smaller syringe pump (Fig. P–38) can be attached directly to the lowest port on the IV tubing for immediate infusion of medication.

It is important to be familiar with the type of infusion pump used at your institution. Be sure to set controls for both the amount of fluid to be infused and the rate of infusion.

Preparation for Hanging Fluids

Before hanging any fluids, check the bag or bottle for leaks, expiration date, impurities, or color changes.

Select tubing for either a pump or gravity drip. Make sure that the tubing is clamped off. Remove the protective covering from the insertion piece. Place the insertion piece into the entry port of the bag or bottle. Invert the bag or bottle and hang it on a pole. Pinch the drip chamber (it should be no more than one half full). Direct the distal end of the tubing into a clean receptacle. Open the clamp and let the fluid run through the length of the tubing. Tap the tubing at each port to remove any trapped air. Close the clamp, and check the entire length of tubing for air bubbles. The tubing is now primed and ready for use.

If a Soluset or Metriset is used, attach it to the bag or bottle (as above). Close the clamp that is closest to the fluid and the one that is distal to the Soluset. Open the top clamp. Let about 50 mL into the Soluset and then close the clamp. Pinch the drip chamber as above. Open the distal clamp, and continue to purge the tubing.

If you are using a pump, check the manufacturer's guidelines for purging the tubing.

Guidelines for Dripping of IV Fluids

Rules for determining flow rate for instilling IV fluids via gravity are based on the drip factor of the IV tubing being used.

Microdrip Tubing

Manufacturer	Drops /mL
All major manufacturers	60 drops (gtt) = 1 mL

FORMULA
mL/hr = gtt/min

EXAMPLE
$$\frac{1000 \text{ mL}}{8 \text{ hr}} = 125 \text{ mL/hr} = 125 \text{ gtt/min}$$

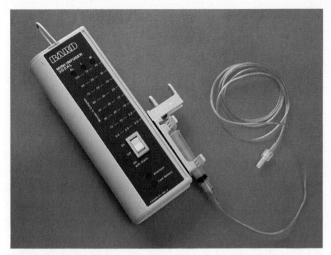

FIGURE P–38 Syringe pump.

Macrodrip Tubing

Manufacturer	Drops /mL
AVI	20 gtt = 1 mL
McGaw/Abbot	15 gtt = 1 mL
Travenol	10 gtt = 1 mL

FORMULA
$$\frac{\text{Total volume} \times \text{Drop factor}}{\text{Infusion time in minutes}} = \text{Drops/minute}$$

EXAMPLE
$$\frac{1000 \text{ mL} \times 10 \text{ (Travenol)}}{8 \text{ hr (480 min)}} = 21 \text{ gtt/min}$$

Blood Administration

To safely administer blood or blood products to the infant or child, be aware of the protocols followed at your institution.

Selected Equipment

Blood product
Tubing plus bag of normal saline (if Y set is being used)
Normal saline flush solution
Needle

Preparation

Identify the bag to be used and compare it with the requisition (type, Rh factor, patient number, blood donor number) and the child's identification bracelet. Do this step with another nurse at the bedside. Both nurses are responsible for signing the slips as the transfusers.

Check the blood for any bubbles, dark areas, or sediment.

Ask the child or family about previous transfusions, especially any history of allergic reaction.

Take the child's vital signs, including pulse, respiratory rate, temperature, and blood pressure.

When estimating preparation time, keep in mind that blood must be hung within 20 to 30 minutes after being removed from the blood bank refrigerator. Blood should be administered according to the physician's orders. However, a bag should never remain hanging longer than 4 hours. For trauma patients who need massive transfusions, the bag should be warmed to 37° C (only an approved blood warmer should be used).

Use the correct tubing for the blood product being administered. A Y blood administration set is preferred. If a Y setup is used, hang normal saline at the extra connector.

Selected Equipment

Blood product
Tubing plus bag of normal saline (if Y set is being used)
Normal saline flush solution
Needle

Procedure

- Take the baseline vital signs.
- Attach the blood bag to the tubing and flush the line. Flush the normal saline tubing. Clamp off the tubing, keeping the distal end covered.
- Clamp off the IV tubing. Disconnect it, covering the hub with a sterile needle to keep it sterile. Flush the line with normal saline to ensure its patency. Attach the blood tubing.
- Slowly open the clamp-on tubing, adjusting the flow with the roller. Start the transfusion slowly.
- The flow rate may be increased if no reaction is noted. (Most reactions occur within 20 minutes.)
- Closely monitor the child's vital signs and response. Vital signs should be taken every 5 minutes for the first 15 minutes, every 15 minutes during the first hour, then hourly until the transfusion is complete (*or follow your hospital's protocol*).
- If the child develops any sign of a transfusion reaction (Table P–2), stop the transfusion, change the IV to normal saline, and notify the physician immediately.
- After the administration of blood, flush the line with normal saline and connect IV fluid ordered by the physician. Place the used blood bag and tubing in a plastic bag, seal it, and return it to the blood bank with copies of the transfusion information sheet.
- Document all vital signs, responses, and interventions.

TABLE P–2 Transfusion Reactions

Type of Reaction	Description
Allergic	Caused by immune response to protein in blood; signs and symptoms may include rash, itching, urticaria, wheezing, laryngospasm or edema, and/or anaphylaxis
Febrile or septic	Usually result of contamination of blood; also may be caused by idiopathic conditions; signs and symptoms include chills, fever, headache, decreased blood pressure, nausea and/or vomiting, and leg or back pain
Hemolytic	Caused by incompatibility of child's blood with donor blood, history of multiple transfusions, or infusion with a solution containing dextrose or other additives; signs and symptoms include anxiety or restlessness, fever, chills, chest pain, cyanosis, change in vital signs with increased heart and respiratory rates or with decreased blood pressure and/or hematuria; can progress to shock and anuria if not treated promptly
Circulatory overload	Results from infusion of excessive amounts of fluid or too rapid administration; signs and symptoms include labored breathing, chest or lower back pain, productive cough with rales heard on auscultation, and distended neck-veins; central venous pressure may increase

Total Parenteral Nutrition

Total parenteral nutrition (TPN) is the administration of a nutritionally complete formula into a large central vein. TPN is used for children who cannot tolerate gastrointestinal feeding. Children with disorders such as chronic intestinal obstruction, short bowel syndrome, chronic diarrhea, chemotherapy, or tumors may require TPN. (See also Chapter 15.)

Hyperalimentation solutions (TPN and lipids) are delivered by separate pumps and connector tubes. Usually the child who is receiving TPN has a central venous catheter in place. Solutions and tubes need to be changed every 24 hours using strict aseptic technique. Tips and connecting points need to be sterile. Since the hyperalimentation solution needs to be protected from light, the bottle should be covered. Nursing responsibilities when caring for a child receiving TPN are outlined in Table P–3.

TABLE P–3 Caring for the Child Receiving TPN

- Monitor intake and output. Changes may indicate fluid and electrolyte disturbances.
- Weigh the child daily.
- Assess the IV site. Watch for signs of redness, irritation, or infection. Change the dressing according to hospital protocol (see procedure for central venous catheters).
- Make sure to set each pump correctly, noting the volume and rate of each infusion.
- Check laboratory values, especially glucose, minerals, electrolytes, liver function (bilirubin, alkaline phosphatase), proteins, and triglycerides.
- Note any change in glucose levels:
  1. During the first few days, the high concentration of glucose administration may lead to hyperglycemia. Inform the physician of high blood glucose levels. Insulin may be needed to help the body adjust to the formula.
  2. If hyperalimentation is discontinued abruptly, the child may become hypoglycemic. Be aware of the signs and symptoms of hypoglycemia (see Chapter 19). Notify the physician if blood glucose level is low.

Central Venous Catheters

A central venous catheter is surgically placed when long-term access is needed, such as for total parenteral nutrition, administration of antibiotics, or chemotherapy. Usually the subclavian vein is accessed and the catheter is threaded into the right atrium.

The most common catheter used for children is the Broviac catheter (Fig. P–39), which can have a single, double, or triple lumen.

Site Management

The catheter site is covered with a clear occlusive dressing that should be changed under sterile conditions 2 to 3 times a week according to agency protocol.

Procedure

- Remove the current dressing, working from the edges toward the center.
- If *bloody discharge is present*, clean with sterile half-strength peroxide-saturated cotton swabs in an outward circular motion from the point of entry, using one swab for each motion and then changing to a clean one. Clean the area again with povidone-iodine swabs, using the same technique.
- If *no bloody discharge is noted*, clean the area with povidone swabs only, using the above technique.
- Let dry. Cover with an occlusive dressing. Write the date, time, and your initials on a piece of tape and place it on the dressing.

Withdrawing Blood

Check the physician's order for the blood tests to be done. It is recommended that the catheter be accessed no more than twice a day.

Have an assistant open and close the clamps as necessary and put the blood in tubes while you are flushing the line.

The double stopcock method of accessing central lines has certain advantages. It is a simple procedure and requires very little setup. The most important feature, however, is that the line is not broken by frequent syringe exchanges as occurs with the direct or single-syringe method.

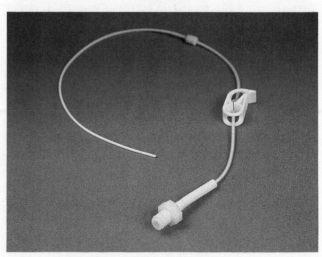

FIGURE P–39 Broviac catheter.

Selected Equipment

Mask
Gown
Appropriate blood collection tubes
19- to 27-gauge needles for transferring blood to tubes
Padded clamp (if a clamp is not attached to tubing)
For each port accessed:
Double stopcock
Syringe filled with 5 to 6 mL of normal saline
Syringe filled with 5 mL of heparin flush solution
5 to 6 mL discard syringe
Syringes for blood samples
Luer-lok or Broviac catheter cap

Preparation

Keeping the equipment sterile, prepare the double stopcock: attach the discard syringe to the access port proximal to the child, the blood-drawing syringe at the next access port, and the normal saline-filled syringe at the distal end.

Procedure

- Put on mask.
- Unpin the catheter from the child's clothes. Remove any tape. Open a sterile 4 x 4 gauze pad to serve as a clean work area. Place the gauze under the catheter connection.
- Clean the connection site with alcohol swabs. Use 3 swabs, and clean for a total of 2 minutes. Let the connection site dry for an additional 20 seconds.
- Make sure that the catheter is clamped. Remove the catheter cap. Attach the prepared double stopcock, making certain that the seal is tight. Unclamp the catheter. Open the stopcock port of the discard syringe, and aspirate 3 to 5 mL of blood. Close the port. Open the next port on the stopcock to obtain the blood samples. Aspirate the amount of blood necessary. Close that port. Remove that syringe and cover with a 19- to 27-gauge needle. Give that syringe to your assistant to fill the blood collection tubes. Meanwhile, attach the syringe filled with heparin flush solution to that port.
- Open the distal port. Gently aspirate to clear the stopcock of air. Tap any bubbles to the top of the saline-filled syringe. Flush the line with 5 mL of normal saline. Close the port. Open the port with the heparin flush solution and flush 5 mL into the catheter.
- Have your assistant clamp the line. Remove the stopcocks. Clean around the edges with sterile gauze or a new alcohol swab. Attach a new Luer-lok or Broviac catheter cap. Tape the connection with double-over tabs that are long enough to pin to the child's clothes. Attach it to the clothing firmly.

Routine Flushing of the Line

Broviac catheters are flushed once a day, both at home and in the hospital, if they are not accessed. For flushing, 5 mL of heparin flush solution is used.

Implanted Ports

Implanted ports are used most often for children and adolescents who require long-term venous access. The stainless steel port has a self-sealing rubber septum and is surgically implanted under the skin over a bony prominence, most often the clavicle. The catheter is then inserted into the vein that leads to the right atrium. Entry is gained by piercing the skin directly over the port with a specially designed needle (Fig. P–40).

The Port-a-Cath is used commonly in pediatrics.

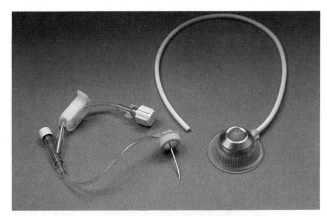

A

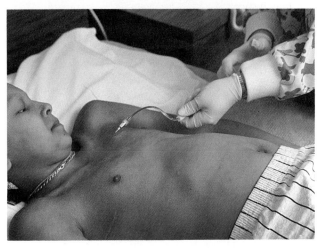

B

FIGURE P–40 A, Huber needle. **B,** Nurse drawing blood from an adolescent with an implantable port.

Administration of Oxygen

When oxygen is to be administered, the concentration ordered and the age of the child are important. To assess response to the therapy, monitor the child's heart rate, respiratory rate and effort, color, pulse oximeter readings, and level of consciousness.

Humidification is often necessary to prevent nasal passages from drying out. This is provided by attaching a sterile water–filled container to the oxygen or flowmeter with a connecting tube.

Safety Precautions

- "No Smoking" and "Oxygen in Use" signs should be posted at the child's doorway and at the bedside.
- Make sure that matches and lighters are not used in the area.
- Use only hospital-approved electrical equipment.
- Do not use flammable or volatile solutions in the child's room.

Delivery Systems

Masks

Several types of masks are available to deliver oxygen. The size of the mask is important. The mask should extend from the bridge of the nose to the cleft of the chin. It should fit snugly on the face but put no pressure on the eyes to avoid stimulating a vagal response.

The *simple face mask* (Fig. P–41) can deliver from 30% to 60% oxygen when a flow rate of 6 to 10 L/min is used.

The *nonrebreather mask* has a reservoir bag attached to deliver higher concentrations of oxygen, up to 95% with a flow of 10 to 12 L/min, when a tight seal is maintained.

Nasal Cannula

A nasal cannula is used to deliver low-flow, low-concentration oxygen. It does not provide humidified oxygen. A flow rate set higher than 6 L/min will irritate the nasopharynx without appreciably improving the child's oxygenation.

The prongs of the cannula are placed in the anterior nares, and the elastic band is placed around the child's head (Fig P–42). Infants, preschool, and school-age children may tolerate this appliance. Toddlers will usually pull the cannula off their face. A face mask or blow-by tubing is often a more appropriate method of oxygen administration for this age group.

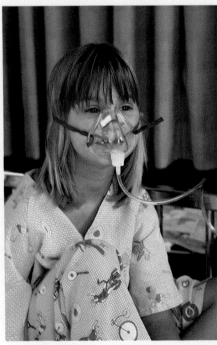

FIGURE P–41 Simple face mask.

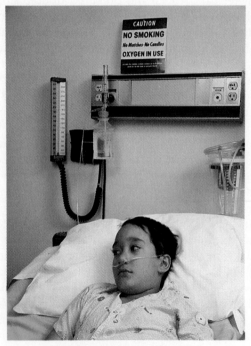

FIGURE P–42 Nasal cannula.

Tent

An oxygen tent (Fig. P–43), in theory, allows for delivery of 50% humidified oxygen, but in practice only 30% humidified oxygen can be achieved. Concentration should be determined with an oxygen analyzer. To avoid air leakage, secure the edges of the tent with blankets.

Access to and visual assessment of the child are difficult when an oxygen tent is used. The child may feel confined, isolated from his or her parents, or claustrophobic when in the tent. The child may respond more favorably to using the mask when awake and the tent while asleep.

Blow-by Cannula

A blow-by cannula may be either a narrow oxygen catheter with small perforations through which oxygen can flow or corrugated oxygen tubing. This device is used when the child will not tolerate other means of oxygen therapy and when low oxygen concentrations with humidification are needed. The parent can hold the child in his or her lap and direct the tubing toward the child's face, moving it as the child moves. This technique reduces the child's anxiety and helps the parent meet the needs of the child.

In the ICU the blow-by method can be used for young infants (Fig. P–44).

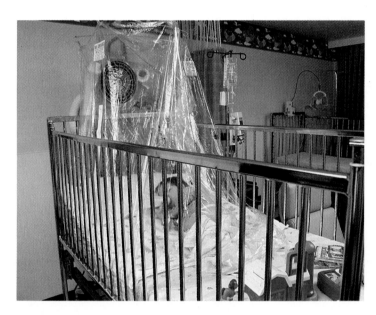

FIGURE P–43 Oxygen tent.

FIGURE P–44 Blow-by cannula.

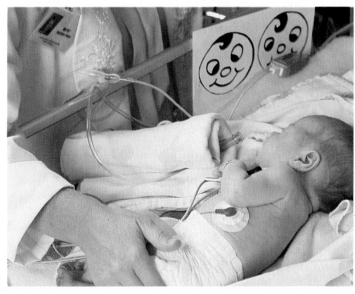

Oropharyngeal Airway

The oropharyngeal airway is commonly used to maintain an airway in children who are unconscious. It is made of plastic and consists of three parts: a flange, a small bite block, and a curved body.

This type of airway is designed to keep the tongue of an unconscious child from falling into the posterior pharynx. It is *never* used for a conscious infant or child because its insertion might stimulate the gag reflex or vomiting.

Pediatric sizes range from 4 to 10 cm in length. It is important that the airway be the correct size. If it is too large, it may obstruct the larynx. If it is too small, it will push the tongue into the posterior pharynx and obstruct the airway. The proper size can be estimated by placing the airway alongside the child's face with the bite block parallel to the hard palate and the flange at the level of the central incisors. The distal end of the airway should reach the angle of the jaw.

An oropharyngeal airway is usually inserted by the physician. The child should be assessed closely during the procedure and suction should be available. Once the airway is in place, the child's head and jaw must be maintained in a neutral position.

Nasopharyngeal Airway

The nasopharyngeal airway provides a passage for air between the tongue and the posterior pharyngeal wall. It is used for a conscious child.

This type of airway is made of soft plastic or rubber and comes in various sizes. The length of the tube is determined by measuring the distance from the tip of the nose to the tragus of the ear. The width must allow for passage through the nares.

The tip of the airway should be lubricated with a water-soluble gel and inserted into the nares in a posterior direction. During insertion, observe for bleeding, which may exacerbate the obstruction and further compromise airway management.

Tracheostomy

A tracheostomy is a surgical procedure in which an opening is made in the trachea to create an airway. It can be performed as an acute life-saving procedure or for management of the child with a chronic disease.

The child with a tracheostomy needs careful observation. Vital signs and respiratory status, including breath sounds, respiratory effort, and airway patency should be routinely checked. Be alert for changes in heart or respiratory rate, blood pressure, color, or level of consciousness.

A neonatal or pediatric tracheostomy tube is made of plastic and has an obturator used for insertion only. The tube is held in place with twill tape tied around the child's neck.

A resuscitation bag, oxygen, and suctioning equipment must be kept at the bedside. Have two prepared tracheostomy tubes ready, one that is the size of the child's current tube and one that is the next size smaller, in case of accidental dislodgment. (See the procedure for tracheostomy care.)

Tracheostomy Collar

The child usually wears a tracheostomy collar (Fig. P–45) ("mist collar") at the stoma site to keep the airway warm and moist. The collar may emit either oxygen or room air, depending on the physician's orders. Watch for condensation in the oxygen tubing and empty it regularly; otherwise, the fluid may drip into the tracheostomy tube, causing the child to aspirate.

When the child is in a crib, put the tubing through, rather than over, the bars to prevent fluid from entering the tracheostomy.

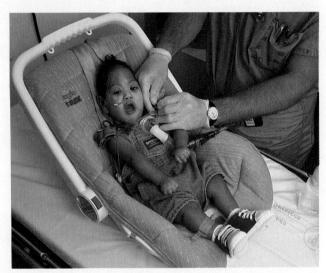

FIGURE P–45 Infant with tracheostomy collar.

Tracheostomy Care

Tracheostomy care is usually performed once per shift. *Always* have an assistant present while doing any tracheostomy care.

Selected Equipment

Towel roll
Precut twill tape
Cotton-tipped applicators (saturated with half-strength hydrogen peroxide)

Cotton-tipped applicators saturated with normal saline
Gauze pads (some moistened with saline and others dry)
Scissors
Suction tray and catheters

This equipment is usually available in a prepackaged kit. Prepared tracheostomy tubes, oxygen, resuscitation bag, and suction tray with catheters should be at the bedside.

Preparation

Have your assistant stand on the opposite side of the bed. Put a towel roll under the child's neck to hyperextend the head.

Procedure

- To make new ties, use two pieces of twill tape. Fold over one end of each piece lengthwise for approximately 1 to 1½ inches. Cut a small hole in the folded area.
- Have your assistant hold the tube in place. Remove the present tape from the flange.
- Attach the twill tape to the flange by first threading the end with the slit through the hole. Place the distal end of the twill tape through the slit and pull it securely.
- Have your assistant repeat this step on the opposite side.
- Put on sterile gloves. Using cotton-tip applicators saturated with half-strength hydrogen peroxide, clean under the tracheostomy at the stoma (Fig. P–46). Rinse the stoma with saline applicators. Wash the area behind the flanges of the tracheostomy and around the neck with damp gauze, observing for redness or skin breakdown. Dry thoroughly.

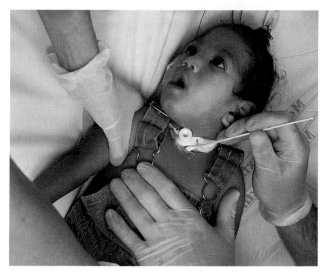

FIGURE P–46 Cleaning of tracheostomy tube.

- Hold the tube while your assistant performs the same care on the opposite side.
- With the tube held in place, tie the tape. The best fit is achieved when the child's neck is slightly flexed. The tape should be tied tightly enough to prevent dislodgment but should still be loose enough so that you can fit one finger between it and the neck. Double-knot or triple-knot the tape for security. Do not place the knot at the back of the neck, since this might cause skin breakdown if the child is supine.

Endotracheal Tube

Endotracheal (ET) tubes are sterile, disposable, and made of a translucent plastic or other synthetic material. The distal end is tapered and has an opening in the side wall (Murphy's eye). The length of the tube is marked in centimeters to serve as a measurement reference point once it is in place. Intubation is usually performed by the physician to protect or maintain the child's airway.

The tubes come in various sizes, both with and without cuffs (Fig. P–47). The uncuffed tube is recommended for the child less than 8 or 9 years old, since the airway is narrowest at the cricoid ring, sealing the airway effectively without a cuff.

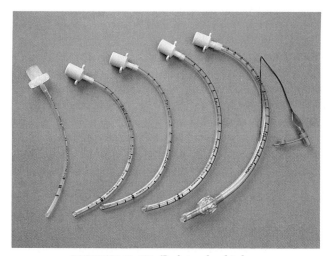

FIGURE P–47 Endotracheal tubes.

The size of the tube can be approximated by comparing it with the diameter of the child's little finger or nares. The formula used for children older than 2 years of age is:

$$\frac{16 + \text{Age in years}}{4} = \text{Size of ET tube}$$

A 3.0 or 3.5 ET tube can usually be used in the full-term newborn. A 4.0 ET tube can be used until the child's first birthday.

Once the tube has been placed by the physician, check for equal breath sounds, symmetry of chest movement, and condensation in the tube. Auscultate over the abdomen to ensure that the tube is not in the esophagus. Listen at the trachea for air leaks. Once correct tube placement is verified, note the centimeter marking at the lip or tooth line and tape the tube in place.

Continuously assess breath sounds, color, heart rate on the monitor, and pulse oximeter readout.

Ventilator

Ventilators are used for children who need assistance in breathing. These children may have a chronic condition, such as neuromuscular disease or persistent lung pathology, or may be acutely ill or injured and need emergency management of ventilation.

To safely provide care for the ventilated child:

1. Be familiar with the ventilator and know which settings have been ordered by the physician, including oxygen concentration, humidity, air temperature, pressure, tidal volume, and inspiratory/expiratory ratio and rate. Identify what the alarms mean, and know how to trouble-shoot problems.
2. Ensure that the child is attached to a cardiorespiratory monitor and pulse oximeter. Always keep a resuscitation bag and mask at the bedside. Oxygen and suction, along with appropriate-size catheters, should also be at hand.
3. Measure arterial blood gases within 15 minutes after the child has been placed on the ventilator and thereafter according to the physician's orders. Assess vital signs every hour, including heart and respiratory rates, blood pressure, temperature, and pulse oximeter reading. Auscultate the lungs in all fields to assess for equal breath sounds. Ensure that the respiratory rate is consistent with the ventilator setting.
4. Suction the ET tube as necessary. Disconnect the ventilator, oxygenate the child once or twice with a resuscitation bag, instill a small amount (1 to 2 mL) of sterile normal saline into the ET tube, apply the bag again, suction for no more than 5 to 10 seconds while watching the heart rate on the monitor and pulse oximeter readout, oxygenate again, and reconnect the ventilator.
5. Protect the ET tube by making sure it is well taped and secure. Support the ventilator tubing to decrease traction on the ET tube by attaching the tubing directly to the bed using a gauze roll and a safety pin. The child may need to have elbow splints applied to prevent him or her from pulling out the tube. Acutely ill or injured children may need to be chemically paralyzed and sedated while

on the ventilator. If the child has been given paralytics, watch for signs that further sedation may be needed (for example, a rise in heart rate and blood pressure or tearing).
6. Listen and look for air leaks. Make sure that the ventilator is firmly attached to the ET tube.
7. Check the reservoir for humidification at least every 8 hours. Refill or replace water as needed. Watch for condensation in the tubing and empty it regularly; otherwise the fluid may drip into the ET tube, causing the child to aspirate.
8. Insert a nasogastric or orogastric tube to keep the child's abdomen decompressed. Check its placement.
9. Tell the child what you are planning to do; for example, "I'm going to wash your face" or "I'm going to move your arms and legs." The child who is sedated or unresponsive may still be able to hear.
10. Support the family by answering their questions. Encourage them to communicate with the child. Have them bring in audio tapes of favorite music or of family members speaking to the child.

Cardiopulmonary Resuscitation*

Cardiopulmonary resuscitation (CPR) is basic life support using techniques to maintain airway, breathing, and circulation (the ABCs). Lay people are routinely taught one-person basic life support. Health care professionals should be skilled in both one- and two-person CPR. The following is the sequence of resuscitation interventions designated by the American Heart Association and the American Academy of Pediatrics.

Infant

Unresponsiveness

Unresponsiveness can be determined by gently tapping the infant on the abdomen or soles of the feet. If the infant does not respond, begin basic life support (BLS).

Provide BLS for 1 minute *before* activating the emergency medical services.

Airway Assessment

Make sure that the airway is patent. Oftentimes, if the infant is unconscious, the tongue will slip into the posterior hypopharynx and cause obstruction. The head needs to be maintained in a neutral position to keep the airway clear. The airway can be opened by using one of two maneuvers:

*Based on Pediatric Basic Life Support (1992). *Journal of the American Medical Association, 268*(16), 2251–2261.

Head Tilt–Chin Lift (Fig. P–48). Place one hand on the infant's forehead to gently tilt the head back into a neutral position. *Do not* hyperextend the neck. Place the fingers of your other hand on the bony prominence of the chin and lift the jaw upward and outward.

Jaw Thrust (Fig. P–49). Standing behind the child's head, place two or three fingers under each side of the jaw at its angle. Lift the jaw upward and outward. This maneuver is performed on all children suspected of having cervical spine injury.

Breathing Assessment

After the airway has been opened, determine whether the infant is breathing (Fig. P–50). Check for the rise and fall of the chest and abdomen, and listen and feel for the flow of expelled air at the mouth.

If no spontaneous breathing is detected, begin rescue breathing, maintaining airway patency by using the head tilt–chin lift or the jaw thrust maneuver.

Mouth-to-Mouth Resuscitation (Fig. P–51). Take a deep breath. Place your mouth over the nose and mouth of the infant to create a tight seal. Give two slow breaths, each lasting 1 to 1½ seconds. After giving the first breath, pause to take a breath to maximize the oxygen content that you can deliver.

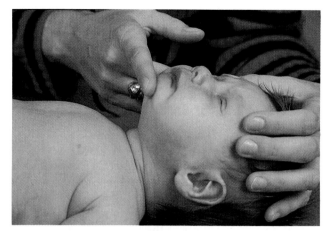

FIGURE P–48 Head tilt–chin lift maneuver.

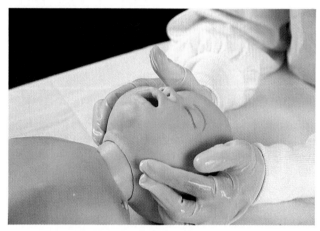

FIGURE P–49 Jaw thrust maneuver.

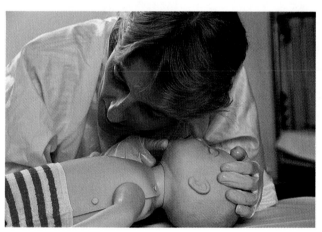

FIGURE P–50 Assessing breathing.

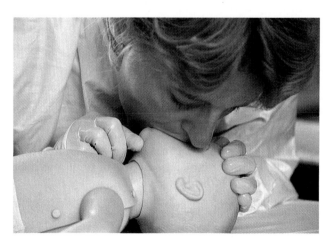

FIGURE P–51 Mouth-to-mouth resuscitation.

Bag and Mask Resuscitation (Fig. P–52). The mask should extend from the bridge of the nose to the cleft of the chin, and should not cover the eyes. A tight seal must be maintained. The bag, with an attached reservoir and hooked up to 100% oxygen, must be the proper size for the infant, usually between 250 mL for the newborn and 500 mL for the older infant. Two breaths are given initially.

Special Considerations. The volume of air, delivered either by mouth-to-mouth or bag and mask resuscitation, should be just enough to produce a visible chest rise. If the chest does not rise, the airway may no longer be patent and the position of the head needs to be readjusted or the breath volume needs to be increased.

Remember that gastric distention can occur with either mouth-to-mouth or bag and mask rescue breathing. This distention compromises ventilation by elevating the diaphragm and decreasing lung size. It may also stimulate vomiting.

Circulation

Once the airway has been opened and two breaths have been given, assess circulation by checking for a brachial pulse (Fig. P–53). The brachial pulse lies on the inside of the upper arm, between the shoulder and the elbow. Assess for 10 seconds before determining pulselessness. If a pulse is palpated, perform rescue breathing every 3 seconds (20 times per minute). If no pulse is felt, begin chest compressions, delivering ventilations between every 5 compressions (Fig. P–54).

Position the infant on a hard surface, with the head in a neutral position to ensure airway patency. (The rescuer may hold the infant, using one arm as the surface.)

- Apply compressions to the lower third of the sternum, which can be located by placing your index finger at the intermammary line and then putting the middle and ring fingers next to it. Keep your other hand on the infant's head to maintain airway patency.
- With 2 or 3 fingers, compress the chest ½ to 1 inch (or approximately one third to one half the depth of the chest) at a rate of at least 100 compressions per minute. With the pause for ventilations, this method will equal about 80 compressions per minute. At the end of each compression, allow the chest to return to the normal position before beginning the next compression.
- Rescue breaths and compressions are performed at a ratio of 1:5 with a pause for ventilations for both one- and two-rescuer CPR.
- Reassess the infant after 20 cycles (one "CPR minute"). Palpate the brachial pulse for 5 seconds. If the pulse is absent, continue the cycle for another 3 to 5 minutes before reassessment.

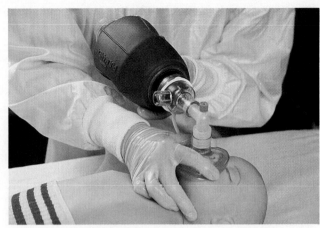

FIGURE P–52 Bag and mask resuscitation.

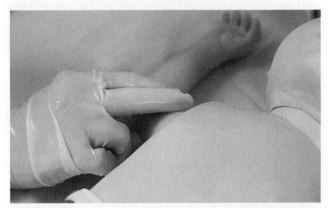

FIGURE P–53 Checking for brachial pulse.

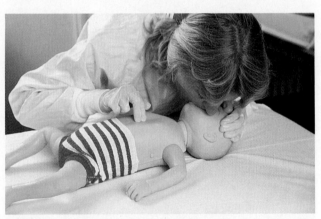

FIGURE P–54 Alternating breathing and chest compressions.

- If the infant has a pulse but is not breathing, continue rescue breathing at a rate of 20 times per minute (once every 3 seconds).
- If the infant has a return of both pulse and respirations and is *not* a trauma victim, place the infant in the "recovery" (side-lying) position. This position is used to protect the airway.

Child Between 1 and 8 Years

Unresponsiveness

Unresponsiveness can be determined by gently tapping the child and speaking loudly enough to get a response. If the child does not respond, begin BLS.

Provide BLS for 1 minute *before* activating the emergency medical services.

Airway and Breathing Assessment

In general, airway and breathing assessment for the child between 1 and 8 years is the same as for the infant.

Mouth-to-Mouth Resuscitation with Mask. Rescue breathing can be performed using a mask with a one-way valve. This method provides an infection-control barrier (Fig. P–55).

Place the mask over the child's nose and mouth, creating a tight seal. Take a deep breath. Give two slow breaths, each lasting 1 to 1½ seconds. After giving the first breath, pause to take a breath to maximize the oxygen content that you are delivering.

Bag and Mask Resuscitation. The mask should be the correct size, extending from the bridge of the nose to the cleft of the chin, and should not cover the eyes. A tight seal must be maintained. The bag, with an attached reservoir and hooked up to 100% oxygen, must be the proper size for the child. Two breaths are given initially.

Special Considerations. The volume of air, either by mouth-to-mask or bag and mask resuscitation, should be just enough to produce a visible chest rise. If the chest does not rise, either the airway is no longer patent and the position of the head needs to be readjusted or the breath volume increased.

Remember that gastric distention can occur with either mouth-to-mask or bag and mask rescue breathing. This distention compromises ventilation by elevating the diaphragm and decreasing lung size. It may also stimulate vomiting.

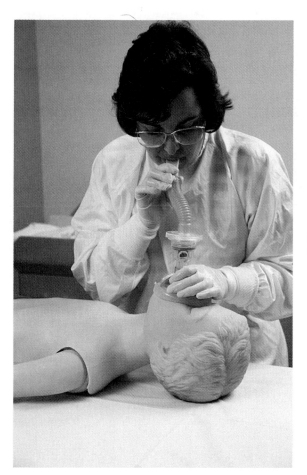

FIGURE P–55 Mouth-to-mouth resuscitation using a mask with a one-way valve.

Circulation

Once the airway has been opened and two breaths have been given, assess circulation by checking for a carotid pulse (Fig. P–56). The carotid pulse lies on the side of the neck between the trachea and the sternocleidomastoid muscle. Assess for 10 seconds before determining pulselessness. If a pulse is palpated, perform rescue breathing every 3 seconds (20 times per minute). If no pulse is felt, begin chest compressions, delivering ventilations between every 5 compressions.

Position the child on a hard surface, with the head in a neutral position to ensure airway patency.

- Apply compressions to the lower third of the sternum while positioned at the child's side.
- Using the middle and index fingers of the hand closest to the child's feet, trace the lower margin of the child's ribs to the notch where the ribs and the sternum meet. Place your middle finger on this notch, and put the index finger adjacent to it on the sternum. Place the heel of one hand on the sternum next to the point where the index finger was located (Fig. P–57). Make sure to keep your fingers off the chest.

- Using the heel of one hand, compress the chest 1 to 1½ inches (approximately one third to one half the depth of the chest) (Fig. P–58) 100 times per minute. With the pause for ventilations, this method will equal about 80 compressions per minute. At the end of each compression, allow the chest to return to the normal position before beginning the next compression. Maintain the head tilt during this time with your other hand.
- Rescue breaths and compressions are performed at a ratio of 1:5 with a pause for ventilations for both one- and two-rescuer CPR.
- Reassess the child after 20 cycles or one "CPR minute." Palpate the carotid pulse for 5 seconds. If the pulse is absent, continue the cycle for another 3 to 5 minutes before reassessment.
- If the child has a pulse but is not breathing, continue rescue breathing at a rate of 20 times per minute (once every 3 seconds).
- If the child has a return of both pulse and respirations and is *not* a trauma victim, place the child in the "recovery" (side-lying) position. This position is used to protect the airway.

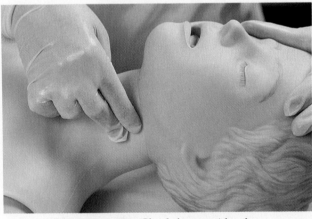

FIGURE P–56 Check for carotid pulse.

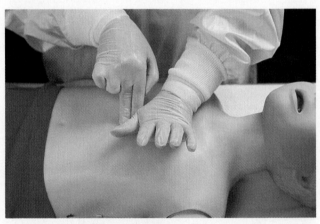

FIGURE P–57 Locating site of chest compressions.

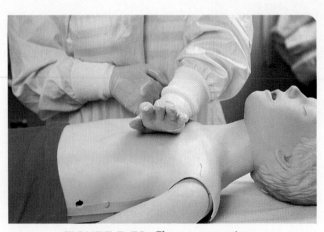

FIGURE P–58 Chest compressions.

Foreign Body Airway Obstruction

Signs and symptoms of airway obstruction may be caused by respiratory disorders (e.g., croup or epiglottitis) or a foreign body.

Attempts to clear the airway should be made in the following situations:

1. *For the witnessed or strongly suspected aspiration of a foreign body.* Encourage the child to continue coughing and breathing as long as the cough is forceful. If the cough becomes ineffective and soundless, if increased respiratory difficulty or stridor is noted, or if the victim loses consciousness, the emergency medical services system must be activated and attempts must be made to remove the obstruction.
2. *When the airway remains obstructed during attempts to provide rescue breathing.*

Infant

Unconscious Infant

- If an infant is found unconscious, begin assessment by using the ABCs.
- If the infant is not breathing, try to ventilate either by mouth-to-mouth resuscitation or with a bag and mask (see CPR guidelines for rescue breathing).
- If the airway is obstructed, reposition the infant's head and attempt to ventilate again.
- If the airway is still obstructed, do not check for the pulse. Instead, perform up to 5 back blows (Fig. P–59), followed by up to 5 chest thrusts with the fingers in the same position used for CPR (Fig. P–60). Then, using a tongue-jaw lift (place index finger on bony prominence of chin and thumb in mouth on tongue; pull up and out to open mouth), look in the infant's mouth for the foreign body and remove it if seen. *Do not* perform a blind sweep. If no object is found, try to ventilate the infant again. If the obstruction is still present, reposition the infant's head and attempt to ventilate once again.
- If the obstruction remains, begin another series of back blows and chest thrusts. Look in the mouth, try to ventilate, reposition the head, and attempt to ventilate again. Continue with this pattern until the airway is clear.
- Once the airway is clear, give two slow full breaths. Check for a pulse. At this point, provide whatever BLS maneuvers are necessary.

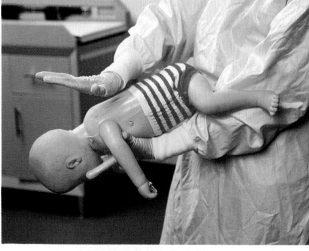

FIGURE P–59 Back blows.

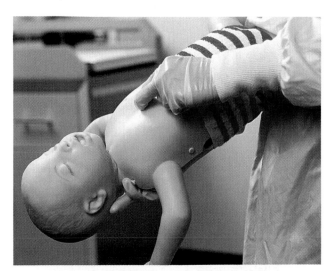

FIGURE P–60 Chest thrusts.

Child Between 1 and 8 Years*

Conscious Child

- Perform abdominal thrusts (Heimlich maneuver) (Fig. P–61) with the child either sitting or standing.
- Stand behind the child, with your arms under the child's axilla and around the chest. Place the thumb of one fist against the abdomen in the midline, below the xiphoid and above the navel. Grasp your fist with your other hand.
- Deliver up to 5 quick upward thrusts. Each thrust should be a distinct effort to remove the obstruction. The series of 5 thrusts should be repeated until the obstruction is cleared or the child becomes unconscious.

Unconscious Child

The child should be placed in a supine position with the rescuer straddling the child at the hips.

- Assess for breathing. If the child is not breathing, try to ventilate either by mouth-to-mouth resuscitation or with a bag and mask (see CPR guidelines for rescue breathing). If the airway is still obstructed, reposition the child's head and attempt to ventilate again.
- If the airway is still obstructed, do not check for a pulse. Instead, place the heel of your hand on the child's abdomen in the midline, between the xiphoid and navel; then place your other hand over the wrist (Fig. P–62). Press into the abdomen, using both hands in quick upward strokes, and deliver up to 5 thrusts. Each thrust should be a distinct attempt to eliminate the obstruction.

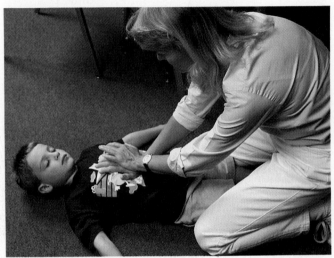

FIGURE P–62 Performing abdominal thrusts on an unconscious child.

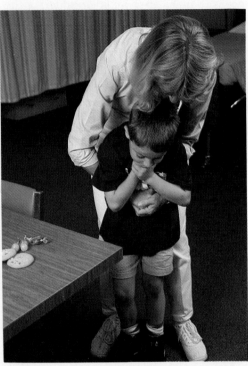

FIGURE P–61 Abdominal thrusts (Heimlich maneuver).

- Using the tongue-jaw lift, look into the mouth for a foreign body and remove it if seen. *Do not* perform a blind sweep. If a foreign body is not visualized, open the airway and attempt to ventilate. If the airway is still obstructed, reposition the child's head and attempt to ventilate once again.
- If the obstruction remains, begin another series of abdominal thrusts, look in the mouth, try to ventilate, reposition the head, and attempt to ventilate again. Continue with this pattern until the airway is clear.
- Once the airway is clear, give two slow full breaths. Check for a pulse. At this point, provide whatever BLS maneuvers are necessary.

---

*In the hospital setting, clean gloves are worn for this procedure.

Suctioning

The nose, mouth, tracheostomy tube, or endotracheal tube may require suctioning. It is important to obtain baseline vital signs before and after the procedure. When suctioning, watch for a decrease in pulse rate, an increase or decrease in respiratory rate, or a change in color. Bradycardia may be a sign of vagal stimulation. If any of these signs occur, stop immediately and give the child oxygen using blow-by, face mask, or resuscitation bag.

The size of the suction catheter depends on the size, age, and weight of the child or on the tube requiring suctioning. Usually a tonsil-tip or Yankauer catheter is used for oral suctioning when copious, thick secretions need to be removed.

Have an assistant gently restrain the child to keep the child's hands out of the way. Your assistant will need to keep the child's head in the midline position. The intubated child is frequently sedated.

A gown, goggles, and mask or face shield should be worn by the nurse for protection.

Nasal/Oral Suctioning

The nose and mouth are suctioned when excess secretions are present or when a decreased level of consciousness interferes with the child's ability to clear normal secretions.

Infant

A bulb syringe is used to remove secretions from an infant's nose or mouth. Care needs to be taken to avoid stimulating the gag reflex.

Procedure
- Deflate bulb.
- Insert the tip of the bulb syringe into the infant's naris (Fig. P–63).
- Release the bulb and remove the syringe from the naris (Fig. P–64).
- Expel the secretions into the proper receptacle.
- Repeat as necessary.

Conscious Child: Awake and Alert

Preparation

Have an assistant help you maintain the child's head in the midline position. The head of the bed should be raised to 30 to 45 degrees. Turn on and set the wall suction to the level ordered by the physician or suggested in your facility's procedure manual.

Procedure
- With your dominant hand, insert the suction catheter into the child's naris and suction for no more than 5 to 10 seconds, gently rotating the catheter. (The depth of insertion depends on the size of the child.)
- Remove and irrigate the catheter.
- Repeat as necessary.

The mouth may also be suctioned for secretions, but care needs to be taken to avoid stimulating the gag reflex.

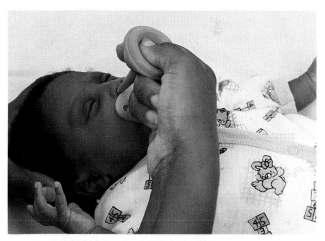

FIGURE P–63 Insertion of bulb syringe.

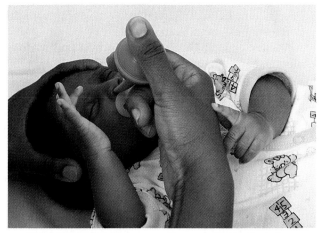

FIGURE P–64 Release and removal of bulb syringe.

Child with Decreased Level of Consciousness

The child with a decreased level of consciousness will likely require deep suctioning to remove secretions.

Preparation

Depending on the level of consciousness noted, you may need an assistant to help maintain the child's head in the midline position. The head of the bed should be raised to 30 to 45 degrees. Turn on and set the wall suction to the level ordered by the physician or suggested in your facility's procedure manual.

Procedure

- Place an oxygen mask on the child's face.
- If possible, encourage the child to cough to make the secretions pool in the hypopharynx.
- Attach the proximal end of the catheter to the wall suction connecting tubing, making sure to keep the distal end sterile.
- Put a sterile glove on the dominant hand and a clean glove on the nondominant hand. Use only the dominant hand to manipulate the catheter.
- Remove the protective sheath from the catheter, and test the suction by placing it in a cup of saline.
- Remove the oxygen mask.

NASAL/ORAL SUCTIONING

- With your dominant hand, insert the catheter into naris or mouth without occluding the suction port.
- Slowly advance the catheter only into the hypopharynx.
- Rotate the catheter, applying intermittent suction.
- Remove the catheter and clear the tubing with sterile saline. Repeat as necessary.

DEEP SUCTIONING

- With your dominant hand, insert the catheter beyond the hypopharynx and into the trachea (the length advanced is determined by the size of the child). *Do not* occlude the suction port.
- When the catheter is in place, gently rotate it during intermittent suction. To prevent hypoxia, *do not* suction for more than 5 to 10 seconds.
- Allow the child to breath normally, and give supplemental oxygen between suctionings.
- Remove the catheter and clear the tubing with sterile saline. Repeat as necessary.

Tracheostomy Tube Suctioning

Preparation

Have the following equipment at the bedside: additional prepared tracheostomy tubes (see the description under tracheostomy care, earlier), resuscitation bag with attached oxygen source, and suction. Place the head of the bed at a 30-degree angle.

Turn on and set the wall suction to the level ordered by the physician or suggested in your facility's procedure manual. Turn on the oxygen source attached to the resuscitation bag to inflate the reservoir bag so it is ready to use.

Procedure

- Put a sterile glove on the dominant hand and a clean glove on the nondominant hand. Use only the dominant hand to manipulate the catheter.
- With your dominant hand, remove the catheter from the paper sheath, keeping it sterile.
- With your nondominant hand, connect the proximal end of the catheter to wall suction connecting tubing.
- Place the distal end of the catheter in a cup of sterile saline to test the suction.
- With your nondominant hand, remove the humidity source from the child's tracheostomy tube. Oxygenate the child before suctioning, using your nondominant hand. Give several breaths.
- Remove the resuscitation bag.
- Using your dominant hand, place the suction catheter into the tube, making sure no suction is being applied at this time. Advance the catheter no farther than 0.5 cm below the edge of the tracheostomy tube.
- Once the catheter is in place, intermittently cover the suction port and rotate the catheter (Fig. P–65).
- Remove the catheter and irrigate it in a cup of sterile saline. To prevent the child from becoming hypoxic, *do not* suction for longer than 5 to 10 seconds.
- Repeat as necessary, oxygenating between suctionings.

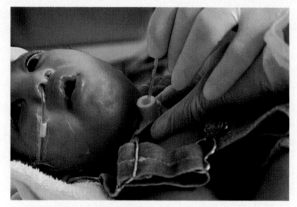

FIGURE P–65 Tracheostomy tube suctioning.

Endotracheal Tube Suctioning

Use extreme care when handling the ET during procedures such as suctioning to avoid dislodging the tube unintentionally. Hold the tube firmly in place while the ventilator is being disconnected, when the resuscitation bag is being attached and removed, during hyperventilation, and during suctioning.

Preparation

Turn on and set the wall suction to the level ordered by the physician or suggested in your facility's procedure manual. Turn on the oxygen source attached to the resuscitation bag to inflate the reservoir bag so it is ready for use.

Procedure

- Put a sterile glove on the dominant hand and a clean glove on the nondominant hand. Use only the dominant hand to manipulate the catheter.
- With your dominant hand, remove the catheter from the paper sheath, keeping it sterile.
- With your nondominant hand, connect the proximal end of the catheter to the wall suction connecting tubing. Place the distal end of the catheter in a cup of sterile saline to test the suction pressure.
- If the child is being ventilated, have an assistant disconnect the ventilator and manually oxygenate the child before suctioning. Give several breaths.
- Remove the resuscitation bag.
- With your dominant hand, place the suction catheter into the ET tube, making sure that no suction is being applied at this time. Advance the catheter no farther than 0.5 cm below the edge of the ET tube. Before inserting the catheter, determine how far the suction catheter can be advanced by making a visual comparison of the airway and the ET tube length.
- Once the catheter is in place, intermittently cover the suction port and rotate the catheter.
- Remove the catheter and irrigate it in a cup of sterile saline. To prevent the child from becoming hypoxic, *do not* suction for longer than 5 to 10 seconds.
- Repeat as necessary, oxygenating the child between suctionings.

If secretions are thick, sterile saline (usually 0.5 to 2 mL) may be instilled and then suctioned.

▥ Chest Physiotherapy/Postural Drainage

In postural drainage, positioning is used to take advantage of gravity in the drainage of secretions. Specific lung areas are drained by gravity, with mucus moving from the affected bronchioles into the bronchi and trachea.

The drainage procedures are usually done before the morning meal, and again at bedtime if the child is subject to nighttime mucus retention, plugging of airways, and/or coughing. With certain conditions, such as cystic fibrosis, drainage is often done before each meal and before bedtime. Bronchodilators are frequently administered by hand nebulizer, intermittent positive pressure breathing (IPPB), or metered-dose aerosols before drainage is performed.

Chest physiotherapy is important for children who have excessive sputum production or retained bronchial secretions. During postural drainage, two maneuvers can be done to aid in drainage: percussion and vibration (see Fig. 10–12).

Percussion

Percussion is performed by clapping the chest wall with cupped hands. This action produces chest vibrations that dislodge retained secretions.

- Cup your hands, holding your fingers together so that the contour of your cupped hand conforms with the chest wall. Keep your wrists loose and flexible, and clap the area with the palm of your hand. Listen for a hollow sound. Alternate hands, clapping the area in a rhythmic pattern for 3 to 5 minutes.
- Alternatively, you can use a round oxygen mask, a baby bottle cap (use only for infants), or a manufactured percussor. Tap the area with the appliance for 3 to 5 minutes.
- Encourage the child to take a deep breath and to cough after percussion.

Vibration

Vibration is the application of a downward vibrating pressure with the flat part of the palm over the area that is being drained. This maneuver is done only during exhalation.
- Tell the child to take deep breaths, inhaling through the nose and exhaling through the mouth.
- Place one of your hands on top of the other on the designated area, keeping your arms and shoulders straight. Vibrate the area by tensing and relaxing your arms for 10 to 15 seconds. Perform these tensing/relaxing actions for 10 to 15 minutes.
- Encourage coughing between vibrations.

After completion, reassess the child's vital signs and respiratory status, noting any changes.

Procedure and Positioning

- Perform a baseline respiratory assessment.
- Place the child in the recommended position and maintain that position for 10 to 15 minutes. (The positions used for each patient are based on the location of mucous obstruction. In generalized obstructive lung disease, the lower lobes are drained first, followed by the middle lobes and lingula, and the upper lobes are drained last. The various positions used for bronchial drainage in a child are described in Table P–3).
- Encourage the child to cough up any sputum.
- Return the child to a normal position.

TABLE P-3 Positions Used for Postural Drainage of the Child

Bronchopulmonary Segments

LOCATION	NO.	COLOR KEY
Right Upper Lobe		
Apical	1	Red ▲
Anterior	2	Light blue ▲
Posterior	3	Green ▲
Right Middle Lobe		
Lateral	4	Purple ▲
Medial	5	Orange ▲
Right Lower Lobe		
Superior	6	Lavender ▲
Medial basal	7	Olive ▲
Anterior basal	8	Yellow ▲
Lateral basal	9	Red ▲
Posterior basal	10	Turquoise ▲
Left Upper Lobe		
Upper apical—		
posterior	1	Red ▲
Anterior	2	Light blue ▲
Lower—lingular		
Superior	4	Purple ▲
Inferior	5	Orange ▲
Left Lower Lobe		
Superior	6	Lavender ▲
Anteromedial	8	Yellow ▲
Lateral basal	9	Red ▲
Posterior basal	10	Turquoise ▲

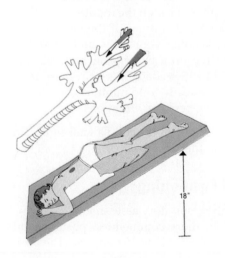

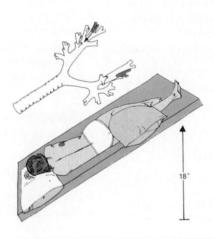

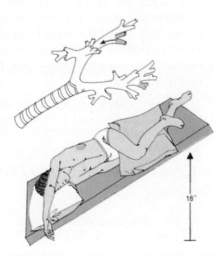

Lower Lobes

▲ *Posterior Basal Segment (10)*

Elevate foot of table or bed 18 inches or 30 degrees. Have child lie prone, head down, with pillow under hips. Upper leg can be flexed over a pillow for support. (Percuss over lower ribs close to spine on each side of chest.)

▲ *Lateral Basal Segment (9)*

Elevate foot of table or bed 18 inches or 30 degrees. Have child lie prone, then rotate ¼ turn upward. Upper leg can be flexed over a pillow for support. (Percuss over uppermost portion of lower ribs.)

▲ *Anterior Basal Segment (8)*

Elevate foot of table or bed 18 inches or 30 degrees. Have child lie on side, head down, pillow under knees. (Percuss over lower ribs just beneath axilla.)

Modified from material provided by Datalizer Slide Charts, Addison, IL.

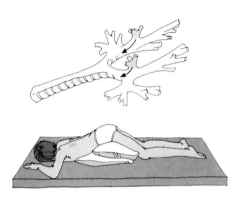

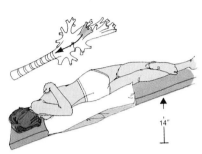

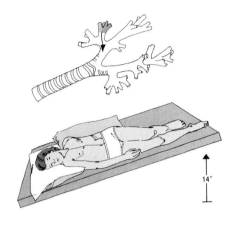

Lower Lobes—cont'd
▲ *Superior Segment (6)*

Place bed or table flat. Have child lie with pillows under hips. (Percuss over middle of back below tip of scapula on either side of spine.)

Right Middle Lobe
▲ *Lateral Segment (4)*
▲ *Medial Segment (5)*

Elevate foot of table or bed 14 inches or about 15 degrees. Have child lie head down on left side and rotate ¼ turn backward. Pillow may be placed behind child from shoulder to hip. Knees should be flexed. (Percuss over right nipple area.)

Left Upper Lobe
▲ *Lingular Segment-Superior (4)*
▲ *Inferior (5)*

Elevate foot of table or bed 14 inches or about 15 degrees. Have child lie head down on right side and rotate ¼ turn backward. Pillow may be placed behind child from shoulder to hip. Knees should be flexed. (Percuss over left nipple area.)

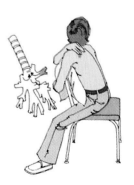

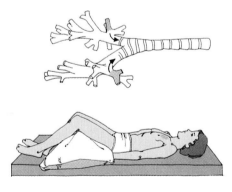

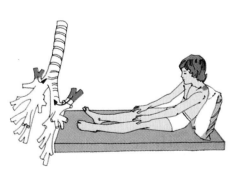

Upper Lobes
▲ *Posterior Segment (3)*

Have child sit up and lean over folded pillow at 30-degree angle. (Percuss over upper back on each side of chest.)

▲ *Anterior Segment (2)*

Place bed or drainage table flat. Have child lie supine with pillow under knees. (Percuss between clavicle and nipple on each side of chest.)

▲ *Apical Segment (1)*

Place bed or drainage table flat. Have child lean back on pillow at 30-degree angle. (Percuss over area between clavicle and top of scapula on each side of chest.)

Procedure for Infant

Lower Lobes

Posterior basal segment:
- Place the infant prone on a pillow on your lap.
- Percuss and vibrate the back at the lower ribs.

Lateral basal segment:
- Place the infant prone on a pillow on your lap at a 30-degree angle.
- Rotate the infant's body slightly so that one side is elevated.
- Percuss and vibrate over the lower ribs.
- Turn and repeat.

Anterior basal segment:
- Extend your legs and keep them slightly flexed (use a chair for support).
- Place the infant, supported on a pillow, in a side-lying position (30-degree angle) with the head down.
- Percuss and vibrate the area over the ribs under the axilla.
- Turn and repeat.

Superior segment:
- Place the infant prone on a pillow on your lap.
- Percuss and vibrate the back.

Upper Lobes

Lateral and medial segments:
- Place the infant on your lap in the prone position.
- Rotate the infant slightly so that the right side is elevated.
- Percuss and vibrate the anterior chest at the nipple.
- Turn the infant and repeat.

Posterior segment:
- Place the infant on your lap in a sitting position and leaning forward on a pillow at about a 30-degree angle.
- Percuss and vibrate both sides of the upper back.

Anterior segment:
- Place the infant supine on your lap.
- Percuss and vibrate the area between the clavicle and the midchest at the nipple line.

Apical segment:
- Place the infant on your lap in a sitting position. Lower the infant to a 30-degree reclining position, using a pillow for support.
- Percuss and vibrate the area between the clavicles and the scapulae.

▉ Placement of ECG Electrodes

The electrocardiogram is a graphic representation of the electricity produced by the heart muscle. The equipment needed is a 12-lead ECG recorder and patches (or suction cups with conductive gel).

Procedure

Electrodes are placed both on the chest and limbs in the following manner.

Chest Leads

V_1—4th intercostal space to right of sternum
V_2—4th intercostal space to left of sternum
V_3—midway between V_2 and V_4
V_4—5th left intercostal space at midclavicular line
V_5—5th left intercostal space at anterior axillary line (midway between V_4 and V_6)
V_6—5th left intercostal space at midaxillary line

Limb Electrodes

Electrodes are placed on the upper extremities slightly above the wrists and on the lower extremities just above the ankles.

NUTRITION

▉ Gastric Tubes

Gastric tubes are used in infants and children to provide a means of alimentation and to decompress or empty the stomach. The size of the nasogastric or orogastric tube is determined by the age, size, and weight of the child.

Orogastric Tubes

Orogastric tubes are used in newborns and young infants who are obligate nose breathers, and in older children who are unconscious, unresponsive, or intubated.

Selected Equipment

Appropriate-size orogastric tube
Suction catheter
Water-soluble lubricant
Stethoscope
20 mL syringe to check tube placement

Preparation

Place the child supine with the head of the bed elevated, unless contraindicated.

Use the tube to measure the distance from the mouth to the tragus of the ear and then to the xiphoid process to determine the distance to the stomach. (Alternatively, use a point midway between the xiphoid and the umbilicus.) Mark the tube with tape.

Procedure

- Have suction at hand. Apply a water-soluble lubricant to the tube.
- Position the child with the neck slightly hyperextended. Open the child's mouth and insert the tube toward the back of the throat. Continue advancing the tube slowly until you reach the mark.
- Check the tube for placement by aspirating the stomach contents or by auscultating over the abdomen while a small amount of air is injected through the tube into the stomach. Assess the child's respiratory status and color. A change in either may indicate that the tube is located in the trachea rather than the esophagus.
- Once assured that the tube is in place, tape it securely to one side of the child's mouth. Place two pieces of tape in a V pattern around the tube at the lip. If necessary, use a third piece of tape over the other two. Clamp the end of the tube if it is not being used for feeding or suction.
- To remove an orogastric tube, instill approximately 10 to 20 mL of air into the tube to remove secretions. Untape the tube, pinch or fold it to prevent fluid leakage, and gently withdraw it. Be sure to have suction available.

Nasogastric Tubes

Nasogastric tubes are used more frequently than orogastric tubes. They are inserted to provide alimentation, to decompress the stomach, or to empty the stomach of its contents in preparation for surgery or lavage.

Selected Equipment

Appropriate-size nasogastric tube
Suction catheter
Water-soluble lubricant
Stethoscope
20 mL syringe to check tube placement

Preparation

The preschool-age child needs to be told what will happen in very simple terms. The school-age child and adolescent need to be given a rationale for the procedure. Since placement of the tube is uncomfortable, allow the child to express his or her feelings and seek the support of family members.

Place the child supine, with the head of the bed ele-

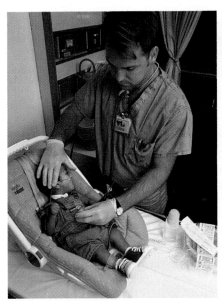
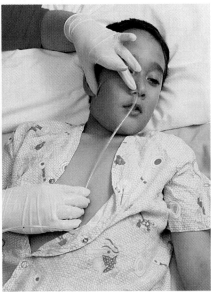

FIGURE P–66 Measuring for nasogastric tube placement in, **A,** infant, and, **B,** child. (A similar technique is used in measuring for orogastric tube insertion. See the discussion above.)

vated to the high Fowler position, if possible. Younger children will need to be restrained because they will fight against the insertion of the tube. An assistant can hold the child's body and arms with his or her body, or the child can be put in a modified mummy restraint. The child's head will need to be held in the midline position.

Use the tube to measure the distance from the tip of the nose to the tragus of the ear and then to the xiphoid process to determine the distance to the stomach (Fig. P–66). (Alternatively, use a point midway between the xiphoid and the umbilicus.) Mark the tube with tape.

Procedure

- Have suction at hand. Apply water-soluble lubricant to the distal end of the tube.
- With the child's neck slightly hyperextended, insert the tube into the child's naris, gently advancing it straight back along the floor of the nasal passages. If resistance is felt at the curve of the nasopharynx, use slight pressure or rotate the tube to continue advancing the tube.
- If the child gags when the tube reaches beyond the oropharynx, flex the child's neck. If the child can take fluids by mouth, have him or her sip water through a straw and swallow it to ease the passage of the tube over the glottis. If the child is not allowed anything by mouth, have him or her swallow.
- After the gag reflex is suppressed, continue advancing the tube slowly until you reach the mark.
- Check the tube for placement by aspirating the stomach contents or by auscultating over the abdomen

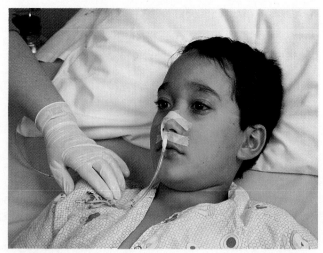

FIGURE P–68 Nasogastric tube taped securely in place.

while a small amount of air is injected through the tube into the stomach (Fig. P–67). Assess the child's respiratory status. A change may indicate that the tube is in the trachea rather than the esophagus.

- Once assured that the tube is in place, tape it securely by placing two pieces of tape in a V pattern around the tube and attaching it to the nose or cheek (Fig. P–68). If necessary, use a second piece of tape over the first.
- To remove the tube, place the child in a Fowler position. Instill approximately 10 to 15 mL of air into the tube to remove any secretions. Unfasten the tape, ask the child to hold his or her breath, pinch the tube, and gently pull out. Have suction available.

Gastrostomy Tubes

Gastrostomy tubes, which are surgically placed in the stomach, are used primarily for gavage feeding. Unless the tube is being used for feeding or decompression, it should remain clamped.

Observe the site for skin breakdown. Keep the area clean and dry. Place a clean dry dressing over the site at every shift. A 2 x 2 or 4 x 4 inch gauze pad can be used. A diagonal cut is made halfway into the square and placed around the tube with tape used at the edges to secure it.

Keep the tube as immobile as possible to prevent unintentional removal or displacement. Tube placement can be checked by aspirating a small amount of gastric contents before each feeding.

The gastrostomy feeding button is a recently developed flexible silicone device that is often used for children who require long-term enteral feedings.

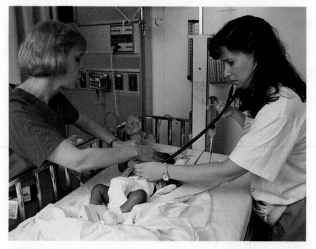

FIGURE P–67 Checking for nasogastric tube placement.

Gavage Feeding

Infants and children require gavage, or tube feeding to counteract absorption disorders, to supply supplemental feedings, and to conserve calories for growth. Feedings can be either continuous or bolus. They can be administered by gravity (Fig. P–69) or by pump. The pump method is preferred because it permits better regulation of the rate and volume of feeding.

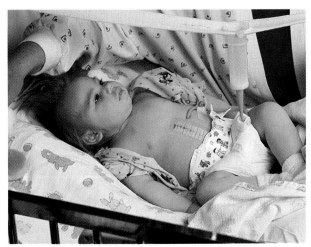

FIGURE P–69 Gavage feeding by gravity.

Selected Equipment

Formula at room temperature (to prevent cramping)
Water for irrigation of the tube
Stethoscope
20 mL syringe to check tube placement

Preparation

If the feeding is to be given by gravity, an IV pole may be used. If the feeding is to be given by pump, gather the necessary bag and tubing. Prime the appropriate tubing, keeping the distal end covered.

Place the child in a semi-Fowler position, if possible. If not, a prone or side-lying position is preferable to the supine position to decrease the risk of aspiration.

Procedure

- Check the placement of the tube before each feeding by aspirating the stomach contents or auscultating over the abdomen while a small amount of air is injected through the tube into the stomach.
- Once assured that the tube is in place, check gastric residuals and proceed with the steps necessary for the feeding.

Bolus Feeding

- Aspirate the stomach contents to check the amount of residual. If the residual is less than half of the previous feeding, return the aspirated contents to the stomach. If the residual is greater, notify the physician.
- Attach the primed tubing from either the pump or the gravity set to the nasogastric/orogastric tube. Start the flow slowly while checking the patency of the tube. Set the rate and volume according to the physician's orders.
- When the feeding has been completed, assess the child's condition. Clamp and disconnect the tubing. Flush the tubing with a small amount of water to clean it.

Continuous Feeding

The procedure for continuous feeding is very similar to that for bolus feeding. However, the formula should hang no longer than 4 hours. When the feeding bag is hung, it should be labeled with the time and date. The feeding set should be changed once per shift or every 8 hours.

Assess the child's condition during the feeding, and monitor the child's respiratory status.

Gastric Suctioning

Both orogastric and nasogastric tubes can be connected to a suctioning device (Fig. P–70) to provide either continuous or intermittent suction.

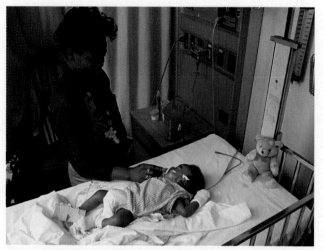

FIGURE P–70 Nasogastric tube attached to suctioning device.

Preparation

Before making the connection:

1. Check the suction equipment.
2. Check that the tube is in proper position by aspirating the stomach contents or auscultating over the abdomen while a small amount of air is injected through the tube into the stomach.
3. Assess the child's respiratory status. Changes may indicate that the tube is in the trachea instead of the esophagus.

Procedure

- Attach the suction to the orogastric or nasogastric tube at its distal end. Tape the connection site.
- Turn the suction to the amount ordered by the physician. Observe the color, amount, and character of the contents suctioned. Record the child's response (vital signs, complaints of abdominal discomfort).

Monitor the child's condition frequently and label the level of the contents collected.

ELIMINATION

Urinary Catheterization

Urinary catheterization is performed to obtain sterile urine for diagnostic purposes, to measure the amount of urine in the bladder accurately, to empty the bladder, or to relieve bladder distention.

Selected Equipment

Sterile urinary catheterization tray (containing gloves, drapes, antiseptic solution, cotton swabs or balls, forceps, lubricant, and container for urine)
Correct size/type of catheter

If a Foley catheter is to be inserted, a syringe filled with normal saline is used to inflate the balloon with the amount noted on the balloon port. Tape and a drainage collection apparatus are also needed. Goggles, a mask, and a gown are worn because of the potential for urine to splash.

Preparation

Check the physician's orders to determine whether intermittent or indwelling catheterization is planned. Determine the size of the catheter based on the child's size, age, and weight.

In the hospital setting urinary catheterization is performed as a sterile procedure. However, it is often performed as a clean procedure on an outpatient basis.

The child needs to be held in position for the catheterization procedure. If the parents wish to stay in the room with the child, encourage them to stand at the head of the bed, talking with the child and holding his or her hand.

Procedure

- Pour the antiseptic over the cotton swabs or balls. Open the tray, maintaining the sterile field. Open the lubricant and squeeze it onto the sterile field.

- Put on sterile gloves. Lubricate the tip of the catheter. Place the distal end in the tray.
- Have your assistant position and restrain the child. Place clean pads under the child's perineum.

Female

- Clean the perineum. With your nondominant hand, hold the labia apart. With your dominant (sterile) hand, pick up the antiseptic-saturated cotton balls with the forceps. Clean the meatus, using one ball for each wipe, in a front-to-back motion along each side of the labia minora, along the sides of the urinary meatus, and finally straight down over the urethral opening.
- Pick up the lubricated catheter tip with your dominant hand, keeping the distal end in the container. Gently insert the tip into the meatus (approximately 2.5 cm in the child) until there is a free flow of urine. If resistance is felt, do not force the catheter. You may try again with another sterile catheter.
- Once the catheter is in place, collect the urine specimen while holding the catheter with your nondominant hand.

Male

- Clean the perineum. With your nondominant hand, hold the penis behind the glans and spread the meatus with your thumb and forefinger. Retract the foreskin if the child is uncircumcised. With your dominant (sterile) hand, pick up the antiseptic-saturated cotton balls with the forceps. Clean the tissue surrounding the meatus using one cotton ball for each wipe in an outward circular fashion.
- Pick up the lubricated catheter tip with your dominant hand, keeping the distal end in the container. Lift the penis, exerting slight traction until it is perpendicular with the body. Insert the catheter steadily into the meatus until there is a free flow of urine. If resistance is felt, do not force the catheter. You may try to insert another sterile catheter.
- Once the catheter is in place, lower the penis and collect the urine specimen while holding the catheter with your nondominant hand.

For Laboratory Specimen

To obtain urine for laboratory analysis, follow the preceding sequence each time urine is to be obtained.

- Drain the bladder of urine.
- Remove the catheter after the specimen has been collected.
- Cap the specimen, label, and send to the lab.

■ Ostomy Care

Ostomies are performed when an infant or child requires fecal or urinary diversion. Infants and children may require an ostomy for several reasons, including necrotizing enterocolitis, Hirschsprung disease, imperforate anus, prune-belly syndrome, inflammatory bowel syndrome, spina bifida, tumor, and trauma. An ileostomy, colostomy, or urinary diversion is performed depending on the disorder and its location.

An adhesive appliance is usually applied just after surgery to measure drainage. If a dressing is applied instead of an adhesive appliance, the drainage can be measured by weighing the dressing both before and after saturation. For each 1-gram increase in weight of the dressing, approximately 30 mL of fluid has drained into it.

In children and infants, ostomies pose special problems because of the fragility of the skin. Care must be taken to prevent skin breakdown at the site.

Dressing Changes for an Infant

Procedure

- After each bowel movement, change the dressing, clean and dry the skin, and apply a nonporous substance.
- To absorb drainage, place gauze with slits cut to fit around the stoma. Use tape to hold the gauze in place. Alternatively, Montgomery straps, an Ace wrap, or a diaper can be used to protect the skin.

Once the stoma has healed and the infant is large enough to wear a pouch, an appliance with a Stomahesive wafer will be used.

Changing a Pouch for an Infant or Child

Procedure

- Empty the pouch when it is one-third to one-half full. Remove the pouch, and place it in a sealable plastic bag for disposal.
- Children will commonly have Stomahesive around the stoma. This is a wafer of protective material to which a pouch can be attached or removed, thus protecting the integrity of the skin. Most wafers need to be changed only once a week.
- Wash the skin and the stoma gently. Note any skin breakdown or signs of infection. Dry the area. Check the condition of the Stomahesive.
- Prepare the new pouch. Place it on the Stomahesive. Press the pouch firmly against the Stomahesive to form a tight seal. Be careful to avoid making any wrinkles. Close the opening of the pouch with the appropriate clamp.

Enemas

There are three important considerations when giving an enema to an infant or a child: the type of fluid, the amount of fluid, and the appropriate distance to insert the tube into the rectum.

It is recommended that isotonic fluid be used for children. This fluid can be either a commercial product, such as a pediatric Fleet enema, or it can be prepared by adding 1 teaspoon of salt to 500 mL water.

Age	Volume (mL)	Distance to Be Inserted (cm)
Infant	50–100	2.5
Toddler	100–200	5.0
Preschool	200–300	5.0
School-Age	300–500	7.5
Adolescent	500–700	10.0

Selected Equipment

Ordered solution (in container with attached tip) *or* enema bag and rectal tube (size 14 to 18 Fr for child; 12 Fr for infant)
Solution container
Ordered fluid

Preparation

Assure the child that a bedpan will be kept at the bedside. If the child is toilet trained, make sure to place him or her in a bed near a bathroom before giving the enema.

Procedure

- Place absorbent pads on the bed. Position the child on his or her left side, with the knees drawn up to the chest. You may need an assistant to hold the child in position.
- If a rectal tube is being used, attach the solution container, add the fluid, and purge the tubing and tube. Lubricate the tip. If a Fleet enema is being used, the tip is prelubricated.
- Gently insert the tip to the recommended distance. Allow the fluid to run in slowly, for at least 10 to 15 minutes. If the child complains of cramping, stop the infusion to allow the child to rest, then continue.
- Infants and children may not be able to retain the fluid. Holding the buttocks together might help.
- When the child is ready or when it is time to expel the contents of the enema, place the bedpan on the bed or escort the child to the bathroom. Provide privacy as requested. Assess for dizziness or weakness before leaving.
- Clean the perineum. The child or parent may choose to perform this step.
- Help the child resume a position of comfort.
- Assess the return for amount and character.

Irrigation of the Ear and Eye

Ear Irrigation

Irrigation of the ear is performed to remove cerumen or a foreign body.

Selected Equipment

Ordered solution, warmed to room temperature
Irrigating syringe (bulb or Asepto)

Procedure

- Check the physician's orders for the type of fluid to be administered.

- Position the child on his or her back. For the child less than 3 years of age, gently pull the pinna straight back and slightly downward to straighten the ear canal. For the older child, pull the pinna back and upward. Place an emesis basin under the ear to be irrigated.
- Draw 20 mL of warm ordered solution into a syringe with the tubing attached. Gently flush the solution into the ear canal, catching the draining fluid with the emesis basin. Repeat according to physician's orders. Dry the child's ear, cheek, and neck.

■ NURSING ALERT

Ear irrigation should not be performed if there is any drainage from the child's ear.

Eye Irrigation

Irrigation of the eye is performed to flush out a foreign body or a chemical irritant (Fig. P–71) .

Preparation

Check the physician's orders for the type of fluid and the volume to be used (most often sterile normal saline).

The child will need to be held in position for this procedure. An assistant can hold the child supine with his or her body over the child's, keeping the child's head turned slightly so that the eye to be irrigated is lower than the other eye. This method is used to avoid cross-contamination of the eye not being irrigated.

Attach the IV tubing to the bag of room temperature normal saline. Purge the line, but keep the tip covered.

Procedure

- Place absorbent pads under the child's head, neck, and shoulders, using towels for extra absorption. Place an emesis basin under the lower eye to catch drainage.
- Using the thumb and forefinger of your dominant hand, gently separate the child's lids. Remove the cover from the IV tubing. Open the clamp midway, pointing the stream of fluid into the lower conjunctival sac from the inner to the outer canthus. Periodically turn off the stream of solution and have the child close the eye so that the solution can also move into the upper conjunctival area.
- When the irrigation has been completed, dry the child's eye gently with gauze or a cotton ball from the inner to the outer canthus.
- Assess the return for color, odor, and character.

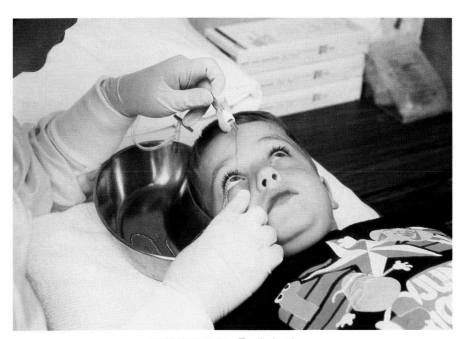

FIGURE P–71 Eye irrigation.

American Heart Association (1992). Guidelines for cardiopulmonary resuscitation and emergency cardiac care. *Journal of the American Medical Association, 268*(16), 2251–2274.

Birdsall, C. (1986). What are dos and don'ts for Hickman/Broviac catheters? *American Journal of Nursing, 16*(4), 385.

Camp, D., & Otten, N. (1990). How to insert and remove nasogastric tubes quickly and easily. *Nursing '90, 20*(9) 59–64.

Carroll, P. (1987). The right way to do chest physiotherapy. *RN, 50*(5), 26–29.

Chameides, L. (Ed.) (1990). *Textbook of pediatric advanced life support.* Dallas: American Heart Association.

Ehrhardt, B., & Graham, M. (1990). Pulse oximetry: An easy way to check oxygen saturation. *Nursing '90, 20*(3), 50–54.

Eichelberger, M., Ball, J., Pratsch, G., et al. (1992). *Pediatric emergencies.* Englewood Cliffs, NJ: Brady.

Engel, J. (1989). *Pocket guide to pediatric assessment.* St. Louis: Mosby–Year Book.

Erickson, R. (1989). Managing the ins and outs of chest drainage, part I. *Nursing '89, 19*(5), 36–44.

Erickson, R. (1989). Managing the ins and outs of chest drainage, part II. *Nursing '89, 19*(6), 46–50.

Frederick, V. (1991). Pediatric IV therapy: Soothing the patient. *RN, 54*(12), 43–48.

Hartsell, M. (1987). Noninvasive oxygen monitoring. *Journal of Pediatric Nursing, 2*(1), 64–65.

Hoekelman, R. (Ed.) (1992). *Primary pediatric care.* (2nd ed.). St. Louis: Mosby–Year Book.

Hoffman, L. (1987). Airway management for the critically ill patient. *American Journal of Nursing, 87*(1), 39–53.

Hoffman, L., Mazzocco, M., & Roth, J. (1987). Fine tuning your chest PT. *American Journal of Nursing, 87*(12), 1566–1572.

Holder, C. (1990). New and improved guide to IV therapy. *American Journal of Nursing, 90*(2), 43–47.

Hower, D. (1987). Blood samples made easy: Using special IV lines at home. *Nursing '87, 17*(7), 56–58.

Lynch, P., Cummings, M.J., Roberts, P., et al. (1990). Implementing and evaluating a system of generic infection precautions: Body substance isolation. *American Journal of Infection Control, 18*(1), 1–12.

Mayo, J. (1987). A nurse's guide to mechanical ventilation. *RN, 50*(8), 18–23.

McAfee, T., Garland, L.R., & McNabb, T.S. (1990). How to safely draw blood from a vascular access device. *Nursing '90, 20*(11), 42–43.

Miracle, V., & Allnutt, D. (1990). How to perform basic airway management. *Nursing '90, 20*(4), 55–60.

Newman, L. (1989). A side-by-side look at two venous access devices. *American Journal of Nursing, 89*(6), 826–835.

Nichols, D., Yaster, M., Lappe, D. et al. (1991). *Golden hour: The handbook of advanced pediatric life support.* St. Louis: Mosby–Year Book.

O'Brien, R. (1991). Starting intravenous lines in children. *Journal of Emergency Nursing, 17*(4), 225–231.

Querin, J., & Stahl, L. (1990). Twelve simple steps for successful blood transfusions. *Nursing '90, 20*(10), 79–81.

Skale, N. (1992). *Manual of pediatric nursing procedures.* Philadelphia: J.B. Lippincott.

Smith, S., & Duell, D. (1992). *Clinical nursing skills (3rd ed.).* Norwalk, CT: Appleton & Lange.

Speer, K.M., & Swann, C.L. (1993). *The Addison-Wesley manual of pediatric nursing procedures.* Menlo Park, CA: Addison-Wesley.

Swearingen, P. (Ed.) (1991). *Photo atlas of nursing procedures* (2nd ed.). Menlo Park, CA: Addison-Wesley.

Thermoscan operator's manual. (1991).

Viall, C.D. (1990). Your complete guide to central venous catheters. *Nursing '90, 20*(2), 34–42.

Zimmerman, S., et al. (1991). *Orientation manual for the emergency medical trauma center, Children's National Medical Center.* Washington, DC: Unpublished.

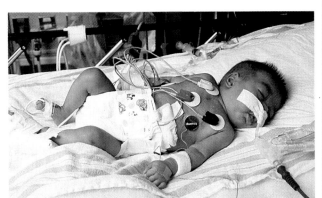
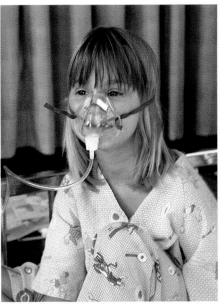
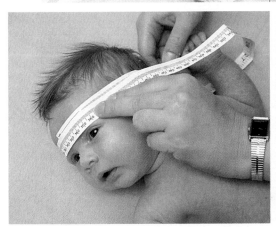
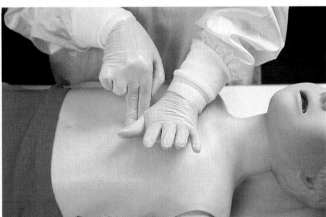
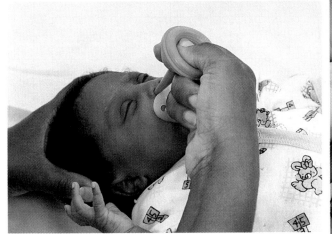
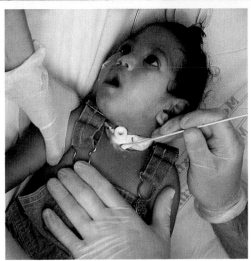

Boys: Birth to 36 Months
Physical Growth
NCHS Percentiles

NAME_____ RECORD #_____

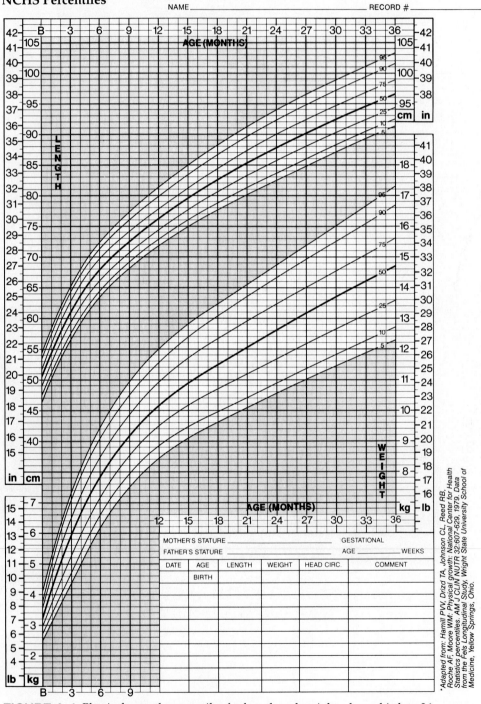

FIGURE A–1 Physical growth percentiles for length and weight—boys: birth to 36 months.

From NCHS Growth Charts, copyright © 1982 Ross Laboratories. Reprinted with permission of Ross Laboratories, Columbus, OH 43216.

Physical Growth Charts

Boys: Birth to 36 Months
Physical Growth
NCHS Percentiles

NAME_____ RECORD #_____

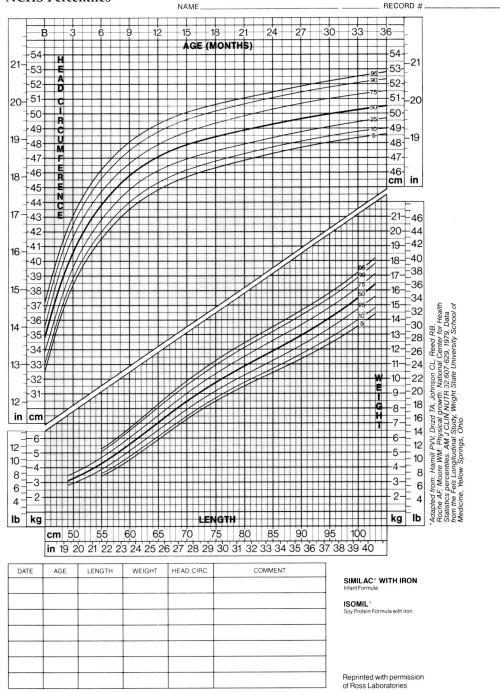

FIGURE A–2 Physical growth percentiles for head circumference, length, and weight—boys: birth to 36 months.

Girls: Birth to 36 Months
Physical Growth
NCHS Percentiles

NAME _____ RECORD # _____

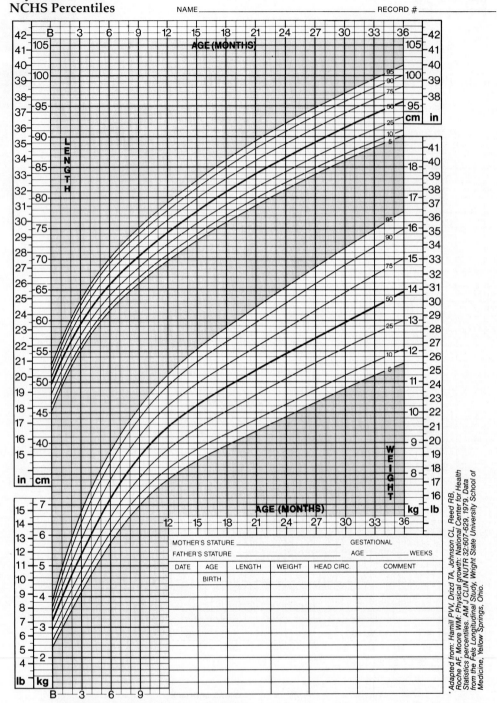

FIGURE A–3 Physical growth percentiles for length and weight—girls: birth to 36 months.

GIRLS: BIRTH TO 36 MONTHS
PHYSICAL GROWTH
NCHS PERCENTILES*

NAME_____ RECORD #_____

FIGURE A–4 Physical growth percentiles for head circumference, length, and weight—girls: birth to 36 months.

From NCHS Growth Charts, copyright © 1982 Ross Laboratories. Reprinted with permission of Ross Laboratories, Columbus, OH 43216.

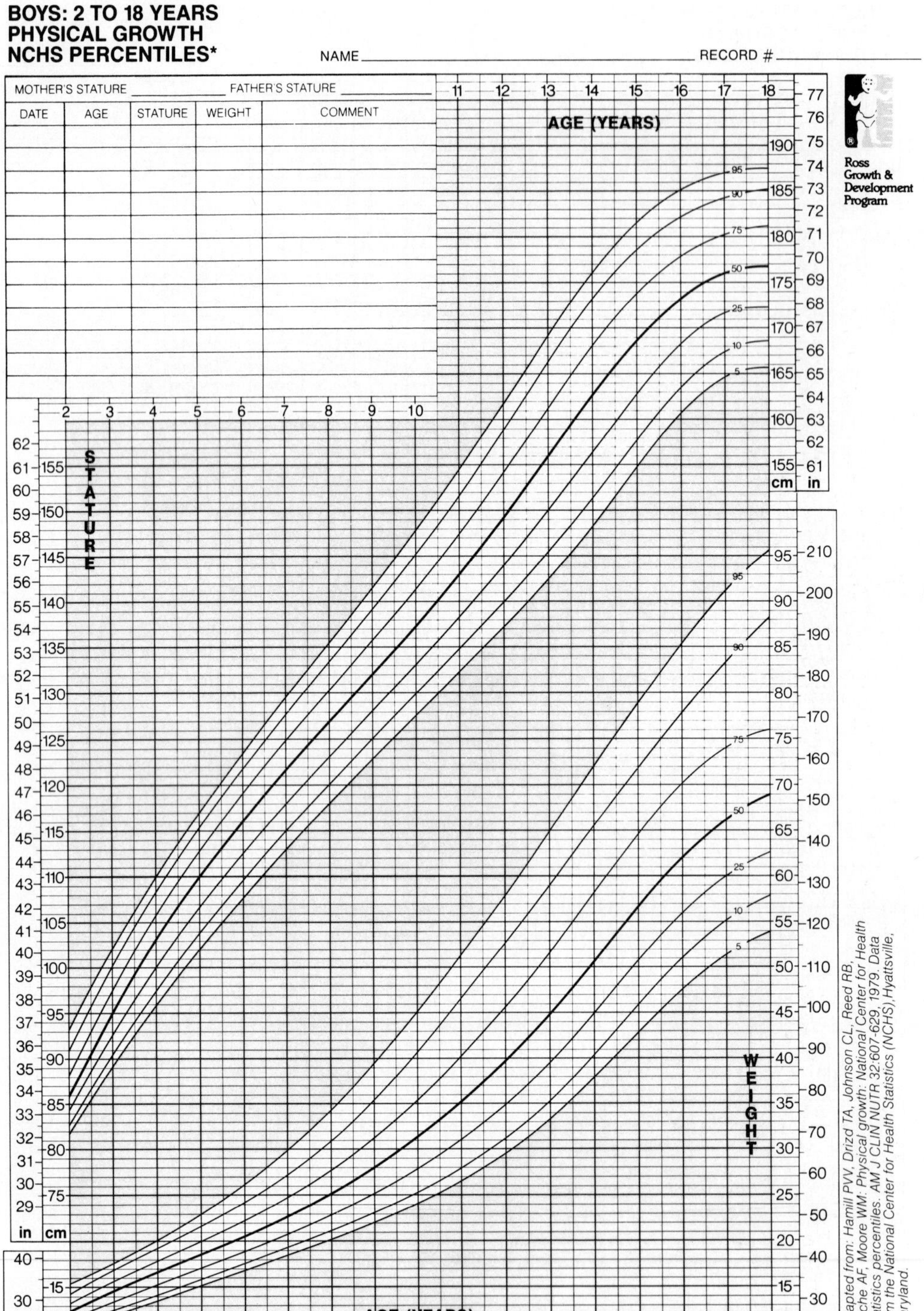

FIGURE A-5 Physical growth percentiles for stature and weight according to age—boys: 2 to 18 years.

From NCHS Growth Charts, copyright © 1982 Ross Laboratories. Reprinted with permission of Ross Laboratories, Columbus, OH 43216.

GIRLS: 2 TO 18 YEARS
PHYSICAL GROWTH
NCHS PERCENTILES*

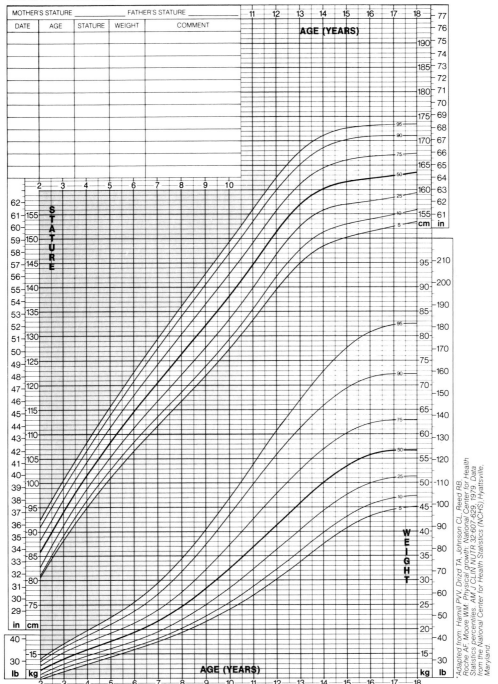

FIGURE A–6 Physical growth percentiles for stature and weight according to age—girls: 2 to 18 years.

From NCHS Growth Charts, copyright © 1982 Ross Laboratories. Reprinted with permission of Ross Laboratories, Columbus, OH 43216.

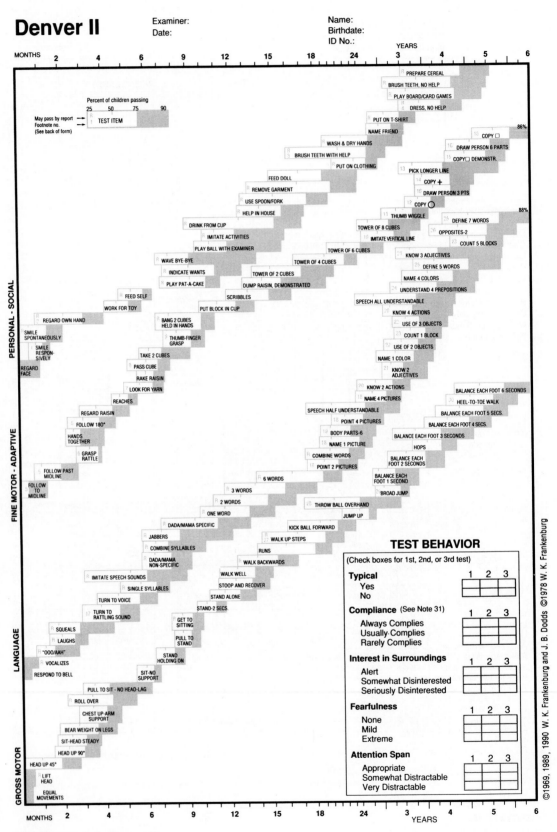

FIGURE B-1 A, Denver II.
From W.K. Frankenburg, Denver, CO.

DENVER II

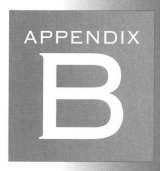

DIRECTIONS FOR ADMINISTRATION

1. Try to get child to smile by smiling, talking or waving. Do not touch him/her.
2. Child must stare at hand several seconds.
3. Parent may help guide toothbrush and put toothpaste on brush.
4. Child does not have to be able to tie shoes or button/zip in the back.
5. Move yarn slowly in an arc from one side to the other, about 8" above child's face.
6. Pass if child grasps rattle when it is touched to the backs or tips of fingers.
7. Pass if child tries to see where yarn went. Yarn should be dropped quickly from sight from tester's hand without arm movement.
8. Child must transfer cube from hand to hand without help of body, mouth, or table.
9. Pass if child picks up raisin with any part of thumb and finger.
10. Line can vary only 30 degrees or less from tester's line.
11. Make a fist with thumb pointing upward and wiggle only the thumb. Pass if child imitates and does not move any fingers other than the thumb.

12. Pass any enclosed form. Fail continuous round motions.

13. Which line is longer? (Not bigger.) Turn paper upside down and repeat. (pass 3 of 3 or 5 of 6)

14. Pass any lines crossing near midpoint.

15. Have child copy first. If failed, demonstrate.

When giving items 12, 14, and 15, do not name the forms. Do not demonstrate 12 and 14.

16. When scoring, each pair (2 arms, 2 legs, etc.) counts as one part.
17. Place one cube in cup and shake gently near child's ear, but out of sight. Repeat for other ear.
18. Point to picture and have child name it. (No credit is given for sounds only.)
    If less than 4 pictures are named correctly, have child point to picture as each is named by tester.

 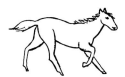   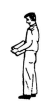

19. Using doll, tell child: Show me the nose, eyes, ears, mouth, hands, feet, tummy, hair. Pass 6 of 8.
20. Using pictures, ask child: Which one flies?... says meow?... talks?... barks?... gallops? Pass 2 of 5, 4 of 5.
21. Ask child: What do you do when you are cold?... tired?... hungry? Pass 2 of 3, 3 of 3.
22. Ask child: What do you do with a cup? What is a chair used for? What is a pencil used for?
    Action words must be included in answers.
23. Pass if child correctly places and says how many blocks are on paper. (1, 5).
24. Tell child: Put block on table; under table; in front of me, behind me. Pass 4 of 4.
    (Do not help child by pointing, moving head or eyes.)
25. Ask child: What is a ball?... lake?... desk?... house?... banana?... curtain?... fence?... ceiling? Pass if defined in terms of use, shape, what it is made of, or general category (such as banana is fruit, not just yellow). Pass 5 of 8, 7 of 8.
26. Ask child: If a horse is big, a mouse is __? If fire is hot, ice is __? If the sun shines during the day, the moon shines during the __? Pass 2 of 3.
27. Child may use wall or rail only, not person. May not crawl.
28. Child must throw ball overhand 3 feet to within arm's reach of tester.
29. Child must perform standing broad jump over width of test sheet (8 1/2 inches).
30. Tell child to walk forward, ⊂⊃⊂⊃⊂⊃⊂⊃➤ heel within 1 inch of toe. Tester may demonstrate.
    Child must walk 4 consecutive steps.
31. In the second year, half of normal children are non-compliant.

OBSERVATIONS:

FIGURE B–1, CONT'D. **B,** Directions for administration of Denver II.

From W.K. Frankenburg, Denver, CO.

Recommended dietary allowances* designed for the maintenance of good nutrition of practically all healthy people in the United States

Category	Age (years) or condition	Weight† (kg)	Weight† (lb)	Height† (cm)	Height† (in)	Protein (g)	Vitamin A (µg RE)‡	Vitamin D (µg)§	Vitamin E (mg/α-TE)ǁ	Vitamin K (µg)
								Fat-soluble vitamins		
Infants	0.0–0.5	6	13	60	24	13	375	7.5	3	5
	0.5–1.0	9	20	71	28	14	375	10	4	10
Children	1–3	13	29	90	35	16	400	10	6	15
	4–6	20	44	112	44	24	500	10	7	20
	7–10	28	62	132	52	28	700	10	7	30
Males	11–14	45	99	157	62	45	1000	10	10	45
	15–18	66	145	176	69	59	1000	10	10	65
	19–24	72	160	177	70	58	1000	10	10	70
	25–50	79	174	176	70	63	1000	5	10	80
	51+	77	170	173	68	63	1000	5	10	80
Females	11–14	46	101	157	62	46	800	10	8	45
	15–18	55	120	163	64	44	800	10	8	55
	19–24	58	128	164	65	46	800	10	8	60
	25–50	63	138	163	64	50	800	5	8	65
	51+	65	143	160	63	50	800	5	8	65
Pregnant						60	800	10	10	65
Lactating	1st 6 months					65	1300	10	12	65
	2nd 6 months					62	1200	10	11	65

From Food and Nutrition Board, National Research Council. (1989). *Recommended dietary allowances* (10th ed.). Washington, DC: National Academy of Sciences. Courtesy of the National Academy Press, Washington, DC.

*The allowances, expressed as average daily intakes over time, are intended to provide for individual variations among most normal persons as they live in the United States under usual environmental stresses. Diets should be based on a variety of common foods in order to provide other nutrients for which human requirements have been less well defined.

†Weights and heights of reference adults are actual medians for the U.S. population of the designated age, as reported by National Health and Nutrition Examination Survey (NHANES) II. The median weights and heights of those under 19 years of age were taken from Hamill, P.V. et al. (1979). Physical growth: National Center for Health Statistics percentiles. *Am J Clin Nutr, 32*, 607–629. The use of these figures does not imply that the height-to-weight ratios are ideal.

‡Retinol equivalent. 1 retinol equivalent = 1 µg retinol or 6 µg β-carotene.

§As cholecalciferol. 10 µg cholecalciferol = 400 IU vitamin D.

ǁ α-Tocopherol equivalents. 1 µg d-α-tocopherol = 1 α-TE.

¶1 NE (niacin equivalent) is equal to 1 mg of niacin or 60 mg of dietary tryptophan.

RECOMMENDED DIETARY ALLOWANCES

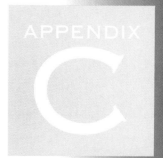

APPENDIX

C

	Water-soluble vitamins						Minerals						
Vita-min C (mg)	Thiamin (mg)	Ribo-flavin (mg)	Niacin (mg NE)¶	Vita-min B_6 (mg)	Folate (µg)	Vita-min B_{12} (µg)	Calcium (mg)	Phos-phorus (mg)	Mag-nesium (mg)	Iron (mg)	Zinc (mg)	Iodine (µg)	Sele-nium (µg)
30	0.3	0.4	5	0.3	25	0.3	400	300	40	6	5	40	10
35	0.4	0.5	6	0.6	35	0.5	600	500	60	10	5	50	15
40	0.7	0.8	9	1.0	50	0.7	800	800	80	10	10	70	20
45	0.9	1.1	12	1.1	75	1.0	800	800	120	10	10	90	20
45	1.0	1.2	13	1.4	100	1.4	800	800	170	10	10	120	30
50	1.3	1.5	17	1.7	150	2.0	1200	1200	270	12	15	150	40
60	1.5	1.8	20	2.0	200	2.0	1200	1200	400	12	15	150	50
60	1.5	1.7	19	2.0	200	2.0	1200	1200	350	10	15	150	70
60	1.5	1.7	19	2.0	200	2.0	800	800	350	10	15	150	70
60	1.2	1.4	15	2.0	200	2.0	800	800	350	10	15	150	70
50	1.1	1.3	15	1.4	150	2.0	1200	1200	280	15	12	150	45
60	1.1	1.3	15	1.5	180	2.0	1200	1200	300	15	12	150	50
60	1.1	1.3	15	1.6	180	2.0	1200	1200	280	15	12	150	55
60	1.1	1.3	15	1.6	180	2.0	800	800	280	15	12	150	55
60	1.0	1.2	13	1.6	180	2.0	800	800	280	10	12	150	55
70	1.5	1.6	17	2.2	400	2.2	1200	1200	320	30	15	175	65
95	1.6	1.8	20	2.1	280	2.6	1200	1200	355	15	19	200	75
90	1.6	1.7	20	2.1	260	2.6	1200	1200	340	15	16	200	75

Normal Values: Blood

Acid-Base Measurements (B)

pH: 7.38–7.42 from 14 minutes of age and older.
PaO_2: 65–76 mm Hg (8.66–10.13 kPa).
$PaCO_2$: 36–38 mm Hg (4.8–5.07 kPa).
Base excess: −2 to +2 mEq/L, except in newborns (range, −4 to −0).

Aldolase (S)

Newborns: 17.5–47.8 IU/L at 37° C.
Children: 8.8–23.9 IU/L at 37° C.
Adults: 4.4–12 IU/L at 37° C.

Aldosterone (P)

First year: 25–140 ng/dL.
Second year: 9–25 ng/dL.

Ammonia (P)

Newborns: 90–150 µg/dL (53–88 µmol/L);
  higher in premature and jaundiced infants.
Thereafter: 0–60 µg/dL (0–35 µmol/L) when
  blood is drawn with proper precautions.

Alkaline Phosphatase (S)

Values in IU/L at 37° C using p-nitrophenol
  phosphate buffered with AMP (kinetic).

Group	Males	Females
Newborns (1–3 d)	95–368	95–368
2–24 mo	115–460	115–460
2–5 yr	115–391	115–391
6–7 yr	115–460	115–460
8–9 yr	115–345	115–345
10–11 yr	115–336	115–437
12–13 yr	127–403	92–336
14–15 yr	79–446	78–212
16–18 yr	58–331	35–124
Adults	41–137	39–118

α_1-Antitrypsin (S)

1–3 mo: 127–404 mg/dL.
3–12 mo: 145–362 mg/dL.
1–2 yr: 160–382 mg/dL.
2–15 yr: 148–394 mg/dL.

Bicarbonate, Actual (P)

Calculated from pH and $PaCO_2$.
Newborns: 17.2–23.6 mmol/L.
2 mo–2 yr: 19–24 mmol/L.
Children: 18–25 mmol/L.
Adult males: 20.1–28.9 mmol/L.
Adult females: 18.4–28.8 mmol/L.

Bilirubin (S)

Values in mg/dL (µmol/L).
Levels after 1 mo are as follows:
Conjugated: 0–0.3 mg/dL (0–5 µmol/L).
Unconjugated: 0.1–0.7 mg/dl (2–12 µmol/L).

Peak Newborn Level	Newborns (Birth Weight) Exceeding Peak Level (%)		
	<2001 g	2001–2500 g	>2500 g
20 (342)	8.2	2.6	0.8
18 (308)	13.5	4.6	1.5
16 (274)	20.3	7.6	2.6
14 (239)	33.0	12.0	4.4
11 (188)	53.8	23.0	9.3
8 (137)	77.0	45.4	26.1

Bleeding Time (Simplate)

2–9 min.

Blood Volume

Premature infants: 98 mL/kg.
At 1 yr: 86 mL/kg (range, 69–112 mL/kg).
Older children: 70 mL/kg (range, 51–86 mL/kg).

Modified from Hathaway, W.E., Hay, W.W., Groothuis, J.R., & Paisley, J.W. (1993). *Current pediatric diagnosis and treatment* (11th ed.). Norwalk, CT: Appleton & Lange.
NOTE: Values may vary with the procedure employed.
(S), Serum; (B), whole blood; (P), plasma; RBC, red blood cells.

NORMAL LABORATORY VALUES

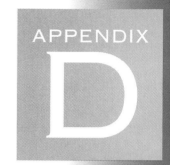
Normal Values: Blood—Continued

Calcium (S)

Premature infants (first week): 3.5–4.5 mEq/L (1.7–2.3 mmol/L).
Full-term infants (first week): 4–5 mEq/L (2–2.5 mmol/L).
Thereafter: 4.4–5.3 mEq/L (2.2–2.7 mmol/L).

Carbon Dioxide, Total (S, P)

Cord blood: 15–20.2 mmol/L.
Children: 18–27 mmol/L.
Adults: 24–35 mmol/L.

Carotene (S, P)

0–6 mo: 0–40 µg/dL (0–0.75 µmol/L).
Children: 50–100 µg/dL (0.93–1.9 µmol/L).
Adults: 100–150 µg/dL (1.9–2.8 µmol/L).

Chloride (S, P)

Premature infants: 95–110 mmol/L.
Full-term infants: 96–116 mmol/L.
Children: 98–105 mmol/L.
Adults: 98–108 mmol/L.

Cholesterol, Total (S, P)

Values in mg/dL (mmol/L)

Group	Males	Females
6–7 yr	115–197 (2.97–5.09)	126–199 (3.25–5.14)
8–9 yr	112–199 (2.89–5.14)	124–208 (3.20–5.37)
10–11 yr	108–220 (2.79–5.68)	115–208 (2.97–5.37)
12–13 yr	117–202 (3.02–5.21)	114–207 (2.94–5.34)
14–15 yr	103–207 (2.66–5.34)	102–208 (2.68–5.37)
16–17 yr	107–198 (2.76–5.11)	106–213 (2.73–5.50)

Coagulation Time (Test Tube Method)

3–9 min.

Complement (S)

C3: 96–195 mg/dL.
C4: 15–20 mg/dL.

Creatine (S, P)

0.2–0.8 mg/dL (15.2–61 mmol/L).

Creatine Kinase (S, P)

Newborns (1–3 d): 40–474 IU/L at 37° C.
Adult males: 30–210 IU/L at 37° C.
Adult females: 20–128 IU/L at 37° C.

Creatinine (S, P)

Values in mg/dL (µmol/L).

Group	Males	Females
Newborns (1–3 d)*	0.2–1.0 (17.7–88.4)	0.2–1.0 (17.7–88.4)
1 yr	0.2–0.6 (17.7–53.0)	0.2–0.5 (17.7–44.2)
2–3 yr	0.2–0.7 (17.7–61.9)	0.3–0.6 (26.5–53.0)
4–7 yr	0.2–0.8 (17.7–70.7)	0.2–0.7 (17.7–61.9)
8–10 yr	0.3–0.9 (26.5–79.6)	0.3–0.8 (26.5–70.7)
11–12 yr	0.3–1.0 (26.5–88.4)	0.3–0.9 (26.5–79.6)
13–17 yr	0.3–1.2 (26.5–106.1)	0.3–1.1 (26.5–97.2)
18–20 yr	0.5–1.3 (44.2–115.0)	0.3–1.1 (26.5–97.2)

*Values may be higher in premature newborns.

Creatinine Clearance

Values show great variability and depend on specificity of analytical methods used.
Newborns (1 d): 5–50 mL/min/1.73 m² (mean, 18 mL/min/1.73 m²).
Newborns (6 d): 15–90 mL/min/1.73 m² (mean, 36 mL/min/1.73 m²).
Adult males: 85–125 mL/min/1.73 m².
Adult females: 75–115 mL/min/1.73 m².

Fibrinogen (P)

200–500 mg/dL (5.9–14.7 µmol/L).

Galactose (S, P)

1.1–2.1 mg/dL (0.06–0.12 mmol/L).

Continued.

Galactose-1-Phosphate (RBC)

Normal: 1 mg/dL of packed erythrocyte lysate; slightly higher in cord blood.
Infants with congenital galactosemia on a milk-free diet: <2 mg/dL.
Infants with congenital galactosemia taking milk: 9–20 mg/dL.

Galactose-1-Phosphate Uridyltransferase (RBC)

Normal: 308–475 mIU/g of hemoglobin.
Heterozygous for Duarte variant: 225–308 mIU/g of hemoglobin.
Homozygous for Duarte variant: 142–225 mIU/g of hemoglobin.
Heterozygous for congenital galactosemia: 142–225 mIU/g of hemoglobin.
Homozygous for congenital galactosemia: <8 mIU/g of hemoglobin.

Glucose (S, P)

Premature infants: 20–80 mg/dL (1.11–4.44 mmol/L).
Full-term infants: 30–100 mg/dL (1.67–5.56 mmol/L).
Children and adults (fasting): 60–105 mg/dL 3.33–5.88 mmol/L).

Glucose 6-Phosphate Dehydrogenase (RBC)

150–215 units/dL.

Glucose Tolerance Test Results in Serum*

	Glucose		Insulin	
Time	mg/dL	mmol/L	μU/mL	pmol/L
Fasting	59–96	3.11–5.33	5–40	36–287
30 min	91–185	5.05–10.27	36–110	258–789
60 min	66–164	3.66–9.10	22–124	158–890
90 min	68–148	3.77–8.22	17–105	122–753
2 hr	66–122	3.66–6.77	6–84	43–603
3 hr	47–99	2.61–5.49	2–46	14–330
4 hr	61–93	3.39–5.16	3–32	21–230
5 hr	63–86	3.50–4.77	5–37	36–265

*Normal levels based on results in 13 normal children given glucose, 1.75 g/kg orally in one dose, after 2 weeks on a high-carbohydrate diet.

Glycohemoglobin (Hemoglobin A_{1c})(B)

Normal: 6.3–8.2% of total hemoglobin.
Diabetic patients in good control of their condition ordinarily have levels <10%.
Values tend to be lower during pregnancy; they also vary with technique.

Growth Hormone (GH)(S)

After infancy (fasting specimen): 0–5 ng/mL.
In response to natural and artificial provocation (e.g., sleep, arginine, insulin, hypoglycemia): >8 ng/mL.
During the newborn period (fasting specimen): GH levels are high (15–40 ng/mL) and responses to provocation variable.

Hematocrit (B)

At birth: 44–64%.
14–90 d: 35–49%.
6 mo–1 yr: 30–40%.
4–10 yr: 31–43%.

Hemoglobin (P)

No more than 0.5 mg/dL (0.3 μmol/L).

Hemoglobin A_{1c}

See Glycohemoglobin.

Hemoglobin Electrophoresis (B)

A_1 hemoglobin: 96–98.5% of total hemoglobin.
A_2 hemoglobin: 1.5–4% of total hemoglobin.

Hemoglobin, Fetal (B)

At birth: 50–85% of total hemoglobin.
At 1 yr: <15% of total hemoglobin.
Up to 2 yr: Up to 5% of total hemoglobin.
Thereafter: <2% of total hemoglobin.

Immunoglobulins (S)

Values in mg/dL.

Group	IgG	IgA	IgM
Cord blood	766–1693	0.04–9	4–26
2 wk–3 mo	299–852	3–66	15–149
3–6 mo	142–988	4–90	18–118
6–12 mo	418–1142	14–95	43–223
1–2 yr	356–1204	13–118	37–239
2–3 yr	492–1269	23–137	49–204
3–6 yr	564–1381	35–209	51–214
6–9 yr	658–1535	29–384	50–228
9–12 yr	625–1598	60–294	64–278
12–16 yr	660–1548	81–252	45–256

Iron (S, P)

Newborns: 20–157 μg/dL (3.6–28.1 μmol/L).
6 wk–3 yr: 20–115 μg/dL (3.6–20.6 μmol/L).
3–9 yr: 20–141 μg/dL (3.6–25.2 μmol/L).
9–14 yr: 21–151 μg/dL (3.8–27 μmol/L).
14–16 yr: 20–181 μg/dL (3.6–32.4 μmol/L).
Adults: 44–196 μg/dL (7.2–31.3 μmol/L).

Iron-Binding Capacity (S, P)

Newborns: 59–175 μg/dL (10.6–31.3 μmol/L).
Children and adults: 275–458 μg/dL (45–72 μmol/L).

Lactate Dehydrogenase (LDH) (S, P)

Values using lactate substrate (kinetic).
Newborns (1–3 d): 40–348 IU/L at 37° C.
1 mo–5 yr: 150–360 IU/L at 37° C.
5–8 yr: 150–300 IU/L at 37° C.
8–12 yr: 130–300 IU/L at 37° C.
12–14 yr: 130–280 IU/L at 37° C.
14–16 yr: 130–230 IU/L at 37° C.
Adult males: 70–178 IU/L at 37° C.
Adult females: 42–166 IU/L at 37° C.

Normal Values: Blood—Continued

Lead (B)
<30 μg/dL (<1.4 μmol/L).

Lipoprotein Cholesterol, High-Density (HDL) (S)
Values in mg/dL (mmol/L).

Group	Males	Females
6–7 yr	35–77 (0.90–1.98)	24–76 (0.62–1.96)
8–9 yr	31–80 (0.80–2.06)	34–77 (0.87–1.98)
10–11 yr	34–81 (0.87–1.09)	30–74 (0.77–1.91)
12–13 yr	30–82 (0.77–2.11)	33–73 (0.85–1.88)
14–15 yr	26–72 (0.67–1.86)	29–73 (0.74–1.88)
16–17 yr	25–66 (0.64–1.70)	27–78 (0.69–2.01)

Lipoprotein Cholesterol, Low-Density (LDL) (S)
Values in mg/dL (mmol/L).

Group	Males	Females
6–7 yr	56–134 (1.44–3.46)	52–149 (1.34–3.85)
8–9 yr	52–129 (1.34–3.33)	57–143 (1.47–3.69)
10–11 yr	45–149 (1.16–3.85)	56–140 (1.44–3.61)
12–13 yr	55–135 (1.42–3.48)	58–138 (1.49–3.56)
14–15 yr	48–143 (1.24–3.69)	47–140 (1.21–3.61)
16–17 yr	53–134 (1.36–3.36)	44–147 (1.13–3.79)

Osmolality (S, P)
270–290 mosm/kg.

Oxygen Capacity (B)
1.34 mL/g of hemoglobin.

Oxygen Saturation (B)
Newborns: 30–80% (0.3–0.8 mol/mol of venous blood).
Thereafter: 65–85% (0.65–0.85 mol/mol of venous blood).

Partial Thromboplastin Time (P)
Children: 42–54 sec.

Phenylalanine (S, P)
0.7–3.5 mg/dL (0.04–0.21 mmol/L).

Potassium (RBC)
87.2–97.6 mmol/L.

Potassium (S, P)
Premature infants: 4.5–7.2 mmol/L.
Full-term infants: 3.7–5.2 mmol/L.
Children: 3.5–5.8 mmol/L.
Adults: 3.5–5.5 mmol/L.

Prostaglandin E (P)
Newborns: 1000–1730 pg/mL.
2–3 d: 60–150 pg/mL.
1–6 yr: 125–200 pg/mL.
6–14 yr: 160–340 pg/mL.
Adults: 450–550 pg/mL.

Proteins in Serum*

Group	Total Protein	Albumin	α_1-Globulin
At birth	4.6–7.0	3.2–4.8	0.1–0.3
3 mo	4.5–6.5	3.2–4.8	0.1–0.3
1 yr	5.4–7.5	3.7–5.7	0.1–0.3
>4 yr	5.9–8.0	3.8–5.4	0.1–0.3

Group	α_2-Globulin	β-Globulin	λ-Globulin
At birth	0.2–0.3	0.3–0.6	0.6–1.2
3 mo	0.3–0.7	0.3–0.7	0.2–0.7
1 yr	0.5–1.1	0.4–1.0	0.2–0.9
>4 yr	0.4–0.8	0.5–1.0	0.4–1.3

*Values are for cellulose acetate electrophoresis and are in g/dL. SI conversion factor: g/dL × 10 = g/L.

Prothrombin (Factor II) (P)
Children: 81–123 units/dL.

Prothrombin Time (P)
Children: 11–15 sec.

Protoporphyrin, "Free" (FEP, ZPP) (B)
Values for free erythrocyte protoporphyrin (FEP) and zinc protoporphyrin (ZPP) are 1.2–2.7 μg/g of hemoglobin.

Sedimentation Rate (Micro) (B)
<2 yr: 1–5 mm/hr.
>2 yr: 1–8 mm/hr.

Serotonin (S, P)
Children: 127–187 ng/mL.
Adults: 119–171 ng/mL.

Sodium (S, P)
Children and adults: 135–148 mmol/L.

Thrombin Time (P)
Children: 12–16 sec.

Thyroid-Stimulating Hormone (TSH) (S)
Levels increase shortly after birth to levels as high as 30–40 μIU/mL. Levels return to the adult normal range (1.6–10.9 μIU/mL) by about 10–14 days.

Continued.

Normal Values: Blood—Continued

Thyroxine (T₄) (S)

1–2 d: 11.4–25.5 μg/dL (147–328 nmol/L).
3–4 d: 9.8–25.2 μg/dL (126–324 nmol/L).
1–6 yr: 5–15.2 μg/dL (64–196 nmol/L).
11–13 yr: 4–13 μg/dL (51–167 nmol/L).
>18 yr: 4.7–11 μg/dL (60–142 nmol/L).

Throxine, "Free" (Free T₄) (S)

1–2.3 ng/dL.

Throxine-Binding Globulin (TBG) (S)

1–7 mo: 2.9–6 mg/dL.
7–12 mo: 2.1–5.9 mg/dL.
Prepubertal children: 2–5.3 mg/dL.
Pubertal children and adults: 1.8–4.2 mg/dL.

Triglyceride (S, P)

Fasting (>12 hr) values in mg/mL (mmol/L).

Group	Males	Females
6–7 yr	32–79 (0.36–0.89)	24–128 (0.27–1.44)
8–9 yr	28–105 (0.31–1.18)	34–115 (0.38–1.29)
10–11 yr	30–115 (0.33–1.29)	39–131 (0.44–1.48)
12–13 yr	33–112 (0.37–1.26)	36–125 (0.40–1.41)
14–15 yr	35–136 (0.39–1.53)	36–122 (0.40–1.37)
16–17 yr	38–167 (0.42–1.88)	34–136 (0.38–1.53)

NOTE: Lower values represent 5th percentile, whereas upper values are calculated from mean + 2 SD.

Triiodothyronine (T₃) (S)

1–3 d: 89–405 ng/dL.
1 wk: 91–300 ng/dL.
1–12 mo: 85–250 ng/dL.
Prepubertal children: 119–218 ng/dL.
Pubertal children and adults: 55–170 ng/dL.

Urea Clearance

Premature infants: 3.5–17.3 mL/min/1.73 m².
Newborns: 8.7–33 mL/min/1.73 m².
2–12 mo: 40–95 mL/min/1.73 m².
≥2 yr: >52 mL/min/1.73 m².

Urea Nitrogen (S, P)

1–2 yr: 5–15 mg/dL (1.8–5.4 mmol/L).
Thereafter: 10–20 mg/dL (3.5–7.1 mmol/L).

Uric Acid (S, P)

Males:
0–14 yr: 2–7 mg/dL (119–416 μmol/L).
>14 yr: 3–8 mg/dL (178–476 μmol/L).

Females:
All ages: 2–7 mg/dL (119–416 μmol/L).

Normal Values: Urine

Addis Count

Red cells (12-hr specimen): <1 million.
White cells (12-hr specimen): <2 million.
Casts (12-hr specimen): <10,000.
Protein (12-hr specimen): <55 mg.

Albumin

First mo: 1–100 mg/L.
Second mo: 0.2–34 mg/L.
2–12 mo: 0.5–19 mg/L.

Aldosterone

Newborns: 0.5–5 μg/24 hr (20–140 μg/g of creatinine).
Prepubertal children: 1–8 μg/24 hr (4–22 μg/g of creatinine).
Adults: 3–19 μg/24 hr (1.5–20 μg/g of creatinine).

Ammonia

2–12 mo: 4–20 μEq/min/m².
1–16 yr: 6–16 μEq/min/m².

Calcium

4–12 yr: 4–8 mEq/L (2–4 mmol/L).

Catecholamines (Norepinephrine, Epinephrine)

Values in μg/24 hr (nmol/24 hr).

Group	Total Catechol-amines	Norepinephrine	Epinephrine
<1 yr	20	5.4–15.9 (32–94)	0.1–4.3 (0.5–23.5)
1–5 yr	40	8.1–30.8 (48–182)	0.8–9.1 (4.4–49.7)
6–15 yr	80	19.0–71.1 (112–421)	1.3–10.5 (7.1–57.3)
>15 yr	100	34.4–87.0 (203–514)	3.5–13.2 (19.1–72.1)

Normal Values: Urine—Continued

Chloride

Infants: 1.7–8.5 mmol/24 hr.
Children: 17–34 mmol/24 hr.
Adults: 140–240 mmol/24 hr.

Corticosteroids (17-Hydroxycorticosteroids)

0–2 yr: 2–4 mg/24 hr (5.5–11 µmol).
2–6 yr: 3–6 mg/24 hr (8.3–16.6 µmol).
6–10 yr: 6–8 mg/24 hr (16.6–22.1 µmol).
10–14 yr: 8–10 mg/24 hr (22.1–27.6 µmol).

Creatine

18–58 mg/L (1.37–4.42 mmol/L).

Creatinine

Newborns: 7–10 mg/kg/24 hr.
Children: 20–30 mg/kg/24 hr.
Adult males: 21–26 mg/kg/24 hr.
Adult females: 16–22 mg/kg/24 hr.

Homovanillic Acid

Children: 3–16 µg/mg of creatinine.
Adults: 2–4 µg/mg of creatinine.

Mucopolysaccharides

Acid mucopolysaccharide screen should yield negative results. Positive results after dialysis of the urine should be followed up with a thin-layer chromatogram for evaluation of the acid mucopolysaccharide excretion pattern.

Osmolality

Infants: 50–600 mosm/L.
Older children: 50–1400 mosm/L.

Phosphorus, Tubular Reabsorption

78–97%.

Porphyrins

δ-Aminolevulinic acid: 0–7 mg/24 hr (0–53.4 µmol/24 hr).
Porphobilinogen: 0–2 mg/24 hr (0–8.8 µmol/24 hr).
Coproporphyrin: 0–160 µg/24 hr (0–244 nmol/24 hr).
Uroporphyrin: 0–26 µg/24 hr (0–31 nmol/24 hr).

Potassium

26–123 mmol/L.

Sodium

Infants: 0.3–3.5 mmol/24 hr (6–10 mmol/m^2).
Children and adults: 5.6–17 mmol/24 hr.

Testosterone

Prepubertal children: 0.2–2.3 µg/24 hr (0.3–5 µg/g of creatinine).
Adult males: 40–130 µg/24 hr.
Adult females: 2–11 µg/24 hr.

Urobilinogen

<3 mg/24 hr (<5.1 µmol/24 hr).

Vanillylmandelic Acid (VMA)

Because of the difficulty in obtaining an accurately timed 24-hour collection, values based on microgram per milligram of creatinine are the most reliable indications of VMA excretion in young children.
1–12 mo: 1–35 µg/mg of creatinine (31–135 µg/kg/24 hr).
1–2 yr: 1–30 µg/mg of creatinine.
2–5 yr: 1–15 µg/mg of creatinine.
5–10 yr: 1–14 µg/mg of creatinine.
10–15 yr: 1–10 g/mg of creatinine (1–7 mg/24 hr; 5–35 µmol/24hr).
Adults: 1–7 µg/mg of creatinine (1–7 mg/24 hr; 5–35 µmol/24 hr).

Normal Values: Feces

Fat, Total

2–6 mo: 0.3–1.3 g/d
6 mo–1 yr: <4 g/d.
Children: <3 g/d.
Adolescents: <5 g/d.
Adults: <7 g/d.

Normal Values: Sweat

Electrolytes

Values for sodium or chloride or both. Elevated values in the presence of a family history or clinical findings of cystic fibrosis are diagnostic of cystic fibrosis.
Normal: <55 mmol/L.
Borderline: 55–70 mmol/L.
Elevated: >70 mmol/L.

Example

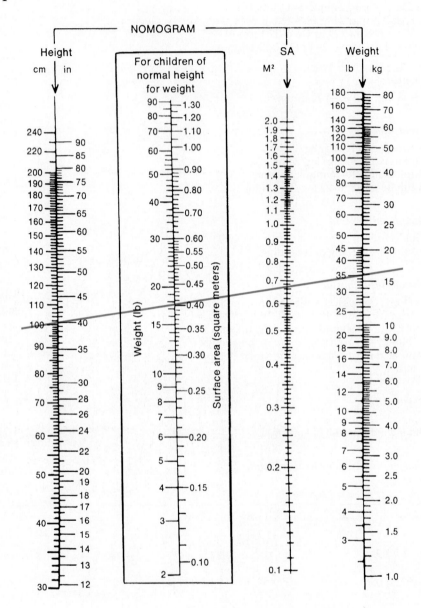

NOMOGRAM

Pediatric doses of medications are generally based on body surface area (BSA) or weight. To calculate a child's BSA, draw a straight line from the height (in the lefthand column) to the weight (in the righthand column). The point at which the line intersects the surface area (SA) column is the BSA (measured in square meters [m²]). If the child is of roughly normal proportion, BSA can be calculated from the weight alone (in the enclosed area).

The following formula can then be used to estimate the pediatric drug dose:

$$\frac{\text{BSA of child}}{\text{Mean BSA of adult}} \times \text{Adult dose} = \text{Estimated pediatric dose}$$

WEST NOMOGRAM FOR CALCULATION OF BODY SURFACE AREA

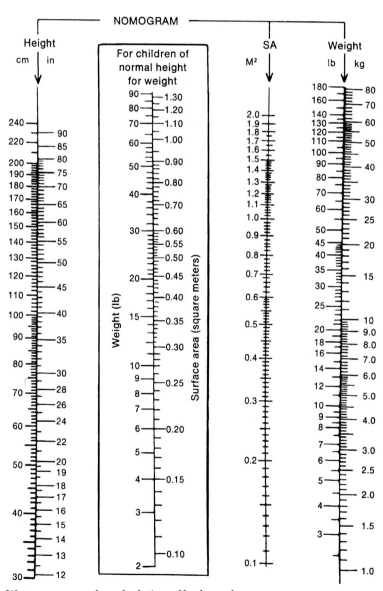

West nomogram for calculation of body surface area.

Nomogram modified from data of E. Boyd by C.D. West; from Behrman, R.E., Vaughan, V.C. (Eds.) (1992). *Nelson's textbook of pediatrics* (14th ed.). Philadelphia: W.B. Saunders.

CHAPTER 4
Nursing Considerations for the Family: Hospital and Home

Association for the Care of Children's Health (ACCH)
7910 Woodmont Ave., Suite 300
Bethesda, MD 20814
(301) 654–6549

National Head Injury Foundation
1776 Massachusetts Ave. NW, Suite 100
Washington, DC 20036
(202) 296–6443

CHAPTER 6
The Child with a Life-Threatening Illness or Injury

Candlelighter's Childhood Cancer Foundation
(for parents of children with cancer)
1901 Pennsylvania Ave. NW, Suite 101
Washington, DC 20006
(202) 659–5136

Children's Hospice International
(for care of the terminally ill)
700 Princess St., Lower Level
Alexandria, VA 22314
(800) 24–CHILD or (703) 684–0330

The Compassionate Friends
(for bereaved parents)
P.O. Box 3696
Oak Brook, IL 60522–3696
(708) 990–0010; fax: (708) 990–0246

The Compassionate Friends
685 Williams Ave.
Winnipeg, Manitoba
CANADA R3E 0Z2
(204) 787–4896

The Ronald McDonald House
419 E. 86th St.
New York, NY 10028
(212) 639–0100

CHAPTER 9
Alterations in Immune Function

AIDS Hotline
(800) 342–2437

The American Juvenile Arthritis Organization
1314 Spring St.
Atlanta, GA 30309
(404) 872–7100 or (800) 283–7800 (9 AM to 7 PM EST)

American Lupus Society
3914 Del Amo Blvd.
Torrance, CA 90503
(800) 331–1802 or (310) 542–8891

Arthritis Society
250 Bloor St. E, Suite 401
Toronto, Ontario
CANADA M4W 3P2
(416) 967–5679

Organizations and Resources

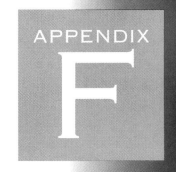

The Lupus Foundation of America
4 Research Pl., Suite 180
Rockville, MD 20850
(800) 558–0121 or (301) 670–9292

CHAPTER 10
Alterations in Respiratory Function

Allergy and Asthma Network/Mothers of
    Asthmatics, Inc.
3554 Chain Bridge Rd.
Fairfax, VA 22030–2709
(800) 878–4403 or (703) 385–4403 (call dur-
    ing business hours)

American Lung Association
1740 Broadway
New York, NY 10010
(212) 315–8700
(check phone book for local chapter ad-
    dress/phone number)

Canadian Cystic Fibrosis Foundation
222 Young St., Suite 601
Toronto, Ontario
CANADA M4S 2B4
(416) 485–9149

Canadian Lung Association
75 Albert St., Suite 908
Ottawa, Ontario
CANADA K1P 5E7
(613) 237–1208

Council of Guilds for Infant Survival
(has 12 guilds in 7 states)
P.O. Box 3841
Davenport, IA 52808
(319) 322–4870

Cystic Fibrosis Foundation
6931 Arlington Rd., Suite 200
Bethesda, MD 20814
(800)–FIGHTCF or (301) 951–4422

The Lung Association
573 King St. E, Suite 201
Toronto, Ontario
CANADA M5A 4L3
(416) 864–1112

SIDS Alliance
10500 Little Patuxent Pkwy., Suite 420
Columbia, MD 21044
(800) 221–7437 or (410) 964–8000

CHAPTER 11
Alterations in Eye, Ear, Nose, and Throat Function

American Federation for the Blind
15 W. 16th St.
New York, NY 10011
(212) 620–2000

Canadian Hearing Society
271 Spadina Rd.
Toronto, Ontario
CANADA M5R 2V3
(416) 964–9595

Canadian National Institute for the Blind
1931 Bayview Ave.
Toronto, Ontario
CANADA M4G 4C8
(416) 486–2500

Low Vision Association of Canada
145 Adelaide St. W
Toronto, Ontario
CANADA M5H 3H4
(416) 921–6609

National Association for the Visually
  Handicapped
22 W. 21st St.
New York, NY 10010
(212) 889–3141

National Federation of the Blind
1800 Johnson St.
Baltimore, MD 21230
(410) 659–9314

National Society to Prevent Blindness
500 E. Remington Rd.
Schaumburg, IL 60173
(708) 843–2020

Woodbine House
5615 Fishers Lane
Rockville, MD 20852
(800) 843–7323
Choices in Deafness: A Parents' Guide
  (1987); $14.95

CHAPTER 12
Alterations in Cardiovascular Function

American Heart Association
7272 Greenville Ave.
Dallas, TX 75231
(214) 373–6300 or (800) AHA–USA1 (to
  reach local chapter)

CHAPTER 13
Alterations in Hematologic Function

Aplastic Anemia Foundation of America
P.O. Box 22689
Baltimore, MD 21203

Canadian Hemophilia Society
1450 City Councillors
Bureau 840
Montreal, Quebec
CANADA H3A 2E6
(514) 848–0503

Cooley's Anemia Foundation
105 E. 22nd St., Suite 911
New York, NY 10010
(800) 221–3571 or (800) 522–7222 (in New
  York); (212) 598–0911

National Association of Sickle Cell Disease
4221 Wilshire Blvd.
Los Angeles, CA 90010
(213) 736–5455

National Hemophilia Foundation
110 Greene St., Suite 303
New York, NY 10012
(800) 424–2634 (resource center) or
  (212) 219–8180

Sickle Cell Association of Ontario
1076 Bathurst St., Suite 305
Toronto, Ontario
CANADA M5R 3G9
(416) 789–2855

CHAPTER 14
Alterations in Neurologic Function

Association for the Rehabilitation of the
  Brain-Injured (ARBI)
3412 Sprue Dr. SW
Calgary, Alberta
CANADA T3C 3A4
(403) 242–7116

Epilepsy Canada
1470 Peel St., Suite 745
Montreal, Quebec
CANADA H3A 1T1
(514) 845–7855

Epilepsy Foundation of America
4351 Garden City Dr.
Landover, MD 20785
(800)EFA–1000 or (301) 459–3700

National Hydrocephalus Foundation
Route 1, River Rd., Box 210
Joliet, IL 60436
(815) 467–6548

Ontario Federation for Cerebral Palsy
163160 Burns W, Suite 104
Toronto, Ontario
CANADA M6L 1C5
(416) 244–9686

Spina Bifida Association of America
3901 Woodhaven Ln., Suite 205
Bowie, MD 20715
(301) 805–0213

United Cerebral Palsy Association, Inc.
710 Penn Plaza, Suite 804
New York, NY 10001
(800) USA–1UCP

CHAPTER 15
Alterations in Gastrointestinal Function

American Celiac Society
58 Musano Ct.
West Orange, NJ 07052
(201) 325–8837

American Cleft Palate Association
1218 Grandview Ave.
Pittsburgh, PA 15211
(800) 24–CLEFT or (412) 481–1376

Canadian Celiac Association, Inc.
6519 B Mississauga Rd.
Mississauga, Ontario
CANADA L5N 1A6
(416) 567–7195

Canadian Foundation for Ileitis and Colitis
21 St. Clair Ave. E, Suite 301
Toronto, Ontario
CANADA M4TL 1L9
(416) 920–5035

Celiac Sprue Association/United States of
    America
P.O. Box 31700
Omaha, NE 68103–0700
(402) 558–0600

Children's Memorial Hospital
707 W. Fullerton
Chicago, IL 60614
(312) 880–4000

Crohn's Colitis Foundation
444 Park Ave. S
New York, NY 10016
(212) 685–3440

La Leche League
P.O. Box 1209
Franklin Park, IL 60131–8209
(708) 455–7730 (24-hour service)
(800) LA–LECHE (for local number or cata-
    log; 9 AM to 3 PM)

La Leche League International, Inc.
495 Main St.
Winchester, Ontario
CANADA K0C 2K0
(613) 774–2850

National Safe Kids Campaign
Children's National Medical Center
111 Michigan Ave. NW
Washington, DC 20010
(202) 884–4993

United Ostomy Association
36 Executive Park, Suite 120
Irvine, CA 92714–6744
(800) 826–0826 or (714) 660–8624

United Ostomy Association, Canada
4 Hamilton Ave.
Hamilton, Ontario
CANADA L8V 2S3
(416) 389–8822

CHAPTER 16
Alterations in Cellular Growth

American Cancer Society
1599 Clifton Rd. NE
Atlanta, GA 30329
(800) ACS–2345
(check phone book for local chapter ad-
    dress/phone number)

Candlelighter's Childhood Cancer Founda-
    tion
(see Chapter 6 for complete listing)

CHAPTER 17
Alterations in Musculoskeletal Function

Muscular Dystrophy Association of
   America
810 Seventh Ave.
New York, NY 10019
(212) 586–0808

Muscular Dystrophy Association of
   Canada
150 Eglinton Ave. E, Suite 400
Toronto, Ontario
CANADA M4P 1E8
(416) 488–0030

National Scoliosis Foundation
72 Mount Auburn St.
Watertown, MA 02172
(617) 926–0397; fax: (617) 926–0398

Osteogenesis Imperfecta Foundation, Inc.
   (OIF)
5005 W. Laurel St., Suite 210
Tampa, FL 33607
(813) 282–1161

Scoliosis Association, Inc.
P.O. Box 811705
Boca Raton, FL 33481–1705
(800) 800–0669

Scoliosis Research Society
6300 N. River Rd., Suite 727
Rosemont, IL 60018–4226
(708) 698–1627

CHAPTER 18
Alterations in Genitourinary Function

Kidney Foundation of Canada
5160 Boulevard Decarie
Bureau 780
Montreal, Quebec
CANADA H3X 2H9
(800) 361–7494 or (514) 369–4806

National Kidney Foundation
30 E. 33rd St.
New York, NY 10016
(800) 622–9010 or (212) 889–2210

CHAPTER 19
Alterations in Endocrine Function

American Diabetes Association, Inc.
1660 Duke St.
Alexandria, VA 22314
(800) 232–3472

Canadian Diabetes Association
78 Bond St.
Toronto, Ontario
CANADA M5B 2J8
(416) 362–4440

Human Growth Foundation
P.O. Box 3090
7777 Leesburg Pike, Suite 2028
Falls Church, VA 22043
(800) 451–6434

Short Stature Foundation
P.O. Box 5356
Huntington Beach, CA 92615
(800) 24–DWARF (help line)

Turner Syndrome Society
768–214 Wayzata Oaks Center
15500 Wayzata Blvd.
Wayzata, MN 55391
(612) 475–9944

Turner Syndrome Society of Canada
7777 Keele St., Floor 2
Concord, Ontario
CANADA L4K XYF

CHAPTER 21
Alterations in Psychosocial Function

Al-Anon
(check Yellow Pages under Health Agencies or Social Services)

Ala-Teen
(check Yellow Pages under Health Agencies or Social Services)

Alcoholics Anonymous
(check Yellow Pages under Health Agencies or Social Services)

American Anorexia and Bulimia Association, Inc.
418 E. 76th St.
New York, NY 10021
(212) 734–1114

Association for Retarded Citizens
500 E. Border St.
Arlington, TX 76010
(800) 433–5255 or (817) 261–6003

Autism Society of America
8601 Georgia Ave., Suite 503
Silver Spring, MD 20910
(301) 565–0433

Nar-Anon
(check Yellow Pages under Health Agencies or Social Services)

Narcotics Anonymous
(check Yellow Pages under Health Agencies or Social Services)

National Anorectic Aid Society, Inc.
1925 E. Dublin-Granville Rd.
Columbus, OH 43229
(614) 436–1112

National Association of Anorexia Nervosa & Associated Disorders, Inc.
Box 7
Highland Park, IL 60035
(312) 831–3438

National Down Syndrome Society
666 Broadway
New York, NY 10012
(800) 221–4602

USA Mainstream
1200 15th St., N.W., Suite 403
Washington, D.C. 20005
(202) 234–4636

acellular vaccine Uses proteins from the microorganism to stimulate the process of active immunity.

acidemia Decreased blood pH.

acidosis Condition caused by too much acid in the blood.

active immunization Stimulation of antibody production without causing clinical disease.

acute pain Sudden pain of short duration that is associated with a tissue-damaging stimulus.

advance directives A patient's living will or appointed durable power of attorney for health care decisions.

affect Outward manifestation of feeling or emotion; the tone of a person's reaction or response to people or events.

airway resistance The effort or force needed to move oxygen through the trachea to the lungs.

aldosterone A hormone secreted by the adrenal cortex that causes the renal tubules to reabsorb saline (sodium and water) and retain it in the body.

alkalemia Increased blood pH.

alkalosis Condition caused by too little acid in the blood.

allergen An antigen capable of inducing hypersensitivity.

alveolar hypoventilation The condition in which the volume of air entering the alveoli during gas exchange is inadequate to meet the body's metabolic needs.

anemia Reduction in the number of red blood cells, the quantity of hemoglobin, and the volume of packed red cells per 100 mL of blood to below-normal levels.

antibody A protein that is capable of reacting specifically to an antigen.

anticipatory guidance The process of understanding upcoming developmental needs and then teaching caretakers to meet those needs.

antidiuretic hormone A hormone released by the posterior pituitary gland that causes the renal tubules to reabsorb water and retain it in the body.

antigen A foreign substance that triggers an immune response.

apnea Cessation of respiration lasting longer than 20 seconds.

areflexic No reflex response to verbal, sensory, or pain stimulation.

assent A child's voluntary agreement to participate in a research project or to accept treatment.

assessment The process of collecting information about a child and family to develop the nursing diagnoses. The assessment process includes the patient history, physical examination, and analysis of the collected data to identify relevant information.

associative play A type of play that emerges in preschool years when children interact with one another, engaging in similar activities and participating in groups.

atopy A hereditary allergic tendency.

audiography A test used to assess hearing in which sounds of various pitches and intensity are presented to children through earphones.

aura Subjective sensation, often olfactory or visual in nature, that is an early sign of a seizure.

auscultation The technique of listening to sounds produced by the airway, lungs, stomach, heart, and blood vessels to identify their characteristics. Auscultation is usually performed with the stethoscope to enhance the sounds heard.

GLOSSARY

azotemia Accumulation of nitrogenous wastes in the blood.

behavior modification A technique used to reinforce desirable behaviors, helping the child to replace maladaptive behaviors with more appropriate ones.

benign A growth that does not endanger life or health.

body fluid The body water with substances (solutes) dissolved in it.

bone marrow suppression Reduction in the activity of the bone marrow stem cells, which leads to a reduction in the number of blood cells produced by the bone marrow.

bone marrow transplantation The receipt of own (treated) or matched bone marrow by intravenous route following destruction of own bone marrow by chemotherapy and radiation.

buffer Related acid-base pair that gives up or takes up hydrogen ions as needed to prevent large changes in pH of a solution.

carbonic acid H_2CO_3; excreted by the lungs in the form of carbon dioxide and water.

carcinogens Chemicals or processes that, when combined with genetic traits and in interaction with one another, cause cancer.

case manager Person who coordinates health care to prevent gaps or overlaps.

cephalocaudal development The process by which development proceeds from the head downward through the body and toward the feet.

chemotherapy Treatment that involves substances taken orally, intravenously, intrathecally, or by injection to combat cancer.

child life specialist Trained professional who plans therapeutic activities for hospitalized children.

chondrolysis The breaking down and absorption of cartilage.

chronic pain Persistent pain lasting longer than 6 months, generally associated with a prolonged disease process.

clinical judgment Analyzing and synthesizing data from the patient history, physical examination, screening tests, and laboratory studies to make decisions about the child's health problems. This is also called diagnostic reasoning.

clonic Alternating muscular contraction and relaxation; often used to describe seizure activity.

cognitive therapy A therapeutic approach that attempts to help the person recognize automatic thought patterns that lead to unpleasant feelings.

collective monologue A type of speech demonstrated when two people talk about separate subjects, wait for each other to speak, and do not respond to each other's topics; common during preschool years.

coma State of unconsciousness in which the child cannot be aroused, even with powerful stimuli.

communicable disease Illness that is directly or indirectly transmitted from one person to another.

compensation Process that tends to restore blood pH to normal by making either the partial pressure of carbon dioxide (PCO_2) or the bicarbonate ion concentration abnormal. Compensation does not fix the cause of the acid-base imbalance.

compliance Amount of distention or expansion that ventricles can achieve to increase stroke volume.

conductive hearing loss Hearing loss caused by inadequate conduction of sound from the outer to the middle ear.

confusion   Disorientation to time, place, or person.

conscious sedation   Light sedation during which the child maintains airway reflexes and responds to verbal stimuli.

constipation   Difficult and infrequent defecation with passage of hard, dry stool.

continuum of care   The system of care for ill and injured children that includes each of the following elements: illness or injury prevention, acute care in the hospital, and restorative care in either the home or a rehabilitation center until the child is reintegrated into the family, school, and community.

cooperative play   A type of play that emerges in school years when children join into groups to achieve a goal or play a game.

correction   Process that tends to restore blood pH to normal by fixing the cause of the acid-base imbalance.

culture   The socially learned beliefs, life-styles, and values that are characteristic of the family and community.

Cushing triad   Reflex response associated with increased intracranial pressure or compromised blood flow to the brainstem; characterized by hypertension, increased systolic pressure with wide pulse pressure, bradycardia, and irregular respirations.

death anxiety   A feeling of apprehension or fear of death.

death imagery   Any reference to death or death-related topics, such as going away, separation, funerals, and dying, given in response to a picture or story that would not usually stimulate other children to discuss death-related topics.

debridement   Removal of dead tissue to speed the healing process.

decibels   Units used to measure the loudness of sounds.

deep sedation   A controlled state of depressed consciousness or unconsciousness in which the child may experience partial or complete loss of protective reflexes.

defense mechanisms   Techniques used by the ego to unconsciously change reality, thereby protecting itself from excessive anxiety.

delirium   State characterized by confusion, fear, agitation, hyperactivity, or anxiety.

dermatophytoses   Fungal infections that affect primarily the skin but may affect the hair and nails.

desaturated blood   Blood with a lower than normal oxygen level resulting when a heart defect causes oxygenated and unoxygenated blood to mix.

development   An increase in capability or function.

dialysate   The solution used in dialysis.

diarrhea   Frequent passage of abnormally watery stool.

digitalization   Process of giving a higher than normal dose of digoxin initially to speed response to the drug.

direct transmission   Passage of infectious disease by physical contact between source of pathogen and new host.

dislocation   Displacement of a bone from its normal articulation with a joint.

distraction   The ability to focus attention on something other than pain, such as an activity, music, or a story.

dramatic play   A type of play in which a child lives out the drama of daily life.

dysphonia   Muffled, hoarse, or absent voice sounds.

dysplasia   Abnormal development resulting in altered size, shape, and cell organization.

dyspnea   Shortness of breath; difficulty in breathing.

ecchymosis   A bruise.

effective communication   Information exchanged between the nurse, parent, and child that is clearly understood by all persons involved in the conversation.

ego   The realistic part of the personality that struggles for acceptable behavior and balances the id and superego.

electroanalgesia   Transcutaneous electrical nerve stimulation (TENS), which competes with pain stimuli for transmission to the spinal cord.

electrolytes   Substances that are charged particles when they are dissolved.

emancipated minors   Self-supporting adolescents under 18 years of age who are not subject to parental control.

equianalgesic dose   The amount of drug, whether administered orally or parenterally, needed to produce the same analgesic effect.

equinus   A condition that limits dorsiflexion to less than normal; usually associated with clubfoot.

erythropoiesis   Formation of red blood cells.

eschar   Slough or layer of dead skin or tissue.

escharotomy   Incision into constricting dead tissue of a burn injury to restore peripheral circulation.

ethics   The philosophic study of morality, moral judgments, and moral problems.

expressive jargon   Use of unintelligible words with normal speech intonations as if truly communicating in words; common in toddlerhood.

extracellular fluid   The fluid in the body that is outside the cells.

extravasation   Damage that occurs when a chemotherapeutic drug leaks into soft tissue surrounding the infusion site.

family-centered care   A philosophy of care that integrates the family's values and potential contributions in the plans for and provision of care to the child.

family crisis   An event occurring when a family encounters problems that for a time seem insurmountable and with which the family is unable to cope in its usual ways.

filtration   Movement into or out of capillaries as the net result of several opposing forces.

focal   Specific area of the brain; often used to describe seizures or neurologic deficits.

glycosuria   Abnormal amount of glucose in the urine.

goiter   Enlargement of the thyroid gland.

graft-versus-host disease Series of immunologic responses mounted by the host of a transplanted organ with the purpose of destroying the transplant cells.

growth An increase in physical size.

hemarthrosis Bleeding into joint cavities.

hematopoiesis Blood cell production.

hemodynamics Pressures generated by blood and passage of blood through the heart and pulmonary system.

hemoglobinopathy Disease characterized by abnormal hemoglobin.

hemosiderosis Increased deposition of iron in body tissues associated with diseases involving destruction of red blood cells.

hernia Protrusion or projection of a body part or structure through the muscle wall of the cavity that normally contains it.

hormone A chemical substance that is produced by a gland or organ and carried in the bloodstream to another part of the body where it has a regulatory effect on particular cells.

hospice A philosophy of care that focuses on helping persons with short life expectancies to live their remaining lives to the fullest—without pain and with choices and dignity.

hydronephrosis Collection of urine in renal pelvis as a result of obstructed outflow.

hypercapnia Greater than normal amounts of carbon dioxide in the blood.

hypersensitivity response An overreaction of the immune system, responsible for allergic reactions.

hypertonic fluid Fluid that is more concentrated than normal body fluid.

hyperventilation Condition in which more air than normal is moved in and out of the lungs.

hypotonic fluid Fluid that is more dilute than normal body fluid.

hypoxemia Abnormally decreased arterial blood oxygen concentration.

hypoxia Lower than normal amounts of oxygen in the blood.

id A basic sexual energy that is present at birth and drives the individual to seek pleasure.

immune therapy Cancer treatment that uses immune system modifiers to influence the response of the body.

immunodeficiency A state of the immune system in which it cannot cope effectively with foreign antigens.

immunoglobulins A protein that functions as an antibody. Immunoglobulins are responsible for humoral immunity.

indirect transmission Passage of infectious disease involving survival of pathogens outside humans before invasion of new host.

individualized education plan Assessment of a child and formulation of a specific learning approach for a child with a physical or mental handicap.

infant mortality Deaths of infants during the first year of life.

infectious disease Illness, caused by a microorganism, that is commonly communicated from one host (human or otherwise) to another.

informed consent A formal preauthorization for an invasive procedure or participation in research.

inspection The technique of purposeful observation by carefully looking at the characteristics of the child's physical features and behaviors. Physical feature characteristics include size, shape, color, movement, position, and location.

interstitial fluid That portion of the extracellular fluid that is between the cells and outside the blood and lymphatic vessels.

intracellular fluid The fluid in the body that is inside the cells.

intracranial pressure Force exerted by brain tissue, cerebrospinal fluid, and blood within the cranial vault.

isotonic fluid Fluid that has the same osmolality as normal body fluid.

karyotype A microscopic display of the 46 chromosomes in the human body lined up from the largest to the smallest. The human female is 46,XX and the human male is 46,XY.

killed virus vaccine Contains the microorganism that has been killed but is still capable of inducing the human body to produce antibodies to the disease.

laryngospasm Spasmodic vibrations of the larynx, which create sudden, violent, unpredictable, involuntary contraction of airway muscles.

leukocytosis Higher than normal leukocyte count.

leukopenia A low white blood cell count.

level of consciousness General description of cognitive, sensory, and motor response to stimuli.

lichenification Thickening of the skin.

live virus vaccine Contains the microorganism in live but attenuated, or weakened, form.

malignant The progressive growth of a tumor that will, if not checked by treatment, result in death.

mature minors Adolescents of 14 and 15 years of age who are able to understand treatment risks and who in some states can consent to or refuse treatment.

metastasis Movement of cancer cells to additional sites in the body.

moral dilemma A conflict of social values and ethical principles that supports different courses of action.

morbidity An illness or injury that limits activity, requires medical attention or hospitalization, or results in a chronic condition.

myringotomy Making an incision in the tympanic membrane to drain fluid.

nature The genetic or hereditary capability of an individual.

neoplasms Cancerous growths.

nonverbal behavior The use of facial expression, eye contact, touch, tone of voice, posture, and body movements that communicate feelings during a conversation.

nosocomial infection Infection acquired in the hospital, not present at the time of admission.

NSAIDs The nonsteroidal antiinflammatory drugs used for pain treatment.

nurture The effects of the environment on an individual's performance.

object permanence The knowledge that an object or person continues to exist when not seen, heard, or felt.

obtunded Diminished level of consciousness with minimal response to stimuli.

occult blood Blood that is present in minute quantities and can be seen only on microscopic examination or through chemical testing.

oliguria Diminished urine output (less than 0.5 to 1 mL/kg/hr).

oncogene A portion of the DNA that is altered and, when duplicated, causes uncontrolled cellular division.

opioids Natural and synthetic narcotic drugs used for pain treatment.

opportunistic infection An infection that is often caused by normally nonpathogenic organisms in persons who lack normal immunity.

osmolality The "concentratedness" of a fluid; technically, the number of moles of particles per kilogram of water.

osmosis Movement of water across a semipermeable membrane into an area of higher particle concentration.

ossification Formation of bone from fibrous tissue or cartilage.

osteotomy Surgical cutting of bone.

ostomy An artificial opening into the urinary or gastrointestinal canal that diverts urine or fecal matter to provide an outlet for it.

pain An unpleasant sensory and emotional experience associated with actual or potential tissue damage. Pain exists when the patient says it does.

palliative procedure Intervention that reduces or relieves symptoms but does not provide a cure; used for children with potentially lethal heart defects.

palpation The technique of touch to identify characteristics of the skin, internal organs, and masses. Characteristics include texture, moistness, tenderness, temperature, position, shape, consistency, and mobility of masses and organs.

pancytopenia A decreased number of blood cell components.

parallel play A type of play that emerges in toddlerhood when children play side by side with similar or different toys, demonstrating little or no social interaction.

passive immunization Immunity produced through introduction of specific antibodies to the disease, which are usually obtained from the blood serum of immune persons and animals. *Does not confer lasting immunity.*

patient-controlled analgesia A method for administration of an intravenous analgesic, such as morphine, using a computerized pump that the patient controls.

percussion The technique of striking the surface of the body, either directly or indirectly, to set up vibrations that reveal the density of underlying tissues and borders of internal organs.

periodic breathing Pauses in respiration lasting less than 20 seconds; a normal breathing pattern in infancy and childhood.

peristalsis A progressive, wavelike movement that occurs involuntarily throughout the gastrointestinal tract.

petechiae Pinpoint red lesions, usually indicative of a bleeding disorder.

pH Negative logarithm of the hydrogen ion concentration; used to monitor the acidity of body fluid.

physiologic anorexia A decrease in appetite manifested when the extremely high metabolic demands of infancy slow to keep pace with the more moderate growth rate of toddlerhood.

play therapy Therapeutic intervention often used with preschool and school-aged children. The child reveals conflicts, wishes, and fears on an unconscious level while playing with dolls, toys, clay, and other objects.

polycythemia Above-normal increase in the number of red cells in the blood.

polydipsia Excessive thirst.

polyphagia Excessive or voracious eating.

polyuria Passage of a large volume of urine in a given period.

postictal period Period after seizure activity during which the level of consciousness is decreased.

posturing Abnormal position assumed after injury or damage to the brain that may be seen as extreme flexion or extension of the limbs.

preload Volume of blood in the ventricle at the end of diastole that stretches the heart muscle before contraction.

primary immune response The process in which B lymphocytes produce antibodies specific to a particular antigen on first exposure.

projectile vomiting Vomiting in which the stomach contents are ejected with great force.

protooncogene A gene with the latent ability to change normal cells into cancer cells.

proximodistal development The process by which development proceeds from the center of the body outward to the extremities.

pseudohermaphroditism Ambiguous development of the external genitalia.

puberty Period of life when the ability to reproduce sexually begins; characterized by maturation of the genital organs, development of the secondary sex characteristics, and (in females) the onset of menstruation.

pulmonary hypertension Condition resulting from a chronic blood volume overload through the pulmonary arteries. It is often irreversible and leads to a life-threatening increase in pulmonary vascular resistance.

purpura Condition characterized by bleeding into the tissues, particularly beneath the skin and mucous membranes, and lesions that vary from red to purple.

quality assurance A process for monitoring the procedures and outcomes of care that uses indicators to measure compliance with standards of care.

radiation Cancer treatment using unstable isotopes that release varying levels of energy to destroy cells.

range of motion The direction and extent to which a particular joint is capable of moving, either independently or with assistance.

rehabilitation Treatment and education of a disabled child to maximize function.

retractions A visible drawing in of the skin of the neck and chest, which occurs on inhalation in infants and young children in respiratory distress.

review of systems A comprehensive interview to identify and record the parent's or child's health concerns and health problems by body system that provides an overview of the child's health status.

risk management A process established by a health care institution to ensure compliance with standards of care and thereby reduce the institution's liability.

rooming in Practice in which parents stay in the child's hospital room and care for the child.

sensorineural hearing loss Hearing loss caused by damage to the inner ear structures or the auditory nerve.

separation anxiety Behaviors observed in young children separated from their parents.

shunt Movement of blood between heart chambers through an abnormal anatomic or surgically created opening.

stent A device used to maintain patency of the urethral canal after surgery.

stereotypy Repetitive, obsessive, machine-like movements, commonly seen in autistic or schizophrenic children.

stranger anxiety Wariness of strange people and places, often shown by infants between 6 and 12 months of age.

stridor An abnormal, high-pitched musical respiratory sound caused when air moves through a narrowed larynx or trachea.

stupor Diminished level of consciousness with response only to vigorous stimulation.

subluxation Partial or complete dislocation of a joint.

superego A moral system that develops in childhood and includes a set of values and a conscience.

support systems The extended network of family, friends, and religious and community contacts that provide nurturance, emotional support, and direct assistance to parents.

tachypnea An abnormally rapid rate of respiration.

therapeutic play Planned play techniques that provide an opportunity for children to deal with their fears and concerns related to illness or hospitalization.

thrombocytopenia A low platelet count.

tonic Continuous muscular contraction; often used to describe seizure activity.

toxoid Toxin that has been treated (by heat or chemical) to weaken its toxic effects but retain its antigenicity.

trigger A stimulus that initiates an asthmatic episode; a substance or condition, including exercise, infection, allergy, irritants, weather, or emotions.

tumor suppressor genes Genetic material that controls the growth of cells.

tympanostomy tubes Small Teflon tubes inserted surgically into the tympanic membrane to promote fluid drainage and ventilate the middle ear.

uremia Toxicity resulting from the buildup of urea and nitrogenous waste in the blood.

valgus An abnormal position of a limb that involves bending away from the midline of the body.

varus An abnormal position of a limb that involves bending toward the midline of the body.

vascular fluid That portion of the extracellular fluid that is in the blood vessels.

vaso-occlusion Blockage of a blood vessel.

vesicoureteral reflux The backflow of urine from the bladder into the ureters during voiding.

INDEX

Brain; *see also* Nervous system
    anatomy of, 434
    hypoxic-ischemic injury to,
        479–480
    pediatric anatomy and physiology
        of, 435
    sickle cell anemia and, 419
    tumor of, 563–566
Brainstem glioma, 563–564
Breast
    assessment of, 113–115
    precocious puberty and, 661
Breast feeding, 45
    cleft lip and palate and, 490
Breath sounds, 111–113
    heart failure and, 383
    laryngotracheobronchitis and, 313
Breath test, hydrogen, 525–526
Breathing; *see also* Airway;
        Respiratory system
    burn injury and, 713
    cardiopulmonary resuscitation
        and, in infant, 835–836
    disorders of, 308
    nasal patency and, 100–101
    periodic, 299
    scoliosis surgery and, 601
Brittle bone disease, 605–607
Bronchial asthma, 320–326
Bronchial/tracheal breath sounds, 111
Bronchiole
    anatomy of, 302
    bronchopulmonary dysplasia and,
        328
Bronchiolitis, 329–333
Bronchitis, 329
Bronchodilator, 323
Bronchophony, 112
Bronchopulmonary dysplasia,
    328–329
Bronchovesicular breath sound, 111
Brown recluse spider bite, 719
Bruise
    age of, 84
    color of, 84
Bryant traction, 592, 614
Buccal mucosa, 105
Buck traction, 614
Buffer
    acid-base balance and, 264–265
    definition of, 263
Bulb syringe, 841
Bulimia nervosa, 740–742
    DSM-III-R criteria for, 741
Bulla, 87
Bullet wound to head, 475
Buprenorphine, 189
Burn injury, 705–716
    etiology of, 706
    to eye, 354
    medical management of, 706–711

Burn injury—*cont'd*
    nursing assessment of, 711
    nursing care plan for, 712–714
    nursing management of, 711–712,
        715–716
    prevention of
        in infant, 48
        in preschool child, 61
        in school-age child, 67
        in toddler, 54
    smoke inhalation and, 344–345
    sunburn and, 716
Butorphanol, 189

C

Cachexia, 543
Calcium, 250–254
    hypercalcemia and, 250–252
    hypocalcemia and, 252–254
    normal blood levels of, 867
    renal failure and, 635
    in urine, 870
Calcium gluconate, 636
Calculation
    of body surface area, 873
    of drug dosage, 822, 872
Calories, deficiency of, 146
Canadian Celiac Association, Inc., 877
Canadian Cystic Fibrosis
        Foundation, 875
Canadian Diabetes Association, 878
Canadian Foundation for Ileitis and
        Colitis, 877
Canadian Hearing Society, 875
Canadian Hemophilia Society, 876
Canadian Lung Association, 875
Canadian National Institute for the
        Blind, 876
Canal
    atrioventricular, 387
    ear, injury to, 357
    inguinal, 128
        assessment of, 128
    urethral, hypospadias and, 622
Cancer; *see* Malignancy
Candida albicans
    diaper dermatitis and, 693
    skin infection with, 699
Candlelighter's Childhood Cancer
        Foundation, 874
Cannula
    blow-by, 831
    nasal, 830
Cap, heparin lock, 824–825
Capillary dynamics, 239
Capillary puncture, 814
Capillary refill, 86, 120
Capital femoral epiphysis, slipped,
    595–596

Car seat
    for infant, 48
    for toddler, 55
Carbon dioxide
    normal blood levels of, 867
    partial pressure of, 265–266
        cyanosis and, 398
Carbon monoxide, 344
Carbonic acid, 263, 264, 265–266
    metabolic acidosis and, 274
    metabolic alkalosis and, 275
Carcinogen, 541, 543–544
Cardiac arrest
    cardiopulmonary resuscitation
        for, 834–838
    hypoxemia and, 377
Cardiac catheterization, 390–392
Cardiac disorder; *see* Heart *entries*
Cardiac output, 377
    heart failure and, 383
Cardiogenic shock, 411
Cardiopulmonary resuscitation
        (CPR), 834–838
    of infant, 834–836
    near-drowning and, 343
    of older child, 837–838
Cardiorespiratory monitoring, 811
Cardiovascular system, 375–412
    acquired heart disease and,
        401–404
    congenital heart disease and,
        385–401; *see also* Heart
        disease
    congestive heart failure and,
        377–385; *see also* Heart failure,
        congestive
    dysrhythmia and, 403–404
    encephalitis and, 456
    head injury and, 472
    infective endocarditis and,
        402–403
    injury of, 407–412
        myocardial contusion and,
            411–412
        shock and, 407–411
    pediatric anatomy and physiology
        of, 376–377
    rheumatic fever and, 401–402
    vascular disease and, 404–407
Carey-Revised Infant Temperament
        Questionnaire, 148
Caries, nursing, 45
Carotene, 867
Case manager, 151
    nurse as, 3
    parent as, 176
Cast
    care of, 586
    hip dysplasia and, 592
    for scoliosis, 603
Cataract, 353

Catecholamine, 870
Catheter
  central venous, 828–829
  urinary, 850–851
  vascular access and, 823
Catheterization, cardiac, 390,
    391–392
Celiac disease, 524–525
Celiac Sprue Association/United
    States of America, 877
Cell
  blood
    leukemia and, 573–576
    types of, 416–417
  osmosis and, 224
  potassium and, 246
Cellular growth alterations, 541–581;
    see also Malignancy
Cellulitis, 701–702
  periorbital, 351
Centers for Disease Control and
    Prevention
  AIDS and
    definition of, 287
    home care for, 289
  sexually transmitted disease and,
    649
Central nervous system; see Nervous
    system
Central venous catheter, 828–829
Centration, 59
Cephalocaudal development, 19,
    21–22
Cerebellar function, 136–138
Cerebral concussion, 473–474
Cerebral contusion, 475
Cerebral edema, 475
  meningitis and, 450
  Reye syndrome and, 453
Cerebral palsy, 465–469
  categories of, 466
  clinical manifestations of, 466
  medical management of, 466–467
  nursing management of, 468–469
  pathophysiology of, 466
Cerebrospinal fluid, meningitis and,
    449, 450
Cervical spinal injury, 478
Chain of infection, 766
Chelation therapy for lead
    poisoning, 537
Chemical burn, 705
Chemotherapy, 545–546
  brain tumor and, 564, 565
  definition of, 541
  neuroblastoma and, 568, 569
  osteosarcoma and, 572
  side effects of, 548
  Wilms tumor and, 570
CHEOPS, 186
Chess, Stella, 35

Chest
  blunt trauma to, 345
  circumference of, 807
  examination of, 108–113
Chest compression
  in infant, 836
  in older child, 838
Chest leads for electrocardiogram,
    846
Chest physiotherapy, 843–846
  cystic fibrosis and, 338, 339
Chest wall, palpation of, 110
Chickenpox, 776–777
Chief complaint, 79
Child abuse, 754–761; see also Abuse
Child life specialist, 160
Child's rights, 13
Children's Hospice International,
    874
Children's Memorial Hospital, 877
Chin lift, in CPR, 835
Chinese culture
  cupping and, 758
  foods in, 26
Chlamydia trachomatis, 650
  conjunctivitis caused by, 351
Chloramphenicol, epiglottitis and,
    316
Chloride, 867
Choanal atresia, 101
Choking
  foreign body and, 341–343
  prevention of, in infant, 49
Cholesterol
  hyperlipidemia and, 405–407
  normal values for, 867
Choline magnesium trisalicylate,
    190
Chordee, 126
Chorea, Syndenham, 401
Christmas disease, 426
Chromosomal abnormality, 23, 24
  cancer and, 544
  sex, 682–684
Chronic pain, 179
Chvostek sign, 271
  hypocalcemia and, 253
  hypomagnesemia and, 257
Circular reactions, 33
Circulation
  cardiopulmonary resuscitation
    and
    of infant, 836
    of older child, 838
  fetal, 376–377
Circumference
  of chest, 807
  of head
    growth charts for, 857, 859
    measurement of, 807
Cirrhosis, 531–532

Cisplatin, 546
Citrate, 235
Clean-catch urine collection, 815
Cleft lip and/or palate, 485–493
  clinical manifestations of, 485
  medical management of, 486
  nursing assessment of, 486
  nursing care plan for, 488–493
  nursing management of, 486–488
  pathophysiology of, 485
Clinical judgment, 75
Clinical practice, role of nurse in, 2–3
Clonic phase of seizure, 433, 441, 442
Closed fracture, 611
Closed pneumothorax, 346
Clostridium tetani, 794–795
Clotting disorder; see Coagulation
    disorder
Clubbing of fingers, 399
Clubfoot, 585–589
Coagulation disorder, 426–430
  disseminated intravascular, 429
    cancer and, 549
    meningitis and, 450
  hemophilia as, 426–428
  idiopathic thrombocytopenic
    purpura as, 429–430
  Von Willebrand disease, 428–429
Coarctation of aorta, 389
Codeine, 189
Cognitive development
  of adolescent, 69
  assessment of, 135–136
  of infant, 39
  play and, 20
  of preschool child, 57
  of school-age child, 64
  of toddler, 50–51
Cognitive therapy, 723, 747
Cold
  application of, for pain, 195
  common, 361
Cold injury, 717–718
Colic, 522
Colitis, ulcerative, 508–510
Collapse of lung, 345–346
Collar, tracheostomy, 832
Collection, specimen, 813–816
Collective monologue, 19, 62
Colloid osmotic pressure, 241
Color
  of bruise, 84
  eye, 92
  of gums, 104
  of mouth and throat, 103
  of nasal mucosa, 101
  respiratory distress and, 300
  skin, 84
  of tympanic membrane, 98
  of urine, 638
Coma, 433, 435

Lymph node
  inguinal, 124
  of neck, 106–107
Lymph node syndrome,
      mucocutaneous, 404–405
Lymphatic system, 240, 241
Lymphocyte, 416, 417
  combined immunodeficiency and,
      284–285
  immune disorders and, 283–284
Lymphocytic leukemia, 573–574
Lysis, tumor, 549

M

Macrodrip tubing, 826
Macula, 96
Macule, 87
Magnesium
  hypermagnesemia and, 254–256
  hypomagnesemia and, 256–258
Malabsorption, 524–525
Male genitalia, 126–128
Malformation; *see* Congenital
      disorder
Malignancy
  of bone, 571–573
  bone marrow transplantation and,
      549
  brain tumor and, 563–566
  causes of, 543–545
  chemotherapy for, 545–547
  clinical manifestations of, 543
  immune therapy for, 547–548
  incidence of, 542–543
  leukemia and, 573–576
  medical management of, 545–550
  nephroblastoma and, 569–571
  neuroblastoma as, 566–568
  nursing care for, 550–562
    assessment and, 552–555
    home care plan for, 561–562
    hospital care plan for, 559–560
    management of, 555–558
  pathophysiology of, 543–545
  radiation for, 547
  retinoblastoma and, 576–577
  rhabdomyosarcoma and, 576
  soft tissue tumors and, 576–579
  surgery for, 545
  Wilms tumor and, 569–571
Management, risk, 1
Manager, case
  definition of, 151
  parent as, 176
Maneuver, Gower, 609
Marijuana, 744
Mask
  mouth-to-mouth resuscitation
      with, 837

Mask—*cont'd*
  oxygen administration and, 830
  use of, in isolation, 804
Mass, abdominal, 123
Mass media, effects of, 25
Maturation
  sexual, 68, 124–128, 655–656
  of wound, 692
Mature minor, 13
Maxillary sinus, 102
McCarthy Scales of Children's
      Abilities, 148
Measles, 792–793
  German, 790–791
  immunization schedule for, 770
Measles vaccine, 793
  information summary on, 772
  reportable events about, 774
Meatus, urethral, 126–127
Mechanical restraint, 801
Mechanical ventilation
  bronchopulmonary dysplasia and,
      329
  procedure for, 834
Meckel diverticulum, 507–508
Meconium, anal patency and, 129
Media, mass, effects of, 25
Medulloblastoma, 563
  treatment of, 565
Megacolon, aganglionic, 501–502
Membrane
  mucous, nasal, 101–102
  tympanic
    examination of, 97–98
    pressure on, 358
    rupture of, 357
Memory, 135
Menarche, 681
Mendelian inheritance, 23
Meningitis
  bacterial, 446–452
    clinical manifestations of,
      446–447
    medical management of, 447–448
    nursing care plan for, 449–451
    nursing management of,
      448–452
    pathophysiology of, 447
  viral, 452
Meningocele, 462
Menstruation
  lack of, 681–682
  painful, 682
Mental combinations, 33
Mental retardation, 735–736
Meperidine, 189
Mercury poisoning, 534
Metabolic acidosis, 268, 272–275
  diabetes mellitus and, 672
Metabolic alkalosis, 268, 275–277
Metabolic emergency in cancer, 549

Metabolism, inborn errors of, 684–686
Metastasis, 541
Methimazole, Graves disease and, 665
Methylphenidate, for hyperactivity,
      732
Methylxanthines, 323
Mexican-American culture
  critical illness and, 214
  foods in, 26
Microdrip tubing, 826
Micturition, involuntary, 628–630
Middle Eastern person, eye contact
      and, 78
Milestones
  balance, 136
  developmental
    for adolescent, 68
    for infant, 40–43
    for preschool child, 58
    for school-age child, 64
    for toddler, 51
  gross motor, 130
Milk
  allergy to, 523
  calcium and, 254
  galactosemia and, 685–686
  lactose intolerance and, 525–526
Milwaukee brace, 598
Minerals, deficiency of, 146
Minimal change nephrotic
      syndrome, 630–634
  clinical manifestations of, 631
  medical management of, 631–632
  nursing management of, 632–634
  pathophysiology of, 631
Minor
  emancipated, 1
  mature, 13
Minor burn, 708–709
Mist tent, 313
Mite infestation, 698–699
Mitotic inhibitor, 546
Mixed acid-base imbalance, 276
Mobility
  arthritis and, 295
  burn injury and, 714
  cancer and, 560
  cerebral palsy and, 468
  fracture and, 613
  scoliosis surgery and, 603
  of tongue, 105
Moiré photography, 597
Mongolian slant of eyelid, 91–92
Mongolian spots, 84
Moniliasis, oral, 699
Monitoring, cardiorespiratory, 811
Monocyte, 416
Monologue, collective, 19, 62
Mons pubis, 124
Moral development, 34
Moral dilemma, 1

Morbidity
    definition of, 1
    statistics on, 7–8
Moro reflex, 140
Morphine, 189
Mortality, infant, 6–7
    definition of, 1
Mosquito bite, 719
Motor development
    of adolescent, 68
    of infant, 40–43
    of preschool child, 58
    of school-age child, 64
    of toddler, 51
Motor function
    assessment of, 68
    cerebral palsy and, 465–469
    coma assessment and, 437
Motor vehicular accident; *see*
        Vehicular accident
Mourning, 211–212, 217–220
Mouth
    AIDS and, 289, 291
    assessment of, 103–105
    cancer and, 559
    candidiasis and, 699
    chemotherapy and, 548
    cleft lip and/or palate and, 485–493;
        see also Cleft lip and/or palate
    oral medications and, 817
    temperature measurement and, 809
Mouth breathing, in infant, 302
Mouth odor, 104
Mouth-to-mouth resuscitation
    of infant, 835
    near-drowning and, 343
    of older child, 837
Movement; *see also* Mobility
    abdominal, 120, 121
    of chest, 110
    chorea and, 402
    extraocular, 93
    musculoskeletal examination and,
        129–134
Mucocutaneous lymph node
        syndrome, 404–405
Mucopolysaccharides, 871
Mucosa
    buccal, 105
    dehydration and, 234
    nasal, 101–102
    nasopharyngitis and, 361
Mucus
    chest physiotherapy to drain,
        843–846
    cystic fibrosis and, 337
Mummy restraint, 802
Mumps, 784–785
    immunization schedule for, 770
Mumps vaccine, 785
    information summary on, 772
    reportable events about, 774

Munchausen syndrome by proxy,
        760–761
Murmur, heart, 118
Muscle; *see also* Musculoskeletal
        system
    abdominal, 121
    black widow spider bite and, 719
    calcium and, 253
    eye, 92–93
    Guillain-Barré syndrome and,
        454–455
    hypermagnesemia, 254
    magnesium and, 256
    pediatric anatomy of, 584
    potassium and, 246, 249
    rectus, 120
    respiratory, 303
    tetanus and, 457
Muscular dystrophy, 607–609
Muscular Dystrophy Association of
        America, 878
Muscular Dystrophy Association of
        Canada, 878
Musculoskeletal system; *see also* Muscle
    allergy and, 295
    disorders of, 584–617
        of bones and joints, 604–607
        of hip, 590–596
        of lower extremities, 584–590
        muscular dystrophy and, 607–609
        spinal, 597–603
    examination of, 129–134
        by inspection, 129
        lower extremities and, 133–134
        by palpation, 129
        posture and spinal alignment
            and, 131–132
        range of motion and, 130
        upper extremities and, 132
    injury to, 610–616
    pediatric anatomy and physiology
        of, 584
Music, therapeutic play and, 164
Mustard procedure, 390
Mycobacterium tuberculosis, 334–335
Myelogenous leukemia, 573
Myelomeningocele, 462
Myocardium
    contusion of, 411–412
    heart failure and, 381
Myoclonic seizure, 442
Myringotomy, 349, 356
Myxovirus infection, 784–785

N

Nails, 132
Nalbuphine, 189
Naproxen, 190
Nar-Anon, 879

Narcotic analgesic, 179
    dosages of, 189
Narcotic withdrawal in newborn,
        465
Narcotics Anonymous, 879
Nasal administration of drug, 821
Nasal anatomy, 350–351
Nasal cannula, 830
Nasal disorder, 359–361
Nasal examination, 100–102
Nasal suctioning, 841
Nasogastric tube, 847–848
Nasolabial fold, 100
Nasopharyngeal airway, 832
Nasopharyngitis, 361
National Anorectic Aid Society, Inc.,
        879
National Association for the
        Visually Handicapped, 876
National Association of Anorexia
        Nervosa & Associated
        Disorders, Inc., 879
National Association of Sickle Cell
        Disease, 876
National Down Syndrome Society,
        879
National Federation of the Blind, 876
National Head Injury Foundation, 874
National Hemophilia Foundation, 876
National Hydrocephalus
        Foundation, 877
National Kidney Foundation, 878
National Organ Transplant Act,
        13–14
National Safe Kids Campaign, 877
National Scoliosis Foundation, 600,
        878
National Society to Prevent
        Blindness, 876
Native American culture
    eye contact in, 78
    toilet training and weaning in, 51
Natural immunity, 282
Nature, 22
Nausea; *see* Vomiting
Near-drowning, 343–344, 479–480
    hypothermia and, 717
Necator americanus, 520
Neck, assessment of, 106–108
Necrosis
    avascular, of femoral head, 593–595
    brown recluse spider bite and, 719
    renal tubular, as cause of acute
        renal failure, 635
Necrotizing enterocolitis, 507
Needle stick, 61
Negative feedback, endocrine, 654
Neglect, 755–756
Neisseria gonorrhoeae, 650
    conjunctivitis caused by, 351
Neisseria meningitidis, 447, 448

Rectus muscle, 121
  assessment of, 120
Recurrent illness or condition
  abdominal pain as, 751–752
  cancer and, 557
  Munchausen syndrome by proxy
    and, 760–761
  otitis media as, 355, 356
Red blood cells
  illustrations of, 417
  normal values for, 417
Red reflex, 95
Reduction of fracture, 613
Refill, capillary, 86, 120
  cardiac assessment and, 120
Reflex
  Babinski, 139
  cremasteric, 127–128
  developmental stage and, 33
  gag, 106
  head injury and, 469
  of infant, 40–41
  light
    corneal, 93
    of tympanic membrane, 98
  primitive, 139, 140–141
  red, 95
  unconsciousness and, 438
Reflux
  gastroesophageal, 498–499
  vesicoureteral, 619, 626
Regression, 29
Regulation
  Baby Doe, 14–15
  of nursing practice, 10–11
  organs for transplantation and, 16
Regurgitation, rumination and, 524;
    see also Vomiting
Rehabilitation, 158
  definition of, 151
Rehydration, oral, 234–235
Relapse of cancer, 557
Relaxation techniques, for pain, 195
Religion
  Jehovah's Witness and, 554
  Jewish culture and, 26
Renal failure
  acute, 630, 634–640
    clinical manifestations of, 634
    diagnosis of, 636
    medical management of, 635–638
    nursing assessment of, 638–639
    nursing management of, 639–640
    pathophysiology of, 634–635
  chronic, 630, 640–644
    clinical manifestations of, 640–641
    medical management of, 641–642
    nursing management of, 643–644
    pathophysiology of, 641
  fluid and electrolyte imbalance
    and, 260

Renal failure—cont'd
  hypermagnesemia and, 256
  potassium and, 247
Renal system
  acid-base balance and, 266–267
    respiratory acidosis and, 269
    respiratory alkalosis and, 271
  diabetes insipidus and, 660
  disorders of, 630–649
  palpation of kidney and, 123
  sickle cell anemia and, 419
  urethral uropathy and, 625
  Wilms tumor and, 568–571
Renal transplantation, 642
Repellent, insect, 720
Reportable condition
  child abuse as, 758–759
  confidentiality and, 14
  immunization reactions as, 774
  tuberculosis as, 334
Repression, 29
Reproductive system
  ambiguous genitalia and, 668–670
  amenorrhea and, 681–682
  dysmenorrhea and, 682
  gynecomastia and, 681
  pediatric anatomy and physiology
    of, 620
  sexually transmitted diseases and,
    649–651
  urinary tract infection and, 627
Rescue breathing, for CPR, 835–836,
  837
Resilience, of skin, 85
Resistance
  airway, 299, 301
  vascular, fetal circulation and, 376
Resonance
  abdominal percussion and, 122
  vocal, 112, 113
Resources, listing of, 874–879
Respiratory acidosis, 268–270
Respiratory alkalosis, 268, 270–272
Respiratory distress
  management of, 327–328
  signs of, 120
  status asthmaticus and, 326–327
Respiratory effort
  assessment of, 110
  consciousness level and, 438–439
Respiratory failure, 307–310
Respiratory rate
  assessment of, 110, 807
  normal, 110, 807
  opioid overdose and, 197
  respiratory distress and, 300
Respiratory syncytial virus, 330
Respiratory system, 299–347
  acid-base balance and, 265–266
  AIDS and, 288–289
  allergy and, 295

Respiratory system—cont'd
  apnea and, 305
  appendicitis and, 506
  asthma and, 320–326
    clinical manifestations of, 320
    medical management of, 322
    nursing management of, 322–326
    pathophysiology of, 321–322
    status asthmaticus and, 326–327
  chest physiotherapy of, 843–846
  croup syndromes of, 310–320
    epiglottitis and, 315–318
    laryngotracheobronchitis and,
      312–315, 318–319
    tracheitis and, 320
  dialysis and, 638
  diaphragmatic hernia and,
    503–504
  heart failure and, 380, 383
  injury to, 341–346
    airway obstruction and, 341–343
    blunt trauma and, 345
    near-drowning and, 343–344
    pneumothorax and, 345–346
    pulmonary contusion and, 345
    smoke inhalation causing,
      344–345
  lower airway disorders of, 327–341
    bronchiolitis and, 329–333
    bronchitis and, 329
    bronchopulmonary dysplasia
      and, 328–329
    cystic fibrosis and, 335–341
    pneumonia and, 333–334
    respiratory distress syndrome
      and, 327–328
    tuberculosis and, 334–335
  pediatric anatomy and physiology
    of, 301–303
  secretion, cultures of, 816
  urgent disorders of
    apnea and, 303–306
    respiratory failure and, 307–310
    sudden infant death syndrome
      and, 306–307
Restraint
  for ear examination, 97
  types of, 800–803
Resuscitation, cardiopulmonary,
  834–838
  of infant, 834–836
  of older child, 837–838
Retardation, mental, 735–736
Retina, 94–95
Retinoblastoma, 576–577
Retinopathy of prematurity, 354
Retractions, respiratory, 299, 303, 309
Reverse isolation, 805
Review of systems
  definition of, 75
  in patient history, 80, 81

Sensorimotor stage, 30, 32, 33
Sensorineural hearing loss, 349, 369
Sensory function
  of adolescent, 68
  assessment of, 138–139
  conversion reaction and, 754
  impairment of
    auditory, 369–373
    visual, 366–369
  of infant, 40–43
  of preschool child, 58
  of school-age child, 64
  of toddler, 51
Separation anxiety, 151, 152, 153,
      203–204, 750–751
Sepsis
  cellulitis and, 702
  signs of, 507
Septal defect
  atrial, 386
  ventricular, 387
Septic arthritis, 605, 606
Septic shock
  cancer and, 549
  mechanism of, 410–411
Septum, nasal, 102
Serotonin, 869
Settings for nursing care, 4–5
Severe combined immunodeficiency
      disease, 284–285
Sex chromosome abnormality, 682–684
Sexual abuse, 756
  manifestations of, 757
  signs of, 126
Sexual development, abnormal
  ambiguous genitalia and, 668–670
  amenorrhea and, 681–682
  dysmenorrhea and, 682
  gynecomastia and, 681
  precocious puberty and, 661
Sexual differentiation, 655, 657
Sexual maturation, 68, 124–128,
      655–656
Sexuality, of adolescent, 72
Sexually transmitted disease, 649–651
  urinary tract infection and, 627
Shock
  cardiogenic, 411
  distributive, 410–411
  hypovolemic, 407–410
  meningitis and, 450
  obstructive, 411
  as parents' reaction, 209–210
  septic
    cancer and, 549
    mechanism of, 411
  types of, 407–411
Short bowel syndrome, 526
Short stature, 658–659
Short Stature Foundation, 878
Short stay admission, 157

Shunt
  cardiac, 375, 389
  ventriculoperitoneal, 459
Sibilant rhonchus, 112
Sibling
  of critically ill child, 214–215
  of dying child, 217–218
  of child with spinal cord injury, 479
Sickle cell anemia, 418–423
  clinical manifestations of, 418
  medical management of, 420
  nursing care plan for, 422–423
  nursing management of, 420–423
  pathophysiology of, 418–420
Sickle Cell Association of Ontario, 876
SIDS Alliance, 875
Sign(s)
  Chvostek
    hypocalcemia and, 253
    hypomagnesemia and, 257
  encephalitis and, 455
  Gower, 130
  of respiratory distress, 120
  of sepsis, 507
  of sexual abuse, 126
  Trousseau, 271
    hypomagnesemia and, 257
Simian crease, 132
Simple partial seizure, 441, 443
Sinus arrhythmia, 116
Sinus, assessment of, 102
Skeletal system, 129–134
Skeletal traction, 615
Skeletal tuberculosis, 606
Skene gland, 126
Skin, 688–721
  accessory structures of, 690, 691
  assessment of, 83–87
  burn injury to, 705–716
  contusion of, 720
  cutaneous stimulation of, for pain,
      195
  dehydration and, 234
  disorders of, 688–721
  drug reactions and, 694
  edema and, 229, 242, 243
  fluid loss through, 226
  fungal infections of, 699–701
  infections of, 697–701
  injuries to, 705–720
  lesions of
    primary, 86–87
    secondary, 691–692
  pediatric anatomy and physiology
      of, 690–691
  wound healing and, 692
Skin traction, 614
  Bryant, 592, 614
Skinner, B.F., 35
Skull, 88–90
  fracture of, 474

Slant of eye, 91–92
Sleep
  cancer and, 559
  pain and, 197
  sudden infant death syndrome
      and, 47
Slipped capital femoral epiphysis,
      595–596
Slow-to-warm-up child, 37
Small-vein filling time, 86
Smell, assessment of, 101
Smoke inhalation
  breathing and, 713
  injury from, 344–345
  passive, 320
    asthma and, 320
    bronchitis and, 329
Smooth muscle, respiratory, 303
Snellen E chart, 812
Social aspects of play, 57, 59
Social learning theory, 35
Social skills, 147
Socialization of visually impaired
      child, 367
Socioeconomic factors, 25
Sodium
  cultural considerations and, 640
  deficit of, 230–231
  edema and, 238–243
  excess of, 226–230
  hypernatremia and, 232–236
  hyponatremia and, 237–238
  normal values for, 869
  renal failure and, 634, 635
Sodium bicarbonate
  metabolic acidosis and, 274, 275
  renal failure and, 636
Sodium nitroprusside, 636
Soft tissue tumor, 576–577
Solid food, introduction of, 46
Sonorous rhonchus, 112
Sore throat
  pharyngitis causing, 361–362
  tonsillitis causing, 362–366
Sounds
  bowel, 121
  breath, 111–113
    laryngotracheobronchitis and,
      313
  conduction of, 99, 100
  heart, 115–118
Southeast Asian culture, head
      examination and, 89
Space, intercostal, 108
Space-occupying lesion, 550
Spasmodic laryngitis, 310, 311
Special needs child, 160
Specialist, child life, 160
Specific gravity of urine, of infant,
      231
Specimen collection, 813–816

Approved Nursing Diagnoses
North American Nursing Diagnosis Association

Activity intolerance
Activity intolerance, high risk for
Adjustment, impaired
Airway clearance, ineffective
Anxiety
Aspiration, high risk for
Body image disturbance
Body temperature, high risk for altered
Breastfeeding, effective
Breastfeeding, ineffective
Breastfeeding, interrupted
Breathing pattern, ineffective
Cardiac output, decreased
Caregiver role strain
Caregiver role strain, high risk for
Communication, impaired verbal
Constipation
Constipation, colonic
Constipation, perceived
Coping, defensive
Coping (family), ineffective: Compromised
Coping (family), ineffective: Disabling
Coping (family), potential for growth
Coping (individual), ineffective
Decisional conflict (specify)
Denial, ineffective
Diarrhea
Disuse syndrome, high risk for
Diversional activity deficit
Dysreflexia
Family Processes, altered
Fatigue
Fear
Fluid volume deficit (1)
Fluid volume deficit (2)
Fluid volume deficit, high risk for
Fluid volume excess
Gas exchange, impaired
Grieving, anticipatory
Grieving, dysfunctional
Growth and development, altered
Health maintenance, altered
Health-seeking behaviors (specify)
Home maintenance management, impaired
Hopelessness
Hyperthermia
Hypothermia
Incontinence, bowel
Incontinence, functional (urinary)
Incontinence, reflex (urinary)
Incontinence, stress (urinary)
Incontinence, total (urinary)
Incontinence, urge (urinary)
Infant feeding pattern, ineffective
Infection, high risk for
Injury, high risk for

Knowledge deficit (specify)
Management of therapeutic regimen, ineffective
Mobility, impaired physical
Noncompliance (specify)
Nutrition, altered: less than body requirements
Nutrition, altered: more than body requirements
Nutrition, altered: high risk for more than body requirements
Oral mucous membrane, altered
Pain
Pain, chronic
Parental role conflict
Parenting, altered
Parenting, high risk for altered
Peripheral neurovascular dysfunction, high risk for
Personal identity disturbance
Poisoning, high risk for
Post-trauma response
Powerlessness
Protection, altered
Rape-trauma syndrome
Rape-trauma syndrome: compound reaction
Rape-trauma syndrome: silent reaction
Relocation stress syndrome
Role performance, altered
Self-care deficit, bathing/hygiene (specify level)
Self-care deficit, dressing/grooming (specify level)
Self-care deficit, feeding (specify level)
Self-care deficit, toileting (specify level)
Self-esteem, chronic low
Self-esteem disturbance
Self-esteem, situational low
Self-mutilation, high risk for
Sensory/perceptual alterations (specify): visual, auditory,
    kinesthetic, gustatory, tactile, olfactory
Sexual dysfunction
Sexuality patterns, altered
Skin integrity, impaired
Skin integrity, high risk for impaired
Sleep pattern disturbance
Social interaction, impaired
Social isolation
Spiritual distress (distress of the human spirit)
Suffocation, high risk for
Swallowing, impaired
Thermoregulation, ineffective
Thought processes, altered
Tissue integrity, impaired
Tissue perfusion, altered (specify type): renal, cerebral,
    cardiopulmonary, gastrointestinal, peripheral
Trauma, high risk for
Unilateral neglect
Urinary elimination, altered patterns of
Urinary retention
Ventilation, inability to sustain spontaneous
Ventilatory weaning response, dysfunctional
Violence, high risk for: self-directed or directed at others